Pathology
of the
Lungs

Commissioning Editor: *Michael Houston*
Development Editor: *Ben Davie*
Editorial Assistant: *Rachael Harrison*
Project Manager: *Gopika Sasidharan*
Design: *Charles Gray*
Illustration Manager: *Gillian Richards*
Marketing Manager (UK): *Richard Jones*

Pathology
of the
Lungs

THIRD EDITION

Bryan Corrin MD FRCPath

Emeritus Professor of Pathology
London University

Honorary Senior Clinical Research Fellow
National Heart and Lung Institute
Imperial College London

Honorary Consultant Pathologist
Royal Brompton Hospital
London, UK

Andrew G. Nicholson DM FRCPath

Consultant Histopathologist
Royal Brompton and Harefield NHS Foundation Trust

Professor of Respiratory Pathology
National Heart and Lung Institute
Imperial College London
London, UK

Contributors:

Margaret Burke MB FRCPath

Honorary Consultant Histopathologist
Royal Brompton and Harefield NHS Foundation Trust
London, UK

Alexandra Rice FRCPath

Consultant Histopathologist
Royal Brompton and Harefield NHS Foundation Trust

Honorary Senior Lecturer
Imperial College
London, UK

CHURCHILL
LIVINGSTONE

ELSEVIER

Edinburgh   London   New York   Oxford   Philadelphia   St Louis   Sydney   Toronto   2011

CHURCHILL
LIVINGSTONE
ELSEVIER

CHURCHILL LIVINGSTONE is an imprint of Elsevier Limited.

First edition 1999
Second edition 2006
Third edition 2011

Notices

Knowledge and best practice in this field are constantly changing. As new research and experience broaden our understanding, changes in research methods, professional practices, or medical treatment may become necessary. Practitioners and researchers must always rely on their own experience and knowledge in evaluating and using any information, methods, compounds, or experiments described herein. In using such information or methods they should be mindful of their own safety and the safety of others, including parties for whom they have a professional responsibility.

With respect to any drug or pharmaceutical products identified, readers are advised to check the most current information provided (i) on procedures featured or (ii) by the manufacturer of each product to be administered, to verify the recommended dose or formula, the method and duration of administration, and contraindications. It is the responsibility of practitioners, relying on their own experience and knowledge of their patients, to make diagnoses, to determine dosages and the best treatment for each individual patient, and to take all appropriate safety precautions.

To the fullest extent of the law, neither the Publisher nor the authors, contributors, or editors, assume any liability for any injury and/or damage to persons or property as a matter of products liability, negligence or otherwise, or from any use or operation of any methods, products, instructions, or ideas contained in the material herein.

ISBN: 978-0-7020-3369-8

British Library Cataloguing in Publication Data
A catalogue record for this book is available from the British Library

Library of Congress Cataloging in Publication Data
A catalog record for this book is available from the Library of Congress

 your source for books,
journals and multimedia
in the health sciences
www.elsevierhealth.com

Working together to grow
libraries in developing countries

www.elsevier.com | www.bookaid.org | www.sabre.org

The publisher's policy is to use **paper manufactured from sustainable forests**

Printed in China
Last digit is the print number: 9 8 7 6 5 4 3 2 1

Contents

Preface

This book is aimed primarily at the practising diagnostic histopathologist. However, the clinical, functional and radiological consequences of the structural changes described are not neglected and the resultant clinicopathological correlation should be of interest to thoracic clinicians, radiologists and surgeons as well as general histopathologists. The intention has been to cover lung disease in as comprehensive yet succinct a manner as possible.

We have collaborated closely on each chapter and believe that this has resulted in a uniform style and proper balance between chapters, minimized repetition and avoided the delays that often render obsolete parts of some multi-author works. Indeed the opportunity has been taken to update both text and references at the latest possible point in the production schedule.

We thank our medical colleagues at the Brompton and Harefield hospitals, in particular Margaret Burke and Alexandra Rice, who have expertly revised the transplantation chapter, and David Hansell, who provided many radiographic images and took time to show us what they represent. We also thank the many pathologists who have provided illustrations or referred cases that expanded our knowledge of lung pathology. They are, Dr I. Abdalsamad, Dr H. Aziz, Dr B.J. Addis, Dr M. Antoine, Dr T. Ashcroft, Dr M. Ashworth, Dr G.S. Balasubramaniam, Professor J. Bignon, Dr M.M. Burke, Mrs D. Bowes, the late Dr A.H. Cameron, Professor F. Capron, Dr V. Chrystal, Dr T.V. Colby, Professor P. Cole, Dr P.M. Cury, Dr C. Danel, Miss A. Dewar, Dr Duboucher, Dr J. DeGaetano, Dr K. Dhaene, Professor D. Denison, Dr D. Dinsdale, Dr R.V.P. Dissanayake, Dr W. Downey, Dr W.G.J. Edwards, Dr B. Fox, Dr Gaafar, Dr W. Geddie, Dr A. Gibbs, Dr M. Goddard, Dr J.T. Gmelich, Dr N. Gubbay, Professor D.M. Hansell, the late Professor B.E. Heard, Professor D. Henderson, Dr A. Herbert, Dr K. Hiroshima, Dr A. Hislop, Professor F. Ho, Professor M. Hodson, Professor L.J. Holloway, Dr G. Hulman, Dr Nassif Ibrahim, Dr M. Jagusch, Professor P.K. Jeffery, Dr T. Jelihovsky, Dr M. Kambouchner, Dr B. Kazzaz, Dr M. Kearney, Dr W. Kenyon, Dr I. Kerr, Dr P. King, Dr M. Kitaichi, the late Professor R.E. Lane, Dr S. Lantuejoul, Professor D.A. Levison, the late Dr A.A. Liebow, Dr J. Longbottom, the late Dr G. Manning, Dr S. McGrath-Morrow, Dr D. Melcher, Dr Max Millard, Professor W. Mooi, Professor B. Nemery, Dr M. Neyra, Dr D. Owen, Dr A. Paiva-Correia, Professor F.D. Pooley, Dr D. Rassl, Dr F. Roberts, Dr A.V. Rogers, Professor V.L. Roggli, the late Dr N. Rossouw, Dr G.A. Russell, Dr R.M.E. Seal, Dr C.A. Seldenrijk, Dr J.W. Seo, Dr C.G.B. Simpson, Dr R. Steele, Dr G. Taylor, Dr J.A. Thomas, Dr J.F. Tomashefski junior, Dr G. Valesini, Dr Sj Sc Wagenaar, Dr J.H.L. Watson, Professor T.J. Williams, Dr M. Wineberg, Dr A.C. Wotherspoon, Dr C. Wright and Professor D.H. Wright.

We are also indebted to our laboratory and secretarial staff for their unstinting support and help, in particular Richard Florio, David Butcher, Ann Dewar, Andrew Rogers, Anne-Marie Campbell, Angela Fenelon, Shehnaaz Ghazali, Matthew Pynegar, James Croud, Joy Sills, Asha Velani, Antony Phillips and Christian Archer, and also the many staff at Elsevier for their excellent support, notably Michael Houston, Ben Davie, Louise Cook, Rachael Harrison, Gillian Richards and Gopika Sasidharan.

BC thanks his wife Sheila for her support and is pleased to acknowledge the debt he owes to his teachers, in particular Winston Evans, who first steered him towards a career in pathology, Hugh Cameron, Colin Campbell, Herbert Spencer and Averill Liebow.

AGN gratefully acknowledges several pathologists, in particular Tom Colby, Bill Travis, Elisabeth Brambilla, Cyril Fisher and Bryan himself, for providing friendship and tutelage in the art of pulmonary pathology over the years. However, his biggest thank you goes to family and friends outside medicine who keep his life in perspective – Jimmy, Betty, Iain, Caroline, James, Tess and Robbie Nicholson, the Garnham family and most of all, Francesca, for her love and support.

Bryan Corrin
Andrew G Nicholson
London

vi

Chapter | 1 |

The structure of the normal lungs

ANATOMY OF THE LUNGS AND AIRWAYS

The trachea starts in the neck and extends downwards from the larynx to enter the thorax at about its midpoint. It terminates by bifurcating into the main bronchi at about the level of the manubriosternal joint and the upper border of the fifth vertebral body. From its origin in the midline it inclines slightly to the right and is angled backwards by up to 30°. Posteriorly the trachea is related to the oesophagus and azygos vein while arrayed around it anteriorly and laterally are the innominate artery, the left common carotid artery, the arch of the aorta, the brachiocephalic veins and the superior vena cava.

The right main bronchus follows more closely the direction of the trachea and, because it branches earlier, is only half the length of the left. The right main bronchus is wider than the left and carries 55% of each breath. It enters the lung behind the right pulmonary artery and is said to be 'eparterial' whereas the left main bronchus crosses behind the left pulmonary artery to enter the lung below it and is therefore said to be 'hyparterial' (Fig. 1.1).

The two lungs, enclosed within the visceral pleura, fill their respective pleural cavities. Tissue is reduced to a minimum in the interests of gas exchange. At mid-inspiration over 80% of lung volume is air, 10% is blood, 3% comprises conductive airways and blood vessels and only 3% is alveolar tissue. The normal combined weight of the

©2010 Elsevier Ltd
DOI: 10.1016/B978-0-7020-3369-8.00001-X

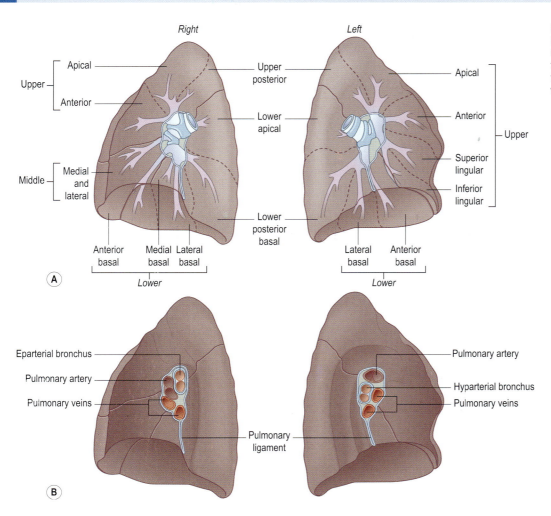

Figure 1.1 Medial aspects of the lungs. (A) The arrangement and nomenclature of the lobes and their segments. (B) The positions of the main bronchi, arteries and veins at the hila.

lungs averages 850 g in men and 750 g in women. Lung weights in children are given in Table 1.1.[1]

The lungs abut the mediastinum medially, rest on the diaphragm below and elsewhere are enclosed by the ribcage. On their medial surface the main bronchovascular structures connect the hilum of the lung with the mediastinum and here the visceral pleura is reflected off the lung to become the parietal pleura. The pleural reflection also extends from the inferior aspect of the hilum to the medial border of the base of the lung at what is termed the pulmonary ligament (see Fig. 1.1B) The pleura is described in more detail in Chapter 13.

Oblique fissures divide the lungs into upper and lower lobes and on the right a transverse fissure separates off a middle lobe. The main bronchi divide in a corresponding manner to give five lobar bronchi. The next division supplies the lung segments, of which there are 19, a segment being the smallest bronchopulmonary unit that can be distinguished and excised separately by a surgeon. The airways branch repeatedly and there may be as many as 23 divisions before alveoli furthest from the trachea are reached, as opposed to alveoli nearer the hilum of the lung which are reached after as few as eight divisions. The pattern of branching is one of asymmetrical dichotomy, meaning that each airway has two branches that often differ in diameter or length.

The airways of the first four generations are individually named and the pathologist must be familiar with the terminology of the 19 lung segments and their bronchi so that lesions can be localised accurately and the pathological findings correlated with those of radiologists and surgeons. Figure 1.2 illustrates the trachea, main, lobar and segmental bronchi diagrammatically, using an internationally recommended nomenclature.[2] A plastic cast of the proximal airways coloured according to the lung segments is shown in Figure 1.3. It will be noted that the following anatomical features are common to the two lungs:

- Each upper lobe has apical, anterior and posterior segments.
- Each lower lobe has an apical segment and anterior, lateral and posterior basal segments.

The two lungs differ in the following respects:

- After giving off the upper lobe bronchus, the right main bronchus continues through a lower (intermediate) part to supply the middle and lower lobes, whereas the left main bronchus continues as the left lower lobe bronchus.
- The right lung has a middle lobe served by a branch of the lower (intermediate) part of the main bronchus, whereas the lingula of the left lung, which is the homologue of the right middle lobe, is served by a lingular division of the upper-lobe bronchus, the other branch of which is known as the upper or superior division.
- The two segments of the right middle lobe are medial and lateral whereas the two segments of the lingula are superior and inferior.
- The right lower lobe has an extra segment, known as the medial or cardiac segment.

Table 1.1 Lung weights in children[1]

Age	Body length (cm)	Right lung (g)	Left lung (g)
Birth–3 days	49	21	18
3–7 days	49	24	22
1–3 weeks	52	29	26
3–5 weeks	52	31	27
5–7 weeks	53	32	28
7–9 weeks	55	32	29
3 months	56	35	30
4 months	59	37	33
5 months	61	38	35
6 months	62	42	39
7 months	65	49	41
8 months	65	52	45
9 months	67	53	47
10 months	69	54	51
11 months	70	59	53
12 months	73	64	57
14 months	74	66	60
16 months	77	72	64
18 months	78	72	65
20 months	79	80	74
22 months	82	83	75
24 months	84	88	76
3 years	88	89	77
4 years	99	90	85
5 years	106	107	104
6 years	109	121	122
7 years	113	130	123
8 years	119	150	140
9 years	125	174	152
10 years	130	177	166
11 years	135	201	190

Table 1.2 The Weibel model of the bronchial tree[3]

Number of branches	Generation	Diameter (mm)	Length (mm)	Structure
1	0	18.0	120.0	Trachea
2	1	12.2	47.6	B
4	2	8.3	19.0	B
8	3	5.6	7.6	B
16	4	4.5	12.7	B
32	5	3.5	10.7	B
64	6	2.8	9.0	B
128	7	2.3	7.6	B
256	8	1.86	6.4	B
512	9	1.54	5.4	MB
1024	10	1.30	4.6	MB
2048	11	1.09	3.9	MB
4096	12	0.95	3.3	MB
8192	13	0.82	2.7	MB
16384	14	0.74	2.3	MB
32768	15	0.66	2.0	MB
65536	16	0.60	1.65	TB
131072	17	0.54	1.41	RB
262144	18	0.50	1.17	RB
524288	19	0.47	0.99	RB
1048576	20	0.45	0.83	AD
2097152	21	0.43	0.70	AD
4194304	22	0.41	0.59	AD
8388608	23	0.41	0.50	AD

B, bronchi; MB, membranous bronchioles; TB, terminal bronchioles; RB, respiratory bronchioles; AD, alveolar ducts. The data are based on a combination of morphometry and assumption.

Beyond the segmental bronchi, individual airways are unnamed but a distinction is drawn between bronchi, which have glands and cartilage in their wall, and bronchioles, which do not. Transition from bronchus to bronchiole takes place in airways approximately 1 mm in diameter. The first orders of bronchioles, which are known as membranous bronchioles, are purely conductive. The last order of these bronchioles is known as terminal bronchioles, despite them leading into further orders of bronchioles. These further bronchioles have alveoli opening directly off them and are known as respiratory bronchioles; they both conduct gas and participate in gas exchange. Such airways form what is termed a transitional zone between the purely conductive airways and the alveoli. It comprises about three generations of respiratory bronchioles and two to nine generations of alveolar ducts, the last of which terminate in alveolar sacs; all these structures have increasing numbers of alveoli opening off their walls. The subdivisions and structure of the intrapulmonary airways are represented diagrammatically in Figure 1.4 and numerical data appertaining to individual orders (generations) of airways are shown in Table 1.2.[3]

The lung substance is divided into primary and secondary lobules. The primary lobule is that portion of the lung supplied by one respiratory bronchiole but it is seldom referred to today and the unqualified term 'lobule' generally equates to the secondary lung lobule. The secondary lobule is a portion of lung surrounded by fibrous septa that are visible on the cut surface of the lung (Figs 1.5 and 1.6) and

Trachea

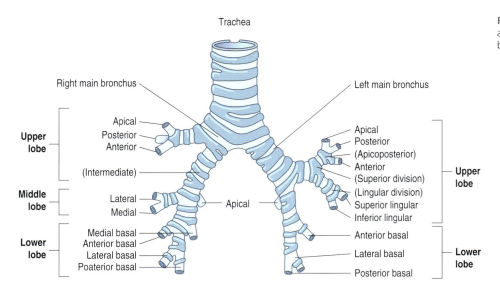

Right main bronchus

Left main bronchus

Upper lobe
Apical
Posterior
Anterior

(Intermediate)

Middle lobe
Lateral
Medial

Apical

Lower lobe
Medial basal
Anterior basal
Lateral basal
Poaterior basal

Apical
Posterior
(Apicoposterior)
Anterior
(Superior division)
(Lingular division)
Superior lingular
Inferior lingular

Upper lobe

Anterior basal

Lateral basal

Posterior basal

Lower lobe

Figure 1.3 Posterior view of a plastic cast of the proximal airways with individual segments distinguished by colour.

through the visceral pleura, particularly when their contained lymphatics are outlined by dust or tumour (Fig. 1.7). However, the fibrous septa that demarcate the secondary lobules are unevenly developed. They are quite well represented laterally in the lower lobes (where they appear as Kerley B lines when thickened by interstitial oedema) but are poorly represented medially and deep in the lungs. The lobules they demarcate are polyhedral. In the adult lung, each lobule measures 1–2 cm across and is in turn made up of about 3–10 acini, an acinus being that portion of the lung supplied by one terminal bronchiole. The volume of a lobule is approximately 2 ml and that

of an acinus approximately 0.2 ml. An acinus is 0.5–1 cm long,[4] so that the bronchi and purely conductive bronchioles make up all but this length of the total gas pathway. Each acinus contains about 2000 alveoli and it is estimated that the two lungs together contain about 300 million alveoli.[5] The edges of adjacent acini interdigitate without any intervening septa and it is impossible to detect where one acinus ends and the next begins, either with the naked eye or the microscope. However, in adult lungs, the centres of the acini are generally 'tattooed' with carbon for it is here that lymphatics commence and dust-laden cells accumulate in what Macklin termed 'dust sumps' (see Figs 1.7 and 7.1.12, p. 339).[6]

The term 'terminal respiratory unit' has been applied to an imprecise number of bronchioles and the alveoli they supply, mainly by embryologists and more recently by pathologists and molecular biologists interested in the histogenesis of adenocarcinomas composed of bronchiolar Clara cells and type II alveolar cells (see below and p. 553).[7,8] This is because these cells ubiquitously express the regulatory thyroid transcription factor-1 (TTF-1), which is potentially a lineage-specific survival oncogene of some lung adenocarcinomas.[9,10]

Each generation of airways is shorter than its predecessor and, whereas individual members of each generation are narrower than their parents, beyond the segmental bronchi the summed cross-sectional area for each generation progressively increases logarithmically (Fig. 1.8),[3,11] and at the periphery resistance to airflow is negligible. Because of this, gas flow velocity falls rapidly in the respiratory bronchioles and gas mixing in the last few airways is largely by diffusion. Diffusion across tissue is less efficient than in the gas phase but at the surface of the alveolar walls gas transfer is maximised as the inspired gas is spread over an area of about 70 m².[12] There is therefore considerable reserve in the conductive capacity of the peripheral airways, large numbers of which may be obliterated before there is any appreciable shortness of breath; for this reason the finer airways have been termed the 'silent area of the lung'.

Lambert's canals are tubular communications approximately 30 μm in diameter that connect terminal and respiratory bronchioles with adjacent peribronchiolar alveoli, thus bypassing the main pathway.[13] They represent accessory air inlets to, or outlets from, the more distant alveoli. In coal miners, these canals and their associated alveoli are early sites of dust cell accumulation, whilst in fibrotic lung disease,

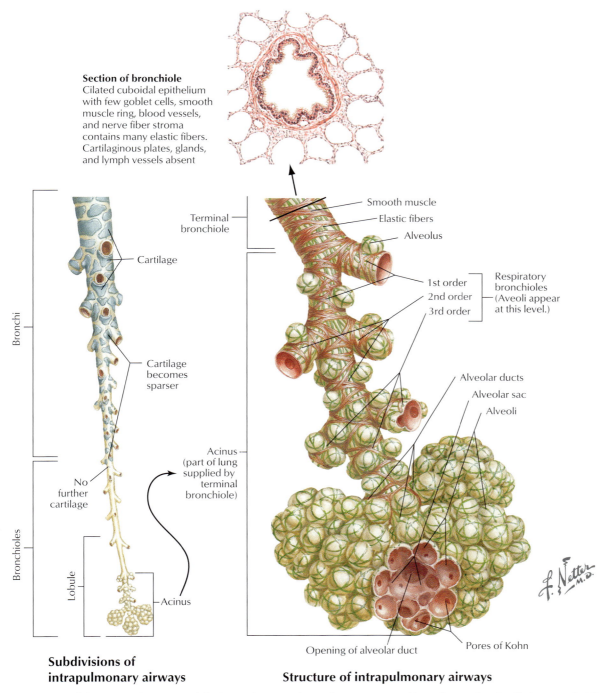

Section of bronchiole
Cilated cuboidal epithelium with few goblet cells, smooth muscle ring, blood vessels, and nerve fiber stroma contains many elastic fibers. Cartilaginous plates, glands, and lymph vessels absent

Smooth muscle
Elastic fibers
Alveolus

Terminal bronchiole

Cartilage

1st order
2nd order
3rd order

Respiratory bronchioles (Aveoli appear at this level.)

Cartilage becomes sparser

Alveolar ducts
Alveolar sac
Alveoli

Bronchi

Acinus (part of lung supplied by terminal bronchiole)

No further cartilage

Lobule

Acinus

Bronchioles

Opening of alveolar duct

Pores of Kohn

Subdivisions of intrapulmonary airways

Structure of intrapulmonary airways

Figure 1.4 Subdivisions and structure of the intrapulmonary airways from a segmental bronchus to the alveoli. *(Netter medical illustration used with permission of Elsevier. All rights reserved.)*

cuboidal bronchiolar epithelial cells often extend through them to line the peribronchiolar alveoli, a metaplastic process that is termed alveolar bronchiolisation, peribronchiolar metaplasia or lambertosis (Figs 1.9 and 3.37A, p. 121).[14]

To what extent the 30-μm diameter Lambert's canals provide collateral circulation is uncertain. They appear to offer a better anatomical pathway than the 2–13-μm diameter pores of Kohn, described below, but may be less effective than certain interconnecting respiratory bronchioles that measure 120 μm in diameter,[15] and the 200-μm diameter interacinar and 80–150-μm diameter intersegmental connections that have been demonstrated using injection techniques[16] and corrosion casts[17] respectively.

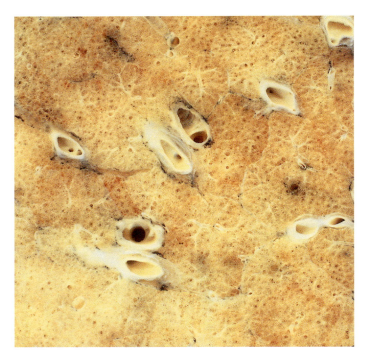

Figure 1.5 Poorly demarcated fibrous septa incompletely separate the lung lobules. The pulmonary arteries accompany the airways in the centres of the lung acini whereas the pulmonary veins are situated at the periphery of the lung lobules in the interlobular septa.

Figure 1.6 A lung lobule demarcated by the pleura and interlobular septa, which are stained red in this elastin van Gieson preparation, as are the periarterial cuffs of connective tissue. The arteries (and poorly stained accompanying airways) mark the centres of the lung acini while the veins are situated in the interlobular septa.

The two main pulmonary arteries arise from the bifurcation of the pulmonary trunk shortly after its origin from the right ventricle and divide to follow the lobar bronchi. Segmental and subsegmental pulmonary arteries continue alongside their corresponding airways and in the periphery of the lungs most small pulmonary arteries enter an acinus with the terminal bronchiole and are thus found at the centre of the acinus (Figs 1.10 and 1.11). As well as these axial vessels there are also small supernumerary branches which do not accompany airways.[18] The pulmonary arteries divide to supply the pulmonary capillaries, which form a meshwork situated in the alveolar walls, regrouping at the periphery of the acinus to form pulmonary veins (Fig. 1.12). In the periphery of the lung the pulmonary veins run in the interlobular septa and are thus separate from the artery and airway in the centre of the acinus (see Figs 1.6 and 1.10), but they take up a position alongside the artery and bronchus proximal to the entry of these structures into the lung lobule.

MICROSCOPY OF THE AIRWAYS

The bronchial wall consists of a thin mucosa and a more substantial submucosal coat, outside which there is the peribronchial sheath of loose connective tissue that also surrounds the accompanying pulmonary artery. The mucosa consists of respiratory epithelium resting on a basement membrane and beneath that a supportive connective tissue layer rich in elastin fibres. There is no clear boundary between the mucosa and the submucosa but muscle, glands and cartilage are conventionally regarded as belonging to the submucosal coat (Fig. 1.13).

In the extrapulmonary bronchi and trachea the cartilage forms irregular, sometimes branching, rings that are incomplete dorsally, the gaps being bridged by smooth muscle. In intrapulmonary bronchi the intercartilaginous gaps are more numerous and haphazardly distributed but in large bronchi at least the cartilage plates are numerous enough to be found in any cross-section. In small bronchi, the cartilage is less abundant and may be missed in some sections. Airways that completely lack cartilage and glands are termed bronchioles.

Smooth muscle, present only in the dorsal intercartilaginous gaps of the trachea, completely encircles the intrapulmonary bronchi, internal to the cartilage. It comprises two sets of fibres that wind around the bronchial tree as opposing spirals, thereby appearing incomplete in individual cross-sections. The arrangement is such that, as the muscle contracts, the airway both shortens and constricts. The muscle forms a more complete ring in the membranous bronchioles than in bronchi or respiratory bronchioles. When respiratory bronchioles are encountered in longitudinal section, the muscle is seen only

Figure 1.7 A Gough–Wentworth paper-mounted whole-lung section of a city-dweller's lung in which the interlobular septa and centriacinar structures are particularly well seen because of dust in the lymphatics.

Figure 1.9 Canal of Lambert in organising pneumonia. (A) The canal (arrow) provides a direct connection between bronchiole and alveolus. (B) Fibronopurulent debris tracks directly between airway and alveolus.

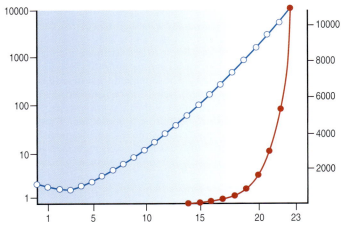

Figure 1.8 Summed cross-sectional area (cm²) plotted against airway generation. Logarithmic scale on the left (open circles), linear scale on the right (solid circles). Note the striking increase in total cross-sectional area of the peripheral airways. The arithmetic plot is often duplicated in mirror-image fashion to illustrate a classic trumpet-shaped concept of the increasing airway cross-sectional area in the paired lungs. *Weibel's data[3] redrawn from Horsfield (1974).[11]*

as small knobs between the mouths of the numerous alveoli that open off these airways.

If the trachea and main bronchi are opened from the front, longitudinal mucosal corrugations or ridges are evident on the posterior wall.[19] Most of those in the trachea pass into the right main bronchus but there is an equal number in the left main bronchus where they commence anew beyond the carina. In the trachea and main bronchi the ridges are limited to the membranous parts but distal to the lobar bronchi the ridges are distributed all around the walls of the airways. They represent longitudinal bundles of elastin fibres situated in the subepithelial mucosal lamina propria (Fig. 1.14). Although the bundles become progressively thinner they persist throughout the bronchial tree and link up with spiral elastin fibres described in the alveolar ducts[20] and with the elastic tissue of the alveolar walls. They are thought to contribute to elastic recoil during expiration and are more prominent in men, older subjects, smokers and asthmatics.[21]

Figure 1.10 A plastic cast showing that the pulmonary arteries (red) accompany the airways (white) and that pulmonary veins (blue) are separate.

Figure 1.11 Bronchioles and pulmonary arteries lie alongside each other in the centres of the lung acini, sharing a connective tissue sheath.

Transverse ridges are also evident in the bronchial mucosa; these lack elastin fibres and probably represent folds produced by muscular shortening of the airways.

Around the pulmonary arteries and to a lesser extent the airways there is a sheath of loose connective tissue (see Fig. 1.11). This connects with the visceral pleura at the hilum and distally with the delicate connective tissue of the respiratory bronchioles and the alveolar interstitium, and through the latter with the interlobular septa and the visceral pleura. The periarterial sheath carries nerves and lymphatic vessels and is expanded considerably in oedema, acting as an interstitial sump for extravascular fluid and thus protecting against this spilling over into the alveoli.

The epithelium of the main airways is pseudostratified, meaning that all its cells rest on the basement membrane but not all reach

the airway lumen (Figs 1.15 and 1.16). Most epithelial cells are columnar and ciliated but these are interspersed with mucous cells, finely granulated neuroendocrine cells, basal cells, brush cells, nerve terminals and migratory lymphocytes and mast cells.[22–24] The airway epithelium decreases in height distally, becoming cuboidal in the bronchioles. The mucous cells decrease in number as the bronchioles are approached and in these small airways Clara[25] and serous[26] cells are found amongst the ciliated cells.[27] Major histocompatibility antigens of both class I (HLA-A, B and C) and II (HLA-DR) are expressed by bronchial, bronchiolar and alveolar epithelium.[28] All airway epithelial cells express cytokeratin 19 while the basal cells also express cytokeratin 17.[29] In contrast to pleural mesothelium, cytokeratins 5 and 6 are not expressed by airway epithelium and rarely by its malignant derivatives, providing a useful point of distinction between pulmonary adenocarcinoma and epithelioid mesotheliomas (see p. 724).[30]

In the main airways there is a surface layer of mucus supported by an aqueous hypophase (Fig. 1.17). More distally, the bronchial mucous layer is discontinuous.[31] In the smaller bronchioles there is a continuous surface layer similar to that lining the alveoli (see below).[32]

The thickness of the surface layer is of considerable importance. In its proximal movement, the surface layer is constantly being added to by airway secretions yet this material has all to be accommodated on a progressively reducing surface area (see Fig. 1.8). Despite losses through evaporation, and clearance being faster proximally (Fig. 1.18),[33] the larger airways would be occluded by the bronchial secretions if these were not concentrated by an epithelial ion exchange mechanism. This vital function is under the control of an epithelial transmembrane regulator, faults in which underlie the development of cystic fibrosis (see p. 65). The same control mechanism operates in reverse in panting dogs to facilitate heat loss. The thickness of the aqueous hypophase is also of crucial importance to ciliary function (see below).

The various epithelial cells are held together by desmosomes, gap junctions and near the lumen by terminal bars that prevent excessive fluid movement across the epithelium.[34] However, irritants such as tobacco smoke, sulphur dioxide and mast cell mediators render the terminal bar permeable to particulate markers placed in the lumen.[35–37]

The epithelial cells rest on a basement membrane that consists of three layers: a lamina lucida, which makes contact with overlying epithelial cells, a lamina densa and a lamina reticularis. The last of these consists of fine fibrillary collagen and is only present in adults. It is not considered to be part of the 'true' basement membrane but it is this layer that is thickened in asthma and, to a lesser extent, a variety of other airway diseases. The laminae lucida and densa comprise the 'true' basement membrane. They each measure 50 nm in thickness, well below the resolution of the light microscope. They are made up of type IV collagen, laminin and fibronectin. They have a negative charge, due to sulphate and carboxyl moieties, which partly contributes to their permeability. This is relatively high; the basement membrane is a relatively poor barrier to the movement of macromolecules and even cells.

Surface epithelial cells are replaced only slowly, less than 1% being in division at any one time, although the mitotic index increases in response to various forms of injury.[38] The role of the basal cell as the sole progenitor has been questioned following recognition that other non-ciliated cells, notably the mucous, Clara and neuroendocrine cells, have an important stem cell function.[38–45]

Approximately 10 000 litres of air are inhaled each day and considerable amounts of potentially harmful environmental agents escape the filtering action of the nose to reach the lower respiratory tract. The

Figure 1.12 Intra-acinar pulmonary blood circulation. *(Netter medical illustration used with permission of Elsevier. All rights reserved.)*

Labels in figure:

Terminal bronchiole
Bronchial artery (from left heart via thoracic aorta)
Pulmonary vein (to left heart)
Pulmonary artery (from right heart)
Respiratory bronchioles
Capillary plexuses within alveolar wall
Pulmonary vein (to left heart)
Septum
Septum
Visceral pleura and subpleural capillaries
Capillary bed within alveolar wall (cut away in places)

Pulmonary arteries and their branches distribute segmentally with the bronchi.
Pulmonary veins and their tributaries drain intersegmentally.

Ciliated cells

Ciliated cells[49] possess numerous mitochondria and two types of surface projection: stubby microvilli about 0.4 μm in length and long slender cilia up to 6 μm in length. There are 200–300 cilia per cell, each beating at about 20 times a second. The rate at which the cilia beat falls with temperature[50] and the upper respiratory tract plays an important role in warming and moistening the inspired air. The ciliary beat consists of a straight-armed effective stroke followed by a curling return stroke.[51] Ciliated cells are arranged in groups within which the cilia beat in a co-ordinated fashion, probably governed by contact with the overlying mucus. The beating appears to be spontaneous. It is independent of nervous control and persists for several hours after death.

The cilia beat in a low viscosity layer beneath the surface mucus and move the overlying mucus only by their tips, which possess minute terminal hooklets (see Fig. 1.17).[52] The depth of the aqueous hypophase is crucial to ciliary action: too much and the mucus is lifted off the tips of the cilia, too little and the cilia become clogged by mucus. The periciliary fluid is thought to derive from the airway epithelial cells under the control of the transmembrane regulator referred to above. The cell surface available for fluid transport is greatly increased by its microvilli, which are akin to the brush border of the intestinal epithelium.

The fine structure of cilia has become of medical importance with the recognition of the ciliary dyskinesia syndromes (see p. 63). Cilia have an axial central pair of microtubules with an outer ring of nine double microtubules (9 + 2 structure) (see Fig. 2.44, p. 64). Small dynein side arms extend from one doublet towards the next and spokes connect each doublet with the central microtubules. All the microtubules fuse together near the tip while near the cell the central pair disappears and the doublets become triploid and fuse together as a cylinder which extends into the cytoplasm as the ciliary basal body. Cilia beat when the microtubules, powered by adenosine triphosphate elaborated in the dynein arms, slide past each other.

Basal cells

Basal cells are found particularly in the large airways but, although they diminish in number peripherally, they reach down as far as the bronchioles. They have only sparse cytoplasm, which often contains bundles of cytokeratin tonofilaments that lead into prominent hemidesmosomes.[53] The basal cell was formerly thought to be the main stem cell of the airways but with the recognition that Clara, mucous and neuroendocrine cells are important in this respect,[38–40,42,45] this view has had to be modified. Although they continue to be recognised as progenitor cells,[54] adhesion of the columnar cells to the basement membrane is now thought to be an additional major function of basal cells.[55,56]

Mucous cells

Mucous cells[24,49] vary in appearance with a cycle of secretory activity that culminates in the discharge of mucus into the airways. Devoid of mucus, they are slender and possess abundant endoplasmic reticulum and well-developed Golgi apparatus. As they synthesise mucus, electronlucent mucous granules accumulate, enlarge and fuse together to produce a large secretion vacuole that distends the apical cell cytoplasm, giving the mature cell its characteristic wine glass or goblet shape. Discharge takes place by further fusion involving the secretion vacuole and apical cell membranes.

Mucins are high-molecular-weight glycoproteins in which oligosaccharide side chains are attached to an elongated protein core.[57] The

Figure 1.13 Normal bronchus, showing surface epithelium resting on elastin-rich connective tissue (these elements constitute the mucosa: see Fig. 1.14), beneath which are the submucosal glands and cartilage. The glands are of mixed seromucous type. The apparent absence of submucosal muscle at this point is attributable to its double spiral arrangement.

respiratory epithelium provides the first line of defence against these.[46] It does this in three ways:

1. by providing an intact surface barrier comparable to the skin and the epithelium of the alimentary tract
2. by secreting an array of substances that act against physical and biological agents
3. by co-ordinating secretory and ciliary function so that there is effective mucociliary clearance.

Nevertheless, immune reactions are constantly at play in the lungs and if these were allowed to proceed unchecked, inflammation would be a permanent feature of the airways. That this is not the case is due at least in part to an inhibitory action that airway epithelial cells exert on dendritic cells within the epithelial milieu.[47,48]

The morphology and function of the individual epithelial cells will now be considered in turn.

Figure 1.14 (A) If the trachea is opened from the front, longitudinal ridges are evident in the posterior membranous portion. The ridges continue into the right main bronchus whilst others commence in the left main bronchus. (B) Microscopy shows that the ridges consist of longitudinal bands of elastic tissue staining black (top). Together with the surface epithelium, not evident in this preparation, this elastin-rich connective tissue constitutes the bronchial mucosa. The bronchial cartilage is also darkly stained but the intervening submucosal glands and muscle are poorly stained. Elastin van Gieson stain.

Figure 1.15 Bronchial epithelium composed of pseudostratified columnar ciliated cells interspersed with occasional mucus-secreting (goblet) cells.

mucous granules of the surface mucous cells contain an acidic mucin, with sialic acid or sulphate groups at the end of the oligosaccharide side chains of the peptide core. The amount and viscoelasticity of the mucus are important to airway clearance and the chemical structure of the mucus probably influences its physical properties and hence the ease with which it is cleared by ciliary activity or coughing. Out of the nine different mucin genes identified in human tissues, seven are expressed in the respiratory tract: MUC1–MUC4, MUC5AC, MUC5B and MUC7.[58,59] While MUC5B and MUC7 expression is predominantly restricted to cells of the submucosal glands,[60] MUC2 and MUC5AC mucins are located more in the surface epithelium.[61] The predominant components of respiratory mucus are MUC5AC and MUC5B,[62] and these are upregulated by various stimuli such as air pollutants or bacteria and also in asthma and cystic fibrosis.[63,64] The number of mucous cells increases in response to irritation. This also induces inflammation and, although the viscosity of mucus is primarily dependent on its glycoprotein content, it is markedly augmented by DNA released from effete inflammatory cells. It is impossible to state at exactly what point goblet cell hyperplasia begins as numbers

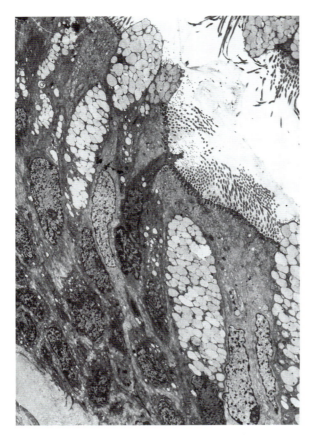

Figure 1.16 Bronchial epithelium. Transmission electron micrograph showing basal, ciliated and mucous cells. The electron-lucent mucus granules fuse together before discharge. Most of the surface is formed of ciliated cells. *(Courtesy of Mrs D Bowes, Midhurst, UK.)*

Figure 1.17 (A) Scanning electron micrograph of the bronchial surface showing mucus (top) resting on the tips of the cilia. The cilia beat in an aqueous hypophase. (B) High-power transmission electron microscopy shows that the tips of the cilia are equipped with hooklets. *(Courtesy of Professor PK Jeffery, Brompton, UK.)*

vary dependent on the site of the biopsy, but a crude figure is more than 3 per 10 cells at any point in the respiratory tract.

Apart from the mucus secreted by mucous cells in the surface epithelium and submucosal glands (see below), non-secretory cells such as the ciliated cells have a thin mucoid glycocalyx forming the outer part of their cell membrane.[57] This differs chemically from the main mucous lining and is probably formed by the cell of which it forms the outermost part. The glycocalyx of the cilia differs chemically from that of the microvilli on the same cell, whilst in the alveolus, different lining cells have chemically different forms of glycocalyx.[65]

Submucosal glands

The submucosal glands far exceed the secretory elements of the surface epithelium in cell mass and are the major source of bronchial secretion. They are situated between the muscle coat and the cartilage (see Fig. 1.13), and between individual cartilage plates, their ducts piercing the muscle coat and mucosa to reach the lumen. They are mixed seromucous glands, and the secretory acini are arranged so that the serous secretion has to pass through the mucous tubules.[66] The two secretions are therefore well mixed before they reach the bronchial lumen. Serous and mucous cells both have abundant rough endoplasmic reticulum and Golgi apparatus but the secretory granules of the serous cells are electron-dense, small and discrete, whereas mucous granules are electron-lucent, large and confluent (Fig. 1.19).[67] The serous granules often show zonal variations in their fine structure,

implying a variety of secretory products. The mucous cells contain large amounts of both acid and neutral glycoprotein whilst the serous cell granules contain smaller amounts of these glycoproteins[65,68] together with lysozyme,[67] lactoferrin[68] and a small-molecular-weight antiprotease specific to the airways.[69] The demonstration of carbonic anhydrase in serous cells implicates them in the production of a watery non-viscous secretion that could facilitate transport of the more viscous mucus secreted downstream.[66] The serous cells are also

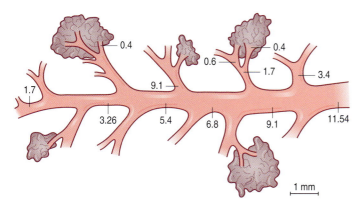

Figure 1.18 Velocity of mucus transport in the airways of a rat. The figures indicate the velocity of transport in millimetres per minute at a particular site at 37°C. From left to right the velocity increases sevenfold. *(Reproduced from Iravani & van As (1972)[33] by permission of the editor of the Journal of Pathology.)*

Figure 1.20 A seromucinous gland showing oncocytic metaplasia.

Figure 1.19 Bronchial gland composed of serous cells (top) which have discrete electron-dense granules, and mucous cells (bottom) in which the secretory granules are electron-lucent and fuse together before discharge. In close proximity to the serous cells is a group of plasma cells (centre right). Immunoglobulin A is produced by plasma cells that lie close to the bronchial glands: it passes through the serous cells to reach the lumen and in so doing acquires its secretory component which is synthesised by the serous cells. Transmission electron micrograph. *(Reproduced from Bowes & Corrin (1977)[67] with permission of the editor of Thorax.)*

the major site of the secretory component of IgA[70–72] and of epithelial peroxidase.[73]

Collecting-duct cells are devoid of secretory granules but often have the characteristics of oncocytes, their cytoplasm being packed with numerous mitochondria. The oncocytes increase in number with age and may form metaplastic nodules (Fig. 1.20).[74] A fluid-regulating role has been suggested for them but similar cells present in several other organs are considered to be degenerative. Glandular secretion is assisted by myoepithelial cells which are situated between the secretory and duct lining cells and the basement membrane. Neuroendocrine cells similar to those in the surface epithelium are also found in this situation, whilst unmyelinated nerve axons are observed in close association with serous, mucous, collecting-duct and myoepithelial cells.[75]

Neuroendocrine cells

Neuroendocrine cells, which are also known as Kultschitsky-type cells, Feyrter cells and APUD cells, are found in the basal layer of the surface epithelium and in the bronchial glands.[75,76] In the surface epithelium they occur singly and in groups, the latter known as neuroepithelial bodies.[77,78] Single neuroendocrine cells are basally situated but send a thin cytoplasmic process to the surface. They are found throughout the airways from the main bronchi to the bronchioles but are only rarely found in the terminal bronchioles and alveoli.[79,80] Neuroepithelial bodies extend from the basement membrane to the surface. They are found particularly at airway bifurcations and have sensory neuronal connections but are less numerous in humans than in many laboratory animals.[78,81–85] Adjacent capillaries have a fenestrated endothelium, as found in many endocrine organs.

Neuroendocrine cells are characterised by numerous small granules, 70–150 nm in diameter, consisting of a round electron-dense central core separated from an outer membrane by a clear halo (Fig. 1.21). In the fetus, two other morphological varieties of granule have been described.[77] The granules are scattered throughout the cytoplasm, but are often concentrated near the basal cell membrane. The neuroendocrine cells only occasionally display argyrophilia or formaldehyde-induced fluorescence but these reactions, indicative of biogenic amines, may be enhanced by prior incubation with precursor substances such as 5-hydroxytryptophan and dihydroxyphenylalanine.[86] Immunohistochemistry shows that both single neuroend-

Figure 1.21 Bronchial neuroendocrine cell granules consist of a dense central core separated from an investing membrane by a thin electron-lucent zone. Transmission electron micrograph. *(Courtesy of Miss A Dewar, Brompton, UK.)*

Figure 1.22 Terminal bronchiole showing non-ciliated Clara cells protruding above the adjacent cilia. Scanning electron micrograph. *(Courtesy of Professor PK Jeffery, Brompton, UK.)*

ocrine cells and the neuroepithelial bodies may contain L-amino acid decarboxylase[87] and 5-hydroxytryptamine,[88] general neuroendocrine markers such as neuron-specific enolase,[89] chromogranin A,[80,90] synaptophysin[91] and neural cell adhesion molecule (CD56)[92] and peptides such as human bombesin (gastrin-releasing peptide),[80,93–96] calcitonin,[80,94,97,98] leu-encephalin,[94] substance P,[99] guanine nucleotide-binding protein[100] and adrenocorticotrophic hormone.[95] Chromogranin, a constituent of the granules, and CD56 are probably the most sensitive and specific immunocytochemical markers.[80,92,101,102]

The main function of the pulmonary neuroendocrine system in humans is thought to concern the control of growth and development of the lungs in utero and thereafter the regulation of pulmonary regeneration and repair. Neuroendocrine cells are more numerous in the fetal than the adult lung and one of their products, human bombesin, has trophic properties in regard to the other cells. Hyperplasia of neuroendocrine cells has been described during epithelial repair,[42,103,104] following asbestos exposure[105] and in pulmonary fibrosis,[106] infantile bronchopulmonary dysplasia,[107] pulmonary arterial disease,[108] bronchiectasis associated with tumourlets[95] and bronchi bearing carcinomas of all cell types.[109] Neuroendocrine hyperplasia plays a role in the development of carcinoids and is thus regarded as a preneoplastic condition.

A subsidiary function of the neuroendocrine cells, which appears to be better developed in lower species, concerns the pulmonary response to hypoxia. Animal experiments have demonstrated that neuroendocrine cells increase in number and degranulate in hypoxic conditions, suggesting a chemoreceptor function.[110–113] In the case of the neuroepithelial bodies this function is modulated by intrapulmonary axon reflexes.[82] However, the relevance of these observations to humans is uncertain.

Clara cells

These cells are named after the Austrian histologist Max Clara who provided a detailed description of them in 1937.[25] They are most

numerous in the terminal bronchioles where they protrude above the ciliated cells (Fig. 1.22). The region immediately above the nucleus contains many large mitochondria with unusually sparse cristae. The apical portion is notable for a rich smooth endoplasmic reticulum network and, immediately beneath the luminal cell membrane, small electron-dense secretory granules of about 500 nm diameter. The granules are angulated in humans but round in many species. There is considerable species variation in the internal structure of Clara cells. The nature of the secretory product of the Clara cell and its precise mode of secretion are uncertain, but the major constituent of the granules is a 10-kDa protein (CC10) that inhibits several inflammatory cytokines and is therefore thought to be important in modulating bronchiolar inflammation and protecting the lung against emphysema[69]; mice that are deficient in this protein are more susceptible to the damaging effects of hyperoxia.[114] Cytochrome P-450-dependent mixed-function oxidase activity[115] has also been identified in Clara cells. Mixed-function oxidases are involved in metabolising many environmental chemicals, including carcinogens that require catalytic activation. Intracellular levels of glutathione are important in protecting the Clara cells from injury by reactive intermediates produced by the metabolism of xenobiotics such as 3-methylindole, trichloroethylene and naphthylamine.[41,116,117] Clara cell secretion of endothelin, a powerful bronchoconstrictor and vasoconstrictor, has also been demonstrated.[118] The Clara cell also has stem-cell potentiality and in response to irritation gives rise to both ciliated and mucous cells.[39,41,44]

Brush cells

Brush cells occur infrequently at all levels of the airways from the trachea to the alveoli, where they have been called type III pneumocytes.[119,120] They have a brush border of closely packed stubby microvilli up to 2 μm in length, the axial filaments of which continue into the cell without ending in a terminal web. A resemblance to intestinal cells has led to a belief that they are concerned in fluid absorption but their function remains obscure.[121]

Figure 1.23 A terminal bronchiole dividing into alveolated respiratory bronchioles, representing the termination of the purely conductive membranous bronchioles, the commencement of the transitional zone of the lung and the apex of a pulmonary acinus. A pulmonary artery is seen alongside the bronchiole. Artery and bronchiole are of roughly the same calibre. Between them is a lymphoreticular aggregate, marking the point at which lymphatics commence.

Figure 1.24 The cut surface of part of a lung lobule, showing some of the branches of an acinus. TB, terminal bronchiole; RB 1, 2 and 3, successive orders of respiratory bronchioles; AD, alveolar duct. The fibrous septa that border the lobule are also seen. *(Reproduced from Heard and Izukawa (1964)[122] with permission of the late Professor B E Heard and the editor of the* Journal of Pathology.*)*

MICROSCOPY OF THE ALVEOLAR TISSUE

Beyond the terminal bronchioles, which constitute the last of the purely conductive airways, alveoli are found in progressively increasing numbers through three orders of respiratory bronchioles and two to nine orders of alveolar ducts (Figs 1.23 and 1.24).[122] The walls of the alveolar ducts consist only of a thin spiral band of collagen and elastin, between which are the mouths of the alveoli, also arranged in a spiral fashion.[20] The arrangement is like the coils of a spring, lengthening in inspiration and closing up in expiration. The alveolar openings usually have four straight sides whilst the alveolar walls consist of flat pentagonal or hexagonal plates arranged as a polyhedron. The alveoli are thus like boxes with one open side[123]: if the alveoli were spherical, their walls would stretch on inspiration and the alveolar capillaries would close. The alveolar duct system and the polyhedral shape of the alveoli act together like a concertina and thereby permit changes in volume without alterations in surface area.

The human adult lungs contain about 300–500 million alveoli,[5,124] each measuring about 250 µm in diameter when expanded, although gravitational forces result in them being bigger in the upper than the lower parts of the lung.[125] The size of the alveoli and the surface tension of their lining layer are the major determinants of distensibility and hence elastic recoil of the lungs; tissue components such as elastin and collagen contribute to a lesser degree.[126] The Laplace equation indicates that the collapsing force acting on the lungs is proportional to alveolar surface tension and inversely proportional to alveolar size. Surface tension is reduced, and expansion of the lung thereby facilitated, by certain lipids, collectively known as pulmonary surfactant, that are secreted by alveolar lining cells (see below).

Small holes, the pores of Kohn, are found in the alveolar walls of many species, including humans (Fig. 1.25). Their diameter ranges from 2 to 13 µm and there are from one to seven in each alveolus. The pores are absent at birth and only develop after the first year of life. For this reason some argue that they are abnormal and represent the beginnings of emphysema. Others believe that they are normal and provide collateral ventilation, although perfusion fixation, which

Figure 1.25 Scanning electron micrograph of normal mouse lung. The small holes in the alveolar walls are the pores of Kohn. *(Courtesy of the late Professor B E Heard, Brompton, UK.)*

Figure 1.27 Parts of two alveolar walls, the lower and upper respectively showing the thin and thick portions of the air–blood barrier respectively. The upper alveolar wall is lined by the nucleated portion of a type I cell (solid arrow) and a type II (open arrow) cell, the former partly covered by an alveolar macrophage (M). Abundant connective tissue is seen beneath these epithelial cells, in contrast to the thin part of the air–blood barrier where the interstitum consists of no more than the fused epithelial and endothelial basement membranes. A, air space; C, capillary lumen. Transmission electron micrograph. *(Courtesy of Mrs D Bowes, Midhurst, UK.)*

Figure 1.26 An immunocytochemical preparation of normal alveolar tissue shows that epithelial cells are plentiful but by light microscopy it is not apparent that the epithelial lining is complete. Immunoperoxidase for cytokeratin.

preserves the alveolar lining layer, demonstrates that the pores are normally plugged by this layer.[127] In pneumonia, however, threads of fibrin can sometimes be seen passing through the pores from one alveolus to another. Transmission electron microscopy shows the edge of the pores to be lined by an intact epithelium.

Under the light microscope the alveolar wall is evidently rich in blood capillaries but it is not generally clear whether cells bordering the capillaries are endothelial, epithelial or interstitial. Cytokeratin immunocytochemistry shows that epithelial cells are plentiful but by light microscopy the alveolar epithelium appears to be incomplete (Fig. 1.26). It was not until 1953 that electron microscopy clarified an age-old dispute concerning the nature of the alveolar lining layer, showing that a complete simple epithelium extends throughout all alveoli (Figs 1.27 and 1.28).[128] It is continuous with that of the airways. The lining epithelium is separated from the underlying connective tissue by a supportive basement membrane.

On one side of the alveolar wall the capillary is closely applied to the alveolar epithelium. Here the endothelial and epithelial basement membrane fuse and the air–blood barrier is at its thinnest, about 0.15 μm. On the opposite side of the alveolar wall, interstitial tissue separates endothelium from epithelium; this is known as the thick side of the air–blood barrier (see Figs 1.27 and 1.28). The alveolar epithelium, interstitium and capillary endothelium constitute about 30%, 40% and 30% respectively of the air–blood barrier.[129]

The alveolar epithelium consists of two principal cell types, variously known as I and II, A and B, small and large, non-vacuolated

Figure 1.29 Two type II alveolar epithelial cells with surface microvilli and two surface pits through which surfactant has been secreted from vacuoles within the cytoplasm. Scanning electron micrograph. *(Courtesy of Dr J H L Watson, Detroit, USA.)*

Figure 1.28 Alveolar wall with the nuclear portion of a type I cell and the thin part of the air–blood barrier on the right-hand side. The interstitium contains bundles of collagen surrounding very electron-dense elastin. Transmission electron micrograph. *(Courtesy of Miss A Dewar, Brompton, UK.)*

and vacuolated, squamous and granular respectively, which will now be considered.

Type I alveolar epithelial cells

These cells have few cytoplasmic organelles but are remarkable for their attenuated cytoplasm, which extends long distances from the nuclear zone of the cell (see Figs 1.27 and 1.28) and may even penetrate the alveolar wall so that one cell contributes to the lining of more than one alveolus.[130] They each cover up to 5000 μm^2 of the alveolar surface yet generally measure no more than 0.2 μm in thickness.[131] Their function is to provide a complete but thin covering, preventing fluid loss but facilitating rapid gas exchange. Type I cells are connected to each other and to type II cells by tight junctions, and the alveolar epithelium provides the major barrier to fluid movement into and out of the alveolus. Nevertheless, a variety of proteins known as aquaporins that facilitate water transport across epithelia have been identified in the cell membrane of type I alveolar cells.[132] Following large-volume alveolar lavage for lipoproteinosis (see p. 318) it has been found that about 53% of the residual fluid is absorbed within 1 hour.[133] Numerous small pinocytotic vesicles are seen within the type I cells and macromolecules are absorbed from the alveolus by this route.[134] Very fine particles reach the interstitium from the alveolar lumen by the same vesicular transport mechanism.[135,136] Such absorption is probably important in sensitising the host to inhaled antigens

but as a clearance pathway the alveolar epithelium is of trifling importance compared with the alveolar macrophages.

The long thin cytoplasmic processes of the type I epithelial cells are extremely sensitive to damage by various injurious agents. Together with the capillary endothelium these cells represent the component of the lung most vulnerable to damage (see Chapter 4).

Type II alveolar epithelial cells

These cells are taller and twice as numerous as the type I cells but they cover only 7% of the alveolar surface.[131] They usually occupy the corners of alveoli and often all but the apex of the cell is covered by neighbouring type I cells. The free surface has blunt microvilli and the cytoplasm includes mitochondria, endoplasmic reticulum, Golgi apparatus and characteristic osmiophilic lamellar structures which represent the secretory vacuoles of pulmonary surfactant (Figs 1.29 and 1.30). These appear in fetal life at the time when surfactant can first be identified and an extrauterine existence first becomes possible. Their role in surfactant secretion has been established by experimental ultrastructural autoradiography, tracing the incorporation of surfactant precursors in a sequential fashion through secretory organelles and into the lamellar structures.[137-140] Cell separation techniques enabling pure type II cell suspensions to be studied in vitro support the role of these cells as secretors of surfactant.[141] Lysosomal enzymes identified in the lamellar structures are derived from multivesicular bodies which fuse with them.[142,143] One of these hydrolases, phosphatidic acid phosphatase, controls an essential step in surfactant synthesis.[144] Further vesicles and multivesicular bodies located immediately beneath the cell membrane are concerned in the secretion of certain surfactant-specific proteins, which are described below.[145]

After injury there are found occasional alveolar epithelial cells that possess features of both type I and type II cells (see Fig. 4.10, p. 139).

Figure 1.32 An alveolar macrophage with prominent lysosomal dense bodies and pseudopodia is seen close to the alveolar wall. Transmission electron micrograph. *(Courtesy of Professor P K Jeffery, Brompton, UK.)*

Figure 1.33 Two alveolar macrophages near a pore of Kohn. Unstained electron micrograph to show the electron-dense reaction product of lysosomal acid phosphatase, thus confirming the lysosomal nature of the cytoplasmic dense bodies. *(Reproduced from Corrin et al. (1969)[143] by permission of the editor of the Journal of Anatomy.)*

stimulated T lymphocytes, they are important in presenting antigen to lymphocytes, and are aided in this by the presence of immunoglobulin and complement receptors on their surface.[188] Furthermore, alveolar macrophages appear to modulate the expression of immune reactions in the lung for in differing circumstances they appear either to enhance or to suppress the proliferation, differentiation and function of antigen-stimulated lymphocytes.[191]

The alveolar macrophages are normally situated within the alveolar lining film, but are floated off into the alveolar lumen during immersion fixation. They are irregular in outline and have prominent pseudopodial cytoplasmic extensions (Fig. 1.32). The cytoplasm contains many dense bodies rich in lysosomal enzymes (Fig. 1.33).[142,143] Phagosomal vacuoles and multiloculated phagolysosomes are also numerous.

The alveolar macrophage is avidly phagocytic[135,136,192] (Fig. 1.34) and represents an important defence mechanism against inhaled bacteria. It also provides the major means of clearing the alveolus of inhaled dust. In smokers, the phagolysosomal inclusions are more plentiful and pleomorphic and contain characteristic 'tar bodies' or minute kaolinite crystals (see Fig. 7.2.3, p. 374).[193] Lung lining material is a chemotactant for alveolar macrophages[194] and the phagocytic action of alveolar macrophages is potentiated by the surfactant-associated proteins SP-A and SP-D.[155,195] Conversely, alveolar macrophages provide one means of removing spent surfactant.[158]

Phagocytosis involves a process of membrane fusion concerning first the cell membrane and then those of the phagosome and lysosomes. In addition to acid hydrolases, alveolar macrophages contain catalase and a peroxidase distinct from myeloperoxidase, but which in the presence of iodide and peroxide has similar antibacterial properties.[196,197] Superoxide production by alveolar macrophages is characterised by a burst in oxygen consumption and glycogenolysis that is stimulated by the phagocytosis of a variety of inhaled pollutants.[198] Another powerful antibacterial agent formed in macrophages, and other phagocytic cells, is nitric oxide.[199–201] The antibacterial activity of alveolar macrophages is depressed by hypoxia, hyperoxia, cold,

alcohol, cigarette smoke, metabolic acidosis and viral infections[202–207] and is defective in chronic granulomatous disease (see p. 484 [systemic diseases]). Bacteria killed within macrophages are digested by the action of lysosomal acid hydrolases.

Although primarily concerned with intracellular digestion, lysosomal enzymes are known to be released during phagocytosis. This was initially thought to represent inadvertent leakage due to premature membrane fusion, but it is now appreciated that macrophages actively secrete certain substances and the release of acid hydrolases during phagocytosis may not be fortuitous.[208,209] Indeed, the bulk of the lysozyme within macrophages appears to be destined for secretion outside the cell rather than intracellular digestion; its secretion is independent of phagocytic activity. Other antimicrobial factors secreted by macrophages include interferon. The excessive release of reactive oxygen metabolites, nitric oxide and lysosomal enzymes from macrophages may have deleterious results, possibly contributing to lung injury in processes such as septic shock (see p. 143). Macrophages can also be an abundant source of matrix metalloproteinases such as collagenase, gelatinase and elastase, the release of which is implicated in the development of emphysema.[210,211]

Other macrophage factors of interest are those influencing the activity of other host cells and the identification of a fibroblast-stimulating substance is clearly relevant to fibrotic lung disease.[212–215] Transformation of macrophages into epithelioid and multinucleated giant cells is particularly associated with the development of organelles more associated with secretory than phagocytic cells, e.g. Golgi apparatus and vesicles (see Fig. 6.1.32, p. 286). This is associated with the secretion of an array of cytokines.

Figure 1.34 Unstained electron micrograph of rat lung injected with finely divided electron-dense tracer particles via the trachea. Numerous large phagosomes are evident in an alveolar macrophage (M) but are scanty and minute in the alveolar epithelium (arrows). II, type II pneumocyte. *(Reproduced from Corrin (1970) by permission of the editor of Thorax.[135])*

Figure 1.35 A pulmonary arteriogram produced by injecting the arteries of an excised lung with a molten barium–gelatine mixture.

BLOOD SUPPLY OF THE LUNGS

The pulmonary vasculature is unique in that it receives the whole of the cardiac output, but it perfuses rather than nourishes the lungs, this latter function being undertaken by the bronchial vasculature. The pulmonary circulation is a low-pressure system. At rest a mean pressure of only 10 mmHg is sufficient to distribute the cardiac output through the lungs. This barely counteracts gravity and in the upright position blood flow through the apices of the lungs is minimal at rest. Cardiac output may double without any increase in pulmonary artery pressure because closed capillaries in the underperfused upper zones of the lungs are first recruited. Thus there is considerable reserve in the pulmonary vascular bed and many vessels may be lost in disease or surgically without incurring a significant rise in pulmonary vascular resistance. The full extent of the pulmonary arterial system is shown in Figure 1.35.

Pulmonary arteries

The anatomy of the main pulmonary arteries and the relationship of their branches to the airways have been described above (see p. 6). The major pulmonary arteries are elastic vessels and at birth the pattern of their elastic laminae closely resembles that of the aorta. Within the first few months of life there is fragmentation of the elastic fibres and an irreversible 'adult pattern' is reached by about the age of 6 months (see Fig. 8.2.8, p. 423).

There is a sharp transition from elastic to muscular pulmonary arteries at a level of the bronchovascular tree where bronchi give way to bronchioles (such airways having a diameter close to 1 mm and the accompanying arteries being of similar or slightly smaller size). Muscular pulmonary arteries have well-defined internal and external elastic laminae enclosing their muscular media. The whole wall is very thin compared with systemic arteries of comparable diameter, reflecting the different pressures in the two circulations. In normal uninjected lungs, the medial thickness of muscular pulmonary arteries is about 5% of the external diameter compared with 15–20% in systemic arteries.[216] Injection of the pulmonary arteries with fixative or contrast medium yields lower values. Despite blood flow being greater in the base of the lung than the apex, there is normally no quantitative difference in pulmonary artery structure between these zones (although such differences develop when venous pressure is raised).

The muscle of the media thins progressively as the arteries narrow with repeated branching, and in vessels between 100 and 30 μm in diameter the muscle coat is represented only by a spiral, so that in cross-section, arteries of this size are only muscularised for part of their circumference. Below 30 μm diameter, precapillary vessels have no muscle in their walls, which consist only of fibroelastic tissue. The existence of partially muscularised blood vessels obscures the distinction between arteries and arterioles. For this reason many workers prefer to call all precapillary vessels arteries.

The pulmonary artery endothelium has many fine cytoplasmic projections which increase the surface area considerably.[217] Myofilaments are found in the endothelium of pulmonary arteries and precapillaries, but not capillaries.[218] Distinctive inclusions first found in the endothelium of pulmonary arteries have subsequently been identified in systemic arteries and are occasionally also observed in alveolar capillaries. They consist of parallel microtubules forming rod-shaped membrane-bound granules up to 3 μm in length and are frequently termed Weibel–Palade bodies after those who first described them.[219] Their function is uncertain but it has been shown that they contain von Willebrand protein.[220]

Ventilation–perfusion matching

The muscular pulmonary arteries are unique in contracting in response to hypoxia and an important consequence of defective ventilation of the lung is that it induces a corresponding fall in pulmonary perfusion. This mechanism operates at the local level. There is a remarkably fine local matching of pulmonary perfusion to ventilation, brought about by vasoconstriction in poorly ventilated areas.[221,222] It is important that such a mechanism should operate, for blood leaving the lungs is normally fully saturated with oxygen and, if poorly ventilated lung tissue was perfused, hypoxaemia would inevitably result (Fig. 1.36). Local perfusion/ventilation matching minimises the danger of hypoxaemia. This is an important adaptive mechanism and beneficial when there is focal ventilatory impairment, as with an inhaled foreign body, but if airflow limitation is generalised, as in chronic bronchitis and emphysema, there is widespread pulmonary vasoconstriction, which causes right-heart strain and eventual failure. The immediate cause of the pulmonary vasoconstriction is low oxygen tension in the inspired air but how this operates has been the subject of much debate. The rise in pulmonary vascular resistance is virtually unaffected by vagotomy, indicating that it is a local response. Mechanisms that have been suggested include a local axon reflex, paracrine activity by neuroendocrine cells in the airway mucosa (see p. 13) and a direct vascular response to the low oxygen tension.[223] The last of these mechanisms has most support; arterial endothelia synthesise and secrete various vasoactive substances, notably the vasoconstrictor, endothelin[224] and the relaxing factor, nitric oxide. In the lungs hypoxia has the effect of increasing the release of endothelin and inhibiting the release of nitric oxide.[225] The resultant vasoconstriction is most profound in small muscular pulmonary arteries of about 30–50 μm diameter.[221,222] Generalised pulmonary vasoconstriction imposes a considerable burden on the right side of the heart, which counters by releasing atrial natriuretic factor. This decreases pulmonary vasoconstriction, as well as opposing the action of renin and aldosterone on the kidney and promoting diuresis.[226]

Alveolar capillaries

The alveolar capillaries form a tightly matted network of short intersecting tubules (Fig. 1.37).[227] There are about 1000 such capillary segments per alveolus[228] and a blood cell passing through the lungs would have to traverse about 60.[229] The capillary wall consists merely of endothelium of the usual continuous type and a basement membrane (see Figs 1.27 and 1.28).

Pinocytotic vesicles are numerous in the endothelial cells. They open as caveolae on to both the luminal and interstitial aspects, but are more noticeable on the former where many of them have a special structure, being 'sealed' by a thin single membrane or diaphragm (Fig.

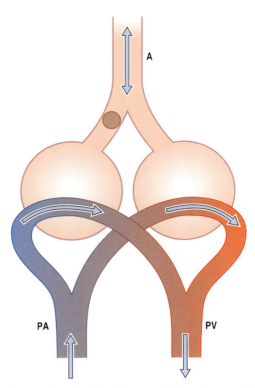

Figure 1.36 The blood leaving the lungs is normally fully oxygenated and perfusion of any poorly ventilated areas (as on the left) would inevitably result in hypoxaemia. This is prevented by matching perfusion to ventilation through arteriolar constriction at the local level, which is probably mediated by reduced nitric oxide release from the endothelium in response to low oxygen tension. A, airway; PA, pulmonary artery; PV, pulmonary vein.

1.38). Where the caveolar membrane, diaphragm and cell membrane fuse, dense knobs are found, possibly representing a ring structure that may maintain the patency of the stoma and the integrity of the diaphragm. Nucleotide-splitting enzymes thought to minimise the risk of thrombosis have been localised within these caveolae.[230]

The capillary diameter is about 5 μm, less than that of the blood cells, but erythrocytes at least are fairly deformable. White blood cells are less deformable and transit of these cells through the alveolar capillaries is slower than that of erythrocytes.[231] This delay is increased in pulmonary inflammation. The alveolar capillaries are the vessels involved in neutrophil sequestration and migration,[232] in contrast to the systemic circulation where these processes take place in venules.

The endothelial cell is similar to the type I epithelial cell in thickness (see Fig. 1.27) but covers only one-third the area and the alveolar wall contains many more endothelial than type I epithelial cells.[131] In contrast to the alveolar epithelium the endothelial cell junctions readily permit the passage of small-molecular-weight proteins and the basement membrane similarly offers no barrier to fluid transport.[233] Larger molecules such as albumin are retained by the intercellular junctions but small amounts of albumin cross the endothelium to reach the interstitium by pinocytotic transport.[234] Alveolar capillaries are attended by pericytes, elongated contractile cells rich in cytoplasmic filaments and which are ensheathed by the endothelial basement membrane.[166] The role of pericytes and myofibroblasts in controlling perfusion is discussed above (see alveolar interstitium, p. 18).

Figure 1.37 The alveolar capillaries (which are unduly prominent in this congested lung) form many short, interconnecting segments. Scanning electron micrograph. *(Courtesy of Professor PK Jeffery, Brompton, UK.)*

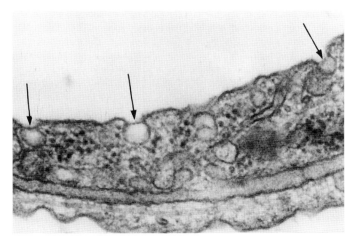

Figure 1.38 The air–blood barrier showing three caveolae (arrows) in the surface of the capillary endothelium, each sealed by a thin single membrane. Transmission electron micrograph. *(Courtesy of Mrs D Bowes, Midhurst, UK.)*

Pulmonary veins

The walls of the intrapulmonary veins consist largely of multiple irregular elastic laminae and collagen with little intervening muscle. However, with increased venous pressure, they may acquire a muscular media and become 'arterialised' (see Fig. 8.2.16, p. 428). In disease states therefore the structure of the vessel wall is not a wholly reliable criterion in distinguishing veins from arteries. More valuable is an assessment of the location of the vessel, remembering that pulmonary veins are found at the periphery of the lung lobule and in the interlobular septa. Intralobular veins less than 30 μm in diameter are identical in structure to arteries of comparable size and are distinguishable from them only by their connections to larger veins. Pulmonary veins are not valved but sphincters have been described in the pulmonary veins of rats.[235]

Sometimes small cellular collections are observed adjacent to the pulmonary veins. They have been likened to chemoreceptor tissue but ultrastructural studies show that they have a remarkable resemblance to meningeal arachnoid cells. Some authors refer to them as arachnoid nodules and suggest that, like those in the meninges that transfer interstitial fluid to the dural veins, those in the lungs may transfer interstitial lung fluid to the pulmonary veins and so minimise the danger of pulmonary oedema.[236] These structures are described more fully in the section dealing with lung tumours (see multiple minute meningothelioid nodules, p. 700).

The intrapulmonary veins join to form extrapulmonary vessels connecting the lungs to the left atrium. There are generally four of these vessels, the right and left superior and inferior pulmonary veins, but they may number three or five.[237] Immediately before the pulmonary veins enter the left atrium they acquire a sheath of myocardium, which varies from 0.2 to 1.7 cm in length.[237] Ectopic foci within these myocardial sleeves communicate with the cardiac conducting system and are now believed to be the commonest cause of atrial fibrillation (see p. 76).[238-240]

Pulmonary arteriovenous shunts

Shunts that bypass the capillary bed have been demonstrated in experimental animals by perfusing glass spheres 20–40 times the diameter of the capillaries.[241] In humans, these shunts have been shown to be at the entry to the bronchopulmonary segments, the entry to the acini and within the visceral pleura.[242] They normally conduct little of the pulmonary blood flow but widen when small pulmonary vessels are narrowed.

Non-chromaffin paraganglia

Non-chromaffin paraganglia ('glomera') were identified widely distributed throughout an infant's lung in a search of 5250 serial sections, being found particularly at the branching point of pulmonary arteries in close relation to nerves.[243] In fine structure they resembled chemoreceptors and a regulatory role in respiration and pulmonary blood flow was proposed. The possibility that non-chromaffin paragangliomas arise from these structures is discussed on page 638.

Metabolic functions of the pulmonary endothelium

It is now recognised that many serum factors, including certain drugs and hormones, are modified as they pass through the lung, and that the pulmonary endothelium is not just a smooth inert vascular lining. Some substances are merely bound to the endothelium and may be dislodged by others. For example, imipramine is a drug for which the lung has a high affinity but no metabolic capability and further infusions of imipramine or chlorpromazine will displace imipramine previously accumulated in the lung.[244] Other substances are taken up by the endothelium and actively metabolised, either on the surface or within the cytoplasm of the endothelial cell, resulting in the serum factor being either activated or inactivated. For example, angiotensin is activated and bradykinin inactivated by a peptidase* that is distributed uniformly along the endothelial cell surface.[230] Substances taken up and metabolised within the endothelial cells include 5-hydroxytryptamine (by monoamine oxidase), noradrenaline (norepinephrine: by catechol-o-methyl transferase) and prostaglandins of the E and F series (by 14-hydroxyprostaglandin dehydrogenase). 5-Hydroxytryptamine is taken up by endothelial cells throughout the pulmonary circulation, whereas noradrenaline is preferentially taken up by small pre- and postcapillary vessels and by veins.[245,246] Some substances that the endothelium is capable of metabolising pass through the pulmonary circulation unchanged because there is no uptake mechanism. For example, despite the presence within the pulmonary endothelial cells of peptidases capable of splitting oxytocin, vasopressin and substance P, these substances are unchanged on passage through the pulmonary circulation because there is no uptake. Similarly histamine and prostaglandin A pass through the lung unchanged despite the presence of intracellular imidazole-N-methyl transferase and 14-hydroxyprostaglandin dehydrogenase, again because of the low affinity the lung has for these substances.[247]

Prostacyclin synthetase is found particularly in relation to the arterial intima.[248] Prostacyclin is spontaneously released from the lungs and it has been proposed that this represents active secretion by the endothelium.[249] Prostacyclin is vasodilatory and, in regard to platelets, antiaggregatory: in particular, prostacyclin is antagonistic to thromboxane, the platelet-aggregating factor released from platelets themselves. Prostacyclin therefore plays an important role in minimising pulmonary thrombosis. Nucleotidases found in the endothelial caveolae described above are also thought to minimise the risk of thrombosis. However, thrombogenic factors are also found in the endothelium: for example, von Willebrand protein has been localised to Weibel–Palade bodies, which are widely distributed in vascular endothelium,[220] and factor VIII-related antigen is strongly represented in pulmonary endothelium.

The endothelium lining pulmonary arteries, and to a lesser extent pulmonary veins, also secretes potent vasoactive substances outwards, that is, away from the lumen towards the smooth muscle in the medial coat of the vessel. Two substances are of note here, endothelin,[224,250] which is a particularly powerful vasoconstrictor, and nitric oxide,[199,200,251] which was known as endothelium-derived relaxing factor before its simple chemical structure was appreciated. Enhanced nitric oxide activity is thought to contribute to the normal decline in pulmonary vascular resistance at birth. Neither of these vasoactive factors is unique to the pulmonary circulation, being formed in endothelia throughout the body. Indeed, neither is confined to blood vessels and both function quite differently in other tissues. In the lung, endothelin is also formed in airway epithelium[118,224] and when administered via the airways has a strong bronchoconstrictor effect. Nitric oxide, which is cytotoxic and has only a very short tissue half-life, is an important neurotransmitter and, in phagocytes, an effective bactericidal agent. In blood vessels, endothelin and nitric oxide have opposing actions and normal vascular tone depends upon them balancing one another. This equilibrium is disturbed in diseases such as

pulmonary hypertension, where there is evidence of excess endothelin activity,[252] and in septic shock, where excess nitric oxide is released from activated neutrophils and macrophages.[201]

The alveolar capillary endothelium also shares antigens with a macrophage subset capable of presenting antigens to lymphocytes, suggesting that it may play a role in the immunological response of the lung.[253]

Megakaryocytes in the pulmonary circulation: the lung as a source of platelets

Megakaryocytes are produced in the bone marrow and some at least are evidently released intact for they are also found in mixed venous blood. The dimensions of megakaryocytes and pulmonary capillaries are such that any megakaryocytes arriving in the lungs would be held there. Occasional megakaryocytes are indeed seen in normal lung, trapped in alveolar capillaries.[254–256] They generally appear as irregular haematoxyphil clumps representing only the condensed nuclei of these platelet precursor cells.[256,257] They are devoid of cytoplasm and have evidently discharged their platelets. The fact that platelets are more numerous in arterial than mixed venous blood whereas the converse applies for megakaryocytes suggests that many platelets are first released from megakaryocytes trapped in the lungs,[258–264] but this does not mean that the lungs are the principal site of platelet production.[256] Megakaryocytes are particularly easy to find in pulmonary capillaries when there is an increased demand for platelets, as in conditions such as shock and carcinomatosis which lead to increased platelet consumption (see Fig. 4.22B, p. 145).[256,265,266]

Bronchial vasculature

Whereas the pulmonary circulation receives the whole venous return of the body, the bronchial circulation is part of the systemic circulation and receives only 1–2% of the output of the left ventricle. The pulmonary circulation is a high-capacity, low-resistance system whereas the bronchial circulation is a low-capacity, high-resistance system.[267,268] In response to hypoxaemia the pulmonary arteries constrict but the bronchial arteries dilate. Bronchial blood flow also increases in response to the inhalation of cold air.

Bronchial arteries

The bronchial arteries supply oxygenated blood to the walls of the airways, the interlobular septa and the visceral pleura. There is usually one bronchial artery on the right, which arises from the third posterior intercostal artery or from the upper left bronchial artery. The left bronchial arteries usually number two and arise from the descending thoracic aorta inferior to the origin of the third posterior intercostal artery. However, bronchial arteries may arise from the thyrocervical trunk, an internal mammary artery, the costocervical trunk, a subclavian artery, a lower intercostal artery, an inferior phrenic artery or even the abdominal aorta. They anastomose with tracheal arteries derived from the inferior thyroid artery. Bronchopulmonary anastomoses are considered below.

Within the lung, bronchial arteries are best seen at the level of the larger bronchi where the pulmonary arteries are still of the elastic type, which contrasts sharply with the muscular structure of the bronchial arteries. Bronchial arteries have a thicker medial coat than pulmonary arteries, commensurate with the higher pressure they have to withstand. They also lack an outer elastic membrane, having only a single internal elastic lamina (Fig. 1.39). Bronchial arteries also lie within the wall of the bronchi whereas pulmonary blood vessels lie alongside.

---

*Since this enzyme cleaves the carboxyl terminal dipeptide from both bradykinin and angiotensin I, it is preferable to use its biochemical name dipeptidyl carboxypeptidase rather than either of its trivial names, kininase or angiotensin converting enzyme.

Figure 1.39 A bronchial artery, which lacks an external elastic lamina and, in comparison to pulmonary arteries, has a thick medial coat. Elastin van Gieson stain.

Normally the bronchial arteries are inconspicuous but the bronchial circulation is greatly expanded in many pathological conditions: lesions as diverse as bronchiectasis and carcinoma are largely supplied by bronchial arteries (Fig. 1.40).[269–272] The bronchial circulation can also make an important contribution to gas exchange in conditions where the pulmonary blood supply is reduced, as in certain forms of congenital heart disease and thromboembolic lung disease.

Small peripheral bronchial arteries sometimes exhibit longitudinal bundles of smooth muscle. These develop both within and outwith the elastic lamina and on occasion are so well developed that they seriously compromise or even completely obliterate the lumen (Fig. 1.41) Such *Sperrarterien* (from the German word *Sperr* meaning dam or valve) are generally thought to represent sphincters controlling the flow through arteriovenous or bronchopulmonary anastomoses (see below).[273] It is postulated that the longitudinal muscle hypertrophy is a response to intermittent stretching,[273] but this is disputed.[274]

Bronchial capillaries

Bronchial capillaries form a profuse subepithelial network, the extent of which reflects the high metabolic rate of an epithelium involved in warming the inspired air, ion exchange and ciliary activity. The subepithelial capillaries are connected to a deeper system of muscularised sinusoidal vessels which are distensible and so influence bronchial wall thickness, thus narrowing the lumen,[275–277] albeit at the expense of ventilation. Bronchial capillaries generally have the usual continuous type of endothelium but a fenestrated type is found in the vicinity of neuroepithelial bodies and submucosal glands, raising the possibility that circulating or endothelial factors may regulate the function of these structures.[278–280] A fenestrated capillary endothelium is also found in many fibrotic disorders of the lung.[278,281]

Bronchial veins

The bronchial veins, usually two on each side, open into the azygos vein on the right and the superior intercostal vein, the superior

Figure 1.40 A bronchial arteriogram showing a greatly hypertrophied artery (right) supplying congeries of new vessels (left) in the wall of a bronchiectactic cavity.

Figure 1.41 A *Sperrarterie* (arrows). These vascular structures, believed to represent valvular arteriovenous or bronchopulmonary anastomoses, are often markedly narrowed by bundles of hyperplastic longitudinal muscle. This one lies next to a pulmonary artery (to its right) but they may be found as far out as the pleura. (A) Haematoxylin and eosin; (B) elastin van Gieson stain.

hemiazygos vein or the innominate vein on the left. They drain only blood supplied to the proximal bronchi, the blood supplied to the distal airways being drained into pulmonary veins via bronchopulmonary anastomoses described below. Thus, part of this systemic blood is destined for the right side of the heart and part for the left.

Bronchopulmonary anastomoses

The bronchial and pulmonary circulations mix through precapillary, capillary and venous bronchopulmonary anastomoses: flow is normally from systemic to pulmonary vessels. At the arterial level mixing is normally very limited but up to two-thirds of the bronchial venous flow escapes the right side of the heart by entering anastomotic channels which connect with the pulmonary veins. By this means up to 4% of the output of the left ventricle consists of blood from the bronchial circulation.[282] When the bronchial circulation expands, as in a variety of lung diseases (see above), new bronchopulmonary anastomoses are established. Large bronchopulmonary anastomoses bypass stenosed pulmonary valves or arteries in congenital heart disease. Similarly, bronchopulmonary anastomoses develop in diseases characterised by thrombotic occlusion of pulmonary arteries.[283] The experimental ligation of a pulmonary artery results in an enormous expansion of thick-walled bronchopulmonary collaterals that is well advanced by 12 weeks.[284] Bronchopulmonary anastomoses minimise the likelihood of full ischaemic necrosis, as does reversed anastomotic flow when there is acute occlusion of a bronchial artery.

At the venous level, pulmonobronchial anastomoses direct oxygenated blood back to the right ventricle in conditions such as mitral stenosis and pulmonary veno-occlusive disease, whilst there may be increased flow in the reverse direction when precapillary causes of pulmonary hypertension lead to right-sided heart failure and vena caval hypertension: blood from the azygos veins may then flow through the bronchial veins into the pulmonary veins and cause cyanosis.[285]

Lymphatic drainage of the lungs

Lymphatics are not found in the alveolar walls but commence in the centriacinar region and in the interlobular septa. They are wide in relation to their wall thickness, and are attached to adjacent connective tissue fibres by special anchoring filaments which hold the lymphatics open when interstitial fluid accumulates, interstitial pressure rises and compression might otherwise be expected.[286] There is considerable reserve in the clearance capability of the pulmonary lymphatics which may increase their load 10-fold when pulmonary oedema threatens.[287] Pulmonary lymphatics are valved structures and, in addition to the above features, their capillaries differ from blood capillaries in that their endothelium has poorly developed junctions. Adjacent endothelial cells often merely overlap and the endothelial basal lamina is discontinuous. Although lymphatics are not found at the alveolar level their commencement near the smallest bronchioles means that no part of the lung is removed from a lymphatic vessel by much more than 2 mm. They accompany the blood vessels to the hilum of the lung, which they also reach by joining a pleural plexus on the outer surface of the lung. At the hila of the lungs they drain into hilar and thence mediastinal lymph nodes.

The lymph nodes of the mediastinum receive most clinical attention in the staging of lung cancer, for which purpose they are grouped as inferior, aortic and superior. The inferior group comprises subcarinal, paraoesophageal and pulmonary ligament nodes, the aortic group comprises subaortic and paraaortic nodes, and the superior group comprises lower paratracheal, pre- and retrotracheal, upper paratracheal and highest mediastinal nodes (see Box 12.1.6, p. 572).[288] A network of lymphatics connects these lymph nodes so that there is free lymphatic communication between the two lungs. Nevertheless, lymph from the left lung largely drains via ipsilateral nodes to the thoracic duct and on to the left subclavian vein while that from the right lung drains via right-sided nodes to the right bronchomediastinal trunk and the right subclavian vein. The evidence for this is based upon studies of the nodal distribution of pulmonary tumour metastases[289] and gainsays an older, widely held view that lymph from the lower lobe of the left lung drains to the right.

The thoracic duct drains lymph from most of the body. It enters the mediastinum through the diaphragmatic aortic hiatus in front of the 12th thoracic vertebral body, between the aorta to its left and the azygos vein to its right, and ascends in front of the vertebral column to reach the neck where it empties into the left subclavian vein.

Regional differences in ventilation and perfusion relevant to the location of lung disease

Gravity affects both ventilation and perfusion and in so doing results in several diseases of the lung having a characteristic upper- or lower-lobe predominance. In our customary upright position pulmonary blood pressure barely matches the hydrostatic pressure difference between the right ventricle and the apices of the lungs so that at rest the apices are hardly perfused at all. They are also less well ventilated because gravity drags on the upper lobes and compresses the bases so that alveoli in the upper lobes are larger than those in the lower, allowing more room for expansion in the lower lobes.[290,291] Inhaled dust particles are therefore preferentially directed to the lower lobes. However, because these regions are also better perfused, lymph flow is greater there and clearance is superior. Thus, although the bases receive more dust, less accumulates there and most pneumoconioses therefore show an upper-lobe predominance.

As with dust, inhaled bacteria are directed preferentially to the lower lobes and many infections consequently commence there. Thus the Ghon focus of primary tuberculosis is found more often in the lower lobes than in the upper. The classic upper-lobe location of postprimary tuberculosis has a more complex basis but this is also entirely dependent upon the regional differences in ventilation and perfusion, as explained on page 207 (see Fig. 5.3.14). A similar mechanism may underlie the upper-lobe predominance of diseases such as sarcoidosis, Langerhans cell histiocytosis and extrinsic allergic alveolitis.

LYMPHOID TISSUE OF THE LUNGS

This section first describes three principal locations within the lung in which lymphoid cells are found and then outlines the important features of the lymphoid cells themselves.

Intrapulmonary lymph nodes

Encapsulated lymph nodes of classic structure are found within the lungs, mainly related to the bifurcations of large bronchi. They are situated in the peribronchial tissues and do not come into direct contact with respiratory epithelium. Although mainly related to bronchi of the first three or four orders they may rarely be found in the peripheral lung, generally close to the visceral pleura of the middle lobe, lingula or lower lobes (see Fig. 12.4.1, p. 654). Although they are not of direct clinical relevance, they are becoming more important in relation to the differential diagnosis of peripheral nodules, especially in relation to computed tomography screening for carcinoma.[292-294]

Figure 1.42 A focus of bronchial mucosa-associated lymphoid tissue shows follicular hyperplasia in a case of follicular bronchiectasis. Note how the lymphoid cells infiltrate the overlying epithelium, which at this point is not ciliated.

Bronchus-associated lymphoid tissue

Certain lymphoid collections are closely related to the bronchial epithelium and because of their resemblance to Peyer's patches (gut-associated lymphoid tissue or GALT) are termed bronchial mucosa-associated lymphoid tissue (MALT).[295,296] Bronchial MALT is not thought to be a normal constituent of the human bronchial tree but acquired in response to various antigenic stimuli.[297–299] It is better represented in children[300] and in smokers,[299,301] and is prominent in certain inflammatory diseases, such as follicular bronchiectasis (Fig. 1.42). It is also better developed in species such as the rabbit and rat where again it may undergo hypertrophy when subjected to antigenic stimulation.[297,302–304] Bronchial MALT is found especially at the airway bifurcations, which is where inhaled antigens are particularly likely to impinge.

In many species bronchial MALT is formed of follicular lymphoid tissue which is closely applied to a distinctive overlying 'lymphoepithelium' consisting of flattened non-ciliated epithelial cells known as microfold or 'M cells', intimately involved with which are lymphocytes that form part of the outer mantle or dome region of the underlying lymphoid follicle (Figs 1.42 and 1.43). Antigen is taken up by the M cells[304] and passed to follicular dendritic cells (see below) within the bronchial MALT.[305] The germinal centres consist of a mesh of follicular dendritic cells that sustain rapidly dividing B lymphocytes and present them with antigenic information. More than half the lymphocytes of the bronchial MALT are B cells, with IgA being the predominant isotope.[72,306] T cells comprise about 18% of lymphocytes in bronchial MALT.

In humans bronchial MALT is not so well organised or so closely applied to the surface epithelium, being better seen in the outer coat of the bronchus[301] and around the bronchial glands.[299] IgA-secreting plasma cells are concentrated about the serous acini of the bronchial glands[299,306] where the secretory component of IgA is synthesised and incorporated into the IgA dimer as this passes across the epithelium to reach the lumen (see Fig. 1.19).[70–72]

After an immune response is induced in the bronchial MALT, lymphocytes enter the blood and travel to mucosal effector sites such as the lamina propria throughout the body where large amounts of IgA are produced.[307] This migratory pathway forms part of a common mucosal immune system in which responses induced in one location can be replicated elsewhere. Similarly, lymphomas arising in

Figure 1.43 The dome region of bronchus-associated lymphoid tissue consisting of a collection of lymphocytes, one of which is located within surface epithelium that at this point is non-ciliated. Transmission electron micrograph. *(Courtesy of Miss A Dewar, Brompton, UK.)*

one part of this system tend to recur in the mucosae of other organs (see p. 659).

Lymphoreticular aggregates

Lymphoreticular aggregates were described before bronchial MALT and today many would probably be classified as such. However, they are more widely distributed, being found throughout the lungs, about bronchi and in alveolar tissue, interlobular septa and the pleura. They are particularly noticeable at the centres of the acini, interposed between the terminal or a respiratory bronchiole and its accompanying artery (see Fig. 1.23).[308] This is the point at which lymphatics commence and the aggregates are well placed to monitor fluid and cells draining from the alveolar tissue in the interstitial plane. They consist of small collections of lymphocytes with a few plasma cells and eosinophils. Reticulin stains show a delicate connective tissue network but the sinusoidal and nodal architecture of a lymph node is lacking. Dust-laden macrophages accumulate in the lymphoreticular aggregates, leading Macklin to refer to the aggregates as 'dust sumps'.[6] On the cut surface of a city-dweller's or smoker's lung they provide a useful marker of the centres of the lung acini (see Fig. 1.7).

Lymphocytes

Lymphocytes of all classes are present in the lung: B and T, T-helper and T-suppressor, and T-helper-1 and -2. The functions of B and T cells in humoral and cellular immunity and hypersensitivity are well known, as are the promoter and suppressor/cytotoxic functions of T-helper (CD4+) and T-suppressor (CD8+) cells. T-helper cells are cytokine secretors whereas T-suppressor cells are mainly cytotoxic killer cells. Their respective roles are dealt with in some detail under various granulomatous diseases, notable tuberculosis (see p. 200) and sarcoidosis (see p. 286). The subsets of T-helper cells (Th1 and Th2) determine whether an immune response is directed towards phagocytosis and bacterial elimination or hypersensitivity reactions characterised by eosinophilia. The former is effected by activated Th1 lymphocytes through the elaboration of cytokines such as interleukin-2 and interferon-γ and the latter by elective activation of the Th2 lymphocytes resulting in interleukin-4, -5, -6 and -10 secretion. Interleukin-4 is responsible for plasma cells forming IgE rather than IgG while interleukin-5 is responsible for tissue eosinophilia. Both cell types produce granulocyte–macrophage colony-stimulating factor. Further T-cell subsets identified in the lungs include alpha beta and gamma delta cells, the former thought to be important for immunological memory while the latter contribute to the early immune response.[309]

Dendritic cells

There are two types of dendritic cells, both of which are described in the lungs: follicular dendritic cells, mentioned above as a component of the bronchial MALT, and interdigitating dendritic cells.[310–316] They are both derived from bone marrow stem cells and reach the lung by the blood stream. Both function as antigen presenters to T lymphocytes. They do this by processing the antigen intracellularly into short peptides before presenting it to T lymphocytes on their surface in association with the HLA-DR histocompatibility complex. Dendritic cells are also activated by endogenous signals such as interferon-α released from virus-infected cells and heat-shock proteins released by dying cells.

Interdigitating dendritic cells are found in T-cell-dependent areas of lymph nodes and are widely distributed in the lung, being found around and within the walls of bronchi and bronchioles, and in alveolar walls, interlobular septa and the pleura. They have long cytoplasmic processes and irregular, convoluted nuclei.[317] In the airways interdigitating dendritic cells form a network at the base of the epithelium that is ideally positioned to sample inhaled antigens (Fig. 1.44).[317] They are not present at birth but develop in the respiratory mucosa after about 1 year of life, probably in response to infection.[318] Interdigitating dendritic cells are also found deeper in the airway wall, outside the muscle coat, and it is here that they interact with T cells.[319]

In addition to the Langerhans cells described below, phenotypically varying subsets of dendritic cells are described: myeloid type 1 expressing CD1c, myeloid type 2 expressing CD141 and plasmacytoid expressing CD303, but whether these are distinct cell types or variations of the same is uncertain.[320–322] However, the experimental evidence suggests that they are capable of a significant degree of plasticity.[323]

Langerhans cells

These cells constitute a subpopulation of dendritic cells, from which they are derived by a process of differentiation.[311] They differ from other dendritic cells by expressing CD1a and langerin (CD207) and by the presence of certain pentalaminar structures known as Birbeck granules[324] (see Fig. 6.1.38, p. 289), which develop in the cytoplasm during the internalisation of surface-bound antigens. They are essentially a cell of the epidermis but small numbers are found in the bronchial epithelium. Proliferation and differentiation of pulmonary

dendritic cells into Langerhans cells are influenced by factors affecting the epithelium, notably smoking and epithelial metaplasia.[317,322,325–327] Like dendritic cells, Langerhans cells do not normally enter the air space but lavage fluid from smokers and patients with bronchial epithelial hyperplasia contains up to 5% Langerhans cells. They are referred to again under the disease Langerhans cell histiocytosis (see p. 288).

Mast cells

There are at least two types of mast cell, mucosal and connective tissue, both of which originate in the bone marrow and are represented in the lung.[328,329] It is not known whether they are interchangeable but this is likely as with an appropriate stimulus their relative proportions may change rapidly.[330] The two types differ in many respects but are usually distinguished by their content of tryptase and chymase, of which only tryptase is found in mucosal mast cells whereas connective tissue mast cells contain both these proteases. Mucosal mast cells predominate in the lungs and are the prevailing type in the airway mucosa and alveoli, whereas connective tissue mast cells are the more numerous in airway muscle and blood vessels.

In the airways mast cells are mainly situated in the subepithelial tissues but some are found in the surface epithelium and may be recovered by bronchoalveolar lavage.[331–337] Airway mast cells progressively increase in number distally so that in the small bronchioles total mast cell numbers are 100–150-fold greater than in the trachea. Mast cells make up about 2% of the cross-sectional area of the alveolar walls, with higher values in disease states.[338]

In both normal and fibrotic lung, mast cells show remarkably close apposition to fibroblasts,[339] and there is evidence that they promote fibrosis.[340–342] However, they are best known for their role in type I allergic reactions and are referred to again under asthma (see p. 114). Various mediators are released when the mast cell degranulates. Preformed mediators include histamine, serine proteases (tryptase, chymase) and eosinophil and neutrophil chemotactic factors. Degranulation also stimulates the generation and release of newly formed mediators, including prostaglandin D_2, platelet-activating factor and leukotrienes C_4 and D_4. Mast cells also produce a variety of cytokines, notably interleukins-1–5, granulocyte–macrophage colony-stimulating factor, interferon-γ and tumour necrosis factor-α.[343] Release is tailored to the stimulus. Lipopolysaccharide, for example, induces cytokine secretion but not degranulation.[344]

INNERVATION OF THE LUNGS

Several nerve bundles enter the lung from a plexus formed at the hilum by parasympathetic fibres derived from the vagus nerve and sympathetic fibres from the upper thoracic ganglia of the sympathetic chain. Peptidergic (non-cholinergic, non-adrenergic) fibres are also included.[345–350]

On entering the lung, the nerves divide into peribronchial and perivascular plexuses, the former further ramifying about the cartilage plates and beneath the surface epithelium. Sensory endings include rapidly adapting receptors within the surface epithelium responding to irritants and promoting the cough reflex, those supplying the neuroepithelial chemoreceptors, slowly adapting stretch receptors associated with muscle and thought to be responsible for the Hering–Breuer reflex, and juxtacapillary (J-type) receptors in the alveolar walls sensitive to rises in pulmonary venous pressure and possibly interstitial oedema.[78,80–85,351–353]

Terminals identified by vital staining in the walls of pulmonary veins and bronchial arteries, but not pulmonary arteries, are probably

Figure 1.44 Bronchial dendritic cells (DC). (A) Transmission electron micrograph of a DC in the mucosa of a normal non-atopic adult with a cytoplasmic extension (pseudopod) which straddles the basement membrane (arrows) with its nucleus within the epithelium. A mast cell (M) and fibroblasts (F) are observed in the subepithelium. Scale bar = 10 μm. (B) Transmission electron micrograph showing a DC in the bronchial mucosa of a stable asthmatic in the epithelium in close proximity to the reticular basement membrane (RBM) with cytoplasmic projections/pseudopodia (arrows) which extend amongst the basal cells (BC). An associated lymphocyte (L) is indicated. The DC exhibits a characteristic electron-lucent cytoplasm and nuclei with a distinctive narrow rim of heterochromatin. Scale bar = 5 μm. (C) Transmission electron micrograph montage of a DC in two consecutive tissue sections from the epithelium of an asthmatic subject. The dotted line indicates the boundary between sections. The cell body extensions or pseudopodia (see outline) observed in this plane of sectioning of the stellate DC extend between the BC. A lymphocyte (L) is present at the RBM. Scale bar = 5 μm. *(Courtesy of Dr AV Rogers, Brompton, UK; reproduced from Rogers et al. (2008).[317])*

further pressor receptors.[354] Histochemical and ultrastructural studies have shown that the whole pulmonary vasculature is innervated by noradrenergic and cholinergic nerves, and that rapid changes take place in these nerves during the postnatal adaptation of the pulmonary circulation.[355] Non-chromaffin paraganglia that possibly act as vascular chemoreceptors are described above (p. 23).

Motor terminals are also found in bronchial glands, muscle and surface epithelium, whilst ganglia containing Kultschitsky-like cells in addition to nerve cells and fibres have been identified in the bronchial submucosa.[75] Neurotransmitters include acetylcholine, catecho-lamines and peptides such as vasoactive intestinal peptide[356] and substance P.[357] Cholinergic innervation appears to be the most important effector drive to bronchial contraction and secretion but may be augmented by the peptide substance P. Inhibition of contraction may be by catecholamines or by peptidergic nerves, particularly those releasing vasoactive intestinal peptide.[358] Cholinergic stimulation also appears to extend to alveolar secretory cells, for bilateral vagotomy in the rat results in atelectasis[359] whilst cholinergic drugs increase the production of type II cell lamellar bodies[360] and the secretion of surfactant.[361]

REFERENCES

Anatomy of the lungs and airways

1. Coppoletta JM, Wolbach SB. Body length and normal weights of more important vital organs between birth and twelve years of age. Am J Pathol 1933;9:55.
2. Thoracic Society. The nomenclature of broncho-pulmonary anatomy. Thorax 1950;5:222–7.
3. Weibel ER. Morphometry of the Human Lung. Berlin: Springer; 1963.
4. Haefeli-Bleuer B, Weibel ER. Morphometry of the human pulmonary acinus. Anat Rec 1988;220:401–14.
5. Dunnill MS. Postnatal growth of the lung. Thorax 1962;17:329–33.
6. Macklin CS. Pulmonary sumps, dust accumulations, alveolar fluid and lymph vessels. Acta Anat 1955;23:1–33.
7. Emery JL, Mithal A. The number of alveoli in the terminal respiratory unit of man during late intrauterine life and childhood. Arch Dis Child 1960;35:544–7.
8. Yatabe Y, Kosaka T, Takahashi T, et al. EGFR mutation is specific for terminal respiratory unit type adenocarcinoma. Am J Surg Pathol 2005;29:633–9.
9. Weir BA, Woo MS, Getz G, et al. Characterizing the cancer genome in lung adenocarcinoma. Nature 2007;450:893–8.
10. Tanaka H, Yanagisawa K, Shinjo K, et al. Lineage-specific dependency of lung adenocarcinomas on the lung development regulator TTF-1. Cancer Res 2007;67:6007–11.
11. Horsfield K. The relation between structure and function in the airways of the lung. Br J Dis Chest 1974;68:145–60.
12. Hasleton PS. The internal surface of the adult human lung. J Anat 1972;112:391–9.
13. Lambert MW. Accessory bronchiole-alveolar communications. J Pathol Bacteriol 1955;70:311–4.
14. Fukuoka J, Franks TJ, Colby TV, et al. Peribronchiolar metaplasia: a common histologic lesion in diffuse lung disease and a rare cause of interstitial lung disease: clinicopathologic features of 15 cases. Am J Surg Pathol 2005;29:948–54.
15. Martin HB. Respiratory bronchioles as the pathway for collateral ventilation. J Appl Physiol 1966;21:1443–7.
16. Raskin SP, Harman PG. Interacinar pathways in the human lung. Am Rev Respir Dis 1975;111:489–95.
17. Andersen JB, Jespersen W. Demonstration of intersegmental respiratory bronchioles in normal human lungs. Eur J Respir Dis 1980;61:337–41.
18. Elliott FM, Reid L. Some new facts about the pulmonary artery and its branching pattern. Clin Radiol 1965;16:193–8.

Microscopy of the airways

19. Monkhouse WS, Whimster WF. An account of the longitudinal mucosal corrugations of the human tracheo-bronchial tree, with observations on those of some animals. J Anat 1976;122:681–95.
20. Whimster WF. The microanatomy of the alveolar duct system. Thorax 1970;25:141–9.
21. Carroll NG, Perry S, Karkhanis A, et al. The airway longitudinal elastic fiber network and mucosal folding in patients with asthma. Am J Respir Crit Care Med 2000;161:244–8.
22. Breeze RJ, Wheeldon EB. The cells of the pulmonary airways. Am Rev Respir Dis 1977;116:705–77.
23. Jeffery PK. Morphologic features of airway surface epithelial cells and glands. Am Rev Respir Dis 1983;128:S14–20.
24. Jeffery PK. Airway mucosa: secretory cells, mucus and mucin genes. Eur Resp J 1997;10:1655–62.
25. Clara M. Zur Histobiologie des Bronchalepithels. Z Forschung 1937;41:321–47.
26. Rogers AV, Dewar A, Corrin B, et al. Identification of serous-like cells in the surface epithelium of human bronchioles. Eur Respir J 1993;6:498–504.
27. Mercer RR, Russell ML, Roggli VL, et al. Cell number and distribution in human and rat airways. Am J Respir Cell Mol Biol 1994;10:613–24.
28. Glanville AR, Tazelaar HD, Theodore J, et al. The distribution of MHC class-I and class-II antigens on bronchial epithelium. Am Rev Respir Dis 1989;139:330–4.
29. Nakajima M, Kawanami O, Jin E, et al. Immunohistochemical and ultrastructural studies of basal cells, Clara cells and bronchiolar cuboidal cells in normal human airways. Pathol Int 1998;48:944–53.
30. Clover J, Oates J, Edwards C. Anti-cytokeratin 5/6: A positive marker for epithelioid mesothelioma. Histopathology 1997;31:140–3.
31. Hulbert WC. Fixation of the respiratory epithelial surface mucus. Lab Invest 1983;48:650–2.
32. Gil J, Weibel ER. Extracellular lining of bronchioles after perfusion-fixation of rat lungs for electron microscopy. Anat Rec 1971;169:185–99.
33. Iravani J, van As A. Mucus transport in the tracheobronchial tree of normal and bronchitic rats. J Pathol 1972;106:81–93.
34. Inoue S, Hogg JC. Intercellular junctions of the tracheal epithelium in guinea pigs. Lab Invest 1974;31:68–74.
35. Richardson JB, Bouchard T, Ferguson CC. Uptake and transport of exogenous proteins by respiratory epithelium. Lab Invest 1976;35:307–14.
36. Vai F, Fournier MF, Lafuma JC, et al. SO$_2$ induced bronchopathy in the rat: abnormal permeability of the bronchial epithelium in vivo after anatomic recovery. Am Rev Respir Dis 1980;121:851–8.
37. Hulbert WC, Walker DC, Jackson A, et al. Airway permeability to horseradish peroxidase in guinea pigs: the repair phase after injury by cigarette smoke. Am Rev Respir Dis 1981;123:320–1.
38. Ayers MM, Jeffery PK. Proliferation and differentiation in mammalian airway epithelium. Eur Respir J 1988;1:58–80.
39. Evans MJ, Cabral-Anderson LJ, Freeman G. Role of the Clara cell in renewal of the bronchiolar epithelium. Lab Invest 1978;38:648–55.
40. Bolduc P, Jones R, Reid L. Mitotic activity of airway epithelium after short exposure to tobacco smoke, and the effect of the anti-inflammatory agent phenylmethyloxadiazole. Br J Exp Pathol 1981;62:461–8.
41. Villaschi S, Giovanetti A, Lombardi CC, et al. Damage and repair of mouse bronchial epithelium following acute inhalation of trichloroethylene. Exp Lung Res 1991;17:601–14.
42. Reynolds SD, Giangreco A, Power JHT, et al. Neuroepithelial bodies of pulmonary airways serve as a reservoir of progenitor cells capable of epithelial regeneration. Am J Pathol 2000;156:269–78.
43. Otto WR. Lung epithelial stem cells. J Pathol 2002;197:527–35.
44. Hayashi T, Ishii A, Nakai S, et al. Ultrastructure of goblet-cell metaplasia from Clara cell in the allergic asthmatic airway inflammation in a mouse model of asthma in vivo. Virchows Arch 2004;444:66–73.
45. Snyder JC, Teisanu RM, Stripp BR. Endogenous lung stem cells and contribution to disease. J Pathol 2009;217:254–64.
46. Thompson AB, Robbins RA, Romberger DJ, et al. Immunological functions of the pulmonary epithelium. Eur Respir J 1995;8:127–49.
47. Mayer AK. Airway epithelial cells modify immune responses by inducing an anti-inflammatory microenvironment. European journal of immunology 2008;38:1689–99.
48. Wang H, Su Z, Schwarze J. Healthy but not RSV-infected lung epithelial cells profoundly inhibit T cell activation. Thorax 2009;64:283–90.
49. Salathe M. Cilia and Mucus From Development to Respiratory Defense. New York: Marcel Dekker; 2001.
50. Iravani J, Melville GN. Mucociliary function in the respiratory tract influenced

by physicochemical factors. Pharmac Ther 1976;2:471–92.

51. Sleigh MA. The nature and action of respiratory tract cilia. In: Brain JD, Proctor DF, Reid LM, editors. Respiratory defense mechanisms. Lung biology in health and disease. Vol 5 (part 1). New York: Marcel Dekker; 1977. p. 247–82.

52. Jeffery PK, Reid LM. New observations of rat airway epithelium: a quantitative electron microscopic study. J Anat 1975;120:295–320.

53. Schlegel R, Banks-Schlegel S, Pinkus GS. Immunohistochemical localization of keratin in normal human tissues. Lab Invest 1980;42:91–6.

54. Hong KU, Reynolds SD, Watkins S, et al. Basal cells are a multipotent progenitor capable of renewing the bronchial epithelium. Amer J Pathol 2004;164:577–88.

55. Evans MJ, Plopper CG. The role of basal cells in adhesion of columnar epithelium to airway basement membrane. Am Rev Respir Dis 1988;138:481–3.

56. Evans MJ, Moller PC. Biology of airway basal cells. Exp Lung Res 1991;17:513–31.

57. Voynow JA, Rubin BK. Mucins, mucus, and sputum. Chest 2009;135:505–12.

58. Gendler SJ, Spicer AP. Epithelial mucin genes. Annu Rev Physiol 1995;57:607–34.

59. Sharma P, Dudus L, Nielsen PA, et al. MUC5B and MUC7 are differentially expressed in mucous and serous cells of submucosal glands in human bronchial airways. Am J Respir Cell Mol Biol 1998;19:30–7.

60. Wickstrom C, Davies JR, Eriksen GV, et al. MUC5B is a major gel-forming, oligomeric mucin from human salivary gland, respiratory tract and endocervix: identification of glycoforms and C-terminal cleavage. Biochem J 1998;334:685–93.

61. Hovenberg HW, Davies JR, Carlstedt I. Different mucins are produced by the surface epithelium and the submucosa in human trachea: identification of MUC5AC as a major mucin from the goblet cells. Biochem J 1996;318:319–24.

62. Davies JR, Herrmann A, Russell W, et al. Respiratory tract mucins: structure and expression patterns. Novartis Found Symp 2002;248:76–88.

63. Groneberg DA, Eynott PR, Oates T, et al. Expression of MUC5AC and MUC5B mucins in normal and cystic fibrosis lung. Respir Med 2002;96:81–6.

64. Boggaram V. Regulation of lung surfactant protein gene expression. Front Biosci 2003;8:d751–64.

65. Spicer SS, Schulte BA, Thomopoulos GN. Histochemical properties of the respiratory tract epithelium in different species. Am Rev Respir Dis 1983;128:S20–6.

66. Meyrick B, Sturgess J, Reid L. Reconstruction of the duct system and secretory tubules of the human bronchial submucosal gland. Thorax 1969;24:729–36.

67. Bowes D, Corrin B. Ultrastructural immunocytochemical localization of lysozyme in human bronchial glands. Thorax 1977;32:163–70.

68. Bowes D, Clark AE, Corrin B. Ultrastructural localisation of lactoferrin and glycoprotein in human bronchial glands. Thorax 1981;36:108–15.

69. Kramps JA, Franken C, Meijer CJLM, et al. Localization of low molecular weight protease inhibitor in serous secretory cells of the respiratory tract. J Histochem 1981;29:712–19.

70. Brandtzaeg P. Mucosal and glandular distribution of immunoglobulin components: immunohistochemistry with a cold ethanol-fixation technique. Immunology 1974;26:1101–13.

71. Goodman JR, Link DW, Brown WR, et al. Ultrastructural evidence of transport of secretory IgA across bronchial epithelium. Am Rev Respir Dis 1981;123:115–19.

72. Pilette C, Ouadrhiri Y, Godding V, et al. Lung mucosal immunity: immunoglobulin-A revisited. Eur Resp J 2001;18:571–88.

73. Christensen TG, Janeczek AH, Gaensler EA, et al. Localisation of endogenous peroxidase in human bronchial submucosal glands. Am Rev Respir Dis 1981;123:222.

74. Matsuba K, Takizawa T, Thurlbeck W. Oncocytes in human bronchial mucous glands. Thorax 1972;27:181–4.

75. Bensch KG, Gordon GB, Miller LR. Studies on the bronchial counterpart of the Kultschitsky (argentaffin) cell and the innervation of bronchial glands. J Ultrastruct Res 1965;12:668–86.

76. Bensch KG, Corrin B, Pariente R, et al. Oat cell carcinoma of the lung: its origin and relationship to bronchial carcinoid. Cancer 1968;22:1163–72.

77. Capella C, Hage E, Solcia E, et al. Ultrastructural similarity of endocrine-like cells of the human lung and some related cells of the gut. Cell Tissue Res 1978;186:25–37.

78. Lauweryns JM, Van Lommel A. The intrapulmonary neuroepithelial bodies after vagotomy: demonstration of their sensory neuroreceptor-like innervation. Experientia 1983;39:1123–4.

79. Tateishi R. Distribution of argyrophil cells in adult human lungs. Arch Pathol 1973;96:198–202.

80. Boers JE, Denbrok JLM, Koudstaal J, et al. Number and proliferation of neuroendocrine cells in normal human airway epithelium. Am J Respir Crit Care Med 1996;154:758–63.

81. Lauweryns JM, Van Lommel AT, Dom RJ. Innervation of rabbit intrapulmonary neuroepithelial bodies. Quantitative and qualitative ultrastructural study after vagotomy. J Neurol Sci 1985;67:81–92.

82. Lauweryns JM, Van Lommel A. Effect of various vagotomy procedures on the reaction to hypoxia of rabbit neuroepithelial bodies: modulation by intrapulmonary axon reflexes? Exp Lung Res 1986;11:319–39.

83. Lauweryns JM, Van Lommel A. Ultrastructure of nerve endings and synaptic junctions in rabbit intrapulmonary neuroepithelial bodies: a single and serial section analysis. J Anat 1987;151:65–83.

84. Van Lommel A, Lauweryns JM, Deleyn P, et al. Pulmonary neuroepithelial bodies in neonatal and adult dogs: histochemistry, ultrastructure, and effects of unilateral hilar lung denervation. Lung 1995;173:13–23.

85. Brouns I, VanGenechten J, Hayashi H, et al. Dual sensory innervation of pulmonary neuroepithelial bodies. Am J Respir Cell Mol Biol 2003;28:275–85.

86. Cutz E, Chan W, Wong V, Conen PE. Endocrine cells in rat fetal lungs. Ultrastructural and histochemical study. Lab Invest 1974;30:458–64.

87. Lauweryns JM, Van Ranst L. Immunocytochemical localization of aromatic L-aminoacid decarboxylase in human, rat, and mouse bronchopulmonary and gastrointestinal endocrine cells. J Histochem Cytochem 1988;36:1181–6.

88. Lauweryns JM, de Bock V, Verhofstad AAJ, et al. Immunohistochemical localization of serotonin in intrapulmonary neuro-epithelial bodies. Cell Tissue Res 1982;226:215–23.

89. Wharton J, Polak JM, Cole GA, et al. Neuro-specific enolase as an immunocytochemical marker for the diffuse neuroendocrine system in human fetal lung. J Histochem Cytochem 1981;29:1359–64.

90. Lauweryns JM, Van Ranst L, Lloyd RV, et al. Chromogranin in bronchopulmonary neuroendocrine cells. Immunocytochemical detection in human, monkey and pig respiratory mucosa. J Histochem Cytochem 1987;35:113–18.

91. Lee I, Gould VE, Moll R, et al. Synaptophysin expressed in the bronchopulmonary tract: neuroendocrine cells, neuroepithelial bodies, and neuroendocrine neoplasms. Differentiation 1987;34:115–25.

92. Lantuejoul S, Moro D, Michalides RJAM, et al. Neural cell adhesion molecules (NCAM) and NCAM-PSA expression in neuroendocrine lung tumors. Am J Surg Pathol 1998;22:1267–76.

93. Wharton J, Polak JM, Bloom SR, et al. Bombesin-like immunoreactivity in the lung. Nature 1978;273:769–70.

94. Cutz E, Chan W, Track NS. Bombesin, calcitonin and leuenkephalin immunoreactivity in endocrine cells of the human lung. Experientia 1981;37:765–6.

95. Tsutsumi Y, Osamura Y, Watanabe K, et al. Immunohistochemical studies on gastrin-releasing peptide and adrenocorticotropic hormone-containing cells in the human lung. Lab Invest 1983;48:623–32.

96. Willey JC, Lechner JR, Harris CC. Bombesin and the C-terminal tetradecapeptide of gastrin-releasing peptide are growth factors for normal human bronchial epithelial cells. Exp Cell Res 1984;153:245–8.

97. Becker KL, Monaghan KG, Silva OL. Immunocytochemical localization of calcitonin in Kulchitsky cells of human lung. Arch Pathol Lab Med 1980;104:196–8.

98. Tsutsumi Y, Osamura Y, Watanabe K, et al. Simultaneous immunohistochemical localization of gastrin-releasing peptide (GPR) and calcitonin (CT) in human bronchial endocrine-type cells. Virchows Arch A Pathol Anat Histopathol 1983;400:163–71.

99. Gallego R, Garciacaballero T, Roson E, et al. Neuroendocrine cells of the human lung express substance-P-like immunoreactivity. Acta Anat 1990;139:278–82.

100. Kato K, Asano T, Kamiya N, et al. Production of the alpha subunit of guanine nucleotide binding protein Go by neuroendocrine tumors. Cancer Res 1987;47:5800–5.

101. Brambilla E, Veale D, Moro D, et al. Neuroendocrine phenotype in lung cancers – comparison of immunohistochemistry with biochemical determination of enolase isoenzymes. Am J Clin Pathol 1992;98:88–97.

102. Gosney JR, Gosney MA, Lye M, et al. Reliability of commercially available immunocytochemical markers for identification of neuroendocrine differentiation in bronchoscopic biopsies of bronchial carcinoma. Thorax 1995;50:116–20.

103. Reznik-Schuller H. Sequential morphologic alterations in the bronchial epithelium of Syrian golden hamsters during N-nitrosomorpholine-induced pulmonary tumorigenesis. Am J Pathol 1977;89:59–66.

104. Peake JL, Reynolds SD, Stripp BR, et al. Alteration of pulmonary neuroendocrine cells during epithelial repair of naphthalene-induced airway injury. Am J Pathol 2000;156:279–86.

105. Johnson NF, Wagner JC, Wills HA. Endocrine cell proliferation in the rat lung following asbestos exposure. Lung 1980;158:221–8.

106. Wilson NJE, Gosney JR, Mayall F. Endocrine cells in diffuse pulmonary fibrosis. Thorax 1993;48:1252–6.

107. Johnson DE, Lock JE, Elde RP, et al. Pulmonary neuroendocrine cells in hyaline membrane disease and bronchopulmonary dysplasia. Pediatr Res 1982;16:446–54.

108. Gosney J, Heath D, Smith P, et al. Pulmonary endocrine cells in pulmonary arterial disease. Arch Pathol Lab Med 1989;113:337–41.

109. Gould VE, Linnoila RI, Memoli VA, et al. Neuroendocrine cells and neuroendocrine neoplasms of the lung. Pathol Annu 1983;18:287–330.

110. Lauweryns JM, Cokelaere M. Intrapulmonary neuroepithelial bodies: hypoxia-sensitive neuro (chemo-) receptors. Experientia 1973;29:1384–6.

111. Moosavi H, Smith P, Heath D. The Feyrter cell in hypoxia. Thorax 1973;28:729–41.

112. Taylor W. Pulmonary argyrophil cells at high altitude. J Pathol 1977;122:137–44.

113. Anand IS. Hypoxia and the pulmonary circulation. Thorax 1994;49:S19–24.

114. Johnston CJ, Mango GW, Finkelstein JN, et al. Altered pulmonary response to hyperoxia in Clara cell secretory protein deficient mice. Am J Respir Cell Mol Biol 1997;17:147–55.

115. Boyd MR. Evidence for the Clara cell as a site of cytochrome P450-dependent mixed-function oxidase activity in lung. Nature 1977;269:713–15.

116. Woods LW, Wilson DW, Schiedt MJ, et al. Structural and biochemical changes in lungs of 3-methylindole-treated rats. Am J Pathol 1993;142:129–38.

117. Plopper CG, VanWinkle LS, Fanucchi MV, et al. Early events in naphthalene-induced acute Clara cell toxicity – II. Comparison of glutathione depletion and histopathology by airway location. Am J Respir Cell Mol Biol 2001;24:272–81.

118. Laporte J, Dorleansjuste P, Sirois P. Guinea pig Clara cells secrete endothelin 1 through a phosphoramidon-sensitive pathway. Am J Respir Cell Mol Biol 1996;14:356–62.

119. Meyrick B, Reid L. The alveolar brush cell in rat lung – a third pneumocyte. J Ultrastruct Res 1968;23:71–80.

120. Hijiya K, Okada Y, Tankawa H. Ultrastructural study of the alveolar brush cell. J Electron Microsc 1977;26:321–9.

121. Reid L, Meyrick B, Antony VB, et al. The mysterious pulmonary brush cell: a cell in search of a function. Am J Respir Crit Care Med 2005;172:136–9.

Microscopy of the alveolar tissue

122. Heard BE, Izukawa T. Pulmonary emphysema in fifty consecutive male necropsies in London. J Pathol Bacteriol 1964;88:423–31.

123. Oderr C. Architecture of the lung parenchyma. Studies with a specially designed X-ray microscope. Am Rev Respir Dis 1964;90:401–10.

124. Ochs M, Nyengaard LR, Lung A, et al. The number of alveoli in the human lung. Amer J Crit Care Med 2004;169:120–4.

125. Glazier JB, Hughes JMB, Maloney JE, et al. Vertical gradient of alveolar size in lungs of dogs frozen intact. J Appl Physiol 1967;23:694–705.

126. Haber PS, Colebatch HJH, Ng CKY, et al. Alveolar size as a determinant of pulmonary distensibility in mammalian lungs. J Appl Physiol 1983;54:837–45.

127. Parra SC, Gaddy LR, Takaro T. Ultrastructural studies of canine interalveolar pores (of Kohn). Lab Invest 1978;38:8–13.

128. Low FN. The pulmonary alveolar epithelium of laboratory mammals and man. Anat Rec 1953;117:241–63.

129. Weibel ER, Knight BW. A morphometric study on the thickness of the pulmonary air–blood barrier. J Cell Biol 1964;21:367–84.

130. Weibel ER. The mystery of 'non-nucleated plates' in the alveolar epithelium of the lung explained. Acta Anat 1971;78:425–43.

131. Crapo JD, Barry BE, Gehr P, et al. Cell characteristics of the normal human lung. Am Rev Respir Dis 1982;125:740–5.

132. Crandall ED, Matthay MA. Alveolar epithelial transport – basic science to clinical medicine. Amer J Crit Care Med 2001;163:1021–9.

133. Chesnutt MS, Nuckton TJ, Golden J, et al. Rapid alveolar epithelial fluid clearance following lung lavage in pulmonary alveolar proteinosis. Chest 2001;120:271–4.

134. Gonzales-Crussi F, Boston RW. The absorptive function of the neonatal lung: ultrastructural study of horseradish peroxidase uptake at the onset of ventilation. Lab Invest 1972;26:114–21.

135. Corrin B. Phagocytic potential of pulmonary alveolar epithelium with particular reference to surfactant metabolism. Thorax 1970;25:110–15.

136. Brody AR, Hill LH, Adkins B, et al. Chrysotile asbestos inhalation in rats: deposition pattern and reaction of alveolar epithelium and pulmonary macrophages. Am Rev Respir Dis 1981;123:670–8.

137. Faulkner CS. The role of the granular pneumonocyte in surfactant metabolism. An autoradiographic study. Arch Pathol 1969;87:521–5.

138. Askin FB, Kuhn C. The cellular origin of pulmonary surfactant. Lab Invest 1971;25:260–8.

139. Massaro GD, Massaro D. Granular pneumocytes. Electron microscopic radioautographic evidence of intracellular protein transport. Am Rev Respir Dis 1972;105:927–31.

140. Chevalier G, Collet AJ. In vivo incorporation of choline-3H , leucine-3H and galactose-3H in alveolar type II pneumocytes in relation to surfactant synthesis. A quantitative radiographic study in mouse by electron microscopy. Anat Rec 1972;174:289–310.

141. Kikkawa Y, Yoneda K, Smith F, et al. The type II epithelial cells of the lung. II

Chemical composition and phospholipid synthesis. Lab Invest 1975;32:295–302.

142. Corrin B, Clark AE. Lysosomal aryl sulphatase in pulmonary alveolar cells. Histochemie 1968;15:95–8.

143. Corrin B, Clark AE, Spencer H. Ultrastructural localisation of acid phosphatase in the rat lung. J Anat 1969;104:65–70.

144. Meban C. Localization of phosphatidic acid phosphatase activity in granular pneumocytes. J Cell Biol 1972;53:249–52.

145. Ochs M, Johnen G, Muller KM, et al. Intracellular and intraalveolar localization of surfactant protein a (SP-A) in the parenchymal region of the human lung. Am J Respir Cell Mol Biol 2002;26:91–8.

146. Evans MJ, Cabral LJ, Stephens RJ, et al. Renewal of alveolar epithelium in the rat following exposure to NO_2. Am J Pathol 1973;70:175–98.

147. Evans MJ, Cabral LJ, Stephens RJ, et al. Transformation of alveolar type 2 cells to type 1 cells following exposure to NO_2. Exp Mol Pathol 1975;22:142–50.

148. Adamson IYR, Bowden DH. Derivation of type 1 epithelium from type 2 cells in the developing rat lung. Lab Invest 1975;32:736–45.

149. Pattle RE. Properties, function and origin of the alveolar lining layer. Proc R Soc B 1958;148:217–40.

150. Hamm H, Kroegel C, Hohlfeld J. Surfactant: a review of its functions and relevance in adult respiratory disorders. Respir Med 1996;90:251–70.

151. Creuwels LAJM, Vangolde LMG, Haagsman HP. The pulmonary surfactant system: biochemical and clinical aspects. Lung 1997;175:1–39.

152. Clements JA, Avery ME. Lung surfactant and neonatal respiratory distress syndrome. Am J Respir Crit Care Med 1998;157:S59–66.

153. Gil J, Weibel ER. Improvements in demonstration of lining layer of lung alveoli by electron microscopy. Respir Physiol 1969;8:13–36.

154. Johansson J, Curstedt T, Robertson B. The proteins of the surfactant system. Eur Respir J 1994;7:372–91.

155. LaForce FM, Kelly WJ, Huber GL. Inactivation of staphylococci by alveolar macrophages with preliminary observations on the importance of alveolar lining material. Am Rev Respir Dis 1973;108:784–90.

156. Restrepo CI, Dong Q, Savov J, et al. Surfactant protein D stimulates phagocytosis of Pseudomonas aeruginosa by alveolar macrophages. Am J Respir Cell Mol Biol 1999;21:576–85.

157. Slade R, Crissman K, Norwood J, et al. Comparison of antioxidant substances in bronchoalveolar lavage cells and fluid from humans, guinea pigs, and rats. Exp Lung Res 1993;19:469–84.

158. Rao RH, Waite M, Myrvik QN. Deacylation of dipalmitoyllecithin by phospholipases A in alveolar macrophages. Exp Lung Res 1981;2:9–15.

159. Jobe A, Ikegami M, Sarton-Miller I. The in vivo labelling with acetate and palmitate of lung phospholipids from developing and adult rabbits. Biochim Biophys Acta 1980;617:65–75.

160. Jacobs H, Jobe A, Ikegami M, et al. The significance of reutilization of surfactant phosphatidylcholine. J Biol Chem 1983;258:4156–65.

161. Stevens PA, Wright JR, Clements JA. Changes in quantity, composition, and surface activity of alveolar surfactant at birth. J Appl Physiol 1987;63:1049–57.

162. Baritussio A, Bellina L, Carraro R, et al. Heterogeneity of alveolar surfactant in the rabbit: composition, morphology, and labelling of subfractions isolated by centrifugation of lung lavage. Eur J Clin Invest 1984;14:24–9.

163. Sirianni FE, Chu FSF, Walker DC. Human alveolar wall fibroblasts directly link epithelial type 2 cells to capillary endothelium. Amer J Respir Crit Care Med 2003;168:1532–7.

164. Kapanci Y, Assimcopoulos A, Irle C, et al. Contractile interstitial cells in pulmonary alveolar septa: a possible regulator of ventilation/perfusion ratio? J Cell Biol 1974;60:375–92.

165. Adler KB, Low RB, Leslie KO, et al. Biology of disease. Contractile cells in normal and fibrotic lung. Lab Invest 1989;60:473–85.

166. Weibel ER. On pericytes, particularly their existence in lung capillaries. Microvasc Res 1974;8:218–35.

167. Adamson IYR, Bowden DH. Role of monocytes and interstitial cells in the generation of alveolar macrophages. II. Kinetic studies after carbon loading. Lab Invest 1980;42:518–24.

168. Crowell RE, Heaphy E, Valdez YE, et al. Alveolar and interstitial macrophage populations in the murine lung. Exp Lung Res 1992;18:435–46.

169. Sebring RJ, Lehnert BE. Morphometric comparisons of rat alveolar macrophages, pulmonary interstitial macrophages, and blood monocytes. Exp Lung Res 1992;18:479–96.

170. Johansson A, Lundborg M, Skold CM, et al. Functional, morphological, and phenotypical differences between rat alveolar and interstitial macrophages. Am J Respir Cell Mol Biol 1997;16:582–8.

171. Wallace WAH, Gillooly M, Lamb D. Intra-alveolar macrophage numbers in current smokers and non-smokers – a morphometric study of tissue sections. Thorax 1992;47:437–40.

172. Bowden DH, Adamson IYR. Role of monocytes and interstitial cells in the generation of alveolar macrophages. I.

Kinetic studies of normal mice. Lab Invest 1980;42:511–13.

173. Takahashi K, Naito M, Takeya M. Development and heterogeneity of macrophages and their related cells through their differentiation pathways. Pathol Int 1996;46:473–85.

174. Vijeyaratnam GS, Corrin B. Origin of the pulmonary alveolar macrophage studied in the iprindole-treated rat. J Pathol 1972;108:115–18.

175. Bowden DH, Adamson IYR. Alveolar macrophage response to carbon in monocyte-depleted mice. Am Rev Respir Dis 1982;126:708–11.

176. Polosukhin VV, Manouilova LS, Romberger DJ, et al. Ultrastructural heterogeneity of the alveolar macrophages from tobacco smokers with chronic bronchitis. Ultrastruct Pathol 2001;25:5–11.

177. Evans MJ, Cabral LJ, Stephens RJ, et al. Cell division of alveolar macrophages in rat lung following exposure to NO_2. Am J Pathol 1973;70:199–206.

178. Shellito J, Esparza C, Armstrong C. Maintenance of the normal rat alveolar macrophage cell population. The roles of monocyte influx and alveolar macrophage proliferation in situ. Am Rev Respir Dis 1987;135:78–81.

179. Cordingley JL, Nicol T. The lung: an excretory route for macromolecules and particles. J Physiol (Lond) 1967;190:7.

180. Nakstad B, Lyberg T, Skjorten F, Boye NP. Subpopulations of human lung alveolar macrophages: ultrastructural features. Ultrastruct Pathol 1989;13:1–14.

181. Spiteri MA, Poulter LW. Characteristics of immune inducer and suppressor macrophages from the normal human lung. Clin Exp Immunol 1991;83:157–62.

182. Schaberg T, Klein U, Rau M, et al. Subpopulations of alveolar macrophages in smokers and nonsmokers: relation to the expression of CD11/CD18 molecules and superoxide anion production. Am J Respir Crit Care Med 1995;151:1551–8.

183. Brain JD. Free cells in the lungs. Arch Intern Med 1970;126:477–87.

184. Policard A, Collet A, Pregermain S, et al. Etude au microscope electronique du granulome pulmonaire silicotique experimental. Presse Med 1957;65:121–4.

185. Harmsen AG, Muggenburg BA, Snipes MB, et al. The role of macrophages in particle translocation from lungs to lymph nodes. Science 1985;230:1277–80.

186. Corry D, Kulkarni P, Lipscomb MF. The migration of bronchoalveolar macrophages into hilar lymph nodes. Am J Pathol 1984;115:321–8.

187. Oren R, Farnham AE, Saito K, et al. Metabolic patterns in three types of phagocytosing cells. J Cell Biol 1963;17:487–501.

188. Reynolds HY, Atkinson JP, Newball HH, et al. Receptors for immunoglobulin and

complement on human alveolar macrophages. J Immunol 1975;114:1813–19.

189. Sone S, Bucana C, Hoyer LC, et al. Kinetics and ultrastructural studies of the induction of rat alveolar macrophage fusion by mediators released from mitogen-stimulated lymphocytes. Am J Pathol 1981;103:234–46.

190. Hocking WG, Golde DW. The pulmonary-alveolar macrophage. N Engl J Med 1979;301:639–45.

191. Kaltreider HB. Alveolar macrophages. Enhancers or suppressors of pulmonary immune reactivity? Chest 1982;82:261–2.

192. Adamson IYR, Bowden DH. Adaptive responses of the pulmonary macrophagic system to carbon. II. Morphological studies. Lab Invest 1978;38:430–8.

193. Brody AR, Craighead JE. Cytoplasmic inclusions in pulmonary macrophages of cigarette smokers. Lab Invest 1975;32:125–32.

194. Schwartz LW, Christman CA. Lung lining material as a chemotactant for alveolar macrophages. Chest 1979;75:284S–8S.

195. Crouch EC. Collectins and pulmonary host defense. Am J Respir Cell Mol Biol 1998;19:177–201.

196. Gee JBL, Vassallo CL, Vogt MT, et al. Peroxidative metabolism in alveolar macrophages. Arch Intern Med 1971;127:1046–9.

197. Davies P, Drath DB, Engel EE, et al. The localization of catalase in the pulmonary alveolar macrophage. Lab Invest 1979;40:221–6.

198. Hatch GE, Gardner GE, Menzel DB. Stimulation of oxidant production in alveolar macrophages by pollutant and latex particles. Environ Res 1980;23:121–36.

199. Moncada S, Palmer RMJ, Higgs EA. Biosynthesis of nitric oxide from L-arginine: a pathway for the regulation of cell function and communication. Biochem Pharmacol 1989;38:1709–15.

200. Kobzik L, Bredt DS, Lowenstein CJ, et al. Nitric oxide synthase in human and rat lung – immunocytochemical and histochemical localization. Am J Respir Cell Mol Biol 1993;9:371–7.

201. Barnes PJ, Belvisi MG. Nitric oxide and lung disease. Thorax 1993;48:1034–43.

202. Green GM, Kass EH. The influence of bacterial species on pulmonary resistance to infection in mice subjected to hypoxia, cold, stress, and ethanolic intoxication. Br J Exp Pathol 1965;46:360–6.

203. Green GH, Carolin D. The depressant effect of cigarette smoke on the in vitro antibacterial activity of alveolar macrophages. N Engl J Med 1967;276:421–7.

204. Goldstein E, Green GM, Seamans C. The effect of acidosis on pulmonary

bactericidal function. J Lab Clin Med 1970;75:912–13.

205. Jakab GJ, Green GM. Defect in intracellular killing of Staphylococcus aureus within alveolar macrophages in Sendai virus-infected murine lungs. J Clin Invest 1976;57:1533–9.

206. Raffin TA, Simon LM, Braun D, et al. Impairment of phagocytosis by moderate hyperoxia (40 to 60 per cent oxygen) in lung macrophages. Lab Invest 1980;42:622–6.

207. Wallaert B, Aerts C, Colombel JF, et al. Human alveolar macrophage antibacterial activity in the alcoholic lung. Am Rev Respir Dis 1991;144:278–83.

208. Unanue ER, Beller DI, Calderon J, et al. Regulation of immunity and inflammation by mediators from macrophages. Am J Pathol 1976;85:465–78.

209. Nathan CF. Secretory products of macrophages. J Clin Invest 1987;79:319–26.

210. Gibbs DF, Warner RL, Weiss SJ, et al. Characterization of matrix metalloproteinases produced by rat alveolar macrophages. Am J Respir Cell Mol Biol 1999;20:1136–44.

211. Gibbs DF, Shanley TP, Warner RL, et al. Role of matrix metalloproteinases in models of macrophage-dependent acute lung injury – evidence for alveolar macrophage as source of proteinases. Am J Respir Cell Mol Biol 1999;20:1145–54.

212. Leibovich SJ, Ross R. A macrophage-dependent factor that stimulates the proliferation of fibroblasts in vitro. Am J Pathol 1976;84:501–14.

213. Lemaire I, Beaudoin H, Masse S, et al. Alveolar macrophage stimulation of lung fibroblast growth in asbestos-induced pulmonary fibrosis. Am J Pathol 1986;122:205–11.

214. Osorniovargas AR, Bonner JC, Badgett A, et al. Rat alveolar macrophage derived platelet-derived growth factor is chemotactic for rat lung fibroblasts. Am J Respir Cell Mol Biol 1990;3:595–602.

215. Denholm EM. Continuous secretion of monocyte chemotactic factors and fibroblast growth factors by alveolar macrophages following a single exposure to bleomycin invitro. Am J Pathol 1992;141:965–71.

Blood supply of the lungs

216. Hattano S, Strasser T. Primary pulmonary hypertension. Geneva: World Health Organization; 1975.

217. Smith U, Ryan JW, Michie DD, et al. Endothelial projections as revealed by scanning electron microscopy. Science 1971;173:925–7.

218. Bensch KG, Gordon GB, Miller LR. Fibrillar structures resembling leiomyofibrils in endothelial cells of mammalian pulmonary blood vessels.

Zeitschrift fur Zellforschung 1964;63:759–66.

219. Weibel ER, Palade GE. New cytoplasmic components in arterial endothelia. J Cell Biol 1964;23:101–12.

220. Wagner DD, Olmsted JB, Marder VJ. Immunolocalization of von Willebrand protein in Weibel–Palade bodies of human endothelial cells. J Cell Biol 1982;95:355–60.

221. Kato M, Staub NC. Response of small pulmonary arteries to unilobar hypoxia and hypercapnia. Circ Res 1966;19:426–39.

222. Nagasaka Y, Bhattacharya F, Nanjo S, et al. Micropuncture measurement of lung microvascular pressure profile during hypoxia in cats. Circ Res 1984;54:90–5.

223. Brij SO, Peacock AJ. Cellular responses to hypoxia in the pulmonary circulation. Thorax 1998;53:1075–9.

224. Michael JR, Markewitz BA. Endothelins and the lung. Am J Respir Crit Care Med 1996;154:555–81.

225. Kourembanas S, Bernfield M. Hypoxia and endothelial smooth muscle cell interactions in the lung. Am J Respir Cell Mol Biol 1994;11:373–4.

226. Perreault T, Gutkowska J. Role of atrial natriuretic factor in lung physiology and pathology. Am J Respir Crit Care Med 1995;151:226–42.

227. Guntheroth WG, Luchtel DL, Kawabori I. Pulmonary microcirculation: tubules rather than sheet and post. J Appl Physiol 1982;53:510–15.

228. Weibel ER. Lung cell biology. In: Handbook of physiology. The respiratory system. American physiology society. Bethesda: Maryland; 1984. p. 47–91.

229. Hogg JC. Neutrophil kinetics and lung injury. Physiol Rev 1987;67:1249–95.

230. Ryan US, Ryan JW, Whitaker C, et al. Localization of angiotensin converting enzyme (kininase II). II. Immunocytochemistry and immunofluorescence. Tissue Cell 1976;8:125–46.

231. Macnee W, Selby C. Neutrophil kinetics in the lungs. Clin Sci 1990;79:97–107.

232. Downey GP, Worthen GS, Henson PM, et al. Neutrophil sequestration and migration in localized pulmonary inflammation – capillary localization and migration across the interalveolar septum. Am Rev Respir Dis 1993;147:168–76.

233. Schneeberger-Keeley EE, Karnovsky MJ. The ultrastructural basis of alveolar-capillary membrane permeability to peroxidase used as a tracer. J Cell Biol 1968;37:781–93.

234. Feldmann G, Chahinian P, Leturcq E, et al. Localisation ultrastructurale par anticorps couples à la peroxydase de l'albumine extra-vasculaire dans le poumon de rat. Comptes rendus de l'Academie des Sciences 1973;277:251.

235. Schraufnagel DE, Patel KR. Sphincters in pulmonary veins. An anatomic study in rats. Am Rev Respir Dis 1990;141: 721–6.

236. Heath D, Williams D. Arachnoid nodules in the lungs of high altitude Indians. Thorax 1993;48:743–5.

237. Ho SY, Sanchez-Quintana D, Cabrera JA, et al. Anatomy of the left atrium: implications for radiofrequency ablation of atrial fibrillation. J Cardiovasc Electrophysiol 1999;10:1525–33.

238. Nathan H, Eliakim M. The junction between the left atrium and the pulmonary veins. An anatomic study of human hearts. Circulation 1966;34:412–22.

239. Haissaguerre M, Jais P, Shah DC, et al. Spontaneous initiation of atrial fibrillation by ectopic beats originating in the pulmonary veins. N Engl J Med 1998;339:659–66.

240. Steiner I, Haíjkova P, Kvasnicìka J, et al. Myocardial sleeves of pulmonary veins and atrial fibrillation: a postmortem histopathological study of 100 subjects. Virchows Archiv 2006;449:88–95.

241. Printzmetal M, Ornitze EM, Simkin B, et al. Arterio-venous anastomoses in liver, spleen and lungs. Am J Physiol 1948;152:48–52.

242. Tobin CE, Zariquiey MD. Arterio-venous shunts in the human lung. Proc Soc Exp Biol Med 1950;75:827–9.

243. Blessing MH, Hora BI. Glomera in der Lunge des Menschen. Zeitschrift fur Zellforschung 1968;87:562–70.

244. Junod AE. Accumulation of ^{14}C-imipramine in isolated perfused rat lungs. J Pharmacol Exp Ther 1972;183:182–7.

245. Strum JM, Junod AF. Radioautographic demonstration of 5-hydroxytryptamine-3H uptake by pulmonary endothelial cells. J Cell Biol 1972;54:456–67.

246. Nicholas TE, Strum JM, Angelo LS, et al. Site and mechanism of uptake of HL-norepinephrine by isolated perfused rat lungs. Circ Res 1974;35:670–80.

247. Ferreira SH, Greene LJ, Salgado MCO, et al. The fate of circulating biologically active peptides in the lungs. In: Ciba foundation, symposium 78: metabolic activities of the lung. Amsterdam: Excerpta Medica; 1980. p. 129–45.

248. Moncada S, Vane JR. Pharmacology and endogenous roles of prostaglandin endoperoxides, thromboxane A₂ and prostacyclin. Pharmacol Rev 1978;30:293–331.

249. Gryglewski RJ, Korbut R, Ocetkiewicz A. Generation of prostacyclin by lungs in vivo and its release into the arterial circulation. Nature 1978;273:765–7.

250. Yanagisawa M, Kurihara H, Kimura S, et al. A novel potent vasoconstrictor peptide produced by vascular endothelial cell. Nature 1988;332:411–15.

251. Moncada S, Palmer RMJ, Higgs EA. Nitric oxide: physiology, pathophysiology and pharmacology. Pharmacol Rev 1991;43:109–42.

252. Cernacek P, Stewart DJ. Immunoreactive endothelin in human plasma: marked elevations in patients in cardiogenic shock. Biochem Biophys Res Commun 1989;161:562–7.

253. Yamamoto M, Shimokata K, Nagura H. An immunohistochemical study on phenotypic heterogeneity of human pulmonary vascular endothelial cells. Virchows Arch A Pathol Anat Histopathol 1988;412:479–86.

254. Brill R, Halpern MM. The frequency of megakaryocytes in autopsy sections. Blood 1948;3:286–91.

255. Aabo K, Hansen KB. Megakarocytes in pulmonary blood vessels. 1. Incidences at autopsy, clinicopathological relations especially to disseminated intravascular coagulation. Acta Pathol Microbiol Scand 1978;86:285–91.

256. Sharma GK, Talbot IC. Pulmonary megakaryocytes: 'missing link' between cardiovascular and respiratory disease? J Clin Pathol 1986;39:969–76.

257. Crow J. Pulmonary haematoxyphil bodies. J Clin Pathol 1982;35:690–1.

258. Scheinin TM, Koivuniemi AP. Megakaryocytes in the pulmonary circulation. Blood 1963;22:82–7.

259. Melamed MR, Cliffton EE, Mercer C, et al. The megakaryocyte blood count. Am J Med Sci 1966;252:301–9.

260. Kallinikos-Maniatis A. Megakaryocytes and platelets in central venous and arterial blood. Acta Haematol 1969;42: 330–5.

261. Tinggaard Pedersen N. The pulmonary vessels as a filter for circulating megakaryocytes in rats. Scand J Haematol 1974;13:225–31.

262. Tinggaard Pedersen N. Occurrence of megakaryocytes in various vessels, and their retention in the pulmonary capillaries of man. Scand J Haematol 1978;21:369–75.

263. Trowbridge EA, Martin JF, Slater DN. Evidence for a theory of physical fragmentation of megakaryocytes, implying that all platelets are produced in the pulmonary circulation. Thromb Res 1982;28:461–75.

264. Slater DN, Trowbridge EA, Martin JF. The megakaryocyte in thrombocytopenia: a microscopic study which supports the theory that platelets are produced in the lungs. Thromb Res 1983;31:163–76.

265. Hardaway RM, Johnson D. Clotting mechanism in endotoxin shock. Arch Intern Med 1963;112:775–82.

266. Soares FA. Increased numbers of pulmonary megakaryocytes in patients with arterial pulmonary tumour embolism and with lung metastases seen at necropsy. J Clin Pathol 1992;45:140–2.

267. Deffebach ME, Charan NB, Lakshminarayan S, et al. The bronchial circulation. Small, but a vital attribute of the lung. Am Rev Respir Dis 1987;135:463–81.

268. Paredi P, Barnes PJ. The airway vasculature: recent advances and clinical implications. Thorax 2009;64:444–50.

269. Hales MR, Liebow AA. Collateral circulation to the lungs in congenital pulmonic stenosis. Bull Assoc Med Mus 1948;28:1–22.

270. Liebow AA, Hales MR, Lindskog GE. Enlargement of the bronchial arteries, and their anastomoses with the pulmonary arteries in bronchiectasis. Am J Pathol 1949;25:211–31.

271. Turner-Warwick M. Pre-capillary systemic-pulmonary anastomoses. Thorax 1963;18:225–37.

272. Charan NB, Baile EM, Pare PD. Bronchial vascular congestion and angiogenesis. Eur Respir J 1997;10:1173–80.

273. Weibel E. Die Entstehung der Langsmuskulatur in den Asten der A. bronchialis. Zeitschrift fur Zellforschung 1958;47:440–68.

274. Wagenaar S, Wagenvoort CA. Experimental production of longitudinal smooth muscle cells in the intima of muscular arteries. Lab Invest 1978;39:370–4.

275. Hill P, Goulding D, Webber SE, Widdicombe JG. Blood sinuses in the submucosa of the large airways of the sheep. J Anat 1989;162:235–47.

276. Laitinen A, Laitinen LA, Moss R, et al. The organisation and structure of tracheal and bronchial blood vessels in the dog. J Anat 1989;165:133–40.

277. Widdicombe JG. Tracheobronchial vasculature. Br Med Bull 1992;48: 108–19.

278. Suzuki Y. Fenestration of alveolar capillary endothelium in experimental pulmonary fibrosis. Lab Invest 1969;21:304–8.

279. Wanner A. Airway circulation. Am Rev Respir Dis 1992;146:S1–2.

280. Renkin EM. Cellular and intercellular transport pathways in exchange vessels. Am Rev Respir Dis 1992;146:S28–31.

281. Kawanami O, Matsuda K, Yoneyama H, et al. Endothelial fenestration of the alveolar capillaries in interstitial fibrotic lung diseases. Acta Pathol Jpn 1992;42:177–84.

282. Fritts HWJr, Harris P, Chidsey CAI, et al. Estimation of flow through bronchial-pulmonary vascular anastomoses with use of T-1824 dye. Circulation 1961;23: 390–8.

283. Heath D, Thompson IM. Bronchopulmonary anastomoses in sickle cell anaemia. Thorax 1969;24:232–8.

284. Liebow AA, Hales MR. Studies on the lung after ligation of the pulmonary artery; anatomical changes. Am J Pathol 1950;26:177–95.

285. Vanderhoeft PJ. Broncho-pulmonary circuits: a synoptic appraisal. Thorax 1963;19:537–40.

286. Lauweryns JM. The blood and lymphatic microcirculation of the lung. Pathol Annu 1971;6:365–415.

287. Staub NC. The pathophysiology of pulmonary edema. Hum Pathol 1970;1:419–32.

288. International Union Against Cancer (UICC). TNM Atlas Illustrated guide to the TNM classification of malignant tumours. 5th ed. Hoboken, New Jersey: Wiley-Liss; 2005.

289. Baird JA. The pathways of lymphatic spread of carcinoma of the lung. Br J Surg 1965;52:868–75.

290. West JB, Dollery CT. Distribution of blood flow and ventilation perfusion ratio in the lung, measured with radioactive CO_2. J Appl Physiol 1960;15:405–10.

291. West JB. Ventilation/Blood Flow and Gas Exchange. 3th ed. Oxford: Blackwell; 1977. p. 30.

Lymphoid tissue of the lungs

292. Trapnell DH. Recognition and incidence of intrapulmonary lymph nodes. Thorax 1964;19:44–50.

293. Kradin RI, Spirn PW, Mark EJ. Intrapulmonary lymph nodes. Clinical, radiologic and pathologic features. Chest 1985;87:662–7.

294. Oshiro Y, Kusumoto M, Moriyama N, et al. Intrapulmonary lymph nodes: thin-section CT features of 19 nodules. J Comput Assist Tomogr 2002;26:553–7.

295. Bienenstock J, Johnston N, Perey DYE. Bronchial lymphoid tissue I morphologic characteristics. Lab Invest 1973;28:686–92.

296. Bienenstock J, Johnston N, Perey DYE. Bronchial lymphoid tissue II functional characteristics. Lab Invest 1973;28:693–8.

297. Pabst R, Gehrke I. Is the bronchus-associated lymphoid tissue (BALT) an integral structure of the lung in normal mammals, including humans? Am J Respir Cell Mol Biol 1990;3:131–6.

298. Gould SJ, Isaacson PG. Bronchus-associated lymphoid tissue (BALT) in human fetal and infant lung. J Pathol 1993;169:229–34.

299. Richmond I, Pritchard GE, Ashcroft T, et al. Bronchus associated lymphoid tissue (BALT) in human lung – its distribution in smokers and non-smokers. Thorax 1993;48:1130–4.

300. Tschernig T, Kleemann WJ, Pabst R. Bronchus-associated lymphoid tissue (BALT) in the lungs of children who had died from sudden infant death syndrome and other causes. Thorax 1995;50:658–60.

301. Bosken CH, Hards J, Gatter K, et al. Characterization of the inflammatory reaction in the peripheral airways of cigarette smokers using immunocytochemistry. Am Rev Respir Dis 1992;145:911–17.

302. McDermott MR, Befus AD, Bienenstock J. The structural basis for immunity in the respiratory tract. Int Rev Exp Pathol 1982;23:47–112.

303. Rudzik R, Clancy RL, Perey DYE, et al. Repopulation with IgA-containing cells of bronchial and intestinal lamina propria after transfer of homologous Peyer's patch and bronchial lymphocytes. J Immunol 1975;114:1599–604.

304. Fournier M, Vai F, Derenne JP, et al. Bronchial lymphoepithelial nodules in the rat. Morphologic features and uptake and transport of exogenous proteins. Am Rev Respir Dis 1977;116:685–94.

305. Matsuura Y, Matsuoka T, Fuse Y. Ultrastructural and immunohistochemical studies on the ontogenic development of bronchus-associated lymphoid tissue (BALT) in the rat – special reference to follicular dendritic cells. Eur Respir J 1992;5:824–8.

306. Soutar CA. Distribution of plasma cells and other cells containing immunoglobulin in the respiratory tract of normal man and class of immunoglobulin contained therein. Thorax 1976;31:158–66.

307. Sato J, Chida K, Suda T, et al. Migratory patterns of thoracic duct lymphocytes into bronchus-associated lymphoid tissue of immunized rats. Lung 2000;178:295–308.

308. Emery JL, Dinsdale F. The postnatal development of lymphoreticular aggregates and lymph nodes in infants' lungs. J Clin Pathol 1973;26:539–45.

309. Hayday AC, Roberts S, Ramsburg E. Gamma delta cells and the regulation of mucosal immune responses. Am J Respir Crit Care Med 2000;162:S161.

310. Holt PG, Schon-Hegrad MA, Oliver J, et al. A contiguous network of dendritic antigen-presenting cells within the respiratory epithelium. Int Arch Allergy Appl Immunol 1990;91:155–9.

311. Hance AJ. Pulmonary immune cells in health and disease – dendritic cells and Langerhans cells. Eur Respir J 1993;6:1213–20.

312. Vanhaarst JMW, Dewit HJ, Drexhage HA, et al. Distribution and immunophenotype of mononuclear phagocytes and dendritic cells in the human lung. Am J Respir Cell Mol Biol 1994;10:487–92.

313. Austyn JM. Antigen-presenting cells – experimental and clinical studies of dendritic cells. Am J Respir Crit Care Med 2000;162:S146.

314. Holt PG. Antigen presentation in the lung. Am J Respir Crit Care Med 2000;162:S151–6.

315. Lambrecht BN, Prins JB, Hoogsteden HC. Lung dendritic cells and host immunity to infection. Eur Resp J 2001;18:692–704.

316. Vermaelen K, Pauwels R. Pulmonary Dendritic Cells. Am J Respir Crit Care Med 2005;172:530–51.

317. Rogers AV, Adelroth E, Hattotuwa K, et al. Bronchial mucosal dendritic cells in smokers and ex-smokers with COPD: an electron microscopic study. Thorax 2008;63:108–14.

318. Tschernig T, Debertin AS, Paulsen F, et al. Dendritic cells in the mucosa of the human trachea are not regularly found in the first year of life. Thorax 2001;56:427–31.

319. Veres TZ, Shevchenko M, Krasteva G, et al. Dendritic cell-nerve clusters are sites of T cell proliferation in allergic airway inflammation. Am J Pathol 2009;174:808–17.

320. Demedts IK, Bracke KR, Maes T, et al. Different roles for human lung dendritic cell subsets in pulmonary immune defense mechanisms. Am J Respir Cell Mol Biol 2006;35:387–93.

321. Tsoumakidou M, Tzanakis N, Papadaki HA, et al. Isolation of myeloid and plasmacytoid dendritic cells from human bronchoalveolar lavage fluid. Immunol Cell Biol 2006;84:267–73.

322. Tsoumakidou M, Demedts IK, Brusselle GG, et al. Dendritic cells in chronic obstructive pulmonary disease: new players in an old game. Am J Respir Crit Care Med 2008;177:1180–6.

323. Tsoumakidou M, Kemp SJ, Thorley AJ, et al. Expression of blood dendritic cell antigens (BDCAs) by CD1a+ human pulmonary cells. Respiratory Medicine 2009;103:935–8.

324. Birbeck MS, Breathnach AS, Everall JD. An electron microscopic study of basal melanocytes and high level clear cells (Langerhans' cell) in vitiligo. J Invest Dermatol 1961;37:51.

325. Soler P, Valeyre D, Georges R, et al. The role of epithelial abnormality in recruiting Langerhans cells to the lower respiratory tract. Am Rev Respir Dis 1986;133:A-243.

326. Hosokawa S, Shinzato M, Kaneko C, et al. Migration and maturation of Langerhans cells in squamous metaplasia of the rat trachea induced by vitamin A deficiency. Virchows Arch B Cell Pathol 1993;63:159–66.

327. Casoloro MA, Bernaudin J-F, Saltini C, et al. Accumulation of Langerhans' cells on the epithelial surface of the lower respiratory tract in normal subjects in association with cigarette smoking. Am Rev Respir Dis 1988;137:406–11.

328. Irani AA, Schechter NM, Craig SS, et al. Two types of human mast cells that have distinct neutral protease compositions. Proc Natl Acad Sci U S A 1986;83:4464–8.

329. Andersson CK, Mori M, Bjermer L, et al. Novel site-specific mast cell subpopulations in the human lung. Thorax 2009;64:297–305.

330. Hsieh FH, Sharma P, Gibbons A, et al. Human airway epithelial cell determinants of survival and functional phenotype for primary human mast cells. Proceedings of the National Academy of Sciences of the United States of America 2005;102:14380–5.

331. Guerzon GM, Pare PD, Michoud M-C, et al. The number and distribution of mast cells in monkey lungs. Am Rev Respir Dis 1979;119:59–66.

332. Lamb D, Lumsden A. Intra-epithelial mast cells in human airway epithelium: evidence for smoking-induced changes in their frequency. Thorax 1982;37:334–42.

333. Heard BE. Histochemical aspects of the staining of mast cells with particular reference to heterogeneity and quantification. In: Kay AB, editor. Asthma. Clinical Pharmacology and Therapeutic Progress. Oxford: Blackwell; 1986. p. 286–94.

334. Heard BE, Nunn AJ, Kay AB. Mast cells in human lungs. J Pathol 1989;157:59–63.

335. Heard BE, Dewar A, Nunn AJ, et al. Heterogeneous ultrastructure of human bronchial mast cells: morphometric subdivision of cell types and evidence for a degranulation gradient. Am J Respir Cell Mol Biol 1990;3:71–8.

336. Djukanovic R, Wilson JW, Britten KM, et al. Quantitation of mast cells and eosinophils in the bronchial mucosa of symptomatic asthmatics and healthy control subjects using immunohistochemistry. Am Rev Respir Dis 1990;142:863–71.

337. Bradley BL, Azzawi M, Jacobson M, et al. Eosinophils, T-lymphocytes, mast cells, neutrophils, and macrophages in bronchial biopsy specimens from atopic subjects with asthma: comparison with biopsy specimens from atopic subjects without asthma and normal controls subjects and relationship to bronchial hyperresponsiveness. J Allergy Clin Immunol 1991;88:661–74.

338. Fox B, Bull TB, Guz A. Mast cells in the human alveolar wall: an electronmicroscopic study. J Clin Pathol 1981;34:1333–42.

339. Heard BE, Dewar A, Corrin B. Apposition of fibroblasts to mast cells and lymphocytes in normal human lung and in cryptogenic fibrosing alveolitis – ultrastructure and cell perimeter measurements. J Pathol 1992;166:303–10.

340. Chanez P, Lacoste JY, Guillot B, et al. Mast cells' contribution to the fibrosing alveolitis of the scleroderma lung. Am Rev Respir Dis 1993;147:1497–502.

341. Qu ZH, Liebler JM, Powers MR, et al. Mast cells are a major source of basic fibroblast growth factor in chronic inflammation and cutaneous hemangioma. Am J Pathol 1995;147:564–73.

342. Inoue Y, King TE, Tinkle SS, et al. Human mast cell basic fibroblast growth factor in pulmonary fibrotic disorders. Am J Pathol 1996;149:2037–54.

343. Lane SJ, Lee TH. Mast cell effector mechanisms. J Allergy Clin Immunol 1996;98:S67–71.

344. Varadaradjalou S. Toll-like receptor 2 (TLR2) and TLR4 differentially activate human mast cells. European journal of immunology 2003;33:899–906.

Innervation of the lungs

345. Barnes PJ. Neural control of human airways in health and disease. Am Rev Respir Dis 1986;134:1289–314.

346. Barnes PJ. Modulation of neurotransmission in airways. Physiol Rev 1992;72:699–729.

347. Barnes PJ, Baraniuk JN, Belvisi MG. Neuropeptides in the respiratory tract 1. Am Rev Respir Dis 1991;144:1187–98.

348. Barnes PJ, Baraniuk JN, Belvisi MG. Neuropeptides in the respiratory tract 2. Am Rev Respir Dis 1991;144:1391–9.

349. Jeffery PK. Innervation of the airway mucosa: structure, function and changes in airway disease. In: Goldie R, editor. Handbook of Immunopharmacology of Epithelial Barriers. London: Academic Press; 1994. p. 85–118.

350. Belvisi MG. Overview of the innervation of the lung. Curr Opin Pharmacol 2002;2:211–5.

351. Fox B, Bull TB, Guz A. Innervation of alveolar walls in the human lung: an electron microscopical study. J Anat 1980;131:683–92.

352. Laitinen A. Ultrastructural organisation of intraepithelial nerves in the human airway tract. Thorax 1985;40:488–92.

353. Larson SD, Schelegle ES, Hyde DM, et al. The three-dimensional distribution of nerves along the entire intrapulmonary airway tree of the adult rat and the anatomical relationship between nerves and neuroepithelial bodies. Am J Respir Cell Mol Biol 2003;28:592–9.

354. Spencer H, Leof D. The innervation of the human lung. J Anat 1964;98:599–609.

355. Wharton J, Haworth SG, Polak JM. Postnatal development of the innervation and paraganglia in the porcine pulmonary arterial bed. J Pathol 1988;154:19–27.

356. Uddman R, Alumeta J, Densert O, et al. Occurrence and distribution of VIP nerves in the nasal mucosa and tracheobronchial wall. Acta Otolaryngol (Stockh) 1978;86:443–8.

357. Wharton J, Polak JM, Bloom SR, et al. Substance P-like immunoreactive nerves in mammalian lung. Invest Cell Pathol 1979;2:3–10.

358. Barnes PJ. The third nervous system in the lung: physiology and clinical perspectives. Thorax 1984;39:561–7.

359. Goldenberg VE, Buckingham S, Sommers SC. Pulmonary alveolar lesions in vagotomized rats. Lab Invest 1967;16:693–705.

360. Goldenberg VE, Buckingham S, Sommers SC. Pilocarpine stimulation of granular pneumocyte secretion. Lab Invest 1969;20:147–58.

361. Delahunty TJ, Johnston JM. Neurohumoral control of pulmonary surfactant secretion. Lung 1979;157:45–51.

Chapter 2

Development of the lungs; perinatal and developmental lung disease

The traditional division of disease into congenital and acquired is less useful in the case of the lungs than one that considers developmental as opposed to non-developmental disorders. This is because lung development continues long after birth. Developmental disease may therefore be acquired well into the postnatal period. Conversely some congenital lung disease is non-developmental but acquired in utero, a good example of which is congenital pneumonia. Other abnormalities may be acquired in utero because of adjacent developmental anomalies, one example of which is a defect in the diaphragm admitting abdominal viscera into the thorax and thereby causing pulmonary hypoplasia.

Knowledge of embryology is often helpful in understanding developmental diseases but, except for a few conditions such as tracheo-oesophageal fistula and anomalous pulmonary veins, this is hardly true of the lungs as the embryological basis of most developmental lung disease is poorly understood. Nor is the pathogenesis of most pulmonary malformations at all clear.

DEVELOPMENT OF THE LUNGS

Airway development

Human lung development is first marked by a longitudinal groove that appears on the ventral side of the primitive foregut 26 days after fertilisation. This separates from the foregut, first at its caudal end,

©2010 Elsevier Ltd
DOI: 10.1016/B978-0-7020-3369-8.00002-1

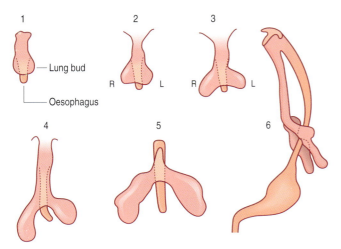

Figure 2.1 Development of the human lungs from the 26th to the 33rd day of gestation. l. At 26 days a bud appears at the lower end of the laryngopharyngeal sulcus. 2–4. The bud elongates to form a primitive trachea and lungs. 5. At 33 days there is early lobation of the lungs. 6. The primitive lungs extend dorsally on either side of the oesophagus.

Figure 2.2 Cross-section of a human embryo at 44 days' gestation. At this stage the pleural, pericardial and peritoneal cavities have separated from the primitive coelomic cavity and the main and lobar bronchi have formed. A vertebral body is seen at the top and anterior to this lie the dorsal aorta, the oesophagus, the lungs in their pleural cavities and the heart, of which the two thin-walled structures represent the atria and the more solid lower part the ventricles. Immunoperoxidase stain for the cell junction marker vinculin. *(Courtesy of Dr Alison Hislop, London, UK.)*

and then progressively forward until a connection is retained only at the cranial end. This bud then bifurcates and grows on either side of the foregut as the embryonic lungs, with successive branching giving rise to the lobar (about 33 days), segmental and further divisions of the airways (Fig. 2.1).[1] The developing lungs protrude into the coelomic cavity, the mesothelial lining of which forms from the mesoderm about the 14th day of gestation. With the development of the diaphragm and a pleuropericardial membrane the lungs become confined to the pleural cavities (Fig. 2.2).

The phases of lung development and the major events therein are summarised in Table 2.1. The embryonic stage of lung development lasts until 6 weeks' gestation, by which time the lungs have acquired a pseudoglandular appearance (Fig. 2.3). At this time the primitive potential air spaces are widely separated by abundant mesenchyme and lined by a vacuolated columnar or cuboidal epithelium rich in glycogen. The glycogen is particularly plentiful in the budding terminal epithelium where mitoses are most frequent. The pseudoglandular stage of development lasts until 16 weeks by which time division of the conductive airways down to the terminal bronchiole is complete.[2] This is followed by a canalicular stage marked by the appearance of further air spaces which have an attenuated lining epithelium (Fig. 2.4). During this period the epithelium loses its glycogen and differentiates into the type I and II cells seen in adult alveoli. Although no proper alveoli are yet present, respiration is possible towards the end of the canalicular period around 28 weeks. Substantial amounts of connective tissue still separate the air spaces at this time but in the saccular stage of intrauterine lung development the connective tissue progressively diminishes by an apoptotic mechanism[3] as new air spaces called terminal sacs develop. These resemble adult alveoli but are shallower and their walls still have enough connective tissue to separate the capillaries abutting air spaces into two layers. The development of true alveoli, first apparent at 36 weeks' gestation, is characterised by infolding of one of the two capillary layers, further thinning of the connective tissue and the eventual fusion of the double capillary layer into one.[4]

Alveoli develop mainly in the first year of extrauterine life and lung disease in infancy seriously impairs this. At birth, there are about 24 million terminal sacs and alveoli, compared to the adult figure of about 300 million alveoli. In the first year of life there is a fivefold increase in alveolar number with continued but slower increase thereafter, up to about 8 years of age and perhaps well into adolescence.[5] There is also remodelling of airways in the first year of life. This entails an increase in length of all airway generations, further branching of alveolar ducts to give more generations, transformation of distal respiratory bronchioles into alveolar ducts by increasing alveolisation of their walls, and transformation of terminal into respiratory bronchiole by centripetal alveolisation.[6–8] An important facet of postnatal lung development is that events in infancy and childhood may predispose to pulmonary disease in adult life. Thus, an increased frequency of respiratory infections in childhood has been identified in adults with chronic airflow obstruction.[9–11]

All the epithelial tissues of the lung, down to and including the alveoli, are of endodermal origin and all the interstitial elements are mesodermal in origin. This is contrary to older views on the development of the lung which envisaged the peripheral parts being purely mesodermal, but is demonstrated quite conclusively by electron microscopic studies of the developing mammalian lung. These show that the epithelial cells of the primitive endodermal bud extend continuously down to the smallest air spaces and that the epithelial lining of these spaces is not contributed to by any mesodermal elements.[12–14]

Table 2.1 Major events during lung development

Phase	Gestation	Major events
Embryonic	Up to 6 weeks	Lung buds form Segmental airways appear (6 weeks)
Pseudoglandular	6–16 weeks	Bronchial smooth muscle appears (7 weeks) Neuroendocrine cells and submucosal glands appear (8 weeks) Bronchial cartilages appear (10 weeks) Airway branching complete (16 weeks)
Canalicular	17–28 weeks	Basal cells appear (17 weeks) Clara cells appear (25 weeks) Basic structure of the acinus develops Mesenchyme starts to regress Blood vessels grow into acinar mesenchyme Type II alveolar cells appear (22 weeks)
Saccular	29–35 weeks	Subdivision of saccules Further thinning of mesenchyme
Alveolar[a]	36 weeks to term	Terminal air spaces lined by flat epithelial cells Inconspicuous interstitium Double layer of alveolar capillaries fuses to give a single layer
	Birth	Lung liquid rapidly cleared

[a]Alveolar multiplication continues from 36 weeks well into childhood.

Figure 2.4 The canalicular stage of lung development at 20 weeks' gestation. Further air spaces have developed and the lining epithelium is more attenuated.

Vascular and neural development

The blood supply to the developing lung buds is derived from the sixth pair of aortic arches. On the right, the ventral part of this arch persists as the right pulmonary artery whilst the dorsal part disappears. On the left, the ventral part persists as the ductus arteriosus. Within the lung buds blood vessels are formed by two processes. Angiogenesis (the sprouting of new from pre-existing vessels) underlies the formation of proximal lung vessels whilst vasculogenesis within the mesenchyme (the formation of vascular lakes by precursor angioblasts) contributes the peripheral vascular component, the two ultimately fusing by a lytic process.[15,16] The pulmonary arteries develop alongside newly formed airways, the latter seemingly acting as templates for the arteries.[17] A well-defined branching pattern is apparent by 14 weeks' gestation and all preacinar arteries are present by 16 weeks. At 20 weeks the branching pattern resembles that of adults. However, many peripheral arteries develop after birth (Fig. 2.5).[18]

The processes of vasculogenesis and angiogenesis are also involved in the development of the pulmonary veins.[19] Veins and arteries both first develop close to the primitive lung bud but the veins gradually take up a more peripheral position and by the time that the lung has a lobular structure the primitive veins are found in their adult position between the lobules. They initially enter a plexus around the foregut but later switch to a primary pulmonary vein that grows from the developing left atrium towards the lung buds. Incorporation of the primary pulmonary vein and its first two orders of branches into the wall of the left atrium results in two pulmonary veins from each lung entering the left atrium separately. Failure of the intrapulmonary veins to switch from the enteric venous plexus to the primary pulmonary vein underlies the congenital condition of anomalous pulmonary venous drainage (see p. 76).

Lymphatic development is first seen in the lung from about the eighth gestational week and by 14 weeks the pulmonary lymphatics are well established.

Neural tissue derived from the vagus nerve extends into the growing tips of the fetal airways and bronchial smooth muscle, which develops from 7 weeks' gestation, contracts in response to nervous stimulation from early gestation.[20]

Factors controlling lung development

Molecular mechanisms play an important role throughout lung development from the early induction of tracheal separation from the

Figure 2.3 The pseudoglandular stage of lung development at 12 weeks' gestation showing air spaces widely separated by abundant mesenchyme and lined by columnar epithelium showing marked subnuclear vacuolation.

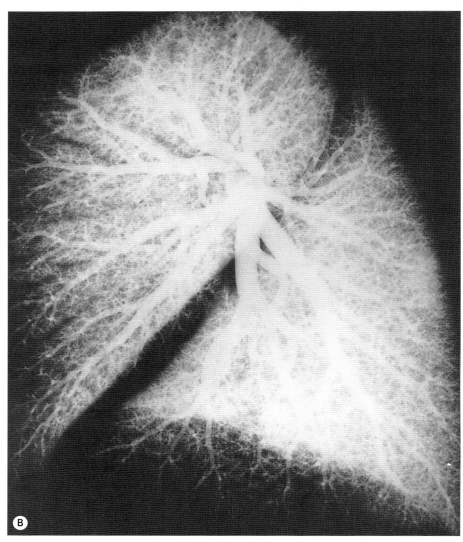

Figure 2.5 Pulmonary arteriograms showing the development of the pulmonary circulation after birth. (A) Life-size pulmonary arteriogram of the left lung of a baby at term. The arterial branching pattern is complete but there is little background haze as there are as yet few peripheral arteries. (B) Life-size pulmonary arteriogram of the left lung of an infant aged 18 months. The branching pattern is similar to that seen at birth but there is now a dense background haze made up of numerous peripheral arteries that have grown in the alveolar region of the lung after birth and that are too small to be identified individually. *(Reproduced with permission from Jeffery and Hislop (2003).[18])*

embryonic oesophagus to the appearance of cells specific to the lung such as the bronchiolar Clara cell and the alveolar pneumocytes. Various members of the forkhead homologue hepatocyte nuclear factor-3 (HNF-3) family are essential for the formation of the foregut endoderm and derivative organs, including the lung, while the induction of tracheal budding is dependent upon the simultaneous expression of the transcription marker Nkx2.1 (also known as thyroid transcription factor-1 or TTF-1).[21-23] TTF-1 is expressed throughout the embryonic lung in the early stages of its development but later becomes restricted to the more distal elements where growth is most active. It is particularly involved in epithelial cell differentiation.

The endodermal and mesodermal elements of the lung are each important to the proper development of the other with the basement membrane, cell adhesion factors such as fibronectin and integrin, and a variety of growth factors all playing a role in this interaction.[24-30] Growth factors include epithelial signalling molecules such as bone morphogenetic factor, transforming growth factor and sonic hedgehog that influence the underlying mesenchyme while the mesen-

chyme expresses signalling molecules such as fibroblast growth factor that are important in pulmonary epithelial development. Contacts between interstitial and type II epithelial cells have been identified in the newborn and shown to diminish during a postnatal proliferative phase.[31] Experiments demonstrate that respiratory epithelium has an inhibitory effect on the growth of the underlying mesenchyme,[32,33] whilst in fetal organ culture, intestinal mesoderm will induce bronchial budding but not branching, bronchial mesoderm will induce the tracheal endoderm to branch, and tracheal mesoderm will inhibit bronchial branching.[34] Furthermore, whilst the bronchial mesoderm of one species will induce the endoderm of another to branch, the pattern of endodermal branching is that of the species contributing the mesoderm. These experiments clearly demonstrate the interdependence of mesoderm and endoderm in pulmonary development. They are reinforced by the arrested development of endodermal lung buds within ectopic neuroglia (see p. 73).

The fetal air spaces are filled by a chloride-rich fluid secreted by their lining epithelium, which makes a substantial contribution to the production of amniotic fluid.[35] Its presence in the airways appears to be important to fetal lung growth for this is retarded if the fluid is drained.[36] Conversely, ligation of the trachea results in large lungs.[37]

Neuroendocrine cells are particularly numerous in the respiratory epithelium of the developing airways[38–42] and at least one of their products, gastrin-releasing peptide (human bombesin), is known to stimulate lung growth and maturation during the later stages of development.[43] The expression of gastrin-releasing peptide receptor gene peaks at a time and at sites of most rapid airway growth and development.[44]

Respiratory movements take place in utero and these too are thought to be important for fetal lung growth and maturation.[45] Section of the cervical cord above, but not below, the phrenic nucleus leads to severe pulmonary hypoplasia.[46]

Hormones are also important in lung development. The lungs bear steroid receptors, and maturation, but not growth, is promoted by glucocorticosteroids and probably other hormones. Glucocorticoid treatment of the fetus accelerates epithelial glycogen depletion, differentiation into type I and II cells, the appearance of lamellar bodies in type II cells, and their release into the air spaces.[47] This is utilised in clinical practice to minimise the risk of respiratory distress in premature infants (see below): a decreased incidence of the respiratory distress syndrome and increased survival are reported in premature infants exposed to maternal steroid therapy.[48] The steroids appear to act, at least in part, by stimulating lung fibroblasts to produce an oligopeptide known as fibroblast pneumonocyte factor which in turn stimulates surfactant synthesis by the type II cells, an example of paracrine activity.[49]

PERINATAL DISORDERS

Meconium aspiration

The expulsion of meconium into the amniotic fluid occurs as a response to fetal stress from a wide range of causes and its aspiration may cause a chemical or infective fetal pneumonia,[50] described below under neonatal pneumonia. Fetal stress also increases the normal respiratory excursions that take place before birth and may result in the airways being obstructed by numerous fetal squames and mucus (Fig. 2.6). Pathologists are likely to encounter only fatal cases but the lungs are inherently normal and the obstruction is potentially

Figure 2.6 Meconium aspiration. Fetal hypoxia has led to excessive respiratory movements in utero, resulting in the alveoli being filled with amniotic squamous cells.

reversible. The natural clearance mechanisms can be augmented with suction but such treatment may need to be prolonged, in which case oxygenation of the blood has to be maintained with an extracorporeal device; mechanical ventilation would only impair clearance. The mortality remains high, although corticosteroid and surfactant treatment are of some benefit.[51–53]

Massive pulmonary haemorrhage

This is a fairly common finding in perinatal necropsies and has several causes. In some cases of apparent pulmonary haemorrhage the findings are due to heavy blood-staining of oedema fluid rather than true haemorrhage and in these patients shock and left ventricular failure are important contributory factors. A coagulopathy, usually acquired, may cause true haemorrhage but the commonest cause is asphyxia. Cerebral oedema and haemorrhage are often also present and probably represent further manifestations of asphyxial damage. The condition is disproportionately frequent among preterm babies with very low birth weights[54] and it is postulated that abnormal alveolar surface forces may contribute to the bleeding.[55]

Neonatal pneumonia

Pulmonary infection in the neonate may be due to transplacental transmission from the mother, aspiration of either infected amniotic fluid before birth or infected material during birth, or environmental contacts after birth.

With transplacental transmission the pneumonia is only part of a generalised infection. Causative agents include cytomegalovirus, rubella virus, herpes simplex virus, varicella virus, mycoplasmas, *Listeria monocytogenes*, *Treponema pallidum*, *Mycobacterium tuberculosis* and *Toxoplasma gondii*. Many of these microbes elicit specific reactions that are dealt with in later chapters. However, it may be mentioned here that eosinophilic nuclear inclusions that represent parvovirus may be found in the lungs and other organs of premature stillbirths and neonates with non-immune hydrops.[56]

Pneumonia acquired by aspiration of infected amniotic fluid is known as congenital or intrauterine pneumonia. It is particularly likely if there is prolonged rupture of the membranes. Chorioamnionitis suggests this mechanism and examination of the placenta and its membranes is therefore helpful. Vaginal group B haemolytic streptococci or *Candida albicans* may be responsible, as may bowel bacteria such as *Escherichia coli*, klebsiellae and *Pseudomonas aeruginosa*. The air spaces contain polymorphonuclear leukocytes and fibrin but neither of these is as prominent as in an adult with pneumonia (Fig. 2.7). The distribution of the process is that of a bronchopneumonia. In some cases there is a combination of hyaline membrane disease and pneumonia. Bacteria may then be seen in the hyaline membranes, rendering them haematoxyphilic. It is possible that in such cases the bacteria promote the formation of the membranes by damaging the alveolar epithelium. Acute pneumonia and hyaline membranes may also result from the chemical toxicity of the bilirubin in aspirated meconium.[50] The fact that atelectasis is minimal helps to distinguish pneumonia with hyaline membranes from the infantile respiratory distress syndrome, which is dealt with next.[57] The combination of pneumonia and hyaline membranes is also seen in immature babies requiring ventilator support when there is secondary infection.[58,59]

Infantile respiratory distress syndrome (hyaline membrane disease)

By 28 weeks' gestation, the alveolar epithelium has differentiated into type I and type II pneumocytes, surfactant can be detected and an

Figure 2.7 Fetal (intrauterine) pneumonia. Neutrophils are evident in the alveoli but they are not as numerous as in fatal bacterial pneumonia in an adult.

Figure 2.9 Infantile respiratory distress syndrome (hyaline membrane disease). The interlobular septa are broadened by oedema and lymphatics within them are dilated. Alveoli have collapsed and air is confined to the bronchioles.

Figure 2.8 The lungs of a premature infant dying of the infantile respiratory distress syndrome (hyaline membrane disease) are dark and airless.

Figure 2.10 Infantile respiratory distress syndrome (hyaline membrane disease). Hyaline membranes separate collapsed alveoli from aerated bronchioles.

extrauterine existence is possible. With modern intensive care, an increasing number of babies born before 28 weeks are surviving, but without it the chances of successful respiration at this age are slim. By 34–36 weeks, premature birth is generally followed by successful respiration but the capacity of type II pneumocytes to replenish spent stocks of surfactant is frequently inadequate, in which case respiratory distress becomes evident within a few hours of birth.[60] This is apparent as grunting, indrawing of the intercostal tissues on inspiration and hypoxia. Radiographically there is opacification of the whole lung fields except for an 'air bronchogram'. Without respiratory support the death rate in the first few days is high.

Pathological findings

At necropsy the lungs are heavy, dark and airless (Fig. 2.8). Microscopy confirms the atelectasis, with air limited to the bronchioles (Fig. 2.9). There is also lymphatic distension and interstitial oedema, best seen in the perivascular connective tissue sheaths (see Fig. 2.9). Alveolar collapse and interstitial oedema are the expected consequences of high surface tensive forces acting on the alveolar walls. Hyaline membranes are found at the boundary of the air-filled bronchioles and the collapsed alveoli (Fig. 2.10). They are not found when death occurs in the first few hours of life and they are no longer thought to play a causal role in the alveolar collapse. The hyaline membranes represent compacted plasma exudates and cellular debris. They do not stain for fibrin with conventional histological stains but fibrin can be demon- strated in them by immunocytochemistry and epithelial necrosis by electron microscopy.[61] The hyaline membranes are yellow if there has also been unconjugated hyperbilirubinaemia (Fig. 2.11).[62,63]

Hyaline membranes are not specific to premature babies and may be found in term infants who die of birth asphyxia some hours later. Virtually identical pathological changes are seen in the adult respiratory distress syndrome (see p. 135). Hyaline membrane disease is evidently a consequence of non-specific injury to the bronchiolar and alveolar lining. In premature infants the injury is likely to be physical;

Figure 2.11 Yellow hyaline membranes in a premature infant with hyperbilirubinaemia.

ventilatory efforts in the surfactant-deficient lung put undue shear forces on the epithelium at the air–liquid interface, which at end-expiration is at the bronchiolar level, the alveoli having collapsed completely. Such mechanical stress operates during each ventilatory cycle so that it is repeated several thousand times in the first few hours of extrauterine life.[61]

Therapy and its complications

If premature birth is expected, or induction of premature labour planned, the risks of respiratory distress can be reduced by administering corticosteroids to the mother.[48] This promotes maturation of the fetal lung, including surfactant secretion.[47] It is a preventive measure that is only feasible when premature birth can be anticipated.

After birth, mechanical respiratory support with oxygen enrichment is the main means of maintaining oxygenation. This is being increasingly supplemented by the insufflation of natural or synthetic surfactant into the infant's airways.[64] Such surfactant therapy is proving very successful but, if the infant does come to autopsy, the exogenous surfactant is seen in the air spaces as a yellow birefringent material. Another useful measure is the administration of nitric oxide gas in low concentrations (less than 80 parts per million) to induce pulmonary arterial dilatation and improve ventilation/perfusion matching. Extracorporeal oxygenation of the infant's blood may also be undertaken but results are best in babies greater than 37 weeks' gestation: preterm babies weighing less than 2 kg have blood vessels that are too fragile to withstand the damage from cannulae and are at risk of ventricular haemorrhage from the heparinised circuits.

With these measures the survival rate of preterm infants who develop respiratory distress has been greatly increased and hyaline membrane disease is now seen far less frequently. However, there are cardiopulmonary complications of such treatment. Immediate complications of positive-pressure ventilation include interstitial emphysema and pneumothorax (see below), while patency of the ductus arteriosus and cardiac failure (persistent fetal circulation, see below) may dominate the clinical picture after a few days. Some infants who survive the first weeks of life on ventilator support develop diffuse lung disease and die in the succeeding months from extensive bronchopulmonary dysplasia (see below). Long-term survivors tend to have impaired lung function for some months[65,66] and a high incidence of bronchiolitis and pneumonia in infancy.[67] Babies who recover spontaneously from the respiratory distress syndrome do so completely and suffer none of these pulmonary complications.

Figure 2.12 Bronchopulmonary dysplasia. (A) A bronchiole is lined by atypical regenerative epithelium. Hyaline membranes are seen in the bronchiolar lumen. Adjacent alveolar tissue shows interstitial fibroblast proliferation. (B) A bronchiole shows mucosal thickening by cellular fibrosis and there is squamous metaplasia.

Bronchopulmonary dysplasia and chronic lung disease of prematurity

Bronchopulmonary dysplasia is the condition found in premature infants who are enabled with the help of artificial ventilation to survive the respiratory distress syndrome but die in the first few months of life.[68,69] As infants who recover spontaneously do not develop this condition it must be attributed to the respirator support but it is controversial whether oxygen toxicity or barotrauma is mainly responsible.[70,71] Other factors that have been incriminated include prematurity, infection, tracheal intubation, patency of the ductus arteriosus and fluid overload.

It represents disordered prolongation of the healing phase of hyaline membrane disease in which the original damage is augmented by the supportive therapy. Interstitial oedema persists and granulation tissue develops in the walls of the airways and alveoli, progressing to interstitial fibrosis. The air–blood barrier is thickened and the alveolar capillaries are reduced in number. There is also organisation of the hyaline membranes, and intraluminal fibrosis leads to the obliteration of many bronchioles. Regenerative hyperplasia is evident in the epithelium of alveoli, bronchioles and bronchi, often with metaplastic changes (Fig. 2.12). Distal air spaces are lined by cuboidal type II pneumocytes or atypical elongated cells which represent type II cells

Figure 2.13 Bronchopulmonary dysplasia. Solid areas of collapse and fibrosis alternate with lighter distended areas. *(Courtesy of Dr W Geddie, formerly of Toronto, Canada.)*

differentiating into type I. Severe squamous metaplasia is often evident in the larger airways. The epithelial changes resolve with time and in babies who survive longer than 3 months the changes are more marked in the lung parenchyma. The changes are often patchy and consist of fibrotic airless areas of lung tissue alternating with distended or even emphysematous areas (Fig. 2.13). Fibrosis predominates in babies who die in the first 2 months and emphysema in those who survive a year or more.[72] Long-term survivors generally have impaired lung function.[73] They also show hypertrophy of the right ventricle.[74]

These may be considered the classic features of bronchopulmonary dysplasia, as described in infants born at about 32 weeks' gestation. However, with improved therapy most such babies now survive and autopsy is today largely limited to extremely immature infants, those born at about 24–26 weeks' gestation. The pathological findings in these children differ sufficiently from the classic picture described above to warrant the introduction of a new term, chronic lung disease of prematurity. That the features differ from the classic ones described above should occasion no surprise given the dramatic changes that take place in the normal lung between 22 and 32 weeks' gestation. This period encompasses the change from the canalicular to the saccular phase of lung development and the changes represent disrupted alveolar and capillary development.

Chronic lung disease of prematurity is characterised by large simple air spaces lined by undifferentiated cuboidal cells and separated by cellular fibroelastic septa of even thickness. Mean linear intercept counts are low, indicating reduced numbers of air spaces and arrested alveolar development. The squamous metaplasia and alternating areas of collapse and overinflation seen in bronchopulmonary dysplasia are not well represented in chronic lung disease of prematurity (Box 2.1).[75,76]

Surfactant dysfunction disorders

The surfactant deficiency underlying the great majority of cases of the infantile respiratory distress syndrome (hyaline membrane disease) is attributable to immaturity of the lung but the syndrome is also seen in a few mature babies who have an inherited defect in surfactant production.[77] To date, three such conditions have been identified in humans, respectively involving surfactant proteins B and C and an integral membrane protein known as ABCA3 (Table 2.2).[78]

The best known is that involving faults in surfactant protein B synthesis.[79–82] Various mutations of the surfactant protein B gene have been identified, resulting in considerable molecular and phenotypic variability.[83–85] These babies may die with hyaline membrane disease or bronchopulmonary dysplasia or survive the neonatal period only to develop changes that resemble pulmonary alveolar proteinosis, desquamative interstitial pneumonia or cholesterol pneumonitis together with type II cell hyperplasia, features that overlap with those of chronic pneumonitis of infancy, described below.[79,86] It seems likely

Table 2.2 Surfactant dysfunction disorders[78]

	Surfactant apoprotein-B	Surfactant apoprotein-C	ABCA3	Others?
Genetic inheritance	Autosomal recessive	Autosomal dominant, sporadic	Autosomal recessive	Unrecognised
Chromosome	2p12-11.2	8p21	16p13.3	Unrecognised
Clinical features	Neonatal respiratory failure and death	Infants and older children with respiratory failure	Neonatal and early infantile respiratory failure. Some cases reported of older children with pattern similar to adult desquamative interstitial pneumonia	Unexplained neonatal or infantile respiratory failure
Lung histology	Alveolar type II cell hyperplasia and alveolar proteinosis, interstitial inflammation and fibrosis	Variety of patterns including desquamative, usual or non-specific interstitial pneumonia	Alveolar type II cell hyperplasia, accumulation of macrophages and proteinaceous material in air spaces	Endogenous lipid pneumonia, cholesterol pneumonitis, alveolar proteinosis, chronic pneumonitis of infancy, desquamative interstitial pneumonia or non-specific interstitial pneumonia

that in protein B deficiency the alveolar proteinosis is due to excessive amounts of surfactant being secreted in order to compensate for its defective protein content. As in autoimmune alveolar proteinosis, there is an initial stage of endogenous lipid pneumonia, representing macrophage ingestion of the excess surfactant. Electron microscopy shows abnormal type II cell inclusions: these lack their normal whorled lamellae and resemble those described in mice in which the surfactant protein B gene has been disrupted.[87,88] The diagnosis of surfactant protein B deficiency may be established by immunostaining bronchoalveolar lavage material or lung tissue for the various surfactant proteins and thereby demonstrating an absence of surfactant protein B and increased amounts of surfactant protein A.

Abnormalities involving surfactant protein C have also been reported,[89] again with considerable phenotypic variation.[90] Most patients have been neonates or infants but some have been older children or adults. Young children generally show the changes of chronic pneumonitis of infancy described below,[91] but some show alveolar proteinosis whilst other cases have been adults displaying histological patterns of usual desquamative or non-specific interstitial pneumonia.[90]

An absence of surfactant lamellar bodies from type II alveolar cells in term infants who develop respiratory distress soon after birth represents a further genetic error in surfactant production, one involving an integral membrane protein known as ABCA3.[92-95] This is an ATP-binding cassette protein, one of several concerned in transmembrane delivery of a variety of substances, including lipids. In the lung it has been localised to the limiting membrane of the surfactant lamellar bodies. ABCA3 deficiency is associated with a histological pattern of desquamative interstitial pneumonia, non-specific interstitial pneumonia, endogenous lipid pneumonia, alveolar proteinosis or, rarely, usual interstitial pneumonia.[92,93,96,97] A variant of ABCA3 deficiency is characterised by the presence of abnormal lamellar bodies that have been likened to fried eggs.[98] Genetic studies have subsequently identified ABCA3 deficiency in older children and young adults with a variety of obscure interstitial lung diseases.[95,99]

It is likely that children reported in the older literature as showing a combination of endogenous lipid pneumonia, cholesterol granulomas and alveolar proteinosis of obscure etiology represented further cases of abnormal surfactant production, possibly due to as-yet unrecognised defects.[100-105] Deficiency of surfactant protein A has not yet been firmly established in humans but may be represented by the Hermansky–Pudlak syndrome described on page 491, and the pale ear mouse, which provides an animal model of the human syndrome, where it appears that faulty production of surfactant protein A leads to the development of giant lamellar bodies and pulmonary fibrosis.[106,107]

Chronic pneumonitis of infancy

Chronic pneumonitis of infancy represents a pattern of disease first described in full-term infants of either sex whose mothers experienced uncomplicated pregnancies and deliveries.[108] The infants are normal at birth but cough, respiratory distress and a failure to thrive develop at ages varying from 2 weeks to 11 months (average 3.6 months). Radiographs show a predominantly interstitial pattern of opacification. The prognosis is variable: some of the children recover spontaneously whereas others die of respiratory failure within 3 months of the onset of symptoms.

The aetiology is unknown and may be multifactorial. It has been suggested that the condition represents recurrent or poorly cleared infection[108] but there is no firm evidence of this. The changes within the air spaces often resemble those of alveolar proteinosis, suggesting that causes of this disease in infancy such as surfactant protein B or C deficiency, as described above, and lysinuric protein intolerance[109-111] may be responsible. Gastro-oesophageal reflux with aspiration is another possibility.

Biopsy shows alveolar wall thickening with a variety of air space abnormalities. There is little inflammation. The alveolar wall thickening is due to interstitial spindle cell proliferation and type II epithelial cell hyperplasia. Collagen is not a feature in the early stages but the disease may progress to interstitial fibrosis. Within the alveolar lumen, macrophages are increased and there is often an accumulation of granular eosinophilic material in which acicular cholesterol crystal clefts may be seen. The macrophages may have foamy cytoplasm (Fig. 2.14).

Cellular interstitial pneumonitis and pulmonary interstitial glycogenosis

Cellular interstitial pneumonitis shows less marked interstitial thickening, type II cell hyperplasia and alveolar filling than chronic

Figure 2.14 Chronic pneumonitis of infancy. The alveolar walls are thickened by immature connective tissue cells; there is little interstitial inflammation. Type II pneumocytes are hyperplastic and there is focal proteinaceous debris in alveoli.

Figure 2.15 Pulmonary interstitial glycogenosis. The alveolar interstitium is expanded by cytologically bland round cells with clear cytoplasm. These changes are seen in other paediatric disorders and pulmonary interstitial glycogenosis is only diagnosed if these interstitial changes predominate.

pneumonitis of infancy and appears to have a better prognosis. However, whether this means that the two represent separate conditions[91] or are variations of one[112,113] is debatable.

Some of those that distinguish cellular interstitial pneumonitis and chronic pneumonitis of infancy equate the former with what has been described as pulmonary interstitial glycogenosis,[91] a term that was coined when vacuoles in the interstitial cells were shown to represent glycogen (Fig. 2.15).[114] Such glycogenosis appears to be self-limiting[115] and may be merely an epiphenomenon, as interstitial cells with clear cytoplasm are not infrequently seen in association with other disorders such as antibody deficiency[116] and alveolar capillary dysplasia.[117] The term 'glycogenosis' is unfortunate as it usually refers to an inborn error of glycogen metabolism due to enzyme deficiency for which there is no evidence in this condition: the term 'pulmonary interstitial glycogen accumulation disorder' is therefore preferred by some authors.[118]

Interstitial emphysema

This condition is a form of barotrauma and in infancy is often a complication of mechanical ventilation. High ventilatory pressures rupture the alveolar walls and permit air to enter the interstitial tissue. The air is seen particularly in the abundant connective tissue that surrounds the pulmonary artery and bronchiole in the centre of the acinus and forms the interlobular septa. Lines of bubbles are seen through the pleura, outlining the lung lobules. Blebs may project from the pleura, and cyst-like spaces up to 3 cm in diameter are found on the cut surface of the lung (Figs 2.16 and 2.17).[119–121] Pneumothorax and surgical emphysema of the mediastinum and neck frequently accompany interstitial emphysema. The air may track into the other serosal cavities causing pneumopericardium or pneumoperitoneum. Rarely, large subpleural cysts develop.[122] In some cases the changes resolve spontaneously whereas in others they persist and may require excision of affected tissue.[123,124]

Microscopically the differential diagnosis is from congenital lymphangiectasia (see p. 77). This can be extremely difficult, not least because the air tracks within lymphatics as well as the surrounding connective tissue.[125] It is therefore helpful if the nature of the content of the cysts, gaseous or fluid, is ascertained at necropsy. If the emphysema has been present for a few days before death the diagnosis is simplified by the development of a foreign-body giant cell reaction to the air (Fig. 2.18). The presence of interstitial emphysema has been used forensically as evidence of live birth.[126]

Persistent tachypnoea of infancy associated with neuroendocrine cell hyperplasia

Neuroendocrine cell hyperplasia was identified by immunostaining for bombesin when it was decided to review the archival tissue of a group of infants less than 2 years of age who had presented with persistent tachypnoea, hypoxia, rib retraction or respiratory crackles, and had had a lung biopsy reported as showing seemingly insignificant non-specific changes (Fig. 2.19). These infants showed an increased number of neuroendocrine cells compared to a group of controls.[127] The mean onset of symptoms was 3.8 months (range, 0–11 months). Radiographs demonstrated hyperinflation, interstitial markings and ground-glass densities. Oxygen was initially required for prolonged periods, and medication trials did not eliminate symptoms. After a mean of 5 years, no deaths had occurred, and the patients' condition had improved. It was suggested that these infants represented a distinct group of patients defined by the absence of known lung diseases, the clinical signs and symptoms of interstitial lung disease and idiopathic neuroendocrine cell hyperplasia of infancy. More reports are awaited.

Persistent fetal circulation (persistent pulmonary hypertension of the newborn)

In this condition the high pulmonary blood pressure of the fetus fails to fall at birth and right-to-left shunting through the foramen ovale

Figure 2.17 Interstitial emphysema. Air-filled spaces are seen in the interlobular septa.

Figure 2.18 Interstitial emphysema. Within a few days the cysts are lined by a foreign-body giant cell reaction to the air.

Figure 2.16 Interstitial emphysema. (A) Lines of air bubbles are seen through the pleura, outlining the lung lobules. (B) Cyst-like spaces are seen on the cut surface of the lung.

and ductus arteriosus continues in neonatal life.[128] The incidence of the condition is about one in 1000 live births and prior to the introduction of nitric oxide therapy the mortality was about 50%. Autopsy studies show that the muscular pulmonary arteries have a thickened media and that muscle extends into small peripheral arteries that are not normally muscular.[129] The condition may be idiopathic or secondary to a wide variety of neonatal cardiopulmonary disorders, including hyaline membrane disease, asphyxia, meconium aspiration and diaphragmatic hernia. The idiopathic cases are poorly understood but autopsy has shown that some are secondary to alveolar capillary dysplasia (see p. 50) that was undetected until autopsy,[130,131] whilst others show alveolar dysplasia with good capillary growth.[117] All these underlying causes reduce the stimuli that normally initiate pulmonary vascular dilatation at birth, namely pulmonary expansion, raised pulmonary oxygen tension and lowered pulmonary carbon dioxide tension. Notable amongst the agents that mediate the vasodilatation is nitric oxide (endothelium-derived relaxation factor – see p. 22), and the inhalation of low levels of this gas appears to reverse the hypoxaemia of persistent pulmonary hypertension of the newborn.[132,133]

Diffuse developmental lung disorders

Three conditions come under this heading: congenital acinar dysplasia, congenital alveolar dysplasia and alveolar capillary dysplasia with misalignment of pulmonary veins. The abnormality in each is one of arrested development, the first at the pseudoglandular phase of

Figure 2.19 Neuroendocrine cell hyperplasia of infancy. (A) A small airway showing only minimal chronic inflammation on routine staining but (B) staining for bombesin shows increased numbers of neuroendocrine cells within the surface epithelium.

development, the second at the canalicular or early saccular phase and the third involving the vascularisation of the acinus so that capillaries remain close to their supplying artery in the centre of the acinus and veins also develop in this position rather than in the interlobular septa.[117,134]

These disorders of development have to be distinguished from several other conditions that affect the neonatal lungs in a diffuse manner. A useful classification of them has recently been promulgated by a North American consortium, dividing them into the diffuse developmental disorders now to be considered, acquired growth abnormalities, specific conditions of undefined etiology and surfactant dysfunction disorders (Table 2.3).[134]

Congenital acinar dysplasia

Congenital acinar dysplasia is the rarest and most severe condition of the diffuse developmental lung disorders, being characterised by a complete absence of acinar development. The affected babies, who may be born at term or premature, are cyanosed from birth and survive only a few hours.[136-138] They usually have other abnormalities, such as cardiovascular anomalies, dermal hypoplasia and renal hypoplasia. The lungs are small and firm throughout. Microscopically, bronchial-type airways that have cartilage, smooth muscle and glands are separated by abundant mesenchymal tissue. No alveoli are seen (Fig. 2.20).[139] An absence of TTF-1, which is implicated in respiratory epithelial differentiation, is reported and occasionally siblings are affected, suggesting that the condition has a genetic basis. It is referred to again on page 59.

Congenital alveolar dysplasia

Congenital alveolar dysplasia was first described in 1948, since when there have been few further reports.[140] The condition is characterised by poorly developed air spaces separated by varying degrees of undifferentiated mesenchyme that may histologically resemble pulmonary intersitital glycogenosis. Features of persisitent pulmonary hypertension may also be present. It is generally incompatible with an extra-uterine existence but some children survive the neonatal period despite severe respiratory embarrassment.[117]

Alveolar capillary dysplasia with misalignment of pulmonary veins

Alveolar capillary dysplasia with misalignment of pulmonary veins represents a failure of capillaries and veins to migrate away from the centres of the primitive lung acini. It is an unusual cause of persistent pulmonary hypertension and respiratory distress of the newborn.[117,130,141–146] Cases reported to date have all been fatal, with survival generally not exceeding a few hours. Many cases show associated gastrointestinal or genitourinary malformations. Occasionally, siblings are affected and an autosomal-recessive genetic abnormality has been demonstrated in some cases.[145,147]

The pulmonary lobules are small and radial alveolar counts are decreased. The alveolar septal connective tissue is increased and alveolar capillaries are greatly reduced (Figs 2.21 and 2.22). Those present are in poor contact with the alveolar epithelium, which shows type II cell hyperplasia.[117] The pulmonary veins accompany small pulmonary arteries in the centres of the acini rather than occupying their normal

Table 2.3 Diffuse parenchymal disorders of infancy[134]

Disorders	
Primary disorders of lung development (aberration in primary molecular mechanism of lung and/or pulmonary vascular development) Congenital acinar dysplasia Congenital alveolar dysplasia Alveolar capillary dysplasia with misalignment of pulmonary veins	5.8%
Growth abnormalities reflecting deficient alveolarisation (usually secondary) Pulmonary hypoplasia Chronic lung disease of prematurity	24.6%
Specific conditions of undefined aetiology Pulmonary interstitial glycogenosis Neuroendocrine cell hyperplasia of infancy	3.2% 9.6%
Surfactant dysfunction disorders Surfactant protein B mutations Surfactant protein C mutations ABCA3 mutations Histology consistent with surfactant dysfunction but as yet without a recognised genetic etiology: Alveolar proteinosis Chronic pneumonitis of infancy Desquamative interstitial pneumonia Non-specific interstitial pneumonia	9.6%
Miscellaneous (e.g. systemic disease processes, immunocompromised states)	35.5%
Unclassified	11.7%

Figure 2.21 Persistent pulmonary hypertension of the newborn in a case of alveolar capillary dysplasia. A pulmonary artery showing marked medial hypertrophy (arrow) is seen within underdeveloped alveoli. The vessel next to the artery is a pulmonary vein: misalignment of pulmonary vessels is a major feature of alveolar capillary dysplasia.

position in the interlobular septa (see Figs 2.21 and 2.22B). The pulmonary arteries are decreased in number and show increased muscularisation. These changes are more easily appreciated if immunostains that localise vascular markers such as CD34 are employed.

Tracheobronchomalacia acquired in infancy

Tracheobronchomalacia (softening of the major airways) may be congenital or acquired but the two are often confused because the condition is most commonly acquired as a complication of congenital lung disease or its treatment, notably intubation.[148] This section is concerned with acquired disease. Congenital tracheobronchomalacia is dealt with below. The acquired disease is seen most commonly in premature babies who are intubated because of respiratory distress. Airway infection may also contribute to tracheobronchomalacia being acquired in infancy. Other causes include pressure from congenital abnormalities such as pectus excavatum, bronchogenic cyst or an aberrant artery. Whatever its cause, tracheobronchomalacia causes undue collapsibility of the airways and, hence, respiratory obstruction. Histopathological examination shows fibrous replacement of the tracheobronchial cartilages.

FURTHER DISORDERS OF DEVELOPMENT AND GROWTH

Anomalies of the larynx and trachea

Laryngeal atresia

This condition is usually due to cartilaginous overgrowth just below the vocal cords leaving only a narrow channel between the

Figure 2.20 Acinar dysplasia. The lung lobules are composed of irregular air spaces lined throughout by ciliated columnar epithelium and separated by abundant loose stroma. (Reproduced from Current Diagnostic Pathology by permission of Dr C Wright, Newcastle-upon-Tyne, UK.[139])

Figure 2.22 Alveolar capillary dysplasia. (A) There is a low density of alveoli. (B) High power shows alveolar septal thickening, scarcity of alveolar capillaries and misalignment of pulmonary vessels, both artery (A) and vein (V) lying alongside an airway.

pharynx and trachea that is insufficient to permit respiration. Viewed from above the larynx appears normal but attempts at intubation are unsuccessful and the baby quickly asphyxiates. In utero diagnosis may be possible because the airway obstruction often causes the lungs to be hyperplastic[149] and therefore hyperechogenic, in which case an immediate tracheostomy undertaken before the cord is clamped may prove life-saving. However, the condition is often associated with other congenital abnormalities, notably those comprising Fraser's syndrome. The identification of pulmonary hyperplasia should therefore lead to a search for additional malformations. Pulmonary hyperplasia is described in more detail on page 70.

Laryngeal webs may also be congenital, the majority involving the anterior glottis. They show a strong association with the velocardiofacial syndrome (chromosome 22q11.2 deletion).

Figure 2.23 Tracheal stenosis due to segmental absence of the posterior membranous portion so that the cartilaginous plates form complete rings (associated in this patient with an aberrant left pulmonary artery forming a sling round the trachea, the two abnormalities making a 'ring–sling' complex). (Courtesy of Dr M Kearney, Tromso, Norway.)

Tracheal aplasia

With total or partial absence of the trachea, the main bronchi either communicate only with each other, in which case the lungs are hyperplastic, or with the oesophagus.[150] A minor degree of tracheal hypoplasia, with both the sagittal and coronal diameters being reduced, may be seen in Down's syndrome.[151] The normal diameters of the adult trachea are given on page 63 under Mounier-Kuhn's syndrome of tracheobronchomegaly, a genetic disorder which generally becomes evident in adult life.

Tracheal stenosis

Tracheal stenosis may result from intrinsic or extrinsic lesions, which may be congenital or acquired. Congenital intrinsic stenosis may take the form of a gradual tapering, an isolated segmental narrowing or a membranous web, or be due to a nodule of ectopic oesophageal tissue.[154] Congenital extrinsic compression may be due to various anomalies of the great vessels forming (vascular) rings or a sling around the trachea (see p. 481). The left pulmonary artery sling syndrome may form part of a (tracheal) ring–sling complex in which the tracheal cartilages form complete rings, the left bronchus is short and the right is long (bronchial pseudoisomerism).[152] The complete cartilage rings represent an absence of the posterior membranous part of the trachea (Fig. 2.23) and the abnormally long trachea is consequently narrowed, the stenosis generally being funnel-shaped. This abnormality is difficult to correct surgically and the prognosis is poor. The trachea normally has 22 cartilages. More are generally seen in the ring–sling complex and fewer in infants with a congenitally short neck. A congenitally short trachea may not be recognised until the seventh decade.[153]

Figure 2.24 Tracheo-oesophageal fistula. The oesophagus has been opened from the rear to show the orifice of a tracheo-oesophageal fistula towards its lower end.

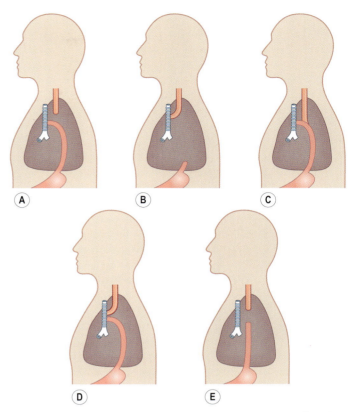

Figure 2.25 Tracheo-oesophageal fistula. (A) The arrangement found in 87% of cases where the upper oesophagus ends blindly and the lower oesophagus joins the trachea. (B–D) Rare variants of tracheo-oesophageal fistula. (E) Oesophageal atresia without fistula.

Tracheo-oesophageal fistula

The mesodermal separation of those parts of the primitive foregut destined to become oesophagus and trachea may be incomplete, resulting in a tracheo-oesophageal fistula (Fig. 2.24). Separation of trachea and oesophagus normally proceeds in a cephalad direction and if this is incomplete the two may communicate. Usually the proximal part of the oesophagus ends in a blind sac and the distal part takes origin from the lower part of the trachea, but the anatomy varies (Fig. 2.25). Histological examination shows that abnormalities in the wall of the trachea extend beyond the fistula; there is often widespread loss of cartilage and squamous metaplasia.[154,155] Tracheal communication with remnants of the branchial clefts (branchial cysts) is also recorded.[156] Occasionally it is a bronchus that communicates with the oesophagus.[157] Tracheo-oesophageal fistula sometimes forms part of a so-called VACTERL association, which represents a non-random grouping of birth defects involving mesodermal structures for which no genetic basis has yet been identified, VACTERL being a mnemonic for vertebral, anal, cardiovascular, tracheo-esophageal, renal and limb abnormalities.

Congenital tracheobronchomalacia

Tracheobronchomalacia (softening of the major airways) may be congenital or acquired but the two are often confused because the condition is most commonly acquired as a complication of congenital disease (e.g., cardiovascular abnormalities compressing the airways) or its treatment, notably intubation.[148,158,159] Acquired tracheobronchomalacia has been dealt with above (see p. 51) and this section is confined to congenital tracheobronchomalacia, a condition in which there is softening of the airway cartilages, often as part of a generalised chondrodystrophy seen in several skeletal dysplasia syndromes, e.g. Kneist dysplasia.[160] The trachea and bronchi may be affected alone or in combination. Other causes of congenital tracheobronchomalacia include the presence of oesophageal remnants in the wall of the trachea, which is generally seen in association with oesophageal atresia and tracheo-oesophageal fistula.[154]

Tracheobronchomalacia causes undue collapsibility of the airways and, hence, respiratory obstruction. However, as a cause of respiratory obstruction congenital tracheobronchomalacia is less common than focal absence of airway cartilages, the supposed basis of both congenital bronchiectasis (Williams–Campbell syndrome, see p. 62) and infantile lobar emphysema (see p. 72).

Anomalies of the bronchi and bronchioles

Abnormal bronchial branching and pulmonary lobation

The main bronchi may be displaced so that one or both whole lungs arise from the alimentary tract rather than the trachea (Fig. 2.26).[150] This often accompanies tracheal agenesis and probably represents a variety of tracheo-oesophageal fistula, but a bronchobiliary fistula (connecting the biliary and tracheobronchial trees, usually near the carina) may be part of a duplication of the upper alimentary tract from the level of the fistula to the ampulla of Vater.[161,162] Bile causes intense inflammation of the bronchial tree and in infancy the combination of cough with bile-stained sputum forms a distinctive clinical picture indicative of this type of fistula. An unusual case of bronchial diverticulosis possibly represents abnormal bronchial branching.[163]

Abnormalities of the lobar bronchi include a tracheal right upper-lobe bronchus, either displaced or supernumerary (Fig. 2.27), a double upper-lobe bronchus and an accessory cardiac lobe bronchus arising from the intermediate bronchus. There is a high incidence of tracheal upper-lobe bronchus in association with the tetralogy of Fallot.[164] A 'bridging bronchus' crossing the mediastinum from left to right represents origin of the right lower-lobe bronchus from the left bronchial tree.[165]

Abnormalities of segmental bronchi include double bronchi to the apical segment of either upper lobe, origin of the apical segmental bronchus of the right upper lobe from the trachea, either displaced or

Figure 2.26 Origin of main bronchus from the oesophagus. The lungs, oesophagus and stomach viewed from behind to show the right main bronchus arising from the lower oesophagus. *(Courtesy of the late Dr AH Cameron, Birmingham, UK.)*

Table 2.4 Relative frequency of abnormalities of pulmonary lobation[172]

Right		Left	
Deficient transverse fissure	25%	Lingular fissure	25%
Superior accessory fissure	18%	Superior accessory fissure	2%
Medial basal fissure	10%	Medial basal fissure	18%
Other	2%		

The abnormalities may be complete or partial and in 20% of cases they are multiple.

of the right or left upper lobes by the azygos and hemiazygos veins respectively. Absence of a lobe (and its bronchus) is rare.

Bronchopulmonary isomerism represents symmetry of the lungs and bronchi, with both sides having the pattern of either the normal right lung or the normal left lung. As emphasised above, lobation is an unreliable indicator of whether a lung is 'right' or 'left'. This can however be assessed by examining the extrapulmonary bronchi and pulmonary arteries. It will be remembered that the right main bronchus is shorter than the left and enters the lung behind the pulmonary artery whereas the longer left main bronchus is 'hyparterial', crossing behind the main left pulmonary artery to enter the lung below the artery. Bronchopulmonary isomerism is often associated with atrial isomerism, anomalous pulmonary veins and abnormalities of the spleen and liver (Fig. 2.29).[164,173] The Ivemark asplenia syndrome consists of bilateral right-sidedness with two morphologically right lungs, absence of the spleen, a symmetrical liver, malrotation of the gut and a variety of cardiac abnormalities including a common ventricle, totally anomalous pulmonary veins and bilateral superior venae cavae and right atria.[174] Bilateral morphologically left lungs are found in association with multiple minute spleens (polysplenia), a symmetrical liver, malrotation of the gut, partially anomalous pulmonary venous drainage and cardiac septal defects. Either right- or left-sided bronchopulmonary isomerism may be associated with multiple spleens of varying size (anisopolysplenia). Although non-familial, Ivemark's syndrome is confined to males whereas the other isomerism syndromes may affect either sex.

Bronchogenic cyst

Bronchogenic cysts, recognisable by cartilage and glands in their wall and a lining of respiratory epithelium (Fig. 2.30), are a variety of foregut duplication cyst, related to oesophageal and gastroenteric cysts. They are usually situated in the mediastinum close to the carina (51%) but may be found in the right paratracheal region (19%), alongside the oesophagus (14%), the hilum of the lung (9%) or a variety of other locations (7%), including the substance of the lungs, and even beneath the diaphragm.[175–181] Occasionally air–fluid levels are demonstrated radiographically suggesting a connection with the airways. Cysts lined by respiratory epithelium but lacking cartilage in their walls should be regarded as undifferentiated foregut cysts (also termed simple congenital cysts). These differ from type I congenital cystic adenomatoid malformations as the latter show polypoid infoldings, mucous cell hyperplasia and disordered parenchymal growth with smaller cysts resembling bronchioles (see p. 59). Congenital lung cysts are often not discovered until adult life, either as an incidental radiographic finding or because of complications, which include infection, haemorrhage and, in rare instances, neoplastic transformation.[182]

supernumerary, an absent right upper-lobe apical segmental bronchus and separate origin of the apical segmental bronchus of the left lower lobe from the main bronchus. A crossover lung segment is one with bronchial and arterial connections from the other side.[166–168] Usually the crossover is from right to left, the right lung is hypoplastic and the venous drainage anomalous, a variant of the 'scimitar' syndrome (see p. 76). These are features that crossover lung segment shares with the equally rare condition 'horseshoe' lung, where there is fusion of the lungs behind the heart and in front of the oesophagus.[168–171] However, unlike 'horseshoe' kidney, there is no fusion of the lungs; there are separate pleural cavities and the crossover segment lies in a pleural recess behind the heart that communicates with the pleural cavity on the side from which the segment derives.[167,168]

Abnormal lobation of the lungs does not imply an abnormal pattern of bronchial branching: lack or incomplete development of one or more interlobar fissures is common despite the presence of five lobar bronchi. Extra fissures separating segments off as extra lobes are also common, particularly the lingula and the medial basal and apical segments of the lower lobes (Table 2.4 and Fig. 2.28).[172] Fissures accommodating blood vessels may also be found, so that an azygos lobe may be formed by the parasagittal separation of the medial part

Figure 2.27 (A) Anomalous origin of the right upper-lobe bronchus from the trachea (which has been opened anteriorly), an arrangement that is normal in the pig, sheep, goat and ox. *(Courtesy of the late Dr AH Cameron, Birmingham, UK.)* (B) Three-dimensional computed tomography scan of the same condition TB, tracheal bronchus; C, carina. *(Courtesy of Dr Sharon McGrath-Morrow, Baltimore, USA.)*

Figure 2.28 Abnormal lobation of the left lung. Extra fissures partly separate the apical segments of both lobes and the complete posterior basal segment of the lower lobe. *(Courtesy of the late Dr AH Cameron, Birmingham, UK.)*

Other varieties of lung cyst encountered in childhood are listed in Box 2.2.[183]

Bronchial atresia

This anomaly is generally detected radiographically in an asymptomatic individual: the age range is therefore wide, with the average age

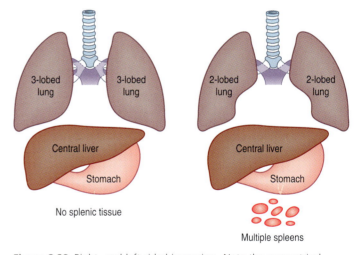

Figure 2.29 Right- and left-sided isomerism. Note the symmetrical extrapulmonary bronchoarterial anatomy (compared with the normal asymmetrical arrangement – see Figs 1.1B, p. 2 and 10.11, p. 482).

being 17 years.[184–187] The radiological appearances are virtually diagnostic, consisting of an ovoid hilar opacity, most commonly in the left upper lobe, with branches radiating out into a distal area of hyperinflation.

The opacity represents a distended, mucus-filled bronchus that is continuous with the distal airways but has no connection with the more proximal airways, the corresponding one of which ends blindly. Infection may result in inflammation and fibrosis. The interruption to the airway may take the form of a membrane, a fibrous cord or a gap. The distal hyperinflation is due to collateral ventilation and air-trapping. Failure to identify the atresia may lead to the mucous plugging being wrongfully identified as allergic bronchopulmonary aspergillosis or plastic bronchitis. Bronchial atresia differs from

Figure 2.30 An intrapulmonary bronchogenic cyst. (A) Gross appearances. On the left the cyst is filled by mucus. On the right the mucus has been removed to show the cyst wall. *(Courtesy of Dr M Jagusch, formerly of Auckland, New Zealand.)* (B) Microscopy shows respiratory epithelium, cartilage and seromucous glands.

Figure 2.31 Aberrant systemic artery supplying an intralobar sequestration. A systemic artery (lower right) enters the lateral aspect of the lung to supply a well-demarcated partly solid and partly cystic intralobar sequestration. A cystically dilated airway is seen centrally, consistent with lack of communication with the bronchial tree.

Box 2.2 Pulmonary 'cysts' in infancy and childhood[183]

Developmental	Non-developmental
Bronchogenic cyst[a]	Pneumatocoele
Sequestration	Bronchiectasis
Congenital cystic adenomatoid malformation	Interstitial emphysema
Lobar 'emphysema'	Low-grade cystic pleuropulmonary blastoma
Bronchial atresia	
Lymphangiectasia	
Birt–Hogg–Dubé syndrome	

[a]Generally mediastinal rather than pulmonary. Other mediastinal cysts include thymic, pericardial, lymphatic (cystic hygroma), oesophageal, gastroenteric, neurenteric and teratomatous ('dermoid') cysts.

---

infantile lobar emphysema in that it is focal and does not affect a whole lobe. The continuity of the cyst with the distal airways and the hyperinflation of the distal lung distinguish bronchial atresia from bronchogenic cyst, but the two conditions are occasionally associated.[188]

Sequestration

The term 'sequestration' indicates that a portion of lung exists without appropriate bronchial and vascular connections. Classically, no airway connects the lesion to the tracheobronchial tree and the blood supply is systemic (Figs 2.31 and 2.32), but the separation may be purely vascular.[189] Alternatively, an 'airway' may connect the sequestration to the oesophagus or stomach in a complex 'bronchopulmonary–foregut malformation',[190] or ectopic pancreatic tissue may be present within the sequestration.[191,192] Sequestrations may be associated with a variety of other malformations such as foregut duplications[180,192,193] and venous anomalies such as the scimitar syndrome while the histological features may be those of a congenital adenomatoid malformation (Fig. 2.33).[194–196] There is therefore a spectrum of abnormalities associated with pulmonary sequestration.[197–199] Pathologists dealing with these malformations should report on all their connections (bronchial, arterial and venous) and on the presence of any associated abnormalities.

Two forms of sequestration are recognised: extralobar, which has its own covering of visceral pleura, and intralobar, which is embedded in otherwise normal lung (Fig. 2.34). The first was called an accessory lobe until Pryce[200] described the intralobar variety, related it embryologically to accessory lobe and coined the term 'sequestration'. Intralobar sequestrations are much the commoner. The major differences between the two types are summarised in Table 2.5.

Figure 2.33 Pulmonary sequestration. The sequestered lung tissue is poorly developed and resembles a type 2 cystic congenital adenomatoid malformation.

Figure 2.32 Arterial supply to an intralobar sequestration. (A) A systemic artery forms the predominant blood supply, and a pulmonary artery (left) shows fibrous obliteration. (B) The same stained for elastin (elastin van Gieson stain).

Table 2.5 Pulmonary sequestration

	Intralobar sequestration	**Extralobar sequestration**
Age at diagnosis	50% over 20 years (15% asymptomatic)	60% less than 6 months (10% asymptomatic)
Sex ratio (M:F)	1.5:1	4:1
Typical site	Posterior basal segment of the left lower lobe	Between the left lower lobe and the diaphragm
Arterial supply	Systemic	Systemic
Venous drainage	Pulmonary	Systemic
Associated anomalies	Uncommon (6–12%)	Common (50–70%)
Aetiology	Uncertain whether developmental or acquired	Developmental anomaly

Extralobar sequestration is generally detected in infancy because of associated malformations and affects males four times more frequently than females. In contrast, intralobar sequestration is often an isolated anomaly and therefore escapes recognition until adult life, and has a male-to-female ratio of only 1.5:1.[201]

Intralobar sequestrations are typically located in the posterior basal segment of the left lower lobe and extralobar sequestrations beneath the left lower lobe. There is often a defect in the diaphragm and about 15% of extralobar sequestrations are abdominal. The veins leaving an extralobar sequestration generally join the azygos or other systemic veins whereas an intralobar sequestration usually has normal pulmonary venous connections.

The embryological basis of pulmonary sequestration is poorly understood. Indeed, some workers believe that the intralobar variety is an acquired condition in which the aberrant artery is a dilated systemic collateral to a focus of infection, basing this on the relative sparcity of malformations associated with this type of sequestration and its rarity in perinatal autopsies.[202,203] However, although the incidence of associated anomalies is lower than with extralobar sequestrations (50–70%), it is still appreciable (6–12%),[204] and the rarity of the condition in neonates may be because it is easily overlooked until there is cystic degeneration or infection. Advocates of a congenital aetiology generally propose that accessory lung buds are fundamental to both forms of pulmonary sequestration and liken them to intestinal duplications,[199] but are undecided whether the aberrant systemic arteries play a causative role by pulling on the developing lung[200] or are merely compensatory to a primary failure of the pulmonary arteries.[205] The absence of a bronchial connection has led some to link sequestration to bronchial atresia, bronchogenic and simple congenital lung cysts, infantile lobar emphysema and congenital cystic adenomatoid malformation,[197–199] whilst on the basis of cases in which there is communication with the oesophagus or stomach it has been proposed that the lesions are congenital foregut malformations,[190,206] attributable to a fault within embryonic organiser centres.[207]

Figure 2.34 Pulmonary sequestration. (A) Extralobar sequestration. The left lung has been reflected to the right to reveal a separate nodule of lung tissue lying against the ribs. The sequestration is completely detached from the rest of the lung but has a thin pedicle containing systemic blood vessels through which it is supplied from the aorta. *(Courtesy of Dr GA Russell, Tunbridge Wells, UK.)* (B) Intralobar sequestration in which the sequestered lung tissue is cystically dilated. *(Courtesy of the late Dr AH Cameron, Birmingham, UK.)*

Although there is no bronchial connection, small bronchi may be found within the sequestration (see Fig. 2.33). The lung tissue in the lesion is often poorly developed and cystically dilated (see Fig. 2.34b). The cysts are lined by columnar or cuboidal epithelium, or the sequestered lung may be entirely composed of structures resembling bronchioles surrounded by alveolar ducts and alveoli, histologically resembling a type 2 congenital adenomatoid malformation in up to 60% of cases (see Fig. 2.33).[204,208] Mucus distends the multiple intercommunicating spaces and the lesion appears solid radiographically, unless air enters through a bronchial connection or, in the case of intralobar sequestration, by collateral ventilation, when fluid levels are often seen. Features of pulmonary hypertension are also frequently present within sequestrations, but this appears to be of no clinical significance.[208] In the absence of associated anomalies, detection is unlikely unless a radiograph is undertaken for some other reason or infection ensues, this being most likely when there is air entry. When operation is contemplated for any cystic or suppurative lesion of the lungs it is important that sequestration be consid-

ered and the possibility of unusual blood vessels investigated angiographically. Inadvertent severance of anomalous systemic arteries has led to fatal haemorrhage, whilst ligation of anomalous veins from adjacent non-sequestered lung has led to infarction of potentially salvable tissue.

Congenital cystic adenomatoid malformation (congenital pulmonary airway malformation)

The term 'congenital cystic adenomatoid malformation' encompasses a spectrum of conditions, the interrelationship of which is contentious. The aetiology of the condition is obscure but a maturation defect is envisaged.[209–211]

Early reports date from 1897[212] and only in 1949 was the term 'congenital adenomatoid malformation' introduced.[213] It was applied to a newborn infant's greatly enlarged and apparently airless left lower lobe, which microscopically consisted solely of bronchiole-like structures so that it had an adenomatoid appearance. Subsequently, cystic

Table 2.6 Congenital cystic adenomatoid malformation (congenital pulmonary airway malformation)

Stocker type[217]	Proportional incidence	Gross appearance	Microscopy	Other features
0	1–3%	Solid	Pseudostratified ciliated cells, cartilage, glands, mucous cells	Neonates Other malformations Poor prognosis Also known as congenital acinar dysplasia
1	60–70%	Large cysts (up to 10 cm)	Pseudostratified ciliated cells, often with rows of mucous cells	Presentation may be late Resectable Good prognosis except for rare carcinomatous change
2	10–15%	Small cysts (up to 2 cm)	Simple columnar epithelium Striated muscle in 5%	Neonates Other malformations Poor prognosis Rare rhabdomyosarcomatous change
3	5%	Solid	Simple cuboidal epithelium	Male neonates Poor prognosis
4	15%	Large cysts (up to 10 cm)	Flattened epithelium	Neonates, infants Good prognosis Uncertain relation to pleuropulmonary blastoma

and intermediate (microcystic) varieties were described and the name changed to congenital cystic adenomatoid malformation.[209,214–216] These were initially numbered I–III but with the addition of two further lesions the numbering switched to 0–4, it being envisaged that the spectrum represented malformations of five successive groups of airways, type 0 being tracheobronchial and type 4 alveolar.[214,217] This is not wholly convincing because, except for type 4, which tends to be peripheral, the lesions are not obviously distributed along the bronchial pathway. Types 0 and 3 tend to affect a whole lobe or lung. Furthermore, although cartilaginous airways are a prominent feature of the type 0 ('tracheobronchial') lesion, the complete absence of bronchioles and alveoli cannot be overlooked. Previous workers concentrated upon the undifferentiated stroma that separates the cartilaginous airways and preferred the term 'acinar dysplasia', implying a developmental error affecting the periphery of the lung rather than the central airways, a view with which we concur.[136,218,219]

A further development is the proposed introduction of the term 'congenital pulmonary airway malformation' in place of congenital cystic adenomatoid malformation. This is advocated because only types 1, 2 and 3 are adenomatoid and only types 1, 2 and 4 are cystic.[217]

An alternative view is that types 0, 3 and 4 all represent different pathogenetic processes: congenital acinar dysplasia (type 0), pulmonary hyperplasia (type 3) and regressed type 1 pleuropulmonary blastoma (type 4).[220,221] This reduces the five types to two, the commoner types 1 and 2, for which the term 'congenital cystic adenomatoid malformation' remains appropriate. Many examples of these have now been reported.[209,214,215,222–226]

Some workers envisage an even wider 'sequestration spectrum' encompassing both sequestration and congenital cystic adenomatoid malformation[199] and others extend this by adding bronchial atresia, bronchogenic cysts, simple foregut cysts and infantile lobar emphysema.[198] Congenital cystic adenomatoid malformation is also associated with abnormalities of the bronchial tree on occasion.[227] Examples of extralobar sequestrations containing tissue with the distinctive features of congenital cystic adenomatoid malformation strengthen the proposed link between these two conditions (see Fig. 2.33).[194,195,228]

The five types are compared in Table 2.6 and will now be considered individually. Despite the above contentions regarding their interrelationships and appropriate classification, their distinction is important because certain varieties carry an albeit low risk of malignant transformation.

Type 0 congenital pulmonary airway malformation (acinar dysplasia)

This rare form of the anomaly is incompatible with life, being seen in term or premature babies who are cyanosed at birth and survive only a few hours.[136–138] It is described on page 50 under its older title of congenital acinar dysplasia.

Type 1 congenital pulmonary airway malformation (cystic type of congenital cystic adenomatoid malformation)

This is the commonest type and the one with the best prognosis as it is a localised lesion that typically affects only part of a lobe and lends itself to surgical resection. The boundary between the lesion and the adjacent normal lobe is sharply delineated but there is no capsule. Presentation usually takes the form of neonatal respiratory distress but the condition may be detected in utero by ultrasonography[229] and surgery undertaken soon after birth. Alternatively, recurrent infections in older children or even young adults may prompt initial investigation.[230] Radiographically, air-filled cysts that are usually limited to one lobe compress the rest of the lung, depress the diaphragm and cause mediastinal shift.

The cysts range in size from 1 to 10 cm (Figs 2.35 and 2.36). The relevant bronchus is often atretic,[198,222,223,227,231,232] yet the cysts are usually radiolucent, presumably due to collateral ventilation. They are lined by pseudostratified ciliated columnar epithelium, sometimes interspersed with rows of mucous cells (Fig. 2.37).[217] The type 1 adenomatoid malformation is occasionally complicated by malignant change, nearly always to a mucous adenocarcinoma of lepidic pattern.[233–239] Mucous cell proliferation within the cyst is regarded as

Figure 2.35 Congenital cystic adenomatoid malformation – type 1 cystic variety. The right lung is enlarged, causing mediastinal shift to the left and hypoplasia of the left lung. *(Courtesy of Dr GA Russell, Tunbridge Wells, UK.)*

Figure 2.36 Congenital cystic adenomatoid malformation – type 1 cystic variety. *(Courtesy of Professor LJ Holloway, formerly of Wellington, New Zealand.)*

Figure 2.37 Congenital cystic adenomatoid malformation – type 1 cystic variety. In places the respiratory epithelium is replaced by a row of mucous cells.

hyperplasia whereas extensions of this process into the adjacent alveoli, where it assumes a lepidic growth pattern, is taken to represent carcinoma (Fig. 2.38).[226] However, this division is wholly arbitrary and genetic studies have shown chromosomal aberrations in the mucous cells both within and beyond the cyst similar to those seen in adenocarcinomas encountered in non-smokers.[238,240] As would be expected of a localised adenocarcinoma of lepidic pattern, survival following excision is good and metastasis is exceptional.[241] Numbers are too small to give a precise estimate of the risk of malignant transformation but extension of the mucinous cells beyond the cyst wall is probably seen in no more than 1–2% of cases.

The complex cystic nature of the malformation and sparsity of bronchial cartilage in the walls of cystic spaces distinguish this lesion from bronchogenic cyst. The distinction from intralobar sequestration may be difficult but a systemic blood supply indicates sequestration.

Type 2 congenital pulmonary airway malformation (intermediate type of congenital cystic adenomatoid malformation)

This is the second most frequent type. It generally involves only one lobe but nevertheless usually causes respiratory distress in the first month of life. Associated anomalies such as renal agenesis, cardiovascular defects, diaphragmatic hernia and syrenomelia often have a further adverse effect on the prognosis but occasional cases present later in childhood with infection.[230] It is often identified within extralobar sequestrations (Figs 2.33, 2.39).[194,196,228] The lesion is sponge-like, consisting of multiple small cysts measuring up to 2 cm and solid pale tumour-like tissue (Fig. 2.39). Microscopically the cysts are seen to comprise an excess of dilated structures resembling bronchioles separated by poorly developed alveoli or alveolar ducts (Fig. 2.40).[217] Occasional examples contain striated muscle, which if extensive has been termed rhabdomyomatous dysplasia.[217,242,243]

Type 3 congenital pulmonary airway malformation (solid type of congenital cystic adenomatoid malformation)

This uncommon type occurs almost exclusively in male babies. Some consider it to be the original congenital adenomatoid malformation described in 1949[213,217] whereas others view it as a form of pulmonary hyperplasia similar to that seen in laryngeal atresia.[220] It is a large, bulky lesion that typically involves and expands a whole lobe, the others being compressed and the mediastinum displaced. The result-

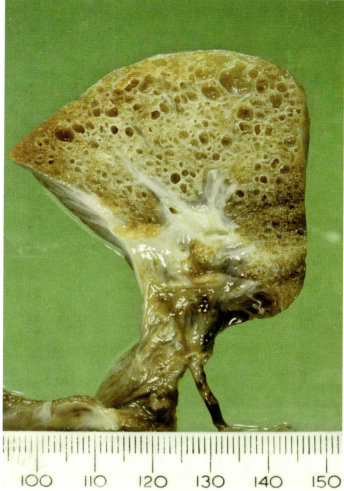

Figure 2.39 An extralobar sequestration with the structure of a congenital cystic adenomatoid malformation – type 2 microcystic variety. The sequestered lobe has the spongy appearance of this pattern of adenomatoid malformation. The cord-like structure entering from bottom right is an aberrant systemic artery from the descending aorta. *(Reproduced from* Current Diagnostic Pathology *by permission of Dr C Wright, Newcastle-upon-Tyne, UK.[139])*

Figure 2.38 Adenocarcinoma complicating congenital cystic adenomatoid malformation – type 1 cystic variety. (A) A high-resolution computed tomograph of a long-standing type 1 congenital adenomatoid malformation shows foci of consolidation in the ipsilateral lung adjacent to the cyst, with additional nodules of consolidation on the opposite (right) side. (B) Biopsy of the right side shows mucinous adenocarcinoma of lepidic pattern.

ant venous compression usually causes the mother to suffer from hydramnios and the baby from generalised anasarca.[229] It also results in hypoplasia of the remaining pulmonary tissue. The prognosis is dependent upon the amount of unaffected lung and hence on the size of the lesion. Microscopically, bronchiolar structures separated by air spaces that are small, have a cuboidal lining and resemble late fetal lung, are seen (Fig. 2.41). There are virtually no arteries within the lesion.[217] Unlike the preceding types there is little or no cystic change.

Type 4 congenital pulmonary airway malformation

This relatively uncommon type typically presents as infantile respiratory distress or repeated pneumonia in childhood, but may occasionally present in adult life.[226] Radiographically, large air-filled cysts are seen with compression of the other thoracic structures and occasionally pneumothorax. The cysts are peripheral and thin-walled. They are lined by alveolar or bronchiolar epithelial cells resting upon loose mesenchymal tissue (Fig. 2.42). Occasionally the stroma is focally hypercellular and one underwent malignant change to recur as a high-grade pleuropulmonary blastoma.[244] At present the interrelationship of these two conditions is uncertain and some now advocate classifying lesions of type 4 congenital cystic adenomatoid malformation morphology with any degree of hypercellularity as type 1 pleuropulmonary blastomas,[226,245] with those lacking any blastematous component being viewed as regression of the malignant elements of the tumour.[221]

Figure 2.40 Congenital cystic adenomatoid malformation – type 2. There is an excess of bronchioles, which are separated by poorly developed alveolar tissue. This pattern is also sometimes seen in sequestrations (see Figs 2.33 and 2.39).

Figure 2.42 Congenital pulmonary airway malformation type 4. The cysts are thin-walled and multiloculated. They are lined by alveolar or bronchiolar cells resting upon loose mesenchymal tissue.

Figure 2.41 Congenital cystic adenomatoid malformation – type 3 solid variety. Densely packed irregular air spaces are lined by cuboidal epithelium. *(Reproduced from* Current Diagnostic Pathology *by permission of Dr C Wright, Newcastle-upon-Tyne, UK.[139])*

Fetal surgery for congenital cystic adenomatoid malformation

Uterine ultrasound is now routine in many obstetric practices and on occasion it detects a chest mass. Such lesions are prone to change character with time and even regress[246] but those that enlarge are often referred for fetal surgery because they lead to mediastinal shift, cardiac compression and hydrops. Many are cystic but pathologists dealing with the excised lesions report difficulty in applying the above five-part classification.[247,248] Subdivision of these fetal lesions does not appear warranted at present.

Congenital peribronchial myofibroblastic tumour

This rare lesion is found in the newborn, sometimes causing heart failure or hydrops fetalis.[249,250] It forms a localised mass that shows a characteristic peribronchial infiltrate of spindle cells of mixed smooth muscle and fibroblast phenotype. The proliferation spreads from the

bronchoarterial bundles to involve the pleura and interlobular septa. It is suggested that it develops from the condensed mesenchyme that surrounds the proximal bronchi at about the 12th week of intra-uterine development. The condition is probably akin to other organ-specific lesions that are collectively termed fibromatoses of early infancy,[249] rather than representing a neoplasm or hamartoma, as implied by some of the other terms that have been applied – congenital leiomyosarcoma, bronchopulmonary fibrosarcoma, massive congenital mesenchymal malformation. The lesion has no metastatic capability and outcome depends entirely upon resectability.

The histological appearances are characteristic. They show interlacing bundles of spindle cells surrounding the bronchovascular bundles and extending into the interlobular septa and occasionally the pleura (Fig. 2.43). Foci of hypercellularity, necrosis, calcification and cartilaginous differentiation may be seen but there is no atypia. Immunohistochemistry is positive for vimentin and may be focally positive for smooth-muscle actin, muscle-specific actin and desmin. Electron microscopy supports a myofibroblastic derivation.

Congenital bronchiectasis

Several congenital defects lead to the development of bronchiectasis after birth. These are dealt with in the next section. Conditions characterised by bronchiectasis at birth are less numerous but the Williams–Campbell syndrome possibly falls into this category.

Williams–Campbell syndrome

This syndrome is characterised by bilateral diffuse cylindrical bronchiectasis associated with deficiency of bronchial cartilage.[252–254] There is also panlobular alveolar distension. The deficiency is similar to that found in infantile lobar emphysema (see p. 72) but more widespread. Secondary infection leads to chronic inflammation and bronchiolitis obliterans, and hence confusion with the Swyer–James or Macleod syndrome of hyperlucent lung which, as explained on page 73, is probably postinfective. The occasional association of other congenital abnormalities,[255] its early onset and rare instances of the disease in siblings all favour a congenital deficiency.[256,257] The most convincing cases are those in which there is only minimal inflammation.

Figure 2.43 Congenital peribronchial myofibroblastic tumour (A and B). Interlacing bundles of myofibroblasts surround the bronchovascular bundles and extend into the interlobular septa. *(Courtesy of Dr M Ashworth, London, UK.)*

Anomalies promoting bronchiectasis in later life

Certain familial diseases predispose to recurrent respiratory infections and hence bronchiectasis. The bronchiectasis develops after birth but the basic defect is congenital. These conditions are tracheobronchomegaly (Mounier-Kuhn's syndrome), Kartagener's and other primary ciliary dyskinesia syndromes (including polycystic kidney disease), Young's syndrome and cystic fibrosis. Apart from these conditions, which will now be considered, bronchiectasis may be caused by many of the primary immune deficiencies[258] and is recorded in a young adult with homozygous α_1-antitrypsin deficiency,[259] which is more often associated with emphysema.

Mounier-Kuhn's syndrome (tracheobronchomegaly or trachiectasis)

In this rare disease the major airways are dilated by saccular bulges between the cartilages, and bronchial clearance is impaired, resulting in recurrent respiratory infection.[260–265a] It becomes manifest between the ages of 30 and 50 years, and occurs predominantly in males.[266] A congenital connective tissue defect with autosomal-recessive inheritance is suggested.[267] This is supported by the occasional association of Mounier-Kuhn's syndrome with Ehler–Danlos syndrome,[268] cutis laxa[269] or Kenny–Caffey syndrome.[270] When considering the diagnosis it is useful to know that in the normal adult the maximum transverse diameters of the trachea and main bronchi are 20 and 14.5 mm respectively.[271]

Kartagener's syndrome and primary ciliary dyskinesia

The triad of situs inversus, bronchiectasis and sinusitis was first described in 1904[272] but its usual eponym, Kartagener's syndrome, derives from the Swiss paediatrician who described four cases with these features in 1933.[273] The syndrome was given a firm pathogenetic basis when it was recognised that in many cases the respiratory infections were the consequence of a developmental anomaly consisting of a reduced number of ciliary dynein arms (Fig. 2.44).[274] Roughly half the patients with dynein arm defects do not have situs inversus, indicating random lateralisation of the viscera, which is attributed to

absence of the embryonic nodal monocilia that normally control the direction of flow of extraembryonic fluid.[275,276] The term 'immotile cilia syndrome' was introduced to encompass all patients with a developmental ciliary defect, regardless of their visceral anatomy, but later the term 'primary ciliary dyskinesia' was substituted because the cilia show some movement although they do not beat effectively.[277–279] The condition is inherited as an autosomal recessive with variable penetrance and to date two gene mutations that result in dynein arm defects have been identified, one affecting the DNA11 gene located on bands 9p13 to 9p21 and the DNAH5 gene located on chromosome 5p.[280,281] A third gene defect, involving the DNAH11 gene on band 7p21, has been identified in patients with primary ciliary dyskinesia whose cilia show no ultrastructural abnormalities but are inflexible.[282,282a]

As well as dynein arm defects, primary ciliary dyskinesia may be caused by absence of ciliary spokes, transposition of one of the outer microtubular doublets of the cilium to replace the central pair, random ciliary orientation or abnormally long cilia (Fig. 2.44B–D).[283–288] The relative frequency of these abnormalities is shown in Table 2.7. These primary ciliary defects must not be confused with acquired ciliary abnormalities, such as compound or cystic cilia, which commonly result from infection or chemical injury (Fig. 2.44E).[289] More recently described primary ciliary defects[289–291] require further evaluation.

Sperm tails have a similar structure to cilia and dynein arm defects often result in affected males being infertile due to immotility of their spermatozoa.[292,293] Female fertility also appears to be impaired, but the incidence of ectopic pregnancy does not appear to be increased.[294] Some patients are more concerned with their infertility than their respiratory problems, which may be relatively minor.

The various primary abnormalities are not clearly evident in every ciliary profile and their recognition requires rather tedious electron microscopic quantitation.[295–298] This is only justified if functional studies are abnormal. These include (i) the saccharine test, in which a saccharine particle is placed on the anterior end of the inferior turbinate and the time taken for the patient to notice the taste is recorded, (ii) in vitro assessment of ciliary beat frequency, suitable cells for which may be obtained by brushing the back of the nose; and (iii) the assessment of nitric oxide emanating from the nasal sinuses; low levels of this gas in the exhaled breath are characteristic of primary

Figure 2.44 Ciliary ultrastructure. (A) Normal: an axial pair of microtubules is connected by radiating spokes to nine outer double microtubules (9 + 2 arrangement). Small dynein arms extend from one outer microtubule to one in the adjacent pair. The dynein arms are involved in the outer double microtubules sliding on each other and thereby causing the cilium to beat. (B–D) Ciliary dyskinesia syndromes: (B) absent dynein arms; (C) absent spokes; (D) transposition of one of the nine outer doublets to replace the central pair of microtubules, which is absent, so that there are only eight doublets in the outer ring. (E) Compound cilia, a secondary focal abnormality that is to be distinguished from the diffuse congenital abnormalities of the ciliary dyskinesia syndromes. *(Courtesy of Professor P Cole and Miss A Dewar, Brompton, UK.)*

Table 2.7 Abnormal ciliary ultrastructure identified in 275 patients with primary ciliary dyskinesia at the Brompton Hospital 1988–2008 (unpublished data provided by Dr Amelia Shoemark, Brompton, UK)

Ciliary defect	n	%
Outer dynein arm defect	105	38
Outer and inner dynein arm defect	57	21
Inner dynein arm defect	30	11
Transposition defect	28	10
Radial spoke defect	22	8
No ultrastructural abnormality	33	12

Table 2.8 Frequency of cystic fibrosis and the carrier state in different populations

Race	Homozygotes	Heterozygotes
UK white	1:2500	1:25
US white	1:3500	1:30
Sweden	1:7700	1:45
US black	1:14 000	1:60
US Asian	1:25 500	1:80

ciliary dyskinesia.[278,299–302] Where possible, ultrastructural studies should be conducted on more than one occasion or on ciliated cells from different organs,[303] whilst in adult men, sperm tail ultrastructure may demonstrate a primary abnormality.[292,293]

Autosomal-dominant polycystic kidney disease

Autosomal-dominant polycystic kidney disease (ADPKD) is a relatively common disease with several extrarenal manifestations but until recently no known pulmonary features. However, the renal cysts have been attributed to dysfunction of primary cilia and the cilia-associated proteins polycystin-1 and -2, and this prompted one group to examine respiratory cilia in these patients. Immunostaining revealed polycystin-1 in the airway epithelia of non-ADPKD patients while autopsy material from one of five patients showed histological evidence of bronchiectasis. This led to a review of computed tomography scans for evidence of bronchiectasis in 95 ADPKD patients and an equal number of non-ADPKD chronic kidney disease patients, which revealed a threefold increased prevalence of radiographic bronchiectasis in ADPKD (37% versus 13%).[304]

Cystic fibrosis

Incidence and inheritance

Fifty years ago, four out of five patients with cystic fibrosis died in the first year of life, whereas today most can expect to survive until the fourth decade. The predicted median survival for babies born in the UK in the twenty-first century now exceeds 50 years.[305] This improvement in survival is attributable to a combination of earlier diagnosis, better management of meconium ileus, dietary control, pancreatic enzyme supplementation, physiotherapy, the introduction of potent antibiotics, and the development of specialist centres.

Cystic fibrosis has been reported in all racial groups but is commonest in white people (Table 2.8). In Great Britain it is the commonest lethal genetic disorder, affecting 1 in 2500 live births with the gene responsible for the condition being carried by 1 in 25 of the Caucasian population. About 1 in 400 marriages involves two carriers and, because transmission is by an autosomal-recessive gene, the children of such marriages have a 1 in 4 chance of having the disease. The carriers are entirely normal and, apart from the siblings of an affected child, a family history of cystic fibrosis is unusual. Because the homozygotes have only recently survived to sexual maturity and the males are generally infertile due to agenesis of the vasa deferentia,

persistence of the condition is puzzling. It suggests that there is either a high mutation rate or the heterozygotes carry some advantage, either in reproductive fitness or resistance to other diseases. One possibility is that the defect minimises dehydration when severe diarrhoeal diseases are contracted.[306]

The gene responsible for cystic fibrosis is located on the long arm of chromosome 7,[307–309] and DNA probes now provide a test by which, in families having an affected infant, it is possible to identify the abnormality in further pregnancies as early as the first trimester.[310] This test has also enabled the identification of carrier status in the healthy siblings of an affected person or in couples contemplating parenthood.[311–313] Although more than 800 cystic fibrosis mutations have been identified, one (ΔF508) accounts for about 70% of alleles[314] and another (G551D) for a further 5%.[315] The identification of specific genetic defects has led to trials of gene therapy involving the insufflation of the airways with preparations of the normal gene carried within liposomes or on a viral vector.[316]

Pathogenesis[317]

Cystic fibrosis is thought to depend upon abnormal secretions, as indicated by its alternative name 'mucoviscidosis', although this term has no direct relevance to the abnormally salty sweat that characterises the condition. Furthermore, the hyperviscous mucus is not the primary abnormality. Ciliary beat frequency and ultrastructure are normal,[318,319] and claims that there is a serum factor that inhibits ciliary function in vivo offer no explanation for the intestinal and pancreatic lesions of the disease. It is now known that an abnormality of chloride ion transport underlies both the sweat hypersalinity and the mucus hyperviscosity.[320,321] The genetic abnormalities referred to above affect a protein named the cystic fibrosis transmembrane conductance regulator (CFTR) that acts as a cyclic adenosine monophosphate-regulated chloride channel and thereby controls ion and hence water movement across the cell membrane.[322,323] This protein is made up of 1480 amino acids, of which the 508th from the N-terminus (phenylalanine) is deleted when there is ΔF508 gene homozygosity. The abnormal protein is trapped in the endoplasmic reticulum leading to defective ion transport at the apical cell membrane.[324,325] Another variant, G551D, is properly transported to the plasma membrane but is unresponsive to cyclic adenosine monophosphate.[325] Such defects result in excessive reabsorption of water and hence hyperviscosity of mucus and hypersalinity of sweat and mucosal secretions. About 96% of male patients are infertile due to congenital absence or focal atresia of the vas deferens.[326] The cause of this is uncertain but it has been attributed to obstruction in early fetal life rather than anomalous development.[326,327] Female fertility is slightly impaired, probably because the cervical mucus is unduly viscid.

In the airways, hypersalinity impairs the antibacterial action of constituents such as lactoferrin and lysozyme,[328,329] and this, coupled

Table 2.9 Extrapulmonary manifestations of cystic fibrosis

Cardiac		Cor pulmonale Fibrosis of left ventricle Enlarged carotid bodies
Gastrointestinal	Upper	Barrett's oesophagus Varices (due to cirrhosis)
	Lower	Meconium ileus (leading to obstruction, perforation, prolapse) Appendicitis Fibrosing colonopathy (due to treatment)
	Liver	Sclerosing cholangitis Biliary cirrhosis
	Gallbladder	Cholecystitis and microgallbladder
	Pancreas	Pancreatic insufficiency (steatorrhoea) Chronic pancreatitis Diabetes mellitus
Kidney		Nephrolithiasis Diabetic glomerulopathy Immune complex-mediated glomerulonephritis
Genital tract	Male	Atresia of vas deferens
	Female	Multiple follicular cysts Cervicitis, mucous gland hyperplasia, vaginitis Reduced fertility
Musculoskeletal		Osteoporosis Muscle wasting Hypertrophic pulmonary osteoarthropathy Clubbing
Skin		Salty sweat, hyponatraemia Acrodermatitis Dilation of eccrine and apocrine glands
General		Malnutrition Vitamin deficincies (E, K,[a] B$_{12}$) Amyloidosis

[a]Vitamin K deficiency at birth may lead to bleeding.

with the difficulty in clearing hyperviscous mucus, inevitably leads to permanent infection and inflammation of the respiratory tract. A deficiency of surfactant apoproteins A and D is a further factor promoting continued bacterial infection.[330] Deoxyribonucleic acid released in large amounts from effete neutrophils[331] polymerises with glycoprotein to exacerbate the hyperviscosity of the mucus. Further neutrophil and bacterial products damage the bronchial wall, resulting in bronchiectasis.

Cystic fibrosis patients benefit from lung transplantation[332] and it is relevant to the pathogenesis that the donor lungs maintain normal membrane ion transport[333] and do not develop the changes found in the explanted lungs.

The phenotypic spectrum associated with mutations of the CFTR gene is now known to extend beyond the classic features of cystic fibrosis and includes several monosymptomatic diseases such as isolated forms of pancreatitis, lung disease,[334] nasal polyposis[335] and atresia of the vasa deferentia (which is responsible for 6% of obstructive aspermia and 1–2% of male infertility).[326,327,336]

Clinical features

Despite improvements in patient care, repeated pulmonary infection remains the major clinical problem in cystic fibrosis. Bronchopulmonary infection, respiratory failure and cor pulmonale are the usual causes of death in adults,[337] but there are also many extrapulmonary features (Box 2.3 and Table 2.9).[326,327] Advanced age is no bar to a new diagnosis of cystic fibrosis[338–340] but in most cases the diagnosis is made in the first year of life, often through newborn screening.

The diagnosis may also be made before birth by chorionic villous sampling or amniocentesis, which is performed in high-risk families or following the identification of intestinal abnormalities by ultrasound. After birth several countries screen all newborns using the Guthrie blood spot test to detect raised concentrations of immunoreactive trypsinogen.[341] Bronchoalveolar lavage shows infection and inflammation to be already established in a substantial proportion of affected but asymptomatic neonates diagnosed by newborn screening.[342] The diagnosis is generally confirmed by a skin test that detects high sodium levels in the sweat, but some mutations are associated with normal sweat salinity.[334] Alternative diagnostic procedures include recognition of an unduly negative potential difference across a mucosal surface, such as that lining the nose,[343,343a] and genetic

testing. Once the diagnosis has been confirmed, other family members may be offered screening. All siblings need this while asymptomatic adult relatives may wish to be screened for carrier status.

Bacteriology

The episodic attacks of airway infection represent acute exacerbations of a permanent colonisation of the lower respiratory tract by *Staphylococcus aureus*, *Haemophilus influenzae* or *Pseudomonas aeruginosa*, which defies eradication with long-term antibiotics. This is associated with the emergence of mucoid alginate-producing mutants that develop into bacterial microcolonies embedded in exopolysaccharide biofilms on the bronchial mucosa, leading to an exaggerated tissue-damaging immune response.[344–346]

More recently, *Burkholderia* (formerly *Pseudomonas*) *cepacia* infection has also proved troublesome in cystic fibrosis.[347] This plant pathogen was previously regarded as a harmless commensal in humans but is

Figure 2.45 Cystic fibrosis. The earliest changes in the lungs consist of plugs of viscid mucus distending bronchial gland ducts.

Figure 2.46 Cystic fibrosis. In advanced cases the bronchi are dilated and filled with pus.

now recognised to attack the lungs of patients with cystic fibrosis and hasten their deterioration. *B. cepacia* is resistant to most antibiotics. Acquisition is by person-to-person transmission and advice based on this that the infected should not mix with other cystic fibrosis patients is very distressing to individuals who derive much comfort from mutual support groups.[348] *Chlamydia pneumoniae* and opportunistic mycobacteria have also been identified as troublesome pathogens in cystic fibrosis.

Immunological abnormalities

Atopy and immunological abnormalities are common in cystic fibrosis but it is uncertain whether these are primary or secondary. They include circulating immune complexes, which are deposited in the respiratory and intestinal tracts and could conceivably contribute to the tissue damage there.[349] These complexes presumably also underlie the cutaneous vasculitis and arthritis that are occasionally encountered in cystic fibrosis.[350] Bronchial hyperactivity is common, possibly due to easier penetrance of the damaged epithelium by common environmental allergens. Serum immunoglobulins are generally raised and there is a high prevalence of positive skin reactions (type I and III) to common allergens such as *Aspergillus fumigatus*.[337,351] The incidence of allergic bronchopulmonary aspergillosis is markedly increased in cystic fibrosis.[352,353] Aspergillomas are rare but the increasing use of immunosuppressive and antipseudomonal drugs in cystic fibrosis has led to an increase in invasive aspergillosis.

Structural changes in the respiratory tract

The earliest histological change in the respiratory tract in cystic fibrosis is mucous plugging of the tracheobronchial glands (Fig. 2.45).[354] This is found in infants who succumb to meconium ileus or its complications and who show no bronchopulmonary inflammation,[355] indicating that it is a primary change. The plugging develops to obstruct bronchi and infection invariably follows (Fig. 2.46), resulting in recurrent attacks of bronchitis, bronchiolitis and ultimately pneumonia. The bronchitis is characterised by secondary hyperplasia of the bronchial glands indistinguishable from that seen in the chronic bronchitis of cigarette smokers.[356,357] There may also be papillary hyperplasia of the bronchial mucosa. The bronchiolitis is accompanied by peribronchiolar fibrosis, which constricts these airways.[358] An obstructive pneumonitis consisting of interstitial inflammation and fibrosis develops.[359] There may also be evidence of organising pneumonia, air-trapping and collapse. The chronic sepsis leads to bronchial ulceration, destruc-

tion of the bronchial cartilage and bronchiectasis.[360] At necropsy, pus-filled bronchiectatic cavities, abscesses and areas of pneumonic consolidation are found throughout the lungs (Figs 2.47 and 3.32A, p. 122). The upper lobes are generally more severely affected than the lower.[361] Lymphoid follicles often develop in relation to the bronchiectatic cavities.[356] Air cysts are another frequent finding in older patients.[362] Some of these are bronchiectatic cysts, some have multiple communications with bronchi showing that they are pneumatoceles derived from former abscesses, some represent interstitial emphysema and others are emphysematous bullae. Their rupture largely accounts for the high incidence of pneumothorax that is seen in adults with cystic fibrosis.[362,363] Attenuated and shortened interalveolar septa may be evident microscopically, resulting in appearances resembling panacinar emphysema but probably representing retarded postnatal lung growth.[358] In older patients pulmonary hypertension and cor pulmonale may develop.[364,365] Large haemoptyses may occur,[337] probably from the highly vascularised granulation tissue that lines the bronchiectatic cavities and which is supplied by systemic arteries. Nasal polyps are common in cystic fibrosis, but they differ from those of atopic subjects in that they lack eosinophils.[366]

Extrapulmonary disease (Table 2.9)

The many extrapulmonary effects of cystic fibrosis include serious consequences before birth, notably meconium ileus obstructing the fetal bowel to such a degree that the intestine ruptures in utero, leading to a sterile chemical peritonitis and severe ascites, which may prolong labour. If the child dies during delivery, the deficiency in the bowel wall may have healed but extensive peritoneal calcification is often present and this gives a clue to the nature of the peritonitis. More often meconium ileus causes constipation or intestinal obstruction after birth. If bowel is resected or autopsy undertaken, the intestine is found to be obstructed by hard rubbery meconium and the appropriateness of the term 'mucoviscidosis' can be readily appreciated. Older children and even adults may be similarly affected by a 'meconium ileus-equivalent'. Microscopy shows the bowel to be filled and the crypts of Lieberkuhn distended by mucus (Fig. 2.48). Mucus may also plug the ducts of salivary and labial glands.

Pancreatic disease is a further manifestation of cystic fibrosis. Indeed, the term 'cystic fibrosis' was coined specifically for the late changes in the pancreas. The first change is mucous plugging of the pancreatic ducts, which leads to atrophy and fatty replacement of the exocrine portion of the gland. Low-grade inflammation is common

Figure 2.47 Cystic fibrosis. At necropsy the lungs are largely replaced by pus-filled bronchiectatic cavities and abscesses, more marked in the upper lobe.

Figure 2.49 Cystic fibrosis. Pancreas. The exocrine portion is reduced to dilated ducts in a fibrous stroma or shows fatty replacement. Islets of Langerhans survive, but these too may eventually atrophy.

Figure 2.50 Cystic fibrosis. Liver. Small bile ducts are plugged by eosinophilic secretions.

Figure 2.48 Cystic fibrosis. Meconium ileus-equivalent in an adult patient. The crypts of Lieberkuhn are distended by mucus, which also forms a thick coat on the surface.

and this leads to fibrosis (Fig. 2.49) while the obstructed ducts become cystically dilated. The administration of pancreatic enzymes is possibly responsible for an increasing incidence of colonic strictures. The endocrine portion of the gland is initially spared but eventually even the islets of Langerhans atrophy; diabetes mellitus is a common late result, generally preceded by years of malabsorption.

Hepatic disease has a similar basis to that in the pancreas. Initially small bile ducts are plugged by mucus (Fig. 2.50), leading to biliary cirrhosis (Figs 2.51 and 2.52).

Renal disease includes diabetic glomerulopathy, amyloidosis and immune complex-mediated glomerulonephritis. There is also an increase in urinary oxalate excretion, which is linked to the malabsorption and results in microscopic nephrocalcinosis[367] and urolithiasis.[368,369] Cardiac disease includes cor pulmonale and focal myocardial necrosis, suggested causes of which include malnourishment and hypovitaminosis.[370,371]

The vasa deferentia are frequently atretic and the patient is consequently sterile.[326,327] At autopsy, the epididymes and testes show

Figure 2.51 Cystic fibrosis. Liver, showing well-established cirrhosis.

Figure 2.53 Cystic fibrosis. Epididymis, showing glandular dilatation and stromal fibrosis.

Figure 2.52 Cystic fibrosis. Liver, showing the gross appearances of macronodular biliary cirrhosis.

Figure 2.54 Cystic fibrosis. Testis, showing basement membrane thickening but normal spermatogenesis.

obstructive features (Figs 2.53 and 2.54) and the vasa cannot be identified or are represented by thin fibrous bands. The female genital tract is anatomically normal and patients reach the menarche, although this may be delayed by chronic pulmonary sepsis. However, cervical mucus is abnormal and cervicitis, cervical erosions and cervical mucous gland hyperplasia are commonly found. Nevertheless, pregnancy is possible and with improved support is now becoming more frequent.

Generalised changes include all those classically associated with the secondary effects of cystic fibrosis, including malnutrition, systemic amyloidosis and the immunological abnormalities referred to above. Thus there may be generalised muscle wasting and osteoporosis. Other changes include hypertrophic pulmonary osteoarthropathy and clubbing, and the craniofacial alterations seen in children with nasal obstruction.[372]

Young's syndrome

Young's syndrome consists of sinusitis, bronchiectasis and obstructive oligospermia caused by mucociliary dysfunction in the respiratory tract and epididymes. Spermatozoa accumulate in the head of the epididymis, which is markedly dilated. Ciliary ultrastructure and beat frequency in vitro are both normal,[373,374] yet in vivo tracer studies show impaired mucociliary clearance.[375] The basic defect in Young's syndrome is obscure but it may be hyperviscosity of the respiratory and epididymal secretions.

Pulmonary aplasia (agenesis)

Absence of one lung (Fig. 2.55) is not uncommon but absence of a lobe (as distinct from left-sided isomerism – see above) or of both lungs is distinctly rare. The bronchi may also be absent or there may be a rudimentary stump, an important point in unilateral aplasia as secretions tend to pool in the stump, become infected and spill over to infect the sole lung.[376] Also in unilateral aplasia the single lung is

Figure 2.55 Left-sided pulmonary aplasia. The left chest cavity contains only the heart which is partly overlapped by the anterior border of the right lung. *(Courtesy of the late Dr AH Cameron, Birmingham, UK.)*

Figure 2.56 Bilateral pulmonary agenesis. The larynx is well formed but the trachea is short and the bronchi are blind-ending. *(Reproduced from Current Diagnostic Pathology by permission of Dr C Wright, Newcastle-upon-Tyne, UK.[139])*

enlarged and contains twice the normal number of alveoli, but the bronchi are normal.[377] Nevertheless there is a significant reduction in vital capacity and exercise tolerance.[378] In bilateral pulmonary aplasia the trachea or proximal bronchi end blindly (Fig. 2.56) and the pulmonary artery joins the aorta. Aplasia is often associated with other malformations and, if the aplasia is unilateral, these are often on the same side of the body.[378–380] They include anomalous pulmonary venous drainage.[381]

Pulmonary hypoplasia

Hypoplastic lungs are small but normal in form and it is possible that some cases are misdiagnosed as atelectasis. Hypoplasia of the lungs signifies that the alveoli are reduced in number or size. This may be assessed by counting the intercepts made by alveolar walls on a line from the terminal bronchiole to the interlobular septum.[382,383] Alternatively, the lungs may be weighed. Normal right and left lung weights at term are 21 and 18 g respectively (see Table 1.1, p. 3) but hypoplasia is best considered to be present in term babies when the lung-to-body weight ratio is less than 0.012.[384] The reduction in alveoli may be associated with fewer airway generations, the degree

of loss depending upon how early lung development was impaired. Development of airways down to the terminal bronchioles is complete by 16 weeks and the whole gas conductive system is complete by birth, unlike the alveoli and alveolar ducts, which continue to grow throughout infancy and into childhood. It follows that correction after birth of such causes of hypoplasia as diaphragmatic hernia may permit growth of alveoli but not airways.[385]

Hypoplasia of the lungs is seldom an isolated finding. It is usually associated with a variety of other abnormalities.[386] These include diaphragmatic defects, renal anomalies, extralobar pulmonary sequestration and severe musculoskeletal disorders. Most of these associations have a causal relationship (see below) but some, such as that with Down's syndrome[387] and the low-set ears of Potter's syndrome (see below), are not readily explained. Lung growth before birth is dependent upon blood supply, availability of space, respiratory movements taking place in utero and fluid filling the airways. The causes of pulmonary hypoplasia therefore include the following:

1. Congenital abnormalities of blood vessels supplying the lungs, as in pulmonary valve stenosis.
2. Compression of the lungs by intrathoracic masses, as with herniation of abdominal viscera through a congenital diaphragmatic defect (Figs 2.57 and 2.58) or cystic malformation of the contralateral lung.
3. Compression of the lungs due to deformities of the thorax such as Jeune's asphyxiating thoracic dystrophy (see p. 80). Because the lungs continue to grow after birth, infantile scoliosis may also cause postnatal hypoplasia.[388,389]
4. Lack of respiratory movements due to the antenatal onset of neuromuscular diseases such as myotonic dystrophy.

Figure 2.57 Pulmonary hypoplasia due to diaphragmatic hernia. Loops of bowel and the stomach fill much of the left side of the chest, compressing the thoracic viscera. *(Courtesy of Dr GA Russell, Tunbridge Wells, UK.)*

Figure 2.58 Pulmonary hypoplasia due to diaphragmatic hernia. The left lung, seen as a small nodule (arrow) between the right lung and the heart, is hypoplastic.

Figure 2.59 Potter facies consisting of low-set ears and a small hooked nose is seen in association with renal agenesis and pulmonary hypoplasia. *(Courtesy of the late Dr AH Cameron, Birmingham, UK.)*

5. Oligohydramnios, caused by either chronic leakage or deficient production of amniotic fluid. The mechanism whereby oligohydramnios causes pulmonary hypoplasia could again be compression of the lungs, but manometry shows that amniotic pressure is reduced rather than raised in oligohydramnios.[390] Loss of lung liquid is probably more important, being implicated by the demonstration that experimental tracheal ligation prevents the adverse pulmonary effects of oligohydramnios,[391] and by the observation that human fetuses with renal agenesis do not develop pulmonary hypoplasia if there is also laryngeal atresia.[392] Indeed, laryngeal atresia is recorded in association with pulmonary hyperplasia rather than hypoplasia.[149] Lung liquid therefore appears to act as a stent and thereby provide internal support essential to proper lung development. Fetal urine contributes greatly to amniotic fluid and renal agenesis and urethral stricture are important causes of oligohydramnios-associated pulmonary hypoplasia. The Potter syndrome consists of abnormal facies (Fig. 2.59), pulmonary hypoplasia and renal agenesis: oligohydramnios due to the renal

Figure 2.60 Pulmonary hyperplasia due to laryngeal atresia. The heart is enveloped by the voluminous lungs. *(Reproduced from* Current Diagnostic Pathology *by permission of Dr C Wright, Newcastle-upon-Tyne, UK.[139])*

agenesis is generally thought to be the cause of the pulmonary abnormality,[393] although a lack of renal metabolites has also been proposed.[37]

Hypoplasia is evident on antenatal scans and some of these causes are amenable to various surgical interventions before birth. Thus, diaphragmatic herniae have been repaired in utero, the fetal trachea has been occluded by the insertion of a balloon catheter (to retain lung liquid) and lung cysts have been drained into the amniotic cavity by the insertion of a catheter.

Pulmonary hyperplasia

It is mentioned above that lung fluid is important to lung growth, that deficient liquid within the lungs leads to hypoplasia and that obstruction to fluid outflow, as in laryngeal atresia, leads to overgrowth.[149] The latter takes the form of pulmonary hyperplasia, which is the exact opposite of pulmonary hypoplasia in that it is characterised by hyperalveolisation. This is manifest in the linear intercepts described above as being greater than normal and in the lungs being heavy. Hyperplastic lungs are voluminous, envelop the heart and show a pleural pattern of rib indentation (Fig. 2.60). They depress the diaphragm and compress veins, causing ascites and hydrops. Airway atresia at a lower level

than the larynx is more easily overlooked and probably accounts for seemingly inexplicable localised areas of pulmonary hyperplasia, which may not be recognised as such and therefore thought to represent a form of congenital cystic adenomatoid malformation or new forms of congenital 'emphysema', e.g. polyalveolar lobe.

Congenital 'emphysema'

Emphysema is defined in a later chapter as enlargement of air spaces distal to the terminal bronchiole due to breakdown of their walls. This is not found at birth: so-called congenital emphysema is a miscellany of other conditions in which the lungs are light and airy. A single segment, a lobe, a whole lung or all the lung tissue may be so affected in the neonatal period. Most of these conditions represent alveolar distension rather than destruction. Familial α_1-antitrypsin deficiency causes true emphysema and is congenital but the onset of the emphysema is not until adult life and this condition is therefore considered later in Chapter 3.

Alveolar distension may be compensatory to collapse or hypoplasia of the adjacent lung,[394] or it may be obstructive.[395] If the obstructed airway supplies a segment of a lobe or less, inflation of the distal lung may be by collateral ventilation, but if a lobar or main bronchus is affected collateral ventilation is not possible and a check valve mechanism is generally invoked to explain the distension. Bronchial atresia typically affects a segmental bronchus, and any distension is focal and due to collateral ventilation, in contrast to infantile lobar emphysema.

Infantile lobar emphysema (congenital lobar emphysema)

Infantile lobar emphysema is due to partial obstruction of the lobar bronchus leading to air-trapping. The other lobes are thereby compressed and mediastinal structures displaced causing severe respiratory distress, which generally necessitates early surgical resection. The condition generally affects neonates but cases occasionally come to light in adult life.[396,397] Males are affected more than females but the condition is not familial. The condition affects the left upper lobe in about half the cases, with the right middle and right upper lobes being involved in most of the remainder and the lower lobes in less than 10%.

The obstruction may be caused by intrinsic abnormalities of the bronchus, such as mucosal flaps, mucous plugs or twisting of the lobe on its pedicle, or by external compression from causes such as a bronchogenic cyst or abnormal blood vessels.[395,398] In the absence of such causes, a deficiency of bronchial cartilage is generally postulated. This may be demonstrated in the resected lobe by dissecting out the bronchi, staining the cartilage with toluidine blue and clearing the specimen with potassium hydroxide or an organic solvent such as cedarwood oil or xylol (Fig. 2.61).[399–401]

In practice the cause is frequently not identified. Explanations based on simple air-trapping are possibly too facile as the lobe is not only distended to its normal maximum but hyperinflated. This implies a connective tissue defect at the alveolar level,[402] although none has been convincingly demonstrated so far. About 20% of patients also have congenital cardiac anomalies and it is possible that the relationship is causal.[403] The bronchi supplying the lobes that are predominantly affected (the left upper and right middle lobes) are in particularly close proximity to pulmonary arteries and, if these are distended, as in acyanotic congenital heart disease, they are liable to be compressed; the narrow, pliable bronchi of neonates are particularly susceptible (see Fig. 10.9, p. 481).

The causes of external compression cannot be identified by examining the excised lobe and it is therefore essential that as well as paying

Figure 2.61 Infantile lobar emphysema. A fatal case in which the bronchi have been dissected out, their cartilages stained with toluidine blue and the tissues cleared. Bronchi to the right are devoid of cartilage. *(Courtesy of the late Professor BE Heard, Brompton, UK.)*

Figure 2.62 Swyer–James syndrome. A chest radiograph shows hyperlucency of the right lung due to diminished vascularity. *(Courtesy of Professor DM Hansell, Brompton, UK.)*

particular attention to the lobar bronchus the pathologist is aware of the clinical, radiological and surgical findings.

Polyalveolar lobe

A polyalveolar lobe has a normal number of conductive airways but an increased number of alveoli in each acinus.[404] The affected lobe is enlarged, light and airy but individual alveoli are not increased in size. The number of alveoli in an acinus is best assessed by counting the intercepts made by alveolar walls on a line from the terminal bronchiole to the interlobular septum.[382] The number of alveoli depends on the age of the child, but in general, fetuses have a radial count of 2–5, infants have a count of 5–10 and children a few years old have a count of 10–12. These figures are increased by as much as three to five times in a polyalveolar lobe.

Clinically, polyalveolar lobe resembles infantile lobar emphysema and often the true diagnosis only becomes apparent on examination of the excised specimen.[405] Affected babies are dyspnoeic and chest radiographs show lobar enlargement with displacement of the other thoracic viscera. The prognosis following surgery is good, and it may be preferable to operate early rather than late to maximise compensatory lung growth.

Hyperlucent lung (hypertransradiant lung; Swyer–James or Macleod syndrome)

This is a condition in which the normal radiographic markings of the lungs, which predominantly represent the pulmonary blood vessels, are diminished (Fig. 2.62). The syndrome was originally thought to be due to unilateral hypoplasia of the pulmonary artery but vascular shutdown in response to hypoventilation caused by postinfective obliterative bronchiolitis is now the favoured explanation.[406,407] The airway obstruction may add an element of distension but, in contrast to the forms of overinflation discussed above, the affected lung is not enlarged. This is compatible with an infective aetiology as this could well impair the normal postnatal growth of the lung at the alveolar level.

Ectopia

Two categories of ectopia need to be considered – ectopia of nonpulmonary tissues in the thorax and ectopia of lung tissue outside the thoracic cavity. Pleural endometriosis and splenosis, teratomas of the lung and traumatic embolism of bone marrow, liver or brain tissue to the lung are dealt with separately.

Ectopia of adrenocortical tissue,[408] thyroid (lacking C cells)[409] and liver[410] has been described in the lung and pancreatic tissue has been noted within intralobar sequestrations with gastrointestinal connections.[191,192] Ectopic striated muscle is recorded in sequestered and hypoplastic lungs[242,411,412] and occasionally as an isolated pulmonary abnormality,[413] sometimes tumour-like.[414] Rarely, a whole kidney may be found above the diaphragm but outside the lung.[415]

Ectopia of glial tissue within the lung is well recognised.[416–422] Nodules of glial tissue may be implanted in the embryonic lung by aspiration of amniotic fluid in some cases of anencephaly[416,418,419] and in the absence of anencephaly by embolisation due to intrauterine trauma[421] or, with small macerated fetuses, merely normal uterine contractions.[422] The ectopic glial tissue lacks neurones but may contain cysts lined by ciliated epithelium: devoid of their normal mesenchyme these primitive lung buds fail to develop bronchial cartilage and muscle or differentiate into alveoli. Two patients with unexplained glial ectopia survived surgery for neonatal respiratory distress to reach adult life, one with mental retardation[417] and one without.[420]

Ectopia of lung tissue in the neck, the abdomen or the chest wall is often termed herniation but is probably due neither to raised

Figure 2.63 Ectopia of the lungs. The diaphragm and abdominal contents are viewed from above. The left hemidiaphragm is largely absent and through this deficiency dark unaerated lung tissue and abdominal viscera can be seen. *(Courtesy of the late Dr AH Cameron, Birmingham, UK.)*

intrathoracic pressure nor deficiencies in the thoracic boundaries, as often proposed, for the one causes pulmonary hypoplasia and the other leads to herniation of structures into, rather than from, the thorax. Although it is often associated with skeletal or diaphragmatic abnormalities (Fig. 2.63), it appears to represent genuine ectopia. Some examples of abdominal pulmonary ectopia represent extralobar sequestration as well as ectopia.[423]

Hamartomas

Hamartomas represent abnormal mixtures of tissue elements, or an abnormal proportion of a single element normally present in an organ resulting in changes that are tumour-like but not neoplastic. Pleuropulmonary examples include vascular malformations, and mesenchymal malformation of the chest wall. However, the so-called (chondroid) hamartoma shows an increasing incidence with age and is probably a true neoplasm. It is therefore dealt with in the tumour section. It is also debatable whether the so-called mesenchymal cystic hamartoma is a valid entity. It was first described in 1986,[424] since when only a few more cases have been reported.[425–429] Some appear to have represented metastases of either endometrial stromal sarcoma or cellular fibrous histiocytoma,[430,432] while others have resembled the type 4 congenital cystic adenomatoid malformation or a type 1 pleuropulmonary blastoma.

The condition of so-called benign metastasising leiomyoma is generally considered to represent metastasis from an occult extrapulmonary tumour and is dealt with in Chapter 12.6, but some suggest that the condition represents hamartomatous growth, showing that some of the lesions are polyclonal.[433] However, other molecular studies support the concept of metastatic growth.[434]

The term 'muscular hamartoma' is often applied to small focal proliferations of smooth muscle that are occasionally observed inci-

dentally in the lung. They are generally stellate in outline and almost always the muscle is intermingled with fibrous tissue. Such lesions more likely represent old scars in which there is prominent reactive smooth-muscle hyperplasia. Diffuse changes of this nature are often seen in end-stage diffuse pulmonary fibrosis and the term 'muscular cirrhosis of the lung' has been used for this. Genuine examples of smooth-muscle hamartomas are reported in the lung, sometimes associated with similar lesions in the bowel and liver,[435] but they are much rarer than focal scars.

Anomalies of the pulmonary blood vessels

The condition known as alveolar capillary dysplasia with misalignment of lung vessels represents arrested development in the canalicular stage of lung development and is accordingly described with other diffuse developmental disorders of infancy on page 50. The left pulmonary artery sling syndrome is also described elsewhere – on page 481, together with the various ring anomalies of systemic vessels that may similarly result in compression of the major airways in infancy.

Unilateral absence of a pulmonary artery

Absence of one of the main pulmonary arteries leads to the lung on that side receiving only systemic blood, through either anomalous arteries or enlarged bronchial arteries.[436,437] Either lung may be affected and the defect may be isolated or associated with other cardiovascular anomalies, typically the tetrad of Fallot with an absent left pulmonary artery and a patent ductus arteriosus with an absent right pulmonary artery.[436] Patients with an isolated anomaly of this type may lead a normal life or symptoms may not arise until adult life, when they are generally attributable to pulmonary infection or to bleeding from bronchopulmonary anastomoses.[438–442] Clinically, the condition may be difficult to distinguish from embolic occlusion but an association with other congenital vascular defects would support the diagnosis.[438] Only a short segment of the artery may be lacking and surgical correction may be possible.[443] In other cases, pulmonary arteries may be difficult to identify in lung sections, where they tend to be overshadowed by hypertrophied bronchial arteries, sometimes showing plexiform lesions.[441] Pulmonary hypertension develops in 18% of patients with an isolated defect and more often when there are other vascular anomalies. Relevant to this is the observation that ligation of one main pulmonary artery, for example during pneumonectomy, has little effect on the contralateral vasculature in adults but when the ligation is conducted in the perinatal period the high fetal pulmonary pressure is maintained.[436]

Pulmonary artery stenosis and Fallot's tetrad

Stenosis may affect the main pulmonary artery or any of its branches. There may be multiple constrictions and, as with absence of a pulmonary artery, the condition may be isolated or associated with other vascular anomalies. Stenosis of the main pulmonary artery is the dominant factor in the tetrad of Fallot, in which it is combined with a ventricular septal defect, an overriding aorta and right ventricular hypertrophy. It leads to a right-to-left ventricular shunt, the clinical features of which – cyanosis, polycythaemia and clubbing – develop in infancy, in contrast to Eisenmenger's syndrome in which cyanosis develops later. In all patients with cyanotic congenital heart disease, but particularly those with Fallot's tetrad, a sudden reduction in systemic resistance or increase in pulmonary resistance leads to episodes of more profound cyanosis and hypoxaemia, which can be fatal. With pulmonary stenosis, the attenuation of the pulmonary artery walls that normally takes place after birth proceeds apace so that the normal medial thinning is greatly exaggerated, in contrast to Eisenmenger's syndrome in which the pulmonary arteries are hypertrophied. Following the experimental ligation of a pulmonary artery there occurs an enormous expansion of thick-walled bronchial collaterals that is well advanced by 12 weeks.[444]

Congenital anomalies characterised by direct communication between the two circulations

Some of the more severe pulmonary effects of cardiovascular disease are caused by congenital abnormalities that establish a direct communication between the systemic and pulmonary circulations – anomalies such as septal defects, patent ductus arteriosus, transposition of the great arteries and variants of the tetrad of Fallot in which there is little obstruction to right ventricular outflow. These all lead to shunting of oxygenated blood back into the lesser circulation.

With atrial septal defects the principal effect is that the output of the right ventricle is greater than that of the left. In many cases the increased flow is accommodated by underperfused vessels being recruited. This lowers pulmonary artery resistance so that there is no rise in pressure. However, with large defects hyperkinetic pulmonary hypertension eventually develops, a complication that occurs much earlier with communications at the ventricular or aortic level than with atrial septal defects. Hyperkinetic pulmonary hypertension is characterised by plexogenic arteriopathy (see p. 420). The major pulmonary arteries are distended and, where they are in close proximity to bronchi, the latter may be compressed, particularly in young infants in whom the bronchial cartilages are still soft and pliable, as explained above (see Fig. 10.9, p. 481).[403] The result is pulmonary collapse, or if the obstruction is partial, infantile lobar emphysema. Eventually the right ventricle becomes dominant and the left-to-right shunt is reversed, causing cyanosis, a process known as Eisenmenger's reaction or syndrome. Eisenmenger's own case combined a ventricular septal defect with an overriding aorta, an arrangement that is termed Eisenmenger's complex. Eisenmenger attributed the cyanosis to the biventricular origin of the aorta but cardiac catheter studies have subsequently shown that acquired pulmonary hypertension is the responsible factor.

Dieulafoy's disease

This vascular malformation is best known in the gastrointestinal tract but a few cases affecting bronchial arteries have been described.[445–447] The patients generally present with massive haemoptysis and are found to have an isolated aneurysmally dilated bronchial artery that has bled into a bronchus (Fig. 2.64).

Anomalous systemic arteries

Anomalous systemic arteries to the lung are an essential feature of pulmonary sequestration. They are also found with pulmonary artery aplasia and arteriovenous malformations, or they may be an isolated abnormality. They are usually small but sometimes the right pulmonary artery arises from the aorta.[448] As well as these congenital anomalies, conditions such as bronchiectasis often acquire a systemic blood supply, usually via enlarged bronchial arteries but also from intercostal or mediastinal arteries if there are pleural adhesions.[449]

Anomalous pulmonary veins

Anomalous pulmonary veins result in blood from the lungs returning to the right side of the heart rather than entering the left atrium. The embryological basis is a failure of the veins within the primitive lungs to switch from draining into channels around the foregut to a new

Figure 2.64 Dieulafoy's disease. (A) Rupture of an aneurysmally dilated mucosal artery proved to be the cause of intractable haemoptysis that necessitated lobectomy. (B) An elastin stain highlights the eroded bronchial artery. *(Courtesy of Dr MM Burke, Harefield, UK.)*

primary pulmonary vein which grows from the developing left atrium toward the lung buds. The anomalous veins may join the inferior vena cava or hepatic, portal or splenic veins below the diaphragm, or above the diaphragm they may drain into the superior vena cava or its tributaries, the coronary sinus or the right atrium (Table 2.10). The anomaly may be total or partial, unilateral or bilateral, and isolated or associated with other cardiopulmonary developmental defects. These include bronchopulmonary isomerism, dextrocardia, asplenia, pulmonary stenosis, patent ductus arteriosus and a small interatrial communication.[450] The type of isomerism gives a good indication as to whether the anomaly is total or partial; right-sided isomerism suggests totally anomalous veins and left-sided isomerism suggests a partial anomaly.[164] Occasionally the anomalous vein runs much of its course buried within the lung substance.[451] Anomalous pulmonary venous connections are often narrow and this may cause pulmonary hypertension of the relatively mild, reversible venous variety.[452] Occasional

Table 2.10 Anomalous pulmonary veins. Venous drainage in 27 cases of totally anomalous pulmonary venous drainage documented by the late Dr AH Cameron at the Birmingham Children's Hospital over a 15-year period (excluding cases of asplenia and situs inversus)

Tributaries of the superior vena cava	9
Right atrium	8
Coronary sinus	4
Portal vein	3
Hepatic vein	1
Splenic vein	1
Inferior vena cava	1

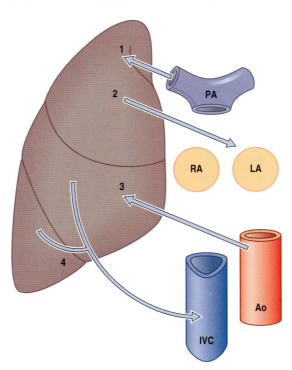

Figure 2.65 Scimitar syndrome. 1. The right upper lobe is often supplied by a hypoplastic pulmonary artery (PA). 2. The blood from the upper part of the lung drains into the left atrium (LA). 3. The remainder of the right lung is supplied by vessels arising from the aorta (Ao). 4. The blood from a variable part of the right lung drains by a prominent vein (evident radiologically as a curved, scimitar-shaped linear opacity) which joins the inferior vena cava (IVC) below the diaphragm. Less frequently, the drainage of the lower part of the right lung is by veins which pass directly to the right atrium (RA). *(Redrawn from Brewis RAL, Corrin B, Geddes DM et al. Respiratory Medicine, 2nd edn. London: Saunders, 1995.)*

reports of plexogenic pulmonary hypertension probably reflect the association with a patent ductus arteriosus.[450]

Atresia of the pulmonary veins[453,454] or narrowing of their ostia entering the left atrium (collectively termed pulmonary vein stenosis[453]) does not in itself constitute anomalous drainage but similarly results in pulmonary venous obstruction and may be associated with partial anomalous pulmonary venous drainage. The atresia may be unilateral or bilateral but in either case severe hypertensive changes develop in both lungs. Small capillary-sized vessels may be found within all coats of the thickened arteries, or congeries of them may be seen alongside the larger blood vessels. They represent abortive anastomotic attempts at bypassing the obstruction, which are doomed to failure because the obstruction is extrapulmonary. They bear some resemblance to plexiform lesions but the necrotising arteritis that leads to plexogenic arteriopathy is not a feature. There is a closer resemblance to pulmonary capillary haemangiomatosis, supporting the view that this supposedly neoplastic condition merely represents a reaction to pulmonary venous occlusion (see p. 429). Congenital pulmonary vein atresia carries a very poor prognosis; few children with the condition survive longer than a year.

Partial anomalous pulmonary venous drainage is an essential feature of the scimitar syndrome, in which an anomalous right pulmonary vein descending to join the inferior vena cava just below the diaphragm gives a characteristic, supposedly scimitar-like, vertical radiographic opacity parallel to the right side of the heart (Fig. 2.65). The right pulmonary artery is hypoplastic and the arterial supply of the right lung is often largely from the aorta, so that there is some overlap with pulmonary sequestration. Due to the deficient pulmonary artery supply the right lung is hypoplastic with consequent mediastinal shift to the right. The vascular connections of the left lung are normal. Cardiovascular, diaphragmatic, gastrointestinal and other pulmonary anomalies are often found. The syndrome can be familial with an autosomal-dominant pattern of inheritance. Some patients are asymptomatic and the lesion is detected only on routine radiographs. Others suffer from recurrent pneumonia, breathlessness or haemoptysis.[455,456] The anomaly represents a left-to-right shunt and surgical correction may be required if this is large.

Pulmonary vein stenosis and atrial fibrillation

Atrial fibrillation is the commonest form of cardiac dysrhythmia and one that is associated with significant morbidity and mortality. The condition is multifactorial but it appears that in most patients the fibrillation is triggered by ectopic foci in the muscular sleeves that surround the pulmonary veins immediately prior to their entry into the left atrium, prompting attempts to ameliorate the dysrhythmia by catheter ablation.[457,458] The commonest technique aims to isolate the source of these ectopic beats by delivering radiofrequency energy at the junctions of the four veins and the atrium. Whilst it can succeed in curing the dysrhythmia several patients have developed pulmonary venous stenosis.[458a,459]

Arteriovenous fistula

Arteriovenous fistulas may be developmental or acquired. The latter result from injuries such as penetrating chest wounds or they may complicate liver disease. This account will be confined to the developmental variety, which was first reported in 1897,[460] since when many further cases have been reported.[461–466] The lesion is a vascular hamartoma resulting from persistence of anastomotic fetal capillaries. This results in abnormal communication between pulmonary arteries and veins, bypassing the normal pulmonary capillary bed. More rarely the lesion connects systemic and pulmonary vessels.[467–470] The lesions may be single or multiple and often increase in size with age.[471] About 70% of patients have hereditary haemorrhagic telangiectasia (Rendu–Osler–Weber disease), which is an autosomal-dominant condition (see p. 481).[463,472,473] Conversely, about 15% of patients with hereditary haemorrhagic telangiectasia have pulmonary arteriovenous fistulae.[474] This association portends an increased risk of multiple fistulae and progressive symptoms, which is important as surgical correction is only possible with limited disease. Patients with multiple fistulae are more suitable for treatment by balloon occlusion or embolisation. However, migration of a coil embolus into a bronchus is recorded.[475] The role of lung transplantation is controversial.[476,477]

Clinical features

Although the lesion is a developmental anomaly, it may remain asymptomatic until late in life. The average age at presentation is about 40 years but the condition has been first identified in both the newborn and the very old.[462,463,468] Fistulae with an appreciable arteriovenous shunt cause cyanosis, clubbing of the fingers, breathlessness, polycythaemia and an extracardiac murmur. Haemorrhage from the lungs, as opposed to nasal telangiectasia, is an uncommon but potentially fatal complication.[478] The proximity of most malformations to the pleura explains the occasional complication of haemothorax. Systemic complications may be caused by hypoxaemia, thrombosis secondary to the polycythaemia, haemorrhage due to associated hereditary telangiectasia, and paradoxical embolism or metastatic abscesses due to loss of the filtering effect of the pulmonary capillaries or, rarely, infective endarteritis within the fistula. Cerebral abscess is reported in 20% of patients, stroke in 18% and transient ischaemic attacks in 37%.[472] Sarcomatous change has been reported[479] but is very rare.

Pathology

The lower lobes are most commonly affected but any lobe may be involved. The lesions are multiple in one-third of cases and in one-sixth the condition is bilateral. Resected lesions will almost certainly have been demonstrated angiographically before operation (Fig. 2.66A, B). If not, the pathologist may do this with a barium gelatin mixture before fixing the specimen but the results are rarely better than the images produced in vivo. The lesion is usually peripheral and visible as a bluish swelling beneath the visceral pleura. It consists of vascular channels of various size and wall thickness, with little supportive tissue, separated by normal lung tissue (Fig. 2.66C, D). Individual vessels may be narrowed by intimal fibrosis or there may be dilatation associated with medial atrophy. Without prior angiography, arteriovenous communication can only be demonstrated by semi-serial sections.

Anomalies of the pulmonary lymphatics

Congenital pulmonary lymphangiectasia

Congenital pulmonary lymphangiectasia may be caused by obstruction to pulmonary lymphatic or venous drainage or be 'primary', the latter either limited to the lung or part of generalised lymphangiectasia.[480] There is a high association of primary pulmonary lymphangiectasia with other congenital abnormalities, particularly asplenia[481] and cardiac anomalies. When the other abnormalities entail impaired pulmonary venous drainage there is obviously a causal relationship, but this is not always the case.[481,482]

Primary pulmonary lymphangiectasia is presumed to result from developmental failure of the pulmonary lymphatics to link with the main drainage channels. It causes severe respiratory distress and is generally fatal in the neonatal period, but some children survive, albeit with respiratory impairment,[483] and presentation may be delayed until adult life.[484–486]

The macroscopic findings can be very instructive diagnostically. The microscopic distinction of lymphangiectasia from interstitial emphysema can be extremely difficult and it is regrettable that sure macroscopic distinctions are often omitted from the autopsy report. In lymphangiectasia the lungs are heavy but this is often also the case in

interstitial emphysema because of some underlying disease which necessitated artificial respiration. In both conditions the interlobular septa are widened and on the visceral pleural surface there is a pronounced reticular pattern of small cysts which accentuates the lobular architecture of the lungs. Pricking the cysts gives invaluable evidence of their content; clear serous fluid will run out in lymphangiectasia. On slicing the lungs, further fluid runs from the cut surfaces, which show a microcystic pattern (Fig. 2.67A). The cysts measure up to 5 mm in diameter and are situated in the interlobular septa and about the bronchovascular bundles. Near the hila of the lungs the cysts are elongated.[487]

Microscopy confirms that the cysts are located in connective tissue under the pleura, in the interlobular septa and about the bronchioles and arteries (Fig. 2.67B). Serial sections show that they are part of an intricate network of intercommunicating channels which vary greatly in width and are devoid of valves.[487] The cysts are lined by an attenuated simple endothelium, an appearance which may be mimicked by compressed connective tissue cells in interstitial emphysema. Never seen in lymphangiectasia is the foreign-body giant cell reaction to air which develops after a few days in interstitial emphysema (see Fig. 2.18). Apart from this the two conditions can be virtually indistinguishable microscopically, which is understandable as in interstitial emphysema the air is contained within lymphatics as well as dissecting the interstitial tissues.[125] Interstitial emphysema rather than lymphangiectasia may also be suspected if there is some other underlying disease that necessitated ventilator support.

It is important not to confuse lymphangiectasia with artefactual expansion of the interlobular septa by overzealous injection of formalin.

Klippel–Trenaunay syndrome

This congenital condition is characterised by varicosities of systemic veins, cutaneous haemangiomas, soft-tissue hypertrophy and pleuro-pulmonary abnormalities that include pulmonary lymphatic hyperplasia, pleural effusions, pulmonary thromboembolism and pulmonary vein varicosities.[488,489]

Yellow-nail syndrome

Lymphatic hypoplasia of varied distribution underlies this syndrome, which is characterised by lymphoedema accompanied by discoloration of the nails and pleural effusions. Although widely regarded as representing a hereditary disorder, the family history is generally negative and the condition is not usually manifest until adult life (see also p. 709).

Anomalies of the thoracic cage

Diaphragmatic anomalies

The diaphragm forms from the fetal septum transversum, which grows across the common coelomic cavity to divide the peritoneal from the pleural and pericardial cavities. The posterolateral portions containing the foramina of Bochdalek are the last to form and arrested development here results in widened foramina through which herniation of abdominal viscera is prone to occur, particularly on the left, resulting in mediastinal shift to the right.[490] Hernias of this type are among the commonest congenital defects. They occur in about 1 in 2000 fetuses but many of these have other major anomalies, in particular cardiac abnormalities, and are stillborn. Chromosomal abnormalities are only common when there are other anomalies. Most isolated congenital diaphragmatic hernias appear to be sporadic. Several teratogens, including phenmetrazine, thalomide, quinine, nitrofen and vitamin A deficiency, have been identified. If the infant is suitable for surgical

Figure 2.66 Arteriovenous aneurysm of the right lung demonstrated angiographically (A, B: (B) shows delayed emptying) and after lobectomy when unusually large thin-walled blood vessels were evident on the cut surface of the lung (C). *(A–C courtesy of Dr M Jagusch, formerly of Auckland, New Zealand.)* The lobectomy specimen from another patient is shown in (D). *(d courtesy of Dr T Jelihovsky, Sydney, Australia.)*

Figure 2.67 Congenital pulmonary lymphangiectasia. (A) Cystically dilated lymphatics are evident on the cut surface of the lung. *(Courtesy of Dr M Jagusch, formerly of Auckland, New Zealand.)* (B) Lymphatics in the interlobular septa are markedly dilated.

Figure 2.68 Asphyxiating thoracic dystrophy (Jeune's syndrome). Deformity of the chest wall reduces the thoracic cavity to a narrow funnel and thereby causes pulmonary hypoplasia. *(Courtesy of the late Dr AH Cameron, Birmingham, UK.)*

tration. The whole diaphragm may be affected but more often the defect is unilateral.

Posterolateral herniation and eventration are both commoner on the left and affect boys twice as often as girls. Anterior and para-oesophageal hernias each account for only 5% of the total, while total absence of half or the whole diaphragm is very unusual.[491] All these diaphragmatic defects result in abdominal viscera moving into a pleural space and compromising lung development (see pulmonary hypoplasia, p. 70). Hepatopulmonary fusion is a much rarer association.[491a]

Duplication of the diaphragm results in a fibromuscular septum dividing one pleural cavity in two, usually between the right upper and middle lobes. Associated anomalies of the heart and lungs are frequent.

Pectus excavatum (funnel chest)

This condition is relatively common, being found in approximately 1 child in 400. Males are affected more commonly than females. The condition appears soon after birth and is occasionally associated with

correction, respiratory insufficiency and persistent fetal circulation are frequent postoperative problems. The foramina are normally sealed at about 8 weeks' gestation by the pleural and peritoneal membranes so that hernias forming after this time tend to be enclosed in a serosal sac.

The diaphragmatic muscle is formed between the pleural and peritoneal membranes and if it is deficient the diaphragm is reduced to a thin membrane, which rises into the thorax, a process known as evenkyphosis, scoliosis or mitral valve prolapse. It may be familial or associated with Marfan's syndrome, the Ehlers–Danlos syndrome and hyperflexibility of the joints. It may also be acquired in infancy by upper-airway obstruction from enlargement of the tonsils and adenoids necessitating an increase in the force of the respiratory movements. Initially the condition is reversible but it may become permanent. The respiratory effects are minor but the heart may be compressed between the depressed sternum and the spine so that cardiac filling is impaired.[492] Surgical correction is sometimes undertaken, largely for cosmetic or psychological reasons as it confers only marginal functional benefit. It is best deferred until the growth spurt of puberty is over as the basic fault of both pectus excavatum and pectus carinatum is an overgrowth of the costal cartilages, causing the sternum to buckle inwards in the former condition and outwards in the latter.

Pectus carinatum (pigeon breast)

In this condition the sternum protrudes anteriorly and may lie obliquely if the excessive growth of the ribs is asymmetrical. It may be present at birth but usually becomes prominent during adolescence. About 1 in 1500 children are so affected. Respiratory function is normal as there is no loss of lung volume and little interference with rib movement.

Asphyxiating thoracic dystrophy (Jeune's syndrome)

This is a rare disorder of the ribs, which are shortened and the ribcage narrowed so that lung development is retarded and there is pulmonary hypoplasia (Fig. 2.68).[493,494] Less severe degrees are compatible with life but respiratory movements are entirely abdominal and respiratory failure often develops in infancy or childhood. Although rare, Jeune's syndrome is the commonest of several generalised skeletal disorders that result in a small chest. In many of them the thoracic deformity is associated with short limbs, syndactyly or polydactyly.[495]

Scoliosis

Scoliosis (lateral curvature of the spine) is generally accompanied by rotation of the spine. If the condition is present at birth there is often a recognisable congenital abnormality of the spine, such as hemivertebra, and other congenital skeletal abnormalities such as absent or fused ribs may also be present. However, most cases are idiopathic. Some idiopathic cases present in infancy. These tend to progress to respiratory failure in later life.[388,389] However, it is commoner for idiopathic scoliosis to appear during adolescence and not progress in this way. Scoliosis may also be secondary to neuromuscular disorders, both hereditary and acquired.

REFERENCES

Development of the lungs

1. Jeffery PK. The development of large and small airways. Am J Respir Crit Care Med 1998;157:S174–80.

2. Bucher U, Reid L. Development of the intrasegmental bronchial tree: The pattern of branching and development of cartilage at various stages of intra-uterine life. Thorax 1961;16:207–18.

3. Scavo LM, Ertsey R, Chapin CJ, et al. Apoptosis in the development of rat and human fetal lungs. Am J Respir Cell Mol Biol 1998;18:21–31.

4. Zeltner TB, Burri PH. The postnatal development and growth of the human lung. II. Morphology. Respir Physiol 1987;67:269–82.

5. Thurlbeck WM, Angus GE. Growth and aging of the normal human lung. Chest 1975;67:3S–7S.

6. Hislop A, Reid L. Development of the acinus in the human lung. Thorax 1974;29:90–4.

7. Thurlbeck WM. Postnatal growth and development of the lung. Am Rev Respir Dis 1975;111:803–44.

8. Thurlbeck WM. Postnatal human lung growth. Thorax 1982;37:564–71.

9. Burrows B, Knudson RJ, Lebowitz MD. The relationship of childhood respiratory illness to adult obstructive airway disease. Am Rev Respir Dis 1977;115:751–60.

10. Shaheen S, Barker DJP. Early lung growth and chronic airflow obstruction. Thorax 1994;49:533–6.

11. Johnston IDA, Strachan DP, Anderson HR. Effect of pneumonia and whooping cough in childhood on adult lung function. N Engl J Med 1998;338:581–7.

12. Campiche MA, Gautier A, Hernandez EI, et al. An electron microscope study of the fetal development of human lung. Pediatrics 1963;32:976–94.

13. Leeson TS, Leeson CR. A light and electron microscope study of developing respiratory tissue in the rat. J Anat 1964;98:183–93.

14. O'Hare KH, Sheridan MN. Electron microscopic observations on the morphogenesis of the albino rat lung, with special reference to pulmonary epithelial cells. Am J Anat 1970;127:181–205.

15. Demello DE, Sawyer D, Galvin N, et al. Early fetal development of lung vasculature. Am J Respir Cell Mol Biol 1997;16:568–81.

16. Demello DE, Reid LM. Embryonic and early fetal development of human lung vasculature and its functional implications. Pediatr Dev Pathol 2000;3:439–49.

17. Hall SM, Hislop AA, Pierce CM, et al. Prenatal origins of human intrapulmonary arteries formation and smooth muscle maturation. Am J Respir Cell Mol Biol 2000;23:194–203.

18. Jeffery PK, Hislop AA. Embryology and Growth. In: Gibson GJ, Geddes DM, Costabel U, et al, editors. Respiratory Medicine. 3rd ed. Edinburgh: Saunders; 2003. p. 51–63.

19. Hall SM, Hislop AA, Haworth SG. Origin, differentiation, and maturation of human pulmonary veins. Am J Respir Cell Mol Biol 2002;26:333–40.

20. Weichselbaum M, Sparrow MP. A confocal microscopic study of the formation of ganglia in the airways of fetal pig lung. Am J Respir Cell Mol Biol 1999;21:607–20.

21. Perl AK, Whitsett JA. Molecular mechanisms controlling lung morphogenesis. Clin Genet 1999;56:14–27.

22. Warburton D, Bellusci S, De Langhe S, et al. Molecular mechanisms of early lung specification and branching morphogenesis. Pediatr Res 2005;57:26R–37R.

23. Groenman F, Unger S, Post M. The molecular basis for abnormal human lung development. Biol Neonate 2005;87:164–77.

24. Adamson IYR, Young L, King GM. Reciprocal epithelial–fibroblast interactions in the control of fetal and adult rat lung cells in culture. Exp Lung Res 1991;17:821–35.

25. Virtanen I, Laitinen A, Tani T, et al. Differential expression of laminins and their integrin receptors in developing and adult human lung. Am J Respir Cell Mol Biol 1996;15:184–96.

26. Arai H, Hirano H, Mushiake S, et al. Loss of EDB+ fibronectin isoform is associated with differentiation of alveolar epithelial cells in human fetal lung. Am J Pathol 1997;151:403–12.

27. Shannon JM, Deterding RR. Epithelial-mesenchymal interactions in lung

development. In: McDonald JA, editor. Lung Growth and Development. New York: Marcel Dekker; 1997. p. 81–118.

28. Warburton D, Schwarz M, Tefft D, et al. The molecular basis of lung morphogenesis. Mech Dev 2000;92: 55–81.

29. Cardoso WV. Molecular regulation of lung development. Annu Rev Physiol 2001;63:471–94.

30. Bartram U, Speer CP. The role of transforming growth factor beta in lung development and disease. Chest 2004;125:754–65.

31. Adamson IYR, King GM. Epithelial–mesenchymal interactions in postnatal rat lung growth. Exp Lung Res 1985;8:261–74.

32. Terzaghi M, Nettesheim P, Williams ML. Repopulation of denuded tracheal grafts with normal, preneoplastic and neoplastic epithelial cell populations. Cancer Res 1978;38:4546–53.

33. Caniggia I, Tseu I, Rolland G, et al. Inhibition of fibroblast growth by epithelial cells in fetal rat lung. Am J Respir Cell Mol Biol 1995;13:91–8.

34. Taderera JV. Control of lung differentiation in vitro. Dev Biol 1967;16:489–512.

35. Olver RE, Strang LB. Ion fluxes across the pulmonary epithelium and the secretion of lung liquid in the foetal lamb. J Physiol (Lond) 1974;241:327–57.

36. Symchurch PS, Winchester P. Animal model: amniotic fluid deficiency and fetal lung growth in the rat. Am J Pathol 1978;90:779–82.

37. Hislop A, Hey E, Reid L. The lungs in congenital bilateral renal agenesis and dysplasia. Arch Dis Child 1979;54: 32–8.

38. Cutz E, Chan W, Wong V, et al. Endocrine cells in rat fetal lungs. Ultrastructural and histochemical study. Lab Invest 1974;30:458–64.

39. Wharton J, Polak JM, Cole GA, et al. Neuro-specific enolase as an immunocytochemical marker for the diffuse neuroendocrine system in human fetal lung. J Histochem Cytochem 1981;29:1359–64.

40. Stahlman MT, Gray ME. Ontogeny of neuroendocrine cells in human fetal lung. I. An electron microscopic study. Lab Invest 1984;51:449–63.

41. Stahlman MT, Kasselberg AG, Orth DN, et al. Ontogeny of neuroendocrine cells in human fetal lung. II. An immunohistochemical study. Lab Invest 1985;52:52–60.

42. Van Lommel A, Lauweryns JM, Deleyn P, et al. Pulmonary neuroepithelial bodies in neonatal and adult dogs: histochemistry, ultrastructure, and effects of unilateral hilar lung denervation. Lung 1995;173:13–23.

43. Aguayo SM, Schuyler WE, Murtagh JJ, et al. Regulation of lung branching morphogenesis by bombesin-like peptides and neutral endopeptidase. Am J Respir Cell Mol Biol 1994;10:635–42.

44. Wang DS, Yeger H, Cutz E. Expression of gastrin-releasing peptide receptor gene in developing lung. Am J Respir Cell Mol Biol 1996;14:409–16.

45. Gutierrez JA, Ertsey R, Scavo LM, et al. Mechanical distention modulates alveolar epithelial cell phenotypic expression by transcriptional regulation. Am J Respir Cell Mol Biol 1999;21:223–9.

46. Wigglesworth JS, Desai R. Effects on lung growth of cervical cord section in the rabbit fetus. Early Hum Dev 1979;3: 51–65.

47. Ballard PL, Benson BJ, Brehier A. Glucocorticoid effects in fetal lung. Am Rev Respir Dis 1977;115.

48. Liggins GC, Howie RN. A controlled trial of antepartum glucocorticoid treatment for prevention of the respiratory distress syndrome in premature infants. Pediatrics 1972;50:515–25.

49. Monkhouse WS. Characterization of proteoglycans synthesized by fetal rat lung type II pneumocytes in vitro and the effects of cortisol. Exp Lung Res 1987;12:253–64.

Perinatal disorders

50. Burgess AM, Hutchins GM. Inflammation of the lungs, umbilical cord and placenta associated with meconium passage in utero – review of 123 autopsied cases. Pathol Res Pract 1996;192:1121–8.

51. Finer NN. Surfactant use for neonatal lung injury: beyond respiratory distress syndrome. Paediatr Respir Rev 2004;5:S289–97.

52. Salvia-Roiges MD, Carbonell-Estrany X, Figueras-Aloy J, et al. Efficacy of three treatment schedules in severe meconium aspiration syndrome. Acta Paediatr 2004;93:60–5.

53. Keenan WJ. Recommendations for management of the child born through meconium-stained amniotic fluid. Pediatrics 2004;113:133–4.

54. Lin TW, Su BH, Lin HC, et al. Risk factors of pulmonary hemorrhage in very-low-birth-weight infants: a two-year retrospective study. Acta Paediatr Taiwan 2000;41:255–8.

55. Esterly JR, Oppenheimer WH, Rowe S, et al. Massive pulmonary haemorrhage in the newborn. J Pediatr 1966;69:3–20.

56. Franciosi RA, Tattersall P. Fetal infection with human parvovirus B19. Hum Pathol 1988;19:489–91.

57. Ablow RC, Driscoll SG, Effman EL, et al. A comparison of early onset group B streptococcal neonatal infection and the respiratory distress syndrome of the newborn. N Engl J Med 1976;294:65–70.

58. Cordero L, Ayers LW, Miller RR, et al. Surveillance of ventilator-associated pneumonia in very-low-birth-weight infants. Am J Infect Control 2002;30:32–9.

59. Apisarnthanarak A, Holzmann-Pazgal G, Hamvas A, et al. Ventilator-associated pneumonia in extremely preterm neonates in a neonatal intensive care unit: characteristics, risk factors, and outcomes. Pediatrics 2003;112:1283–9.

60. Clements JA, Avery ME. Lung surfactant and neonatal respiratory distress syndrome. Am J Respir Crit Care Med 1998;157:S59–66.

61. Robertson B. Pathology of neonatal surfactant deficiency. In: Rosenberg HS, Bernstein J, editors. Respiratory and Alimentary Tract Diseases Vol 11 Perspectives in Pediatric Pathology. Basel: Karger; 1987. p. 6–46.

62. Doshi N, Klionsky B, Fujikura T, et al. Pulmonary yellow hyaline membranes in neonates. Hum Pathol 1980;11:520–7.

63. Morgenstern B, Klionsky B, Doshi N. Yellow hyaline membrane disease. Identification of the pigment and bilirubin binding. Lab Invest 1981;44:514–8.

64. Kresch MJ, Lin WH, Thrall RS. Surfactant replacement therapy. Thorax 1996;51:1137–54.

65. Bryan MH, Hardie MJ, Reilly BJ, et al. Pulmonary function studies during the first year of life in infants recovering from the respiratory distress syndrome. Pediatrics 1973;52:169–78.

66. Baraldi E, Filippone M, Trevisanuto D, et al. Pulmonary function until two years of life in infants with bronchopulmonary dysplasia. Am J Respir Crit Care Med 1997;155:149–55.

67. Kamper J. Long term prognosis of infants with severe idiopathic respiratory distress syndrome. Acta Paediatr Scand 1978;67:71–6.

68. Northway WH, Rosan RC, Porter DY. Pulmonary disease following respirator therapy of hyaline membrane disease. Bronchopulmonary dysplasia. N Engl J Med 1967;276:357–68.

69. Edwards DK, Dyer WM, Northway WH. Twelve years experience with bronchopulmonary dysplasia. Pediatrics 1977;59:839–46.

70. Taghizadeh A, Reynolds EOR. Pathogenesis of bronchopulmonary dysplasia following hyaline membrane disease. Am J Pathol 1976;82:241–64.

71. Chang LYL, Subramaniam M, Yoder BA, et al. A catalytic antioxidant attenuates alveolar structural remodeling in bronchopulmonary dysplasia. Am J Respir Crit Care Med 2003;167:57–64.

72. Erickson AM, de la Monte SM, Moore GW, et al. The progression of morphologic changes in bronchopulmonary dysplasia. Am J Pathol 1987;127:474–84.

73. Jacob SV, Lands LC, Coates AL, et al. Exercise ability in survivors of severe bronchopulmonary dysplasia. Am J Respir Crit Care Med 1997;155:1925–9.

74. Anderson WR, Engel RR. Cardiopulmonary sequelae of reparative stages of

bronchopulmonary dysplasia. Arch Pathol Lab Med 1983;107:603–8.

75. Chambers HM, van Velzen D. Ventilator-related pathology in the extremely immature lung. Pathology 1989;21: 79–83.

76. Coalson JJ. Pathology of new bronchopulmonary dysplasia. Semin Neonatol 2003;8:73–81.

77. Boggaram V. Regulation of lung surfactant protein gene expression. Front Biosci 2003;8:d751–64.

78. McFetridge L, McMorrow A, Morrison PJ, et al. Surfactant metabolism dysfunction and childhood interstitial lung disease (chILD). Ulster Med J 2009;78:7–9.

79. Nogee LM, Demello DE, Dehner LP, et al. Brief report – deficiency of pulmonary surfactant protein-B in congenital alveolar proteinosis. N Engl J Med 1993;328: 406–10.

80. Nogee L, Garnier G, Dietz H, et al. A mutation in the surfactant protein B gene responsible for fatal neonatal respiratory disease in multiple kindreds. J Clin Invest 1994;93:1860–3.

81. Demello DE, Heyman S, Phelps DS, et al. Ultrastructure of lung in surfactant protein B deficiency. Am J Respir Cell Mol Biol 1994;11:230–9.

82. Ball R, Chetcuti PAJ, Beverley D. Fatal familial surfactant protein B deficiency. Arch Dis Child 1995;73:F53.

83. Demello DE, Nogee LM, Heyman S, et al. Molecular and phenotypic variability in the congenital alveolar proteinosis syndrome associated with inherited surfactant protein B deficiency. J Pediatr 1994;125:43–50.

84. Nogee LM, Wert SE, Proffit SA, et al. Allelic heterogeneity in hereditary surfactant protein B (SP-B) deficiency. Am J Respir Crit Care Med 2000;161:973–81.

85. Dunbar AE, III, Wert SE, Ikegami M, et al. Prolonged survival in hereditary surfactant protein B (SP-B) deficiency associated with a novel splicing mutation. Pediatr Res 2000;48:275–82.

86. Mildenberger E, Demello DE, Lin ZW, et al. Focal congenital alveolar proteinosis associated with abnormal surfactant protein B messenger RNA. Chest 2001;119:645–7.

87. Clark JC, Wert SE, Bachurski CJ, et al. Targeted disruption of the surfactant protein B gene disrupts surfactant homeostasis, causing respiratory failure in newborn mice. Proc Natl Acad Sci U S A 1995;92:7794–8.

88. Stahlman MT, Gray MP, Falconieri MW, et al. Lamellar body formation in normal and surfactant protein B-deficient fetal mice. Lab Invest 2000;80:395–403.

89. Nogee LM, Dunbar AE, III, Wert SE, et al. A mutation in the surfactant protein C gene associated with familial interstitial lung disease. N Engl J Med 2001;344:573–9.

90. Thomas AQ, Lane K, Phillips J, et al. Heterozygosity for a surfactant protein C gene mutation associated with usual interstitial pneumonitis and cellular nonspecific interstitial pneumonitis in one kindred. Am J Respir Crit Care Med 2002;165:1322–8.

91. Fan LL, Langston C. Pediatric interstitial lung disease – Children are not small adults. Am J Respir Crit Care Med 2002;165:1466–7.

92. Cutz E, Wert SE, Nogee LM, et al. Deficiency of lamellar bodies in alveolar type II cells associated with fatal respiratory disease in a full-term infant. Am J Respir Crit Care Med 2000;161:608–14.

93. Tryka AF, Wert SE, Mazursky JE, et al. Absence of lamellar bodies with accumulation of dense bodies characterizes a novel form of congenital surfactant defect. Pediatr Dev Pathol 2000;3:335–45.

94. Shulenin S, Nogee LM, Annilo T, et al. ABCA3 gene mutations in newborns with fatal surfactant deficiency. N Engl J Med 2004;350:1296–303.

95. Garmany TH, Moxley MA, White FV, et al. Surfactant composition and function in patients with ABCA3 mutations. Pediatr Res 2006;59:801–5.

96. Doan ML, Guillerman RP, Dishop MK, et al. Clinical, radiological and pathological features of ABCA3 mutations in children. Thorax 2008;63:366–73.

97. Young LR, Nogee LM, Barnett B, et al. Usual interstitial pneumonia in an adolescent with ABCA3 mutations. Chest 2008;134:192–5.

98. Bruder E, Hofmeister J, Aslanidis C, et al. Ultrastructural and molecular analysis in fatal neonatal interstitial pneumonia caused by a novel ABCA3 mutation. Mod Pathol 2007;20:1009–18.

99. Bullard JE, Wert SE, Whitsett JA, et al. ABCA3 mutations associated with pediatric interstitial lung disease. Am J Respir Crit Care Med 2005;172:1026–31.

100. Buchta RM, Park S, Giammona ST. Desquamative interstitial pneumonia in a 7-week-old infant. Am J Dis Child 1970;120:341–3.

101. Bhagwat AG, Wentworth P, Conen RE. Observation on the relationship of desquamative interstitial pneumonia and pulmonary alveolar proteinosis in childhood: A pathologic and experimental study. Chest 1970;58:326–32.

102. Wigger HJ, Berdon WE, Ores CN. Fatal desquamative interstitial pneumonia in an infant. Arch Pathol Lab Med 1977;101:129–32.

103. Fisher M, Roggli V, Merten D, et al. Coexisting endogenous lipoid pneumonia, cholesterol granulomas, and pulmonary alveolar proteinosis in a pediatric population: a clinical, radiographic, and pathologic correlation. Pediatr Pathol 1992;12:365–83.

104. McDonald JW, Roggli VL, Bradford WD. Coexisting endogenous and exogenous lipoid pneumonia and alveolar proteinosis in a patient with neurodevelopmental disease. Pediatr Pathol 1993;14:505–11.

105. Sato K, Takahashi H, Amano H, et al. Diffuse progressive pulmonary interstitial and intra-alveolar cholesterol granulomas in childhood. Eur Respir J 1996;9:2419–22.

106. Nakatani Y, Nakamura N, Sano J, et al. Interstitial pneumonia in Hermansky–Pudlak syndrome: significance of florid foamy swelling/degeneration (giant lamellar body degeneration) of type-2 pneumocytes. Virchows Archiv 2000;437:304–13.

107. Tang X, Yamanaka S, Miyagi Y, et al. Lung pathology of pale ear mouse (model of Hermansky–Pudlak syndrome 1) and beige mouse (model of Chediak–Higashi syndrome): Severity of giant lamellar body degeneration of type II pneumocytes correlates with interstitial inflammation. Pathology International 2005;55: 137–43.

108. Katzenstein ALA, Gordon LP, Oliphant M, et al. Chronic pneumonitis of infancy: a unique form of interstitial lung disease occurring in early childhood. Am J Surg Pathol 1995;19:439–47.

109. Parto K, Maki L, Pelliniemi LJ, et al. Abnormal pulmonary macrophages in lysinuric protein intolerance: ultrastructural, morphometric, and X-ray microanalytic study. Arch Pathol Lab Med 1994;118:536–41.

110. Parto K, Kallajoki M, Aho H, et al. Pulmonary alveolar proteinosis and glomerulonephritis in lysinuric protein intolerance: case reports and autopsy findings of four pediatric patients. Hum Pathol 1994;25:400–7.

111. McManus DT, Moore R, Hill CM, et al. Necropsy findings in lysinuric protein intolerance. J Clin Pathol 1996;49:345–7.

112. Schroeder SA, Shannon DC, Mark EJ. Cellular interstitial pneumonitis in infants. A clinicopathologic study. Chest 1992;101:1065–9.

113. Boyce JA, Mark EJ, Bramson RT, et al. A four-month-old girl with chronic cyanosis and diffuse pulmonary infiltrates. Cellular interstitial pneumonitis. N Engl J Med 1999;341:2075–83.

114. Canakis AM, Cutz E, Manson D, et al. Pulmonary interstitial glycogenosis – A new variant of neonatal interstitial lung disease. Am J Respir Crit Care Med 2002;165:1557–65.

115. Deutsch GH, Young LR. Histologic resolution of pulmonary interstitial glycogenosis. Pediatr Dev Pathol 2009;12:475–80.

116. Becker BA, Demello DE, Noyes BE. Selective antibody deficiency in two children with pulmonary interstitial glycogenosis. J Allergy Clin Immunol 2005;115:S159.

117. Melly L, Sebire NJ, Malone M, et al. Capillary apposition and density in the diagnosis of alveolar capillary dysplasia. Histopathology 2008;53:450–7.

118. Smets K, Dhaene K, Schelstraete P, et al. Neonatal pulmonary interstitial glycogen accumulation disorder. European Journal of Pediatrics 2004;163:408–9.

119. Stocker JT, Madewell JE. Persistent interstitial pulmonary emphysema: another complication of the respiratory distress syndrome. Pediatrics 1977;59:847–57.

120. Brewer LL, Moskowitz PS, Carrington CB, et al. Pneumatosis pulmonalis. A complication of the idiopathic respiratory distress syndrome. Am J Pathol 1979;95:171–90.

121. Wilson JM, Mark EJ, Connolly SA, et al. A preterm newborn female triplet with diffuse cystic changes in the left lung – Pulmonary interstitial emphysema, localized, persistent. N Engl J Med 1997;337:916–24.

122. Deroux SJ, Prendergast NC. Large sub-pleural air cysts: an extreme form of pulmonary interstitial emphysema. Pediatr Radiol 1998;28:981–3.

123. Donnelly LF, Lucaya J, Ozelame V, et al. CT findings and temporal course of persistent pulmonary interstitial emphysema in neonates: a multiinstitutional study. AJR Am J Roentgenol 2003;180:1129–33.

124. Belcher E, Abbasi MA, Hansell DM, et al. Persistent interstitial pulmonary emphysema requiring pneumonectomy. J Thorac Cardiovasc Surg 2009;138:237–9.

125. Wood BP, Anderson VM, Mauk JE, et al. Pulmonary lymphatic air: locating 'pulmonary interstitial emphysema' of the premature infant. Am J Roentgenol 1982;138:809–14.

126. Lavezzi WA, Keough KM, Der'Ohannesian P, et al. The use of pulmonary interstitial emphysema as an indicator of live birth. Am J Forensic Med Pathol 2003;24:87–91.

127. Deterding RR, Pye C, Fan LL, et al. Persistent tachypnea of infancy is associated with neuroendocrine cell hyperplasia. Pediatr Pulmonol 2005;40:157–65.

128. Morin FC, Stenmark KR. Persistent pulmonary hypertension of the newborn. Am J Respir Crit Care Med 1995;151:2010–32.

129. Haworth SG, Reid L. Persistent fetal circulation: newly recognized structural features. J Pediatr 1976;88:614–20.

130. Boggs S, Harris MC, Hoffman DJ, et al. Misalignment of pulmonary veins with alveolar capillary dysplasia: affected siblings and variable phenotypic expression. J Pediatr 1994;124:125–8.

131. Gutierrez C, Rodriguez A, Palenzuela S, et al. Congenital misalignment of pulmonary veins with alveolar capillary dysplasia causing persistent neonatal pulmonary hypertension: report of two affected siblings. Pediatr Dev Pathol 2000;3:271–6.

132. Roberts JD, Polaner DM, Lang P, et al. Inhaled nitric oxide in persistent pulmonary hypertension of the newborn. Lancet 1992;340:818–9.

133. Kinsella JP, Neish SR, Shaffer E, et al. Low-dose inhalational nitric oxide in persistent pulmonary hypertension of the newborn. Lancet 1992;340:819–20.

134. Deutsch GH, Young LR, Deterding RR, et al. Diffuse lung disease in young children: application of a novel classification scheme. Am J Respir Crit Care Med 2007;176:1120–8.

135. Reference removed in text.

136. Rutledge JC, Jensen P. Acinar dysplasia: a new form of pulmonary maldevelopment. Hum Pathol 1986;17:1290–3.

137. Moerman P, Vanhole C, Devlieger H, et al. Severe primary pulmonary hypoplasia ('acinar dysplasia') in sibs: a genetically determined mesodermal defect? J Med Genet 1998;35:964–5.

138. Gillespie LM, Fenton AC, Wright C. Acinar dysplasia: a rare cause of neonatal respiratory failure. Acta Paediatr 2004;93:712–13.

139. Wright C. Congenital malformations of the lung. Current Diagnostic Pathology 2006;12:191–201.

140. MacMahon HE. Congenital alveolar dysplasia of the lungs. Am J Pathol 1948;24:919–31.

141. Janney CG, Askin FB, Kuhn C. Congenital alveolar capillary dysplasia – an unusual cause of respiratory distress in the newborn. Am J Clin Pathol 1981;76:722–7.

142. Wagenvoort CA. Misalignment of lung vessels: a syndrome causing persistent neonatal pulmonary hypertension. Hum Pathol 1986;17:727–30.

143. Cater G, Thibeault DW, Beatty EC, et al. Misalignment of lung vessels and alveolar capillary dysplasia: a cause of persistent pulmonary hypertension. J Pediatr 1989;114:293–300.

144. Oldenburg J, Vanderpal HJH, Schrevel LS, et al. Misalignment of lung vessels and alveolar capillary dysplasia. Histopathology 1995;27:192–4.

145. Vassal HB, Malone M, Petros AJ, et al. Familial persistent pulmonary hypertension of the newborn resulting from misalignment of the pulmonary vessels (congenital alveolar capillary dysplasia). J Med Genet 1998;35:58–60.

146. Eulmesekian P, Cutz E, Parvez B, et al. Alveolar capillary dysplasia: a six-year single center experience. J Perinat Med 2005;33:347–52.

147. Sen P, Thakur N, Stockton DW, et al. Expanding the phenotype of alveolar capillary dysplasia (ACD). J Pediatr 2004;145:646–51.

148. Carden KA, Boiselle PM, Waltz DA, et al. Tracheomalacia and tracheobronchomalacia in children and adults: an in-depth review. Chest 2005;127:984–1005.

Further disorders of development and growth

149. Silver MM, Thurston WA, Patrick JE. Perinatal pulmonary hyperplasia due to laryngeal atresia. Hum Pathol 1988;19:110–13.

150. Hopkinson JM. Congenital absence of the trachea. J Pathol 1972;107:63–7.

151. Aboussouan LS, Odonovan PB, Moodie DS, et al. Hypoplastic trachea in Down's syndrome. Am Rev Respir Dis 1993;147:72–5.

152. Berdon WE, Baker DH, Wung J-T, et al. Complete cartilage-ring tracheal stenosis associated with anomalous left pulmonary artery: the ring–sling complex. J Radiol 1984;152:57–64.

153. Ravenna F, Caramori G, Panella GL, et al. An unusual case of congenital short trachea with very long bronchi mimicking bronchial asthma. Thorax 2002;57:372–3.

154. Wailoo MP, Emery JL. The trachea in children with tracheo-oesophageal fistula. Histopathology 1979;3:329–38.

155. Emery JL, Haddadin AJ. Squamous epithelium in the respiratory tract of children with tracheo-oesophageal fistula. Arch Dis Child 1971;46:236–42.

156. Tanaka H, Igarashi T, Teramoto S, et al. Lymphoepithelial cysts in the mediastinum with an opening to the trachea. Respiration 1995;62:110–13.

157. Deb S, Ali MB, Fonseca P. Congenital bronchoesophageal fistula in an adult. Chest 1998;114:1784–6.

158. Jacobs IN, Wetmore RF, Tom LW, et al. Tracheobronchomalacia in children. Arch Otolaryngol Head Neck Surg 1994;120:154–8.

159. Boogaard R, Huijsmans SH, Pijnenburg MWH, et al. Tracheomalacia and bronchomalacia in children: incidence and patient characteristics. Chest 2005;128:3391–7.

160. Hicks J, De Jong A, Barrish J, Zhu SH, Popek E. Tracheomalacia in a neonate with Kniest dysplasia: histopathologic and ultrastructural features. Ultrastruct Pathol 2001;25:79–83.

161. Stigol LC, Traversaro J, Trigo ER. Carinal trifurcation with congenital tracheobiliary fistula. Pediatrics 1966;37:89–91.

162. de Carvalho CRR, Barbas CSV, Guarnieri RDDG, et al. Congenital bronchobiliary fistula: first case in an adult. Thorax 1988;43:792–3.

163. Barbato A, Novello A, Zanolin D, et al. Diverticulosis of the main bronchi – a rare cause of recurrent bronchopneumonia in a child. Thorax 1993;48:187–8.

164. Bloor CM, Liebow AA. In: Sonnenblick E, Parmley WW, editors. The Pulmonary and Bronchial Circulations in Congenital Heart Disease. New York: Plenum; 1980.

165. Gonzalez-Crussi F, Padilla L-M, Miller JK, et al. 'Bridging bronchus', a previously undescribed airway anomaly. Am J Dis Child 1976;130:1015–18.

166. Clements BS, Warner JO. The crossover lung segment: congenital malformation associated with a variant of scimitar syndrome. Thorax 1987;42:417–19.

167. Warner JO, Clements BS. The crossover lung segment: congenital malformation associated with a variant of scimitar syndrome. Thorax 1987;42:992.

168. Kelly DR, Mroczek EC, Galliani CA, et al. Horseshoe lung and crossover lung segment: a unifying concept of fusion events in the lungs and other paired organs. In: Askin FB, Langston C, Rosenberg HS, et al. eds. Pulmonary Disease. Basel: Karger; 1995. p. 183–213.

169. Frank JL, Poole CA, Rosas G. Horseshoe lung: clinical, pathologic, and radiologic features and a new plain film finding. AJR Am J Roentgenol 1986;146:217–26.

170. Kramer MS. 'Horseshoe' lung: report of five new cases. Am J Roentgenol 1986;146:211–5.

171. Ersoz A, Soncul H, Gokgoz L, et al. Horseshoe lung with left lung hypoplasia. Thorax 1992;47:205–6.

172. Langlois SLP, Henderson DW. Variant pulmonary lobation. Australas Radiol 1980;24:255–61.

173. Landing BH, Lawrence TYK, Payne VC, et al. Bronchial anatomy syndromes with abnormal visceral situs, abnormal spleen and congenital heart disease. Am J Cardiol 1971;28:456–62.

174. Ivemark BI. Implications of agenesis of the spleen on the pathogenesis of cono-truncus anomalies in childhood. An analysis of the heart malformations in the splenic agenesis syndrome. With fourteen new cases. Acta Paediatrica Scand 1955;44:1–110.

175. Maier HC. Bronchogenic cysts of mediastinum. Ann Surg 1948;127:476–502.

176. Aktogu S, Yuncu G, Halilcolar H, et al. Bronchogenic cysts: clinicopathological presentation and treatment. Eur Respir J 1996;9:2017–21.

177. Haddadin WJ, Reid R, Jindal RM. A retroperitoneal bronchogenic cyst: a rare cause of a mass in the adrenal region. J Clin Pathol 2001;54:801–2.

178. Kim NR, Kim HH, Suh YL. Cutaneous bronchogenic cyst of the abdominal wall. Pathol Int 2001;51:970–3.

179. Ingu A, Watanabe A, Ichimiya Y, et al. Retroperitoneal bronchogenic cyst – A case report. Chest 2002;121:1357–9.

180. Matsubayashi J, Ishida T, Ozawa T, et al. Subphrenic bronchopulmonary foregut malformation with pulmonary-sequestration-like features. Pathol Int 2003;53:313–6.

181. Pradeep KE. Cutaneous bronchogenic cyst: an under-recognised clinicopathological entity. J Clin Pathol 2009;62:384.

182. Okada Y, Mori H, Maeda T, et al. Congenital mediastinal bronchogenic cyst with malignant transformation: an autopsy autopsy. Pathol Int 1996;46:594–600.

183. Soosay GN, Baudouin SV, Hanson PJV, et al. Symptomatic cysts in otherwise normal lungs of children and adults. Histopathology 1992;20:517–22.

184. Simon G, Reid L. Atresia of an apical bronchus of the left upper lobe – report of three cases. Br J Dis Chest 1963;57:126–32.

185. Meng RL, Jensik RJ, Faber LP, et al. Bronchial atresia. Ann Thorac Surg 1978;25:184–92.

186. Jederlinic PJ, Sicilian LS, Baigelman W, et al. Congenital bronchial atresia. A report of 4 cases and a review of the literature. Medicine (Baltimore) 1986;65:73–83.

187. Rossoff LJ, Steinberg H. Bronchial atresia and mucocele: a report of two cases. Respir Med 1994;88:789–91.

188. Williams AJ, Schuster SR. Bronchial atresia associated with a bronchogenic cyst. Evidence of early appearance of atretic segments. Chest 1985;87:396–8.

189. Gustafson RA, Murray GF, Wardon HE, et al. Intralobar sequestration. A missed diagnosis. Ann Thorac Surg 1989;47:841–7.

190. Gerle RD, Jaretzkia A, Ashley CA, et al. Congenital bronchopulmonary-foregut malformation: pulmonary sequestration communicating with the gastrointestinal tract. N Engl J Med 1968;278:1413–19.

191. Beskin CA. Intralobar enteric sequestration of the lung containing aberrant pancreas. J Thorac Cardiovasc Surg 1961;41:314–17.

192. Corrin B, Danel C, Allaway A, et al. Intralobar pulmonary sequestration of ectopic pancreatic tissue with gastro-pancreatic duplication. Thorax 1985;40:637–8.

193. Flye MW, Izant RJ. Extralobar pulmonary sequestration with esophageal communication and complete duplication of the colon. Surgery 1972;71:744–52.

194. Aulicino MR, Reis ED, Dolgin SE, et al. Intra-abdominal pulmonary sequestration exhibiting congenital cystic adenomatoid malformation – report of a case and review of the literature. Arch Pathol Lab Med 1994;118:1034–7.

195. Fraggetta F, Cacciaguerra S, Nash R, et al. Intra-abdominal pulmonary sequestration associated with congenital cystic adenomatoid malformation of the lung: Just an unusual combination of rare pathologies? Pathol Res Pract 1998;194:209–11.

196. Samuel M, Burge DM. Management of antenatally diagnosed pulmonary sequestration associated with congenital cystic adenomatoid malformation. Thorax 1999;54:701–6.

197. Sade RM, Clouse M, Ellis Jr FH. The spectrum of pulmonary sequestration. Ann Thorac Surg 1974;18:644–55.

198. Demos NJ, Teresi A. Congenital lung malformations. A unified concept and a case report. J Thorac Cardiovasc Surg 1975;70:260–4.

199. Heithoff KB, Sane SM, Williams HJ, et al. Bronchopulmonary foregut malformations. A unifying etiological concept. Am J Roentgenol 1976;126:46–55.

200. Pryce DM. Lower accessory pulmonary artery with intralobar sequestration of lung: a report of seven cases. J Pathol Bacteriol 1946;58:457–67.

201. Carter R. Pulmonary sequestration. Ann Thorac Surg 1969;7:68–85.

202. Gebauer PW, Mason CB. Intralobar pulmonary sequestration associated with anomalous pulmonary vessels. Dis Chest 1959;35:282–8.

203. Stocker JT, Malczak HT. A study of pulmonary ligament arteries. Relationship to intralobar sequestration. Chest 1984;86:611–5.

204. Stocker JT. Sequestration of the lung. Semin Diagn Pathol 1986;3:106–21.

205. Smith RA. A theory of the origin of intralobar sequestration of lung. Thorax 1956;11:10–24.

206. Hruban RH, Shumway SJ, Orel SB, et al. Congenital bronchopulmonary foregut malformations: intralobar and extralobar pulmonary sequestrations communicating with the foregut. Am J Clin Pathol 1989;91:403–9.

207. Baar HS, d'Abreu AL. Duplications of the foregut. Superior accessory lung (2 cases); epiphrenic oesophageal diverticulum; intrapericardial teratoid tumour; and oesophageal cyst. Br J Surg 1949;37:220–30.

208. Desai S, Dusmet M, Ladas G, et al. Secondary vascular changes in pulmonary sequestrations. Histopathology 2010;57:121–7.

209. Van Dijk C, Wagenvoort CA. The various types of congenital adenomatoid malformation of the lung. J Pathol 1973;110:131–4.

210. Cangiarella J, Greco MA, Askin F, et al. Congenital cystic adenomatoid malformation of the lung: insights into the pathogenesis utilizing quantitative analysis of vascular marker CD34 (QBEND-10) and cell proliferation marker MIB-1. Mod Pathol 1995;8:913–18.

211. Morotti RA, Cangiarella J, Gutierrez MC, et al. Congenital cystic adenomatoid malformation of the lung (CCAM): Evaluation of the cellular components. Hum Pathol 1999;30:618–25.

212. Stoerk O. Ueber angeborene blasige mis-bildung der lung. Wien Klin Wschr 1897;10:25–31.

213. Ch'in KY, Tang MY. Congenital adenomatoid malformation of one lobe of a lung with general anasarca. Arch Pathol 1949;48:221–9.

214. Stocker JT, Madewell JE, Drake RM. Congenital cystic adenomatoid

malformation of the lung. Hum Pathol 1977;8:155–71.

215. Ostor AG, Fortune DW. Congenital cystic adenomatoid malformation of the lung. Am J Clin Pathol 1978;70: 595–604.

216. Bale PM. Congenital cystic malformation of the lung. A form of congenital bronchiolar ('adenomatoid') malformation. Am J Clin Pathol 1979;71:411–20.

217. Stocker JT. Congenital pulmonary airway malformation – a new name for an expanded classification of congenital cystic adenomatoid malformation of the lung. Histopathology 2002;41:424–58.

218. Chambers HM. Congenital acinar aplasia – an extreme form of pulmonary maldevelopment. Pathology 1991;23:69–71.

219. Davidson LA, Batman P, Fagan DG. Congenital acinar dysplasia: a rare cause of pulmonary hypoplasia. Histopathology 1998;32:57–9.

220. Langston C. New concepts in the pathology of congenital lung malformations. Semin Pediatr Surg 2003;12:17–37.

221. Hill DA, Jarzembowski JA, Priest JR, et al. Type I pleuropulmonary blastoma: pathology and biology study of 51 cases from the international pleuropulmonary blastoma registry. Am J Surg Pathol 2008;32:282–95.

222. Dempster AG. Adenomatoid hamartoma of the lung in a neonate. J Clin Pathol 1969;22:401–6.

223. Miller RK, Sieber WK, Yunis EJ. Congenital adenomatoid malformation of the lung. A report of 17 cases and review of the literature. In: Sommers SC, Rosen PP, editors. Pathology Annual Vol 15 Part 1. New York: Appleton-Century-Crofts; 1980. p. 387–406.

224. Avitabile AM, Hulnick DH, Greco MA, et al. Congenital cystic adenomatoid malformation of the lung in adults. Am J Surg Pathol 1984;8:193–202.

225. Kinane TB, Mark EJ, Connolly SA, et al. A newborn triplet with episodes of respiratory distress and a pulmonary mass – congenital cystic adenomatoid malformation of the lung. N Engl J Med 1996;334:1726–32.

226. MacSweeney F, Papagiannopoulos K, Goldstraw P, et al. An assessment of the expanded classification of congenital cystic adenomatoid malformations and their relationship to malignant transformation. Am J Surg Pathol 2003;27:1139–46.

227. Imai Y, Mark EJ. Cystic adenomatoid change is common to various forms of cystic lung diseases of children: a clinicopathologic analysis of 10 cases with emphasis on tracing the bronchial tree. Arch Pathol Lab Med 2002;126:934–40.

228. Ajitsaria R, Awad WI, Jaffe A, et al. Congenital lung abnormality in a 1-yr old

– congenital intradiaphragmatic cystic lung abnormality, Stocker's classification type 2. Eur Resp J 2004;23:348–51.

229. Mendoza A, Wolf P, Edwards DK, et al. Prenatal ultrasonographic diagnosis of congenital adenomatoid malformation of the lung. Arch Pathol Lab Med 1986;110:402–4.

230. Lujan M, Bosque M, Mirapeix RM, et al. Late-onset congenital cystic adenomatoid malformation of the lung – embryology, clinical symptomatology, diagnostic procedures, therapeutic approach and clinical follow-up. Respiration 2002;69:148–54.

231. Cachia R, Sobonya RE. Congenital cystic adenomatoid malformation of the lung with bronchial atresia. Hum Pathol 1981;12:947–50.

232. Moerman P, Fryns JP, Vandenberghe K, et al. Pathogenesis of congenital cystic adenomatoid malformation of the lung. Histopathology 1992;21:315–21.

233. Sheffield EA, Addis BJ, Corrin B, et al. Epithelial hyperplasia and malignant change in congenital lung cysts. J Clin Pathol 1987;40:612–14.

234. Ribet ME, Copin MC, Soots JG, et al. Bronchioloalveolar carcinoma and congenital cystic adenomatoid malformation. Ann Thorac Surg 1995;60:1126–8.

235. Kaslovsky RA, Purdy S, Dangman BC, et al. Bronchioloalveolar carcinoma in a child with congenital cystic adenomatoid malformation. Chest 1997;112:548–51.

236. Ota H, Langston C, Honda T, et al. Histochemical analysis of mucous cells of congenital adenomatoid malformation of the lung: Insights into the carcinogenesis of pulmonary adenocarcinoma expressing gastric mucins. Am J Clin Pathol 1998;110:450–5.

237. Ioachimescu OC, Mehta AC. From cystic pulmonary airway malformation, to bronchioloalveolar carcinoma and adenocarcinoma of the lung. Eur Respir J 2005;26:1181–7.

238. Lantuejoul S, Nicholson AG, Sartori G, et al. Mucinous cells in type 1 pulmonary congenital cystic adenomatoid malformation as mucinous bronchioloalveolar carcinoma precursors. Am J Surg Pathol 2007;31:961–9.

239. Lantuejoul S, Ferretti GR, Goldstraw P, et al. Metastases from bronchioloalveolar carcinomas associated with long-standing type 1 congenital cystic adenomatoid malformations. A report of two cases. Histopathology 2006;48:204–6.

240. Stacher E, Ullmann R, Halbwedl I, et al. Atypical goblet cell hyperplasia in congenital cystic adenomatoid malformation as a possible preneoplasia for pulmonary adenocarcinoma in childhood: a genetic analysis*1. Human Pathology 2004;35:565–70.

241. Prichard MG, Brown PJ, Sterrett GF. Bronchioloalveolar carcinoma arising in

longstanding lung cysts. Thorax 1984;39:545–9.

242. Fraggetta F, Davenport M, Magro G, et al. Striated muscle cells in non-neoplastic lung tissue: a clinicopathologic study. Hum Pathol 2000;31:1477–81.

243. Lienicke U, Hammer H, Schneider M, et al. Rhabdomyomatous dysplasia of the newborn lung associated with multiple congenital malformations of the heart and great vessels. Pediatr Pulmonol 2002;34:222–5.

244. Papagiannopoulos KA, Sheppard M, Bush A, et al. Pleuropulmonary blastoma: is prophylactic resection of congenital lung cysts effective? Ann Thorac Surg 2001;72:604–5.

245. Hill DA, Dehner LP. A cautionary note about congenital cystic adenomatoid malformation (CCAM) type 4. Am J Surg Pathol 2004;28:554–5.

246. LaBerge JM, Flageole H, Pugash D, et al. Outcome of the prenatally diagnosed congenital cystic adenomatoid lung malformation: a Canadian experience. Fetal Diagn Ther 2001;16:178–86.

247. Cha I, Adzick NS, Harrison MR, et al. Fetal congenital cystic adenomatoid malformations of the lung: A clinicopathologic study of eleven cases. Am J Surg Pathol 1997;21:537–44.

248. Kreiger PA, Ruchelli ED, Mahboubi S, et al. Fetal pulmonary malformations: defining histopathology. Am J Surg Pathol 2006;30:643–9.

249. McGinnis M, Jacobs G, Elnaggar A, et al. Congenital peribronchial myofibroblastic tumor (so-called congenital leiomyosarcoma) – a distinct neonatal lung lesion associated with nonimmune hydrops-fetalis. Mod Pathol 1993;6:487–92.

250. Alobeid B, Beneck D, Sreekantaiah C, et al. Congenital pulmonary myofibroblastic tumor: A case report with cytogenetic analysis and review of the literature. Am J Surg Pathol 1997;21:610–14.

251. Maguire CP, Hayes JP, Hayes M, et al. Three cases of pulmonary aspergilloma in adult patients with cystic fibrosis. Thorax 1995;50:805–6.

252. Williams H, Campbell P. Generalized bronchiectasis associated with deficiency of cartilage in the bronchial tree. Arch Dis Child 1960;35:182–91.

253. Williams HE, Landau LI, Phelan PD. Generalized bronchiectasis due to extensive deficiency of bronchial cartilage. Arch Dis Child 1972;47:423–8.

254. Mitchell RE, Bury RG. Congenital bronchiectasis due to deficiency of bronchial cartilage (Williams–Campbell syndrome). J Pediatr 1975;87:230–4.

255. Lee P, Bush A, Warner JO. Left bronchial isomerism associated with bronchomalacia, presenting with intractable wheeze. Thorax 1991;46:459–61.

256. Wayne KS, Taussig LM. Probable familial congenital bronchiectasis due to cartilage deficiency (Williams–Campbell syndrome). Am Rev Respir Dis 1976;114:15–22.

257. Jones VF, Eid NS, Franco SM, et al. Familial congenital bronchiectasis: Williams–Campbell syndrome. Pediatr Pulmonol 1993;16:263–7.

258. Notarangelo LD, Plebani A, Mazzolari E, et al. Genetic causes of bronchiectasis: primary immune deficiencies and the lung. Respiration 2007;74:264–75.

259. Rodriguez-Cintron W, Guntupalli K, Fraire AE. Bronchiectasis and homozygous (piZZ) α1-antitrypsin deficiency in a young man. Thorax 1995;50:424–5.

260. Mounier-Kuhn P. Dilatation de la trachée; constatations radiographiques et bronchoscopiques. Lyon Med 1932;150:106–9.

261. Al-Mallah Z, Quantock OP. Tracheobronchomegaly. Thorax 1968;23:320–4.

262. Himalstein MR, Gallagher JC. Tracheobronchomegaly. Ann Otol Rhinol Laryngol 1973;82:223–7.

263. Van Schoor J, Joos G, Pauwels R. Tracheobronchomegaly – the Mounier–Kuhn syndrome: report of two cases and a review of the literature. Eur Respir J 1991;4:1303–6.

264. Schwartz M, Rossoff L. Tracheobronchomegaly. Chest 1994;106:1589–90.

265. Schwarz MI. A 60-year-old man with recurrent pneumonias – The underlying pathologic finding is poorly formed or absent bronchial cartilage. Chest 2001;119:1590–2.

265a. Noori F, Abduljawad S, Suffin D, et al. Mounier-kuhn syndrome: a case report. Lung 2010:188:353–4.

266. Vidal C, Pena F, Mosquera MR, et al. Tracheobronchomegaly associated with interstitial pulmonary fibrosis. Respiration 1991;58:207–10.

267. Johnston RF, Green RA. Tracheobronchiomegaly: Report of five cases and demonstration of familial occurrence. Am Rev Respir Dis 1965;91:35–50.

268. Aaby GV, Blake HA. Tracheobronchiomegaly. Ann Thorac Surg 1966;2:64–70.

269. Wanderer AA, Ellis EF, Goltz RW, et al. Tracheobronchiomegaly and acquired cutis laxa in a child. Pediatrics 1969;44: 709–15.

270. Sane AC, Effmann EL, Brown SD. Tracheobronchiomegaly – the Mounier–Kuhn syndrome in a patient with the Kenny–Caffey syndrome. Chest 1992;102:618–19.

271. Katz I, Levine M, Herman P. Tracheobronchiomegaly: the Mounier–Kuhn syndrome. AJR Am J Roentgenol 1962;88:1084–93.

272. Siewert A. Uber einem Fall von Bronchiektasien bei einem Patienten mit situs inversus viscerum. Klin Wochenschr 1904;41:139–41.

273. Kartagener M. Zur Pathogenese der Bronchiektasien. I Mitteilung Bronchiektasien bei situs viscerum inversus. Beitr Klin Tuberk 1933;83:489–501.

274. Camner P, Mossberg B, Afzelius BA. Evidence for congenitally non-functioning cilia in the tracheobronchial tract in two subjects. Am Rev Respir Dis 1975;112:807–9.

275. Nonaka S, Tanaka Y, Okada Y, et al. Randomization of left–right asymmetry due to loss of nodal cilia generating leftward flow of extraembryonic fluid in mice lacking KIF3B motor protein. Cell 1998;95:829–37.

276. Afzelius BA. Cilia-related diseases. J Pathol 2004;204:470–7.

277. Eliasson R, Mossberg B, Camner P, et al. The immotile-cilia syndrome. A congenital ciliary abnormality as an etiologic factor in chronic airway infections and male sterility. N Engl J Med 1977;297:1–6.

278. Afzelius BA. Immotile cilia syndrome: past, present, and prospects for the future. Thorax 1998;53:894–7.

279. Rossman CM, Forrest JB, Lee RMKW, et al. The dyskinetic cilia syndrome. Ciliary motility in immotile cilia syndrome. Chest 1980;78:580–2.

280. Storm van's GK, Omran H. Primary ciliary dyskinesia: clinical presentation, diagnosis and genetics. Ann Med 2005;37:439–49.

281. Hornef N, Olbrich H, Horvath J, et al. DNAH5 mutations are a common cause of primary ciliary dyskinesia with outer dynein arm defects. Am J Respir Crit Care Med 2006;174:120–6.

282. Schwabe GC, Hoffmann K, Loges NT, et al. Primary ciliary dyskinesia associated with normal axoneme ultrastructure is caused by DNAH11 mutations. Hum Mutat 2008;29:289–98.

282a. Pifferi M, Michelucci A, Conidi ME, et al. New DNAH11 mutations in primary ciliary dyskinesia with normal axonemal ultrastructure. Eur Respir J 2010;35: 1413–16.

283. Sturgess JM, Chao J, Wong J, et al. Cilia with defective radial spokes. A cause of human respiratory disease. N Engl J Med 1979;300:53–6.

284. Sturgess JM, Chao J, Turner JAP. Transposition of ciliary microtubules: another cause of impaired ciliary motility. N Engl J Med 1980;303:318–22.

285. Rutland J, Deiongh RU. Random ciliary orientation – a cause of respiratory tract disease. N Engl J Med 1990;323:1681–4.

286. Niggemann B, Muller A, Nolte A, et al. Abnormal length of cilia – a cause of primary ciliary dyskinesia – a case report. Eur J Pediatr 1992;151:73–5.

287. Rayner CFJ, Rutman A, Dewar A, et al. Ciliary disorientation alone as a cause of primary ciliary dyskinesia syndrome. Am J Respir Crit Care Med 1996;153:1123–9.

288. Plesec TP, Ruiz A, McMahon JT, et al. Ultrastructural abnormalities of respiratory cilia: a 25-year experience. Arch Pathol Lab Med 2008;132:1786–91.

289. Pifferi M, Cangiotti AM, Caramella D, et al. 'Cyst-like' structures within the ciliary shafts in children with bronchiectasis. Eur Respir J 2004;23:857–60.

290. Tsang KWT, Tipoe G, Sun J, et al. Severe bronchiectasis in patients with 'cystlike' structures within the ciliary shafts. Am J Respir Crit Care Med 2000;161:1300–5.

291. Kovesi T, Sinclair B, MacCormick J, et al. Primary ciliary dyskinesia associated with a novel microtubule defect in a child with Down's syndrome. Chest 2000;117: 1207–9.

292. Afzelius BA, Eliasson R, Johnsen O, et al. Lack of dynein arms in immotile human spermatozoa. J Cell Biol 1975;66:225–32.

293. Munro NC, Currie DC, Lindsay KS, et al. Fertility in men with primary ciliary dyskinesia presenting with respiratory infection. Thorax 1994;49:684–7.

294. Afzelius BA, Eliasson R. Male and female infertility problems in the immotile-cilia syndrome. Eur J Respir Dis 1983;64:144–7.

295. Greenstone MA, Dewar A, Cole PJ. Ciliary dyskinesia with normal ultrastructure. Thorax 1983;38:875–6.

296. Greenstone M, Rutman A, Dewar A, et al. Primary ciliary dyskinesia: cytological and clinical features. Q J Med 1988;253: 405–30.

297. Mierau GW, Agostini R, Beals TF, et al. The role of electron microscopy in evaluating ciliary dysfunction – report of a workshop. Ultrastruct Pathol 1992;16:245–54.

298. Deiongh RU, Rutland J. Ciliary defects in healthy subjects, bronchiectasis, and primary ciliary dyskinesia. Am J Respir Crit Care Med 1995;151:1559–67.

299. Rutland J, Cole PJ. Non-invasive sampling of nasal cilia for measurement of beat frequency and study of ultrastructure. Lancet 1980;2:564–5.

300. Rutland J, Dewar A, Cox T, et al. Nasal brushing for the study of ciliary ultrastructure. J Clin Pathol 1982;35:357–9.

301. Bush A, Cole P, Hariri M, et al. Primary ciliary dyskinesia: diagnosis and standards of care. Eur Resp J 1998;12:982–8.

302. Narang I, Ersu R, Wilson NM, et al. Nitric oxide in chronic airway inflammation in children: diagnostic use and pathophysiological significance. Thorax 2002;57:586–9.

303. Rutland J, Cox T, Dewar A, et al. Transitory ultrastructural abnormalities of cilia. Br J Dis Chest 1982;76:185–8.

304. Driscoll JA, Bhalla S, Liapis H, et al. Autosomal dominant polycystic kidney

disease is associated with an increased prevalence of radiographic bronchiectasis. Chest 2008;133:1181–8.

305. Dodge JA, Lewis PA, Stanton M, et al. Cystic fibrosis mortality and survival in the UK: 1947–2003. Eur Respir J 2007;29:522–6.

306. Clausiusz J. Hidden benefits. Available online at: http://www.people.virginia.edu/~rjh9u/cysfib.html 1997.

307. Wainwright BJ, Scambler PJ, Schmidtke J, et al. Localization of cystic fibrosis locus to chromosome 7cen-q22. Nature 1985;318:384–5.

308. Tsui LC, Buchwald M, Barker D, et al. Cystic fibrosis locus defined by a genetically linked polymorphic DNA marker. Science 1985;230:1054–7.

309. Davidson DJ, Porteous DJ. The genetics of cystic fibrosis lung disease. Thorax 1998;53:389–97.

310. Farral M, Law HY, Rodek CH, et al. First-trimester prenatal diagnosis of cystic fibrosis using linked DNA probes. Lancet 1986;i:1402–4.

311. Wald NJ. Couple screening for cystic fibrosis. Lancet 1991;338:1318–20.

312. Grody WW. Cystic fibrosis – Molecular diagnosis, population screening, and public policy. Arch Pathol Lab Med 1999;123:1041–6.

313. Lyon E, Miller C. Current challenges in cystic fibrosis screening. Arch Pathol Lab Med 2003;127:1133–9.

314. Kerem B-S, Rommens JM, Buchanan JA, et al. Identification of the cystic fibrosis gene: genetic analysis. Science 1989;245:1073–80.

315. Cutting GR, Kasch LM, Rosenstein BJ, et al. A cluster of cystic fibrosis mutations in the first nucleotide-binding fold of the cystic fibrosis conductant regulator protein. Nature 1990;346:366–9.

316. Davies JC, Alton EW. Airway gene therapy. Adv Genet 2005;54:291–314.

317. Koch C, Hoiby N. Pathogenesis of cystic fibrosis. Lancet 1993;341:1065–9.

318. Rutland J, Cole PJ. Nasal mucociliary clearance and ciliary beat frequency in cystic fibrosis compared with sinusitis and bronchiectasis. Thorax 1981;36:654–8.

319. Katz SM, Holsclaw DS. Ultrastructural features of respiratory cilia in cystic fibrosis. Am J Clin Pathol 1980;73:682–5.

320. Quinton PM. Chloride impermeability in cystic fibrosis. Nature 1983;301:421–2.

321. Welsh MJ, Liedtke CM. Chloride and potassium channels in cystic fibrosis airway epithelia. Nature 1986;322:467–70.

322. Tsui LC. The cystic fibrosis transmembrane conductance regulator gene. Am J Respir Crit Care Med 1995;151:S47–53.

323. Frizzell RA. Function of the cystic fibrosis transmembrane conductance regulator protein. Am J Respir Crit Care Med 1995;151:S54–8.

324. Puchelle E, Gaillard D, Ploton D, et al. Differential localization of the cystic

fibrosis transmembrane conductance regulator in normal and cystic fibrosis airway epithelium. Am J Respir Cell Mol Biol 1992;7:485–91.

325. Yang Y, Engelhardt JF, Wilson JM. Ultrastructural localization of variant forms of cystic fibrosis transmembrane conductance regulator in human bronchial epithelia of xenografts. Am J Respir Cell Mol Biol 1994;11:7–15.

326. Valman HB, France NE. The vas deferens in CF. Lancet 1969;ii:566–7.

327. Chillon M, Casals T, Mercier B, et al. Mutations in the cystic fibrosis gene in patients with congenital absence of the vas deferens. N Engl J Med 1995;332:1475–80.

328. Smith JJ, Travis SM, Greenberg EP, et al. Cystic fibrosis airway epithelia fail to kill bacteria because of abnormal airway surface fluid [published erratum appears in Cell 1996;87:following 355]. Cell 1996;85:229–36.

329. Goldman MJ, Anderson GM, Stolzenberg ED, et al. Human beta-defensin-1 is a salt-sensitive antibiotic in lung that is inactivated in cystic fibrosis. Cell 1997;88:553–60.

330. Postle AD, Mander A, Reid KBM, et al. Deficient hydrophilic lung surfactant proteins A and D with normal surfactant phospholipid molecular species in cystic fibrosis. Am J Respir Cell Mol Biol 1999;20:90–8.

331. Lethem MI, James SL, Marriott C, et al. The origin of DNA associated with mucus glycoproteins in cystic fibrosis sputum. Eur Respir J 1990;3:19–23.

332. Yacoub MH, Banner NR, Khaghani A, et al. Heart–lung transplantation for cystic fibrosis and subsequent domino heart transplantation. J Heart Transplant 1990;9:459–67.

333. Tsang VT, Alton EWFW, Hodson ME, et al. In vitro bioelectric properties of bronchial epithelium from transplanted lungs in recipients with cystic fibrosis. Thorax 1993;48:1006–11.

334. Bronsveld I, Bijman J, Mekus F, et al. Clinical presentation of exclusive cystic fibrosis lung disease. Thorax 1999;54:278–81.

335. Drake-Lee AB, Pitcher-Wilmott RW. The clinical and laboratory correlates of nasal polyps in cystic fibrosis. Int J Pediatr Otorhinolaryngol 1982;4:209.

336. Anguiano A, Oates RD, Amos J. Congenital absence of the vas deferens – a primary genital form of cystic fibrosis. JAMA 1992;267:1794.

337. Penketh ARL, Wise A, Mearns MB, et al. Cystic fibrosis in adolescents and adults. Thorax 1987;42:526–32.

338. van Biezen P, Overbeek SE, Hilvering C. Cystic fibrosis in a 70-year-old woman. Thorax 1992;47:202–3.

339. Rosenbluth D, Goodenberger D. Cystic fibrosis in an elderly woman. Chest 1997;112:1124–6.

340. Gilljam M, Bjorck E. Cystic fibrosis diagnosed in an elderly man. Respiration 2004;71:98–100.

341. Southern KW, Munck A, Pollitt R, et al. A survey of newborn screening for cystic fibrosis in Europe. J Cyst Fibros 2007;6:57–65.

342. Sly PD, Brennan S, Gangell C, et al. Lung disease at diagnosis in infants with cystic fibrosis detected by newborn screening. Am J Respir Crit Care Med 2009;180:146–52.

343. Alton E, Currie D, Logan-Sinclair R, et al. Nasal potential difference: a clinical diagnostic test for cystic fibrosis. Eur Respir J 1990;3:922–6.

343a. Sermet-Gaudelus I, Girodon E, Roussel D, et al. Measurement of nasal potential difference in young children with an equivocal sweat test following newborn screening for cystic fibrosis. Thorax 2010;65:539–44.

344. Donlan RM. Biofilms: microbial life on surfaces. Emerg Infect Dis 2002;8:881–90.

345. Donlan RM, Costerton JW. Biofilms: survival mechanisms of clinically relevant microorganisms. Clin Microbiol Rev 2002;15:167–93.

346. Starner TD, Zhang N, Kim G, et al. Haemophilus influenzae forms biofilms on airway epithelia: implications in cystic fibrosis. Am J Respir Crit Care Med 2006;174:213–20.

347. Stableforth DE, Smith DL. Pseudomonas cepacia in cystic fibrosis. Thorax 1994;49:629–30.

348. Govan JRW, Brown PH, Maddison J, et al. Evidence for transmission of Pseudomonas cepacia by social contact in cystic fibrosis. Lancet 1993;342:15–19.

349. McFarlane H, Holzel A, Brenchley P, et al. Immune complexes in cystic fibrosis. BMJ 1975;1:423–8.

350. Finnegan MJ, Hinchcliffe J, Russell-Jones D, et al. Vasculitis complicating cystic fibrosis. Q J Med 1989;72:609–22.

351. Hodson M. Immunological abnormalities in cystic fibrosis: chicken or egg? Thorax 1980;35:801–6.

352. Geller DE, Kaplowitz H, Light MJ, et al. Allergic bronchopulmonary aspergillosis in cystic fibrosis – Reported prevalence, regional distribution, and patient characteristics. Chest 1999;116:639–46.

353. Mastella G, Rainisio M, Harms HK, et al. Allergic bronchopulmonary aspergillosis in cystic fibrosis. A European epidemiological study. Eur Resp J 2000;16:464–71.

354. Bedrossian CWM, Greenberg SD, Singer DB, et al. The lung in cystic fibrosis. A quantitative study of pathologic findings amongst different age groups. Hum Pathol 1976;7:195–204.

355. Oppenheimer EH, Esterly JR. Pathology of cystic fibrosis. Review of the literature and comparison with 146 autopsied cases. Perspect Pediatr Pathol 1975;2:241–78.

356. Esterly JR, Oppenheimer EH. Observations in cystic fibrosis of the pancreas. II. Pulmonary lesions. Johns Hopkins Med J 1968;122:94–101.

357. Lamb D, Reid L. The tracheobronchial submucosal glands in cystic fibrosis: a qualitative and quantitative histochemical study. Br J Dis Chest 1972;66:239–47.

358. Esterly JR, Oppenheimer EH. Cystic fibrosis of the pancreas: structural changes in peripheral airways. Thorax 1968;23:670–5.

359. Tomashefski JF Jr, Konstan MW, Bruce MC, et al. The pathologic characteristics of interstitial pneumonia in cystic fibrosis. A retrospective autopsy study. Am J Clin Pathol 1989;91:522–30.

360. Ogrinc G, Kampalath B, Tomashefski JF. Destruction and loss of bronchial cartilage in cystic fibrosis. Hum Pathol 1998;29:65–73.

361. Tomashefski JF, Bruce M, Goldberg HI, et al. Regional distribution of macroscopic lung disease in cystic fibrosis. Am Rev Respir Dis 1986;133:535–40.

362. Tomashefski JF, Bruce M, Stern RC, et al. Pulmonary air cysts in cystic fibrosis: relation of pathologic features to radiologic findings and history of pneumothorax. Hum Pathol 1985;16:253–61.

363. Flume PA, Strange C, Ye X, et al. Pneumothorax in cystic fibrosis. Chest 2005;128:720–8.

364. Wentworth P, Gough J, Wentworth JE. Pulmonary changes and cor pulmonale in mucoviscidosis. Thorax 1968;23:582–9.

365. Ryland D, Reid L. The pulmonary circulation in cystic fibrosis. Thorax 1975;30:285–92.

366. Oppenheimer EH, Rosenstein BJ. Differential pathology of nasal polyps in cystic fibrosis and atopy. Lab Invest 1979;40:445–9.

367. Couper R, Bentur L, Kilbourn JP, et al. Immunoreactive calmodulin in cystic fibrosis kidneys. Aust N Z J Med 1993;23:484–8.

368. Turner MA, Goldwater D, David TJ. Oxalate and calcium excretion in cystic fibrosis. Arch Dis Child 2000;83:244–7.

369. Perez-Brayfield MR, Caplan D, Gatti JM, et al. Metabolic risk factors for stone formation in patients with cystic fibrosis. J Urol 2002;167:480–4.

370. Wiebicke W, Artlich A, Gerling I. Myocardial fibrosis – a rare complication in patients with cystic fibrosis. Eur J Pediatr 1993;152:694–6.

371. Zebrak J, Skuza B, Pogorzelski A, et al. Partial CFTR genotyping and characterisation of cystic fibrosis patients with myocardial fibrosis and necrosis. Clin Genet 2000;57:56–60.

372. Hellsing E, Brattstrom V, Strandvik B. Craniofacial morphology in children with cystic fibrosis. Eur J Orthod 1992;14:147–51.

373. Hendry WF, Knight RK, Whitfield HN, et al. Obstructive azoospermia: respiratory function tests, electron microscopy and the results of surgery. Br J Urol 1978;50:598–604.

374. Deiongh R, Ing A, Rutland J. Mucociliary function, ciliary ultrastructure, and ciliary orientation in Young's syndrome. Thorax 1992;47:184–7.

375. Pavia D, Agnew JE, Bateman JRM, et al. Lung mucociliary clearance in patients with Young's syndrome. Chest 1981;80:892–5.

376. Borja AR, Ransdell HT, Villa S. Congenital developmental arrest of the lung. Ann Thorac Surg 1970;10:317–26.

377. Ryland D, Reid L. Pulmonary aplasia – a quantitative analysis of the development of the single lung. Thorax 1971;26:602–9.

378. Booth JB, Berry CL. Unilateral pulmonary agenesis. Am J Dis Child 1967;42:361–74.

379. Cunningham ML, Mann N. Pulmonary agenesis: A predictor of ipsilateral malformations. Am J Med Genet 1997;70:391–8.

380. Cunningham ML, Mann N. Pulmonary agenesis: a predictor of ipsilateral malformations. Am J Med Genet 1997;70:391–8.

381. Finci V, Beghetti M, Kalangos A, et al. Unilateral total and contralateral partial pulmonary agenesis associated with total anomalous pulmonary venous drainage. J Pediatr 1999;134:510–12.

382. Emery JL, Mithal A. The number of alveoli in the terminal respiratory unit of man during late intrauterine life and childhood. Arch Dis Child 1960;35:544–7.

383. Nakamura Y, Yamamoto I, Fukuda S, et al. Pulmonary acinar development in diaphragmatic hernia. Arch Pathol Lab Med 1991;115:372–6.

384. Reale FR, Esterly JR. Pulmonary hypoplasia: a morphometric study of the lungs of infants with diaphragmatic hernia, anencephaly, and renal malformations. Pediatrics 1972;51:91–6.

385. Hislop A, Reid L. Persistent hypoplasia of the lung after repair of congenital diaphragmatic hernia. Thorax 1976;31:450–5.

386. Page DV, Stocker JT. Anomalies associated with pulmonary hypoplasia. Am Rev Respir Dis 1982;125:216–21.

387. Cooney TP, Thurlbeck WM. Pulmonary hypoplasia in Down's syndrome. N Engl J Med 1982;307:1170–3.

388. Davies G, Reid L. Effect of scoliosis on growth of alveoli and pulmonary arteries and on right ventricle. Arch Dis Child 1971;46:623–32.

389. Boffa P, Stovin P, Shneerson J. Lung developmental abnormalities in severe scoliosis. Thorax 1984;39:681–2.

390. Nicolini U, Fisk NM, Rodeck CH, et al. Low amniotic pressure in oligohydramnios – Is this the cause of pulmonary hypoplasia? Am J Obstet Gynecol 1989;161:1098–101.

391. Adzick NS, Harrison MR, Glick PL, et al. Experimental pulmonary hypoplasia and oligohydramnios: Relative contributions of lung fluid and fetal breathing movements. J Pediatr Surg 1984;19:658–65.

392. Wigglesworth JS, Hislop A, Desai R. Fetal lung growth in congenital laryngeal atresia. Pediatr Pathol 1987;7:515–25.

393. Thomas IT, Smith DW. Oligohydramnios, cause of the non-renal features of Potter's syndrome, including pulmonary hypoplasia. J Pediatr 1974;84:811–14.

394. Henderson R, Hislop A, Reid L. New pathological findings in emphysema of childhood: 3. Unilateral congenital emphysema with hypoplasia – and compensatory emphysema of the contralateral lung. Thorax 1971;26:195–205.

395. Hislop A, Reid L. New pathological findings in emphysema in childhood: 2. Overinflation of a normal lobe. Thorax 1971;26:190–4.

396. Critchley PS, Forrester-Wood CP, Ridley PD. Adult congenital lobar emphysema in pregnancy. Thorax 1995;50:909–10.

397. Sedivy R, Bankl HC, Stimpfl T, et al. Sudden, unexpected death of a young marathon runner as a result of bronchial malformation. Mod Pathol 1997;10:247–51.

398. Khemiri M, Ouederni M, Mansour FB, et al. Bronchogenic cyst: An uncommon cause of congenital lobar emphysema. Respiratory Medicine 2008;102:1663–6.

399. Stovin PGI. Congenital lobar emphysema. Thorax 1959;14:254–62.

400. Warner JO, Rubin S, Heard BE. Congenital lobar emphysema: a case with bronchial atresia and abnormal bronchial cartilages. Br J Dis Chest 1982;76:177–84.

401. MonforteMunoz H, Walls RL. Intrapulmonary airways visualized by staining and clearing of whole-lung sections: the transparent human lung. Modern Pathol 2004;17:22–7.

402. Leape LL, Longino LA. Infantile lobar emphysema. Pediatrics 1964;34:246–55.

403. Stanger P, Lucas RV, Jr., Edwards JE. Anatomic factors causing respiratory distress in acyanotic congenital cardiac disease. Special reference to bronchial obstruction. Pediatrics 1969;43:760–9.

404. Hislop A, Reid L. New pathological findings in emphysema in childhood: 1. Polyalveolar lobe with emphysema. Thorax 1970;25:682–90.

405. Mani H, Suarez E, Stocker JT. The morphologic spectrum of infantile lobar emphysema: a study of 33 cases. Paediatr Respir Rev 2004;5:S313–20.

406. Reid L, Simon G. Unilateral lung transradiancy. Thorax 1962;17:230–9.

407. Stokes D, Sigler A, Khouri NF, et al. Unilateral hyperlucent lung (Swyer–James

syndrome) after severe *Mycoplasma pneumoniae* infection. Am Rev Respir Dis 1978;117:145–52.

408. Armin A, Castelli M. Congenital adrenal tissue in the lung with adrenal cytomegaly. Case report and review of the literature. Am J Clin Pathol 1984;82:225–8.

409. Bando T, Genka K, Ishikawa K, et al. Ectopic intrapulmonary thyroid. Chest 1993;103:1278–9.

410. Mendoza A, Voland J, Wolf P, et al. Supradiaphragmatic liver in the lung. Arch Pathol Lab Med 1986;110:1085–6.

411. Aterman K, Patel S. Striated muscle in the lung. Am J Anat 1970;128:341–58.

412. Remberger K, Hubner G. Rhabdomyomatous dysplasia of the lung. Virchows Arch A Pathol Anat Histopathol 1974;363:363–9.

413. Hardisson D, Garcia Jimenez JA, Jimenez Heffernan JA, et al. Rhabdomyomatosis of the newborn lung unassociated with other malformations. Histopathology 1997;31:474–9.

414. Ramaswamy A, Weyers I, Duda V, et al. A tumorous type of pulmonary rhabdomyomatous dysplasia. Pathol Res Pract 1998;194:639–42.

415. Burke EC, Wenzl JE, Utz DC. The intrathoracic kidney. Report of a case. Am J Dis Child 1967;113:487–90.

416. Kanbour AJ, Barmada MA, Klionsky B, et al. Anecephaly and heterotopic central nervous tissue in lungs. Arch Pathol Lab Med 1979;103:116–8.

417. Gonzalez-Crussi F, Boggs JD, Raffensperger JG. Brain heterotopia in the lungs. Am J Clin Pathol 1980;73:281–5.

418. Chen WJ, Kelly MM, Shaw CM, et al. Pathogenic mechanisms of heterotopic neural tissue associated with anencephaly. Hum Pathol 1982;13:179–82.

419. Rakestraw MR, Masood S, Ballinger WE. Brain heterotopia and anenecephaly. Arch Pathol Lab Med 1987;111:858–60.

420. Fuller C, Gibbs AR. Heterotopic brain tissue in the lung causing acute respiratory distress in an infant. Thorax 1989;44:1045–6.

421. Kershisnik MM, Kaplan C, Craven CM, et al. Intrapulmonary neuroglial heterotopia. Arch Pathol Lab Med 1992;116:1043–6.

422. Langlois NEI, Gray ES. Scatterbrain fetus. J Pathol 1992;168:347–8.

423. Lager DJ, Kuper KA, Haake GK. Subdiaphragmatic extralumbar pulmonary sequestration. Arch Pathol Lab Med 1991;115:536–8.

424. Mark EJ. Mesenchymal cystic hamartoma of the lung. N Engl J Med 1986;315:1255–9.

425. Hedlund GL, Bisset GSI, Bove KE. Malignant neoplasms arising in cystic hamartomas of the lung in childhood. Radiology 1989;173:77–9.

426. Mushtaq M, Ward SP, Hutchison JT, et al. Multiple cystic pulmonary hamartomas. Thorax 1992;47:1076–7.

427. Leroyer C, Quiot JJ, Dewitte JD, et al. Mesenchymal cystic hamartoma of the lung. Respiration 1993;60:305–6.

428. van Klaveren RJ, Hassing HHM, Wiersma-van Tilburg JM, et al. Mesenchymal cystic hamartoma of the lung: a rare cause of relapsing pneumothorax. Thorax 1994;49:1175–6.

429. Cottin V, Thomas L, Loire R, et al. Mesenchymal cystic hamartoma of the lung in Cowden's disease. Resp Med 2003;97:188–91.

430. Chadwick SL, Corrin B, Hansell DM, et al. Fatal haemorrhage from mesenchymal cystic hamartoma of the lung. Eur Respir J 1995;8:2182–4.

431. Abrams J, Talcott J, Corson JM. Pulmonary metastases in patients with low-grade endometrial stromal sarcoma. Clinicopathologic findings with immunohistochemical characterization. Am J Surg Pathol 1989;13:133–40.

432. Chang KL, Crabtree GS, Lim-Tan SK, et al. Primary uterine endometrial stromal neoplasms. A clinicopathologic study of 117 cases. Am J Surg Pathol 1990;14:415–38.

433. Sugawara M, Kato N, Endo M, et al. Clonal expansion of multiple pulmonary leiomyomatous hamartoma: 12-year follow-up. Pathol Int 2009;59:828–30.

434. Tietze L, Gunther K, Horbe A, et al. Benign metastasizing leiomyoma: A cytogenetically balanced but clonal disease. Hum Pathol 2000;31:126–8.

435. Rosenmann E, Maayan C, Lernau O. Leiomyomatous hamartosis with congenital jejunoileal atresia. Isr J Med Sci 1980;16:775–9.

436. Pool PE, Vogel JHK, Blount SG. Congenital unilateral absence of a pulmonary artery. Am J Cardiol 1962;10:706–32.

437. Brassard JM, Johnson JE. Unilateral absence of a pulmonary artery – data from cardiopulmonary exercise testing. Chest 1993;103:293–5.

438. Arriero JM, Gil J, Martin C, et al. Unilateral absence of a pulmonary artery – congenital disease or embolic occlusion. Eur Respir J 1991;4:1299–300.

439. Morales P, Miravet L, Marco V. Agenesis of the right pulmonary artery in a young asymptomatic girl. Eur Respir J 1991;4:1301–2.

440. Ko T, Gatz MG, Reisz GR. Congenital unilateral absence of a pulmonary artery: Report of two adult cases. Am Rev Respir Dis 1990;141:795–8.

441. Maeda S, Suzuki S, Moriya T, et al. Isolated unilateral absence of a pulmonary artery: Influence of systemic circulation on alveolar capillary vessels. Pathol Int 2001;51:649–53.

442. TenHarkel ADJ, Blom NA, Ottenkamp J. Isolated unilateral absence of a pulmonary artery – A case report and review of the literature. Chest 2002;122:1471–7.

443. Presbitero P, Bull C, Haworth SG, et al. Absent or occult pulmonary artery. Br Heart J 1984;52:178–85.

444. Liebow AA, Hales MR. Studies on the lung after ligation of the pulmonary artery; anatomical changes. Am J Pathol 1950;26:177–95.

445. Sweerts M, Nicholson AG, Goldstraw P, et al. Dieulafoy's disease of the bronchus. Thorax 1995;50:697–8.

446. Stoopen E, Baquera Heredia J, Cortes D, et al. Dieulafoy's disease of the bronchus in association with a paravertebral neurilemoma. Chest 2001;119:292–4.

447. Pomplun S, Sheaff MT. Dieulafoy's disease of the bronchus: an uncommon entity. Histopathology 2005;46:598–9.

448. Nashef SAM, Jamieson MPG, Pollock JCS, et al. Aortic origin of right pulmonary artery: successful surgical correction in three consecutive patients. Ann Thorac Surg 1987;44:536–8.

449. Liebow AA, Hales MR, Lindskog GE. Enlargement of the bronchial arteries, and their anastomoses with the pulmonary arteries in bronchiectasis. Am J Pathol 1949;25:211–31.

450. Petersen RC, Edwards WD. Pulmonary vascular disease in 57 necropsy cases of total anomalous pulmonary venous connection. Histopathology 1983;7:487–96.

451. Wang JK, Chiu IS, How SW, et al. Anomalous pulmonary venous pathway traversing pulmonary parenchyma: diagnosis and implication. Chest 1996;110:1363–6.

452. Haworth SG, Reid L. Structural study of pulmonary circulation and of heart in total anomalous pulmonary venous return in early infancy. Br Heart J 1977;39:80–92.

453. Sun CC, Doyle T, Ringel RE. Pulmonary vein stenosis. Hum Pathol 1995;26:880–6.

454. Omasa M, Hasegawa S, Bando T, et al. A case of congenital pulmonary vein stenosis in an adult. Resp Med 2004;71:92–4.

455. Honey M. Anomalous pulmonary venous drainage of right lung to inferior vena cava ('scimitar syndrome'): clinical spectrum in older patients and role of surgery. Q J Med 1977;184:463–83.

456. Dupuis C, Charaf LA, Breviere GM, et al. 'Infantile' form of the scimitar syndrome with pulmonary hypertension. Am J Cardiol 1993;71:1326–30.

457. Steiner I, Haíjkova P, Kvasniċika J, et al. Myocardial sleeves of pulmonary veins and atrial fibrillation: a postmortem histopathological study of 100 subjects. Virchows Archiv 2006;449:88–95.

458. Lubitz SA, Fischer A, Fuster V. Catheter ablation for atrial fibrillation. BMJ 2008;336:819–26.

458a. Yang HM, Lai CK, Patel J, et al. Irreversible intrapulmonary vascular changes after pulmonary vein stenosis complicating catheter ablation for atrial fibrillation. Cardiovasc Pathol 2007;16: 51–5.

459. Kojodjojo P, Wong T, Wright AR, et al. Pulmonary venous stenosis after treatment for atrial fibrillation. BMJ 2008;336:830–2.

460. Churton T. Multiple aneurysms of pulmonary artery. Br Med J 1897;i:1223.

461. Le Roux BT. Pulmonary arteriovenous fistulae. Q J Med 1959;28:1–19.

462. Utzon F, Brandup F. Pulmonary arteriovenous fistulas in children. Acta Paediatr Scand 1973;62:422–32.

463. Dines DE, Arms RA, Bernatz PE, et al. Pulmonary arteriovenous fistulas. Mayo Clin Proc 1974;49:460–5.

464. Przybojewski JZ, Maritz F. Pulmonary arteriovenous fistulas. A case presentation and review of the literature. S Afr Med J 1980;57:366–73.

465. Prager RL, Laws KH, Bender Jr HW. Arteriovenous fistula of the lung. Ann Thorac Surg 1983;36:231–9.

466. Gossage JR, Kanj G. Pulmonary arteriovenous malformations – A state of the art review. Am J Respir Crit Care Med 1998;158:643–61.

467. Grishman A, Poppel MH, Simpson RS, et al. The roentgenographic and angiocardiographic aspects of (1) aberrant insertion of pulmonary veins associated with interatrial septal defect and (2) congenital arteriovenous aneurysm of the lung. Am J Roentgenol 1949;62:500–8.

468. Gomes MR, Bernatz PE, Dines DE. Pulmonary arteriovenous fistulas. Ann Thorac Surg 1969;7:582–93.

469. Pouwels HMM, Janevski BK, Penn OCKM, et al. Systemic to pulmonary vascular malformation. Eur Respir J 1992;5:1288–91.

470. Akahane T, Yaegashi H, Kurokawa Y, et al. Systemic-to-pulmonary vascular malformation of lung visualized by computer-assisted 3-D reconstruction. Histopathology 1997;31:252–7.

471. Hoffman R, Rabens R. Evolving pulmonary nodules: multiple pulmonary arteriovenous fistulas. AJR Am J Roentgenol 1974;120:861–4.

472. Hughes JMB. Intrapulmonary shunts: coils to transplantation. J R Coll Physicians Lond 1994;28:247–53.

473. Shovlin CL, Letarte M. Hereditary haemorrhagic telangiectasia and pulmonary arteriovenous malformations: issues in clinical management and review of pathogenic mechanisms. Thorax 1999;54:714–29.

474. Hodgson CH, Burchell HB, Good CA, et al. Hereditary hemorrhagic telagiectasia and pulmonary arteriovenous fistula. Survey of a large family. New Engl J Med 1959;261:625–36.

475. Abad J, Villar R, Parga G, et al. Bronchial migration of pulmonary arterial coil. Cardiovasc Intervent Radiol 1990;13:345–6.

476. Reynaud-Gaubert M, Thomas P, Gaubert JY, et al. Pulmonary arteriovenous malformations: lung transplantation as a therapeutic option. Eur Resp J 1999;14:1425–8.

477. Faughnan ME, Lui YW, Wirth JA, et al. Diffuse pulmonary arteriovenous malformations – Characteristics and prognosis. Chest 2000;117:31–8.

478. Ference BA, Shannon TM, White RI, et al. Life-threatening pulmonary hemorrhage with pulmonary arteriovenous malformations and hereditary hemorrhagic telangiectasia. Chest 1994;106:1387–90.

479. Wang N-S, Seemayer TA, Ahmed MN, et al. Pulmonary leiomyosarcoma associated with an arteriovenous fistula. Arch Pathol 1974;98:100–5.

480. Faul JL, Berry GJ, Colby TV, et al. Thoracic lymphangiomas, lymphangiectasis, lymphangiomatosis, and lymphatic dysplasia syndrome. Am J Respir Crit Care Med 2000;161:1037–46.

481. Esterly JR, Oppenheimer EH. Lymphangiectasis and other pulmonary lesions in the asplenia syndrome. Arch Pathol 1970;90:553–60.

482. Reference deleted in text.

483. Barker PM, Esther CR, Jr., Fordham LA, et al. Primary pulmonary lymphangiectasia in infancy and childhood. Eur Respir J 2004;24:413–9.

484. Wagenaar SS, Swierenga J, Wagenvoort CA. Late presentation of primary pulmonary lymphangiectasis. Thorax 1978;33:791–5.

485. White JES, Veale D, Fishwick D, et al. Generalised lymphangiectasia: pulmonary presentation in an adult. Thorax 1996;51:767–8.

486. Okumura Y, Takeda S, Sawabata N, et al. Pulmonary lymphangiectasis in an asymptomatic adult. Respiration 2006;73:114–6.

487. Laurence KM. Congenital pulmonary lymphangiectasis. J Clin Pathol 1959;12:62–9.

488. Joshi M, Cole S, Knibbs D, et al. Pulmonary abnormalities in Klippel–Trenaunay syndrome – a histologic, ultrastructural, and immunocytochemical study. Chest 1992;102:1274–7.

489. Gianlupi A, Harper RW, Dwyre DM, et al. Recurrent pulmonary embolism associated with Klippel–Trenaunay–Weber syndrome. Chest 1999;115:1199–201.

490. Clugston RD, Klattig J, Englert C, et al. Teratogen-induced, dietary and genetic models of congenital diaphragmatic hernia share a common mechanism of pathogenesis. Am J Pathol 2006;169:1541–9.

491. Sheehan JJ, Kearns SR, McNamara DA, et al. Adult presentation of agenesis of the hemidiaphragm. Chest 2000;117:901–2.

491a. Gander JW, Kadenhe-Chiweshe A, Fisher JC, et al. Hepatic pulmonary fusion in an infant with a right-sided congenital diaphragmatic hernia and contralateral mediastinal shift. J Pediatr Surg 2010;45: 265–8.

492. Theerthakarat R, El Halees W, Javadpoor S, et al. Severe pectus excavatum associated with cor pulmonale and chronic respiratory acidosis in a young woman. Chest 2001;119:1957–61.

493. Jeune M, Carron R, Beraud C, et al. Polychondrodystrophie avec blocage thoracique d'évolution fatale. Pediatrie, Lyon 1954;9:390–2.

494. Jeune M, Beraud C, Carron R. Dystrophie thoracique asphyxiante de charactère familial. Arch Fr Pediatrie 1955;12:886–91.

495. Greenough A. Abnormalities of the skeleton. In: Greenough A, Milner AD, editors. Neonatal Respiratory Disorders. 2nd ed. London: Arnold; 2003. p. 505–18.

Chapter | 3 |

Diseases of the conductive airways

The function of the airways is to conduct gas in and out of the lungs and all airway diseases are liable to impede this, resulting in 'obstructive lung disease', as opposed to the 'restrictive lung disease' that is caused by many diseases of the lung parenchyma. Airway obstruction has important effects on the lung parenchyma and this chapter first considers one of these, pulmonary collapse. Another important consequence of airway obstruction is obstructive pneumonia, which is dealt with on page 315, while if airway obstruction is not relieved, distal infection is almost inevitable.

ATELECTASIS AND PULMONARY COLLAPSE

The term 'atelectasis' means imperfect expansion, and is applied specifically to failure of the lungs to expand fully at birth. This may be due to congenital airway obstruction or pulmonary compression, and is of course found in stillbirths. Once the lungs have expanded, return to the airless state is sometimes referred to as secondary atelectasis, but is more widely known as pulmonary collapse. Two types of pulmonary collapse are recognised, one due to pressure changes and the other to absorbed alveolar gas not being replenished.

Pressure collapse may result from external forces exerted by air or fluid in the pleural cavity, enlargement of the heart or mediastinum, or a thoracic tumour. Alternatively, pressure collapse may be due to a rise in alveolar surface tension from depletion of pulmonary surfactant, as in the infantile and adult respiratory distress syndromes.

Absorption collapse is likely when bronchial obstruction prevents free entry of air into the lungs. The causes are listed in Box 3.1. Mucus frequently collects during anaesthesia, when respiratory movements are reduced and the cough reflex suppressed, whilst mucus plugging is a cardinal feature of asthma, allergic bronchopulmonary aspergillosis and plastic bronchitis. The inhalation of a foreign body is especially common in children while the narrow, pliable bronchi of infants are particularly liable to be compressed by distended pulmonary arteries at points where they are in close anatomical proximity

©2010 Elsevier Ltd
DOI: 10.1016/B978-0-7020-3369-8.00003-3

(see Fig. 10.9, p. 481) or by abnormally located systemic arteries. In time, the alveolar air – first the oxygen and later the nitrogen – is removed by the blood that passes through the affected area and the alveoli then progressively collapse.

Pulmonary collapse has been seen quite commonly in the crew of high-performance aircraft. An important cause is breathing pure oxygen, which washes nitrogen from the alveoli and is more rapidly absorbed into the blood. Parts of the lung filled with oxygen but temporarily closed off by increased gravitational forces distorting airways are liable to absorption collapse. These forces operate whenever the pilot makes a tight turn at high speed or pulls out of a steep dive. Clothing designed to protect the aviator from burst lung (see p. 369) increases the adverse effect on the basal parts of the lungs by raising the diaphragm and reducing lung volume.

Pathological findings

Whatever the cause, collapsed lungs are small and firm, and have a deeply wrinkled pleural surface. Portions of collapsed lungs tend to sink when dropped into water but this is not an infallible test of airlessness. Where part of a lung has recently collapsed, the immediately adjacent, pale pink, aerated lobules are sharply separated from the dark red depressed areas of collapse by zigzag lines that correspond to the interlobular septa (see Fig. 4.3, p. 137). The collapse involves alveoli and bronchioles but bronchial cartilage maintains the patency of these larger airways. Subsequent changes differ according to whether the collapse is due to absorption or compression. With absorption collapse the affected lung resembles splenic tissue, both grossly and microscopically.[1] Alveolar walls are in apposition and their capillaries are greatly dilated so that the bulk of the collapsed lung no longer consists of air space but of sinusoidal vessels engorged with blood, although the circulation may be reduced. The interlobular septa are thickened but there is little fibrosis of the alveolar tissue. The changes are irreversible, suggesting that there is fusion of the apposed alveolar walls. With pressure collapse congestion is less marked and fibrosis of both the alveolar tissue and overlying pleura is more marked (Fig. 3.1). In either case, reinflation is prevented.

Collateral ventilation

When obstruction to an airway is only partial, permitting inspiration but hindering expiration, air is retained in the affected area and there is full inflation rather than collapse (see infantile lobar emphysema, p. 72). Absorption collapse may also be prevented by collateral ven-

Figure 3.1 Chronic pulmonary collapse due to long-standing pleural effusion. On the right pleuropulmonary fibrosis has developed, preventing the lung from ever expanding.

tilation, a process by which one portion of lung is ventilated through another via the pores of Kohn and other peripheral communications (see p. 15). Collateral ventilation is best developed at the acinar level, being hindered by the interlobular septa and prevented by interlobar fissures, but because interlobular septa are incomplete, it may prevent whole segments undergoing absorption collapse. However, air flow through the tortuous bypass channels afforded by many pores of Kohn is poor and collateral ventilation plays little part in gas exchange.[2] Its function is to maintain inflation of alveoli when their supplying airways are obstructed by secretions or a foreign body. This is essential to the cough mechanism, dependent upon which is the expulsion of the obstructive material and the restoration of bronchial patency.

Middle-lobe syndrome

The term 'middle-lobe syndrome' was coined to describe a condition of chronic or recurrent absorption collapse of the right middle lobe that was originally described in 1937.[3] The collapse was most frequently caused by tuberculous involvement of lymph nodes compressing the right middle-lobe bronchus. Tuberculosis is less common today but any disease enlarging these lymph nodes may have the same effect. Predilection for involvement of the middle lobe was considered to be the result of a combination of factors: the prominent collar of nodes about its bronchus, the lymphatic drainage of these nodes being from much of the right lung and parts of the left, and the

Bronchiectasis involving the middle lobe or lingula of middle-aged women has also been termed the Lady Windermere syndrome, based upon the belief that such a fastidious person as the eponymous person in Oscar Wilde's play *Lady Windermere's Fan* would refrain from expectorating and thereby retain any infected bronchial secretions.[6] However, the bronchi to these portions of the lungs extend forwards so that unless the person spent a considerable time in the prone position the middle lobe and lingula are the least likely parts of the lungs to be affected by aspiration (see Fig. 5.2.14, p. 189).[7] Infection (or colonisation) by *Mycobacterium avium-intracellulare* is frequently identified in this 'syndrome'.

OBSTRUCTION OF THE UPPER AIRWAYS

Obstruction of the upper airways may be complete, and cause rapid asphyxial death, or incomplete, when there is stridor or wheezing, or distal complications such as obstructive pneumonia may ensue. Foreign bodies are an important cause, especially in children and edentulous adults. Tumours are another important cause. Rare causes include amyloid tumours, Wegener's granulomatosis[8] and tracheo-bronchomalacia. In infancy the airways are unduly pliable and may be compressed by distended arteries, particularly where the two are in close contact (see Fig. 10.9, p. 481). Anomalous arteries may also compress airways in infancy, as in the vascular sling and ring syndromes (see Figs 10.10 and 10.11, pp. 481, 482).

Obstructive sleep apnoea

Obstructive sleep apnoea is characterised by repeated periods during which the patient stops breathing for 10 or more seconds whilst asleep. The patient may not waken but is repeatedly aroused so that the quality of the sleep is poor and daytime sleepiness is consequently excessive.[9] Snoring is a common accompaniment. The patient is generally obese and it is postulated that cervical fat pads obstruct the upper airway.[10] Other family members are often similarly affected, possibly because of similarities in cervicofacial structure. Charles Dickens was evidently familiar with such individuals, portraying one in his novel *The Pickwick Papers*. Such patients have therefore been termed 'pickwickian', although the Dickens character was the 'fat boy' rather than Mr Pickwick himself. Defects in the secretion of testosterone and growth hormone may also be identified.[11] These are reversible and are probably due to the central effects of sleep fragmentation and hypoxaemia.

The principal problem in obstructive sleep apnoea is the daytime tiredness, which leads to poor performance at work and a tendency to fall asleep at inappropriate moments. The consequences of this can be very serious if, for example, the patient drives. The periods of apnoea result in hypoxaemia, which in turn causes pulmonary hypertension. The apnoeic episodes are also accompanied by systemic hypertension and death may be caused by biventricular cardiac failure.[12] The pulmonary blood vessels show the usual changes found with hypoxia, principally hypertrophy of the arterial media (see p. 424). Pulmonary haemorrhage and haemosiderosis are further features, possibly attributable to the left ventricular failure. Pronounced capillary proliferation resembling capillary haemangiomatosis (see p. 429) is also described.[13] Continuous positive airway pressure provides effective treatment.[14]

Obstructive sleep apnoea is to be distinguished from a central variety of apnoea known as Ondine's curse. In German legend, the water nymph Ondine, having been jilted by her mortal lover, took from him all automatic functions, requiring him to remember to breathe. When he finally fell asleep, he died. Central apnoea has been

Figure 3.2 Middle-lobe syndrome. (A) The middle lobe is collapsed and its bronchi are dilated. (B) In this patient the syndrome was caused by a bronchiolith (arrow) blocking the lobar bronchus.

relatively narrow calibre and possibly undue compressibility of the middle-lobe bronchus. A further possible factor is the limited capacity for collateral ventilation (see above) within the middle lobe: this stems from the fact that its two segments have relatively large proportions of their surfaces covered by pleura and, together with the inferior segment of the lingula, are the only ones that abut no more than one other segment.[4]

Patients with the middle-lobe syndrome complain of chronic cough, haemoptysis, chest pain and dyspnoea, and the diseased lobe may be removed to relieve this. Pathological changes in the resected lobe include bronchiectasis, chronic bronchitis and bronchiolitis, lymphoid hyperplasia, organising pneumonia and abscess formation, in addition to collapse (Fig. 3.2).[5] A similar syndrome may affect the lingula.

Figure 3.3 Tracheobronchopathia osteochondroplastica. (A) Bronchoscopic view. The nodules affect all but the posterior membranous portion of the trachea, compatible with them arising from the tracheal cartilages. (B) Extensive roughening of the tracheal mucosa is seen at necropsy. *(Courtesy of Dr Sj Sc Wagenaar, Utrecht, Netherlands.)*

encountered with bulbar poliomyelitis and it is likely that the syndrome results from damage to the medullary CO_2 receptor. Airway patency is maintained but respiratory drive is weak, especially during sleep.

Tracheobronchopathia osteochondroplastica

The first descriptions of this condition date back to the middle of the nineteenth century,[15,16] since when it has continued to arouse interest because of its apparent rarity and disputed aetiology.[17,18] It is confined to the trachea and bronchi and does not infiltrate surrounding tissues or metastasise but it endangers life through airway obstruction.[19] It affects men more often than women, and is seldom recognised before the age of 50. Symptomatic cases are rare but it is possible that mild cases are overlooked[20]: four cases were reported in one series of 500 bronchoscopies.[21]

Tracheobronchoscopy reveals multiple mucosal nodules and relevant to both the diagnosis and aetiology of the condition is the observation that the membranous portion of the trachea is spared (Fig. 3.3).[22] This suggests that the condition is related to the airway cartilage and that the lesions represent exostoses (as suggested by Virchow) rather than submucosal metaplasia (as suggested by

Aschoff).[16,23] A superficial resemblance to tracheobronchial amyloidosis (which is prone to ossify) has led to erroneous suggestions that these two conditions are related.[24–26] Growth factors that induce new bone formation have been demonstrated about the ossifying nodules but not about those composed of mature lamellar bone.[27]

Pathology

At necropsy the tracheobronchial mucosa is roughened by numerous nodular excrescences (see Fig. 3.3B). Microscopy shows that the nodules consist of cartilage, which, like the normal cartilage of the airways may calcify and ossify.[19,22,28–30] These osseocartilaginous nodules are situated between the normal cartilage and the surface epithelium of the airway, causing the mucosa to protrude into and compromise the lumen. The new cartilage differs from that normally found in the airways only in its abnormal position. Cytologically it is quite normal and in a small fibreoptic biopsy is likely to be mistaken for the normal cartilage of the large airways. It generally appears to have no connection with the normal cartilage but step sections show that there is indeed continuity through narrow pedicles,[22,30] supporting the view that the condition represents multiple ecchondroses of the tracheobronchial cartilages,[28] as originally proposed by Virchow.[16]

Figure 3.4 Relapsing polychondritis. The bronchial cartilage is cuffed (A) and its edge eroded (B) by a heavy lymphoid infiltrate. (C) The burnt-out stage. The inflammation has resolved but the bronchial cartilage is disrupted by fibrosis.

Treatment consists of nibbling the nodules away endoscopically as often as proves necessary.

Relapsing polychondritis

This condition is characterised by recurrent inflammation of cartilaginous structures and other tissues rich in glycosaminogycans.[31–35] Immunoglobulins and complement have been identified at the chondrofibrous junction,[36] and the presence of circulating anticartilage immunoglobulin and the ability of cartilage antigens to transform lymphocytes from these patients provide evidence that the disease has a tissue-specific autoimmune basis.[37]

Clinical features

The disease affects patients of both sexes and any age but the maximum frequency is in the fourth decade. It typically causes distortion of the pinnae and collapse of the nose. Other tissues involved include the larynx, trachea, bronchi, joints, eyes, inner ears and blood vessels. The trachea and bronchi are involved in 21% of patients but very rarely are they affected in isolation.[38–42] Tracheobronchial involvement is characterised by airflow obstruction due to airway collapse, manifest as breathlessness, cough, hoarseness and stridor.[38–40] Less commonly there is bronchorrhoea.[43] The arthritis has a predilection for thoracic

joints and may further contribute to respiratory difficulties. Blood vessel involvement is characterised by vasculitis involving vessels of all sizes and leading to aneurysms of major arteries. Occasionally, medium-sized arteries develop aneurysms and the changes are then those of polyarteritis nodosa.[44] Glomerulonephritis may also develop.[45]

Pathology

The affected bronchi may feel soft. Microscopically, the appearances vary according to the degree of inflammatory activity. In the active stage of the disease, the tracheobronchial cartilage is less basophilic than normal, reflecting loss of acidic proteoglycans, which may appear in the urine.[33] The tracheal and bronchial cartilages are cuffed by a chronic inflammatory infiltrate of lymphocytes, plasma cells and occasional multinucleate histiocytes that is limited to the edge of the cartilage, which is ragged and evidently under attack (Fig. 3.4A, B).[32] In the late stages of the disease the inflammation may have resolved, leaving collagen surrounding and intersecting the cartilage matrix, which at this stage is fibrillary rather than amorphous and shows increased basophilia (Fig. 3.4C).[33,38,40] Other components of the airway appear normal and there is generally no evidence of vasculitis in the airways. These features are characteristic but not specific, being seen for example in a postintubation tracheal stricture.

Idiopathic tracheal stenosis

Idiopathic tracheal stenosis is reputedly rare but one group was able to review 63 such patients who had required surgery at one hospital over a 19-year period.[46] The patients were all middle-aged women (mean age 49 years), one-third of whom gave a history of gastro-oesophageal reflux. None had evidence of rheumatoid disease, systemic lupus erythematosus or polychondritis and ANCA testing was uniformly negative. The stenosis affected the subglottis or upper one-third of the trachea and showed extensive keloid formation with dilatation of the tracheal glands. A form of fibromatosis was postulated.

ACUTE TRACHEOBRONCHITIS AND BRONCHIOLITIS

Acute inflammation of the conductive airways is common, especially among young children and the elderly, and a number of factors, environmental and microbial, may contribute to its causation. There is a marked seasonal incidence. In the summer months the mortality is low, but from early winter the death rate rises steadily to reach a peak in the late winter or early spring. The time of greatest mortality varies considerably from year to year, and depends partly on the severity of the weather and partly on the prevalence of epidemic respiratory diseases such as influenza.

In the normal person, the defensive mechanisms of the respiratory tract usually destroy or remove any inhaled microbes that may be caught on its mucus-covered surface. But if the combined defences of mucus, ciliated epithelium and the cough reflex are weakened from any cause, such as exposure to cold, irritant dust or vapours, or certain specific infections, the potentially pathogenic bacteria that are ordinarily resident in the nose and pharynx may succeed in temporarily colonising the mucosa of the trachea and bronchi. In the pathogenesis of acute tracheobronchitis, therefore, these potentiating factors are of particular significance, for without them the responsible organisms might be unable to establish themselves in these portions of the respiratory tract, which are normally sterile.

Environmental causes

Atmospheric pollution by hydrocarbon combustion products is common in many cities, and from time to time, often in particular meteorological conditions, the level of pollution may rise to values that cause an attack of acute tracheobronchitis. Los Angeles, Liège and London have been notorious for their smogs but in recent years they have been overtaken in this respect by such rapidly growing conurbations as Athens and São Paulo. In some cities, smoke control has reduced the levels of visible particulates and sulphur dioxide but not pollution by ozone and oxides of nitrogen, which are chiefly derived from internal combustion engines.

In men engaged in industries in which irritant gases or dusts may be inhaled, the mucous membrane of the trachea and bronchi may become acutely inflamed, and occasionally noxious gases such as ammonia, oxides of nitrogen and sulphur dioxide may be breathed in such concentrations that widespread injury to the respiratory mucosa may follow. Silo-filler's disease, described on page 356 [ch 7.1], is one such example. The use of thermal lances on steel is ordinarily safe but if special alloys of steel are attacked with these tools the inhalation of beryllium, cadmium and other hot metal fumes may cause acute bronchiolitis and diffuse alveolar damage. In the First World War, the military use of chlorine and phosgene as poisonous gases was often followed by destructive lesions throughout the respiratory tracts of the exposed troops.

The damage inflicted by soluble noxious gases and fumes is liable to be concentrated on the main airways whereas less soluble gases are prone to damage more distal air spaces, including alveoli as well as the finer conductive airways (see Fig. 7.2.2 and Table 7.2.2, p. 372).[47] Examples of the former include chlorine and ozone, whilst the latter include beryllium, mercury and cadmium fumes, oxides of nitrogen and high concentrations of oxygen.

Microbial causes

In recent decades, great changes have taken place in the relative importance of bacteria and viruses in the aetiology of acute tracheo-bronchitis.[48] Prophylactic immunisation against measles, diphtheria and pertussis, and the availability of antibiotics effective against the bacterial causes of secondary pneumonia, particularly pneumococci, have together greatly lessened the frequency of both the primary diseases and the respiratory complications. Most of these microbial diseases are dealt with in the chapters devoted to viral and bacterial infections (Chapters 5.1–5.3) but diphtheria and whooping cough will now be described.

Diphtheria

Diphtheria is caused by infection with the bacterium *Corynebacterium diphtheriae*. It formerly cost many lives each year but immunisation programmes have been highly successful and the disease is now very rare. It is characteristic of diphtheria that the bacteria responsible inhabit a surface membrane of fibrin and necrotic epithelium and that much of the ill effects are due to powerful exotoxins that are distributed throughout the body by the blood stream, typically causing myocardial degeneration and peripheral neuropathy. Infection is generally limited to the pharynx and only occasionally does it spread down to cause acute laryngitis, tracheitis and bronchitis. The typical membrane may obstruct the larynx and cause death from asphyxia. More often the primary injury to the respiratory mucosa by the locally released toxin lays the lungs open to invasion by various other organisms, among them *Haemophilus influenzae* and the pyogenic cocci.

Whooping cough (pertussis)

Whooping cough is a highly infectious bacterial disease of childhood caused by the bacterium *Bordetella pertussis*. It is spread by droplet infection. The incubation period is 7–10 days and a case is infectious from 7 days after exposure to 3 weeks after the onset of typical paroxysms. An initial catarrhal stage is the most infectious period. An irritating cough then develops and gradually becomes paroxysmal, which is responsible for the typical 'whoop'. Whooping cough may be complicated by bronchopneumonia, post-tussive vomiting and cerebral hypoxia, most commonly in infants under 6 months of age.

At one time, whooping cough was one of the commonest causes of death in children, and its decline in the developed countries of the world since the Second World War represents one of the notable contributions of prophylaxis to public health. In the UK, for example, widespread immunisation resulted in a 30-fold reduction in the number of notifications, and deaths became rare. Understandably, complacency followed, and when publicity was given to cerebral complications of the vaccine in 1974, its acceptance rate dropped dramatically, followed in 1977 by the biggest epidemic for 20 years (Fig. 3.5). Subsequent studies showed that the risk of permanent brain damage was very small – 1 in 310 000 injections. Increased vaccine uptake resulting from a return of public confidence cut short an expected

Figure 3.5 Whooping cough notifications and vaccine coverage, England and Wales 1940–2003.

epidemic in 1986 and in 1991, when uptake had risen to 88%, an anticipated epidemic failed to materialise.

B. pertussis has a marked tendency to attach itself to respiratory epithelium.[49] In fatal cases, *B. pertussis* can be recovered from the lungs, and the organisms can be seen microscopically in large numbers in the thick mucopurulent film that covers the mucosa of the trachea and the bronchi. The mucus may be so viscous that it obstructs the passage of air and so leads to segmental lung collapse. Spread of the infection via the airways results in bronchopneumonia. In recent years intractable pulmonary hypertension has been recognised in some fatal cases, with large collections of leukocytes being found within the pulmonary vessels in such cases.[50]

Although *B. pertussis* itself seems to be capable of establishing an acute inflammatory reaction in the lower respiratory passages, it would appear from bacteriological studies at necropsy that the terminal, fatal bronchopneumonia is more often caused by *Haemophilus influenzae* or by one of the pyogenic cocci; these are enabled to enter the lungs by the damage caused by the *Bordetella*, which impairs the tracheobronchial defence mechanisms. In infants this complication is the chief cause of death in whooping cough, which in many countries is still one of the most fatal infectious diseases in the first 2 years of life. Bronchiectasis is a notable complication amongst survivors.

Necrotising sialometaplasia

Throughout the lower respiratory tract regenerative processes may be so atypical that carcinomatous transformation has to be considered in the differential diagnosis. This impression is often augmented by excessive mitotic activity and metaplasia. Thus, at the alveolar level necrotising lesions such as infarcts and the granulomatoses may be bordered by foci of atypical squamous hyperplasia that are easily mistaken for squamous cell carcinoma. Similarly, damage to the bronchial epithelium is often followed by atypical regeneration that is easily mistaken for carcinoma,[51] particularly when exfoliated cells are being examined. Bronchoscopy inevitably involves bronchial injury and cytopathologists have to be aware of the atypicalities that follow this procedure. Necrotising lesions of the larynx are sometimes accompanied by atypical regeneration that involves both the surface epithelium and the submucosal glands: the term 'necrotising sialometaplasia'[52,53] has been applied to this and to a similar process involving the trachea in patients with herpetic tracheitis undergoing repeated intubation.[54,55] Microscopically there is coagulative necrosis of the tracheal glands with the ghost outlines of the acinar cells retaining a

lobular distribution. There is often mucous extravasation and a mixed acute and chronic inflammatory infiltrate. Regenerative hyperplasia, often with squamous metaplasia, is usually first evident in the gland ducts. The changes are benign and self-limiting but in small biopsies may be mistaken for those of squamous cell carcinoma or muco-epidermoid carcinoma. Identification of the investing myoepithelial cells by staining for smooth-muscle actin favours sialometaplasia as these cells are soon destroyed by invasive growths.[56] Low immuno-reactivity for p53 also favours this benign process.[53]

CHRONIC OBSTRUCTIVE PULMONARY DISEASE[57]

The term 'chronic obstructive pulmonary disease' (COPD) encompasses three quite distinct conditions that have much in common: chronic bronchitis, emphysema and one that was formerly thought to be a subtype of chronic bronchitis but is now increasingly recognised as a separate disease. No specific name exists for this condition but it is generally known as small-airway disease or chronic obstructive bronchiolitis. It is important to understand how these three diseases differ and what features they share. One obvious difference is that chronic bronchitis and small-airway disease involve conducting airways of differing size whereas emphysema involves the alveoli. Another is that, whilst chronic bronchitis is hypersecretory in nature, small-airway disease is essentially obstructive, and emphysema is a purely destructive process. However, they are related in their causation. The most important aetiological factors in all are cigarette smoking and atmospheric pollution, and for this reason they frequently coexist. They all show airflow limitation to some degree and can therefore be difficult to distinguish clinically, although the ventilatory defect is based on very different structural abnormalities. In chronic bronchitis the airflow limitation is due to inflammatory thickening of the wall and intermittent luminal plugging; in small-airway disease, to inflammatory thickening of the wall and peribronchiolar fibrosis; and in emphysema to premature closure of inherently normal or atrophic airways because of diminished pulmonary elastic recoil.

Morbidity and mortality

COPD is the fourth leading cause of death in Europe and North America and with the increase in smoking in developing countries it is expected to become the third leading cause of death worldwide by 2020.[58] Death comes many years after the onset of the disease and COPD is therefore also a major cause of sickness and incapacity for work. The social gradient of the disease is steep; the death rate in the poorest section of the population is some five times that in the most prosperous. Death is due to respiratory insufficiency, often complicated by bronchopneumonia, cardiac failure or pulmonary thromboembolism.[59] There is also a four- to fivefold increased risk of lung cancer in patients with COPD, as compared with controls matched for cigarette smoking.[60,61]

Clinical features

Patients with COPD are generally current or former smokers over 35 years of age. The sex ratio reflects recent smoking patterns so that in the UK, for example, the disease formerly showed a marked male predominance but is now becoming less common in men and more common in women. Whether or not there is a sex difference in susceptibility is uncertain.[61a]

Patients complain of breathlessness, impaired exercise tolerance and cough. Wheeze is more suggestive of asthma but the conditions may coexist. The cough is particularly likely to be productive in chronic bronchitis. The sputum is typically mucoid and white but the disease is marked by episodes of acute bronchitis when the sputum becomes purulent and yellow. Later the sputum may become purulent continuously; it accumulates in the bronchi during sleep and causes severe obstruction of the airways until it is coughed up in the morning. Whilst a change from white to yellow sputum usually signifies infection it should be noted that large numbers of eosinophils also render the sputum yellow, a potential pitfall in the clinical distinction of bronchitis and asthma.

Microbiological examination of the sputum in chronic bronchitis has shown that the most frequent and important pathogens are *Haemophilus influenzae, Streptococcus pneumoniae, Branhamella (Moraxella) catarrhalis* and *Chlamydia pneumoniae*.[62–67] Purulent sputum usually contains one or more of these organisms in abundance: they tend to disappear after antimicrobial therapy when the sputum becomes mucoid again.

The productive cough appears at first only in the winter months; later it is present all through the year, characteristically with acute exacerbations in winter that are usually precipitated by a viral infection.[68,69]

The majority of patients with COPD suffer from both obstructive airway disease and emphysema but a minority of patients have only one of these conditions. Two clinical syndromes, types A ('pink puffer') and B ('blue bloater'), have been described with the former thought to indicate emphysema and the latter chronic bronchitis.[70,71] The association of the type A syndrome with emphysema is fairly well established but the association of type B with chronic bronchitis is not well substantiated morphologically. Type A patients show rapid shallow breathing and this maintains near normal blood gases at the cost of subjective breathlessness. They are usually thin and because their blood gases are not severely deranged they tend not to develop polycythaemia or cor pulmonale. Type B patients on the other hand are hypoxic and therefore suffer from polycythaemia and repeated bouts of congestive cardiac failure. They are usually obese and oedematous and have a productive cough but they are seldom severely breathless. It is important to realize that most patients with chronic airflow limitation do not fit neatly into one or other of these types. Nor do these two types reflect pure bronchitis or pure emphysema.[72] The fundamental difference between type A and type B patients may be in the brain rather than the lungs: type B patients seem to have a respiratory centre that is relatively unresponsive to the usual stimuli, an abnormality that may be genetically determined.

Chronic bronchitis

Definition

Chronic bronchitis is defined in clinical terms as a persistent or recurrent excess of secretion in the bronchial tree on most days for at least 3 months in the year, over at least 2 years.[73] The secretions of the normal human respiratory tract are believed to total less than 100 ml in 24 hours, all of which is swallowed without the conscious need to clear the throat or cough so that the normal person produces no sputum. The diagnosis of chronic bronchitis may be made only when other conditions that cause expectoration, such as tuberculosis and bronchiectasis, have been excluded.

Chronic bronchitis was formerly subdivided into simple mucoid bronchitis, mucopurulent bronchitis and obstructive bronchitis.[74] It was widely thought that these subdivisions represented successive phases of the disease but a strong counterargument to this was advanced by British epidemiologists.[75] These workers showed that,

while simple mucoid bronchitis progresses to the mucopurulent variety, this does not progress in turn to the obstructive form. In line with this, neither bronchial gland size nor sputum production is significantly related to airflow limitation.[76] The view that the development of obstructive bronchitis is independent of the repeated respiratory infections that characterise mucopurulent bronchitis has been challenged[77] but the obstructive form of the disease is now nevertheless widely recognised as a separate condition – small-airway disease.

Aetiology

Chronic bronchitis affects mainly the middle-aged and elderly and is commoner in men; cigarette smoking is by far the most important cause.[58,78,79] The influence of cigarette smoke often begins in infancy when the child is exposed passively to parental cigarette smoke. This is generally augmented by active cigarette smoking when the child emulates parents or schoolmates and acquires the habit, often becoming addicted for life. However, as with lung cancer, many indulge in smoking with impunity, indicating that susceptibility to disease varies considerably,[57] probably reflecting genetic differences in the control of factors such as the balance of helper and cytotoxic T lymphocytes.[80] Marijuana smoke is likely to be recognised as a further aetiological agent as it has similar morphological effects on the airways as tobacco smoke.[81]

Other factors contributing to chronic bronchitis include general air pollution, which accounts for the higher prevalence of the disease in urban communities, domestic air pollution, which is important in many poor communities due to the combustion of biomass,[82–84a] occupational dust exposure,[85,86] fog, and a damp, cold climate. The morbidity from the disease rises every winter, and remains high throughout the colder, damper months. The occurrence of fog, especially that form known as smog in which the water vapour becomes heavily contaminated with smoke and sulphurous gases, causes a prompt increase in both morbidity and mortality among older people. The heavy 4-day smog in London in 1952 is believed to have precipitated 4000 deaths.

Infections by respiratory viruses and bacteria are also of importance in both initiating and promoting chronic bronchitis.[87] Some patients may recall a liability in their earlier years for head colds to go to their chest.[88] Relatives are often similarly affected. An increased frequency of respiratory infection in childhood has been identified in adults with chronic bronchitis.[89]

These various irritants initiate mucus secretion by a combination of direct action on the mucous cells and nervous reflexes involving sensory nerve endings in the airway epithelium and both local peptidergic and spinal cholinergic pathways. Upregulation of the mucin (MUC) genes is involved and epidermal growth factor is a key mediator in the mucous cell hyperplasia.

Morbid anatomy

When the lungs of a patient with chronic bronchitis are dissected at necropsy, the exposed bronchi, especially those in the lower lobes, are typically filled with a mixture of mucus and pus. When the purulent material is washed away from bronchi that have been opened longitudinally, the underlying mucous membrane is seen to be a dusky red. The calibre of the main bronchi may remain unchanged but distal bronchi characteristically are slightly dilated: when they are opened with fine scissors, the dilation is found to reach almost to the pleura (Fig. 3.6).[90] Some consider the dilation to be due to atrophy of the bronchial wall and describe it in association with emphysema rather than as a feature of chronic bronchitis.[91,92] Others have described degenerative changes in the bronchial cartilage

Figure 3.6 Chronic bronchitis. The bronchi do not show the normal peripheral narrowing; their calibre is maintained until they approach the pleura. *(Courtesy of the late Professor BE Heard, Brompton, UK.)*

Figure 3.7 Chronic bronchitis. The bronchial glands are greatly enlarged; the Reid index measures 0.6, double the normal. The bronchial glands are also almost entirely mucous in type.

Figure 3.8 (A) Normal bronchus. (B) Chronic bronchitis. As well as enlargement of the submucosal glands, chronic bronchitis is characterised by a shift in the nature of the glands from the normal mixed seromucous pattern to one that is almost entirely mucous, while within the mucous acini there is a shift from mixed neutral and acidic (red/blue) mucus to purely acidic (blue) mucus. A further shift within the acidic mucus, one from sialomucin to sulphomucin, is not apparent with this Alcian blue-periodic acid–Schiff stain.

in chronic bronchitis and emphysema and have correlated this with the degree of inflammation.[93] The lung substance is often emphysematous in patients with chronic bronchitis and there may be bronchopneumonia.

Histological appearances

The main features of chronic bronchitis become apparent only when the lungs are examined histologically. The submucosal glands are much enlarged, and there is a shift in gland type from mixed seromucous to pure mucous (Figs 3.7 and 3.8).[94] The enlargement is primarily a hyperplastic change.[95] Furthermore the usual mixture of neutral and acidic glycoprotein in bronchial mucus changes to one that is largely acidic and within the acidic mucins sulphomucin increases at the expense of sialomucin, alterations that possibly increase sputum viscosity. The mucous acini and their ducts become distended with retained mucus.[94,96]

It is possible to correlate the clinical history of chronic bronchitis with the size of the bronchial glands. This may be done by measuring the ratio of the thickness of the gland layer to the thickness of the wall between the base of the surface epithelium and the internal limit of the cartilage plates. The fraction occupied by the glands is known as the Reid index.[94] In chronic bronchitis this may double from the normal value of 0.3 (see Figs 3.7 and 3.8). The Reid index takes no account of the glands situated between the cartilaginous plates and a more accurate method of assessing the size of the glands is to estimate their cross-sectional area as a percentage of that of all the bronchial wall components.[97,98] This is now greatly facilitated by the use of a computerised digitising tablet rather than relying on the accurate but tedious method of point counting.

As well as the glands, the epithelium that lines the bronchi shows signs of increased mucus production, the proportion of goblet cells being increased at the expense of the ciliated cells (Fig. 3.9).[99] Also,

Figure 3.9 Chronic bronchitis. In the surface epithelium, goblet cells are increased at the expense of the ciliated cells.

the surface epithelium may undergo patchy squamous metaplasia. The accompanying loss of cilia, which ordinarily clear bacteria and dust particles from the lower respiratory tract, predisposes to infection.

The fall in the proportion of serous to mucous acini in the bronchial glands may also be expected to promote infection as the serous cells are a major source of the antibacterial agents lysozyme and lactoferrin[100,101]; however, these antibacterial agents continue to be detectable in patients' sputum.[102] The serous cells also contribute the secretory piece to immunoglobulin A, so protecting it from proteolytic degradation. Reduced expression of this secretory piece has been demonstrated in severe COPD.[103] The serous cells are also a major source of secretory leukocyte protease inhibitor.[104] This factor can be identified in the sputum of patients with chronic bronchitis but normal values have not been established: a diminution could help explain why chronic bronchitis and emphysema are so commonly associated.

Mucus accumulates in the airways and may completely fill their lumen. With infection, neutrophil leukocytes are added to the mucus and the airway wall is swollen by oedema and an acute inflammatory infiltrate; between acute attacks, the wall of the airways is infiltrated by lymphocytes and macrophages and its blood vessels are congested. The lymphocytes are largely CD8-positive (cytotoxic/suppressor) T cells, in contrast to the CD4-positive Th2 cells found in asthma.[99,105,106] Thus, although essentially hypersecretory, chronic bronchitis is also a truly inflammatory disease (Fig. 3.10).[107] Furthermore, it appears that the inflammation in turn promotes hypersecretion,[108,109] a process envisaged by an older generation of pathologists when they spoke of catarrhal inflammation. A vicious cycle is thus set in motion in chronic bronchitis, as in bronchiectasis (see p. 119). In contrast to bronchiectasis, however, the musculature and cartilage of the bronchial walls remain intact in chronic bronchitis.[90]

'Wheezy' bronchitis

Hyperplasia of bronchial muscle in chronic bronchitis is reported by some observers[110] but not by others.[111] The explanation for this discrepancy may be that some patients have features of both asthma and bronchitis. The amount of muscle in the airways of these 'wheezy bronchitics' is intermediate between the normal amounts found in

Figure 3.10 Chronic bronchitis with superadded infection. The submucosal glands are enlarged, a gland duct is plugged by mucus, mucus has accumulated in the bronchial lumen and as a consequence of secondary infection there is also pus in the lumen and chronic inflammation of the bronchial wall.

purely bronchitic subjects and the increased amount found in atopic asthmatics.[112]

Constitutional factors, in particular bronchial hyperactivity, may contribute to airflow limitation in certain cigarette smokers who develop 'chronic asthmatic bronchitis'.[113] This concept is embodied in what has become known as the 'Dutch hypothesis' – that smokers with progressive airflow limitation have increased bronchial reactivity and atopic features similar to, but less marked than, those observed in asthma.[114] The observation that cigarette smokers have elevated serum immunoglobulin E levels raises the possibility that some of the adverse effects of smoking might be immunologically mediated.[115] However the elevated serum immunoglobulin E in smokers does not appear to be specific for the common seasonal aeroallergens. Chronic bronchitis and asthma are compared in Table 3.1.[116]

Small-airway disease (chronic obstructive bronchiolitis)

The aetiological differences between chronic bronchitis and small-airway disease are as yet unclear but cigarette smoking is undoubtedly important in both. The latter condition is met more often in those

Table 3.1 Comparison of chronic bronchitis and asthma[116]

	Chronic bronchitis	Asthma
Age	Over 35 years	Any
Smoking history	Almost invariable	Possible
Cough	Persistent and productive	Intermittent and non-productive
Breathlessness	Progressive and persistent	Intermittent and variable
Nocturnal symptoms	Uncommon	Common
Family history	Uncommon unless family members also smoke	Common
Concomitant eczema or allergic rhinitis	Uncommon	Common
Airflow obstruction	Fixed and irreversible	Variable and reversible
Sputum	Macrophages Neutrophils	Eosinophils Charcot–Leyden crystals Creola bodies Curschmann's spirals
Postmortem appearances	Excess mucus Bronchial dilatation Associated emphysema	Mucous plugs Hyperinflation but no emphysema
Airway inflammation	CD8+ T cells Neutrophils periodically	CD4+ T cells Eosinophils Mast cells
Airway congestion and oedema	Present	Present
Airway epithelium	Intact Goblet cell hyperplasia Squamous metaplasia	Fragile with stripping Goblet cell hyperplasia Squamous metaplasia
Basement membrane reticular layer thickening	Mild-to-moderate	Marked
Bronchial glands	Marked enlargement of the mucous acini	Moderate enlargement of both mucous and serous acini
Mucin histochemistry	Shift from neutral to acid and within the acid mucins from sialo- to sulpho-	Unchanged
Airway muscle	May show hypertrophy	Marked hypertrophy
Major complications	Cor pulmonale	Allergic bronchopulmonary aspergillosis

Figure 3.11 Peribronchiolitis and fibrosis in small-airway disease.

patients whose breathlessness steadily increases with the years and in whom there is progressive deterioration in exercise tolerance leading to inability to continue working.

Postmortem studies have shown that in chronic obstructive lung disease the major site of airflow obstruction is in airways of about 2 mm diameter or less.[117] Airways of this calibre, which correspond to those of approximately the eighth generation, have subsequently become generally known as 'small airways'. They include both small bronchi and proximal bronchioles.

Such small-calibre airways are numerous and in health they have a large collective cross-sectional area so that they normally contribute little to total airflow resistance (see Fig. 1.8, p. 7). Many may be lost before there is any appreciable impairment of airflow. It is likely therefore that many cigarette smokers are progressively developing obstructive airway disease long before they notice any significant reduction in their respiratory capabilities. For this reason the periphery of the lung has become known as its 'silent zone'.

Histopathology

Small-airway disease is characterised by bronchiolar goblet cell hyperplasia.[118] This takes place at the expense of Clara cells,[119] which, together with the serous cells of the bronchial glands, secrete an airway-specific low-molecular-weight protease inhibitor (antileukoprotease), which is a potent protective factor against the development of emphysema.[104,120–123] There is also inflammation in the smaller bronchi and bronchioles. Similar chronic inflammatory changes to those affecting the larger airways in chronic bronchitis are observed in the walls and adjacent tissues of bronchioles and small bronchi, the predominant cell again being the CD8-positive T lymphocyte.[124] Wall thickening[125] and fibrosing peribronchiolitis[126] (Fig. 3.11) lead to the lumen becoming severely reduced: this causes irreversible obstruction and severe airflow limitation. The narrowing takes the form of focal stenoses.[127] Proximal to the stenoses the bronchioles are often dilated. Bronchographic medium pools in the dilated segments, giving what has been described as a 'mimosa flower' effect,[128] and there is an absence of peripheral filling.[129] The focal stenoses are difficult to identify in random sections but are well demonstrated in plastic casts of the airways (Fig. 3.12).[130,131] Alternatively, quantitative methods may be employed: these show both organic narrowing and mucus plugging of small airways.[132] It is likely that cases of small-airway disease were included among the patients with chronic lung diseases studied by McLean.[133–135] In many smokers peribronchiolar

Figure 3.12 Small-airway disease. Plastic cast of some small airways of a patient dying of chronic obstructive bronchiolitis, showing a focal stenosis. (*Courtesy of Professor J Bignon, Creteil, France.*)

inflammation and fibrosis involve the more distal respiratory bronchioles and thicken the walls of adjacent alveoli so that there is restrictive as well as obstructive lung disease. This so-called respiratory bronchiolitis-associated interstitial lung disease overlaps with yet another effect of cigarette smoking, namely desquamative interstitial pneumonia, and is dealt with on page 313.

Complications

Patients with small-airway disease are prone to develop cor pulmonale, mainly as a result of widespread hypoxic pulmonary vasoconstriction and the consequent rise in pulmonary vascular resistance. Hypoxic pulmonary hypertension is dealt with on page 424. A further consequence of the hypoxia is a compensatory polycythaemia, the resultant haemoconcentration adding to the increased cardiac burden. Whilst death from small-airway disease is usually due to right-sided heart failure, obstructive respiratory failure and bronchopneumonia also contribute. These conditions are often present in combination.

Emphysema

Emphysema denotes pathological inflation of the affected tissue. Two fundamentally different forms are recognised, vesicular and interstitial (or surgical). The first affects spaces that normally contain air whilst the second represents the ingress of air into the normally airless interstitial planes of the lung and contiguous connective tissues outside the lung. The distinction between vesicular and interstitial emphysema was first made by Laennec in 1819 but pathological descriptions of the condition have been traced back to as early as 1679.[136] The adjective vesicular has fallen into disuse and may be inferred when the term 'emphysema' is used without qualification. Although interstitial emphysema does not fall within current definitions of emphysema the term 'interstitial (or surgical) emphysema' persists and the condition is described as such on pp. 48 and 108.

Vesicular emphysema is a common condition. A consecutive series of 50 male necropsies in London identified emphysema in more than trace amounts in 37, although few of the patients had respiratory symptoms.[137] Similar findings have been reported in other English cities.[138]

Airways may be normal in emphysema. Alternatively, they may be atrophic and dilated but prone to collapse prematurely,[91,92] unless there is also chronic bronchitis with its characteristic thickening of the airway wall by glandular hyperplasia and inflammatory oedema.

Definition

Emphysema was defined in 1959 as a condition of the lung characterised by increase beyond the normal in the size of air spaces distal to the terminal bronchiole either from dilatation or from destruction of their walls.[73] Subsequently, this was modified by excluding purely distensive forms of pulmonary enlargement so that the definition became: 'an abnormal increase in the size of air spaces beyond the terminal bronchioles with destruction of air space walls'.[139] This seems to be the most sensible definition. However, in some patients the destruction is secondary to scarring and it has been suggested that this type of air space enlargement should also be excluded from the definition. The American Thoracic Society accepted this recommendation and adopted the following definition: 'abnormal, permanent enlargement of the air spaces distal to the terminal bronchioles, accompanied by destruction of their walls and without obvious fibrosis'.[140,141] The exclusion of fibrosis is unfortunate for two reasons. Firstly the term 'scar emphysema' is a useful one and secondly those forms of emphysema that are not secondary to scarring do entail some degree of fibrosis, albeit slight.[142-144] More severe centriacinar fibrosis is being increasingly recognised in smokers in association with what is described as air space enlargement, a term that is used in place of the term 'emphysema' because of the fibrosis. This combination of centriacinar air space enlargement and fibrosis is often termed smoking-associated interstitial lung disease and is considered again under this title on page 373.

Pathology

Early emphysematous changes can only be detected microscopically: these include an increase in the size and number of fenestrae (pores of Kohn) in the alveolar walls.[145] When the destruction is moderate in degree, there is loss of alveolar walls, resulting in fewer alveolar attachments to bronchioles and the consequent premature closure of these airways on expiration.[72,146-148] Quantitation of the microscopic changes in the lung substance can best be achieved by the application of an image analyser set to calculate factors such as mean linear intercept[149,150] or the air space wall surface area per unit volume.[151,152] More severe changes are characterised by complete loss of most of the wall of the air spaces, bronchiolar as well as alveolar, leaving only a network of blood vessels and some interlobular septa.

These gross changes are better appreciated by the macroscopic study of whole lung slices rather than microscopy. If the lungs are fixed by distension with aqueous formalin at a pressure of 25–30 cm of water before slicing, the emphysema can be appreciated much better than in the collapsed fresh lung. Fixation overnight is adequate and if time presses a few hours' fixation is beneficial. If the fixed slices are impregnated with barium sulphate, deficiencies in the lung substance are highlighted and the amount of destruction and the type of emphysema can be better appreciated.[153] Barium sulphate impregnation is simply achieved by gently squeezing a slice of lung in a saturated solution of sodium sulphate and then immersing it in one of barium nitrate. Paper-mounted whole lung sections can be prepared if a permanent record is desired.[154] Various ways of quantitating the gross changes have been recommended[155] but none is as accurate or as easy as computerised image analysis.[156]

Several morphological types of emphysema are distinguished according to the part of the acinus that is affected, as observed in whole lung slices or paper-mounted whole lung sections. Three of

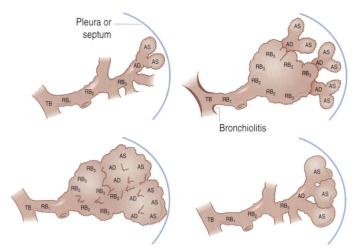

Figure 3.13 Morphological types of emphysema in relation to the acinar architecture of the lung. Upper left: The normal acinus. Upper right: Centriacinar emphysema, in which third-order respiratory bronchioles are predominantly involved. Lower left: Panacinar emphysema in which there is destructive enlargement of all air spaces distal to the terminal bronchiole, and the acinus is affected uniformly. Lower right: Paraseptal emphysema. TB, terminal bronchiole; RB, three orders of respiratory bronchioles; AD, alveolar duct; AS, alveolar sac. For simplicity only one order of alveolar duct and one of alveolar sac are drawn and they are not to scale.

these types, centriacinar, paraseptal and panacinar, are illustrated diagrammatically in Figure 3.13. The fourth type, scar or irregular emphysema, bears no relation to the acinar architecture of the lung.

Centriacinar emphysema

This form of emphysema is characterised by focal lesions confined to the centres of the acini (Fig. 3.14). They are often pigmented with dust. The changes are more marked in the upper lobes, a feature that has been attributed to the greater gravitational forces there, consequent upon our upright posture, and also upon the support afforded to the lower lobes by the diaphragm. Spaces that exceed 1 cm in size are known as bullae and may be seen in severe cases. The alveolar walls are lost; only some pulmonary vessels survive to cross the spaces as seemingly bare strands radiating outward from their parent arteries to supply the alveoli of the periphery of the acini (see Fig. 3.14). Although centriacinar emphysema affects the upper lobes of the lungs more severely than the lower, any part may be involved and centriacinar emphysema is quite often accompanied by panacinar emphysema. Severe centriacinar emphysema may be difficult to distinguish from the panacinar form but an upper-lobe predominance suggests that the lesions were originally confined to the centres of the acini, as does the presence of an obviously centriacinar form of emphysema in the less severely affected portions of the lung.

Panacinar emphysema

Panacinar emphysema involves all the air spaces beyond the terminal bronchiole more or less equally (Fig. 3.15). Most classic descriptions of emphysema refer to this variety. It affects all zones or is worse in the lower lobes. There may be a remarkable degree of parenchymal destruction. The lungs have a doughy feel, pit on pressure, do not collapse when the chest is opened and overlap the heart because of their great size. They appear very pale because of loss of substance; air-filled bullae, several centimetres across, may be seen.

Paraseptal emphysema

This form of emphysema affects air spaces adjacent to septa or to the pleura, thus involving only the periphery of the lung lobules (Fig. 3.16B). It may result from forces pulling on the septa and perhaps also from inflammation. It may occur alone or in association with other forms of emphysema.

Particularly large solitary bullae are apt to form in paraseptal emphysema (Fig. 3.16A). On inspiration, emphysematous portions of the lung in general and large bullae in particular are preferentially inflated, in accordance with Laplace's law, which states that a distending force is proportional to surface tension and inversely proportional to diameter. Inflation of these large useless air sacs prevents the expansion of adjacent normal lung and their excision may be beneficial. Subpleural bullae that are liable to rupture and cause pneumothorax are also particularly common in paraseptal emphysema. Giant bullae may be multilocular or crossed by fibrous bands containing the remnants of blood vessels.

Some bullae have oedematous papillary infoldings which bear a superficial histological resemblance to chorionic villi and this has given rise to the somewhat bizarre terms placental transmogrification of the lung and bullous placentoid lesion or, if fat is also present, pulmonary lipomatosis (see p. 703).

Irregular, scar or cicatricial 'emphysema'

This term has been used to describe permanent enlargement of air spaces distal to terminal bronchioles caused by fibrosis, a category of enlargement that is specifically excluded from the latest definitions of emphysema (see above). This type of air space enlargement does not affect the lungs in any regular pattern in relation to the acini or lobules, but occurs in focal areas near scars. It is a consequence of the scars and is therefore often known as scar or cicatricial 'emphysema'. Diffuse pulmonary fibrosis is often accompanied by widespread irregular 'emphysema', which together with bronchiolectasis gives a characteristic gross appearance known as 'honeycombing' that reflects end-stage fibrosis, typically in idiopathic pulmonary fibrosis (see Fig. 6.10A). Apical foci of cicatricial 'emphysema' with bulla formation are found in 6% of healthy young adults and are the probable cause of many cases of spontaneous pneumothorax (see p. 711).

Aetiology and pathogenesis of emphysema

Better knowledge of the anatomical types of emphysema has improved our understanding of its aetiology. So too have discoveries concerning the control of tissue proteolysis.

Centriacinar emphysema is related to cigarette smoking[157] and has long been thought to be the result of airway inflammation.[126,158] Particular blame is attached to elastases released by neutrophil leukocytes during episodes of acute inflammation. That proteases can have this effect is shown by the experimental induction of a non-inflammatory panacinar form of emphysema by the intratracheal injection of the proteolytic enzyme papain.[159]

Panacinar emphysema, in contrast, is recognised as being that form associated with an inherited deficiency of α_1-antitrypsin, which is normally the chief component of plasma α_1-globulin.[160–161a] Deficiency of this protein results in leukocyte elastases acting unopposed on the connective tissues of the lungs.

α_1-Antitrypsin deficiency is inherited through an autosomal-recessive gene which exhibits polymorphism, the variants being classified alphabetically in a Pi (protease inhibitor) nomenclature according to their electrophoretic mobility. For example, $PiBB$ is the homozygote for an anodal variant and $PiZZ$ for a cathodal variant, with $PiMM$ representing the homozygote for the normal M allele. There are over

Figure 3.14 Centriacinar emphysema. (A) Paper-mounted whole lung section. (B) Inflation fixation and barium sulphate precipitation. Dust-pigmented deficiencies in the lung substance are confined to the centres of the acini. As well as using barium sulphate to emphasise the emphysema, the pulmonary arteries have been injected with a barium gelatine preparation for angiography.

70 different variants. Those of particular medical relevance are the Z and S mutants.[162-164] The frequency of Pi types in England and Wales and the corresponding serum levels of α_1-antitrypsin are shown in Table 3.2. Although α_1-antitrypsin deficiency was first identified in Sweden, subsequent studies have shown that it affects all races.[165] Madeira is reputed to have the highest prevalence.[166]

PiZZ homozygotes are prone to suffer hepatitis, cirrhosis or emphysema, the liver being the site of synthesis of the enzyme and the lung an important site of its action.[167] α_1-Antitrypsin deficiency accounts for about 6% of all clinically significant emphysema (*PiZZ* 5%, *PiSS* and *PiSZ* 1%). It is debatable whether *PiM* heterozygotes (*PiMS* and *PiMZ*) have an increased risk of emphysema but it appears unlikely, particularly if they do not smoke.[168,169]

The emphysema associated with α_1-antitrypsin deficiency develops unusually early in life, typically in the third or fourth decade. The condition is familial and patients may have seen an older relative die of the same disease. The probability of survival to age 50 years is estimated to be 52% and to age 60 years 16%.[170] Mortality is reported to be 2% a year.[171] The bases of the lungs are particularly affected because their greater blood flow, which is attributable to gravity, brings more leukocytes to these regions.[167] Although emphysema is the predominant respiratory abnormality, radiographic changes sug-

Table 3.2 Serum α_1-antitrypsin concentrations (expressed as percentage of normal level) and frequencies of the commoner phenotypes in the UK[162,163]

Phenotype	Serum concentration	Frequency
MM	100	86
MS	75	9
MZ	57	3
SS	52	0.25
SZ	37	0.2
ZZ	16	0.03

gesting bronchiectasis are also described.[172] Rarely, several family members suffer from either α_1-antitrypsin deficiency or idiopathic pulmonary fibrosis.[173]

α_2-Macroglobulin is another antiprotease that is synthesised in the liver but it is of too large a molecular size to leave the circulation.

Figure 3.15 Panacinar emphysema. The whole of lung acinus is affected uniformly. (A) Paper-mounted whole lung section. (B) Barium sulphate precipitation.

However, as well as antiproteases that reach the lungs from the blood, antiproteases specific to the lung have been identified, notably in the serous acini of the bronchial glands and in the Clara cells of the bronchioles.[104,120–122] A reported increase in Clara cells in small-airway disease[123] possibly represents a compensatory response to inactivation of antiproteases by irritants such as cigarette smoke[174,175] and to the increased release of proteases that cigarette smoke elicits from phagocytic cells.[176] Others report that the bronchiolar goblet cell proliferation seen in smokers takes place at the expense of Clara cells.[119]

Cigarette smokers have a constant increase in alveolar macrophages,[177,178] particularly in the central part of the lung acini.[179] During phagocytosis these cells release proteolytic enzymes[180] and a neutrophil-chemotactic factor,[181] and this process is enhanced by cigarette smoking.[182] The role of cigarette smoking in the development of emphysema was demonstrated in a radiological study of persistent smokers during which foci of ground-glass attenuation probably representing bronchiolocentric aggregates of alveolar macrophages progressed to emphysema over a 5-year period in about 25% of cases.[183]

Neutrophils are an even richer source of proteases than macrophages and large numbers of these cells enter the lungs in the acute exacerbations that characterise chronic bronchitis. An imbalance between proteases and antiproteases is therefore considered to underlie the aetiology of emphysema.[184] The various factors contributing to this imbalance are represented in Figure 3.17. This protease–antiprotease theory may be invoked to explain both centriacinar and panacinar emphysema, which frequently coexist.

The inflammatory component of emphysema is often maintained long after the patient gives up smoking,[185] possibly because peptides derived from degraded connective tissue are chemotactic for inflammatory cells.[186] This suggests that the disease is sometimes self-perpetuating, which may explain the progressive clinical deterioration that is seen in some ex-smokers with obstructive airway disease.

A check-valve mechanism is often envisaged to explain the formation of bullae, but pressure measurements at thoracotomy show that the air in bullae is at the same negative pressure as that in the rest of the lungs, except when they are subjected to positive-pressure ventilation.[187] It would appear that bullae originate in the same way

Figure 3.16 Paraseptal emphysema. (A) Giant bulla formation. (B) Barium sulphate precipitation.

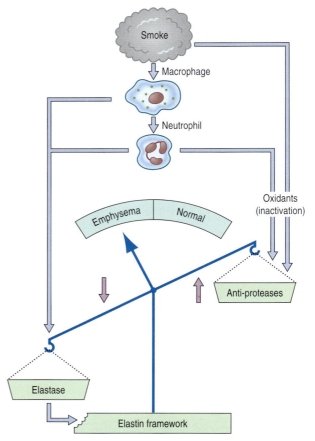

Figure 3.17 The pathogenesis of emphysema, envisaged as a consequence of imbalance between proteases and antiproteases in the lung.

as smaller emphysematous foci, namely by a process of unchecked proteolysis rather than through undue distensive forces.

Cadmium is a further factor involved in the pathogenesis of emphysema. It has been found that occupational exposure to cadmium fumes over long periods can cause emphysema,[188] and this clinical observation has experimental support from the production of emphysema through the introduction of cadmium into the trachea of animals or its inhalation in the form of an aerosol.[189] In humans, the emphysema that is attributable to inhalation of cadmium affects the upper lobes severely and is mainly of the centriacinar type.[190] Cigarette smoke is an important source of inhaled cadmium and there is a significant correlation between the degree of emphysema and the concentration of cadmium in the lungs at necropsy, even in the case of patients who have not been exposed to cadmium fumes at work.[191] A combination of occupational cadmium exposure and cigarette smoking appears to be particularly dangerous.[192]

Functional effects of emphysema

Although much emphasis is placed on elastin digestion in the pathogenesis of emphysema, it is debatable whether the amounts of elastin are reduced in this disease.[143,144,193] Nevertheless, if a piece of elastic material such as a rubber band is cut at merely one point its functional integrity is completely destroyed: focal digestion of alveolar elastin may be expected to have a similar effect without there necessarily being much overall loss of this protein. Experiments inducing emphysema with elastase show that losses in elastin can be made good but that the structural derangement is irreversible.[194]

Although elastic recoil is often attributed to the connective tissue framework of the lung it is markedly reduced when alveolar air is replaced by water, showing that it is surface tensive forces at the tissue–air interface that underlies recoil. These forces are, of course, also weakened when there is loss of alveolar tissue.

Diminished elastic recoil and severance of alveolar attachments to bronchioles result in premature closure of these airways on expiration (Fig. 3.18).[72,146–148] The resultant air trapping is responsible for the overinflation of the lungs and 'barrel chest' that are characteristic of emphysema. Respiration is conducted near maximal lung volume, which severely compromises inspiratory muscle function. Some adaptation to this is achieved by an increase in the proportion of slow ('endurance') fibres in the inspiratory muscles.[195]

Emphysema also results in there being less alveolar surface available for gas exchange but the extent of this is seldom appreciated when lung slices are examined. The relationship of diameter to surface area is logarithmic so that for a given increase in air space diameter there is a much greater loss in surface area. Normal alveoli are about 0.25 mm in diameter, which corresponds to an alveolar surface area of about 24 mm^2/mm^3, whereas by the time emphysema is just visible to the naked eye at an alveolar diameter of 1 mm, three-quarters of the surface area of the lung has been lost, the alveolar surface area being reduced to 6 mm^2/mm^3. Emphysema that is easily recognisable in the postmortem room has air spaces that measure about 4 mm in diameter, when the alveolar surface is less than 10% of normal (Fig. 3.19).

Emphysema is often accompanied by the small-airway disease dealt with in the preceding section. In their different ways, emphysema and small-airway disease both contribute to the airflow limitation that these patients suffer, one permitting premature bronchiolar closure and the other narrowing the bronchioles, but there has been much debate as to which of these mechanisms is the more important.

Treatment of emphysema

The cessation of smoking is essential to minimising progression of the disease but apart from bullectomy there has, until recently, been no effective treatment for emphysema. However, in recent years, the intravenous infusion of α_1-antitrypsin,[196] lung transplantation[197] and lung volume reduction surgery (reduction pneumoplasty)[198–200] have been introduced. In addition, there is potential in techniques that enhance expiratory air flow by inserting bronchial valves or injecting polymers, producing bronchopulmonary fenestrations and the thoracoscopic plication or compression of emphysematous lung.[201–206] In the future there is also the possibility of genetic manipulation to correct α_1-antitrypsin deficiency.

Figure 3.18 Emphysema showing bronchiolar collapse due to loss of alveolar attachments.

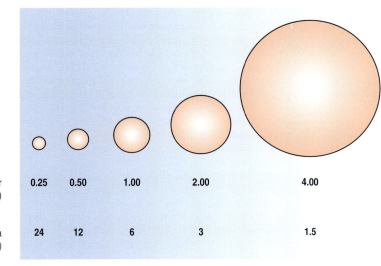

Diameter (mm)	0.25	0.50	1.00	2.00	4.00
Surface area ($mm^2\ mm^{-3}$)	24	12	6	3	1.5

Figure 3.19 Relationship between alveolar diameter and surface area. The normal alveolar diameter is about 0.25 mm. Emphysema is just detectable when the diameter is increased fourfold (to 1 mm), at which time there is a 75% loss of alveolar surface area. At autopsy the emphysematous air spaces commonly have a diameter of 4 mm, representing a loss of alveolar surface of approximately 90%.

Bullectomy is practised to reduce the risk of pneumothorax and to eliminate tissue which, in accordance with Laplace's law is preferentially aerated and compresses comparatively normal adjacent tissue. In contrast to bullectomy, lung volume reduction surgery often involves the resection of much comparatively normal lung tissue as well as the most severely diseased portions, a seemingly paradoxical way to treat someone who has already lost considerable lung tissue. The undoubted success of this operation probably stems from the improved efficiency of the inspiratory muscles when they are no longer operating at maximal stretch.[207,208] Pathological examination of the resected tissue is worthwhile as it occasionally reveals unexpected diseases such as fibrosis, inflammation, lymphangioleiomyomatosis and even carcinoma that adversely affect the postoperative course.[209,210]

Early attempts at treating emphysema by unilateral lung transplantation were unsuccessful and at the time this was attributed to a poor understanding of Laplace's principles, which dictate that the inspired air will enter the large-volume diseased lung rather than the unilateral implant. In retrospect, rejection was the probable cause of the failure. Today, transplantation of one or both lungs is firmly established in the treatment of emphysema; the success of the unilateral procedure probably depends partly upon the improved efficiency of the inspiratory muscles, as in lung volume reduction surgery.

Intervention at the molecular level has great potential in the prevention of emphysema in groups particularly at risk, such as those with α_1-antitrypsin deficiency, and replacement or supplemental therapy using either natural or recombinant antiproteases is being attempted. Unfortunately the half-life of natural α_1-antitrypsin is only 4 days, so weekly infusions are needed. Recombinant α_1-antitrypsin has an even shorter half-life but aerosol trials are in progress. Bronchial antileukoprotease has also been produced by recombinant methods and trials of this are under way. Work is also in progress on the production of synthetic antiproteases.

Emphysema-like conditions

The term 'emphysema' has been applied to several other conditions, none of which falls strictly within the limits of the current definition which requires destruction of respiratory tissue as well as the abnormal enlargement of air spaces.

Senile 'emphysema'

The condition that has been known as senile 'emphysema' is not a true form of the disease because the alterations are neither destructive nor beyond the limits of normal age change. After a developmental period of alveolar multiplication that terminates in adolescence, there is a gradual alteration in the shape of the lungs coupled with progressive diminution in elastic recoil and alveolar surface area, the latter reducing by about 4% in each decade after the age of 30 years.[211] Total lung capacity remains constant throughout adult life but with increasing age the lungs change shape, increasing in height and particularly in anteroposterior distance. There is also a gradual shift in the distribution of air from the alveoli to the alveolar ducts and bronchioles. The alveolar ducts gradually enlarge and the mouths of alveoli opening from them dilate so that the alveoli become more shallow. All these changes may be regarded as part of the normal ageing process and therefore outwith the definition of emphysema. Although the ageing lungs lose some elastic recoil, this is not so great as in true emphysema, and they generally collapse when the chest is opened. This gave rise to the term 'atrophic emphysema' as an alternative to senile emphysema and in contrast to 'hypertrophic emphysema' which was formerly used for true emphysema. The definition of emphysema given on page 102 renders the terms atrophic, senile and hypertrophic emphysema redundant.

Infantile lobar 'emphysema'

Infantile lobar 'emphysema' is described on page 72. It is the result of valvular obstruction to a lobar bronchus and is characterised by extreme distension without destruction.

Compensatory 'emphysema'

This is another condition characterised by distension without destruction. It occurs when parts of the lung collapse or are removed. Pneumonectomy leads to distension of the remaining lung rather than true (destructive) emphysema. Lung cancer is a common reason for pneumonectomy, and with cigarette smoking underlying both lung cancer and emphysema, the remaining lung may well show true emphysema: the relationship between the pneumonectomy and the emphysema is not then a causal one.

Focal 'emphysema'

Focal 'emphysema' and simple pneumoconiosis of coalworkers are terms applied to a distensive bronchiolectasis that closely simulates the milder degrees of centriacinar emphysema.[212] It may represent an early form of centriacinar emphysema but is said to affect more proximal respiratory bronchioles and to be non-destructive. Until recently, the UK pneumoconiosis medical panels have restricted their attention to fibrosis, not attempting to distinguish focal and centriacinar emphysema and attributing both to social factors rather than occupation. Others did not accept this and believed that mine dust causes chronic bronchitis, obstructive bronchiolitis and true emphysema, and in addition to this, focal dilatation of respiratory bronchioles.[213–215] This view has now prevailed so that British miners are now compensated financially if they have these diseases (see also p. 340).

Interstitial emphysema

The fundamental difference between this condition and those described above is outlined on page 102 and may be summarised thus: whereas all other forms of emphysema affect spaces that normally contain air, interstitial emphysema represents the ingress of air into tissues that are normally airless.

Air reaches the interstitial tissues of the lung when abnormal pressure ruptures the alveolar walls. Interstitial emphysema is therefore a form of barotrauma. The rupture may be due to excessively high pressure caused by violent artificial respiration, exposure to the blast of explosions, sudden decompression, or tearing of alveolar walls by fractured ribs or by instruments.

At operation or necropsy, interstitial emphysema is seen as small bubbles of air in the connective tissue immediately beneath the visceral pleura (see Fig. 2.16, p. 49). Large interstitial air bubbles are termed blebs, as distinct from bullae, which represent enlargement of pre-existent air spaces (see Fig. 13.4, p. 711).[139] Air in the interstitial tissues may track along the connective tissue sheaths about the pulmonary vessels to the hila of the lungs, producing mediastinal emphysema; it may then reach the neck and present subcutaneously as surgical emphysema. Systemic air embolism may complicate interstitial emphysema.

Microscopically, minute air bubbles appear as seemingly empty interstitial spaces, particularly in the abundant connective tissue that surrounds the pulmonary artery and airway and forms the interlobular septa. The differential diagnosis on microscopy is from congenital lymphangiectasia and this can be extremely difficult, not least because the air tracks within lymphatics as well as through the surrounding connective tissues. It is therefore helpful if the nature of the contents of the spaces, gaseous or fluid, is ascertained at necropsy. If the emphysema has been present for a few days before death, the diag-

Table 3.3 A comparison of mucoid impaction and plastic bronchitis

	Mucoid impaction	**Plastic bronchitis**
Clinical features	Aggravation of underlying asthma. Progression to hilar bronichectasis	Expectoration of stringy sputum
Cause	Atopy: allergic bronchopulmonary aspergillosis complicating asthma	Unknown. Numerous associations of questionable causal relationship, e.g. heart disease, lymphatic abnormalities, hypogammaglobulinaemia
Gross appearance of expectorate	A short stubby mucoid plug	A long stringy bronchial cast of up to eight airway generations
Microscopic appearance of plug/cast	Alternating layers of mucus and inspissated eosinophils with numerous Charcot–Leyden crystals and scanty *Aspergillus* hyphae	Alternating layers of mucus and fibrin with variable numbers of lymphocytes. No eosinophils. No fungi

Figure 3.20 A 15-cm-long bronchial cast from a patient with plastic bronchitis. Compare with the short, stubby plugs characteristic of allergic bronchopulmonary aspergillosis shown in Fig. 5.4.17, p. 230.

nosis is simplified by the development of a foreign-body giant cell reaction to the air (see Fig. 2.18, p. 49),[216–218] similar to that found in pneumatosis coli and following the experimental injection of gases into the subcutaneous tissues.[216]

PLASTIC BRONCHITIS

Patients with plastic bronchitis are generally well but complain of fits of coughing that often result in them involuntarily expectorating long stringy pieces of sputum, which causes them much social embarrassment.[219–221,223–224] The expectorate represents a bronchial cast of up to eight airway generations (Fig. 3.20). Microscopically the cast is seen to consist of alternating bands of fibrin and mucus, with the fibrin containing variable numbers of lymphocytes.[220,221] The appearances suggest that the cast represents an inspissated fibrinous exudate and the term 'fibrinous bronchitis' is sometimes applied to the condition. Several associated conditions have been described[220,222,224–225] and it is possible that some of these have a causal relationship, notably heart failure and lymphatic abnormalities. Plastic bronchitis is often confused with the mucoid impaction of allergic bronchopulmonary aspergillosis,[226] which is characterised by the expectoration of short stubby gobbets of mucus (see Fig. 5.4.17, p. 230). The two conditions are quite different. They are compared in Table 3.3.[220,227,228]

CHRONIC IDIOPATHIC COUGH

A chronic cough, defined as one lasting for more than 8 weeks, is very common. Usually there is an identifiable cause but this is not always the case and it is postulated that such patients have an intrinsic synaptic excitability in the brainstem, spine or airway innervation that enhances the normal cough reflex and persists after the resolution of the initiating event.[229] Bronchial biopsy shows non-specific changes including goblet cell hyperplasia, increased vascularity and sub-basement membrane fibrosis but nothing that distinguishes these patients from those with cough of known cause.[230]

BRONCHIAL ASTHMA

Bronchial asthma is to be distinguished from the aetiologically distinct condition of cardiac asthma. The latter represents pulmonary oedema consequent upon a failing left heart. Bronchial asthma, hereafter called simply asthma, is a condition in which breathing is periodically rendered difficult by widespread narrowing of the bronchi that changes in severity over short periods of time, either spontaneously or under treatment.[73] The difficulty becomes particularly apparent during expiration because the airways normally collapse during that phase of respiration, and because the expiratory muscles are less powerful than those that act during inspiration. Clinically, the disease is characterised by episodic attacks of wheezing, tightness of the chest, shortness of breath and cough.

Extrinsic and intrinsic forms of asthma

Asthma is said to be 'extrinsic' if allergy to exogenous substances is recognised, and 'intrinsic' if no such exogenous factors can be identified. Extrinsic asthma is the commoner; it usually begins in childhood and is generally paroxysmal, the attack starting suddenly and lasting a few hours or days. Boys are affected about twice as commonly as girls. Extrinsic asthma tends to become less severe as the child grows older, and often ceases during adolescence. However, about 30% of asthmatic children continue to have symptoms in adult life. Extrinsic asthma is often familial and some of the genes responsible have been identified.[231–234] This form of asthma is frequently preceded by flexural infantile eczema and succeeded in adult life by perennial vasomotor rhinitis, although in such families any one of these three diseases may affect some members much more than others. In contrast, intrinsic asthma more often has its onset in adult life, is chronic, with exacerbations and remissions less evident, and tends to worsen with age; also the symptoms are apt to become more severe in winter, when the asthmatic disabilities are likely to be complicated by infection of the respiratory tract. In both types of the disease, the dyspnoea is characteristically accompanied by cough, wheezy breathing, some cyanosis and expectoration. Blood eosinophilia is more prominent in extrinsic asthma but eosinophils are found in the airways in both. Serum immunoglobulin E is often raised in extrinsic asthma and normal or low in intrinsic asthma. There is an increased incidence of nasal polyps in both forms of asthma, but especially in the intrinsic variety and in certain asthmatic patients in whom bronchospasm is triggered by aspirin. Despite these differences the pathological features are similar and an immunological basis may be envisaged in both.[235,236]

Epidemiology

Over the past few decades the prevalence of asthma has increased considerably in most developed countries, where it now stands at about 10%. The reason for this is unclear but it is notable that it has been paralleled by similar increases in the prevalence of allergic rhinitis and eczema.

General atmospheric pollution has been widely incriminated but there is little to support this: the increase has been experienced in countries such as New Zealand which have little atmospheric pollution and in Philadelphia at a time when atmospheric pollution declined.[237] Atmospheric pollution is more likely to aggravate asthma than cause it. Changes in the home that encourage the growth of the principal allergen, the house dust mite (higher temperature and humidity and extensive carpeting), are more likely environmental factors.[238,239]

Another possibility is the decline in childhood infections in the developed countries. Infection induces a Th1 response rather than the Th2 reactions responsible for atopy (see aetiology, below).[240] Indirect support for this possibility comes from studies of family size and birth order. Atopy is less common in children belonging to large families and, within such families, in the younger children – the ones that are most likely to be exposed in infancy to infections brought home by their siblings.[241,242] More direct evidence comes from studies showing less atopy in those who had previously had measles,[243] were seropositive for hepatitis A[244,245] or gave a strong tuberculin reaction.[246] This raises the attractive possibility of preventive immunisation using harmless bacteria.[247]

Mortality figures have fluctuated over the past few decades, apparently being influenced adversely on occasion by the introduction of new drugs, particularly β-agonists.[248,249] The mechanism underlying these fluctuations is not fully understood but overdosage, cardiac dysrhythmia, refractoriness to the bronchodilatory effect of the drug and a false sense of security afforded by carrying an inhaler are all

Figure 3.21 Charcot–Leyden crystals in sputum from an asthmatic patient.

thought to have contributed.[250] The prognosis is worse in late-onset intrinsic asthma. Most asthma deaths occur in the elderly, although asthma accounts for a greater proportion of deaths in the young (0.9% of those under 25 against 0.3% overall).

The sputum in asthma

The sputum is viscous[251] and yellow in asthma. The colour should not be taken as evidence that the sputum is infected. It is due to myeloperoxidase, which is found in both eosinophils and neutrophils. In asthma, the sputum is rich in eosinophils, but not neutrophils unless there is also infection. As well as eosinophils, microscopy shows the presence of certain formed elements: Charcot–Leyden crystals, Curschmann's spirals and Creola bodies.

Charcot–Leyden crystals are found when there are large numbers of eosinophils. They have the shape of a pair of long, narrow, six-sided pyramids placed base to base (Fig. 3.21). Their hexagonal shape can often be seen when they are cut across in histological preparations. Chromatographic studies suggested that they consisted of lysophospholipase derived from the cell membranes of eosinophils[252] but molecular analyses indicate that they represent a β-galactose-binding lectin, galectin-10.[253]

A Curschmann spiral (Fig. 3.22) is a corkscrew-shaped twist of condensed mucus several millimetres long that is usually surrounded by an elongated mass of clear or opalescent material. Curschmann spirals are widely believed to represent bronchial casts, but their calibre is more commensurate with that of a bronchial gland duct or of a peripheral bronchiole. Furthermore they have also been observed in uterine cervical smears, and in peritoneal and pleural effusions, where they have been attributed to myxoid degeneration of the subserosal connective tissue.[254]

Creola bodies (see Fig. 3.22) are compact clumps or strips of columnar epithelial cells shed from the bronchus. They are sometimes found in the sputum of asthmatics and care must be taken not to mistake them for exfoliated adenocarcinoma cells.[255]

Morbid anatomy

No differences are recognised between the structural changes in extrinsic and intrinsic asthma, but most of our knowledge has come from necropsies in cases of status asthmaticus. This has tended to overemphasise the terminal features and the complications of the condition, but from the few biopsy specimens obtained from asthmatics or autopsies performed on asthmatics dying of other diseases, it seems

Figure 3.22 A Curschmann spiral and two Creola bodies in sputum from an asthmatic patient. Methylene blue stain.

Figure 3.24 Status asthmaticus. Tenacious plugs of mucus occlude the airways. *(Reproduced by permission of Dr GA Russell, Tunbridge Wells, UK.)*

Figure 3.23 The lungs of a patient dying of status asthmaticus. After their removal from the chest and exposure to atmospheric pressure the lungs fail to collapse owing to mucus obstructing the airways. *(Reproduced by permission of Dr GA Russell, Tunbridge Wells, UK.)*

that qualitatively similar but less severe lesions are present between attacks: during non-fatal attacks it is assumed that similar lesions of intermediate severity are present. Bronchography has shown that airway plugging is widespread between asthmatic attacks as well as being prominent in patients dying of asthma.[256]

The gross appearances are characteristic. When the chest is opened in cases of death in status asthmaticus, the lungs are found to be greatly distended: they fail to retract as normal lungs do when the negative intrapleural pressure is replaced by atmospheric pressure on opening the pleural cavities (Fig. 3.23). Contrasting with the general distension, small foci of collapse may sometimes be seen as dark, airless, firm areas, depressed below the level of the surrounding lung. The airways are occluded by plugs of thick, tenacious mucus (Fig. 3.24). These are found in airways of all sizes beyond the second-order bronchi[256] but the most striking changes are seen in airways of about 5 mm diameter. When the cut surface of the lung is exposed, the bronchi of this size are seen to be filled with grey plugs of viscous

mucus that can be made to protrude from the lumen by compressing the lungs. Bronchography shows that air can pass the plugs only on inspiration.[256]

Patches of subpleural fibrosis and honeycombing are common, particularly in the upper lobes; these are possibly the sequel of eosinophilic pneumonia which is often most marked in the periphery of the upper lobes. It is notable in asthma that, although the lungs may be fully distended with air at necropsy, very little emphysema is found. Some patients have right ventricular hypertrophy but this is uncommon in the absence of associated bronchiectasis or chronic bronchitis.

The above changes are typically found in patients dying hours after the onset of an asthmatic attack but they have also been found after death in asthmatic patients who have been well seconds earlier.[257,258] Rarely, a patient with asthma dies suddenly and the airways are found to be empty of mucus.[259] Myocardial contraction bands that have been described in such patients[260] are possibly connected with the overuse of β-adrenergic drugs, which may have contributed to these deaths.[261,262] Other such patients have been found to have inflammation of their cardiac conduction system.[263]

Mucous plugging of airways and hyperinflation of the lungs are not confined to patients with a history of asthma. They are also found in patients dying of anaphylaxis initiated by factors such as wasp or bee venom, foodstuffs and drugs.[264]

Histopathology

Microscopically, three major processes are seen to contribute to the airway narrowing: increased amounts of mucus, inflammatory oedema and muscular hypertrophy. These are found principally in bronchi but may also be found in smaller airways, including bronchioles.[265–269] The inflammation may even involve alveoli.[270]

The airway lumen is compromised by the accumulation of mucus and an exudate of eosinophils and desquamated epithelial cells mixed with components derived from the plasma but not including fibrin

Figure 3.25 Asthma showing bronchial plugging by mucus. (A) Haematoxylin and eosin, (B) Alcian blue–periodic acid–Schiff.

Figure 3.26 Asthma showing epithelial desquamation, hypersecretion of mucus, thickening of the epithelial basement membrane and infiltration of the bronchial wall by lymphocytes and eosinophils.

(Figs 3.25 and 3.26).[271,272] The mucus commonly has a concentric or spiral pattern in cross-section, and includes cells that are often aggregated in a corresponding distribution. These cells are mostly eosinophils and desquamated epithelium. There is goblet cell hyperplasia in the surface epithelium and the bronchial glands are enlarged, but not as much as in chronic bronchitis[111,112,265]; in contrast to chronic bronchitis, the serous elements in the submucosal glands are as numerous as the mucous acini.[273] The mucus is consequently less acidic than that in chronic bronchitis.[274] Changes in the bronchioles are less obvious than those in the larger airways but there may be muscle hypertrophy and an increase in goblet cells.[265,268] The bronchioles may also contain mucous plugs and mucus may even be seen in alveolar ducts. How much of this mucus is derived from bronchiolar goblet cells and how much is aspirated from the more proximal airways is unknown.

A characteristic feature of the airways in status asthmaticus is infiltration of the walls of bronchi and proximal bronchioles by eosinophils (Fig. 3.26).[265] It has been shown immunocytochemically that the eosinophils are activated to secrete major basic protein.[275–277] Neutrophils are generally uncommon and when numerous suggest secondary bacterial infection. However, more attention is now being paid to the pathogenetic role of these cells in asthma.[278,279] It is reported that in fatal asthma of sudden onset neutrophils outnumber eosinophils,[280] or even that they are the only polymorphonuclear leukocyte present.[281] Lymphocytes (mainly T-helper cells) are gener-

ally numerous in asthma, making up half the inflammatory cells.[275,276,282] Mast cells are not usually identified in appreciable numbers, but this is only because of degranulation, which can sometimes be recognised in appropiately stained sections by the presence of clusters of free metachromatic granules.[274] Staining for mast cell tryptase shows that these cells are increased in number.[283] Eosinophil degranulation is also evident and degranulation of both eosinophils and mast cells is confirmed by electron microscopy.[284]

The eosinophil inflammation of the airways is accompanied by marked congestion and oedema, and separation and detachment of the more superficial columnar epithelial cells from the underlying basal cells.[285,286] Where such exfoliation has occurred, regeneration may be evident in the form of mitotic division of the basal cells of the epithelium. The loss of ciliated cells contributes to the impaired bronchial clearance. Between attacks, patchy exfoliation of the epithelium may still be recognized,[287] and electron microscopy shows blebbing of the apical cell membrane and bizarre cilia.[288] During the regenerative process the epithelium may show evidence of cell proliferation and squamous metaplasia.[286,289]

Loss of the surface epithelial cells also exposes intraepithelial nerves to inflammatory mediators released in the bronchial lumen: stimulation of these nerves is thought to lead to an axon reflex that is responsible for much of the vasodilatation, oedema, mucus secretion and smooth-muscle contraction that characterises an asthmatic attack.[290]

The epithelial basement membrane is often thickened in asthma. This may be a reflection of the repeated shedding of epithelial cells, for basement membrane thickening is well known in other situations where the cells it supports are rapidly replaced. However, electron microscopy shows that the thickening is confined to the deepest layer of the basement membrane, the collagen and fibronectin-rich lamina reticularis (Figs 3.27 and 3.28),[291–293] which is probably produced by myofibroblasts derived from the epithelium by a process of epithelial–mesenchymal transition.[294,295] Tenascin, a glycoprotein concerned in repair, has been identified in the bronchial basement membrane in asthma but not in controls[296] whereas although plasma proteins, including immunoglobulins, can be demonstrated in the thickened basement membrane they are also present in the bronchial basement membrane of many non-asthmatic patients.[291] Although basement membrane thickening is frequently emphasised as being characteristic of asthma, it is by no means specific for this disease[274,287,297]; lesser degrees are often seen in biopsy specimens from non-asthmatic patients, taken for example because of suspected cancer. Much atten-

Figure 3.27 Asthma showing heavy eosinophil infiltration and marked basement membrane thickening.

Figure 3.28 Bronchial asthma. (A) Transmission electron micrograph showing that the epithelial basement membrane dividing epithelium (above) from connective tissue (below) is greatly thickened. Immediately beneath the basement membrane there is a lymphocyte and a mast cell. (B) Higher magnification shows that the lamina rara and lamina densa (arrows) are normal and that the thickening involves the deepest layer of the basement membrane, the lamina reticularis (LR). (A) ×2500; (B) ×30 000.

tion is paid to the thickening of the basement membrane, with the implication that it makes a considerable contribution to airway narrowing but, as shown in Figure 3.29, its role in this is insignificant compared to that of muscular hypertrophy and inflammatory oedema.

A prominent increase in the amount of airway muscle is a major feature of bronchial asthma and presumably reflects sustained muscular contraction (Fig. 3.29).[110–112,267,298–300] The increase involves airways of all sizes but is most apparent in small bronchi of about 0.5 cm diameter.[110,267,268,298,301] It is attributable to hyperplasia as well as hypertrophy.[110,300] The bronchial smooth muscle is hyperactive in asthma and the peptidergic (non-adrenergic, non-cholinergic) bronchial innervation is probably important here as fatal asthma is characterised by depletion of vasoactive intestinal peptide from bronchial nerve terminals.[302] Hyperplasia of the myoepithelial cells of the bronchial glands is also seen.[303]

The major changes in the airways act together and enhance the effect of each other on airway calibre. Mathematical modelling suggests that a moderate degree of inflammatory thickening of the mucosa, which by itself would have little effect on baseline resistance to gas flow, can profoundly affect the airway narrowing caused by normal smooth-muscle shortening: the various processes narrowing the airways are more than additive in their effect on airway responsiveness.[266,304–306]

It will be evident from the above that asthma and chronic bronchitis have features in common but that there are notable differences. The two diseases are compared in Table 3.1 (p. 101). A possible overlap condition known as 'wheezy bronchitis' is described on page 100.

Pathogenesis and aetiology of asthma

Two major mechanisms operate in both extrinsic and intrinsic asthma, one neurological and the other inflammatory.[290,307,308] The two mechanisms may interact. Thus, inflammatory mediators are prone to trigger nerve reflexes whilst nerve stimuli, or loss of inhibitory activity, may, in addition to causing secretion and contraction, affect vascular permeability and promote oedema.

In both extrinsic and intrinsic asthma there are many non-specific trigger factors. For example, many asthmatics are overresponsive to irritant dusts and to respiratory infection, reacting to either with marked bronchial narrowing. Emotional stress is another non-specific triggering factor in asthma. Exercise has a similar effect in many asthmatic patients, the large amount of cold dry air inhaled during were found to coincide with the unloading of soybean.[316] Occupational factors can be identified as contributing to asthma in about 2% of adult cases (see p. 357). Such asthma occurs in many industries and over 200 aetiological agents have been identified (see Table 7.1.8, p. 356).

Intrinsic asthma usually affects people older than those afflicted with extrinsic asthma. IgE levels are lower than in extrinsic asthma and skin tests are often negative or only weakly positive. It is therefore widely presumed that, in intrinsic asthma, airway inflammation is triggered by non-immunological mechanisms. However, IgE levels and the prevalence of positive skin tests to common allergens decline throughout adult life and some workers find that a high age-corrected IgE level is as good a marker of asthma in the elderly as in the young.[317,318] When these age-related changes are taken into account the traditional separation of intrinsic and extrinsic asthma is less clear.

The reaginic antibodies are largely fixed to cells, particularly to the Fc receptors on the surface of mast cells.[319] Inhalation of the appropriate allergen then leads to an antigen–antibody reaction on the surface of the mast cells; the consequent degranulation releases various chemical mediators from these cells.

The mast cell and the eosinophil leukocyte are central to the pathogenesis of asthma, the former cell being responsible for many of the acute manifestations of the disease and the latter for more of its chronic features. In response to both immunological and non-specific stimuli, the mast cell secretes a range of bioactive substances, whilst the eosinophil secretes substances antagonistic to mast cell mediators but also releases others that are detrimental to the integrity of the respiratory epithelium.

Mast cells are most numerous in relation to airway muscle and glands,[320] but they are also present within the surface epithelium[288,321] and can be recovered in bronchial washes.[322] Inhaled antigens first react with immunoglobulin E bound to mast cells free in the bronchial lumen, and this causes release of mediators from these mast cells and consequent weakening of the tight junctions binding together surface epithelial cells, so facilitating access of the antigen to mast cells in the epithelium. The degranulation of these mast cells further augments epithelial permeability. Penetration of antigen into the rest of the bronchial wall is thus facilitated as successive mast cells are rapidly triggered. Differences between mucosal and connective tissue mast cells are described: the former are smaller and contain heparin and tryptase rather than chymase.[323,324] Both types have been identified in human airways.[323]

Various mediators are released when the mast cell degranulates. Some of these cause immediate effects whilst others are responsible for reactions that come on hours later. Preformed mediators include histamine, exoglycosidases, tryptase, and eosinophil and neutrophil chemotactic factors. Histamine causes dilatation and increased permeability of blood vessels, triggers irritant nerve receptors causing coughing, and stimulates smooth-muscle contraction and mucus secretion, whilst exoglycosidases such as glucuronidase, hexosaminidase and galactosidase together with neutral proteases disrupt the integrity of the bronchial submucosa through their actions on connective tissue ground substance. Histamine release also stimulates the generation and release of newly formed mediators, including prostaglandin D_2, platelet-activating factor and leukotrienes C_4 and D_4, that are responsible for the later effects. Prostaglandin D_2 and leukotriene C_4 respectively enhance vasodilation and vascular permeability, while platelet-activating factor and the leukotrienes C_4 and D_4 cause smooth muscle to contract. Collectively these contribute greatly to the inflammatory oedema, muscular contraction and hypersecretion of mucus that characterise an asthmatic attack. Mast cells also produce a variety of cytokines, notably interleukins-1, 2, 3, 10 and 13, granulocyte–macrophage colony-stimulating factor, interferon-γ and tumour necrosis factor-α.[325]

Figure 3.29 Asthma. The bronchial muscle is greatly hypertrophied.

outdoor exercise probably being the non-specific bronchial irritant. Exercise-induced asthma is rare in the warm, humid atmosphere of an indoor swimming bath. Eosinophilia is not a feature of exercise-induced asthma.[309]

Up to 10% of asthmatic patients are unduly sensitive to aspirin and other non-steroidal anti-inflammatory drugs[310,311]: non-atopic patients with nasal polyps whose asthma is difficult to control are particularly sensitive to aspirin.[312] Aspirin-induced bronchial narrowing is attributed to inhibition of arachidonic acid metabolism by the cyclo-oxygenase pathway and its diversion to the lipoxygenase pathway with the production of bronchoconstrictor leukotrienes C4 and D4 (formerly known collectively as slow releasing factor of anaphylaxis).

Extrinsic asthma is usually associated with atopy, this being a liability to develop excessive amounts of immunoglobulin E (so-called reaginic antibodies) in response to commonplace antigens that the individual repeatedly meets in everyday life. Cutaneous prick tests usually result in an immediate wheal and flare response to a range of allergens. Specific allergens are found in many pollens, feathers, horse dander, fur and, especially, house dust. The most important asthma-causing allergen is probably the house dust mite, *Dermatophagoides pteronyssinus*, which is found worldwide. It feeds on shed human epidermal squames and for this reason is particularly numerous in dust from bedding, especially mattresses. Warm damp houses favour the growth of the mites more than cold dry ones, but very few samples of house dust are completely free of them. A reported increase in asthmatic attacks during thunderstorms may be due to pollen counts rising at such times.[313–315] Many environmental allergens causing asthma probably go undetected but one such agent was identified when periodic outbreaks of asthma in the vicinity of Barcelona's docks

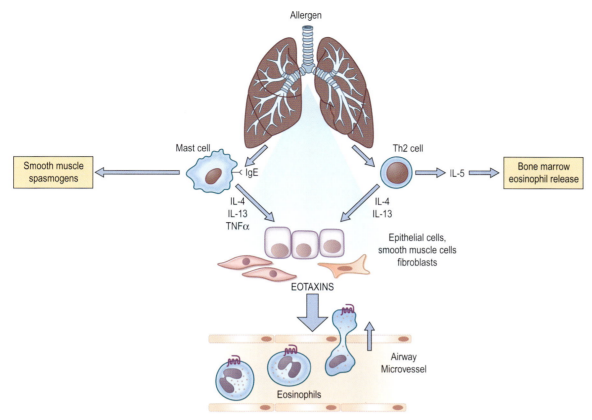

Figure 3.30 Diagrammatic representation of eosinophil production and bronchopulmonary infiltration in response to allergen inhalation. *(Reproduced from* Respiration Research *by permission of Professor TJ Williams, London, UK and BioMed Central Ltd.[326])*

Eosinophil leukocytes are produced in the bone marrow under the control of cytokines secreted by type 2 helper lymphocytes, notably interleukin-5 (Fig. 3.30).[326] They are released into the blood and are drawn into the tissues by chemotactic agents known as eotaxins,[326] of which three are now recognised. These agents are small proteins produced by a variety of cells, which in the lung include bronchial epithelial cells, smooth-muscle cells and fibroblasts, acting under the influence of interleukins derived from type 2 helper lymphocytes and mast cells.[326–328]

Eosinophils counter the action of many of the mast cell mediators described above by secreting degradative enzymes: these include histaminase and aryl sulphatase, which destroy histamine and leukotrienes respectively. However, further substances secreted by the eosinophil aggravate the disease. In helminthic infestation, major basic protein and eosinophil cationic protein derived from the eosinophil are probably beneficial in promoting elimination of the parasites but in asthma they appear to be responsible for the epithelial disintegration that characterises the disease.[329] In vitro, low concentrations of major basic protein impair ciliary motility and cause epithelial disruption, cell shedding and lysis.[329,330] In vivo, there is vacuolation of epithelial cells and the degree to which this occurs correlates with the number of eosinophils.[282] Major basic protein is normally confined to the core of eosinophil granules[331] (see Fig. 9.1, p. 461) but in patients dying of status asthmaticus, it is present within mucous plugs and on damaged epithelial surfaces.[332] Epithelial fragility is likely to enhance the access of allergens and non-specific irritants to mast cells, lymphocytes and nerves in the bronchial wall, thereby aggravating the condition. Nevertheless, a clear disassociation between

eosinophil infiltration of the airways and bronchial hyperresponsiveness is seen in the separate condition of eosinophilic bronchitis, which is considered below.

There is increasing evidence that cellular hypersensitivity is important in asthma, indicating that the T lymphocyte plays an important role in initiating an asthmatic attack (Fig. 3.31). Activated T-helper lymphocytes may be demonstrated in the airways[276,277,333–337] and selective activation of the Th2 subgroup has been identified, resulting in interleukin 4, 5, 9, 10 and 13 secretion.[247,275,338–345] Interleukins-4 and 13 cause plasma cells to form IgE rather than IgG, while interleukin-5 is responsible for increased eosinophil production by the bone marrow and interleukin-10 inhibits the development of Th1 cells. Conversely, Th1 cells produce interferon-γ, which is a potent inhibitor of IgE production.

Both genetic and environmental factors appear to influence the relative activity of Th1 and Th2 cells. Certain infections are characterised by the production of large amounts of interferon-γ but the children of atopic parents have fewer interferon-γ-producing cells in their peripheral blood. It is plausible therefore to envisage repeated viral infections, particularly in early life, selectively enhancing the development of Th1 cells and inhibiting the proliferation of Th2 clones and allergic sensitisation – the so-called hygiene hypothesis that is also touched upon above, under epidemiology. This hypothesis has led to suggestions that vaccines designed to stimulate Th1 cell development could be beneficial in preventing asthma and allied allergic diseases.[247]

Asthma is also characterised by infiltration of the bronchial surface epithelium by Langerhans cells.[338] These non-phagocytic histiocytes

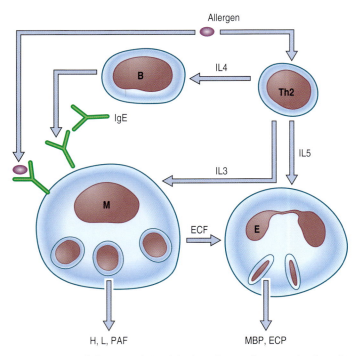

Figure 3.31 Cellular interrelationships in asthma. Allergens stimulate Th2 lymphocytes to release interleukins which activate B lymphocytes, mast cells and eosinophils. Interleukin-5 promotes eosinophil activation while interleukin-4 is responsible for B-lymphocyte maturation, which results in immunoglobulin E production; the adherence of immunoglobulin E to mast cells primes the latter to degranulate on contact with the same allergen. The eosinophil modulates some of the effects of the mast cell by releasing histaminase and aryl sulphatase, which inactivate histamine and leukotrienes respectively, but also damage adjacent tissue by secreting major basic protein and eosinophil cationic protein. Th2, T-helper 2 lymphocyte; B, B lymphocyte; M, mast cell; E, eosinophil; IL, interleukin; IgE, immunoglobulin E; H, histamine; L, leukotrienes; PAF, platelet-activating factor; MBP, major basic protein; ECP, eosinophil cationic protein; ECF, eosinophil chemotactic factor.

are rich in surface receptors and are responsible for the presentation of antigenic information to T lymphocytes: very few Langerhans cells are found in the normal lung, although there is a rich network of the dendritic cells that are their probable precursors.[338,346–348]

The bronchial epithelium also contributes actively to the development of asthma.[307] For example, epithelial expression of the bronchoconstrictor substance endothelin is increased in asthma.[349] Other bronchoconstrictor agents, such as prostacyclins, are also released when bronchial epithelium is damaged.

The association of asthma with nasal polyps and paranasal sinusitis has been ascribed to aspiration of upper respiratory tract secretions but radionuclide tracer studies do not support this.[350] Furthermore asthmatic patients' minor salivary glands show inflammatory changes similar to those in their airways,[351] suggesting that there is generalised mucosal disease affecting both upper and lower airways. The polyps themselves have an oedematous stroma infiltrated by eosinophils. Nasal polyps are common in certain other airway diseases, notably cystic fibrosis and primary ciliary dyskinesia, but in these non-allergic conditions the polyps lack the tissue eosinophilia seen in asthma.

Asthma is also associated with gastro-oesophageal reflux but it is uncertain whether the relationship is causal.[352,353] Contact of the oesophagus or the trachea with hydrochloric acid induces reflex bronchial constriction[354] but it is unclear whether the reflux is the primary

event as hyperinflation of the lungs increases abdominal pressure and thus promotes reflux. Reflux may be asymptomatic[355] and some asthmatics report symptomatic improvement on medical antireflux therapy, but their lung function is generally unchanged.[353] Surgical intervention is currently considered inappropriate.

Some intriguing observations concerning asthma have emanated from transplantation centres. It is reported that the lungs of an asthmatic donor confer asthma on a non-atopic recipient and conversely that an asthmatic recipient receiving lungs from a non-asthmatic donor experiences no further attacks of asthma.[356]

Treatment of asthma

Asthma is largely treated quite successfully by the avoidance of recognised trigger agents coupled with bronchodilator drugs and corticosteroids as required, supplemented on occasion by desensitisation to specific allergens and breathing exercises. Other treatments that have been developed more recently include leukotriene and leukotriene receptor antagonists and antibodies directed against IgE while several asthma genes have recently been identified, suggesting that gene therapy may be introduced at some future date.

Complications of asthma

Asthma is sometimes complicated by allergic bronchopulmonary aspergillosis: it is also a frequent manifestation of the latter (see p. 228). *Aspergillus fumigatus* is the species most commonly concerned in the UK, but other species appear to be relatively more frequent causes in other parts of the world. It is important to note that in this condition the fungus does not invade the tissues. Inhalation of fungal spores sets up a reaction in the sensitised bronchial tree that is characterised by bronchospasm, accumulation of eosinophils and outpouring of abundant, very viscid mucus. The mucus forms a cast which distends the affected segment of the bronchial tree. The cast is colonised by the fungus and the preparation of histological sections of these mucous plugs, expectorated at the end of the acute episode of the illness, permits demonstration of the characteristic hyphae within their substance: silver impregnation methods are very satisfactory for this purpose. It should be noted that the hyphae are usually scanty. Immunological tests have largely superseded histological investigation in the diagnosis of this condition, although the latter is a valuable confirmatory measure and in cases with equivocal immunological results may be the only means of recognising the disease. Immunological tests include the demonstration of precipitating antibodies to *Aspergillus* in the blood, and skin testing with *Aspergillus* antigen which causes both immediate and delayed reactions. Some atopic individuals develop allergic aspergillosis of the paranasal sinuses similar to that in the bronchi.[357]

Bronchocentric granulomatosis (see p. 464) is a further manifestation of allergic bronchopulmonary aspergillosis. So too is eosinophilic pneumonia (see p. 459). In this latter condition, radiological examination of the chest during an attack of asthma reveals scattered opacities which biopsy shows to be foci of eosinophil exudation in the alveoli, with similar infiltration of the bronchiolar and alveolar walls. Such foci appear to be transient but healing of them by fibrosis may contribute to the subpleural honeycombing and bronchiectasis mentioned above.

Non-eosinophilic asthma

Some patients with the clinical features of asthma lack the distinctive sputum eosinophilia of the disease and on biopsy their airways show a non-specific neutrophilic rather than eosinophilic infiltrate and an absence of the usual basement membrane thickening seen in asthma.

They respond poorly to inhaled corticosteroids.[358] The cause is generally unknown and the pathogenesis poorly understood, apart from a possible link to smoking.[359] However, in what has become known as irritant-induced asthma (or reactive airways dysfunction), a similar situation is encountered in non-atopic individuals exposed to a single heavy concentration of a severely irritant gas, fume, smoke or vapour.[360] These patients develop cough, wheezing and dyspnoea within 24 hours of such exposure and their symptoms persist for at least 3 months. They have airflow obstruction and give a positive challenge test but display no eosinophilia. Thus, there are patients who are categorised clinically as having asthma who would not be so recognised by a pathologist.

Eosinophilic bronchitis

Eosinophilic bronchitis is characterised by corticosteroid-responsive cough and eosinophilia but not the variable airflow obstruction, airway hyperresponsiveness or bronchial muscle hypertrophy seen in asthma.[361,362] The inflammatory changes are similar except that mast cells are reportedly better represented in the bronchial muscle in asthma whereas they are best seen in the epithelium in eosinophilic bronchitis.[363,364] Both conditions show thickening of the reticular basement membrane.[362] Exposure to certain occupational allergens has been reported to cause eosinophilic bronchitis.[365]

BRONCHIECTASIS

In literal terms, bronchiectasis means no more than dilatation of the bronchi and it is legitimately used in this restricted sense to describe, for instance, the distensive changes that are commonly encountered distal to a bronchial tumour. More often, however, it is understood to indicate a characteristic clinical condition that has bronchial dilatation and suppuration as its pathological basis. Although such dilatation is traditionally considered to be permanent, radiologists are familiar with early cases reverting to normal with treatment.

Aetiology and clinical features

Prior to the advent of antibiotics and immunisation against the common exanthems of childhood, bronchiectasis usually followed a severe respiratory infection. It was characterised by a chronic cough productive of abundant foul sputum that originated in localised saccular lesions, which were typically located in the lung bases. This form of the disease is now uncommon and has been replaced by, or its reduction has uncovered, an insidious progressive type of bronchiectasis, which is usually more extensive and cylindrical. This is also characterised by persistent purulent sputum production but patients with this form of the disease often give a history of wheezy bronchitis in childhood and have chronic rhinosinusitis.[366] The cause of this form of bronchiectasis is not easily identified and it is often termed idiopathic. Immunological dysfunction is suspected.[367] The idiopathic form has been identified in 14–53% of cases.[368–370] These studies also identified 29–32% of cases as being postinfectious, as well as several rarer causes (Box 3.2).[371–377] A further possible cause is the dysfunction of primary cilia that underlies autosomal-dominant polycystic kidney disease, as discussed on page 65).

An unexplained association of bronchiectasis is that with lymphatic obstruction and pleural effusions in the yellow-nail syndrome (see p. 709). It is also uncertain whether an observed association between bronchiectasis and antitrypsin deficiency is attributable to impaired defence against infection or protease–antiprotease imbalance.[378]

Box 3.2 **Causes of bronchiectasis**

- Infection: measles, pertussis, adenovirus
- Chemical damage: gastric acid, toxic gases
- Diffuse pulmonary fibrosis
- Obstruction: tumour, foreign body, enlarged hilar nodes
- Impaired local defence: cystic fibrosis, ciliary dyskinesia, Young's syndrome
- Impaired systemic immunity: hypogammaglobulinaemia
- Autoimmunity: ulcerative colitis, rheumatoid disease, Sjögren's syndrome, ankylosing spondylitis, relapsing polychondritis, systemic lupus erythematosus, Marfan's syndrome, lung transplant rejection, graft-versus-host disease
- Allergy: allergic bronchopulmonary aspergillosis
- Congenital: Mounier-Kuhn's syndrome, Williams–Campbell syndrome

Bacteriology

In the earlier stages of bronchiectasis, *Haemophilus influenzae* is much the commonest bacterium to be recovered from the sputum. Later, a wide variety of different organisms becomes established in the infected air passages. As well as *H. influenzae*, *Pseudomonas aeruginosa*, *Streptococcus pneumoniae* and *Mycobacterium avium* may be found. Sometimes, various spirochaetes and anaerobes are found and it is through the activities of these organisms that the smell of the sputum is so often offensive. Probably all these bacteria are secondary colonisers rather than the primary causative agent. *P. aeruginosa* is a particularly difficult bacterium to eradicate as it secretes an alginate coating that enables it to live on the mucosal surface esconced within a biofilm where it is protected against phagocytosis and humoral or chemical attack.[379]

Structural changes[366,371]

The terms 'cylindrical' and 'saccular' (Fig. 3.32), alluded to above, are self-explanatory. Follicular is another descriptive term, one that refers to an abundance of lymphoid follicles in the walls of the affected bronchi (Fig. 3.33) which are usually dilated in a cylindrical fashion. The terms 'follicular' and 'cylindrical' are therefore often used interchangeably. Apart from the association of saccular disease with preceding infection and cylindrical/follicular with idiopathic cases, the distribution of the disease within the lungs also gives a clue to the aetiology. Thus, postinfective bronchiectasis tends to be basal, whilst in cystic fibrosis and ciliary dyskinesia the bronchiectasis is generalised but with upper-lobe preponderance and in allergic bronchopulmonary aspergillosis hilar bronchi are particularly affected. Bronchiectasis confined to the right middle lobe is a major feature of the middle-lobe syndrome (see p. 92).

The affected bronchi are most frequently those of the third or fourth order, the first orders being spared because their more substantial cartilage prevents dilatation. By counting the number of generations of the bronchial tree from the hilum it has been shown that subpleural bronchiectatic cavities of the cystic type usually represent dilated proximal airways.[380]

The dilated airways are usually filled with a purulent exudate and their mucosal surfaces are deeply congested. Many of the normal components of the bronchial wall are partly destroyed, particularly the fibromuscular and elastic framework. The bronchial walls may be thin, but more often they are thickened by fibrosis, inflammatory

Figure 3.32 (A) In a patient with cystic fibrosis there is widespread saccular bronchiectasis; almost all segments of the lung are affected. The lung is largely replaced by saccules with thick fibrous walls, sometimes showing the remains of the mucosal folds of the bronchi from which they were derived. (B) In a patient with idiopathic bronchiectasis, the changes are cylindrical. (C and D) In a further patient with bronchoectasis a peanut was identified obstructing the lumen.

oedema and a heavy infiltrate of lymphocytes and plasma cells. Lymphoid follicles may be prominent (see Fig. 3.33). The mucosa may show polypoid hyperplasia and there may be squamous metaplasia. Thin-walled pus-filled bronchiectatic cavities may be mistaken for abscesses: the essential difference is that the latter entail destruction of lung tissue and consequently several airways may communicate with one abscess cavity (Fig. 3.34).

The dilated airways often end blindly, the more distal airways being obliterated by fibrosis (Fig. 3.35). Unless inflation is maintained by collateral ventilation the distal lung then shows absorption collapse. The adjacent lung may be substantially normal or, particularly in fol-

licular bronchiectasis, there may be extensive chronic interstitial pneumonia. Organising pneumonia may be found in relation to the bronchiectasis but this is not an invariable association and when present it is generally difficult to tell whether it has preceded or followed the bronchiectasis.

As with many diseases of the lung, bronchiectasis derives its blood supply chiefly from the bronchial arteries, leading to the development of large bronchopulmonary anastomoses.[381]

The airway neuroendocrine cells are often increased in bronchiectasis, sometimes leading to the formation of multiple tumourlets (see p. 598).

Figure 3.33 Follicular bronchiectasis. Lymphoid follicles are evident in the wall of this dilated airway, which also contains mucopus.

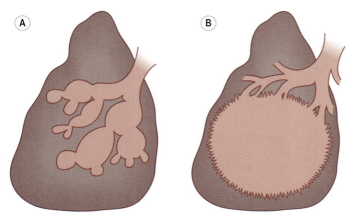

Figure 3.34 Diagrammatic representation of (A) bronchiectasis and (B) lung abscess. In bronchiectasis each space represents a dilated airway that communicates only with its parent and daughter airways, in contrast to an abscess cavity brought about by 'cross-country' necrosis forming a newly formed cavity that communicates with several separate airways. *(Redrawn after Liebow.)*

Figure 3.35 Bronchiolitis in long-standing bronchiectasis (A) shows widespread peribronchiolar inflammation; (B) shows peribronchiolar fibrosis.

Pathogenesis

The pathogenesis of bronchiectasis is complex and several mechanisms have been proposed. It is likely that some of these act in conjunction, establishing a 'vicious cycle' of events.[382,383] This involves initial damage to the bronchial epithelium permitting heavy secondary bacterial colonisation which in turn inhibits ciliary clearance and so promotes continued infection and inflammation. Evidence for this comes from the isolation of a heat-labile bacterial product that attacks ciliated cells and slows ciliary motility. Other bacterial products capable of perpetuating obstructive lung disease include proteinases that stimulate the secretion of mucus into the airways.[108,384] *Pseudomonas aeruginosa* is a particularly troublesome coloniser because it survives within a biofilm on the mucosal surface where it is protected against cellular and humoral attack but is nevertheless responsible for strong antigen–antibody reactions that attract neutrophils.

An undoubtedly important pathogenetic mechanism is inflammatory weakening of the walls of the bronchi, largely stemming from proteolytic enzymes and toxic oxygen radicals released by neutrophils.

The normal tractive forces that operate on the airways in inspiration may then be enough to stretch their walls unduly. Distal to an obstruction, dammed-up secretions exert distensive forces, whilst outside the inflamed airways, increased tractive forces are brought to bear on their weakened walls by processes such as absorption collapse and post-pneumonic fibrosis (Fig. 3.36). Coughing may be dismissed as a possible pathogenetic factor because it entails the sudden closure of airways rather than their distension.

Complications

Notable local complications of bronchiectasis include the development of lung abscess and empyema, the latter being the less common because adhesions often form early and obliterate the pleural cavity. Bronchiectasis is seldom widespread enough to cause severe pulmonary hypertension but cor pulmonale is common in the generalised form of the disease that develops in cystic fibrosis. Old bronchiectatic cavities may be colonised saprophytically by fungi (see p. 231). Distant complications of bronchiectasis include metastatic abscesses, particularly in the brain, generalised amyloidosis and immune complex vasculitis.[385,386]

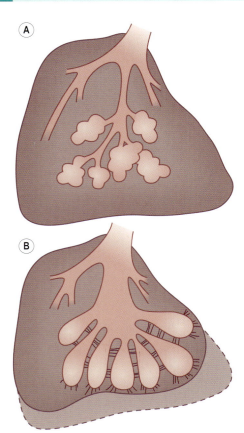

Figure 3.36 Pathogenesis of bronchiectasis. Top: bronchopneumonia. Bottom: the peribronchiolar consolidation has healed by fibrosis, contracture of which exerts a tractive force on airway walls weakened by inflammation. *(Redrawn after Liebow.)*

Treatment and outcome

Bronchiectasis can be treated by pharmacological and non-pharmacological means, the former including antibiotics, mucolytics and anti-inflammatory agents, and the latter physiotherapy and, if the disease is localised, surgical resection. In one group of patients followed for 13 years, 30% died: mortality correlated with the degree of restrictive and obstructive disease, poor gas transfer and chronic *Pseudomonas* infection.[387]

There is also a variety of conditions characterised by small free bodies, calcified or otherwise, that may be detected in sputum or lung tissue. These are mainly found free in the air spaces and are dealt with under alveolar filling defects on pp. 320–322.

BRONCHOLITHIASIS

Occasionally the laboratory is presented with a stony hard object that a patient has coughed up. Such sputum 'liths' (or broncholiths) may derive from many conditions characterised by bronchopulmonary calcification. Analytical electron microscopy and X-ray diffraction may give information on their elemental composition and crystalline structure that can be helpful in identifying the underlying disease.[388] Generally the cause is a heavily calcified bronchial lymph node, representing healed tuberculosis, sarcoidosis or histoplasmosis, that presses upon and gradually ulcerates the wall of a bronchus until it is free in the lumen (see Fig. 3.2B, p. 93). Bronchial obstruction or bleeding may necessitate intervention before the broncholith works itself free.[389] Broncholiths may also cause obstructive pneumonia, mediastinal abscess or broncho-oesophageal fistula.[390]

CHRONIC BRONCHIOLITIS

Bronchiolitis may be acute, chronic or acute on chronic. The more acute forms have been dealt with earlier in this chapter and this section is concerned with the chronic forms, particularly that in which the lumen is compromised, for which the term 'obliterative bronchiolitis' (or bronchiolitis obliterans) is used, in contrast to cellular bronchiolitis, which term is sometimes used when the bronchiole is inflamed but the lumen remains patent.[391]

It is useful to separate those disorders in which bronchiolar disease is the predominant feature from those in which it represents a distal extension of what is primarily a bronchial disorder and those in which it represents a proximal extension of an essentially parenchymal condition (Box 3.3).[392,393] Attention here is confined to the disorders in which bronchiolar disease is the predominant feature.

Chronic bronchiolitis is often non-specific but some forms have distinctive histological patterns. These are dealt with separately: see follicular bronchiolitis (see p. 654), respiratory bronchiolitis (see p. 313) and diffuse panbronchiolitis (see p. 124). Obliterative bronchiolitis is also encountered in diffuse idiopathic neuroendocrine cell hyperplasia (see p. 599) and chronic obstructive bronchiolitis ('small-airways disease') is an important facet of chronic obstructive pulmonary disease (see p. 100).

Clinical features

Chronic bronchiolitis is characterised by cough, wheeze and shortness of breath of varying severity. It becomes life-threatening when there is widespread luminal obliteration. Widely differing orders of bronchioles may be affected, the disease sometimes extending proximally into small bronchi and in other patients extending distally to involve alveoli. For this reason the functional effects are not uniform: whereas obliteration of proximal bronchioles causes an obstructive pattern of impairment, scarring in the region of respiratory bronchioles causes restrictive functional impairment.

Imaging

Imaging shows centrilobular nodules, extending from which there are short branching lines, the so-called 'tree in bud' pattern. This represents thick-walled bronchioles filled with mucus or mucopus. There may also be patchy centrilobular ground-glass opacification representing spread of the bronchiolar inflammation into adjacent alveoli. Focal air-trapping, best seen on expiratory scans, is a further feature. Loss of the normal lung markings may also be observed. This represents vascular shutdown in response to hypoventilation (see ventilation-perfusion matching, p. 22), which in this case is due to obliterative bronchiolitis. Although this is generally patchy, resulting in a mosaic pattern, it may affect a whole segment, lobe or lung.

The Swyer–James or Macleod syndrome of unilateral hypertransradiancy (or hyperlucency) of the lungs[394–397] was once thought to represent congenital unilateral atresia of pulmonary vessels but it is now recognised that arterial constriction in response to hypoventilation underlies the condition. The condition is an acquired one with obliterative bronchiolitis as its pathological basis. The hypertransradiancy (see Fig. 2.62, p. 73) appears soon after an attack of bronchiolitis and is initially due to vascular constriction; later, structural obliteration of the vessels supervenes. Absorption collapse, which would render the lung radiopaque rather than radiolucent, is prevented by collateral ventilation (see p. 92). The syndrome is considered further on page 73.

Pathological features

The bronchiolar wall is thickened by non-specific lymphoplasmacytic inflammation, oedema and a varying degree of fibrosis. All components of the wall are affected – mucosa, muscularis and adventitia. Sometimes the inflammation and fibrosis extend out to affect the adjacent alveoli, resulting in a bronchiolocentric interstitial pneumonia and fibrosis. This may be accompanied by a centrifugal extension of the bronchiolar epithelium through the canals of Lambert (see p. 4) so that peribronchiolar alveolar septa thickened by fibrosis are lined by tall columnar epithelial cells, a process termed bronchiolisation of alveoli, peribronchiolar metaplasia or lambertosis (Fig. 3.37).[398] The epithelial cells are generally ciliated and closely abut each other, in contrast to atypical adenomatous hyperplasia, which involves non-ciliated, low columnar or cuboidal Clara cells and type II pneumocytes separated by gaps representing type I pneumocytes (see Fig. 12.1.3, p. 538). It has become apparent that the epithelial

Figure 3.37 Lambertosis. (A) Centriacinar scarring with bronchiolar epithelial metaplasia. (B) The appearances differ from those of atypical adenomatous hyperplasia in that the cells are mainly of ciliated type, closely abut each other and there is no atypia.

cells contribute directly to the fibrosis by participating in a process of epithelial–mesenchymal transition.[399,400]

If the mucosal fibrosis encroaches upon the bronchiolar lumen the changes are described as obliterative bronchiolitis (or bronchiolitis obliterans). Two major pathological patterns of bronchiolar obliteration are recognised: one characterised by polypoid intraluminal buds of granulation tissue, which is sometimes termed proliferative or intrusive, and a constrictive type. Both forms are the result of epithelial damage but whereas the polypoid type represents healing of damage inflicted at one point in time, the constrictive type is the result of chronic attrition from continuing damage. Thus, the polypoid form is typically seen soon after viral and chemical attack on the bronchioles and the constrictive type with autoimmune disease, lung transplant rejection and graft-versus-host disease (Box 3.4). However, with time the intraluminal buds of granulation tissue seen in the former

Figure 3.38 Bronchiolitis due to intraluminal organisation complicating viral infection. A granulation tissue polyp protrudes into and occupies most of the bronchiolar lumen.

type may become incorporated into the airway wall, resulting in appearances indistinguishable from those of the constrictive type.

The polypoid type of obliterative bronchiolitis results from the organisation of luminal inflammatory exudates and entails the development of granulation tissue polyps that protrude into and obstruct much of the bronchiolar lumen (Fig. 3.38). These are akin to the Masson bodies (*bourgeons conjonctifs*) of organising pneumonia, which may also be present in the distal lung. Alternatively, alveoli beyond the bronchiolar obstruction may contain abundant foamy macrophages, the hallmark of endogenous lipid pneumonia, which should prompt the pathologist to examine the bronchioles.

In the constrictive pattern of obliterative bronchiolitis[401,402] the mucosa is concentrically thickened by chronic inflammatory granulation tissue (Figs 3.39 and 3.40) and in active cases the surface epithelium is destroyed (Fig. 3.39). Sometimes the bronchiole is totally replaced by scar tissue. In this case, the presence of small fibrous scars next to pulmonary arteries that lack their usual accompanying airways should suggest that there has been bronchiolar destruction. Elastin stains may support this by showing a remnant of the bronchiolar wall in the scar, a feature that is often difficult to identify on haematoxylin and eosin staining (Fig. 3.41). The disease is often patchy and may affect only short segments of the bronchioles. More distal airways may therefore appear structurally normal, although they are in fact non-functioning continuations of completely obliterated bronchioles, something that may only be appreciated by studying serial sections. As with the intraluminal pattern peripheral accumulations of foamy alveolar macrophages may be found, suggesting that there is an obstructive pneumonitis and that the bronchioles may therefore be worthy of more detailed examination (Fig. 3.42).

Aetiology

Bronchiolar infection is a major cause of the classic polypoid pattern of obliterative bronchiolitis. The organisation of an acute inflammatory exudate caused by viral infection complicated by bacterial super-infection results in the polypoid intraluminal buds of granulation tissue.[133,135,403,404] The viruses responsible include adenoviruses, respiratory syncytial virus and influenza virus. This pattern of bronchiolar

obstruction may also be found beyond chronic suppurative bronchial diseases, such as bronchiectasis or cystic fibrosis, and in immunocompromised patients.[405,406]

Intraluminal organisation is again seen when the bronchiolitis is caused by the inhalation of noxious gases, fume or smoke, whether the exposure is occupational, environmental or encountered in war. The pathogenesis is identical to that which follows infective bronchiolitis. Examples are provided in Chapters 7.1 and 7.2. They include silo-filler's disease due to oxides of nitrogen (see p. 356), diacetyl, which is encountered by popcorn workers (p. 355) and thionyl chloride used in the manufacture of lithium batteries (see p. 356). War gases such as phosgene and sulphur mustard and indeed many irritant gases or fumes that are inadvertently inhaled are liable to cause a chemical bronchiolitis that may be complicated by luminal organisation.[407] When due to inhaled chemicals this is generally indistinguishable from that caused by infections but nylon flock worker's lung has a distinctive lymphoid pattern (see p. 354). Ingested chemicals may also cause obliterative bronchiolitis: *Sauropus androgynus*, described on page 376, is a notable example; here the damage is perpetuated by repeated ingestion and the resultant obliterative bronchiolitis is consequently of the constrictive variety.

Figure 3.39 Active constrictive obliterative bronchiolitis obliterative in a rheumatoid patient. The epithelium is under constant attack and is consequently unable to regenerate, leading to the build-up of granulation tissue.

Figure 3.40 Constrictive obliterative bronchiolitis in a rheumatoid patient. Internal to the muscle coat there is a thick layer of pale-staining granulation tissue which severely compromises the airway lumen. Surviving bronchiolar epitheium is reduced to a small central nidus. *(Reproduced from Geddes et al. (1977)[402] by permission of the editor of the* Quarterly Journal of Medicine.)

Bronchiolar involvement is often evident in the pneumoconioses. The clearance mechanisms of the alveolus result in inhaled dust being concentrated in and around the terminal bronchiole and its accompanying lymphoreticular aggregates (see Macklin's dust sumps, pp. 27 and 329 and Figs 1.7, p. 7 and 7.1.12, p. 339). This is therefore a site where pneumoconiotic nodules are particularly likely to develop, with inevitable distortion of the bronchiole.[408–410] Peribronchiolar fibrosis is also an early feature of asbestosis,[409,411] probably because much inhaled fibrous dust initially penetrates no further than the bronchioles.

Cigarette smokers are at risk of two forms of bronchiolitis: respiratory bronchiolitis and chronic obstructive bronchiolitis (small-airway disease). The former predominantly affects the peribronchiolar alveoli and is therefore dealt with in Chapter 6.2 (see p. 313) while the latter is considered above under chronic obstructive lung disease (see p. 100).

Obliterative bronchiolitis of constrictive pattern has been described in such autoimmune disorders as rheumatoid disease,[402,412] ankylosing spondylitis, systemic sclerosis[413] and paraneoplastic pemphigus.[414] The disease affects small bronchi as well as bronchioles and is rapidly progressive: affected patients may die of obstructive respiratory impairment within a year of the onset of dyspnoea. Milder but other-wise clinically similar 'cryptogenic' cases have been reported in patients free of connective tissue disease.[415,416] In some cases the changes have been attributed to drugs used to treat the underlying disease (e.g. penicillamine) but the bronchiolar narrowing is recorded in patients who have not been so treated and conversely bronchiolitis obliterans is not recorded in patients who have received these drugs in the treatment of other diseases (e.g. Wilson's disease). It is therefore more likely to be a manifestation of the connective tissue disease than an effect of the drug. Similarly, some cases of obliterative bronchiolitis attributed to chemical fumes have involved rheumatoid patients and may represent rheumatoid airway disease rather than chemical damage.[417] The association of bronchiolar disease and connective tissue disease is discussed further in Chapter 10.

Obstructive pulmonary disease has been recorded in several patients with ulcerative colitis.[418,419] Airways of any size from the trachea to small bronchioles may be affected and there is a spectrum of disease ranging from sclerosing tracheobronchitis to obliterative bronchiolitis

Figure 3.41 Constrictive obliterative bronchiolitis. (A) At low power there are no obvious abnormalities but an elastin stain (B) highlights that what might have been interpreted as an interlobular septum is a bronchiole wholly obliterated by fibrosis. *(Courtesy of Dr G Taylor, Auckland, New Zealand.)*

Figure 3.42 Chronic bronchiolitis. A small airway shows chronic inflammation and intraluminal accumulation of macrophages suggesting proximal obstruction.

DIFFUSE PANBRONCHIOLITIS

The cause of this disease is unknown but it is prevalent in Japan, and, to a lesser extent, Korea and China.[422-426] Only a few cases have been described in the west,[427-430] possibly because of genetic differences. The affected Asians show an increase in certain HLA antigens that do not occur in other races, notably B54 in Japan and A11 in Korea.[431,432] However, environmental factors also appear to be important since the disease is uncommon in persons of Japanese ancestry living abroad. The identification of diffuse panbronchiolitis in a Hispanic man who had visited Japan raises the possibility that a transmissible agent may be involved.[433] As diffuse panbronchiolitis mimics several other obstructive airway diseases,[424] it is possibly masquerading as one or other of these elsewhere and chest physicians and pathologists outside Japan need to be more conversant with the features of this disease.

Clinical features

The disease has a wide age distribution with a peak age incidence between the fourth and seventh decades of life. It does not appear to be related to smoking. Men are affected twice as commonly as women.

Long-standing sinusitis generally precedes the onset of lower respiratory tract disease, which in its early stages is characterised by a productive cough and obstructive respiratory impairment. The term 'sinobronchial syndrome' is often applied. Wheezing may lead to a resemblance to chronic bronchitis or asthma.

of constrictive type, similar to that seen in autoimmune connective tissue disease. As in rheumatoid disease, the airway narrowing is progressive and may prove fatal. The temporal relationship of disease activity in the bowel and airways is a weak one. Indeed, the pulmonary disease may appear years after the patient has undergone colectomy. The changes in the airways are comparable to those that develop in the biliary tree in sclerosing cholangitis, another extraintestinal complication of ulcerative colitis. The association of lung and bowel disease is dealt with further in Chapter 10.

Patients who have undergone lung transplantation are at risk of both forms of obliterative bronchiolitis. In the early posttransplant period they are subject to infection or aspiration, either of which is likely to result in obliterative bronchiolitis of classic polypoid pattern, whereas later they are at risk of graft rejection, a major feature of which is obliterative bronchiolitis of constrictive pattern.[420,421]

Early in the course of the disease sputum cultures are unrevealing. Infection and/or colonisation follows and, in the advanced stages, large amounts of purulent sputum infected by *Haemophilus influenzae* and *Pseudomonas aeruginosa* are produced and dilatation of proximal bronchioles develops. The disease then resembles bronchiectasis, particularly the idiopathic variety, which is also associated with sinusitis. Cold haemagglutinins frequently develop after the disease is established but *Mycoplasma* antibodies are generally lacking. Rheumatoid factor is often present but few patients with diffuse panbronchiolitis have overt rheumatoid disease.

Imaging

Chest radiographs show numerous small nodular opacities scattered throughout both lung fields and, in late cases, bronchiolectasis and bronchiectasis may be demonstrated. High-resolution computed tomography is characteristic but not pathognomonic. The nodular opacities are centrilobular and often extend as short linear opacities ('tree in bud' pattern). Expiratory scans usually show focal air-trapping.

Pathological features

As its name suggests, diffuse panbronchiolitis is an inflammatory disease of small airways that is widely disseminated throughout both lungs, but it especially affects the bases. Numerous yellow nodules measuring up to 4 mm in diameter are seen on the cut surfaces of the lungs. Microscopically, the walls of membranous and respiratory bronchioles are thickened by a lymphoplasmacytic infiltrate and there is prominence of the bronchus-associated lymphoid tissue. The inflammatory changes extend into the peribronchiolar tissues and there is obstructive lipid pneumonia, corresponding to the fine yellow nodules observed grossly (Fig. 3.43).[423,434] Interstitial as well as air space accumulation of foamy macrophages is a striking histological feature.

Differential diagnosis

Diffuse panbronchiolitis bears some resemblance to several diseases familiar to non-Japanese practitioners, notably idiopathic bronchiectasis, chronic bronchitis and obliterative bronchiolitis, but whereas these have their major impact on the bronchi or membranous bronchioles, diffuse panbronchiolitis is centred on the respiratory bronchioles.[435] Nevertheless, the pathological changes of diffuse panbronchiolitis are not specific. In a review of American archival material

Figure 3.43 Diffuse panbronchiolitis. The bronchiolar wall is thickened by a chronic inflammatory infiltrate and the surrounding alveoli contain many foam cells, which also infiltrate the alveolar walls. *(Reproduced by permission of Dr M Kitaichi, Kyoto, Japan.)*

the changes of diffuse panbronchiolitis were identified in 20 (1.5%) of 1336 patients with a variety of other lung diseases, notably cystic fibrosis, bronchiectasis and bronchiolitis.[436] However, diffuse panbronchiolitis is a clinicopathological diagnosis and Japanese physicians are reluctant to make the diagnosis if the patient does not exhibit the appropriate clinical features, especially sinusitis.

Course of the disease

Death from respiratory failure and cor pulmonale was formerly common but erythromycin treatment has improved the prognosis.[437,438]

REFERENCES

Atelectasis and pulmonary collapse

1. MacPherson AMC, Zorab PA, Reid L. Collapse of the lung associated with primary tuberculosis: a review of 51 cases. Thorax 1960;15:346–54.
2. Morrell NW, Roberts CM, Biggs T, et al. Collateral ventilation and gas exchange during airway occlusion in the normal human lung. Am Rev Respir Dis 1993;147:535–9.
3. Brock RC, Cann RJ, Dickinson JR. Tuberculous mediastinal lymphadenitis in childhood; secondary effects on the lungs. Guy Hosp Rep 1937;87:295–317.
4. Inners CR, Terry PB, Traystman RJ, et al. Collateral ventilation and the middle lobe syndrome. Am Rev Respir Dis 1978;118:305–10.
5. Kwon KY, Myers JL, Swensen SJ, et al. Middle lobe syndrome: a clinicopathological study of 21 patients. Hum Pathol 1995;26:302–7.
6. Reich JM, Johnson RE. *Mycobacterium avium* complex pulmonary disease presenting as an isolated lingular or middle lobe pattern. The Lady Windermere syndrome. Chest 1992;101:1605–9.
7. Brock RC, Hodgkiss F, Jones HO. Bronchial embolism and posture in relation to lung disease. Guy Hosp Rep 1942;91:131–9.

Obstruction of the upper airways

8. Schokkenbroek AA, Franssen CF, Dikkers FG. Dilatation tracheoscopy for laryngeal and tracheal stenosis in patients with Wegener's granulomatosis. Eur Arch Otorhinolaryngol 2008;265:549–55.
9. McNamara SG, Grunstein RR, Sullivan CE. Obstructive sleep apnoea. Thorax 1993;48:754–64.
10. Crummy F, Piper AJ, Naughton MT. Obesity and the lung: 2. Obesity and sleep-disordered breathing. Thorax 2008;63:738–46.
11. Meston N, Davies RJ, Mullins R, et al. Endocrine effects of nasal continuous

positive airway pressure in male patients with obstructive sleep apnoea. J Intern Med 2003;254:447–54.

12. Wang H, Parker JD, Newton GE, et al. Influence of obstructive sleep apnea on mortality in patients with heart failure. J Am Coll Cardiol 2007;49:1625–31.

13. Ahmed Q, Chung-Park M, Tomashefski JF. Cardiopulmonary pathology in patients with sleep apnea/obesity hypoventilation syndrome. Hum Pathol 1997;28:264–9.

14. Cross MD, Mills NL, Al-Abri M, et al. Continuous positive airway pressure improves vascular function in obstructive sleep apnoea/hypopnoea syndrome: a randomised controlled trial. Thorax 2008;63:578–83.

15. Wilks W. Ossific deposits on the larynx, trachea and bronchi. Pathol Soc Lond 1857;8:88.

16. Virchow R. Die Krankhaften geschwulste. Berlin: Hirschwald; 1863. p. 443.

17. Jabbardarjani H, Radpey B, Kharabian S, et al. Tracheobronchopathia osteochondroplastica: presentation of ten cases and review of the literature. Lung 2008;186:293–7.

18. bu-Hijleh M, Lee D, Braman S. Tracheobronchopathia osteochondroplastica: a rare large airway disorder. Lung 2008;186:353–9.

19. Vilkman S, Keistinen T. Tracheobronchopathia osteochondroplastica – report of a young man with severe disease and retrospective review of 18 cases. Respiration 1995;62:151–4.

20. Coetmeur D, Bovyn G, Leroux P, et al. Tracheobronchopathia osteochondroplastica presenting at the time of a difficult intubation. Resp Med 1997;91:496–8.

21. Primer G. Osteochondroplastica, tracheobronchopathy. Prax Klin Pneumol 1979;33:1060–3.

22. Pounder DJ, Pieterse AS. Tracheopathia osteoplastica: report of four cases. Pathology 1982;14:429–33.

23. Aschoff L. Uber Tracheopathia osteoplastica. Verh Dtsch Pathol Ges 1910;14:125–7.

24. Sakula A. Tracheobronchopathia osteoplastica. Its relationship to primary tracheobronchial amyloidosis. Thorax 1968;23:105–10.

25. Alroy GG, Lichtig C, Kaftori JK. Tracheobronchopathia osteoplastica: end stage of primary lung amyloidosis? Chest 1972;61:465–8.

26. Jones AW, Chatterji AN. Primary tracheobronchial amyloidosis with tracheobronchopathia osteoplastica. Br J Dis Chest 1977;71:268–72.

27. Tajima K, Yamakawa M, Katagiri T, et al. Immunohistochemical detection of bone morphogenetic protein-2 and transforming growth factor beta-1 in tracheopathia

osteochondroplastica. Virchows Archiv 1997;431:359–63.

28. Baird RB, Macartney JN. Tracheopathia osteoplastica. Thorax 1966;21:321–4.

29. Ashley DJB. Bony metaplasia in trachea and bronchi. J Pathol 1970;102:186–8.

30. Pounder DJ, Pieterse AS. Tracheopathia osteoplastica: a study of the minimal lesion. J Pathol 1982;138:235–9.

31. Pearson CM, Cline HM, Newcomer VD. Relapsing polychondritis. N Engl J Med 1960;263:51–8.

32. Verity MA, Larson WM, Madden SC. Relapsing polychondritis. Report of two necropsied cases with histochemical investigation of the cartilage lesion. Am J Pathol 1963;42:251–69.

33. Kaye RL, Sones DA. Relapsing polychondritis. Clinical and pathological features in 14 cases. Ann Intern Med 1964;60:653–64.

34. Hughes RAC, Berry CL, Seifert M, et al. Relapsing polychondritis. Three cases with a clinico-pathological study and literature review. Q J Med 1972;41:363–80.

35. McAdam LP, O'Hanlan MA, Bluestone R, et al. Relapsing polychondritis: prospective study of 23 patients and a review of the literature. Medicine (Baltimore) 1976;55:193–215.

36. Valenzuela R, Cooperrider PA, Gogate P, et al. Relapsing polychondritis. Immunomicroscopic findings in cartilage of ear biopsy specimens. Hum Pathol 1980;11:19–22.

37. Ebringer R, Rook G, Swana GT, et al. Autoantibodies to cartilage and type II collagen in relapsing polychondritis and other rheumatic diseases. Ann Rheum Dis 1979;40:473–9.

38. Higgenbottam T, Dixon J. Chondritis associated with fatal intramural bronchial fibrosis. Thorax 1979;34:563–4.

39. Rogerson ME, Higgins EM, Godfrey RC. Tracheal stenosis due to relapsing polychondritis in rheumatoid arthritis. Thorax 1987;42:905–6.

40. Sheffield E, Corrin B. Fatal bronchial stenosis due to isolated relapsing chondritis. Histopathology 1992;20:442–3.

41. Ozbay B, Dilek FH, Yalcinkaya I, et al. Relapsing polychondritis. Respiration 1998;65:206–7.

42. Ernst A, Rafeq S, Boiselle P, et al. Relapsing polychondritis and airway involvement. Chest 2009;135:1024–30.

43. Chan HS, Pang J. Relapsing polychondritis presenting with bronchorrhoea. Respir Med 1990;84:341–3.

44. Somers G, Potvliege P. Relapsing polychondritis: relation to periarteritis nodosa. BMJ 1978;2:603–4.

45. Neild GH, Cameron JS, Lessof MH, et al. Relapsing polychondritis with crescentic glomerulonephritis. BMJ 1978;1:743–5.

46. Mark EJ, Meng F, Kradin RL, et al. Idiopathic tracheal stenosis: a clinicopathologic study of 63 cases and comparison of the pathology with chondromalacia. Am J Surg Pathol 2008;32:1138–43.

Acute tracheobronchitis and bronchiolitis

47. Haggard HW. Action of irritant gases upon the respiratory tract. J Indust Hyg 1924;5:390.

48. Andersen P. Pathogenesis of lower respiratory tract infections due to Chlamydia, Mycoplasma, Legionella and viruses. Thorax 1998;53:302–7.

49. Holt LB. The pathology and immunology of Bordetella pertussis infection. J Med Microbiol 1972;5:407–24.

50. Paddock CD, Sanden GN, Cherry JD, et al. Pathology and pathogenesis of fatal Bordetella pertussis infection in infants. Clin Infect Dis 2008;47:328–38.

51. Chandraratnam EA, Henderson DW, Meredith DJ, et al. Regenerative atypical squamous metaplasia in fibreoptic bronchial biopsy sites – a lesion liable to misinterpretation as carcinoma on rebiopsy report of 5 cases. Pathology 1987;19:419–24.

52. Wenig BM. Necrotizing sialometaplasia of the larynx: a report of two cases and a review of the literature. Am J Clin Pathol 1995;103:609–13.

53. Carlson DL. Necrotizing sialometaplasia: a practical approach to the diagnosis. Arch Pathol Lab Med 2009;133:692–8.

54. Benizhak O, Benarieh Y. Necrotizing squamous metaplasia in herpetic tracheitis following prolonged intubation – a lesion similar to necrotizing sialometaplasia. Histopathology 1993;22:265–9.

55. Littman CD. Necrotizing sialometaplasia (adenometaplasia) of the trachea. Histopathology 1993;22:298–9.

56. Rizkalla H, Toner M. Necrotizing sialometaplasia versus invasive carcinoma of the head and neck: the use of myoepithelial markers and keratin subtypes as an adjunct to diagnosis. Histopathology 2007;51:184–9.

Chronic obstructive pulmonary disease

57. Barnes PJ. Medical progress: Chronic obstructive pulmonary disease. N Engl J Med 2000;343:269–80.

58. Anto JM, Vermeire P, Vestbo J, et al. Epidemiology of chronic obstructive pulmonary disease. Eur Resp J 2001;17:982–94.

59. Zvezdin B, Milutinov S, Kojicic M, et al. A postmortem analysis of major causes of early death in patients hospitalized with COPD exacerbation. Chest 2009;136:376–80.

60. Davis AL. Bronchogenic carcinoma in chronic obstructive pulmonary disease. JAMA 1976;235:621–2.

61. Skillrud DM, Offord KP, Miller RD. Higher risk of lung cancer in chronic obstructive pulmonary disease. A prospective, matched, controlled study. Ann Intern Med 1986;105:503–7.

61a. Sorheim I-C, Johannessen A, Gulsvik A, Bakke PS, Silverman EK, DeMeo DL. Gender differences in COPD: are women more susceptible to smoking effects than men? Thorax 2010;65:480–5.

62. Mannion PT. Sputum microbiology in a district general hospital. The role of Branhamella catarrhalis Br J Dis Chest 1987;81:391–6.

63. Murphy TF, Sethi S. Bacterial infection in chronic obstructive pulmonary disease. Am Rev Respir Dis 1992;146:1067–83.

64. Sethi S, Muscarella K, Evans N, et al. Airway inflammation and etiology of acute exacerbations of chronic bronchitis. Chest 2000;118:1557–65.

65. Sethi S, Evans N, Grant BJB, et al. New strains of bacteria and exacerbations of chronic obstructive pulmonary disease. N Engl J Med 2002;347:465–71.

66. Blasi F, Damato S, Cosentini R, et al. Chlamydia pneumoniae and chronic bronchitis: association with severity and bacterial clearance following treatment. Thorax 2002;57:672–6.

67. Murphy TF, Brauer AL, Grant BJB, et al. Moraxella catarrhalis in chronic obstructive pulmonary disease: burden of disease and immune response. Am J Respir Crit Care Med 2005;172:195–9.

68. Stuart-Harris CH, Pownall M, Scothorne CM, et al. The factor of infection in chronic bronchitis. Q J Med 1953;22:121–32.

69. Seemungal T, HarperOwen R, Bhowmik A, et al. Respiratory viruses, symptoms, and inflammatory markers in acute exacerbations and stable chronic obstructive pulmonary disease. Am J Respir Crit Care Med 2001;164:1618–23.

70. Dornhorst AC. Respiratory insufficiency. Lancet 1955;1:1185–7.

71. Fletcher CM, Hugh-Jones P, McNicol MW, et al. The diagnosis of pulmonary emphysema in the presence of chronic bronchitis. Q J Med 1963;32:33–49.

72. Mitchell RS, Stanford RE, Johnson JM, et al. The morphologic features of the bronchi, bronchioles, and alveoli in chronic airway obstruction: a clinicopathologic study. Am Rev Respir Dis 1976;114:137–45.

73. Terminology, definitions, and classification of chronic pulmonary emphysema and related conditions. A report of the conclusions of a CIBA guest symposium. Thorax 1959;14:286–99.

74. Medical Research Council. Definition and classification of chronic bronchitis for clinical and epidemiological purposes. Lancet 1965;1:775–9.

75. Fletcher C, Peto R. The natural history of chronic airflow obstruction. BMJ 1977;1:1645–8.

76. Jamal K, Cooney TP, Fleetham JA, et al. Chronic bronchitis. Correlation of morphologic findings to sputum production and flow rates. Am Rev Respir Dis 1984;129:719–22.

77. Vestbo J, Prescott E, Lange P. Association of chronic mucus hypersecretion with FEV$_1$ decline and chronic obstructive pulmonary disease morbidity. Copenhagen City Heart Study Group. Am J Respir Crit Care Med 1996;153:1530–5.

78. Doll R, Hill AB. Mortality in relation to smoking: ten years' observations of British doctors. BMJ 1964;1:1399–410.

79. Doll R, Hill AB. Mortality in relation to smoking: ten years' observations of British doctors. BMJ 1964;1:1460–7.

80. Amadori A, Zamarchi R, De Silvestro G, et al. Genetic control of the CD4/CD8 T-cell ratio in humans. Nat Med 1995;1:1279–83.

81. Hyashi M, Sornberger GC, Huber GL. A morphometric analysis of the male and female tracheal epithelium after experimental exposure to marijuana smoke. Lab Invest 1980;42:65–9.

82. Kiraz K, Kart L, Demir R, et al. Chronic pulmonary disease in rural women exposed to biomass fumes. Clin Invest Med 2003;26:243–8.

83. Regalado J, Perez-Padilla R, Sansores R, et al. The effect of biomass burning on respiratory symptoms and lung function in rural Mexican women. Am J Respir Crit Care Med 2006;174:901–5.

84. Orozco-Levi M, Garcia-Aymerich J, Villar J, et al. Wood smoke exposure and risk of chronic obstructive pulmonary disease. Eur Respir J 2006;27:542–6.

84a. Hu G, Zhou Y, Tian J, et al. Risk of COPD from exposure to biomass smoke. Chest 2010;138:20–31.

85. Oxman AD, Muir DCF, Shannon HS, et al. Occupational dust exposure and chronic obstructive pulmonary disease – a systematic overview of the evidence. Am Rev Respir Dis 1993;148:38–48.

86. Blanc PD, Iribarren C, Trupin L, et al. Occupational exposures and the risk of COPD: dusty trades revisited. Thorax 2009;64:6–12.

87. Rohde G, Wiethege A, Borg I, et al. Respiratory viruses in exacerbations of chronic obstructive pulmonary disease requiring hospitalisation: a case-control study. Thorax 2003;58:37–42.

88. Oswald NC, Harold JT, Martin WJ. Clinical pattern of chronic bronchitis. Lancet 1953;2:639–43.

89. Burrows B, Knudson RJ, Lebowitz MD. The relationship of childhood respiratory illness to adult obstructive airway disease. Am Rev Respir Dis 1977;115:751–60.

90. Restrepo GL, Heard BE. Air trapping in chronic bronchitis and emphysema.

Am Rev Respir Dis 1964;90:395–400.

91. Wright RR. Bronchial atrophy and collapse in chronic obstructive pulmonary emphysema. Am J Pathol 1960;37:63–77.

92. Thurlbeck WM, Pun R, Toth J, et al. Bronchial cartilage in chronic obstructive lung disease. Am Rev Respir Dis 1974;109:73–80.

93. Haraguchi M, Shimura S, Shirato K. Morphometric analysis of bronchial cartilage in chronic obstructive pulmonary disease and bronchial asthma. Am J Respir Crit Care Med 1999;159:1005–13.

94. Reid L. Measurement of the bronchial mucous gland layer: a diagnostic yardstick in chronic bronchitis. Thorax 1960;15:132–41.

95. Douglas AN. Quantitative study of bronchial mucous gland enlargement. Thorax 1980;35:198–201.

96. Restrepo G, Heard BE. The size of the bronchial glands in chronic bronchitis. J Pathol Bacteriol 1963;85:305–10.

97. Matsuba K, Thurlbeck WM. A morphometric study of bronchial and bronchiolar walls in children. Am Rev Respir Dis 1972;105:908.

98. Takizawa T, Thurlbeck WM. A comparative study of four methods of assessing the morphologic changes in chronic bronchitis. Am Rev Respir Dis 1971;103:774–83.

99. Saetta M, Turato G, Baraldo S, et al. Goblet cell hyperplasia and epithelial inflammation in peripheral airways of smokers with both symptoms of chronic bronchitis and chronic airflow limitation. Am J Respir Crit Care Med 2000;161:1016–21.

100. Bowes D, Corrin B. Ultrastructural immunocytochemical localization of lysozyme in human bronchial glands. Thorax 1977;32:163–70.

101. Bowes D, Clark AE, Corrin B. Ultrastructural localisation of lactoferrin and glycoprotein in human bronchial glands. Thorax 1981;36:108–15.

102. Harbitz O, Jenssen AO, Smidsrod O. Lysozyme and lactoferrin in sputum from patients with chronic obstructive lung disease. Eur J Respir Dis 1984;65:512–20.

103. Pilette C, Godding V, Kiss R, et al. Reduced epithelial expression of secretory component in small airways correlates with airflow obstruction in chronic obstructive pulmonary disease. Amer J Respir Crit Care Med 2001;163:185–94.

104. Kramps JA, Franken C, Meijer CJLM, et al. Localization of low molecular weight protease inhibitor in serous secretory cells of the respiratory tract. J Histochem 1981;29:712–19.

105. O'Shaughnessy TC, Ansari TW, Barnes NC, et al. Inflammation in bronchial biopsies of subjects with chronic bronchitis: inverse relationship of CD8+ T lymphocytes with

FEV₁. Am J Respir Crit Care Med 1997;155:852–7.

106. Saetta M, Turato G, Facchini FM, et al. Inflammatory cells in the bronchial glands of smokers with chronic bronchitis. Am J Respir Crit Care Med 1997;156:1633–9.

107. Mullen JBM, Wright JL, Wiggs BR, et al. Reassessment of inflammation of airways in chronic bronchitis. BMJ 1985;291:1235–9.

108. Klinger JD, Tandler B, Liedtke CM, Boat TF. Proteinases of Pseudomonas aeruginosa evoke mucin release by tracheal epithelium. J Clin Invest 1984:74:1669–78.

109. Mullen JBM, Wright JL, Wiggs BR, et al. Structure of central airways in current smokers and ex-smokers with and without mucus hypersecretion: relationship to lung function. Thorax 1987;42:843–8.

110. Hossain S, Heard BE. Hyperplasia of bronchial muscle in chronic bronchitis. J Pathol 1970;101:171–84.

111. Dunnill MS, Massarella GR, Anderson JA. A comparison of the quantitative anatomy of the bronchi in normal subjects, in status asthmaticus, in chronic bronchitis, and in emphysema. Thorax 1969;24:176–9.

112. Takizawa T, Thurlbeck WM. Muscle and mucous gland size in the major bronchi of patients with chronic bronchitis, asthma, and asthmatic bronchitis. Am Rev Respir Dis 1971;104:331–6.

113. Barter CE, Campbell AH. Relationship of constitutional factors and cigarette smoking to decrease in 1-second forced expiratory volume. Am Rev Respir Dis 1976;113:305–14.

114. Orie NGM, Sluiter HJ, deVries K, et al. The Host Factor in Bronchitis. In: Orie NGM, Sluiter HJ, editors. Bronchitis: an international symposium. Assen: Royal van Gorcum; 1961. p. 44–59.

115. Burrows B, Halonen M, Barbee RA, et al. The relationship of serum immunoglobulin E to cigarette smoking. Am Rev Respir Dis 1981;124:523–5.

116. Jeffery PK. Comparison of the structural and inflammatory features of COPD and asthma. Giles F. Filley Lecture. Chest 2000;117:251S–60S.

117. Hogg JC, Macklem PT, Thurlbeck WM. Site and nature of airway obstruction in chronic obstructive lung disease. N Engl J Med 1968;278:1355–60.

118. Thurlbeck WM, Malaka D, Murphy K. Goblet cells in the peripheral airways in chronic bronchitis. Am Rev Respir Dis 1975;112:65–9.

119. Lumsden AB, McLean A, Lamb D. Goblet and Clara cells of human distal airways: evidence for smoking induced changes in their numbers. Thorax 1984;39:844–9.

120. Mooren HWD, Kramps JA, Franken C, et al. Localisation of a low molecular weight bronchial protease inhibitor in the peripheral human lung. Thorax 1983;38:180–3.

121. Water d, Willems LNA, van Muijen GNP, et al. Ultrastructural localization of bronchial antileukoprotease in central and peripheral human airways by a gold-labelling technique using monoclonal antibodies. Am Rev Respir Dis 1986;133:882–90.

122. Willems LNA, Kramps JA, Water de R, et al. Evaluation of antileukoprotease in surgical lung specimens. Eur J Respir Dis 1986;69:242–7.

123. Willems LNA, Kramps JA, Stijnen T, et al. Antileukoprotease-containing bronchiolar cells. Relationship with morphologic disease of small airways and parenchyma. Am Rev Respir Dis 1989;139:1244–50.

124. Edwards C, Cayton R, Bryan R. Chronic transmural bronchiolitis – a non-specific lesion of small airways. J Clin Pathol 1992;45:993–8.

125. Bosken CH, Wiggs BR, Pare PD, et al. Small airway dimensions in smokers with obstruction to airflow. Am Rev Respir Dis 1990;142:563–70.

126. Leopold JG, Gough J. The centrilobular form of hypertrophic emphysema and its relation to chronic bronchitis. Thorax 1957;12:219–35.

127. Esterly JR, Heard BE. Multiple bronchiolar stenoses in a patient with generalized airways obstruction. Thorax 1965;20:309–16.

128. Duinker NW, Huizinga E. The 'flowers' in bronchography. Thorax 1962;17:175.

129. Reid LM. Correlation of certain bronchographic abnormalities seen in chronic bronchitis with the pathological changes. Thorax 1955;10:199–204.

130. Depierre A, Bignon J, Lebeau A, et al. Quantitative study of parenchyma and small conductive airways in chronic nonspecific lung disease. Use of histologic stereology and bronchial casts. Chest 1972;62:699–708.

131. Bignon J, Depierre A. L'obstruction des petites voies aériennes: Essai de corrélations structure–fonction. Poumon et Coeur 1975;31:233–40.

132. Matsuba K, Thurlbeck WM. Disease of the small airways in chronic bronchitis. Am Rev Respir Dis 1973;107:552–8.

133. McLean KH. The pathology of acute bronchiolitis – a study of its evolution. Part I: The exudative phase. Aust Ann Med 1956;5:254–67.

134. McLean KH. The pathology of acute bronchiolitis – a study of its evolution. Part II: The repair phase. Aust Ann Med 1957;6:29–43.

135. McLean KH. Bronchiolitis and chronic lung disease. Br J Tuberc Dis Chest 1958;52:105–13.

136. Rosenblatt MB. Emphysema: historical perspective. Bull N Y Acad Med 1972;48:823–41.

137. Heard BE, Izukawa T. Pulmonary emphysema in fifty consecutive male necropsies in London. J Pathol Bacteriol 1964;88:423–31.

138. Hasleton PS. Incidence of emphysema at necropsy as assessed by point-counting. Thorax 1972;27:552–6.

139. Heard BE, Khatchatourov V, Otto H, et al. The morphology of emphysema, chronic bronchitis, and bronchiectasis: definition, nomenclature, and classification. J Clin Pathol 1979;32:882–92.

140. Snider GL, Kleinerman J, Thurlbeck WM, et al. The definition of emphysema. Report of a National Heart, Lung and Blood Institute, Division of Lung Diseases Workshop. Am Rev Respir Dis 1985;132:182–5.

141. American Thoracic Society. Standards for the diagnosis and care of patients with chronic obstructive pulmonary disease (COPD) and asthma. Am Rev Respir Dis 1987;136:225–44.

142. Thurlbeck WM. Morphology of emphysema and emphysema-like conditions. In: Thurlbeck WM, editor. Chronic Airflow Obstruction in Lung Disease. Philadelphia: Saunders; 1976. p. 98–9.

143. Cardoso WV, Sekhon HS, Hyde DM, et al. Collagen and elastin in human pulmonary emphysema. Am Rev Respir Dis 1993;147:975–81.

144. Lang MR, Fiaux GW, Gillooly M, et al. Collagen content of alveolar wall tissue in emphysematous and non-emphysematous lungs. Thorax 1994;49:319–26.

145. Wright JL. The importance of ultramicroscopic emphysema in cigarette smoke-induced lung disease. Lung 2001;179:71–81.

146. Linhartova A, Anderson AE, Foraker AG. Affixment arrangements of peribronchiolar alveoli in normal and emphysematous lungs. Arch Pathol Lab Med 1982;106:499–502.

147. Wright JL, Hobson JE, Wiggs B, et al. Airway inflammation and peribronchiolar attachments in the lungs of nonsmokers, current and ex-smokers. Lung 1988;166:277–86.

148. Lamb D, McLean A, Gillooly M, et al. Relation between distal airspace size, bronchiolar attachments, and lung function. Thorax 1993;48:1012–7.

149. Dunnill MS. Quantitative methods in the study of pulmonary pathology. Thorax 1962;17:320–8.

150. Dunnill MS. Evaluation of a simple method of sampling the lung for quantitative histological analysis. Thorax 1964;19:443–8.

151. Gillooly M, Lamb D, Farrow ASJ. New automated technique for assessing emphysema on histological sections. J Clin Pathol 1991;44:1007–11.

152. McLean A, Warren PM, Gillooly M, et al. Microscopic and macroscopic

measurements of emphysema – relation to carbon monoxide gas transfer. Thorax 1992;47:144–9.

153. Heard BE. A pathological study of emphysema of the lungs with chronic bronchitis. Thorax 1958;13: 136–49.

154. Gough J, Wentworth JE. Thin sections of entire organs mounted on paper. In: Harrison CV, editor. Recent Advances in Pathology. 7th ed. London: Churchill; 1960. p. 80–6.

155. Thurlbeck WM, Dunnill MS, Hartung W, et al. A comparison of three methods of measuring emphysema. Hum Pathol 1970;1:215–26.

156. Gevenois PA, Zanen J, Demaertelaer V, et al. Macroscopic assessment of pulmonary emphysema by image analysis. J Clin Pathol 1995;48:318–22.

157. Auerbach O, Hammond EC, Garfinkel L, et al. Relation of smoking and age to emphysema: whole-lung section study. N Engl J Med 1972;286:853–7.

158. Heard BE. Further observations on the pathology of pulmonary emphysema in chronic bronchitics. Thorax 1959;14:58–70.

159. Gross P, Pfitzer EA, Tolker E, et al. Experimental emphysema. Its production with papain in normal and silicotic rats. Arch Env Health 1965;11:50–8.

160. Laurell CB, Eriksson S. The electrophoretic alpha 1-globulin pattern of serum in alpha 1-antitrypsin deficiency. Scand J Clin Lab Invest 1963;15:132–40.

161. Mahadeva R, Lomas DA. Alpha(1)-antitrypsin deficiency, cirrhosis and emphysema. Thorax 1998;53:501–5.

161a. Kelly E, Greene CM, Carroll TP, McElvaney NG, O'Neill SJ. Alpha-1 antitrypsin deficiency. Respiratory Medicine 2010;104:763–72.

162. Lieberman J, Gaidulis L, Garoutte B, et al. Identification and characteristics of the common alpha1-antitrypsin phenotypes. Chest 1972;62:557–64.

163. Cook PJL. Genetic aspects of the Pi system. Postgrad Med J 1974;50:362–4.

164. Demeo DL, Silverman EK. α1-Antitrypsin deficiency 2: Genetic aspects of α1-antitrypsin deficiency: phenotypes and genetic modifiers of emphysema risk. Thorax 2004;59:259–64.

165. deSerres FTJ. Worldwide racial and ethnic distribution of alpha(1)- antitrypsin deficiency – Summary of an analysis of published genetic epidemiologic surveys. Chest 2002;122:1818–29.

166. Spinola C, Bruges-Armas J, Pereira C, et al. Alpha-1-antitrypsin deficiency in Madeira (Portugal): The highest prevalence in the world. Respiratory Medicine 2009;103:1498–502.

167. Tomashefski JF, Crystal RG, Wiedemann HP, et al. The bronchopulmonary pathology of alpha-1 antitrypsin (AAT) deficiency: Findings of the death review committee of the national registry for individuals with severe deficiency of alpha-1 antitrypsin. Human Pathology 2004;35:1452–61.

168. Larsson C, Eriksson S. Smoking and intermediate alpha 1-antitrypsin deficiency and lung function in middle-aged men. BMJ 1977;2:922–5.

169. Silva GE, Sherrill DL, Guerra S, et al. A longitudinal study of alpha(1)-antitrypsin phenotypes and decline in FEV_1 in a community population. Chest 2003;123:1435–40.

170. Brantly ML, Paul LD, Miller BH, et al. Clinical features and history of the destructive lung disease associated with alpha-1-antitrypsin deficiency of adults with pulmonary symptoms. Am Rev Respir Dis 1988;138:327–36.

171. Dawkins P, Wood A, Nightingale P, et al. Mortality in alpha-1-antitrypsin deficiency in the United Kingdom. Respiratory Medicine 2009;103:1540–7.

172. Parr DG, Guest PG, Reynolds JH, Dowson LJ, Stockley RA. Prevalence and impact of bronchiectasis in α1-antitrypsin deficiency. Am J Respir Crit Care Med 2007;176:1215–21.

173. Lane KB, Marney A, Phillips JA, et al. Familial interstitial pulmonary fibrosis and linkage to chromosome 14. Chest 2001;120:75S–6S.

174. Janoff A, Carp H, Lee DK, et al. Cigarette smoke inhalation decreases alpha 1-antitrypsin activity in rat lung. Science 1979;206:1313–14.

175. Carp H, Janoff A. Inactivation of bronchial mucous proteinase inhibitor by cigarette smoke and phagocyte-derived oxidants. Exp Lung Res 1980;1:225–37.

176. Blue M-L, Janoff A. Possible mechanisms of emphysema in cigarette smokers. Release of elastase from human polymorphonuclear leukocytes by cigarette smoke condensate in vitro. Am Rev Respir Dis 1978;117:317–25.

177. Harris JO, Swenson EW, Johnson JE. Human alveolar macrophages: comparison of phagocytic ability, glucose utilization and ultrastructure in smokers and non-smokers. J Clin Invest 1970;49:2086.

178. Cosio MG, Hale KA, Niewoehner DE. Morphologic and morphometric effects of prolonged cigarette smoking on the small airways. Am Rev Respir Dis 1980;122:265–71.

179. Niewoehner DE, Kleinerman J, Rice DB. Pathologic changes in the peripheral airways of young cigarette smokers. N Engl J Med 1974;291:755.

180. de Cremoux H, Hornebeck W, Jaurand MC, et al. Partial characterization of an elastase-like enzyme secreted by human and monkey alveolar macrophages. J Pathol 1978;125:171–7.

181. Rodriguez RJ, White RR, Senior RM, et al. Elastase release from human alveolar macrophages: comparison between smokers and non-smokers. Science 1977;198:313.

182. Russell REK, Culpitt SV, DeMatos C, et al. Release and activity of matrix metalloproteinase-9 and tissue inhibitor of metalloproteinase-1 by alveolar macrophages from patients with chronic obstructive pulmonary disease. Am J Respir Cell Molec Biol 2002;26:602–9.

183. Remy-Jardin M, Edme JL, Boulenguez C, et al. Longitudinal follow-up study of smoker's lung with thin-section CT in correlation with pulmonary function tests. Radiology 2002;222:261–70.

184. Gadek JE, Hunninghake GW, Fells GA, et al. Evaluation of the protease-antiprotease theory of human destructive lung disease. Bull Europ Physiopath Resp 1980;16:27S.

185. Retamales I, Elliott WM, Meshi B, et al. Amplification of inflammation in emphysema and its association with latent adenoviral infection. Am J Respir Crit Care Med 2001;164:469–73.

186. Senior RM, Griffin GL, Mecham RP, et al. Val-Gly-Val-Ala-Pro-Gly, a repeating peptide in elastin, is chemotactic for fibroblasts and monocytes. J Cell Biol 1984;99:870–4.

187. Morgan MD, Edwards CW, Morris J, et al. Origin and behaviour of emphysematous bullae. Thorax 1989;44:533–8.

188. Davison AG, Newman Taylor AJ, Darbyshire J, et al. Cadmium fume inhalation and emphysema. Lancet 1988;1:663–7.

189. Snider GL, Hayes JA, Kerthy AL, et al. Centrilobular emphysema experimentally induced by cadmium chloride aerosol. Am Rev Respir Dis 1973;108:40–8.

190. Smith JP, Smith JC, McCall AJ. Chronic poisoning from cadmium fume. J Pathol Bacteriol 1960;80:287–96.

191. Hirst RN, Perry HM, Cruz MG, et al. Elevated cadmium concentration in emphysematous lungs. Am Rev Respir Dis 1973;108:30–9.

192. Leduc D, Defrancquen P, Jacobovitz D, et al. Association of cadmium exposure with rapidly progressive emphysema in a smoker. Thorax 1993;48:570–1.

193. Pierce JA, Hocott JB, Ebert RV. The collagen and elastin content of the lung in emphysema. Ann Intern Med 1961;55:210–22.

194. Kuhn C, Yu S-Y, Chraplyvy M, et al. The induction of emphysema with elastase. II. Changes in connective tissue. Lab Invest 1976;34:372–80.

195. Levine S, Kaiser L, Leferovich J, et al. Cellular adaptations in the diaphragm in chronic obstructive pulmonary disease. N Engl J Med 1997;337:1799–806.

196. Stoller JK, Fallat R, Schluchter MD, et al. Augmentation therapy with alpha(1)-antitrypsin – Patterns of use and adverse events. Chest 2003;123:1425–34.

197. Mannes GPM, Deboer WJ, Vanderbij W, et al. Lung transplantation and chronic

obstructive pulmonary disease. Respir Med 1993;87:61–5.

198. Davies L, Calverley PMA. Lung volume reduction surgery in chronic obstructive pulmonary disease. J Thorac Cardiovasc Surg 1995;109:106–19.

199. Roue C, Mal H, Sleiman C, et al. Lung volume reduction in patients with severe diffuse emphysema: a retrospective study. Chest 1996;110:28–34.

200. Brenner M, Yusen R, Mckenna R, et al. Lung volume reduction surgery for emphysema. Chest 1996;110:205–18.

201. Maxfield RA. New and emerging minimally invasive techniques for lung volume reduction. Chest 2004;125:777–83.

202. Wan IYP, Toma TP, Geddes DM, et al. Bronchoscopic Lung Volume Reduction for End-Stage Emphysema: Report on the First 98 Patients. Chest 2006;129:518–26.

203. Polkey MI, Hopkinson NS. Bronchoscopic lung volume reduction. European Respiratory Review 2006;15:99–103.

204. Wood DE, McKenna RJ, Jr., Yusen RD, et al. A multicenter trial of an intrabronchial valve for treatment of severe emphysema. J Thorac Cardiovasc Surg 2007;133:65–73.

205. Coxson HO, Nasute Fauerbach PV, Storness-Bliss C, et al. Computed tomography assessment of lung volume changes after bronchial valve treatment. Eur Respir J 2008;32:1443–50.

206. Herth FJ, Gompelmann D, Ernst A, et al. Endoscopic lung volume reduction. Respiration 2010;79:5–13.

207. Hoppin FG. Theoretical basis for improvement following reduction pneumoplasty in emphysema. Am J Respir Crit Care Med 1997;155:520–5.

208. Marchand E, Gayanramirez G, Deleyn P, et al. Physiological basis of improvement after lung volume reduction surgery for severe emphysema: where are we? Eur Resp J 1999;13:686–96.

209. Keller CA, Naunheim KS, Osterloh J, et al. Histopathologic diagnosis made in lung tissue resected from patients with severe emphysema undergoing lung volume reduction surgery. Chest 1997;111:941–7.

210. Duarte IG, Gal AA, Mansour KA, et al. Pathologic findings in lung volume reduction surgery. Chest 1998;113:660–4.

211. Gillooly M, Lamb D. Airspace size in lungs of lifelong non-smokers – effect of age and sex. Thorax 1993;48:39–43.

212. Heppleston AG. The pathogenesis of simple pneumokoniosis in coal workers. J Path Bact 1954;67:51–63.

213. Lyons JP, Ryder RC, Seal RME, et al. Emphysema in smoking and non-smoking coalworkers with pneumoconiosis. Bull Europ Physiopath Resp 1981;17: 75–85.

214. Leigh J, Outhred KG, McKenzie HI, et al. Quantified pathology of emphysema, pneumoconiosis, and chronic bronchitis in coal workers. Br J Ind Med 1983;40:258–63.

215. Ruckley VA, Gauld SJ, Chapman JS, et al. Emphysema and dust exposure in a group of coal workers. Am Rev Respir Dis 1984;129:528–32.

216. Wright AW. The local effect of the injection of gases in the subcutaneous tissues. Am J Pathol 1930;6:87–124.

217. Brewer LL, Moskowitz PS, Carrington CB, et al. Pneumatosis pulmonalis. A complication of the idiopathic respiratory distress syndrome. Am J Pathol 1979;95:171–90.

218. Wood BP, Anderson VM, Mauk JE, et al. Pulmonary lymphatic air: locating 'pulmonary interstitial emphysema' of the premature infant. AJR Am J Roentgenol 1982;138:809–14.

Plastic bronchitis

219. Sleigh Johnson R, Sita-Lumsden EG. Plastic bronchitis. Thorax 1960;15:325–32.

220. Wiggins J, Sheffield E, Jeffery PK, et al. Bronchial casts associated with hilar lymphatic and pulmonary lymphoid abnormalities. Thorax 1989;44: 226–7.

221. Jett JR, Tazelaar HD, Keim LW, et al. Plastic bronchitis – an old disease revisited. Mayo Clin Proc 1991;66:305–11.

222. Nicholson AG, Florio R, Hansell DM, et al. Pulmonary involvement by Niemann-Pick disease. A report of six cases. Histopathology 2006;48:596–603.

223. Park JY, Elshami AA, Kang DS, et al. Plastic bronchitis. Eur Respir J 1996;9:612–14.

224. Castet D, Lavandier M, Asquier E, et al. Moules bronchiques associés à des anomalies lymphatiques pulmonaires. Rev Mal Resp 1998;15:89–91.

225. Nair LG, Kurtz CP. Lymphangiomatosis presenting with bronchial cast formation. Thorax 1996;51:765–6.

226. Sanerkin NG, Seal RME, Leopold JG. Plastic bronchitis, mucoid impaction of the bronchi and allergic broncho-pulmonary aspergillosis, and their relationship to bronchial asthma. Ann Allergy 1966;24:586–94.

227. Morgan AD, Bogomoletz W. Mucoid impaction of the bronchi in relation to asthma and plastic bronchitis. Thorax 1968;23:356–69.

228. Seear M, Hui H, Magee F, et al. Bronchial casts in children: a proposed classification based on nine cases and a review of the literature. Am J Respir Crit Care Med 1997;155:364–70.

Chronic idiopathic cough

229. Chung KF, Pavord ID. Prevalence, pathogenesis, and causes of chronic cough. Lancet 2008;371:1364–74.

230. Niimi A, Torrego A, Nicholson AG, et al. Nature of airway inflammation and remodeling in chronic cough. J Allergy Clin Immunol 2005;116:565–70.

Bronchial asthma

231. Cookson WOCM, Young RP, Sandford AJ, et al. Maternal inheritance of atopic IgE responsiveness on chromosome-11q. Lancet 1992;340:381–4.

232. Sandford AJ, Shirakawa T, Moffatt MF, et al. Localisation of atopy and the beta subunit of the high affinity IgE receptor (FcER1) on chromosome 11q. Lancet 1993;341:332–4.

233. Noguchi E, Shibasaki M, Arinami T, et al. Evidence for linkage between asthma/atopy in childhood and chromosome 5q31-q33 in a Japanese population. Am J Respir Crit Care Med 1997;156:1390–3.

234. Moffatt MF, Kabesch M, Liang L, et al. Genetic variants regulating ORMDL3 expression contribute to the risk of childhood asthma. Nature 2007;448:470–3.

235. Bentley AM, Durham SR, Kay AB. Comparison of the immunopathology of extrinsic, intrinsic and occupational asthma. J Investig Allergol Clin Immunol 1994;4:222–32.

236. Humbert M, Durham SR, Ying S, et al. IL-4 and IL-5 mRNA and protein in bronchial biopsies from patients with atopic and nonatopic asthma: evidence against 'intrinsic' asthma being a distinct immunopathologic entity. Am J Respir Crit Care Med 1996;154:1497–504.

237. Lang DM, Polansky M. Patterns of asthma mortality in Philadelphia from 1969 to 1991. N Engl J Med 1994;331:1542–6.

238. Magnussen H, Jorres R, Nowak D. Effect of air pollution on the prevalence of asthma and allergy – lessons from the German reunification. Thorax 1993;48:879–81.

239. Williamson IJ, Martin CJ, McGill G, et al. Damp housing and asthma: a case-control study. Thorax 1997;52:229–34.

240. Romagnani S. Induction of Th1 and Th2 responses: a key role for the 'natural' immune response? Immunol Today 1992;13:379–81.

241. Strachan DP. Hay fever, hygiene, and household size. BMJ 1989;299:1259–60.

242. Strachan DP. Allergy and family size: a riddle worth solving. Clin Exp Allergy 1997;27:235–6

243. Shaheen SO, Aaby P, Hall AJ, et al. Measles and atopy in Guinea-Bissau. Lancet 1996;347:1792–6.

244. Matricardi PM, Rosmini F, Ferigno L, et al. Cross sectional retrospective study of prevalence of atopy among Italian military students with antibodies against hepatitis A virus. BMJ 1997;314:999–1003.

245. Matricardi PM, Rosmini F, Panetta V, et al. Hay fever and asthma in relation to markers of infection in the United States. J Allergy Clin Immunol 2002;110: 381–7.

246. Shirakawa T, Enomoto T, Shimazu S-I, et al. The inverse association between tuberculin responses and atopic disorder. Science 1997;275:77–9.

247. Holt PG. Immunoregulation of the allergic reaction in the respiratory tract. Eur Respir J 1996;9:S85–9.

248. Lanes SF, Rodriguez LAG, Huerta C. Respiratory medications and risk of asthma death. Thorax 2002;57:683–6.

249. Salpeter SR, Ormiston TM, Salpeter EE. Cardiovascular effects of beta-agonists in patients with asthma and COPD: a meta-analysis. Chest 2004;125:2309–21.

250. Blauw GJ, Westendorp RGJ. Asthma deaths in New Zealand: whodunnit? Lancet 1995;345:2–3.

251. Sheehan JK, Richardson PS, Fung DCK, et al. Analysis of respiratory mucus glycoproteins in asthma: a detailed study from a patient who died in status asthmaticus. Am J Respir Cell Mol Biol 1995;13:748–56.

252. Weller PF, Bach DS, Austen KF. Biochemical characterization of human eosinophil Charcot-Leyden crystal protein (lysophospholipase). J Biol Chem 1984;259:15100–5.

253. Ackerman SJ, Swaminathan GJ, Leonidas DD, et al. Eosinophil proteins: structural biology of Charcot-Leyden crystal protein (Galectin-10): new insights into an old protein. Respiratory Medicine 2000;94:1014–6.

254. Wahl RW. Curschmann's spirals in pleural and peritoneal fluids. Report of 12 cases. Acta Cytol 1985;30:147–51.

255. Naylor B. The shedding of the mucosa of the bronchial tree in asthma. Thorax 1962;17:69–72.

256. Rigler L, Koucky R. Roentgen studies in pathological physiology of bronchial asthma. Am J Roentgenol 1938;39:353–62.

257. Robin ED, Lewiston NJ. Unexpected, unexplained sudden death in young asthmatic subjects. Chest 1989;96:790–3.

258. Kolbe J, Fergusson W, Garrett J. Rapid onset asthma: a severe but uncommon manifestation. Thorax 1998;53:241–7.

259. Reid LM. The presence or absence of bronchial mucus in fatal asthma. J Allergy Clin Immunol 1987;80:415–16.

260. Drislane FW, Samuels MA, Kozakewich H, et al. Myocardial contraction band lesions in patients with fatal asthma: possible neurocardiologic mechanisms. Am Rev Respir Dis 1987;135:498–501.

261. Robin ED, McCauley R. Sudden cardiac death in bronchial asthma, and inhaled beta-adrenergic agonists. Chest 1992;101:1699–702.

262. Ziment I. Infrequent cardiac deaths occur in bronchial asthma. Chest 1992;101:1703–5.

263. Bharati S, Lev M. Conduction system findings in sudden death in young adults with a history of bronchial asthma. J Am Coll Cardiol 1994;23:741–6.

264. Pumphrey RSH, Roberts ISD. Postmortem findings after fatal anaphylactic reactions. J Clin Pathol 2000;53:273–6.

265. Dunnill MS. The pathology of asthma, with special references to the changes in the bronchial mucosa. J Clin Pathol 1960;13:27–33.

266. Kuwano K, Bosken CH, Pare PD, et al. Small airways dimensions in asthma and in chronic obstructive pulmonary disease. Am Rev Respir Dis 1993;148:1220–5.

267. Saetta M, Di Stefano A, Rosina C, et al. Quantitative structural analysis of peripheral airways and arteries in sudden fatal asthma. Am Rev Respir Dis 1991;143:138–43.

268. Roche WR. Inflammatory and structural changes in the small airways in bronchial asthma. Am J Respir Crit Care Med 1998;157:S191–4.

269. Balzar S, Wenzel SE, Chu HW. Transbronchial biopsy as a tool to evaluate small airways in asthma. Eur Resp J 2002;20:254–9.

270. Kraft M, Martin RJ, Wilson S, et al. Lymphocyte and eosinophil influx into alveolar tissue in nocturnal asthma. Am J Respir Crit Care Med 1999;159:228–34.

271. Sanerkin NG, Evans DMD. The sputum in bronchial asthma: pathognomonic patterns. J Pathol Bacteriol 1965;89:535.

272. Sanerkin NG. Causes and consequences of airways obstruction in bronchial asthma. Ann Allergy 1970;28:528.

273. Glynn AA, Michaels L. Bronchial biopsy in chronic bronchitis and asthma. Thorax 1960;15:142–53.

274. Salvato G. Some histological changes in chronic bronchitis and asthma. Thorax 1968;23:168–72.

275. Azzawi M, Bradley B, Jeffery PK, et al. Identification of activated T lymphocytes and eosinophils in bronchial biopsies in stable atopic asthma. Am Rev Respir Dis 1990;142:1407–13.

276. Azzawi M, Johnston PW, Majumdar S, et al. Lymphocytes-T and activated eosinophils in airway mucosa in fatal asthma and cystic fibrosis. Am Rev Respir Dis 1992;145:1477–82.

277. Bentley AM, Menz G, Storz C, et al. Identification of lymphocytes-T, macrophages, and activated eosinophils in the bronchial mucosa in intrinsic asthma – relationship to symptoms and bronchial responsiveness. Am Rev Respir Dis 1992;146:500–6.

278. Jatakanon A, Uasuf C, Maziak W, et al. Neutrophilic inflammation in severe persistent asthma. Am J Respir Crit Care Med 1999;160:1532–9.

279. Douwes J, Gibson P, Pekkanen J, et al. Non-eosinophilic asthma: importance and possible mechanisms. Thorax 2002;57:643–8.

280. Sur S, Crotty TB, Kephart GM, et al. Sudden-onset fatal asthma – a distinct entity with few eosinophils and relatively more neutrophils in the airway submucosa. Am Rev Respir Dis 1993;148:713–9.

281. Wenzel SE, Schwartz LB, Langmack EL, et al. Evidence that severe asthma can be divided pathologically into two inflammatory subtypes with distinct physiologic and clinical characteristics. Am J Respir Crit Care Med 1999;160:1001–8.

282. Ohashi Y, Motojima S, Fukuda T, et al. Airway hyperresponsiveness, increased intracellular spaces of bronchial epithelium, and increased infiltration of eosinophils and lymphocytes in bronchial mucosa in asthma. Am Rev Respir Dis 1992;145:1469–76.

283. Carroll NG, Mutavdzic S, James AL. Increased mast cells and neutrophils in submucosal mucous glands and mucus plugging in patients with asthma. Thorax 2002;57:677–82.

284. Djukanovic R, Wilson JW, Britten KM, et al. Quantitation of mast cells and eosinophils in the bronchial mucosa of symptomatic asthmatics and healthy control subjects using immunohistochemistry. Am Rev Respir Dis 1990;142:863–71.

285. Montefort S, Roberts JA, Beasley R, et al. The site of disruption of the bronchial epithelium in asthmatic and non-asthmatic subjects. Thorax 1992;47:499–503.

286. Montefort S, Roche WR, Holgate ST. Bronchial epithelial shedding in asthmatics and non-asthmatics. Respir Med 1993;87:9–11.

287. Crepea SB, Harman JW. The pathology of bronchial asthma. I. Significance of membrane changes in asthmatic and non-allergic pulmonary disease. J Allergy 1955;26:453–60.

288. Cutz E, Levison H, Cooper DM. Ultrastructure of airways in children with asthma. Histopathology 1978;2:407–21.

289. Laitinen LA, Heino M, Laitinen A, et al. Damage of the airway epithelium and bronchial reactivity in patients with asthma. Am Rev Respir Dis 1985;131:599–606.

290. Barnes PJ. Asthma as an axon reflex. Lancet 1986;ii:242–5.

291. McCarter JH, Vazquez JJ. The bronchial basement membrane in asthma: immunohistochemical and ultrastructural observations. Arch Pathol 1966;82:328–35.

292. Roche WR, Beasley R, Williams JH, et al. Subepithelial fibrosis in the bronchi of asthmatics. Lancet 1989;i:520–4.

293. Brewster CEP, Howarth PH, Djukanovic R, et al. Myofibroblasts and subepithelial fibrosis in bronchial asthma. Am J Respir Cell Mol Biol 1990;3:507–11.

294. Zhang M, Zhang Z, Pan HY, et al. TGF-β_1 Induces human bronchial epithelial cell-to-mesenchymal transition in vitro. Lung 2009;187:187–94.

295. Hackett TL, Warner SM, Stefanowicz D, et al. Induction of epithelial-mesenchymal transition in primary airway epithelial cells from patients with asthma by transforming

growth factor-β1. Am J Respir Crit Care Med 2009;180:122–33.

296. Laitinen A, Altraja A, Kampe M, et al. Tenascin is increased in airway basement membrane of asthmatics and decreased by an inhaled steroid. Am J Respir Crit Care Med 1997;156:951–8.

297. Watanabe K, Senju S, Toyoshima H, et al. Thickness of the basement membrane of bronchial epithelial cells in lung diseases as determined by transbronchial biopsy. Resp Med 1997;91:406–10.

298. Heard BE, Hossain S. Hyperplasia of bronchial muscle in asthma. J Pathol 1972;110:319–31.

299. Ebina M, Yaegashi H, Chiba R, et al. Hyperreactive site in the airway tree of asthmatic patients revealed by thickening of bronchial muscles: a morphometric study. Am Rev Respir Dis 1990;141:1327–32.

300. Ebina M, Takahashi T, Chiba T, et al. Cellular hypertrophy and hyperplasia of airway smooth muscles underlying bronchial asthma: a 3-D morphometric study. Am Rev Respir Dis 1993;148: 720–6.

301. Hossain S. Quantitative measurements of bronchial muscle in men with asthma. Am Rev Respir Dis 1973;107:99–109.

302. Ollerenshaw S, Jarvis D, Woolcock A, et al. Absence of immunoreactive vasoactive intestinal polypeptide in tissue from the lungs of patients with asthma. N Engl J Med 1989;320:1244–8.

303. Green FHY, Williams DJ, James A, et al. Increased myoepithelial cells of bronchial submucosal glands in fatal asthma. Thorax 2010;65:32–8.

304. Moreno RH, Hogg JC, Pare PD. Mechanics of airway narrowing in asthma. Am Rev Respir Dis 1986;133:1171–80.

305. James AL, Pare PD, Hogg JC. The mechanisms of airway narrowing in asthma. Am Rev Respir Dis 1989;139:242–6.

306. Wiggs BR, Bosken C, Pare PD, et al. A model of airway narrowing in asthma and in chronic obstructive pulmonary disease. Am Rev Respir Dis 1992;145:1251–8.

307. Djukanovic R, Roche WR, Wilson JW, et al. Mucosal inflammation in asthma. Am Rev Respir Dis 1990;142:434–57.

308. Barnes PJ. Cytokines as mediators of chronic asthma. Am J Respir Crit Care Med 1994;150:S42–9.

309. Gauvreau GM, Ronnen GM, Watson RM, et al. Exercise-induced bronchoconstriction does not cause eosinophilic airway inflammation or airway hyperresponsiveness in subjects with asthma. Am J Respir Crit Care Med 2000;162:1302–7.

310. Van Arsdel PP. Aspirin idiosyncrasy and tolerance. J Allergy Clin Immunol 1984;73:431–4.

311. Ameisen JC, Capron A, Joseph M, et al. Aspirin-sensitive asthma: abnormal platelet response to drugs inducing asthmatic attacks; diagnostic and physiopathological implications. Int Arch Allergy Appl Immunol 1985;78:438–48.

312. Lee TH. Mechanism of aspirin sensitivity. Am Rev Respir Dis 1992;145:S34–6.

313. Marks GB, Colquhoun JR, Girgis ST, et al. Thunderstorm outflows preceding epidemics of asthma during spring and summer. Thorax 2001;56:468–71.

314. Dales RE, Cakmak S, Judek S, et al. The role of fungal spores in thunderstorm asthma. Chest 2003;123:745–50.

315. Grundstein A, Sarnat SE, Klein M, et al. Thunderstorm associated asthma in Atlanta, Georgia. Thorax 2008;63:659–60.

316. Picado C. Barcelona's asthma epidemics: clinical aspects and intriguing findings. Thorax 1992;47:197–200.

317. Barbee RA, Kaltenhorn W, Lebowitz MD, et al. Longitudinal changes in allergen skin test reactivity in a community population sample. J Allergy Clin Immunol 1987;79:16–24.

318. Burrows B, Martinez FD, Halonen M, et al. Association of asthma with serum IgE levels and skin-test reactivity to allergens. N Engl J Med 1989;320:271–7.

319. Wagenaar SS, Peters A, Westermann CJJ, et al. IgE bound to mast cells in bronchial mucosa and skin in atopic subjects. Respiration 1981;41:258–63.

320. Carroll NG, Mutavdzic S, James AL. Distribution and degranulation of airway mast cells in normal and asthmatic subjects. Eur Resp J 2002;19:879–85.

321. Guerzon GM, Pare PD, Michoud M-C, et al. The number and distribution of mast cells in monkey lungs. Am Rev Respir Dis 1979;119:59–66.

322. Flint KC, Leung KBP, Hudspith BN, et al. Bronchoalveolar mast cells in extrinsic asthma: a mechanism for the initiation of antigen specific bronchoconstriction. BMJ 1985;291:923–6.

323. Heard BE. Histochemical aspects of the staining of mast cells with particular reference to heterogeneity and quantification. In: Kay AB, editor. Asthma Clinical pharmacology and therapeutic progress. Oxford: Blackwell; 1986. p. 286–94.

324. Heard BE, Dewar A, Nunn AJ, et al. Heterogeneous ultrastructure of human bronchial mast cells: morphometric subdivision of cell types and evidence for a degranulation gradient. Am J Respir Cell Mol Biol 1990;3:71–8.

325. Lane SJ, Lee TH. Mast cell effector mechanisms. J Allergy Clin Immunol 1996;98:S67–71.

326. Conroy DM, Williams TJ. Eotaxin and the attraction of eosinophils to the asthmatic lung. Respir Res 2001;2:150–6.

327. Mukae H, Kadota J, Kohno S, et al. Increase of activated T-cells in BAL fluid of Japanese patients with bronchiolitis obliterans organizing pneumonia and chronic eosinophilic pneumonia. Chest 1995;108:123–8.

328. Kita H, Sur S, Hunt LW, et al. Cytokine production at the site of disease in chronic eosinophilic pneumonitis. Am J Respir Crit Care Med 1996;153:1437–41.

329. Gleich GJ, Frigas E, Loegering DA, et al. Cytotoxic properties of the eosinophil major basic protein. J Immunol 1979;123:2925–7.

330. Frigas SE, Loegering DA, Gleich GJ. Cytotoxic effects of the guinea pig eosinophil major basic protein on tracheal epithelium. Lab Invest 1980;42:35–43.

331. Peters MS, Rodriguez M, Gleich GJ. Localization of human eosinophil granule major basic protein, eosinophil cationic protein, and eosinophil-derived neurotoxin by immunoelectron microscopy. Lab Invest 1986;54:656–62.

332. Filley WV, Kephart GM, Holley KE, et al. Identification by immunofluorescence of eosinophil granule major basic protein in lung tissues of patients with bronchial asthma. Lancet 1982;2:11–5.

333. Corrigan CJ, Hartnell A, Kay AB. T-lymphocyte activation in acute severe asthma. Lancet 1988;i:1129–32.

334. Wilson JW, Djukanovic R, Howarth PH, et al. Lymphocyte activation in bronchoalveolar lavage and peripheral blood in atopic asthma. Am Rev Respir Dis 1992;145:958–60.

335. Ollerenshaw SL, Woolcock AJ. Characteristics of the inflammation in biopsies from large airways of subjects with asthma and subjects with chronic airflow limitation. Am Rev Respir Dis 1992;145:922–7.

336. Poston RN, Chanez P, Lacoste JY, et al. Immunohistochemical characterization of the cellular infiltration in asthmatic bronchi. Am Rev Respir Dis 1992;145:918–21.

337. Bradley BL, Azzawi M, Jacobson M, et al. Eosinophils, T-lymphocytes, mast cells, neutrophils, and macrophages in bronchial biopsy specimens from atopic subjects with asthma: comparison with biopsy specimens from atopic subjects without asthma and normal control subjects and relationship to bronchial hyperresponsiveness. J Allergy Clin Immunol 1991;88:661–74.

338. Bellini A, Vittori E, Marini M, et al. Intraepithelial dendritic cells and selective activation of Th2-like lymphocytes in patients with atopic asthma. Chest 1993;103:997–1005.

339. Robinson DS, Hamid Q, Ying S, et al. Predominant Th2-type bronchoalveolar lavage T lymphocyte population in atopic asthma. N Engl J Med 1992;326:298–304.

340. Robinson DS, Durham SR, Kay AB. Cytokines in asthma. Thorax 1993;48:845–53.

341. Hamid Q, Azzawi M, Ying S, et al. Expression of mRNA for interleukin-5 in

mucosal bronchial biopsies from asthma. J Clin Invest 1991;87:1541–6.

342. Hamid Q, Azzawi M, Ying S, et al. Interleukin 5 mRNA in mucosal biopsies from asthmatic subjects. Int Arch Allergy Appl Immunol 1991;94:169–70.

343. Ying S, Durham SR, Corrigan CJ, et al. Phenotype of cells expressing mRNA for TH2-type (interleukin 4 and interleukin 5) and TH1-type (interleukin 2 and interferon gamma) cytokines in bronchoalveolar lavage and bronchial biopsies from atopic asthmatic and normal control subjects. Am J Respir Cell Mol Biol 1995;12:477–87.

344. Renauld JC. New insights into the role of cytokines in asthma. J Clin Pathol 2001;54:577–89.

345. Kips JC. Cytokines in asthma. Eur Resp J 2001;18:24S–33S.

346. Holt PG, Schon-Hegrad MA, Phillips MJ, et al. Ia-positive dendritic cells form a tightly meshed network within the human airway epithelium. Clin Exp Allergy 1989;19:597–601.

347. Holt PG, Schon-Hegrad MA, Oliver J, et al. A contiguous network of dendritic antigen-presenting cells within the respiratory epithelium. Int Arch Allergy Appl Immunol 1990;91:155–9.

348. Holt PG. Regulation of antigen-presenting cell function(s) in lung and airway tissues. Eur Respir J 1993;6:120–9.

349. Springall DR, Howarth PH, Counihan H, et al. Endothelin immunoreactivity of airway epithelium in asthmatic patients. Lancet 1991;337:697–701.

350. Bardin PG, van Heerden BB, Joubert JR. Absence of pulmonary aspiration of sinus contents in patients with asthma and sinusitis. J Allergy Clin Immunol 1990;86:82–8.

351. Wallaert B, Janin A, Lassalle P, et al. Airway-like inflammation of minor salivary gland in bronchial asthma. Am J Respir Crit Care Med 1994;150:802–9.

352. Ayres JG, Miles JF. Oesophageal reflux and asthma. Eur Respir J 1996;9:1073–8.

353. Field SK, Sutherland LR. Does medical antireflux therapy improve asthma in asthmatics with gastroesophageal reflux? A critical review of the literature. Chest 1998;114:275–83.

354. Wu DN, Tanifuji Y, Kobayashi H, et al. Effects of esophageal acid perfusion on airway hyperresponsiveness in patients with bronchial asthma. Chest 2000;118:1553–6.

355. Harding SM, Guzzo MR, Richter JE. The prevalence of gastroesophageal reflux in asthma patients without reflux symptoms. Am J Respir Crit Care Med 2000;162:34–9.

356. Corris PA, Dark JH. Aetiology of asthma – lessons from lung transplantation. Lancet 1993;341:1369–71.

357. Katzenstein A, Sale SR, Greenberger PA. Allergic aspergillus sinusitis: a newly recognised form of sinusitis. J Allergy Clin Immunol 1983;72:89–93.

358. Berry M, Morgan A, Shaw DE, et al. Pathological features and inhaled corticosteroid response of eosinophilic and non-eosinophilic asthma. Thorax 2007;62:1043–9.

359. Camus P, Bonniaud P, Fanton A, et al. Drug-induced and iatrogenic infiltrative lung disease. Clin Chest Med 2004;25:479–519, vi.

360. Newman-Taylor AJ. Respiratory irritants encountered at work. Thorax 1996;51:541–5.

361. Brightling CE, Ward R, Goh KL, et al. Eosinophilic bronchitis is an important cause of chronic cough. Am J Respir Crit Care Med 1999;160:406–10.

362. Brightling CE, Symon FA, Birring SS, et al. Comparison of airway immunopathology of eosinophilic bronchitis and asthma. Thorax 2003;58:528–32.

363. Brightling CE, Bradding P, Symon FA, et al. Mast-cell infiltration of airway smooth muscle in asthma. N Engl J Med 2002;346:1699–705.

364. Birring SS, Berry M, Brightling CE, et al. Eosinophilic bronchitis: clinical features, management and pathogenesis. Am J Respir Med 2003;2:169–73.

365. Quirce S. Eosinophilic bronchitis in the workplace. Curr Opin Allergy Clin Immunol 2004;4:87–91.

Bronchiectasis

366. Whitwell F. A study of the pathology and pathogenesis of bronchiectasis. Thorax 1952;7:213–39.

367. Boyton RJ, Smith J, Ward R, et al. HLA-C and killer cell immunoglobulin-like receptor genes in idiopathic bronchiectasis. Am J Respir Crit Care Med 2006;173:327–33.

368. Pasteur MC, Helliwell SM, Houghton S, et al. An investigation into causative factors in patients with bronchiectasis. Am J Respir Crit Care Med 2000;162:1277–84.

369. Eastham KM, Fall AJ, Mitchell L, et al. The need to redefine non-cystic fibrosis bronchiectasis in childhood. Thorax 2004;59:324–7.

370. Shoemark A, Ozerovitch L, Wilson R. Aetiology in adult patients with bronchiectasis. Respir Med 2007;101:1163–70.

371. Williams H, O'Reilly RN. Bronchiectasis in children: its multiple clinical and pathological aspects. Arch Dis Child 1959;34:192–201.

372. Williams H, Campbell P. Generalized bronchiectasis associated with deficiency of cartilage in the bronchial tree. Arch Dis Child 1960;35:182–91.

373. Butland RJA, Cole P, Citron KM, et al. Chronic bronchial suppuration and inflammatory bowel disease. Q J Med 1981;50:63–75.

374. Moles KW, Varghese G, Hayes JR. Pulmonary involvement in ulcerative colitis. Br J Dis Chest 1988;82:79–83.

375. Takanami I, Imamuma T, Yamamoto Y, et al. Bronchiectasis complicating rheumatoid arthritis. Respir Med 1995;89:453–4.

376. Cleveland RH, Khaw KT, Mark EJ, et al. An eight-year-old boy with bronchiectasis – Aspiration of a foreign body (plastic fastener) into the right lung, with bronchiectasis and pulmonary atelectasis and fibrosis. N Engl J Med 1998;339:1144–51.

377. Cohen M, Sahn SA. Bronchiectasis in systemic diseases. Chest 1999;116:1063–74.

378. Rodriguez-Cintron W, Guntupalli K, Fraire AE. Bronchiectasis and homozygous (piZZ) α_1-antitrypsin deficiency in a young man. Thorax 1995;50:424–5.

379. Tsang KWT, Rutman A, Kanthakumar K, et al. Interaction of *Pseudomonas aeruginosa* with human respiratory mucosa in vitro. Eur Respir J 1994;7:1746–53.

380. Reid LM. Reduction in bronchial subdivision in bronchiectasis. Thorax 1950;5:233–47.

381. Liebow AA, Hales MR, Lindskog GE. Enlargement of the bronchial arteries, and their anastomoses with the pulmonary arteries in bronchiectasis. Am J Pathol 1949;25:211–31.

382. Cole PJ. A new look at the pathogenesis and management of persistent bronchial sepsis: a 'vicious circle' hypothesis and its logical therapeutic consequences. In: Davies RJ, editor. Strategies for the Management of Chronic Bronchial Sepsis. Oxford: Medicine Publishing Foundation; 1984. p. 1–20.

383. Cole P, Wilson R. Host–microbial interrelationships in respiratory infection. Chest 1989;95:217S–21S.

384. Adler KB, Hendley DD, Davis GS. Bacteria associated with obstructive pulmonary disease elaborate extracellular products that stimulate mucus secretion by explants of guinea pig airways. Am J Pathol 1986;125:501–14.

385. Hilton AM, Hasleton PS, Bradlow A, et al. Cutaneous vasculitis and immune complexes in severe bronchiectasis. Thorax 1984;39:185–91.

386. Tanaka E, Tada K, Amitani R, et al. Systemic hypersensitivity vasculitis associated with bronchiectasis. Chest 1992;102:647–9.

387. Loebinger MR, Wells AU, Hansell DM, et al. Mortality in bronchiectasis: a long-term study assessing the factors influencing survival. Eur Respir J 2009;34:843–9.

Broncholithiasis

388. Pritzker KPH, Desai SD, Patterson MC, et al. Calcite sputum lith. Characterization by analytic scanning electron microscopy and X-ray diffraction. Am J Clin Pathol 1981;75:253–7.

389. Nollet AS, Vansteenkiste JF, Demedts MG. Broncholithiasis: rare but still present. Resp Med 1998;92:963–5.

390. Studer SM, Heitmiller RF, Terry PB. Mediastinal abscess due to passage of a broncholith. Chest 2002;121:296–7.

Chronic bronchiolitis

391. Colby TV. Bronchiolitis: Pathologic considerations. Am J Clin Pathol 1998;109:101–9.

392. Ryu JH, Myers J, Swenson SJ. Bronchiolar disorders. Am J Resp Crit Care Med 2003;168:1277–92.

393. Rice A, Nicholson AG. The pathologist's approach to small airways disease. Histopathology 2009;54:117–33.

394. Reid L, Simon G. Unilateral lung transradiancy. Thorax 1962;17:230–9.

395. Reid L, Simon G, Zorab PA, Seidelin R. The development of unilateral hypertransradiancy of the lung. Br J Dis Chest 1967;61:190–2.

396. Stokes D, Sigler A, Khouri NF, Talmo RC. Unilateral hyperlucent lung (Swyer–James syndrome) after severe *Mycoplasma pneumoniae* infection. Am Rev Respir Dis 1978;117:145–52.

397. Avital A, Shulman DL, Bar-Yishay E, et al. Differential lung function in an infant with the Swyer–James syndrome. Thorax 1989;44:298–302.

398. Fukuoka J, Franks TJ, Colby TV, et al. Peribronchiolar metaplasia: a common histologic lesion in diffuse lung disease and a rare cause of interstitial lung disease: clinicopathologic features of 15 cases. Am J Surg Pathol 2005;29:948–54.

399. Guarino M, Tosoni A, Nebuloni M. Direct contribution of epithelium to organ fibrosis: epithelial–mesenchymal transition. Human Pathology 2009;40:1365–76.

400. Borthwick LA, Parker SM, Brougham KA, et al. Epithelial to mesenchymal transition (EMT) and airway remodelling after human lung transplantation. Thorax 2009;64:770–7.

401. Gosink BB, Friedman PJ, Liebow AA. Bronchiolitis obliterans. Roentgenologic–pathologic correlation. Am J Roentgenol 1973;117:816–32.

402. Geddes DM, Corrin B, Brewerton DA, et al. Progressive airway obliteration in adults and its association with rheumatoid disease. Q J Med 1977;46:427–44.

403. McLean KH. The pathology of acute bronchiolitis – a study of its evolution. Part II: The repair phase. Aust Ann Med 1957;6:29–43.

404. Becroft DMO. Bronchiolitis obliterans, bronchiectasis and other sequelae of adenovirus type 21 infection in young children. J Clin Pathol 1971;24:72–82.

405. Diaz F, Collazos J, Martinez E, et al. Bronchiolitis obliterans in a patient with HIV infection. Respir Med 1997;91:171–3.

406. Ito M, Nakagawa A, Hirabayashi N, et al. Bronchiolitis obliterans in ataxia-telangiectasia. Virchows Arch 1997;430:131–7.

407. Dompeling E, Jobsis Q, Vandevijver NMA, et al. Chronic bronchiolitis in a 5-yr-old child after exposure to sulphur mustard gas. Eur Resp J 2004;23:343–6.

408. Churg A, Wright JL. Small-airway lesions in patients exposed to nonasbestos mineral dusts. Hum Pathol 1983;14:688–93.

409. Churg A, Wright JL. Small airways disease and mineral dust exposure. Pathol Annu 1983;18:233–51.

410. Churg A, Wright JL, Wiggs B, et al. Small airways disease and mineral dust exposure. Prevalence, structure and function. Am Rev Respir Dis 1985;131:139–43.

411. Wright JL, Churg A. Morphology of small-airway lesions in patients with asbestos exposure. Hum Pathol 1984;15:68–74.

412. Devouassoux G, Cottin V, Liote H, et al. Characterisation of severe obliterative bronchiolitis in rheumatoid arthritis. Eur Respir J 2009;33:1053–61.

413. Hakala M, Paakko P, Sutinen S, et al. Association of bronchiolitis with connective tissue disorders. Ann Rheum Dis 1986;45:656–62.

414. Hasegawa Y, Shimokata K, Ichiyama S, et al. Constrictive bronchiolitis obliterans and paraneoplastic pemphigus. Eur Resp J 1999;13:934–7.

415. Turton CW, Williams G, Green M. Cryptogenic obliterative bronchiolitis in adults. Thorax 1981;36:805–10.

416. Kraft M, Mortenson RL, Colby TV, et al. Cryptogenic constrictive bronchiolitis. A clinicopathologic study. Am Rev Respir Dis 1993;148:1093–101.

417. Murphy DMF, Fairman RP, Lapp NL, et al. Severe airway disease due to inhalation of fumes from cleansing agents. Chest 1976;69:372–6.

418. Wilcox P, Miller R, Miller G, et al. Airway involvement in ulcerative colitis. Chest 1987;92:18–21.

419. Rickli H, Fretz C, Hoffman M, et al. Severe inflammatory upper airway stenosis in ulcerative colitis. Eur Respir J 1994;7:1899–902.

420. Abernathy EC, Hruban RH, Baumgartner WA, et al. The two forms of bronchiolitis obliterans in heart–lung transplant recipients. Hum Pathol 1991;22:1102–10.

421. Sato M, Keshavjee S. Bronchiolitis obliterans syndrome: alloimmune-dependent and -independent injury with aberrant tissue remodeling. Semin Thorac Cardiovasc Surg 2008;20:173–82.

Diffuse panbronchiolitis

422. Homma H, Yamanaka A, Tanimoto S, et al. Diffuse panbronchiolitis. A disease of the transitional zone of the lung. Chest 1983;83:63–9.

423. Maeda M, Saiki S, Yamanaka A. Serial section analysis of the lesions in diffuse panbronchiolitis. Acta Pathol Jpn 1987;37:693–704.

424. Izumi T. Diffuse panbronchiolitis. Chest 1991;100:596–7.

425. Kitaichi M, Nishimura K, Izumi T. Diffuse panbronchiolitis. In: Sharma OP, editor. Lung Disease in the Tropics. New York: Marcel Dekker; 1991. p. 479–509.

426. Yaegashi H, Takahashi T. The site, severity, and distribution of bronchiolar obstruction in lungs with chronic obstructive pulmonary disease – morphometry and computer-assisted three-dimensional reconstruction of airways. Arch Pathol Lab Med 1994;118:975–83.

427. Poletti V, Patelli M, Poletti G, et al. Diffuse panbronchiolitis observed in an Italian. Chest 1990;98:515–6.

428. Randhawa P, Hoagland MH, Yousem SA. Diffuse panbronchiolitis in North-America – report of three cases and review of the literature. Am J Surg Pathol 1991;15:43–7.

429. Fitzgerald JE, King TE, Lynch DA, et al. Diffuse panbronchiolitis in the United States. Am J Respir Crit Care Med 1996;154:497–503.

430. Fisher MS, Rush WL, Rosado-de-Christenson ML, et al. Diffuse panbronchiolitis: Histologic diagnosis in unsuspected cases involving North American residents of Asian descent. Arch Pathol Lab Med 1998;122:156–60.

431. Sugiyama Y, Kudoh S, Maeda H, et al. Analysis of HLA antigens in patients with diffuse panbronchiolitis. Am Rev Respir Dis 1990;141:1459–62.

432. Park MH, Kim YW, Il Yoon H, et al. Association of HLA class I antigens with diffuse panbronchiolitis in Korean patients. Am J Respir Crit Care Med 1999;159:526–9.

433. Homer RJ, Khoo L, Smith GJW. Diffuse panbronchiolitis in a hispanic man with travel history to Japan. Chest 1995;107:1176–8.

434. Sato A, Chida K, Iwata M, et al. Study of bronchus-associated lymphoid tissue in patients with diffuse panbronchiolitis. Am Rev Respir Dis 1992;146:473–8.

435. Homma S, Sakamoto S, Kawabata M, et al. Comparative clinicopathology of obliterative bronchiolitis and diffuse panbronchiolitis. Respiration 2006;73:481–7.

436. Iwata M, Colby TV, Kitaichi M. Diffuse panbronchiolitis: diagnosis and distinction from various pulmonary diseases with centrilobular interstitial foam cell accumulations. Hum Pathol 1994;25:357–63.

437. Ichikawa Y, Hotta M, Sumita S, et al. Reversible airway lesions in diffuse panbronchiolitis: detection by high-resolution computed tomography. Chest 1995;107:120–5.

438. Koyama H, Geddes DM. Erythromycin and diffuse panbronchiolitis. Thorax 1997;52:915–18.

Chapter 4

Acute alveolar injury and repair

CHAPTER CONTENTS

ACUTE REPIRATORY DISTRESS SYNDROME

Acute alveolar injury may be caused by a wide range of pulmonary insults that at their most severe result in what is termed the acute respiratory distress syndrome (ARDS). This was formerly known as the adult respiratory distress syndrome,[1–3] a term introduced to emphasise its similarity to that seen in premature babies suffering from the effects of deficient pulmonary surfactant production, i.e. the infantile respiratory distress syndrome (see p. 43), but following the recognition that the causes of the adult respiratory distress syndrome may also operate in children, 'adult' has given way to 'acute'. The causes of the syndrome differ markedly in infants and adults but whatever the cause, a common cycle of events is initiated (Fig. 4.1) so that the end-result is the same regardless of the cause. It is a common condition, which carries a high mortality, about 50% overall. Estimations of incidence show considerable international variability but one American study reported it to be 79 per 100 000 population.[4]

ARDS is a fulminant form of respiratory failure characterised by refractory hypoxaemia ($P_aO_2/FIO_2 < 200$) and bilateral radiographic opacification in the absence of any evidence of an elevated left atrial pressure.[5] These features indicate widespread alveolar collapse and exudation that cannot be attributed to left heart failure or other cause of pulmonary venous hypertension. There is generalised ground-glass opacification of the lungs, which is most pronounced in the dependent parts of the lungs. The opacification rapidly becomes increasingly dense until there is frank consolidation (Fig. 4.2).[6] Air is then confined to the bronchi, which therefore appear black on plain radiographs where they stand out against the alveolar 'white-out' (so-called air bronchograms).[7]

Functional studies confirm that little of the lung substance is ventilated. There is initially mild pulmonary hypertension but the pulmonary arterial constriction responsible for this is succeeded by vascular non-responsiveness so that the normal vasoconstrictor response to hypoxia is diminished. The consequent ventilation/perfusion mismatching aggravates the hypoxaemia. Other organs suffer both hypoxia and the effects of inflammatory mediators initiated by the pulmonary injury once these gain access to the general circulation. The end stages of ARDS are therefore frequently associated with multiple organ failure.[8]

Despite the variety of causes, most patients with ARDS show the same pattern of pathological changes, one that is termed diffuse alveolar damage (DAD). Much of this chapter is devoted to this pattern of injury but occasionally patients presenting with ARDS show other changes when subjected to biopsy or coming to autopsy. These are listed in Box 4.1 and are considered in other chapters but their chief pathological features are compared with those of DAD in Table 4.1. Recognition of these other patterns may lead to a change in the patient's management. In that they include infection it is essential that some of the specimen goes to the microbiology department. Lung biopsy is also undertaken to assess the reversibility of the changes.[9,10] The process is potentially reversible in its exudative phase whereas widespread fibrosis with loss of the lung architecture is not.

©2010 Elsevier Ltd
DOI: 10.1016/B978-0-7020-3369-8.00004-5

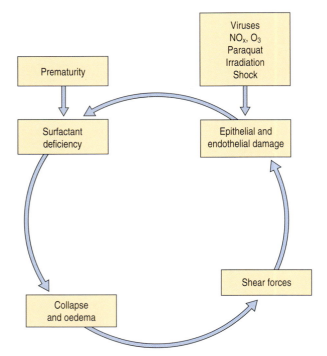

Figure 4.1 The cycle of events in the infantile and acute (formerly adult) respiratory distress syndromes. The infantile syndrome is initiated by the immature fetal lungs being unable to replenish spent surfactant whereas in the acute syndrome the cycle is initiated by a variety of causes that damage the delicate alveolar epithelium.

Figure 4.2 Acute respiratory distress syndrome. High-resolution computed tomography shows dense consolidation of both lungs, especially the dependent regions.

DIFFUSE ALVEOLAR DAMAGE

DAD represents a non-specific pattern of acute alveolar injury caused by a variety of noxious agents.[11–14] It is the chief pathological basis of ARDS. The pathological changes of DAD can be divided into the overlapping phases of exudation, regeneration and repair.[15]

Exudative phase

To facilitate gas exchange the alveolar wall is highly specialised in structure. Unfortunately this specialisation renders it susceptible to injury by a wide variety of agents. The principal cells of the air–blood barrier, the type I alveolar epithelial cell and the capillary endothelial cell are exceptionally thin (see Fig. 1.27, p. 16) and this makes them particularly vulnerable to non-specific damage. Injury to these two cells underlies the development of DAD. At an early stage of alveolar injury the type I epithelial cells show cytoplasmic blebbing, which is soon followed by necrosis resulting in denudation of the basement membrane (see Fig. 7.2.5, p. 376).[16,17] Similar blebbing is seen in the alveolar capillary endothelium but denudation of the endothelial basement membrane is seldom observed, probably because of differences in the ways epithelial and endothelial cells regenerate (see below). The consequences of this damage include the escape of fibrin-rich exudates into the interstitial and air spaces, loss of the surface-active alveolar lining film and pulmonary collapse.

The exudative phase lasts about 1 week, during which the lungs are heavy, often weighing over 1 kg each, dark and airless. The changes are often patchy, with the dorsal and basal regions being most severely affected (Fig. 4.3).[18–20] Slicing shows that they are wet, the cut surface exuding blood or heavily blood-stained watery fluid. Microscopically

Box 4.1 **The pathological basis of the acute respiratory distress syndrome**

1. Diffuse alveolar damage (the typical pattern, considered in this chapter)
2. Other causes (considered elsewhere):
   - Pulmonary oedema due to high-altitude, rapid lung re-expansion or cerebral injury
   - Unusual manifestations of bacterial pneumonia, e.g. streptococcal pneumonia, leptospiral pneumonia
   - Acute fibrinous organising pneumonia
   - Capillaritis/diffuse alveolar haemorrhage
   - Acute eosinophilic pneumonia
   - Unusual forms of malignant disease that affect the lungs diffusely, e.g. adenocarcinoma, intravascular lymphoma, 'lymphangitis carcinomatosis'

there is widespread collapse, intense congestion of the capillaries, interstitial oedema and distension of the lymphatics, a pattern that is sometimes known as congestive atelectasis (Fig. 4.4). Alternatively, there may be haemorrhagic oedema (Fig. 4.5). At the air–tissue interface, which in these collapsed lungs is at the respiratory bronchiole or alveolar duct level, respiratory movements compact a fibrin-rich exudate mixed with necrotic epithelial debris into a thin layer that covers an otherwise denuded epithelial basement membrane (Fig. 4.6), leading to the formation of hyaline membranes (Fig. 4.7)[11–13,21,22]: these are identical to those that paediatric pathologists recognise as the hallmark of the infantile respiratory distress syndrome (compare Fig. 4.3 with Fig. 2.8, p. 44). Similar changes are also seen in acute eosinophilic pneumonia but here the hyaline membranes contain eosinophils, possibly in small focal collections that are easily overlooked (see p. 462).

The congested alveolar capillaries sometimes contain increased numbers of platelets or neutrophil leukocytes. This selective sequestration of formed blood elements in the microvasculature of the lungs

Table 4.1 Histological patterns associated with the acute respiratory distress syndrome

	Diffuse alveolar damage	Acute eosinophilic pneumonia	Acute fibrinous organising pneumonia	Capillaritis/diffuse alveolar haemorrhage
Hyaline membranes	++	+	−	+/−
Eosinophils	−	+	−	−
Fibrin knots	+/−	+/−	++	+/−
Type II cell hyperplasia	++	+/−	+/−	−
Interstitial fibrosis	+	+/−	+/−	−
Capillaritis/haemorrhage	−	−	−	++

Figure 4.3 Shock lung. The lower lobe shows large irregular areas of collapse and congestion. *(Reproduced from Corrin (1980)[18] by permission of the editor of the* Journal of Clinical Pathology.*)*

Figure 4.4 Congestive atelectasis in septic shock. There is severe capillary congestion and alveolar collapse.

Figure 4.5 Haemorrhagic pulmonary oedema in septic shock. The alveolar capillaries are congested and the alveolar spaces are filled by oedema fluid in which there are free erythrocytes.

is particularly noticeable in shock, and is considered in more detail under that heading below.

Regenerative phase

As with any exudative process, healing may be by resolution, which involves fibrinolysis and permits the lungs to return to normal, or repair, which involves fibrosis and leaves the lungs permanently scarred. Resolution and repair are both accompanied by epithelial and endothelial regeneration.

The regenerative (or proliferative) phase becomes prominent 1–2 weeks after the initial injury. It involves proliferation of both epithelial and connective tissue cells. The stem cell concerned in epithelial regeneration is the type II alveolar epithelial cell.[23,24] These cells first proliferate and then differentiate into type I cells, thereby re-epithelialising the denuded basement membranes. The dividing

Figure 4.6 Diffuse alveolar damage. The alveolar epithelium terminates just above centre and from this point (arrow) upwards a mixture of electron-dense fibrin and cell debris (seen at the light microscopic level as a hyaline membrane) is closely applied to the denuded basement membrane. Part of a necrotic cell is seen within the alveolus. Transmission electron micrograph. *(Courtesy of Miss A Dewar, Brompton, UK.)*

Figure 4.7 Diffuse alveolar damage, exudative phase. Hyaline membranes are a conspicuous feature. They often outline alveolar ducts. From a pregnant woman who suffered respiratory arrest due to angioneurotic oedema. She needed to be ventilated for 2 weeks before death and the oxygen concentration in the inspired air constantly increased to prevent hypoxaemia, reaching 70% for the last 8 days of her life. *(Courtesy of Dr D Melcher, Brighton, UK.)*

effete endothelial cell is first undermined by its healthy neighbours and only cast off when these have completely covered the basement membrane.[31] Therefore, although segments of bare basement membrane have been described on the vascular side of the air–blood barrier,[32,33] they are not seen to the same extent as on the epithelial side. Nevertheless, thrombosis may complicate such endothelial damage[21,32] and subsequent organisation of such thrombi is probably responsible for some of the vascular remodelling that is seen in the repair phase of DAD. This remodelling consists of fibrocellular intimal thickening that narrows the lumen of small vessels throughout the lung and can be visualised as decreased background filling on postmortem arteriograms.[34]

Repair phase

If healing is by repair, interstitial connective tissue cells proliferate and, as in any scarring, myofibroblasts are involved at an early stage.[35] Whilst myofibroblast contracture is beneficial when it promotes early closure of an open wound, in the lungs it largely results in harmful distortion of the bronchioloalveolar architecture and shrinkage of the lungs. Possible sources of the proliferating interstitial connective tissues include resting interstitial connective tissue cells, the bone marrow and the alveolar epithelium. Epithelial–mesenchymal transition is being increasingly recognised throughout the body and in the lung in conditions such as idiopathic pulmonary fibrosis, asthma and obliterative bronchiolitis.[36–38]

Whatever the source of the proliferating connective tissue cells, those with a fibroblastic phenotype lay down collagen, leading to the development of interstitial fibrosis.[39,40] Interactions between fibroblasts and the alveolar epithelium through gaps in the basement membrane have been described,[41–45] suggesting that the regenerating epithelial cells play a further role in the underlying process of fibrosis. It is known that these cells synthesise fibrogenic cytokines such as tumour necrosis factor-α; the secretion of tumour necrosis factor-α into the underlying connective tissue would further promote interstitial fibrosis.[46,47]

Fibroblasts also migrate into the alveolar exudates through defects in the epithelial basement membrane to lay down collagen within the

type II cells form a simple cuboidal epithelium (Fig. 4.8), or the alveoli may be lined by plump pleomorphic spindle cells that represent cell forms intermediate between types II and I epithelial cells (Figs 4.9 and 4.10). Eosinophilic cytoplasmic inclusions indicative of cell damage (see Fig. 7.1.25, p. 348) are often present,[25,26] and sometimes there is squamous metaplasia instead of orderly differentiation into type I cells, a change that the unwary pathologist may mistake for neoplasia.[27]

The regenerating epithelium usually grows beneath the exudates lining the denuded basement membrane, casting the hyaline membranes off into the air space (Fig. 4.11), but it may grow over them so that they are incorporated into the interstitium (Figs 4.12 and 4.13),[11–13] where their subsequent organisation contributes to the fibrosis.[22] The regenerating epithelial cells may also bridge the mouths of collapsed alveoli so that these air spaces never re-expand and there is permanent shrinkage of the lung, a process termed atelectatic induration (Figs 4.14 and 4.15).[28–30]

In contrast to the type I epithelial cells, which have no regenerative powers and are replaced by differentiation of proliferating type II cells, endothelial cells are replaced by lateral spread of their own kind. An

Figure 4.9 Diffuse alveolar damage, regenerative phase. Regenerating alveolar epithelial cells are atypical, consisting of plump, elongated forms that represent type II pneumocytes differentiating into type I.

Figure 4.8 Diffuse alveolar damage, regenerative phase. (A) The alveoli have a simple cuboidal epithelial lining. *(Courtesy of Dr D Melcher, Brighton, UK.)* (B) Electron microscopy shows that such cells represent hyperplastic type II pneumocytes, which form a continuous row rather than being scattered singly in the corners of the alveoli. They are readily recognisable by their surface microvilli and the osmiophilic lamellar secretory vacuoles of alveolar surfactant. *(Courtesy of Mrs D Bowes, Midhurst, UK.)*

Figure 4.10 Diffuse alveolar damage, regenerative phase. An alveolar epithelial cell having the squamous form of a type I cell but the microvilli and lamellar vacuoles of a type II cell. Such intermediate cells are indicative of epithelial regeneration.

Figure 4.11 Diffuse alveolar damage, regenerative phase. The regenerating alveolar epithelium grows underneath the hyaline membranes, casting them off into the air space.

Figure 4.13 Diffuse alveolar damage, repair phase. Hyaline membranes, which are stained red, are in the process of being incorporated into the alveolar interstitium. Martius scarlet blue stain.

Figure 4.12 Diffuse alveolar damage, regenerative phase. The regenerating alveolar epithelium may also grow over the hyaline membranes to incorporate them into the alveolar wall. In this electron micrograph the hyaline membranes are largely represented by electron-dense fibrin which is closely applied to previously denuded alveolar epithelial basement membrane and are in turn covered by regenerating epithelium laying down a new basement membrane. *(Courtesy of Miss A Dewar, Brompton, UK.)*

hyaline membranes.[48,49] As epithelial cells grow over the newly formed connective tissue, a new basement membrane is formed, thereby incorporating the collagen into the interstitium,[49] a process known as fibrosis by accretion. Involvement of the alveolar ducts results in these structures being lined by a ring of granulation tissue (Fig. 4.16). Less frequently, the organised exudates retain a predominantly intra-alveolar position, resulting in loose buds of granulation tissue similar to those seen in organising pneumonia due to other causes (see Box 6.2.1, p. 309). However, here they are more widespread and there is more prominent type II cell hyperplasia, interstitial fibroblastic proliferation and interstitial inflammation (Fig. 4.17). Nevertheless, such an organising pneumonia pattern is worth recognising as it carries a better prognosis than interstitial fibrosis.[50] It is claimed that this intra-alveolar pattern of repair is particularly found when generalised sepsis is the cause of the initial damage whereas interstitial fibrosis is more characteristic of injury caused by cytotoxic drugs and the idiopathic cases.[51]

An increase in lung collagen can be detected in patients with ARDS who survive longer than 14 days and this progressively increases with the duration of the disease.[52] The identification of pulmonary fibrosis on transbronchial biopsy is closely related to mortality.[53] Fibrosis can

Figure 4.14 Atelectatic induration. Denuded alveolar epithelial basement membranes are closely apposed (centre). The regenerating alveolar epithelium (top) bridges the mouth of the alveolus, which consequently has little chance of ever re-expanding. *(Courtesy of Miss A Dewar, Brompton, UK.)*

Figure 4.15 Atelectatic induration. Silver staining of the basement membranes shows that what appear to be thickened single alveolar walls represent the closely apposed walls of several collapsed alveoli.

Figure 4.16 'Ring' fibrosis, representing the organisation and incorporation of exudates lining the alveolar ducts into the walls of these airways.

be well established by 2 weeks, at which time the lungs may be contracted and firm with a fine sponge-like pattern on their cut surfaces, representing bronchiolectasis and irregular microcystic distortion of the alveolar architecture (Figs 4.18 and 4.19).[54–57] The changes are similar to those seen in any fibrotic process but are reached remarkably quickly (see Fig. 4.19).[22] However, at this early stage the fibrosis differs from that seen in chronic fibrosis in being more cellular and less collagenous: extensive fibroblast proliferation is evident. With small air cysts alternating with solid areas of fibrosis and foci of squamous metaplasia there is a resemblance to the bronchopulmonary dysplasia seen in the late stages of the infantile respiratory distress syndrome.[55,56] In survivors the granulation tissue undergoes progressive collagenisation and such patients may suffer from debilitating fibrotic lung disease. The pattern is then that of fibrotic non-specific interstitial pneumonia,[58] making it important to determine whether there has been an episode of acute lung injury in such patients.

Causes

The causes of DAD are quite diverse (Box 4.2). So too are the pathways by which the injurious agents reach the lungs. Some enter the lungs directly via the airways, e.g. oxygen in high concentrations, poisonous gases such as phosgene and metallic fumes such as those of mercury and cadmium. Other agents responsible for DAD penetrate the chest wall to damage the lungs (e.g. ionising radiation) and some reach the lungs via the blood stream, having been ingested or injected (e.g. paraquat and cytotoxic chemotherapeutic agents). The blood stream also conveys many of the endogenous factors that underlie the DAD of shock. In numerical terms, septic shock is the most important cause of DAD.[59,60]

Multiple causes may operate in one patient. For example, trauma may be combined with blood loss, fat embolism and sepsis, whilst therapeutic efforts to correct these may themselves be hazardous. The transfusion of stored blood is not without danger, whilst to prevent hypoxaemia, damaged lungs that require rest often have to be forcibly ventilated and subjected to injurious concentrations of oxygen, although it is known that this can only aggravate the injury to the lungs.[22] The damaged lung also appears to be unduly susceptible to infection,[61] partly because of impaired neutrophil migration into the

Figure 4.18 Diffuse alveolar damage, repair phase. The repair process has resulted in interstitial fibrosis.

Figure 4.17 Diffuse alveolar damage, repair phase. (A) A lower lobe seen at autopsy shows diffuse consolidation, with occasional lobules showing more exudative appearances. (B) Microscopy shows diffuse intra-alveolar organisation with abundant interstitial inflammation.

Figure 4.19 Suicidal ingestion of kerosene resulting in advanced pulmonary fibrosis and honeycombing within 2 weeks of the initial injury.

Shock

Shock is a state of prolonged hypotension, generally attributable to trauma, hypovolaemia, cardiac failure, sepsis or anaphylaxis.[63,64] The hypotension leads to inadequate tissue perfusion and, if this is not corrected, multiorgan failure is inevitable. At necropsy, the lungs are the organs most commonly affected.[65–67]

Severe pulmonary injury was well described in patients suffering from shock in the Second World War[68] but it was not until the war in Vietnam that the importance of respiratory failure as a complication

air spaces.[62] It is therefore common in clinical practice for the lungs to be subjected to several injurious agents and since these all contribute to a non-specific pattern of disease it may be difficult for the pathologist to distinguish the initiating factor from the effects of treatment. Consideration of events in the intensive care unit is essential in these circumstances. Many of the causes of DAD listed in Box 4.2 are dealt with elsewhere, leaving only a few to be considered here.

Box 4.2 **Causes of diffuse alveolar damage**

Via the airways

Infection, especially viral

Inhaled smoke, fume and toxic gases, including oxygen in high concentrations

Aspiration of gastric contents

Through the chest wall

X-irradiation

Via the blood stream

Various mediators generated in shock

Reperfusion of ischaemic tissue

Acute pancreatitis

Cardiopulmonary bypass

Transfusion of stored blood

Fat embolism

Paraquat ingestion

Cytotoxic chemotherapeutic agents

of shock was fully appreciated.[69,70] By this time there had been major improvements in medical care. Casualties could be transported rapidly by helicopter to well-equipped field hospitals where intensive care with mechanical ventilatory support was available. Despite this, injured patients often developed fatal respiratory insufficiency, typically after an interval of between 48 and 72 hours. A number of terms graphically described this syndrome – 'shock lung', 'posttraumatic respiratory insufficiency', 'traumatic wet lung' and 'Da Nang lung'. Pathological examination showed congestive atelectasis or haemorrhagic oedema proceeding to fully developed DAD, as described above.

The pathogenesis of 'shock lung' is complex and requires special consideration. In hypovolaemic and cardiogenic shock, compensatory mechanisms such as peripheral vasoconstriction initially maintain cerebral oxygenation, but if the underlying cause is untreated, there follows a state of decompensation characterised by vascular unresponsiveness: vasodilatation develops, the blood pressure plummets and there is widespread hypoxic cell death. Anaphylactic and septic shock are characterised from the outset by such vasodilatation, which is caused by a variety of mediators that are released from inflammatory and other cells.[71] The identification of the same mediators in experimental hypovolaemia[72] suggests that the pathogenesis of shock may be similar regardless of the cause.

In numerical terms, septic shock is the most important cause of diffuse damage.[59,60] It represents the culmination of a clinicopathological continuum of infection-driven sepsis syndromes:

1. Sepsis – the systemic inflammatory response to infection characterised by normal heart rate, temperature, respiratory rate and white blood cell count
2. Severe sepsis – sepsis, as defined in 1, plus multiorgan dysfunction
3. Septic shock – severe sepsis, as defined in 2, plus refractory hypotension.

These terms have replaced 'septicaemia', which proved difficult to define and has now been abandoned. The multiorgan dysfunction is due to inflammatory cytokines released into the circulation from the site of infection, the common sites of which are, in decreasing frequency, lung, blood, intestine and peritoneum, urinary tract and surgical wounds. Gram-positive infections are slightly commoner than

Gram-negative, which are slightly commoner than polymicrobial. The role of lipopolysaccharide derived from the cell walls of Gram-negative bacteria has been particularly well studied in the pathogenesis of septic shock.[73–77] The many effects of this endotoxin include the release of tumour necrosis factor from monocytes, macrophages and polymorphonuclear leukocytes,[74–76,78,79] the production of cytokines such as interleukin-1 and interferon-γ that act synergistically with tumour necrosis factor,[80] the widespread induction of nitric oxide synthesis[81–83] and the activation of both the coagulation and complement cascades.[84] Exotoxins released by Gram-positive bacteria appear to act similarly. Some of the most fulminant forms of shock are seen with group A streptococci causing puerperal sepsis and necrotising fasciitis, meningococci, *Staphylococcus aureus* related to tampon retention and a meticillin-resistant strain that secretes an exotoxin known as Panton–Valentine leukocidin.[85]

Tumour necrosis factor has been demonstrated on the luminal surface of pulmonary endothelium in endotoxin-induced shock.[86] It causes vascular smooth muscle to relax but this action is reduced if the endothelium is removed,[87] indicating that tumour necrosis factor-induced vasodilatation is partially dependent upon the integrity of the endothelium. A factor that causes vascular dilatation has been detected as coming from the vascular endothelium and acting on the medial muscle coat of the vessel. At first termed endothelium-derived relaxing factor, this factor is now known to be nitric oxide, a remarkably simple chemical that has long been recognised to be poisonous.[88] Fortunately, its half-life in the vessel wall is very short, timed in seconds rather than minutes. The enzyme responsible for its production (from L-arginine) is nitric oxide synthase, which is found in endothelium and can be induced in the vascular medial smooth muscle. Both the constitutive and inducible forms of the enzyme are activated by bacterial lipopolysaccharide and it therefore seems likely that in septic shock bacterial products act directly on the vessel wall resulting in the production of excess amounts of nitric oxide. Even momentarily increased levels of nitric oxide might be expected to cause arterial dilatation and hence capillary congestion. It would appear that in septic shock circulating bacterial products such as lipopolysaccharide cause vascular dilatation and possibly increased permeability by direct action on the blood vessels and indirectly through the induction of nitric oxide synthase and the release of the cytokines mentioned in the preceding paragraph. Pulmonary endothelial upregulation is indicated by widespread expression of intercellular adhesion molecule-1 (ICAM-1: CD54) in septic shock. Indeed, positive immunostaining for CD54 is proving to be a useful marker of shock.[89]

Nitric oxide is a powerful vasodilator but it also mediates many other processes throughout the body. In host defence nitric oxide plays a very different and more aggressive role. It enables macrophages to generate free oxygen radicals, the principal means by which these cells eliminate both bacteria and cancer cells, but which, if not inactivated, also damage healthy host cells.[90] Macrophages release much more nitric oxide than endothelial cells but, as in the blood vessels, the amounts released are generally inactivated within seconds. However, overwhelming bacterial infections result in the release of very large amounts of nitric oxide and the overproduction of toxic oxygen radicals. Although the oxygen radicals are countered by the protective action of enzymes such as superoxide dismutase,[91] their excessive release results in oxidation of lipids and protein sulphydryl groups, and DNA damage.[92] Damaged cell membrane phospholipids release free arachidonic acid which in turn is degraded to produce leukotrienes, such as prostaglandins and thromboxane, that are capable of altering vessel calibre and permeability.

The direct vasodilatory action of nitric oxide and the toxic action of the free oxygen radicals that nitric oxide generates account for most of the pathological features of shock but there are other processes in the microvasculature of the lung that contribute to the pulmonary

Figure 4.20 Shock lung. In shock, the alveolar walls are sometimes hypercellular due to the accumulation of neutrophil polymorphonuclear leukocytes.

Figure 4.21 Shock lung. Electron microscopy shows that the neutrophil leukocytes are sequestered in the alveolar capillaries. *(Courtesy of Professor PK Jeffery, Brompton, UK.)*

damage. The vascular engorgement characteristic of shock lung is occasionally accompanied by sequestration of neutrophil polymorphonuclear leukocytes in the pulmonary microvasculature (Figs 4.20 and 4.21).[18,18,93,94] Acting through the complement cascade,[84,95,96] endotoxin activates these cells within the systemic circulation so that they lose their normal deformability and aggregate into microemboli, with the result that they cannot traverse the alveolar capillaries.[73,97,98] Their arrest there is promoted by activated endothelial intercellular adhesion molecules.[99–103] The unique position of the pulmonary capillaries in the circulation is probably responsible for the lungs being the organs most severely affected in shock.[65–67] Trapped in the alveolar capillaries, activated neutrophils damage the alveolar wall by producing reactive oxygen radicals and releasing enzymes such as elastase, collagenase and cathepsins that are able to degrade protein constituents of the wall.[104–110] Impairment of neutrophil migration into the air spaces has been referred to above.[62]

Patients suffering from ARDS frequently have haematological evidence of disseminated intravascular coagulation[111] and it is then generally possible to demonstrate platelet and fibrin thrombi and increased numbers of megakaryocytes in their alveolar capillaries postmortem (Fig. 4.22).[18,112–116] It is uncertain whether intravascular coagulation initiates lung injury,[73,117,118] but histamine released from platelets is likely to increase vascular permeability whilst fibrin degradation products, which are elevated in patients with the respiratory distress syndrome,[119] are known to induce pulmonary oedema.[120] Larger pulmonary thrombi, formed in situ or embolic, are common in patients with ARDS.[34] Any infarction they cause increases the risk of interstitial emphysema and pneumothorax, forms of barotrauma to which all patients on ventilators are prone.

Figure 4.22 Shock lung. Shock is often accompanied by disseminated intravascular coagulation, consumptive coagulopathy and the release of megakaryocytes from the bone marrow. (A) Platelets fill the alveolar capillaries. (B) Megakaryocytes released from the bone marrow are arrested in the pulmonary capillary bed, from whence they release their platelets. Occasional megakaryocytes may be observed in normal lung but they are more noticeable in shock. They are seen as clumps of basophilic nuclear material within alveolar capillaries (centre). To the right a blood vessel contains a globular hyaline microthrombus.

Infection

In assessing the role of infection in causing DAD it is important to distinguish between primary infection of the lung and infection elsewhere in the body. Septic shock has been dealt with above and attention has been drawn to the increased risk of secondary lung infection when the lungs are already damaged.[62] This section is confined to consideration of some primary pneumonias that can produce DAD.

DAD is characteristic of some viral infections, most recently the severe acute respiratory syndrome (SARS)-related coronavirus (see p. 163). Some patients with viral pneumonia succumb during the acute exudative phase and are found to have prominent hyaline membranes, whilst others suffer less severe damage, allowing regeneration and fibrosis. Indications that the disease is viral include the presence of specific inclusions, such as those seen in cytomegalovirus infection, or of syncytial giant cell formation, most typically seen in measles pneumonia.

Figure 4.23 Aspiration of gastric acid (Mendelson's syndrome). There is haemorrhagic oedema and centrally the extravasated blood is discoloured due to the production of brown acid haematin.

The changes of DAD are not typically seen in bacterial pneumonia, but may occur in fulminating infection with organisms such as *Streptococcus pyogenes*. In pneumonic plague and anthrax pneumonia, the overwhelming alveolar damage leads to intensely haemorrhagic pulmonary oedema similar to that sometimes seen in shock. DAD may also accompany miliary tuberculosis and *Pneumocystis* pneumonia, particularly the non-reactive forms seen in the severely immunocompromised.

Aspiration of gastric contents

Pulmonary aspiration of gastric contents is a frequent event in unconscious or semiconscious patients. If the aspirated material is infected it is likely to cause pneumonia and lung abscess but if sterile and highly acid the consequences are liable to be even more dire. Mendelson reported 66 instances of patients aspirating stomach contents during obstetric anaesthesia. The aspiration of abundant solid material resulted in suffocation but Mendelson was more interested in the larger number of patients who aspirated liquids and developed pulmonary oedema. He suspected that the pH of the aspirate was important and confirmed this in experiments on rabbits.[121] The aspiration of gastric acid is now known as Mendelson's syndrome. The mortality is high,[122,123] reaching 94% in some series.[124]

Ultrastructural studies on experimental animals in which fluids of differing pH and osmolarity have been instilled into the lungs show features of alveolar injury that are most severe when the fluid is strongly acid, but even distilled water or saline is able to produce minor damage. Disturbance of the osmotic gradient across the alveolar capillary membrane may therefore be an additional factor. Damage occurs to both epithelial and endothelial cells, which separate from their basement membranes.[125] The most severe changes include necrosis and neutrophil exudation. Pulmonary haemorrhage is generally found and often shows a brown discoloration microscopically, due to the production of acid haematin (Fig. 4.23). The alveolar changes are accompanied by acute bronchitis and bronchiolitis with sloughing of the mucosa. The pathological changes after acid aspiration may be described as those of a severe chemical burn.

Preventive measures include the administration of antacids to postoperative or obstetric patients, but this often results in colonisation of the stomach by Gram-negative bacteria and a bacterial rather than a chemical pneumonia if there is aspiration.[126]

Irradiation

Radiation may be environmental, occupational or employed as a weapon of war and is of course also part of the therapeutic armamentarium. Environmental and occupational exposure carries an increased risk of lung cancer and is dealt with on page 533 while the iatrogenic effects of radiation treatment are dealt with on page 391. This section is concerned with the high-level radiation experienced by the victims of nuclear attack or accident.

Nuclear explosions cause significant acute and long-term damage to the victims. The immediate mortality is high and in such cases it is difficult to separate the direct effects of radiation from those of thermal injury and the secondary effects of bone marrow failure. Nevertheless, by studying the victims of the atomic bombs dropped on Japan in 1945 much was learnt of the effects of large doses of whole-body irradiation. The lungs of victims dying within 2 weeks showed focal collapse and oedema, while those dying between 2 and 6 weeks after exposure had centriacinar areas of necrosis and haemorrhage; and those dying more than 6 weeks afterwards showed broader areas of necrosis with a heavy infiltrate of neutrophils.[127]

Pathogenesis

Radiation generates free radicals in the tissues and its effects are potentiated by the presence of oxygen. Free radicals result in DNA damage and chromosomal abnormalities.[128] At the cellular level, alveolar capillary endothelial cells and type I epithelial cells are most susceptible.

Endothelial injury is believed to be of prime importance in radiation pneumonitis.[129] Severe or prolonged endothelial damage disturbs the normal endothelial–mesenchymal relationships and allows uncoordinated fibroblast proliferation. Endothelial changes are detectable within days of exposure. In rats they are seen within 48 hours after 1100 rads and within 5 days after 650 rads.[130] Endothelial cells become swollen and vacuolated and separate from the basement membrane, resulting in increased capillary permeability and interstitial oedema. Adhesion of platelets to the denuded basement membrane initiates thrombosis and occlusion of the vascular lumen. Proliferation of endothelial cells follows and endothelial basement membrane is reduplicated.[128,130,131] By light microscopy the early vascular changes are evident as thrombosis, which is followed by cellular intimal thickening or even complete occlusion of small arteries and arterioles. In the later fibrotic stage vessels are thick-walled and hyaline.[132]

Epithelial cell damage is also well described in radiation injury. Within 10 days of exposure type I cells become swollen and undergo necrosis and sloughing with the formation of hyaline membranes. Type II cells proliferate and appear swollen and vacuolated.[131] Pleomorphism of regenerating alveolar lining cells is apparent and similar changes are seen in bronchial and bronchiolar epithelium.[133] In many respects therefore the appearances closely resemble those due to cytotoxic drugs (see p. 385).

Pathology

Early radiation changes in human lung include oedematous thickening of the alveolar walls, hyperplasia and swelling of type II cells, and alveolar exudates. The changes are essentially those of DAD, as described above. Fibrosis develops later and is typically interstitial. Type II cells and fibroblasts are often atypical, with large nuclei and prominent nucleoli. Blood vessels are sclerosed and the vasculature

consequently reduced. Irradiation also impairs the bactericidal properties of pulmonary macrophages and predisposes to infection.

Idiopathic acute alveolar injury

In some cases of rapidly progressive DAD no cause is evident. Such patients were described by Hamman and Rich,[134] since when these authors' names have often been applied eponymously to rapidly progressive idiopathic pulmonary fibrosis.[135] Others favour the term 'acute interstitial pneumonia' for such cases and emphasise the differences from chronic interstitial pneumonia,[135,136] but all intermediate stages are encountered. Furthermore, some patients with idiopathic pulmonary fibrosis that for the most part has run a typically chronic course exhibit acute exacerbations. If they die of such a flare-up of their disease autopsy shows the hyaline membranes of DAD superimposed upon long-established collagenous fibrosis (see Fig. 6.1.10, p. 274).[137,138] In a series of 58 patients with DAD diagnosed by surgical biopsy, 21% had no identifiable cause or predisposing condition (i.e. acute interstitial pneumonia) and in 12% the changes represented an acute exacerbation of idiopathic pulmonary fibrosis.[139] Patients with idiopathic pulmonary fibrosis of non-specific interstitial pneumonia pattern may similarly experience acute exacerbations characterised by DAD, while patients with connective tissue disease may develop DAD ab initio or have it complicate pre-existent interstitial fibrosis.[140–142]

Treatment of acute respiratory distress

The treatment of ARDS is based upon minimising whichever of the several causes of the condition are deemed to be operating and achieving a balance between maintaining blood oxygen levels and affording the lungs the rest that all tissues recovering from injury require.[4,143] Ideally, the lungs would be rested completely and the blood oxygenated in some other way. Indeed, this is occasionally attempted by a process of extracorporeal oxygenation in which the systemic blood is diverted through an artificial lung in the form of a membrane oxygenator that sits alongside the patient.[143a–c] This is a major procedure that generally occupies a surgical operating theatre and is often attended by problems with haemostasis and, if prolonged, haemolysis. Lesser procedures involve the insertion of an intravenous oxygenator or the use of an extracorporeal device that removes carbon dioxide from the blood passing through a cannula connecting a femoral artery to its vein, but these only treat a fraction of the blood leaving the heart.

More often, blood oxygenation is maintained by artificial ventilation, sacrificing the optimal conditions for lung recovery in favour of supplying other organs, particularly the brain, with oxygen. Simply allowing the mechanically expanded lung to collapse again several times a minute would establish a pattern of respiration quite unlike the normal and one that would incur further damage to the lungs. With a normal lining of surfactant the alveoli do not collapse completely at the end of expiration. A considerable residual volume of gas is normally retained but, when the alveolar lining film is lost, as in DAD, the alveoli collapse completely at the end of each respiratory excursion and the inspiratory phase commences from a much lower baseline. It is now recognised that this exerts considerable mechanical stress upon the delicate alveolar epithelial lining,[144] the integrity of which is already severely compromised in ARDS. These purely mechanical forces result in the generation and release of a variety of injurious cytokines (e.g. tumour necrosis factor-α) and reactive oxygen species without necessarily involving any inflammation.[145,146] To minimise this, positive pressure is usually maintained throughout the respiratory cycle, a form of ventilation termed positive end-expiratory pressure, frequently referred to as PEEP.[147] If, despite PEEP, hypoxaemia approaches dangerous levels the intensivist has no choice but to raise the concentration of oxygen in the inspired air, although it is recognised that high concentrations of oxygen are themselves injurious to the lung. With severe lung damage a situation is often reached where to prevent cerebral injury increasingly higher concentrations of oxygen have to be employed. The initial damage to the lung is then compounded by a combination of mechanical and chemical injury, resulting in an aggravated form of DAD to which the term 'respirator lung' is often applied.

Nitric oxide, a selective pulmonary vasodilator with anti-inflammatory properties, has been used in acute lung injury but a meta-analysis found that despite limited improvement in oxygenation it confers no mortality benefit and may cause harm.[147a]

A promising technique that is now under experimental investigation follows the recent recognition that bone marrow stem cells are capable of differentiating into a variety of mature cell types, including those that constitute the alveolar epithelium.[148] The successful application of this would hasten the healing process and minimise the likelihood of the damaged lung developing irreversible fibrosis.

Outcome

DAD carries a high mortality rate, around 50% overall but reaching 94% when aspiration of gastric acid is the cause.[124] The DAD associated with septic shock also carries a particularly high mortality rate.[149] Certain polymorphisms of the vascular endothelial growth factor (VEGF) gene have been associated with a higher mortality.[150] Survivors may appear to recover completely but tests of lung function often show that they have a mild restrictive or diffusion defect.[151,152]

PULMONARY FIBROSIS

The healing of DAD by fibrosis leads to a consideration of pulmonary fibrosis in general. This is not an inevitable consequence of injury for, if the damaged tissue is capable of regeneration, healing by resolution is possible and normality is regained. However, if tissue is irretrievably lost, healing can only take place by repair, entailing the replacement of the lost tissue by fibrous tissue and resulting in scar formation. Various patterns of fibrosis are encountered in the lungs and these will now be described.

Focal scars are quite commonly found in the lungs at necropsy, particularly at the apices of the upper lobes where they consist of narrow bands of contracted, often blackened, lung covered by thickened pleura, the so-called apical cap.[153–155a] When such apical scars are accompanied by calcification and pleural adhesions, they have probably followed tuberculosis, but this is now unusual in developed countries. Most apical scars in these countries are probably attributable to the relative ischaemia of the apices of the lungs, which, due to our upright posture, are barely perfused at all for much of the day. Quite minor apical scars are often associated with bullae and rupture of these underlies many spontaneous pneumothoraces (see p. 711). Apical scarring also develops in ankylosing spondylitis (see p. 478). In other parts of the lungs, a focal subpleural scar may be the result of a primary tuberculous lesion or the corresponding primary lesions of fungal infections such as histoplasmosis. Focal scars also result from embolic infarction and pneumonia. In such scars combined stains for elastin and collagen (such as the elastin-van Gieson stain) often show that the alveolar framework of the lung is completely lost, reflecting total destruction of the affected area. Such scars are generally rich in elastin, a feature common to organs such as the lungs and the heart that are subject to repeated movement and one that is not seen to the same degree in scars of organs such as the liver and kidneys that are subjected to less movement.

With more widespread pulmonary fibrosis, elastin stains often show that the framework of the alveolar walls is maintained,[156] and one of three patterns of fibrosis may then be recognised: intra-alveolar, interstitial and obliterative.[157,158] These patterns are not mutually exclusive. For example, interstitial fibrosis may result from the incorporation of organising air space exudates into the alveolar wall,[159,160] as described above in the proliferative phase of DAD. This is particularly likely if the epithelium is lost on a broad front and its regeneration is delayed. Whether the fibrosis has an intra-alveolar, interstitial or obliterative pattern largely depends on the severity and duration of the initial injury. To some extent therefore these patterns are of prognostic significance.

Intra-alveolar fibrosis (organising pneumonia)

Intra-alveolar fibrosis represents organisation of an alveolar exudate.[161] It is characterised by the presence within the alveoli of polypoid knots of myxoid granulation tissue, rich in glycosaminoglycans, fibroblasts and myofibroblasts[162] but containing little polymerised collagen. These intra-alveolar knots of granulation tissue are known as Masson bodies[163] or *bourgeons conjonctifs* (see Figs 4.17B, p. 142, 5.2.4, p. 180 and 6.2.2, p. 310). This is the classic pattern of postpneumonic carnification, found particularly when bacterial pneumonia fails to resolve. It is familiar to all pathologists conducting autopsies and must have been well known to the great morbid anatomists of the nineteenth century. Twentieth-century descriptions date back at least to 1912.[164–166]

Organising pneumonia may also represent incomplete resolution of eosinophilic pneumonia or the fibrin-rich transudate of severe left ventricular failure, or be caused by inhaled irritants,[167] viral infection, including human immunodeficiency virus,[168] drugs,[169,170] radiation[171–173] and connective tissue disease.[174,175] Organising pneumonia is also found in transplanted lungs[176] and is commonly seen around tumours or other localised lung lesions. It is also one of the minor features of extrinsic allergic alveolitis (Box 4.3). Although organising pneumonia is readily recognisable in transbronchial biopsies, such specimens may not include these underlying lesions, which may therefore remain undetected unless a surgical biopsy is obtained.

There is also an idiopathic variety of organising pneumonia, known as cryptogenic organising pneumonia (formerly known as idiopathic bronchiolitis obliterans-organising pneumonia). This is described in Chapter 6.2 (p. 308).

Box 4.3 Causes of intra-alveolar fibrosis

Bacterial pneumonia

Aspiration pneumonia

Eosinophilic pneumonia

Severe left-sided cardiac failure ('congestive consolidation')

Inhaled irritants

Viral infection

Drugs

Radiation

Connective tissue disease

Inflammatory bowel disease

Extrinsic allergic alveolitis

Adjacent lesions such as tumour, abscess, Wegener's granulomatosis

Idiopathic (cryptogenic organising pneumonia)

Figure 4.24 Accidental paraquat poisoning. The patient died from pulmonary fibrosis within 10 days of ingesting a relatively small amount of the chemical. The fibrosis is of the obliterative pattern, resulting from organisation of exudate that flooded many alveoli so that the air spaces are completely obliterated although the alveolar walls can still be identified. (A) Haematoxylin and eosin. (B) Masson stain.

Obliterative fibrosis

Pulmonary fibrosis sometimes effaces the lumen of several adjacent alveoli completely, rendering them totally airless (Fig. 4.24). This obliterative pattern of fibrosis is the result of severe lung injury due to any of the causes of DAD considered above. Intra-alveolar and obliterative pulmonary fibrosis have many causes in common. The pattern of fibrosis depends not so much on the nature of the damage as its severity. With very severe injury the alveolar lumen is flooded with a fibrin-rich exudate, organisation of which completely obliterates the air spaces over broad tracts of lung. Within these areas, however, the framework of the alveolar walls can often still be appreciated, particularly with elastin or basement membrane stains. It is as if the architecture has undergone a form of petrification. The parts of the lung affected by obliterative fibrosis are completely non-functioning. This pattern of fibrosis is unlikely to resolve.

Interstitial fibrosis

This pattern of pulmonary fibrosis involves the interstitial compartment of the alveolar walls and largely spares the air spaces (Fig. 4.25). It often entails the laying down of connective tissue within the

Figure 4.25 Interstitial pulmonary fibrosis.

Box 4.4 Causes of predominantly interstitial pulmonary fibrosis

A 'transudate/exudate' group that affects the dependent parts of the lung	A 'granulomatous' group that tends to spare the bases
Organising diffuse alveolar damage	Sarcoidosis
Idiopathic pulmonary fibrosis (usual interstitial pneumonia)	Extrinsic allergic alveolitis
	Langerhans cell histiocytosis
Chronic oedema	Silicosis
Asbestosis	Chronic berylliosis

The conditions in the left-hand column are ranked on a time scale from organising diffuse alveolar damage, which may progress to fibrosis within 10 days, to asbestosis, which evolves over many years.

---

alveolar walls but it may also be brought about by an accretive process involving incorporation into the interstitium of exudates or connective tissue first formed in air spaces.[159,160,177] The causes are varied but may be divided into two broad groups, one involving the formation of exudates and transudates and the other involving the formation of what may be loosely termed granulomas (Box 4.4). It is particularly notable that the 'exudate and transudate' group of diseases predominantly affects the basal portion of the lungs and the 'granulomatous' group more the upper parts. The reason for this is not well understood but it can be a helpful diagnostic pointer in advanced disease. It requires no great skill in interpreting chest radiographs to assign a patient with widespread reticulonodular opacities to one or other of these two broad groups on the basis of the distribution of the disease. This criterion is also useful when assessing widespread pulmonary fibrosis postmortem.

In the 'exudate and transudate' group many cases are unexplained but some represent the outcome of DAD caused by agents that range from fumes to viruses, irradiation, the aspiration of regurgitated gastric acid and the ingestion of various chemicals (see Box 4.1, p. 136). These causes may also lead to an obliterative pattern of pulmonary fibrosis (see above) but in the present context, instead of exudates flooding alveoli, they line the denuded alveolar walls as hyaline membranes, organisation of which leads to their incorporation into the alveolar interstitium (see Figs 4.12 and 4.13). This augments the activity of interstitial fibroblasts, the two processes combining to cause fibrosis of the alveolar walls. A similar process, albeit at a slower tempo, is envisaged in idiopathic pulmonary fibrosis (usual interstitial pneumonia), which is dealt with in Chapter 6.1. Most of these conditions entail damage to the delicate lining cells of the alveoli and capillaries with consequent exudation. It is perhaps because of this that the subsequent interstitial fibrosis is most marked in the dependent parts of the lungs. This distribution is also seen in the interstitial fibrosis that follows long-standing interstitial oedema in conditions such as mitral stenosis and pulmonary veno-occlusive disease.

The other major group of causes of interstitial fibrosis may be termed 'granulomatous' because focal collections of activated macrophages are involved in the development of the fibrosis. This group includes sarcoidosis, extrinsic allergic alveolitis and Langerhans cell histiocytosis (eosinophilic granuloma), all of which are described in Chapter 6. The fibrosis they cause is predominantly mid- or upper zonal.

The pneumoconioses constitute an important group of diseases causing interstitial pulmonary fibrosis. They are dealt with separately in Chapter 7.1 but it is possible to allocate individual pneumoconioses to one or other of the above two groups (see Box 4.2). Thus, asbestosis resembles the idiopathic cases in having a predominantly basal distribution, whereas others, e.g. silicosis and chronic berylliosis, resemble the granulomatous diseases morphologically (given that early silicotic nodules resemble granulomas) and in their upper zone distribution.

'Honeycomb lung'

In advanced cases of pulmonary fibrosis the normal alveolar architecture is lost and the three patterns just described can no longer be distinguished. At this stage the lung is replaced by a series of cystic spaces giving an appearance that has been termed 'honeycomb lung'. The spaces represent a combination of disrupted alveoli showing bronchiolisation and bronchiolectasis (see Figs 6.1.5 and 6.1.10A, pp. 269 and 274). 'Honeycomb lung' is not a specific disease but represents the final result of many, being an end-stage pattern of injury comparable to the granular contracted kidney and cirrhosis of the liver. Idiopathic pulmonary fibrosis is its commonest cause, particularly those cases with the pattern of usual interstitial pneumonia, and pathologists may see this remodelling microscopically in the absence of changes on high-resolution computed tomography. Other causes include extrinsic allergic alveolitis, Langerhans cell histiocytosis, sarcoidosis and berylliosis. Lymphangioleiomyomatosis also produces widespread cystic change but generally lacks the extensive fibrosis and bronchiolisation seen in these other conditions.

Dystrophic calcification and ossification

Dystrophic calcification is very common in pulmonary scars, particularly those resulting from tuberculosis, chickenpox and histoplasmosis. Pulmonary calcification in the absence of hypercalcaemia also occurs in the tracheobronchial cartilages of the elderly, the cartilaginous nodules of tracheobronchopathia osteochondroplastica and bronchopulmonary amyloid tumours. Pulmonary calcification also accompanies haemosiderin deposition in the lungs and is therefore found in chronic haemorrhagic conditions such as idiopathic haemosiderosis and the postcapillary pulmonary hypertension of mitral stenosis, lymphangioleiomyomatosis and veno-occlusive disease. Pulmonary calcification secondary to hypercalcaemia (metastatic calcification) is described on page 489.

Dystrophic pulmonary ossification takes place in similar circumstances to dystrophic pulmonary calcification: it is found with scarring, ageing of the bronchial cartilages, tracheobronchopathia osteochondroplastica and amyloid tumour formation. Lamellar bone, readily recognisable as such, is laid down, and marrow spaces are often evident. Sometimes branching spicules of bone extend through the lung in a racemose or dendriform manner.[178-183] Isolated foci of laminated bone may also be found within alveoli of otherwise normal appearance (see Fig. 6.2.25, p. 322).

REFERENCES

Acute respiratory distress syndrome

1. Petty TL, Ashbaugh DG. The adult respiratory distress syndrome. Clinical features, factors influencing prognosis and principles of management. Chest 1971;60:233–9.
2. Petty TL. The acute respiratory distress syndrome – historic perspective. Chest 1994;105:S44–7.
3. Ware LB, Matthay MA. Medical progress – The acute respiratory distress syndrome. N Engl J Med 2000;342:1334–49.
4. Rubenfeld GD, Caldwell E, Peabody E, et al. Incidence and outcomes of acute lung injury. N Engl J Med 2005;353:1685–93.
5. Bernard GR, Artigas A, Brigham KL, et al. The American-European Consensus Conference on ARDS. Definitions, mechanisms, relevant outcomes, and clinical trial coordination. Am J Respir Crit Care Med 1994;149:818–24.
6. Desai SR. Acute respiratory distress syndrome: imaging of the injured lung. Clin Radiol 2002;57:8–17.

7. Desai SR, Wells AU, Suntharalingam G, et al. Acute respiratory distress syndrome caused by pulmonary and extrapulmonary injury: a comparative CT study. Radiology 2001;218:689–93.
8. Bone RC, Balk R, Slotman G, et al. Adult Respiratory Distress Syndrome – sequence and importance of development of multiple organ failure. Chest 1992;101:320–6.
9. Bulpa PA, Dive AM, Mertens L, et al. Combined bronchoalveolar lavage and transbronchial lung biopsy: safety and yield in ventilated patients. Eur Resp J 2003;21:489–94.
10. Patel SR, Karmpaliotis D, Ayas NT, et al. The role of open-lung biopsy in ARDS. Chest 2004;125:197–202.

Diffuse alveolar damage

11. Liebow AA. New concepts and entities in pulmonary disease. In: International Academy of Pathology monograph No.8.,

editor. The Lung. Baltimore: Williams & Wilkins; 1967. p. 332–365.
12. Liebow AA. Definition and classification of interstitial pneumonias in human pathology. Prog Resp Res 1975;8:1–33.
13. Katzenstein ALA, Bloor CM, Liebow AA. Diffuse alveolar damage – the role of oxygen, shock and related factors. Am J Pathol 1976;85:210–22.
14. Corrin B. Diffuse alveolar damage. In: Evans TW, Haslett C, editors. ARDS Acute Respiratory Distress in Adults. London: Chapman & Hall Medical; 1996. p. 37–46.
15. Matsubara O. Pathogenesis of diffuse alveolar damage. Histopathology 2002;41:438–41.
16. Vijeyaratnam GS, Corrin B. Experimental paraquat poisoning. J Pathol 1971;103:123–9.
17. Bachofen M, Weibel ER. Alterations of the gas exchange apparatus in adult respiratory insufficiency associated with septicaemia. Am Rev Respir Dis 1977;116:589–615.

18. Corrin B. Lung pathology in septic shock. J Clin Pathol 1980;33:891–4.

19. Yazdy AM, Tomashefski JF, Yagan R, et al. Regional alveolar damage (RAD). A loocalized counterpart of diffuse alveolar damage. Am J Clin Pathol 1989;92: 10–15.

20. Barth PJ, Holtermann W, Muller B. The spatial distribution of pulmonary lesions in severe ARDS – An autopsy study of 35 cases. Pathol Res Pract 1998;194: 465–71.

21. Hill JD, Ratcliff JL, Parrott JCW, et al. Pulmonary pathology in acute respiratory insufficiency: lung biopsy as a diagnostic tool. J Thorac Cardiovasc Surg 1976;71:64–9.

22. Pratt PC, Vollmer RT, Shelburne JD, et al. Pulmonary morphology in a multihospital collaborative extracorporeal membrane oxygenation project. Am J Pathol 1979;95:191–214.

23. Evans MJ, Cabral LJ, Stephens RJ, et al. Renewal of alveolar epithelium in the rat following exposure to NO_2. Am J Pathol 1973;70:175–98.

24. Adamson IYR, Bowden DH. The type 2 cells as progenitor of alveolar epithelial regeneration. Lab Invest 1974;30: 25–42.

25. Warnock ML, Press M, Churg A. Further observations on cytoplasmic hyaline in the lung. Hum Pathol 1980;11:59–65.

26. Yamada T, Uehara K, Kawanishi R, et al. Immunohistochemical detection of ubiquitin-positive intracytoplasmic eosinophilic inclusion bodies in diffuse alveolar damage. Histopathology 2006;48:846–54.

27. Ogino S, Franks TJ, Yong M, et al. Extensive squamous metaplasia with cytologic atypia in diffuse alveolar damage mimicking squamous cell carcinoma: A report of 2 cases. Hum Pathol 2002;33:1052–4.

28. Katzenstein ALA. Pathogenesis of 'fibrosis' in interstitial pneumonia: an electron microscopic study. Hum Pathol 1985;16:1015–24.

29. Burkhardt A. Pathogenesis of pulmonary fibrosis. Hum Pathol 1986;17:971–3.

30. Burkhardt A. Alveolitis and collapse in the pathogenesis of pulmonary fibrosis. Am Rev Respir Dis 1989;140:513–24.

31. Reidy MA, Schwartz SM. Endothelial regeneration. III. Time course of intimal changes after small defined injury to rat aortic endothelium. Lab Invest 1981;44:301.

32. Kapanci Y, Weibel ER, Kaplan HP, et al. Pathogenesis and reversibility of the pulmonary lesions of oxygen toxicity in monkeys. II Ultrastructural and morphometric studies. Lab Invest 1969;20:101–18.

33. Kapanci Y, Tosco R, Eggermann J, et al. Oxygen pneumonitis in man. Chest 1972;62:162–9.

34. Tomashefski JF, Davies P, Boggis C, et al. The pulmonary vascular lesions of the adult respiratory distress syndrome. Am J Pathol 1983;112:112–6.

35. Pache JC, Christakos PG, Gannon DE, et al. Myofibroblasts in diffuse alveolar damage of the lung. Modern Pathol 1998;11:1064–70.

36. Guarino M, Tosoni A, Nebuloni M. Direct contribution of epithelium to organ fibrosis: epithelial–mesenchymal transition. Human Pathology 2009;40:1365–76.

37. Hackett TL, Warner SM, Stefanowicz D, et al. Induction of epithelial–mesenchymal transition in primary airway epithelial cells from patients with asthma by transforming growth factor-β_1. Am J Respir Crit Care Med 2009;180:122–33.

38. Borthwick LA, Parker SM, Brougham KA, et al. Epithelial to mesenchymal transition (EMT) and airway remodelling after human lung transplantation. Thorax 2009;64:770–7.

39. Bachofen M, Weibel ER. Basic pattern of tissue repair in human lungs following unspecific injury. Chest 1974;65:14s–9s.

40. Meduri GU, Chinn A. Fibroproliferation in late adult respiratory distress syndrome – pathophysiology, clinical and laboratory manifestations, and response to corticosteroid rescue treatment. Chest 1994;105:S127–9.

41. Brody AR, Craighead JE. Interstitial associations of cells lining air spaces in human pulmonary fibrosis. Virchows Arch A Pathol Anat Histopathol 1976;372:39–49.

42. Brody AR, Soler P, Basset F, et al. Epithelial–mesenchymal associations of cells in human pulmonary fibrosis and in BHT-oxygen-induced fibrosis in mice. Exp Lung Res 1981;2:207–20.

43. Adamson IYR, Young L, Bowden DH. Relationship of alveolar epithelial injury and repair to the induction of pulmonary fibrosis. Am J Pathol 1988;130:377–83.

44. Adamson IYR, Hedgecock C, Bowden DH. Epithelial cell–fibroblast interactions in lung injury and repair. Am J Pathol 1990;137:385–92.

45. Matsubara O, Tamura A, Ohdama S, et al. Alveolar basement membrane breaks down in diffuse alveolar damage: an immunohistochemical study. Pathol Int 1995;45:473–82.

46. Nash JRG, McLaughlin PJ, Hoyle C, et al. Immunolocalization of tumour necrosis factor-alpha in lung tissue from patients dying with adult respiratory distress syndrome. Histopathology 1991;19:395–402.

47. Pan L-H, Ohtani H, Yamauchi K, et al. Co-expression of TNF alpha and IL-1 beta in human acute pulmonary fibrotic diseases: an immunohistochemical analysis. Pathol Int 1996;46:91–9.

48. Fukuda Y, Ferrans VJ, Schoenberger CI, et al. Patterns of pulmonary structural remodeling after experimental paraquat toxicity. Am J Pathol 1985;118:452–75.

49. Fukuda Y, Ishizaki M, Masuda Y, et al. The role of intraalveolar fibrosis in the process of pulmonary structural remodeling in patients with diffuse alveolar damage. Am J Pathol 1987;126:171–82.

50. Mandal RV, Mark EJ, Kradin RL. Organizing pneumonia and pulmonary lymphatic architecture in diffuse alveolar damage. Hum Pathol 2008;39:1234–8.

51. Kang D, Nakayama T, Togashi M, et al. Two forms of diffuse alveolar damage in the lungs of patients with acute respiratory distress syndrome. Human Pathology 2009;40:1618–27.

52. Zapol WM, Trelstad RL, Coffey JW, et al. Pulmonary fibrosis in severe acute respiratory failure. Am Rev Respir Dis 1979;119:547–54.

53. Martin C, Papazian L, Payan MJ, et al. Pulmonary fibrosis correlates with outcome in adult respiratory distress syndrome: a study in mechanically ventilated patients. Chest 1995;107:196–200.

54. Slavin G, Nunn J, Crow J, et al. Bronchiolectasis: a complication of artificial respiration. BMJ 1982;285: 931–4.

55. Churg A, Golden J, Fligiel S, et al. Bronchopulmonary dysplasia in the adult. Am Rev Respir Dis 1983;127:117–20.

56. Wohl MEB. Bronchopulmonary dysplasia in adulthood. N Engl J Med 1990;323:1834–6.

57. Hert R, Albert RK. Sequelae of the adult respiratory distress syndrome. Thorax 1994;49:8–13.

58. Katzenstein ALA, Fiorelli RF. Nonspecific interstitial pneumonia/fibrosis – histologic features and clinical significance. Am J Surg Pathol 1994;18:136–47.

59. Hudson LD, Milberg JA, Anardi D, et al. Clinical risks for development of the acute respiratory distress syndrome. Am J Respir Crit Care Med 1995;151:293–301.

60. Stapleton RD, Wang BM, Hudson LD. Causes and timing of death in patients with ARDS. Chest 2005;128:525–32.

61. Markowicz P, Wolff M, Djedaini K, et al. Multicenter prospective study of ventilator-associated pneumonia during acute respiratory distress syndrome. Incidence, prognosis, and risk factors. ARDS Study Group. Am J Respir Crit Care Med 2000;161:1942–8.

62. Frevert CW, Warner AE, Kobzik L. Defective pulmonary recruitment of neutrophils in a rat model of endotoxemia. Am J Respir Cell Mol Biol 1994;11:716–23.

63. Parrillo JE. Mechanisms of disease – pathogenetic mechanisms of septic shock. N Engl J Med 1993;328: 1471–7.

64. Evans TJ, Krausz T. Pathogenesis and pathology of shock. In: Anthony PP, MacSween RNM, editors. Recent Advances

in Histopathology, volume 16. Edinburgh: Churchill Livingstone; 1994. p. 21–47.

65. McGovern VJ. Shock. Pathol Annu 1971;6:279–98.

66. McGovern VJ. The pathophysiology of Gram-negative septicaemia. Pathology 1972;4:265–71.

67. McGovern VJ. Hypovolaemic shock with particular reference to the myocardial and pulmonary lesions. Pathology 1980;12:63–72.

68. Moon VH. The pathology of secondary shock. Am J Pathol 1948;24:235–73.

69. Martin AM, Soloway HB, Simmons RL. Pathologic anatomy of the lungs following shock and trauma. J Trauma 1968;8:687–699.

70. Bredenburg CE, James PM, Collins J, et al. Respiratory failure in shock. Ann Surg 1969;169:392–403.

71. Stergiopoulou T, Meletiadis J, Roilides E, et al. Host-dependent patterns of tissue injury in invasive pulmonary aspergillosis. Am J Clin Pathol 2007;127:349–55.

72. Thiemermann C, Szabo C, Mitchell JA, et al. Vascular hyporeactivity to vasoconstrictor agents and hemodynamic decompensation in hemorrhagic shock is mediated by nitric oxide. Proc Natl Acad Sci USA 1993;90:267–71.

73. Clowes GHA. Pulmonary abnormalities in sepsis. Surg Clin North Am 1974;54:993–1013.

74. Stephens KE, Ishizaka A, Larrick JW, et al. Tumor necrosis factor causes increased pulmonary permeability and edema. Am Rev Respir Dis 1988;137:1364–70.

75. Millar AB, Singer M, Meager A, et al. Tumour necrosis factor in bronchopulmonary secretions of patients with adult respiratory distress syndrome. Lancet 1989;ii:712–4.

76. Johnson J, Brigham KL, Jesmok G, et al. Morphologic changes in lungs of anesthetized sheep following intravenous infusion of recombinant tumor necrosis factor-alpha. Am Rev Respir Dis 1991;144:179–86.

77. Monick MM, Hunninghake GW. Activation of second messenger pathways in alveolar macrophages by endotoxin. Eur Resp J 2002;20:210–22.

78. Xing Z, Kirpalani H, Torry D, et al. Polymorphonuclear leukocytes as a significant source of tumor necrosis factor-alpha in endotoxin-challenged lung tissue. Am J Pathol 1993;143:1009–15.

79. Vannhieu JT, Misset B, Lebargy F, et al. Expression of tumor necrosis factor-alpha gene in alveolar macrophages from patients with the adult respiratory distress syndrome. Am Rev Respir Dis 1993;147:1585–9.

80. Martin TR. Lung cytokines and ARDS. Chest 1999;116:2S–8S.

81. Lui SF, Adcock IM, Old RW, et al. Lipopolysaccharide treatment in vivo induces widespread tissue expression of inducible nitric oxide synthase mRNA. Biochemistry and Biophysical Research Communications 1993;196:1208–13.

82. Buttery LDK, Evans TJ, Springall DR, et al. Immunochemical localization of inducible nitric oxide synthase in endotoxin-treated rats. Lab Invest 1994;71:755–64.

83. Ermert M, Ruppert C, Gunther A, et al. Cell-specific nitric oxide synthase-isoenzyme expression and regulation in response to endotoxin in intact rat lungs. Lab Invest 2002;82:425–41.

84. Ward PA. Role of complement in lung inflammatory injury. Am J Pathol 1996;149:1079.

85. Roberts JC, Gulino SP, Peak KK, et al. Fatal necrotizing pneumonia due to a Panton–Valentine leukocidin positive community-associated methicillin-sensitive *Staphylococcus aureus* and influenza co-infection: a case report. Ann Clin Microbiol Antimicrob 2008;7:5.

86. Tanaka N, Kita T, Kasai K, et al. The immunocytochemical localization of tumour necrosis factor and leukotriene in the rat heart and lung during endotoxin shock. Virchows Arch 1994;424:273–7.

87. Hollenberg SM, Cunnion RE, Parrillo JE. The effect of tumour necrosis factor on vascular smooth muscle: in vitro studies using rat aorta rings. Chest 1991;100:1133–7.

88. Moncada S, Palmer RMJ, Higgs EA. Nitric oxide: physiology, pathophysiology and pharmacology. Pharmacol Rev 1991;43:109–42.

89. Tsokos M. Immunohistochemical detection of sepsis-induced lung injury in human autopsy material. Leg Med (Tokyo) 2003;5:73–86.

90. Freeman B. Free radical chemistry of nitric oxide – looking at the dark side. Chest 1994;105:S79–84.

91. Gongora MC, Lob HE, Landmesser U, et al. Loss of extracellular superoxide dismutase leads to acute lung damage in the presence of ambient air: a potential mechanism underlying adult respiratory distress syndrome. Am J Pathol 2008;173:915–26.

92. Rinaldo JE, Rogers RM. Adult respiratory distress syndrome: changing concepts of lung injury and repair. N Engl J Med 1982;306:900–9.

93. Ratliff NB, Wilson JW, Hackel DB, et al. The lung in hemorrhagic shock. II. Observations on alveolar and vascular ultrastructure. Am J Pathol 1970;58:353–73.

94. Kasajima K, Wax SD, Webb WR. Effects of methylprednisolone on pulmonary microcirculation. Surg Gynecol Obstet 1974;139:1–5.

95. Craddock PR, Hammerschmidt DE, White JG, et al. Complement (C5a)-induced granulocyte aggregation in vitro: a possible mechanism of complement-mediated leukostasis and leukopenia. J Clin Invest 1977;60:260–4.

96. Tate RM, Repine JE. Neutrophils and the adult respiratory distress syndrome. Am Rev Respir Dis 1983;128:552–9.

97. Yodice PC, Astiz ME, Kurian BM, et al. Neutrophil rheologic changes in septic shock. Am J Respir Crit Care Med 1997;155:38–42.

98. Drost EM, Kassabian G, Meiselman HJ, et al. Increased rigidity and priming of polymorphonuclear leukocytes in sepsis. Am J Respir Crit Care Med 1999;159:1696–702.

99. Wegner CD, Wolyniec WW, Laplante AM, et al. Intercellular adhesion molecule-1 contributes to pulmonary oxygen toxicity in mice – role of leukocytes revised. Lung 1992;170:267–79.

100. Seekamp A, Mulligan MS, Till GO, et al. Role of beta-2 integrins and ICAM-1 in lung injury following ischemia–reperfusion of rat hind limbs. Am J Pathol 1993;143:464–72.

101. Zimmerman GA, Albertine KH, Carveth HJ, et al. Endothelial activation in ARDS. Chest 1999;116:18S–24S.

102. Doerschuk CM, Mizgerd JP, Kubo H, et al. Adhesion molecules and cellular biomechanical changes in acute lung injury. Chest 1999;116:37S–43S.

103. Laudes IJ, Guo RF, Riedemann NC, et al. Disturbed homeostasis of lung intercellular adhesion molecule-1 and vascular cell adhesion molecule-1 during sepsis. Am J Pathol 2004;164:1435–45.

104. Sacks T, Moldow CF, Craddock PR, et al. Oxygen radicals mediate endothelial cell damage by complement-stimulated granulocytes. J Clin Invest 1978;61:1161–7.

105. Repine JE. Scientific perspectives on adult respiratory distress syndrome. Lancet 1992;339:466–9.

106. Donnelly SC, Haslett C. Cellular mechanisms of acute lung injury – implications for future treatment in the adult respiratory distress syndrome. Thorax 1992;47:260–3.

107. Williams JH, Patel SK, Hatakeyama D, et al. Activated pulmonary vascular neutrophils as early mediators of endotoxin-induced lung inflammation. Am J Respir Cell Mol Biol 1993;8:134–44.

108. Varani J, Fligiel SEG, Till GO, et al. Pulmonary endothelial cell killing by human neutrophils: possible involvement of hydroxyl radical. Lab Invest 1985;53:656–63.

109. Donnelly SC, Macgregor I, Zamani A, et al. Plasma elastase levels and the development of the adult respiratory distress syndrome. Am J Respir Crit Care Med 1995;151:1428–33.

110. Torii K, Iida KI, Miyazaki Y, et al. Higher concentrations of matrix metalloproteinases in bronchoalveolar lavage fluid of patients with adult respiratory distress syndrome. Am J Respir Crit Care Med 1997;155:43–6.

111. Bone RC, Francis PB, Pierce AK. Intravascular coagulation associated with the adult respiratory distress syndrome. Am J Med 1976;61:585–9.

112. Bleyl U, Rossner JA. Globular hyaline microthrombi – their nature and morphogenesis. Virchows Arch A Pathol Anat Histopathol 1976;370:113–28.

113. Hardaway RM. Disseminated intravascular coagulation as possible cause of acute respiratory failure. Surg Gynecol Obstet 1973;137:1–5.

114. Schneider RC, Zapol WM, Carvalho AC. Platelet consumption and sequestration in severe acute respiratory failure. Am Rev Respir Dis 1980;122:445–51.

115. Aabo K, Hansen KB. Megakarocytes in pulmonary blood vessels. 1. Incidences at autopsy, clinicopathological relations especially to disseminated intravascular coagulation. Acta Path Microbiol Scand 1978;86:285–91.

116. Shimamura K, Oka K, Nakazawa M, et al. Distribution patterns of microthrombi in disseminated intravascular coagulation. Arch Pathol Lab Med 1983;107:543–7.

117. Blaisdell FW, Lim RC, Stallone RJ. The mechanism of pulmonary damage following traumatic shock. Surg Gynecol Obstet 1970;130:15–22.

118. Sankey EA, Crow J, Mallett SV, et al. Pulmonary platelet aggregates – possible cause of sudden peroperative death in adults undergoing liver transplantation. J Clin Pathol 1993;46:222–7.

119. Haynes JB, Hyers TM, Giclas PC, et al. Elevated fibrin(ogen) degradation products in adult respiratory distress syndrome. Am Rev Respir Dis 1980;122:841–7.

120. Manwaring D, Thorning D, Currer PW. Mechanisms of acute pulmonary dysfunction induced by fibrinogen degradation product D. Surgery 1978;84:45–53.

121. Mendelson CL. The aspiration of stomach contents into the lungs during obstetric anesthesia. Am J Obstet Gynecol 1946;52:191–205.

122. Ribando CA, Grace WJ. Pulmonary aspiration. Am J Med 1971;50:510–20.

123. Matthay MA, Rosen GD. Acid aspiration induced lung injury: new insights and therapeutic options. Am J Respir Crit Care Med 1996;154:277–8.

124. Fowler AA, Hamman RF, Good JT, et al. Adult respiratory distress syndrome: risk with common predispositions. Ann Intern Med 1983;98:593–7.

125. Alexander IGS. The ultrastructure of the pulmonary alveolar vessels in Mendelson's (acid pulmonary aspiration) syndrome. Br J Anaesth 1968;40:408–14.

126. du Moulin GC, Paterson DG, Hedley-Whyte J, et al. Aspiration of gastric bacteria in antacid-treated patients: a frequent cause of postoperative colonisation of the airway. Lancet 1982;i:242–5.

127. Liebow AA, Warren S, DeCowsey E. Pathology of atomic bomb casualties. Am J Pathol 1949;25:853–940.

128. Gross NJ. The pathogenesis of radiation-induced lung damage. Lung 1981;159:115–25.

129. Adamson IYR, Bowden DH. Endothelial injury and repair in radiation-induced pulmonary fibrosis. Am J Pathol 1983;112:224–230.

130. Adamson IYR, Bowden DH, Wyatt JP. A pathway to pulmonary fibrosis: an ultrastructural study of mouse and rats following radiation to the whole body and hemithorax. Am J Pathol 1970;58:481–98.

131. Madrazo A, Suzuki Y, Churg J. Radiation pneumonitis: ultrastructural changes in the pulmonary alveoli following high doses of radiation. Arch Pathol Lab Med 1973;96:262–8.

132. Warren S, Spencer J. Radiation reaction in the lung. AJR Am J Roentgenol 1940;43:682–701.

133. Warren S, Gates O. Radiation pneumonitis: experimental and pathologic observations. Arch Pathol Lab Med 1940;30:440–60.

134. Hamman L, Rich AR. Acute diffuse interstitial fibrosis of the lungs. Bull Johns Hopkins Hospital 1944;74:177–212.

135. Olson J, Colby TV, Elliott CG. Hamman–Rich syndrome revisited. Mayo Clin Proc 1990;65:1538–48.

136. Katzenstein A-LA, Myers JL, Mazur MT. Acute interstitial pneumonia. A clinicopathologic, ultrastructural, and cell kinetic study. Am J Surg Pathol 1986;10:256–67.

137. Kondo A, Saiki S. Acute exacerbation in idiopathic interstitial pneumonia. In: Harasawa M, Fukuchi Y, Morinari H, editors. Interstitial Pneumonia of Unknown Etiology. Tokyo: University of Tokyo Press; 1989. p. 33–42.

138. Parambil JG, Myers JL, Ryu JH. Histopathologic features and outcome of patients with acute exacerbation of idiopathic pulmonary fibrosis undergoing surgical lung biopsy. Chest 2005;128:3310–5.

139. Parambil JG, Myers JL, Aubry MC, et al. Causes and prognosis of diffuse alveolar damage diagnosed on surgical lung biopsy. Chest 2007;132:50–7.

140. Rice AJ, Wells AU, Bouros D, et al. Terminal diffuse alveolar damage in relation to interstitial pneumonias. An autopsy study. Am J Clin Pathol 2003;119:709–14.

141. Parambil JG, Myers JL, Ryu JH. Diffuse alveolar damage: uncommon manifestation of pulmonary involvement in patients with connective tissue diseases. Chest 2006;130:553–8.

142. Park IN, Kim DS, Shim TS, et al. Acute exacerbation of interstitial pneumonia other than idiopathic pulmonary fibrosis. Chest 2007;132:214–20.

143. Leaver SK, Evans TW. Acute respiratory distress syndrome. BMJ 2007;335:389–94.

143a. Zapol WM, Snider MT, Schneider RC. Extracorporeal membrane oxygenation for acute respiratory failure. Anesthesiology 1977;46:272–85.

143b. Peek GJ, Moore HM, Moore N, et al. Extracorporeal membrane oxygenation for adult respiratory failure. Chest 1977;112:759–64.

143c. Peek GJ, Mugford M, Tiruvoipati R, et al. Efficacy and economic assessment of conventional ventilatory support versus extracorporeal membrane oxygenation for severe adult respiratory failure (CESAR): a multicentre randomized controlled trial. Lancet 2009;374:1351–63.

144. Muscedere JG, Mullen JB, Gan K, et al. Tidal ventilation at low airway pressures can augment lung injury. Am J Respir Crit Care Med 1994;149:1327–34.

145. Steinberg JM, Schiller HJ, Halter JM, et al. Alveolar instability causes early ventilator-induced lung injury independent of neutrophils. Am J Resp Crit Care Med 2004;169:57–63.

146. Bhatia M, Moochhala S. Role of inflammatory mediators in the pathophysiology of acute respiratory distress syndrome. J Pathol 2004;202:145–56.

147. Halter JM, Steinberg JM, Schiller HJ, et al. Positive end-expiratory pressure after a recruitment maneuver prevents both alveolar collapse and recruitment/derecruitment. Am J Respir Crit Care Med 2003;167:1620–6.

147a. Adhikari NKJ, Burns KEA, Friedrich JO, et al. Effect of nitric oxide on oxygenation and mortality in acute lung injury: systemiatic review and meta-analysis. BMJ 2007;334:779–82.

148. Ali NN, Edgar AJ, Samadikuchaksaraei A, et al. Derivation of type II alveolar epithelial cells from murine embryonic stem cells. Tissue Eng 2002;8:541–50.

149. Martin GS, Mangialardi RJ, Wheeler AP, et al. Albumin and furosemide therapy in hypoproteinemic patients with acute lung injury. Crit Care Med 2002;30:2175–82.

150. Zhai R, Gong MN, Zhou W, et al. Genotypes and haplotypes of the VEGF gene are associated with higher mortality and lower VEGF plasma levels in patients with ARDS. Thorax 2007;62:718–22.

151. Hudson LD. What happens to survivors of the adult respiratory distress syndrome. Chest 1994;105:S123–6.

152. Neff TA, Stocker R, Frey HR, et al. Long-term assessment of lung function in survivors of severe ARDS. Chest 2003;123:845–53.

Pulmonary fibrosis

153. Davson J, Susman W. Apical scars and their relationship to siliceous dust

accumulation in non-silicotic lungs. J Path Bact 1937;45:597–612.

154. Butler C, Kleinerman J. The pulmonary apical cap. Am J Pathol 1970;60:205–16.

155. Yousem SA. Pulmonary apical cap – A distinctive but poorly recognized lesion in pulmonary surgical pathology. Am J Surg Pathol 2001;25:679–83.

155a. Yi E, Aubry MC. Pulmonary pseudoneoplasms. Arch Pathol Lab Med 2010;134:417–26.

156. Negri EM, Montes GS, Saldiva PHN, et al. Architectural remodelling in acute and chronic interstitial lung disease: fibrosis or fibroelastosis? Histopathology 2000;37:393–401.

157. Basset F, Ferrans VJ, Soler P, et al. Intraluminal fibrosis in interstitial lung disorders. Am J Pathol 1986;122: 443–61.

158. Usuki J, Fukuda Y. Evolution of three patterns of intra-alveolar fibrosis produced by bleomycin in rats. Pathol Int 1995;45:552–64.

159. Hogg JC. Chronic interstitial lung disease of unknown cause – a new classification based on pathogenesis. Am J Roentgenol 1991;156:225–33.

160. Cohen AJ, King TE Jr, Downey GP. Rapidly progressive bronchiolitis obliterans with organizing pneumonia. Am J Respir Crit Care Med 1994;149:1670–5.

161. Cordier JF. Organising pneumonia. Thorax 2000;55:318–28.

162. Kuhn C, McDonald JA. The roles of the myofibroblast in idiopathic pulmonary fibrosis – ultrastructural and immunohistochemical features of sites of active extracellular matrix synthesis. Am J Pathol 1991;138:1257–65.

163. Masson P, Riopelle JL, Martin P. Poumon rheumatismal. Ann Anat Path 1937;14:359–82.

164. Kidd P. Some moot points in the pathology and clinical history of pneumonia. Lancet 1912;i:1665–70.

165. Floyd R. Organization of pneumonic exudates. Am J Med Sci 1922;163: 527–48.

166. Auerbach SH, Mims OM, Goodpasture EW. Pulmonary fibrosis secondary to pneumonia. Am J Pathol 1952;28: 69–87.

167. Moya C, Anto JM, Taylor AJN, et al. Outbreak of organising pneumonia in textile printing sprayers. Lancet 1994;344:498–502.

168. Allen JN, Wewers MD. HIV-associated bronchiolitis obliterans organising pneumonia. Chest 1989;96:197–8.

169. Camus P, Lombard JN, Perrichon M, et al. Bronchiolitis obliterans organizing pneumonia during treatment with acebutolol and amiodarone. Thorax 1989;44:711–15.

170. Mar KE, Sen P, Tan K, et al. Bronchiolitis obliterans organizing pneumonia associated with massive L-tryptophan ingestion. Chest 1993;104:1924–6.

171. Crestani B, Kambouchner M, Soler P, et al. Migratory bronchiolitis obliterans organizing pneumonia after unilateral radiation therapy for breast carcinoma. Eur Respir J 1995;8:318–21.

172. Bayle JY, Nesme P, Bejui-Thivolet F, et al. Migratory organizing pneumonitis "primed" by radiation therapy. Eur Respir J 1995;8:322–6.

173. Stover DE, Milite F, Zakowski M. A newly recognized syndrome – Radiation related bronchiolitis obliterans and organizing pneumonia. Respiration 2001;68: 540–4.

174. Yousem SA, Colby TV, Carrington CB. Lung biopsy in rheumatoid arthritis. Am Rev Respir Dis 1985;131:770–7.

175. Rees JH, Woodhead MA, Sheppard MN, et al. Rheumatoid arthritis and cryptogenic organising pneumonitis. Respir Med 1991;85:243–6.

176. Yousem SA, Duncan SR, Griffith BP. Interstitial and airspace granulation tissue reactions in lung transplant recipients. Am J Surg Pathol 1992;16:877–84.

177. Spencer H. Interstitial pneumonia. Ann Rev Med 1967;18:423–42.

178. Muller KM, Kriemann J, Stichroth E. Dendriform pulmonary ossification. Pathol Res Pract 1980;168:163–72.

179. Pounder DJ, Pieterse AS. Dendriform pulmonary ossification. Arch Pathol Lab Med 1987;111:1062–4.

180. Joines RW, Roggli VL. Dendriform pulmonary ossification: report of two cases with unique findings. Am J Clin Pathol 1989;91:398–402.

181. Chow LTC, Shum BSF, Chow WH, et al. Diffuse pulmonary ossification – a rare complication of tuberculosis. Histopathology 1992;20:435–7.

182. Ikeda Y, Yamashita H, Tamura T. Diffuse pulmonary ossification and recurrent spontaneous pneumothorax in a patient with bronchial asthma. Resp Med 1998;92:887–9.

183. Lara JF, Catroppo JF, Kim DU, et al. Dendriform pulmonary ossification, a form of diffuse pulmonary ossification: report of a 26-year autopsy experience. Arch Pathol Lab Med 2005;129:348–53.

Infectious diseases

5.1 *Viral, mycoplasmal and rickettsial infections*

VIRAL INFECTIONS

Many viruses infect the lower respiratory tract. They include the orthomyxoviruses (influenza virus), paramyxoviruses (parainfluenza viruses, measles virus and respiratory syncytial virus), adenoviruses, herpesviruses (cytomegalovirus, varicella-zoster virus and herpes simplex virus) and formerly variola virus (smallpox). Many of these viruses are of course also responsible for non-respiratory disease. The role of papillomavirus in neoplasia of the respiratory tract is discussed on page 535 and parvovirus is mentioned as a cause of hydrops fetalis on page 43. The role of herpes-like viruses in Kaposi's sarcoma and body cavity-based lymphomas is discussed on pages 635 and 734 respectively.

Viral infection of the lower respiratory tract occurs in three general situations: infections confined to the respiratory tract, systemic infections that involve the lung and opportunistic infection of the lungs in the immunocompromised (Box 5.1.1).

Respiratory viruses may strike any part or all the respiratory tract but on the whole each tends to affect particular parts and thereby elicit characteristic clinical effects (Fig. 5.1.1). This pattern varies however if there is some predisposing cause. Thus, the rhinoviruses, which usually cause nothing more serious than a cold, are the commonest viral trigger of acute exacerbations of chronic bronchitis, while in the immunodeficient herpes simplex virus and cytomegalovirus are serious pathogens in the lower respiratory tract.

The frequency of these various infections also differs in children and adults. In children, respiratory syncytial virus is the most important viral cause of lower respiratory tract disease, typically causing an obstructive bronchiolitis. Parainfluenza viruses are the most frequent cause of viral pneumonia in children, and the influenza virus in adults. These are followed by the measles and adenoviruses in children and varicella virus in adults, whilst the immunocompromised are also susceptible to cytomegalovirus and herpes simplex virus. A viral aetiology is responsible in 7–15% of adults admitted to hospital with community-acquired pneumonia (see Table 5.2.2, p. 178).

The virus responsible can be cultured from sputum or nasopharyngeal washings and evidence of infection by particular viruses may be provided by the demonstration of a rising titre of specific antibodies in the patient's serum. The advent of monoclonal antibodies has provided specific sensitive and reproducible probes that can be directly conjugated to a fluorescent tag so that the examination of exfoliated cells for viral antigen by immunofluorescent techniques is now the method of choice for the rapid identification of most respiratory

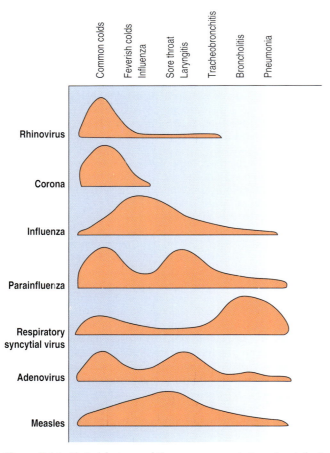

Figure 5.1.1 Clinical features of the common respiratory virus infections.

viruses. In tissue, the particular virus may be identified by immuno-cytochemistry, electron microscopy or gene probes.[1-7]

Most respiratory viral infections end in recovery. In fatal cases, the pathological changes in the lungs are often dominated by the effects of secondary bacterial infection, which is a very frequent complication. Few bacterial species have developed mechanisms for attachment to normal, intact human respiratory epithelium (notable exceptions being *Bordetella pertussis* and *Mycoplasma pneumoniae*) but viral injury to the epithelium permits bacterial attachment to take place and is associated with a greatly increased incidence of bacterial pneumonia.

From the occasional postmortem studies that have been undertaken in uncomplicated cases of viral pneumonia it is apparent that the inflammatory reaction in the lung is mainly lymphocytic and intersti-tial. Neutrophils are numerous only when there is a complicating bacterial infection. At the alveolar level viruses cause an atypical pneumonia characterised by a chronic inflammatory interstitial infiltrate rather than the acute inflammatory exudates that fill the air spaces in the bacterial pneumonias.

The pathology is modified to some extent by the type of virus responsible but infections caused by different viruses have many features in common.[8] In the lungs, as in other organs, some viruses have a cytopathic effect and kill the infected host cells, whilst others stimulate proliferative activity. Thus, influenza, adenovirus, varicella and herpes simplex pneumonia are all characterised by epithelial cell necrosis (Figs 5.1.2 and 5.1.3), whilst respiratory syncytial virus and measles virus stimulate mitotic division and cause characteristic proliferative changes in the bronchioles and alveoli respectively. The distribution of the changes is often characteristic of a particular virus, but not specific. Thus, within the alveoli, influenza tends to affect the epithelium diffusely. The effects of adenovirus, on the other hand, are generally maximal in the region of the terminal bronchioles, whilst varicella pneumonia is also focal but lacks any particular relationship to the acinar architecture. Viral inclusions are evident in certain viral pneumonias, notably measles, adenovirus, cytomegalovirus, varicella and herpes simplex pneumonia, but not in others.

Alveolar epithelial necrosis is a feature of severe viral pneumonia. It causes the formation of hyaline membranes (Fig. 5.1.3) and the pathology of such viral pneumonia is essentially that of diffuse alveo-lar damage (see Chapter 4). The regenerative changes seen in diffuse alveolar damage may be evident, possibly involving epithelial metaplasia.

Much of the damage caused by respiratory viruses is due to a direct cytopathic effect on the infected cells but there may also be indirect injury. The latter may be due to normal immune mechanisms such as cytotoxic T lymphocytes attacking infected host cells, depression of immunity by the virus (facilitating secondary infections) or the development of autoimmunity initiated by the virus.

The possible threat of bioterrorism is a feature of life today and, because of the ease with which they may be widely dispersed, respiratory pathogens figure large in the thinking of defence forces. The US Centers for Disease Control have classified six agents as category A threats. Several of these will be considered in this infectious disease section. The six category A agents are *Bacillus anthracis* (anthrax), *Variola major* (smallpox), *Yersinia pestis* (plague), *Francisella tularensis* (tularaemia), viral haemorrhagic agents and *Clostridium botulinum* toxin. Category B and C agents, which are seen as posing less of a threat, include the repiratory pathogens *Coxiella burnetti* (Q fever), Hantavirus and multidrug-resistant *Mycobacterium tuberculosis*.

Influenza

Microbiology and epidemiology

Influenza is epidemic almost annually in the winter months in many parts of the world and at long intervals the disease occurs in pandemic form, notably in 1889–92, 1918–19, 1957–58, 1968 and 2009. It is estimated that in the pandemic that followed the world war of 1914–18, some 20–30 million people died from the disease in little more

Figure 5.1.2 Necrotising viral bronchiolitis. The bronchiolar epithelium is partly destroyed and the lumen is largely filled with pus due to secondary bacterial infection.

Figure 5.1.3 Viral pneumonia causing necrosis of the alveolar epithelium with the formation of hyaline membranes. The virus responsible in this patient was that of measles but many respiratory viruses have a similar effect, as do several other cytotoxic factors: see diffuse alveolar damage, in Chapter 4. *(Courtesy of Dr V Chrystal, Durban, South Africa.)*

than a year, more than were killed in the war itself. Until 1933 it was widely believed that the disease was caused by the bacterium *Haemophilus influenzae*. The discovery in 1933 that the disease could be transmitted to ferrets by intranasal inoculation of filtered washings from the noses of patients established its viral nature.[9]

There are several types of influenza virus. All are originally bird viruses, some crossing from birds to species such as humans, pigs, horses and seals. Once established in the new species they undergo constant changes in their antigenic makeup, a feature that necessitates the constant manufacture of new vaccines. The strains involved in most serious human infections belong to types A and B, with the former much the more virulent. Outbreaks of infection with influenza A occur most years, with epidemics every 5–15 years. Influenza B also causes epidemics, but less frequently. Influenza C does not appear to cause epidemics. Successive epidemics appear to be decreasing in severity, possibly due to natural selection involving evolutionary changes that favour transmissibility over pathogenicity.[10]

Antigenic lability involves changes in the principal surface antigens of the virus, haemagglutinin and neuraminidase. Minor changes ('antigenic drift') are seen progressively from season to season. Major changes ('antigenic shift') due to acquisition of a new haemagglutinin occur periodically and are responsible for the emergence of new subtypes to which populations have little immunity and which therefore cause epidemics or pandemics. Influenza epidemics generally occur in the winter months and often start in countries south of the equator or in the east, giving northern and western countries time to prepare and distribute appropriate vaccines to those most at risk, notably the infirm. Influenza A viruses are named after their haemagglutinins (H1, H2, etc.), their neuraminidases (N1, N2, N3, etc.), and the place where and year when the strain was first identified. Thus, the 1968 pandemic virus was H3N2 influenza A/Hong Kong/68.

The haemagglutinin molecule enables the virus to attach to host cells prior to infecting them and neuraminidase permits new virus particles to bud from the cell membrane. Although there are considerable differences between the influenza viruses that infect different species, the haemagglutinin molecule's lability occasionally permits its virus to switch from one host species to another, in which the disease is likely to spread in epidemic form. It appears that all the devastating influenza pandemics of the twentieth century, such as Spanish flu in 1918, Asian flu in 1957 and Hong Kong flu in 1968, were caused by viruses that made such a switch from birds to humans.[11]

Recent genomic studies of the H1N1 virus responsible for the 1918 pandemic suggest that it was an avian virus that adapted to humans, rather than developing by a reassortment of avian and human viruses, as in the 1957 and 1968 pandemics.[12]

The switch from animals to humans in the 'wet markets' of the Far East is also relevant to the severe acute respiratory syndrome (SARS), described on page 163.

In 2004, the H5N1 strain of the influenza A virus devastated flocks of poultry in Asia and was responsible for the deaths of some humans from what was termed 'Asian bird flu'.[13,14] This strain was not very infective to humans, possibly because the temperature of the human nose (32°C) is too cold for a virus whose natural host is the avian intestine (temperature 40°C).[15,16] However, when the virus succeeded in infecting humans it was particularly virulent for two reasons. First, it was resistant to the antiviral effects of human interferons and tumour necrosis factor-α, a property acquired by a simple mutation in the non-structural gene resulting in a change from aspartate to glutamate at position 92.[17] Second, it preferentially targeted the alveolar rather than the tracheobronchial epithelium.[18]

The year 2009 saw swine influenza A/H1N1 virus switch to humans and exhibit the ability to spread from case to case, rapidly assuming pandemic proportions. Pigs are unusual in that their respiratory epithelium has receptors for both avian and human influenza viruses so that they can be infected with these viruses simultaneously, providing the ideal environment for genetic reassortment. This appears to have taken place as the 2009 swine influenza virus shows a novel reassortment of genes derived from swine, avian and human influenza viruses, a feature that is probably responsible for this virus being able to infect both pigs and humans. Unlike seasonal influenza, the disease made its first appearance in the northern hemisphere, apparently originating in Mexico, and its first impact was during the summer months. There was much mild disease but again, in contrast to seasonal influenza, severe respiratory failure was seen in young, previously healthy persons, as is often the case in influenza pandemics. This feature is not well explained but it is possible that the healthy mount a more vigorous immune response that is in some way detrimental to the host. Older people were less susceptible but more likely to die when infected.[19] However, one year later it was apparent that the pandemic had not proved as severe as first thought.

Clinical features

The severity of influenza varies from one epidemic to another and from case to case. In its uncomplicated form it is relatively mild, with fever, coryza, headache and body aches as its main features, and recovery after a few days. When the viral infection is followed by invasion of the lungs by staphylococci, pneumococci, streptococci or *Haemophilus influenzae*, the condition assumes a much graver form and the fatality rate may rise alarmingly. Infection rates are highest among schoolchildren and decrease with age but death is commonest in infants, the elderly and those with underlying lung or heart disease, and is generally due to complications.

Primary influenzal pneumonia is generally rare but figured prominently in the 1918–19 pandemic. It carries a high case fatality rate and in the 1918–19 pandemic it was notable that mortality was highest in adults aged 25–34, possibly because older people had been exposed earlier to a similar strain of the virus.[20,21] Primary influenzal pneumonia may be fulminant, leading to the death of a previously healthy person within a few hours of the onset of symptoms.[22]

Recent years have seen the development of effective antiviral agents such as the drugs oseltamivir (Tamiflu) and zanamivir (Relenza) which inhibit viral neuraminidase (in contrast to anti-influenza vaccines, which target viral haemagglutinin).

Pathology of uncomplicated influenza

The cytopathic effect of influenza virus is seen microscopically in characteristic degenerative changes in the epithelial cells of the bronchial and bronchiolar mucosa. These changes involve all cells of the surface epithelium and often the cells lining the bronchial glands: swelling of the cells, vacuolation of their cytoplasm and degeneration of the nucleus proceed to cell loss and frank necrosis (Fig. 5.1.4). Viral inclusions are not evident but the virus can be identified in tissue sections by immunocytochemistry and in situ hybridisation.[23,24] The deeper tissues show oedema, hyperaemia and a moderate to marked accumulation of lymphocytes; neutrophils are present but account for only a small proportion of the cellular infiltrate.

Alveolar involvement is unusual but cases of fulminating influenzal viral pneumonia are occasionally encountered, particularly with the 1918 and more recent H5N1 and H1N1 strains.[14,24,25] Autopsy in such cases shows that the lungs are bulky and deeply congested.[14,22,24a] Blood-stained, frothy fluid oozes freely from the cut surface. Areas of haemorrhage are present and may be extensive. The mucosa of the bronchial tree is very hyperaemic. Microscopically, the alveoli contain

Figure 5.1.4 Influenza. This cytopathic virus has totally destroyed the bronchial epithelium, predisposing to bacterial superinfection.

a fibrin-rich oedema fluid, which is often frankly haemorrhagic. Macrophages may be numerous in the exudate and hyaline membranes are often found lining the alveoli. T lymphocytes are often prominent in the alveolar interstitium while focal necrosis of alveolar walls and thrombosis of capillaries are conspicuous features in the parts most severely affected.[26]

Postmortem examination of two victims of the H5N1 virus showed similar evidence of diffuse alveolar damage but it was also found that viral replication in the respiratory tract had resulted in particularly high levels of cytokines such as interferons and tumour necrosis factor-α, which, with the resultant haemophagocytic syndrome, was considered to be the chief cause of death.[27] Generally, however, H5N1 viral pneumonia shows no special features and it may be difficult to distinguish the changes brought about by the H5N1 virus from those caused by viruses such as that responsible for SARS or by factors such as acid aspiration or oxygen toxicity. More specific tests such as viral isolation, in situ hybridisation and reverse transcription-polymerase chain reaction (RT-PCR) are required to confirm H5N1 infection.

Fulminant uncomplicated influenzal pneumonia is often associated with changes in other parts of the body that indicate the occurrence of influenzal viraemia[14]: among these are haemorrhagic encephalomyelitis, which is an acute infective condition distinct from postinfluenzal encephalomyelopathy, rhabdomyolysis and placentitis.[28,29]

In the healing phase of influenzal pneumonia there is conspicuous swelling of the alveolar lining cells, which proliferate and in places may virtually fill the lumen. The proliferation of alveolar lining cells may be so marked as to produce appearances somewhat resembling a neoplastic state. The changes reach their peak on about the third to fifth day of the disease and then regress, eventually subsiding completely. Also during the phase of recovery, regeneration of the bronchial epithelium may involve squamous metaplasia, but this soon gives place to normal ciliated pseudostratified respiratory tract epithelium.

Bacterial superinfection in influenza

Although pneumonia is the usual cause of death in epidemics of influenza, it is often a secondary bacterial pneumonia that is responsible. Neutrophilic exudates, organising pneumonia and bronchiolitis obliterans are then added to or replace the changes seen in uncomplicated cases.[22,24,30–33] The impact an influenza epidemic has on respiratory death rates in general is shown in Figure 5.1.5.

Before the discovery of the influenza virus in 1933, the changes that are now known to be due to the viral infection were often confused with those of complicating infections, mainly caused by bacteria. *Haemophilus influenzae* was first isolated in the 1889–90 pandemic and so named because its discoverer, Pfeiffer, recovered it from a large proportion of cases and mistook it for the cause of influenza. In the 1918–19 pandemic *H. influenzae* was again found, along with *Streptococcus pneumoniae* and *Staphylococcus aureus.*[32] With the advent of antibiotics, resistant strains of *Staphylococcus aureus* emerged and in the 1957–58 pandemic staphylococcal superinfection of the lungs was the major fatal complication of influenza. In the 1968 epidemic *Streptococcus pneumoniae* was the principal bacterial pathogen in the elderly and *Staphylococcus aureus* in the young.[30]

The relationship of the staphylococcus and the influenza virus has been much studied and there is evidence that each promotes the growth of the other.[34] Thus, certain staphylococci have a protein in their cell wall that binds to the Fc region of immunoglobulin G. In the presence of anti-influenzal serum this protein enhances staphylococcal binding to cells infected by the influenza virus[35] and in this way the staphylococcus takes advantage of the host's immune reaction to the influenza virus. In turn, the staphylococcus aids entry of the

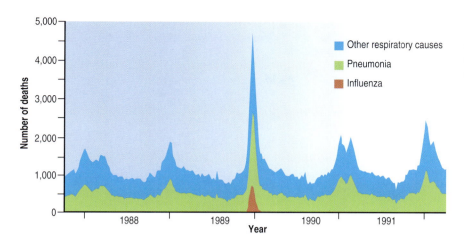

Figure 5.1.5 Weekly deaths from respiratory disease in England and Wales 1987–92, showing the impact of an influenza epidemic in 1989/90 on deaths from other respiratory diseases. *(Data supplied by the Lung and Asthma Information Centre.)*

virus into the host's cell. It does this by secreting a protease that activates a viral surface protein necessary for penetration of the host's cells[36]: normally such proteases are in short supply, so limiting the rate at which influenza virus can infect cells and reproduce. The relationship of influenza and *Streptococcus pneumoniae* infection has been studied in less detail but there is evidence of similar enhancement of bacterial adherence to tracheal epithelium following influenza infection.[37]

Parainfluenza

Parainfluenza is caused by the parainfluenza viruses, not by *Haemophilus parainfluenzae*. It is commoner in children and particularly affects the larynx, causing croup. There may be necrosis of the mucosa as in influenza (Fig. 5.1.6A), and quite frequently small polypoid growths of the bronchial and bronchiolar epithelium develop, similar to those associated with infection by respiratory syncytial virus (see below). In the lung there is hyperplasia of the alveolar epithelium and a serous exudate containing increased numbers of macrophages is seen. In immunosuppressed individuals, parainfluenza type III virus may result in a giant cell pneumonia that is indistinguishable from that of measles except that the inclusion bodies typical of measles pneumonia are not a feature (Fig. 5.1.6B).[38–41]

Respiratory syncytial virus

Epidemiology

Respiratory syncytial virus was first isolated in 1956 from an outbreak of coryza in a colony of chimpanzees and its infectivity for Man was shown when one of the investigators of this epizootic illness contracted the disease. It has since been shown that the virus frequently infects the lower respiratory passages of Man, particularly the young.[42] Specific neutralising antibodies indicative of an earlier infection are found in the serum of almost all children over the age of 5 years in Britain. Most children merely develop a cold but a few suffer from severe bronchiolitis, which in the developing world is an important cause of death in the very young.[42a,b] Those that recover are prone to develop recurrent wheeze later in childhood.[42c] The immunity infection conveys is incomplete and reinfections may occur throughout life.

Respiratory syncytial virus infection shows a marked seasonal pattern, producing annual epidemics each winter in temperate climates and in the hot rainy season in tropical countries. During an incubation period of 3–6 days the virus replicates in the upper

Figure 5.1.6 Parainfluenza in an immunosuppressed patient. (A) The epithelium of the bronchiole seen upper left has been destroyed and giant multinucleate epithelial cells are seen in adjacent alveoli. (B) Higher magnification of the giant cell pneumonia.

respiratory tract, causing fever, cough and coryza. Spread from the upper to the lower respiratory tract may occur, with consequent bronchiolitis and pneumonia.

Particularly important is the bronchiolitis that respiratory syncytial virus is prone to cause in infants. The conductive airways of small infants are quite narrow and easily blocked by relatively small amounts of inflammatory exudate: because of this, fatal asphyxia is liable to follow respiratory syncytial virus infection. This is particularly the case in those who have airflow obstruction as a consequence of prematurity and its treatment. Several epidemics of acute bronchiolitis due to this virus have been described among infants. These outbreaks are often remarkably focal in distribution, affecting only a comparatively small area or community. Infants with bronchopulmonary dysplasia and those who have congenital heart disease or are immunocompromised are particularly at risk and units specialising in these underlying conditions have to guard against nosocomial spread of infection.[43–45] However, most children with respiratory syncytial virus infection have no predisposing factors and even previously healthy children may suffer fatal infection.[42,46]

Figure 5.1.7 Respiratory syncytial virus infection in which the patency of the bronchioles is compromised by epithelial proliferation forming micropolypoid intrusions into the lumen. The bronchiolar lumen is further narrowed by a neutrophil exudate in response to secondary bacterial infection.

Pathogenesis

It is notable that infants under six months of age are particularly prone to respiratory syncytial virus infection. Although this is a period when the infant benefits from the presence of maternal antibodies, placental antibody transmission is selective, being better for immunoglobulin G than A. Breast-feeding protects against respiratory syncytial virus infection,[47] presumably by virtue of breast milk being rich in immunoglobulin A. It has been noted that infants immunized against the virus and subsequently infected naturally, suffer a more severe illness than those not so immunised,[48] suggesting that the damage is mediated immunologically.[49,50] This is supported by the finding that the typical bronchiolitis is characterised by scanty virus whereas in the rarer pneumonic form of the disease the virus is abundant. This is compatible with the bronchiolitis representing an adverse immune reaction and the pneumonia being the result of direct viral damage to the lungs.[51] The cytokine profile suggests that the reaction involved in the bronchiolitis involves a predominantly type 2 response characterised by high interleukin-10/interleukin-12 and interleukin-4/γ-interferon ratios.[52] Suspicion has fallen upon the formaldehyde inactivation of the vaccine creating reactive carbonyl groups on the antigen.[52a] Passive immunisation, conferred by monthly injection, is free of the hazards induced by active immunisation and is recommended for high-risk babies.[53]

Histopathology

The virus infects the bronchiolar epithelium and usually leads to its destruction.[54,55] Occasionally cytoplasmic inclusion bodies may be seen in degenerating bronchiolar epithelial cells or the virus may be demonstrated by immunocytochemistry.[1,55] Regeneration involves the proliferation of poorly differentiated cells which form a stratified non-ciliated epithelium. Occasionally micropolypoid epithelial protrusions are evident (Fig. 5.1.7).[8] The bronchioles are occluded by plugs of mucus, fibrin and epithelial cell debris, and cuffed by an infiltrate of lymphocytes, plasma cells and histiocytes. Except in the immediate vicinity of the bronchioles, alveoli are generally not involved in the inflammatory process. If, however, infection is on a major scale there may be pneumonia with the general features of a viral pneumonia, as described above.[46] In severe immunodeficiency, respiratory syncytial virus may cause giant cell pneumonia,[56] a condition that is more often caused by measles virus.

Metapneumovirus

Metapneumovirus was only discovered in 2001[57] but is now recognised to be ubiquitous; serological evidence of past infection is universal by the age of 5 years. Much of this goes unrecognised but metapneumovirus infection is nevertheless a leading cause of lower respiratory tract illness in young children. In one investigation the virus or its DNA was found in 20% of nasal-wash specimens previously declared virus-negative that had been collected from otherwise healthy infants and children suffering from a lower respiratory tract illness: the infection was associated with bronchiolitis in 59% of cases, pneumonia in 8%, croup in 18% and exacerbation of asthma in 14%, a spectrum of disease similar to that found with respiratory syncytial virus.[58] The pathological changes are not well described.

Measles
Clinical features and epidemiology

Measles (rubeola) is highly infectious and most children are infected soon after their maternal antibodies have waned, the peak incidence being between 1 and 5 years of age. After an incubation period of 1–2 weeks the patient develops coryza, cough and fever. The subsequent development of small red spots with a white centre (Koplik's spots) on the buccal mucosa followed by an erythematous maculopapular rash first involving the face and then the rest of the body facilitates the diagnosis. The infection resolves in about a week, following which the patient enjoys lifelong immunity.

In those parts of the world where measles has been prevalent for centuries the disease is almost invariably mild and, unless complicated by bacterial pneumonia, it has a very low mortality. In contrast, the mortality from measles may be appallingly high in lands to which the virus is newly introduced. When the disease was carried to Fiji from Australia in 1875, almost the whole population contracted it and a quarter of them succumbed. Similar outbreaks have occurred in more recent times, when the infection first reached Greenland for instance.

Measles has been regarded as one of the inevitable infections of childhood but with an effective safe vaccine now available this is no longer necessary (Fig. 5.1.8).[59] In the developed countries first and

Figure 5.1.8 Annual measles notifications and vaccine coverage in England and Wales 1950–1999. *(Adapted by permission from BMJ Publishing Group Limited.[56])*

both adenovirus and herpesvirus pneumonia.[65,66] Secondary pulmonary infection is responsible for about half the mortality in measles.[67] Other causes of death include measles pneumonia and measles encephalitis.

Measles may also be very severe when it affects immunodeficient patients, whether they are suffering from primary immunological defects, acquired diseases such as leukaemia or conditions which require treatment with cytotoxic or immunosuppressant drugs.[68] Such patients may have unpredictable responses to measles virus. They may have a rash but fail to produce antibodies, or they may fail to develop a rash although infected with the virus. Fatal measles pneumonia in a previously healthy adult is very rare.[69]

Pathology of measles pneumonia[70,71]

Death from measles pneumonia occurs typically about 2 weeks after the appearance of the rash. At necropsy, the lungs are heavy and of rubbery consistency, and their cut surface is pale pink. Close examination may show that the small bronchi are cuffed by a greyish zone. Extensive vascular thrombosis has been a feature of some cases.

Microscopically, there are degenerative changes in the epithelium of the bronchi and bronchioles, often accompanied by hyperplasia, particularly in the small airways. As in influenzal pneumonia, squamous metaplasia may occur and mitotic figures may be numerous. Measles pneumonia may take the form of diffuse alveolar damage with hyaline membrane formation (see Fig. 5.1.3), or, more characteristically, multinucleate giant cells may line the alveolar ducts and alveoli (Fig. 5.1.9). Electron microscopy shows that the giant cells are formed from type II alveolar epithelial cells.[71,72] The giant cells contain prominent cytoplasmic and nuclear viral inclusion bodies that are clearly evident in eosin-stained sections. Being epithelial, the pulmonary giant cells are quite different from the Warthin–Finkeldey giant cells that are found in lymphoid tissue throughout the body in measles, particularly in the immediately pre-exanthematous stage.

As well as the epithelial changes, there is a heavy accumulation of macrophages, lymphocytes and plasma cells in the alveolar walls. This cellular infiltrate extends into the connective tissue surrounding the bronchioles and small bronchi, accounting for the pale cuff that is seen around them on naked-eye examination. Neutrophils are not numerous unless there is a secondary bacterial infection. The appearances are closely comparable to those found in the lungs of dogs that have died of distemper (Carré's disease), which is also caused by a paramyxovirus.

Differential diagnosis

Measles is the commonest cause of giant cell pneumonia but occasionally other viruses such as parainfluenza, respiratory syncytial and varicella-zoster viruses are responsible, especially in the immunocompromised (see Fig. 5.1.6).[38,56,73] The diagnosis is usually evident clinically or is made serologically but immunohistochemistry can be performed on tissue sections. Hard-metal disease is also characterised by the presence of alveolar epithelial polykaryons but these are more focal than those of measles, lack viral inclusion bodies and are not accompanied by such severe interstitial pneumonia (see Fig.7.1.25, p. 354).

Adenovirus

Like measles, adenovirus causes a febrile rash and infects the upper respiratory tract much more commonly than the lungs. However, adenovirus may infect the lower respiratory tract at all levels and it is a relatively common cause of pneumonia in malnourished children throughout the world.

more recently in the developing world, immunisation against measles has been promoted vigorously, with spectacular success. Between 2000 and 2007 mortality from measles fell by 74% worldwide and by 89% in Africa, where it was formerly a major cause of death in childhood. The Americas were declared free of endemic measles transmission in 2002 and cases there now occur only as a result of its importation from other countries.[60,61] The disease has not yet been eradicated in the UK, partly because unfounded claims that the vaccine is responsible for autism led to declining vaccine uptake with consequent focal outbreaks of measles.[62] Other European countries still experiencing large outbreaks include the Ukraine, Switzerland and Austria.

Where measles is prevalent, the incidence is usually highest in the early spring, when droplet infections are particularly rife. The epidemics have a remarkably consistent biennial character (see Fig. 5.1.8) and the explanation of this has been the subject of several interesting hypotheses. The one most favoured envisages waning immunity over the succeeding 2 years in those children who had only a subclinical illness in the last epidemic. With the influx of two further entries into infant schools, a new population of susceptible children is formed that is liable to contract overt disease when the seasonal conditions are again favourable for the spread of the virus. In this way a fresh epidemic develops. Overt clinical disease, on the other hand, confers lifelong immunity.

If the lower respiratory tract is infected, the measles virus propagates in the epithelial cells of the main respiratory passages, leading to the destruction of many of the infected cells. In time there is recovery and multiplication of surviving cells, but at the height of the disease the natural defences of the lower respiratory tract are greatly compromised and secondary invading bacteria can successfully establish themselves in the lungs, causing bronchiolitis and pneumonia.

Pneumonia is a rare complication of measles in the western world but is common in malnourished African children, in whom it frequently proves fatal.[63] That pneumonic foci may develop in prosperous countries in the course of severe but non-fatal attacks of measles is shown by the demonstration in some such cases of patchy opacities on chest radiography: in almost all these cases the condition resolves rapidly. The cause is usually one of the common bacterial pathogens but it can be another virus taking advantage of the patient's debility and impaired cellular immunity. Measles virus infection is characterised by both the development of a strong antiviral immune response and abnormalities of immune regulation: there is often a poor skin response to common antigens and helper/suppressor T-cell ratios may be low in both the blood and bronchoalveolar lavage, suggesting that cellular immunity is impaired.[64] Thus, measles has predisposed to

Figure 5.1.9 Measles giant cell pneumonia. There is a syncytial proliferation of type II pneumocytes containing eosinophilic cytoplasmic and nuclear viral inclusions. This response is typical of measles pneumonia but is occasionally encountered with other forms of viral pneumonia (see Fig. 5.1.6).

Adenovirus pneumonia occurs sporadically and in epidemics, particularly in children and young adults, and occasionally complicates measles.[65,66] Adenovirus pneumonia is usually combined with bronchiolitis and the lesions are most severe at the centres of the acini, being concentrated on the bronchioles. The virus causes necrosis of the bronchioles, many of which are totally destroyed or are recognisable only by their muscle coat: hyaline membranes replace the necrotic epithelium (Fig. 5.1.10A). Surviving epithelial cells show nuclear inclusions of varying staining reaction: some are diffusely basophilic or amphiphilic and fill the entire nucleus apart from a rim of chromatin (Cowdry type B) while others are eosinophilic and surrounded by a clear halo (Cowdry type A). The bronchioles are cuffed by a lymphoid infiltrate and may show proliferative epithelial activity, variously interpreted as being the result of viral stimulation or of regeneration.[54,74] The alveolar tissue shows a mononuclear interstitial pneumonia.

The intranuclear viral inclusions measure up to 5 µm and eventually disrupt the nucleus, leaving so-called smudge cells (Fig. 5.1.10B, C). Healing may be by complete resolution or the pneumonia may be complicated by bronchiolitis obliterans or bronchiectasis.[75]

Figure 5.1.10 Adenovirus pneumonia. (A) Bronchioles bear the brunt of the damage and here show necrosis of their lining epithelium. (B) Viable alveolar lining cells contain basophilic nuclear inclusions while others are necrotic, having been reduced to eosinophilic 'smudge cells' by the viral inclusions disrupting the nucleus. (A and B from sections provided by the late Dr N Rossouw, Tygerberg, South Africa and Dr V Chrystal, Durban, South Africa.) (C) Electron microscopy shows that adenovirus particles measure 70–100 nm and have a naked icosahedral structure. (Courtesy of Miss A Dewar, Brompton, UK.)

Severe acute respiratory syndrome

SARS first appeared in southern China in 2002, from where it quickly traversed the globe, facilitated by air travel and coming to international attention particularly after an outbreak in Hong Kong in 2003.[76–81] Cases were subsequently identified in many countries and about 10% of those affected died.[82–85] The cause was a previously unknown coronavirus that had switched from civet cats encountered in Asian food markets and adapted to human transmission.[86,87] Transmission is air-borne but requires close person-to-person contact. There is no evidence of transmission following casual contact. The virus has subsequently been identified in Chinese horseshoe bats and it is likely that these animals represent the natural reservoir of the virus, with the civets merely acting as carriers.[88,89]

Clinical features

The incubation period ranges from 1 to 10 days, following which there is a prodromal fever, cough and dyspnoea. Less common symptoms include headache, diarrhoea, dizziness, myalgia, chills, nausea, vomiting and rigor.[90] There is no apparent sex predilection and the age distribution is wide. Common laboratory features include lymphopenia involving both CD4 and CD8 lymphocytes, thrombocytopenia, prolonged thromboplastin time, elevated alanine transminase, lactate dehydrogenase and creatinine kinase. Positive viral recovery rates from urine, nasopharyngeal aspirate and stool specimen have been reported to be 42%, 68% and 97% respectively on day 14 of illness, whereas serological confirmation may take 28 days to reach a detection rate above 90%. However, quantitative measurement of blood SARS coronavirus RNA using real-time RT-PCR techniques has a detection rate of 80% as early as day 1 of hospital admission.[91]

Radiographic abnormalities include focal, multifocal or diffuse opacities. Computed tomography is more sensitive, sometimes showing extensive consolidation in patients with normal chest radiographs. However, the radiological features are not specific and need to be correlated with the clinical and histological findings.[92]

Pathogenesis

Although pulmonary involvement is the dominant clinical manifestation, extrapulmonary features are common and the virus can often be recovered from faeces and urine, indicating that it is widely distributed in the body. The identification of a specific receptor for the virus is relevant to its tissue distribution. The receptor, a metallopeptidase known as angiotensin-converting enzyme 2, is expressed particularly strongly by pulmonary alveolar and small intestinal epithelia and vascular endothelia.[93–95]

Pathology

The histology varies according to the duration of illness but the predominant pattern is diffuse alveolar damage.[96–100] Cases of less than 10 days' duration show air space oedema and hyaline membranes whereas those of longer duration exhibit type II pneumocyte hyperplasia, squamous metaplasia, multinucleated giant cells and acute bronchopneumonia succeeded by intra-alveolar organisation.[26,96] The alveolar pneumocytes may also show striking cytomegaly with granular amphophilic cytoplasm (Fig. 5.1.11), that sometimes contains eosinophilic inclusions akin to the Mallory bodies of alcoholic hepatitis.[96,97] Less common features include haemophagocytosis and thrombosis.[97,99] The virus can be identified by RT-PCR in fresh or formalin-fixed, paraffin-embedded lung tissue. Electron microscopy may reveal the viral particles in the cytoplasm of epithelial cells.[97–99]

Figure 5.1.11 Severe acute respiratory syndrome. (A) The features of early diffuse alveolar damage are seen, consisting of extravasation of red blood cells, desquamation, an acute and chronic interstitial inflammatory infiltrate and a few hyaline membranes. (B) Regenerating epithelial cells show nuclear atypia.

Treatment and prognosis

Treatment with corticosteroids, broad-spectrum antibiotics and antiviral agents has been beneficial.[98,102] Interferon-α may also have a role.[103] However, infection control is as important as pharmacological therapy in this disease.

In the acute phase, SARS is associated with considerable morbidity and mortality, with a global case fatality rate ranging from 7 to 27% (average about 11%). Adverse prognostic factors include advanced age, coexistent disease, high lactose dehydrogenase levels and high initial neutrophil counts. CT data on the extent of the disease are also useful in assessing prognosis.[104] Clinical follow-up of patients who recover has demonstrated residual abnormalities of varying degree, including abnormal lung function and patchy fibrosis.[105,106] Many survivors also experienced transient pituitary dysfunction.[107]

Herpes simplex[108,109]

Virology and predisposing causes

Herpes simplex virus typically causes mucocutaneous vesiculation, serotype 1 (HSV1) generally affecting the oronasal area and serotype 2 (HSV2) the genital mucosae. As with all herpesviruses, infection is lifelong; the virus remains dormant until immunity weakens, which may be triggered by a variety of factors. In these circumstances either serotype may involve the lower respiratory tract. Respiratory infection by HSV1 is more commonly encountered in adults, the infection spreading from the oropharynx, whereas neonatal respiratory infection is usually due to HSV2 as a component of generalised haematogenous disease.[110,111] Infection of the lower respiratory tract takes the form of tracheobronchitis or pneumonia. Herpes simplex tracheobronchitis is predisposed to by damage to the respiratory epithelium, especially factors that lead to squamous metaplasia, such as endotracheal intubation and burns.[112–116] Risk factors for herpes simplex pneumonia include transplantation,[117] cytotoxic chemotherapy and human immunodeficiency virus (HIV) infection[118]: herpes simplex pneumonia is rare in the immunocompetent.[119]

Pathology

In herpes simplex tracheobronchitis there is extensive mucosal ulceration and pseudomembrane formation. Viral inclusions are most prominent at the periphery of the ulcers and may be identified in exfoliated cells (Fig. 5.1.12). If they are not well developed an immunostain may establish the diagnosis. Long-standing airway infection leads to luminal narrowing and obstructive features. In the lungs the changes are very similar to those of adenovirus pneumonia, including the presence of Cowdry type B ground-glass intranuclear viral inclusions, although these are more eosinophilic than those of adenovirus. Both adenovirus and herpes simplex pneumonia bear a superficial resemblance to bacterial bronchopneumonia but the similarity is in the distribution of the lesions rather than their character: the bronchioles and centriacinar alveoli are mainly affected but the lesions are characterised by necrosis and the accumulation of nuclear

Figure 5.1.12 Herpes simplex virus. Bronchial brushings from an ulcer in the lower trachea show multinucleate epithelial cells with glassy nuclear features. From a patient with oral herpes who had started steroid therapy for asthma.

debris rather than exudation of neutrophils. Occasionally herpes simplex infection takes the form of a focal necrotising pneumonia more typical of varicella infection (see below). Alternatively there may be arterial involvement in herpes simplex pneumonia with a necrotising vasculitis affecting small and medium-sized pulmonary arteries.[120] Sometimes the pneumonia is diffuse: it is suggested that focal disease represents extension of oral mucocutaneous herpesvirus infection down the tracheobronchial tree into the lung whereas diffuse pneumonia is the result of haematogenous spread.[108]

Cytomegalovirus

Virology and epidemiology

Cytomegalovirus is the largest of the herpesviruses and is widespread in most communities, persisting for life, like all herpesviruses. It is transmitted in saliva and blood and by sexual contact and organ transplantation. Seropositivity, taken to indicate carriage of the virus, steadily increases with age. The prevalence of seropositivity in adults is generally over 50% and approaches 100% in homosexual men. However, carriage of the virus does not necessarily equate with disease. The immunocompetent host is unlikely to experience any recognisable clinical effects of cytomegalovirus infection.

Symptomatic cytomegalovirus infection is seen in newborn children infected before birth by virus carried by their mother, and in adults who have undergone organ transplantation or have been infected with HIV. In the newborn the disease presents as an acute fatal infection with jaundice and leukoerythroblastic anaemia.

Cytomegalovirus is a serious pathogen in transplantation recipients,[121] possibly because the virus replicates best in cells that are activated, as in a transplanted organ. The risk is greatest with bone marrow transplantation, intermediate with heart, lung and liver transplantation and lowest with renal transplantation. However, donor and recipient matching for cytomegalovirus status has reduced the incidence of transmission from the donor. Before the introduction of this policy, fatal cytomegalovirus pneumonia or systemic infection was common. Today reactivation of latent infection is a more common problem but it is important to distinguish the mere presence of viral inclusions from pneumonitis. When a lymphoid infiltrate accompanies the viral inclusions it is also important to distinguish an infective pneumonitis from lung allograft rejection: generally, the infiltrate of cytomegalovirus pneumonia lacks the perivascular lymphocyte distribution seen in rejection. As well as causing a pneumonitis that has to be distinguished from rejection, cytomegalovirus may be involved in chronic lung rejection.[122] It has been speculated that cytomegalovirus could promote allograft rejection by stimulating the production of proinflammatory cytokines or increasing the expression of major histocompatibility complex molecules.

The position of cytomegalovirus in regard to pulmonary disease in acquired immunodeficiency syndrome (AIDS) can also be difficult to determine. Cytomegalovirus inclusions are frequently encountered in AIDS but it is often difficult to determine whether pathological changes are due to the virus or to accompanying bacterial or *Pneumocystis* infection. Only occasionally is cytomegalovirus the only pathogen identified in severe pneumonia in AIDS patients.[123] Some investigators claim that cytomegalovirus contributes to the high mortality from pneumonia in AIDS patients[124] while others view it merely as a bystander rather than the primary pathogen in these patients.[125] Sometimes, replication of the virus is unaccompanied by any significant degree of pulmonary inflammation or damage,[126] indicating a poor host response, which, as in other viral infections, largely involves T lymphocytes, cells that are particularly defective in AIDS. The differing roles of cytomegalovirus in AIDS and transplant recipients have led to the view that the pathological changes are not a direct effect of the virus but an immunopathological condition attributable to the T-cell response to the virus.[127]

Pathological features

The pneumonia may be unilateral or bilateral, and generally involves the lower lobes; advanced lesions may appear as reddish purple nodular areas. Two patterns of pulmonary involvement have been described in bone marrow transplant recipients: a fulminant systemic infection characterised by a miliary pattern of disease and a more insidious disease with a more diffuse distribution in the lungs.[121]

Histologically, there is a chronic interstitial pneumonitis and some of the alveolar epithelial cells are enlarged and contain characteristic inclusions. These measure up to as much as 10 μm in diameter and are surrounded by a clear zone inside the nuclear membrane (Fig. 5.1.13). These Cowdry type A intranuclear inclusions have been likened to an owl's eyes. The inclusions represent clumped chromatin and the clear zone the virus. Cytoplasmic inclusions up to 2 μm in diameter are often also present. Severe cases may show a necrotising pneumonia or tracheobronchitis without the inclusions being well developed, in which case immunocytochemistry or in situ hybridisation may be used to advantage as these techniques show that many more cells are infected than those containing the characteristic inclusions (see Fig. 5.1.13D).[6,7,128] Diffuse alveolar damage is a further pattern of disease that is occasionally seen in cytomegalovirus pneumonia.

HIV and AIDS

Virology and means of spread

The HIVs belong to the lentivirus subfamily of the retroviruses and are thought to have originated from chimpanzees, which harbour the closely related simian immunodeficiency virus. They are the cause of AIDS and are transmitted primarily through sexual contact, by anal or vaginal intercourse with an HIV-positive person. Other routes of transmission are by exposure to infected blood, generally through the use of contaminated needles and syringes by drug addicts. Infected blood products and donor tissues are other potential sources of infection. An infected woman can pass the virus to her child in utero, at delivery or through breast-feeding. Occupational acquisition of HIV is unusual but has occurred, chiefly through needlestick injuries. In histopathology departments, particular care is required in handling unfixed tissues, as in preparing frozen sections and conducting autopsies. Fixed tissues do not present a risk of infection. Most national bodies have produced guidelines for safe laboratory practice in the AIDS era.[129] HIV infection is not always recognisable and a practical approach is therefore to treat every cadaver and all unfixed tissue as if it were infectious.

Pathogenesis of AIDS

Following entry into the body and the development of neutralising antibodies, HIV is found in highest concentration within the germinal centres of lymphoid tissue where it can be demonstrated by immunohistochemistry attached to a follicular dendritic cell.[129a] The virus attacks both the follicular dendritic cells and the CD4+ helper T lymphocytes and blood levels of these latter cells below 200/μL are associated with the development of a variety of AIDS-defining conditions. The interferon-γ-secreting Th1 cells that are central to immune defence against a variety of other infections are particularly vulnerable to attack. Once HIV infection has occurred, antibody develops, generally within a month, and after a period that is usually measured in years CD4 counts drop and manifestations of AIDS develop. Concentrations

of virus in the blood and body fluids are particularly high around the time of seroconversion and when AIDS develops.

Epidemiology

AIDS was first recognised in 1981 in Haiti, since when it has spread widely and few countries are now spared its ravages. A quarter of a century after its first recognition AIDS had killed about 25 million people and about 65 million had been infected with HIV. Many of those harbouring HIV do not know they are infected. The number of people infected with HIV is rising, because of population growth and because drug treatment is prolonging life. The epidemic is worst in sub-Saharan Africa and next the Caribbean but it is growing fastest in eastern Europe and central Asia. Worldwide, women make up about half of those infected with HIV, with the largest number in sub-Saharan Africa. Since the introduction of highly active antiretroviral therapy (HAART) mortality rates have declined and life expectancy improved amongst those so treated, but these benefits have so far been largely confined to the industrialised countries.

Pathology

Few organs escape the ravages of fully developed AIDS but the lungs are those most frequently involved in many series.[130,131] AIDS has many pulmonary manifestations, all of which are described in detail under their relevant headings. Most are secondary to the immunodeficiency but it is possible that certain lymphocytic infiltrates reflect HIV infection of the lung. These are generally non-specific T-cell infiltrates, which are largely CD8+ and milder than those that characterise lymphoid interstitial pneumonia[132–136]; HIV has been identified in the lung tissue by in situ hybridisation in a minority of cases.[135] The heavier lymphoid infiltrates of lymphoid interstitial pneumonia seen in HIV-infected children largely comprise CD8+ HIV-specific lymphocytes. Such children have fewer opportunistic infections and survive longer than other HIV-positive children, suggesting that in this setting lymphoid interstitial pneumonia reflects an effective immune response.[137] Experiments in mice suggest that viral persistence and interferon-γ production are involved.[138,139]

The commonest pulmonary manifestations of AIDS are listed in Table 5.1.1.[140–150] Rarer pulmonary manifestations include infection by herpes simplex[118,151] and varicella-zoster[152] viruses, *Blastomyces dermatitidis*,[153] *Candida* species,[152] cryptosporidia,[154] microsporidia[155] and *Strongyloides stercoralis*.[152] There is also an increased incidence of respiratory infection by common pyogenic organisms,[143,156,157] especially *Streptococcus pneumoniae* and *Haemophilus influenzae*,[152] sometimes resulting in obliterative bronchiolitis[158] or unusual diseases such as bacterial tracheitis[159] where the trachea is narrowed by pus or necrotic material containing colonies of mixed bacteria. Tuberculosis has also made an unwelcome resurgence since the advent of AIDS.[160–162] Opportunistic mycobacterial infection,[163] malakoplakia,[164,165] bacillary angiomatosis,[166] secondary alveolar lipoproteinosis,[167] follicular bronchitis and bronchiolitis[149] are also encountered in AIDS patients. However, there are marked geographical differences in the incidences of these manifestations of AIDS: tuberculosis is particularly common in poor countries whereas *Pneumocystis*, non-tuberculous mycobacteriosis and lymphoma are commoner in richer communities. Since the 1990s there has been a trend towards multiple infections, more mycobacterial disease and less *Pneumocystis* infection and Kaposi's sarcoma.[130,142,168]

In most cases the secondary pulmonary infections can be diagnosed from material obtained through the fibreoptic bronchoscope (brushings, washings, lavage or biopsy)[169] or from sputum[170] but occasionally a particular pulmonary manifestation of AIDS is not revealed until open biopsy is undertaken or examination is made postmortem.

Figure 5.1.13 Cytomegalovirus pneumonia. (A) There is a prominent nuclear inclusion in the centre of the field. (B) Electron micrograph of an alveolar epithelial cell infected by cytomegalovirus. Numerous viral particles are evident in both nucleus (above) and cytoplasm (below). As the viral particles leave the nucleus and enter the cytoplasm they acquire a coating derived from the nuclear envelope and consequently enlarge. (C) Low-power electron micrograph of the cell seen in (B), showing that it is greatly enlarged compared with its neighbours. Coated viral particles are evident in the cytoplasm but uncoated particles in the nucleus are too small to be recognised at this magnification. However, characteristic central clumping of the chromatin is evident. (B and C courtesy of Miss A Dewar, Brompton, UK.) (D) Immunocytochemistry shows abundant virus in the cytoplasm as well as the nucleus (immunoperoxidase stain).

Table 5.1.1 The varieties of pulmonary disease described in 131 patients with AIDS.[137,138] **The opportunistic invaders are often present in combination and the inflammatory reaction to them is often atypical: for example, the reaction to mycobacterial infection (frequently *Mycobacterium avium-intracellulare*) is often non-granulomatous, whilst *Pneumocystis jirovecii* may provoke a granulomatous response or diffuse alveolar damage, rather than the usual foamy alveolar exudate**

	Patients (%)
Opportunistic infection	
Pneumocystis jirovecii pneumonia[a]	63
Cytomegalovirus pneumonia	19
Mycobacterial pneumonia	13
Bacterial pneumonia[a]	8
Invasive candidiasis	2
Toxoplasmosis	2
Cryptococcosis	1
Invasive aspergillosis	1
Histoplasmosis	1
Non-infectious diseases	
Diffuse alveolar damage	15
Kaposi's sarcoma	9
Non-specific interstitial pneumonitis[a]	5
Pulmonary haemorrhage	3
Pulmonary lymphoid hyperplasia[b]	0
Lymphoid interstitial pneumonia	2
Lymphoma[a]	2

[a]Since the introduction of highly active antiretroviral therapy (HAART), *P. jirovecii* pneumonia has become less common while bacterial pneumonia and lymphoma have increased.[139–141]

[b]Pulmonary lymphoid hyperplasia is seen particularly in children suffering from acquired immunodeficiency syndrome (AIDS)[142–145] but is also recorded in occasional adults.[146] Together with lymphoid interstitial pneumonia, pulmonary lymphoma and the sicca syndrome,[147] it forms a spectrum of pulmonary lymphoproliferative disease in AIDS and other conditions.

Rapidly progressive plexogenic pulmonary hypertension is also reported in persons infected by HIV but generally not evincing AIDS.[171–176] The lungs are often otherwise normal. The virus has not been identified in the pulmonary vessels but tubuloreticular structures suggestive of cytokine accumulation have been identified there by electron microscopy in HIV-positive individuals.[177] Less frequently, veno-occlusive disease or thrombotic arteriopathy is the basis of HIV-associated pulmonary hypertension. Emboli of foreign particulate material may also be found in the lungs of patients who have acquired their HIV infection through the intravenous injection of drugs formulated for oral use, while a variety of vasculitides affecting various organs including the lungs is described.[178]

As well as the neoplastic manifestations of AIDS listed in Table 5.1.1 (Kaposi's sarcoma and lymphoma), the incidence of carcinoma of the lung is increased in AIDS and the affected patients are younger

than those in the general population.[179–181] All these tumours may present as endobronchial lesions, as may tuberculosis and aspergillosis in AIDS patients.[182] The lymphomas include diffuse large B-cell lymphomas that take the form of mass lesions within the lungs and primary effusion lymphomas affecting the pleura.

Drug toxicity

HAART drug toxicity contributes up to 2% of deaths among HIV-infected patients so treated. The toxicity is mainly hepatic but sarcoid-like nodules have been reported in the lungs,[183] probably reflecting immune restoration.[184] Recovery of immune status may give rise to an active and often dramatic inflammatory response to previously indolent infections, which has been termed the immune reconstitution syndrome (IRIS).[185] It is also suggested that it is HAART rather than HIV that is responsible for the pulmonary hypertension referred to above.[186]

Chickenpox (varicella) and herpes zoster

The manifestations of chickenpox and herpes zoster are generally confined to the skin but visceral involvement occurs on rare occasions.[187,188] Since chickenpox is so common in childhood, most adults are immune. However when chickenpox affects adults, especially pregnant women, it carries a risk of fulminating varicella pneumonia, which can be rapidly fatal. The fetus is also at risk: in the first two trimesters of pregnancy chickenpox may result in embryopathy and in the last trimester it may cause neonatal pneumonia. The immunocompromised, including those receiving systemic corticosteroids, are particularly prone to suffer severe infections, including pneumonia.[189] The severe forms of chickenpox sometimes encountered in otherwise healthy adults may involve the lungs but recognition of this is often retrospective; the healed lesions may produce characteristic radiographic changes, namely innumerable small foci of calcification.[190,191] Such patients are generally cigarette smokers.[192]

Pathological features

The pneumonias of varicella and herpes zoster pneumonia are identical.[193] They represent a focal necrotising condition that lacks any apparent relation to the acinar architecture (Fig. 5.1.14A). It starts as a fibrinous exudate, involving several adjacent alveoli, and goes on to destroy the intervening alveolar walls. Eosinophilic intranuclear viral inclusions may be evident in bronchiolar or alveolar epithelial cells. Giant cell pneumonia is a rare manifestation of varicella-zoster infection.[73]

Healing results in circumscribed fibrous nodules that measure up to 5 mm in diameter and are prone to calcify (Fig. 5.1.14B, C).[190,191] Numerous calcified opacities scattered throughout the lung fields present a radiographic appearance that, outside the USA and other countries where histoplasmosis is endemic, is virtually diagnostic of previous chickenpox pneumonia.

Smallpox (variola)

In 1980 the world was declared free of smallpox and it is to be hoped that this section is only of historical interest. Severe smallpox was often accompanied by acute ulcerative tracheobronchitis and pneumonia. The latter was ordinarily due to secondary bacterial infection, but interstitial lesions of viral type were also found.

A condition described as 'smallpox handler's lung' was also observed. This affected nursing and medical staff attending patients with smallpox. It was characterised by high fever and prostration: radiological examination showed widespread mottling of the lungs

Figure 5.1.14 Chickenpox pneumonia. (A) Lung showing a focus of necrosis similar to that more commonly encountered in the skin. (B) Healed chickenpox pneumonia showing central dystrophic calcification. (C) Healed chickenpox pneumonia evident macroscopically as numerous hard, pale micronodules scattered through the lungs. *(Courtesy of Dr GA Russell, Tunbridge Wells, UK.)*

with shadows up to several millimetres across. Typically, there were no catarrhal symptoms and recovery appeared to be the rule. These patients were well immunised by previous vaccination against small-pox and did not develop a rash. The pulmonary changes may have represented an allergic reaction to smallpox virus inhaled in the dust of scales desquamated by their patients, but it was never possible to study the pathological changes.

Hantavirus pulmonary syndrome

Hantaviruses are best known as the cause of haemorrhagic renal fever but they also cause a (non-haemorrhagic) pulmonary syndrome. This was first recognised in 1993 when an unusual respiratory illness was noted in rural communities in the south-west of the USA and soon identified as a previously unrecognised hantavirus infection.[194–196] As with the previously recognised hantaviruses, that responsible for the pulmonary syndrome is maintained in the wild in a single species of rodent, in this case the deer mouse, *Peromyscus maniculatus*, which is widely distributed across North America. Like other mice they are inclined to impinge on humans in their hunt for food and there had been a marked increase in the number of deer mice in the south-west USA in 1993. Transmission of the virus is believed to be by inhalation

of dried mouse excreta. Further cases have subsequently been identified in other parts of the USA and retrospective studies of archival material have shown that cases existed before 1993, the earliest in 1978.[197] The name Muerto Canyon virus was initially proposed for the hantavirus responsible for the pulmonary syndrome but this has given way to Sin Nombre virus. It is now know to be a member of the *Bunyaviridae* family of RNA viruses.

Cases of hantavirus pulmonary syndrome have subsequently been identified in several South American countries, with one outbreak in southern Argentina being unusual in that there appeared to be person-to-person transmission,[198] a feature that has so far not been observed in any other form of hantavirus infection.

Clinical features

The hantavirus pulmonary syndrome commences with a prodromal illness characterised by fever and myalgia, and perhaps nausea, vomiting, abdominal pain, headache and dizziness.[194,195] After a few days, a cardiopulmonary phase is heralded by progressive cough and shortness of breath. Common physical findings at this stage are tachypnoea, tachycardia, hypotension and fever. Radiographic findings include the rapid development of pulmonary oedema. Most of the original 17 patients with laboratory-confirmed disease required intubation and mechanical ventilation and this led to large volumes of clear proteinaceous fluid being obtained by endotracheal suction. In 13 cases (76%) intractable hypotension terminated in cardiac dysrhythmia and death within 2–16 (median 7) days of the onset of symptoms.

Pathological features

Autopsy shows heavy oedematous lungs and large, serous pleural effusions. Microscopy confirms the oedema and shows interstitial lymphocytic infiltrates.[195,196,199] Hyaline membranes have been described in some studies.[200,201] Neutrophils are scarce and viral inclusions are not found. Despite the profound circulatory failure the heart is normal. Lymphocytosis is evident in the liver, spleen and lymph nodes. Immunocytochemistry shows viral antigen in pulmonary endothelial cells and virus-like particles are evident in these cells on electron microscopy. The target of infection appears to be the capillary endothelium in all organs with particularly heavy involvement of those in the lung, resulting in increased pulmonary vascular permeability.

The diagnosis is now made by serological tests that detect specific IgM antibodies or a fourfold rise in IgG antibodies. Immunocytochemistry and PCR are used to detect the virus in tissue. The danger to mortuary and laboratory staff is unknown but in view of the high mortality rate, full precautionary measures are advocated.[202] Treatment is supportive. Prevention is based on methods that minimise contact with the rodent vectors.

Mycoplasmal pneumonia

Epidemiology and microbiology

During the 1930s, cases of a mild form of pneumonia were reported that clinically were unlike those attributable to bacterial infection. None of the bacteria known to cause pneumonia could be recovered from the sputum, and as long as the condition was uncomplicated by secondary bacterial infection the leukocyte count in the blood showed little tendency to rise. Cases often occurred in small community epidemics in schools, colleges and camps, although even under these conditions, which are usually conducive to the spread of respiratory infections, the disease was not highly contagious. It became known as primary atypical pneumonia.

The aetiology of primary atypical pneumonia attracted much interest and the first advance came in 1944 with the isolation of an organism that became widely known as the 'Eaton agent' after its discoverer. That this agent is specifically concerned with the clinical disease is indicated by the rise in specific antibodies that occurs during the course of the illness. The infection, mainly in subclinical form, has become widely prevalent, as is shown by the frequency with which specific antibodies can be detected in the serum of healthy people in the general population. The clinical disease accounts for 18% of all community-acquired pneumonia requiring admission to hospital, a frequency second only to that of pneumococcal pneumonia.[203]

Because the disease could be transmitted to both experimental animals and human volunteers by filtrates of sputum from cases of primary atypical pneumonia, the Eaton agent was at first regarded as a virus. Later studies indicated instead that it belongs to the group of 'pleuropneumonia-like' organisms (PPLO) – the mycoplasmas which can pass through a coarse bacterial filter. The organism is now known as *Mycoplasma pneumoniae*: it is one of the considerable number of mycoplasmas that have been recognised in humans, animals, plants and soil. Because of their ubiquity in rats and mice, any experiments involving the lungs of these animals are soon bedevilled by the

development of bronchiectasis, pneumonia, lung abscess and empyema, unless specific pathogen-free strains are used.

For a time, *M. pneumoniae* was regarded as the L form of *Streptococcus MG*, a non-haemolytic streptococcus that is agglutinated by the serum of some 10% of patients with *Mycoplasma* pneumonia and that was isolated originally from a case of the latter at necropsy: comparative studies of the nucleic acids of the two organisms have shown that they are in fact unrelated. The explanation of the presence of agglutinins against *Streptococcus MG* is probably a matter of shared antigens. In about half the cases the patient's serum agglutinates group O red blood cells at a temperature between 0 and 5°C (cold haemagglutination test), but the diagnosis is best established by demonstrating antibodies to *M. pneumoniae* in the patient's serum or more recently by PCR assay.[204,205]

Clinical features

The organism generally follows a 4-yearly epidemic cycle and predominantly affects younger patients. There is a wide spectrum of respiratory disease, including sore throat, otitis media, sinusitis, laryngitis, bronchitis, bronchiolitis and pneumonia. The chief clinical features are cough, fever, headache and malaise, sometimes associated with rashes, arthritis and haemolytic anaemia. Pneumonia develops in about 10% of cases and is characterised by a more gradual onset than acute bacterial pneumonia. Chest radiography shows irregular, ill-defined opacities, usually in the hilar region and sometimes bilateral. It is characteristic of the disease that the radiological changes are much more extensive than the comparatively mild clinical manifestations indicate. The case fatality rate is low, of the order of 1 in 1000 patients, and the pulmonary opacities that are conspicuous during the 10 days or so that the illness lasts gradually resolve during the ensuing days of convalescence.

Pathogenesis

The pathogenesis of *M. pneumoniae* infection has been studied in animal models and organ cultures of human respiratory epithelium. The organisms adhere to the respiratory epithelial cells and inhibit ciliary activity. Infected cells show cytoplasmic vacuolation and nuclear swelling, with progression to complete loss of cilia.[206,207] The loss of cilia predisposes the more distal lung to secondary bacterial superinfection but the *Mycoplasma* may also affect the distal parenchyma directly.

Immunodeficient animals show reduced severity of mycoplasmal pneumonia and it is likely that immune mechanisms are involved in the pathogenicity of the disease. Autoantibodies are produced in response to *Mycoplasma* infection, probably as a result of mycoplasmal antigens being shared by host cells; such antibodies could account for many of the bronchopulmonary and extrapulmonary manifestations of the disease.

Histopathology

There have been few opportunities for histological study of the lesions in primary atypical pneumonia but when undertaken it generally discloses widespread bronchiolitis and chronic interstitial pneumonia similar to that caused by many respiratory viruses.[208,209] The bronchiolitis sometimes progresses to epithelial ulceration. Lymphocytic infiltration of the walls of alveolar ducts and alveoli characterises the interstitial pneumonia whilst oedema fluid, red blood cells and macrophages are found in many groups of alveoli, and an occasional alveolus may contain hyaline membranes. Neutrophils are generally less numerous, both in the bronchioles and the alveoli, than in the bacterial forms of pneumonia, but bacterial superinfection is a common complication.[208] The more heavily involved parts may become fibrotic and pleural adhesions may develop. There is nothing pathognomonic about any of these changes. Rarely, *M. pneumoniae* is responsible for fatal respiratory disease, in which case the histological appearances are those of diffuse alveolar damage.[210]

RICKETTSIAL INFECTION

Rickettsia are rod-like or coccobacillary organisms that are similar to but smaller than bacteria. However, rickettsial pneumonia is dealt with in this chapter rather than with the bacterial pneumonias because its clinical and pathological features more closely resemble those of mycoplasmal pneumonia. Of the tribe rickettsiae, three genera contain organisms pathogenic to humans: *Rickettsia*, *Bartonella* (formerly *Rochalimaea*) and *Coxiella*. *Rickettsia* species are responsible for typhus and certain spotted fevers, and whilst pneumonia may occur in several of these,[211-213] the most frequent rickettsial pneumonia is that which occurs in Q fever, the causative organism of which is *Coxiella burnetti*. Respiratory disease is rarely caused by *Bartonella*, but bacillary angiomatosis is one example.

Coxiella burnetti pneumonia (Q fever)[214,215]

Q fever ('query fever') was so named because of its 'questionable' nature prior to the isolation of the causative organism, now recognised to be a *Rickettsia* known as *Coxiella burnetti*. The disease was first recognised in a meat-packing plant in Queensland, Australia, in 1937 and is now known to have a virtually global distribution. It is essentially an infection of cattle, sheep and goats that is transmitted to humans, probably more frequently than is apparent from the incidence of the disease, for many people who have never had Q fever possess circulating antibodies against *C. burnetti*. Among cattle, the disease is sometimes transmitted by ticks, but possibly more frequently by the inhalation of contaminated dust from the floor of milking sheds. The organisms are excreted in milk, urine and faeces, and particularly during calfing when amniotic fluid and placentae are a rich source of infection. In humans, the disease may be acquired by the inhalation of infected dust through close contact with cattle, as in dairy farms, abattoirs and hide factories, or through drinking milk that has been inadequately pasteurised. *C. burnetti* is resistant to drying and may survive exposure to a temperature of 60°C, an important characteristic in regard to the pasteurisation of milk.

Clinical features

Q fever is a disease of sudden onset marked by general malaise, severe frontal or retro-orbital headache, high fever and muscle pain. Men are more often symptomatic than women, despite equal seroprevalence, and there is evidence that sex hormones such as 17β-oestradiol play a protective role.[216] Pneumonia develops in only a very small proportion of those infected. In these patients, chest radiographs at the height of the disease disclose numerous relatively small, but widely distributed, opacities. The symptoms generally subside after about a week and most patients recover completely within a few months without treatment. Chronic Q fever, characterised by infection that persists for more than 6 months, is uncommon but more serious. This form of the disease may also represent a recrudescence of acute Q fever years after apparent recovery. It generally takes the form of endocarditis, usually developing in patients with pre-existent valvular heart disease, transplant recipients or those with cancer. Q fever responds to treatment with doxycycline, quinolones or macrolides.

The organism can generally be recovered during the height of the disease by inoculation of the patient's blood or sputum into guinea pigs but few laboratories offer this test because of the danger of laboratory infection. The detection of specific antibodies is the laboratory test of choice.

Pathology

The case fatality rate in acute Q fever is very low, and few necropsies on cases uncomplicated by bacterial superinfection have been recorded. In these, the lungs show nodular or confluent areas of grey consolidation. The development of an inflammatory pseudotumour is recorded but is a very rare complication.[217]

Microscopically, the changes in the lungs resemble those seen in viral or mycoplasmal pneumonias. There is a diffuse interstitial infiltrate of lymphocytes and plasma cells and an alveolar exudate of fibrinous oedema fluid containing mainly macrophages and only a few neutrophils. Lymphocytic cuffing is seen about the bronchioles and small pulmonary arteries. The bronchioles contain an exudate similar to that in the alveoli and often lose their epithelial lining. Organisation of the exudates may lead to obliterative bronchiolitis and organizing pneumonia.[218]

The causative organisms may be demonstrable: they usually measure about 0.25 × 0.45 μm but bacillary forms measuring up to 1.5 μm in length also occur. The organisms form microcolonies in infected cells,

Figure 5.1.15 Bacillary angiomatosis. (A) There are many capillaries lined by plump endothelial cells, neutrophils and prominent cell debris. (B) Warthin–Starry staining reveals clumps of rickettsial coccibacilli. *(Courtesy of Dr I Abdalsamad, Creteil, France.)*

such as alveolar epithelium, and this facilitates their recognition in Giemsa-stained preparations. *C. burnetti* may also be identified in infected tissues by immunohistochemical staining and DNA detection. If the organisms are not demonstrable the changes are nonspecific and, therefore, in suspected cases, coming to necropsy, blood should be taken for serology. It should be noted that there is a real risk of pathologists and postmortem room staff contracting the disease if precautions to avoid splashing and drying of body fluids are not taken. This infectivity has raised its profile as a potential agent in bioterrorism.[219]

Bacillary angiomatosis

Bacillary angiomatosis is a reactive vascular proliferation that was originally described in the skin and regional lymph nodes of patients infected by HIV.[220,221] Mucosal surfaces may also be involved, sometimes in the absence of cutaneous disease. In the respiratory tract this results in polypoid endobronchial lesions.[166,222] Chest wall involvement with intrathoracic spread is also recorded.[223] The disease has subsequently been described in other forms of immunodeficiency and even in immunocompetent patients, implying that unrecognised cases preceded the AIDS epidemic. The organisms involved have been identified as the rickettsial coccobacilli *Bartonella* (formerly *Rochalimaea*) *henselae* and *B. quintana*,[224,225] These microbes also cause

trench foot and bacillary peliosis hepatis and are responsible for some cases of cat scratch disease (which is also caused by the related bacillus *Afipia felis*).[226]

Histologically, the lesions are likely to be mistaken for granulation tissue or Kaposi's sarcoma. Capillaries lined by plump endothelial cells are separated by neutrophils and cell debris, often surrounding clumps of bacilli (Fig. 5.1.15). The bacilli are easily overlooked in haematoxylin and eosin-stained sections and do not stain well with conventional stains for bacteria. However, aggregates of them are evident in sections stained by the Warthin–Starry or Dieterle silver techniques, predominantly in the extracellular tissue surrounding blood vessels. It should be remembered that these techniques stain many different types of microorganisms and a positive result is only meaningful if conventional methods for bacteria fail to stain the bacilli.

The lesions lack the spindle cells of Kaposi's sarcoma and the endothelial cells are more readily recognisable as such, carrying a wide variety of endothelial markers (CD34, factor VIII-related antigen and *Ulex europaeus* lectin positivity) rather than the more restricted CD34 positivity of Kaposi's sarcoma. Similarly, Weibel–Palade bodies are readily identified on electron microscopy, which is not the case with Kaposi's sarcoma.[227] Bacillary angiomatosis responds well to treatment with erythromycin and its distinction from Kaposi's sarcoma is therefore important.

REFERENCES

1. Wright C, Oliver KC, Fenwick FI, et al. A monoclonal antibody pool for routine immunohistochemical detection of human respiratory syncytial virus antigens in formalin-fixed, paraffin-embedded tissue. J Pathol 1997;182:238–44.

2. Eyzaguirre E, Haque AK. Application of immunohistochemistry to infections. Arch Pathol Lab Med 2008;132:424–31.

3. Unger ER, Budgeon LR, Myerson D, et al. Viral diagnosis by in situ hybridization. Description of a rapid simplified colorimetric method. Am J Surg Pathol 1986;10:1–8.

4. Tomita T, Chiga M, Lenahan M, et al. Identification of herpes simplex virus infection by immunoperoxidase and in situ hybridization methods. Virchows Arch A Pathol Anat Histopathol 1991;419:99–105.

5. Hogg JC, Irving WL, Porter H, et al. In situ hybridization studies of adenoviral infections of the lung and their relationship to follicular bronchiectasis. Am Rev Respir Dis 1989;139:1531–5.

6. Myerson D, Lingenfelter PA, Gleaves CA, et al. Diagnosis of cytomegalovirus pneumonia by the polymerase chain reaction with archived frozen lung tissue and bronchoalveolar lavage fluid. Am J Clin Pathol 1993;100:407–13.

7. Delvenne P, Arrese JE, Thiry A, et al. Detection of cytomegalovirus, *Pneumocystis carinii*, and *Aspergillus* species in bronchoalveolar lavage fluid – a comparison of techniques. Am J Clin Pathol 1993;100:414–18.

8. Zinserling A. Peculiarities of lesions in viral and mycoplasma infections of the respiratory tract. Virchows Arch A Pathol Anat Histopathol 1972;356:259–73.

Influenza

9. Oxford JS, Schild GC. The orthomyxoviridae and influenza. In: Parker MT, Collier LH, editors. Topley and Wilson's Principles of Bacteriology, Virology and Immunity, Volume 4. 8th ed. London: Arnold; 1990. p. 292.

10. Morens DM, Taubenberger JK, Fauci AS. The persistent legacy of the 1918 influenza virus. N Engl J Med 2009;361: 225–9.

11. Gamblin SJ, Haire LF, Russell RJ, et al. The structure and receptor-binding properties of the 1918 influenza hemagglutinin. Science 2004;303:1838–42.

12. Taubenberger JK, Reid AH, Lourens RM, et al. Characterization of the 1918 influenza virus polymerase genes. Nature 2005;437:889–93.

13. Webster RG, Govorkova EA. H5N1 influenza – continuing evolution and spread. N Engl J Med 2006;355: 2174–7.

14. Korteweg C, Gu J. Pathology, molecular biology, and pathogenesis of avian influenza A (H5N1) infection in humans. Am J Pathol 2008;172:1155–70.

15. Wang H, Feng Z, Shu Y, et al. Probable limited person-to-person transmission of highly pathogenic avian influenza A (H5N1) virus in China. Lancet 2008;371:1427–34.

16. Scull MA, Gillim-Ross L, Santos C, et al. Avian Influenza virus glycoproteins restrict virus replication and spread through human airway epithelium at temperatures of the proximal airways. PLoS Pathog 2009;5:e1000424.

17. Seo SH, Hoffmann E, Webster RG. Lethal H5N1 influenza viruses escape host anti-viral cytokine responses. Nat Med 2002;8:950–4.

18. van Riel D, Munster VJ, de Wit E, et al. Human and avian influenza viruses target different cells in the lower respiratory tract of humans and other mammals. Am J Pathol 2007;171:1215–23.

19. Donaldson LJ, Rutter PD, Ellis BM, et al. Mortality from pandemic A/H1N1 2009 influenza in England: public health surveillance study. BMJ 2009;399: b5213.

20. Reid AH, Taubenberger JK. The 1918 flu and other influenza pandemics: 'Over there' and back again. Lab Invest 1999;79:95–101.

21. Luk J, Gross P, Thompson WW. Observations on mortality during the 1918 influenza pandemic. Clin Infect Dis 2001;33:1375–8.

22. Oseasohn R, Adelson L, Kaji M. Clinicopathologic study of thirty-three fatal cases of Asian influenza. N Engl J Med 1959;260:509–18.

23. Guarner J, Shieh WJ, Dawson J, et al. Immunohistochemical and in situ hybridization studies of influenza A virus infection in human lungs. Am J Clin Pathol 2000;114:227–33.

24. Gill JR, Sheng Z-M, Ely SF, et al. Pulmonary pathologic findings of fatal 2009 pandemic influenza A/H1N1 viral infections. Arch Pathol Lab Med 2010;134:235–43.

24a. Shieh WJ, Blau DM, Denison AM, et al. 2009 Pandemic Influenza A (H1N1): Pathology and Pathogenesis of 100 Fatal Cases in the United States. Am J Pathol 2010;177:166–75.

25. Mauad T, Hajjar LA, Callegari GD, et al. Lung pathology in fatal novel human influenza A (H1N1) infection. Am J Respir Crit Care Med 2010;181:72–9.

26. Ng WF, To KF, Lam WWL, et al. The comparative pathology of severe acute respiratory syndrome and avian influenza A subtype H5N1 – a review. Human Pathology 2006;37:381–90.

27. To KF, Chan PK, Chan KF, et al. Pathology of fatal human infection associated with avian influenza A H5N1 virus. J Med Virol 2001;63:242–6.

28. Gerberding JL, Morgan JG, Shepard JA, et al. Case 9–2004 – An 18-year-old man with respiratory symptoms and shock. N Engl J Med 2004;350:1236–47.

29. Gu J, Xie Z, Gao Z, et al. H5N1 infection of the respiratory tract and beyond: a molecular pathology study. Lancet 2007;370:1137–45.

30. Parker MT. Necropsy studies of the bacterial complications of influenza. J Infect 1979;1:9–16.

31. Morens D, Taubenberger J, Fauci A. Predominant role of bacterial pneumonia as a cause of death in pandemic influenza: implications for pandemic influenza preparedness. The Journal of Infectious Diseases 2008;198:962–70.

32. Brundage JF, Shanks GD. Deaths from bacterial pneumonia during 1918–19 influenza pandemic. Emerg Infect Dis 2008;14:1193–9.

33. Yeldandi AV, Colby TV. Pathologic features of lung biopsy specimens from influenza pneumonia cases. Hum Pathol 1994;25:47–53.

34. Loosli CG. Influenza and the interaction of viruses and bacteria in the respiratory tract. Medicine (Baltimore) 1973;52: 369–84.

35. Austin RM, Daniels CA. The role of protein A in the attachment of staphylococci to influenza-infected cells. Lab Invest 1978;39:128–32.

36. Tashiro M, Ciborowski P, Klenk HD, et al. Role of Staphylococcus protease in the development of influenza pneumonia. Nature 1987;325:536–7.

37. Plotkowski MC, Puchelle E, Beck G, et al. Adherence of type I Streptococcus pneumoniae to tracheal epithelium of mice infected with influenza A/PR8 virus. Am Rev Respir Dis 1986;134:1040–4.

38. Weintrub PS, Sullender WM, Lombard C, et al. Giant cell pneumonia caused by parainfluenza type 3 in a patient with acute myelomonocytic leukemia. Arch Pathol Lab Med 1987;111:569–70.

39. Akizuki S, Nasu N, Setoguchi M, et al. Parainfluenza virus pneumonitis in an adult. Arch Pathol Lab Med 1991;115:824–6.

40. Mansell AL, Bramson RT, Shannon DC, et al. An 18-month-old immunosuppressed boy with bilateral pulmonary infiltrates – parainfluenza virus type 3 pneumonia with giant cells (giant-cell pneumonia). N Engl J Med 1996;335:1133–40.

41. Madden JF, Burchette J, Hale LP. Pathology of parainfluenza virus infection in patients with congenital immunodeficiency syndromes*1. Human Pathology 2004;35:594–603.

Respiratory syncytial virus

42. Hall CB, Weinberg GA, Iwane MK, et al. The burden of respiratory syncytial virus infection in young children. N Engl J Med 2009;360:588–98.

42a. Nair H, Nokes DJ, Gessner BD, et al. Global burden of acute lower respiratory infections due to respiratory syncytial virus in young children: a systematic review and meta-analysis. Lancet 2010;375:1545–55.

42b. Hall CB. Respiratory syncytial virus in young children. Lancet 2010;375:1500–2.

42c. Smyth RL, Openshaw PJ. Bronchiolitis. Lancet 2006;368:312–22.

43. Sinnot JT, Cullison JP, Sweery MS, et al. Respiratory syncytial virus pneumonia in a cardiac transplant recipient. J Infect Dis 1989;158:650–1.

44. Harrington SW, Hooton TM, Hackman RC, et al. An outbreak of respiratory syncytial virus in a bone marrow transplant center. J Infect Dis 1989;158:987–93.

45. Kramer MR, Marshall SE, Starnes VA, et al. Infectious complications in heart–lung transplantation. Arch Intern Med 1993;153:2010–6.

46. Kurlandsky LE, French G, Webb PM, et al. Fatal respiratory syncytial virus pneumonitis in a previously healthy child. Am Rev Respir Dis 1988;138:468–72.

47. Downham MAPS, Scott R, Sims DG, et al. Breast-feeding protects against respiratory syncytial virus infections. BMJ 1976;2:274–6.

48. Zapikian AZ, Mitchell RH, Chanock RM, et al. An epidemiologic study of altered clinical reactivity to respiratory syncytial (RS) virus infection in children previously vaccinated with an inactivated RS virus vaccine. Am J Epidemiol 1969;89: 405–21.

49. Openshaw PJM. Immunity and immunopathology to respiratory syncytial virus: the mouse model. Am J Respir Crit Care Med 1995;152:S59–62.

50. Graham BS. Pathogenesis of respiratory syncytial virus vaccine-augmented pathology. Am J Respir Crit Care Med 1995;152:S63–6.

51. Gardner PS, McQuillen J, Court SDM. Speculation on pathogenesis in death from respiratory syncytial virus infection. BMJ 1970;1:327–30.

52. Legg JP, Hussain IR, Warner JA, et al. Type 1 and type 2 cytokine imbalance in acute respiratory syncytial virus bronchiolitis. Amer J Respir Crit Care Med 2003;168:633–9.

52a. Moghaddam A, Olszewska W, Wang B, et al. A potential molecular mechanism for hypersensitivity caused by formalin-inactivated vaccines. Nat Med 2006;12:905–7.

53. The IMpact-RSV study group. Palivizumab, a humanized respiratory syncytial virus monoclonal antibody, reduces hospitalization from respiratory syncytial virus infection in high-risk infants. Pediatrics 1998;102:531–7.

54. Aherne W, Bird T, Court SDM, et al. Pathological changes in virus infections of the lower respiratory tract in children. J Clin Pathol 1970;23:7–18.

55. Johnson JE, Gonzales RA, Olson SJ, et al. The histopathology of fatal untreated human respiratory syncytial virus infection. Mod Pathol 2007;20: 108–19.

56. Delage G, Brochu P, Robillard L, et al. Giant cell pneumonia due to respiratory syncytial virus. Occurrence in severe combined immunodeficiency syndrome. Arch Pathol Lab Med 1984;108: 623–5.

Metapneumovirus

57. van den Hoogen BG, de Jong JC, Groen J, et al. A newly discovered human pneumovirus isolated from young children with respiratory tract disease. Nat Med 2001;7:719–24.

58. Williams JV, Harris PA, Tollefson SJ, et al. Human metapneumovirus and lower respiratory tract disease in otherwise healthy infants and children. N Engl J Med 2004;350:443–50.

Measles

59. Asaria P, MacMahon E. Measles in the United Kingdom: can we eradicate it by 2010? BMJ 2006;333:890–5.

60. de Quadros CA, Izurieta H, Carrasco P, et al. Progress toward measles eradication in the region of the Americas. J Infect Dis 2003;187:S102–10.

61. Vukshich ON, Harpaz R, Redd SB, et al. International importation of measles virus – United States, 1993–2001. J Infect Dis 2004;189:S48–53.

62. Jansen VA, Stollenwerk N, Jensen HJ, et al. Measles outbreaks in a population with declining vaccine uptake. Science 2003;301:804.

63. Morley D. Severe measles in the tropics. BMJ 1969;1:297–300.

64. Myou S, Fujimura M, Yasui M, et al. Bronchoalveolar lavage cell analysis in

measles viral pneumonia. Eur Respir J 1993;6:1437–42.

65. Kipps A, Kaschula ROC. Virus pneumonia following measles. A virological and histological study of autopsy material. S Afr Med J 1976;50:1083–8.

66. Warner JO, Marshall NC. Crippling lung disease after measles and adenovirus infection. Br J Dis Chest 1976;70: 89–94.

67. Miller DC. Frequency of complications of measles. BMJ 1964;2:75–8.

68. Joliat G, Abetel G, Schindler A-M, et al. Measles giant cell pneumonia without rash in a case of lymphocytic lymphosarcoma. Virchows Arch A Pathol Anat Histopathol 1973;358:215–24.

69. Sobonya RE, Hiller FC, Pingleton W, et al. Fatal measles (rubeola) pneumonia in adults. Arch Pathol Lab Med 1978;102:366–71.

70. Becroft DMO, Osborne DRS. The lungs in fatal measles infection in childhood: pathological, radiological and immunological correlation. Histopathology 1980;4:401–12.

71. Rahman SM, Eto H, Morshed SA, et al. Giant cell pneumonia: light microscopy, immunohistochemical, and ultrastructural study of an autopsy case. Ultrastruct Pathol 1996;20:585–91.

72. Archibald RWR, Weller RD, Meadow SR. Measles pneumonia and the nature of inclusion-bearing giant cells: a light- and electron-microscope study. J Pathol 1971;103:27–34.

73. Saito F, Yutani C, Imakita M, et al. Giant cell pneumonia caused by varicella zoster virus in a neonate. Arch Pathol Lab Med 1989;113:201–3.

Adenovirus

74. Becroft DMO. Histopathology of fatal adenovirus infection of the respiratory tract in young children. J Clin Pathol 1967;20:561–9.

75. Becroft DMO. Bronchiolitis obliterans, bronchiectasis and other sequelae of adenovirus type 21 infection in young children. J Clin Pathol 1971;24:72–82.

Severe acute respiratory syndrome (SARS)

76. Webster RG. Wet markets – a continuing source of severe acute respiratory syndrome and influenza? Lancet 2004;363:234–6.

77. Guan Y, Zheng BJ, He YQ, et al. Isolation and characterization of viruses related to the SARS coronavirus from animals in southern China. Science 2003;302: 276–8.

78. Parry J. WHO confirms SARS in Chinese journalist. BMJ 2004;328:65.

79. Chan-Yeung M, Yu WC. Outbreak of severe acute respiratory syndrome in Hong Kong Special Administrative Region: case report. BMJ 2003;326:850–2.

80. Tsang KW, Ho PL, Ooi GC, et al. A cluster of cases of severe acute respiratory syndrome in Hong Kong. N Engl J Med 2003;348:1977–85.

81. Lee N, Hui D, Wu A, et al. A major outbreak of severe acute respiratory syndrome in Hong Kong. N Engl J Med 2003;348:1986–94.

82. Poutanen SM, Low DE, Henry B, et al. Identification of severe acute respiratory syndrome in Canada. N Engl J Med 2003;348:1995–2005.

83. Vu HT, Leitmeyer KC, Le DH, et al. Clinical description of a completed outbreak of SARS in Vietnam, February–May 2003. Emerg Infect Dis 2004;10:334–8.

84. Schrag SJ, Brooks JT, Van Beneden C, et al. SARS surveillance during emergency public health response, United States, March–July 2003. Emerg Infect Dis 2004;10:185–94.

85. Desenclos JC, van der WS, Bonmarin I, et al. Introduction of SARS in France, March–April, 2003. Emerg Infect Dis 2004;10:195–200.

86. Ksiazek TG, Erdman D, Goldsmith CS, et al. A novel coronavirus associated with severe acute respiratory syndrome. N Engl J Med 2003;348:1953–66.

87. Drosten C, Gunther S, Preiser W, et al. Identification of a novel coronavirus in patients with severe acute respiratory syndrome. N Engl J Med 2003;348:1967–76.

88. Li W, Shi Z, Yu M, et al. Bats are natural reservoirs of SARS-like coronaviruses. Science 2005;310:676–9.

89. Lau SK, Woo PC, Li KS, et al. Severe acute respiratory syndrome coronavirus-like virus in Chinese horseshoe bats. Proc Natl Acad Sci U S A 2005;102:14040–5.

90. Tiwari A, Chan S, Wong A, et al. Severe acute respiratory syndrome (SARS) in Hong Kong: patients' experiences. Nurs Outlook 2003;51:212–219.

91. Hui DS, Wong PC, Wang C. SARS: clinical features and diagnosis. Respirology 2003;8:S20–4.

92. Paul NS, Roberts H, Butany J, et al. Radiologic pattern of disease in patients with severe acute respiratory syndrome: the Toronto experience. Radiographics 2004;24:553–63.

93. Ding Y, He L, Zhang Q, et al. Organ distribution of severe acute respiratory syndrome (SARS) associated coronavirus (SARS-CoV) in SARS patients: implications for pathogenesis and virus transmission pathways. J Pathol 2004;203:622–30.

94. Hamming I, Timens W, Bulthuis ML, et al. Tissue distribution of ACE2 protein, the functional receptor for SARS coronavirus. A first step in understanding SARS pathogenesis. J Pathol 2004;203: 631–7.

95. To KF, Lo AW. Exploring the pathogenesis of severe acute respiratory syndrome (SARS): the tissue distribution of the coronavirus (SARS-CoV) and its putative receptor, angiotensin-converting enzyme 2 (ACE2). J Pathol 2004;203:740–3.

96. Franks TJ, Chong PY, Chui P, et al. Lung pathology of severe acute respiratory syndrome (SARS): A study of 8 autopsy cases from Singapore. Hum Pathol 2003;34:743–8.

97. Nicholls JM, Poon LL, Lee KC, et al. Lung pathology of fatal severe acute respiratory syndrome. Lancet 2003;361:1773–1778.

98. Tse GMK, To KF, Chan PKS, et al. Pulmonary pathological features in coronavirus associated severe acute respiratory syndrome (SARS). J Clin Pathol 2004;57:260–5.

99. Chong PY, Chui P, Ling AE, et al. Analysis of deaths during the severe acute respiratory syndrome (SARS) epidemic in Singapore – challenges in determining a SARS diagnosis. Arch Pathol Lab Med 2004;128:195–204.

100. Cheung OY, Chan JWM, Ng CK, et al. The spectrum of pathological changes in severe acute respiratory syndrome (SARS). Histopathology 2004;45:119–24.

102. Chu CM, Cheng VC, Hung IF, et al. Role of lopinavir/ritonavir in the treatment of SARS: initial virological and clinical findings. Thorax 2004;59:252–6.

103. Stroher U, DiCaro A, Li Y, et al. Severe acute respiratory syndrome-related coronavirus is inhibited by interferon-alpha. J Infect Dis 2004;189:1164–7.

104. Paul NS, Chung T, Konen E, et al. Prognostic significance of the radiographic pattern of disease in patients with severe acute respiratory syndrome. AJR Am J Roentgenol 2004;182:493–8.

105. Hui DS, Joynt GM, Wong KT, et al. Impact of severe acute respiratory syndrome (SARS) on pulmonary function, functional capacity and quality of life in a cohort of survivors. Thorax 2005;60:401–9.

106. Ong KC, Ng AW, Lee LS, et al. 1-year pulmonary function and health status in survivors of severe acute respiratory syndrome. Chest 2005;128:1393–400.

107. Leow MK, Kwek DS, Ng AW, et al. Hypocortisolism in survivors of severe acute respiratory syndrome (SARS). Clin Endocrinol (Oxf) 2005;63:197–202.

Herpes simplex

108. Ramsey PG, Fife KH, Hackman RC, et al. Herpes simplex virus pneumonia – clinical, virologic and pathological features in 20 patients. Ann Intern Med 1982;97:813–20.

109. Greenberg SB. Respiratory herpesvirus infections: an overview. Chest 1994;106:S1–2.

110. Francis DP, Herrman KL, MacMahon JR, et al. Nosocomial and maternally acquired herpesvirus hominis infections: a report of four fatal cases in neonates. Am J Dis Child 1975;129:889–93.

111. Greene GR, King D, Romansky SG, et al. Primary herpes simplex pneumonia in a neonate. Am J Dis Child 1983;137:464–5.

112. Schuller D. Lower respiratory tract reactivation of herpes simplex virus – comparison of immunocompromised and immunocompetent hosts. Chest 1994;106:S3–7.

113. Klainer AS, Oud L, Randazzo J, et al. Herpes simplex virus involvement of the lower respiratory tract following surgery. Chest 1994;106:S8–14.

114. Hayden FG, Himel HN, Heggers JP. Herpesvirus infections in burn patients. Chest 1994;106:S15–21.

115. Byers RJ, Hasleton PS, Quigley A, et al. Pulmonary herpes simplex in burns patients. Eur Respir J 1996;9:2313–17.

116. Luyt CE, Combes A, Deback C, et al. Herpes simplex virus lung infection in patients undergoing prolonged mechanical ventilation. Am J Respir Crit Care Med 2007;175:935–42.

117. Smyth RL, Higenbottam TW, Scott JP, et al. Herpes simplex virus infection in heart–lung transplant recipients. Transplantation 1990;49:735–9.

118. Baras L, Farber CM, Vanvooren JP, et al. Herpes simplex virus tracheitis in a patient with the acquired immunodeficiency syndrome. Eur Respir J 1994;7:2091–3.

119. Martinez E, Dediego A, Paradis A, et al. Herpes simplex pneumonia in a young immunocompetent man. Eur Respir J 1994;7:1185–8.

120. Phinney PR, Fligiel S, Bryson YJ, et al. Necrotizing vasculitis in a case of disseminated neonatal herpes simplex infection. Arch Pathol Lab Med 1982;106:64–7.

Cytomegalovirus

121. Beschorner WE, Hutchins GM, Burns WH, et al. Cytomegalovirus pneumonia in bone marrow transplant recipients: miliary and diffuse patterns. Am Rev Respir Dis 1980;122:107–14.

122. Ettinger NA, Bailey TC, Trulock EP, et al. Cytomegalovirus infection and pneumonitis – impact after isolated lung transplantation. Am Rev Respir Dis 1993;147:1017–23.

123. Wallace JM, Hannah J. Cytomegalovirus pneumonitis in patients with AIDS. Findings in an autopsy series. Chest 1987;92:198–203.

124. Waxman AB, Goldie SJ, Brettsmith H, et al. Cytomegalovirus as a primary pulmonary pathogen in AIDS. Chest 1997;111:128–34.

125. Millar AB, Patou G, Miller RF, et al. Cytomegalovirus in the lungs of patients with AIDS. Respiratory pathogen or passenger? Am Rev Respir Dis 1990;141:1474–9.

126. Klatt EC, Shibata D. Cytomegalovirus infection in the acquired immunodeficiency syndrome. Clinical and autopsy findings. Arch Pathol Lab Med 1988;112:540–4.

127. Grundy JE, Shanley JD, Griffiths PD. Is cytomegalovirus interstitial pneumonitis in transplant recipients an immunopathological condition? Lancet 1987;2:996–9.

128. Weiss LM, Movahed LA, Berry GJ, et al. In situ hybridization studies for viral nucleic acids in heart and lung allograft biopsies. Am J Clin Pathol 1990;93:675–9.

Human immunodeficiency viruses

129. Royal College of Pathologists. HIV and the practice of pathology. London: Royal College of Pathologists; 1995.

129a. Moonim MT, Alarcon L, Freeman J, Mahadeva U, van der Walt JD, Lucas SB. Identifying HIV infection in diagnostic histopathology tissue samples – the role of HIV-1 p24 immunohistochemistry in identifying clinically unsuspected HIV infection: a 3-year analysis. Histopathology 2010;56:530–41.

130. Hofman P, SaintPaul MC, Battaglione V, et al. Autopsy findings in the acquired immunodeficiency syndrome (AIDS). A report of 395 cases from the South of France. Pathol Res Pract 1999;195:209–217.

131. Cury PM, Pulido CF, Furtado VMG, et al. Autopsy findings in AIDS patients from a reference hospital in Brazil: Analysis of 92 cases. Pathol Res Pract 2003;199: 811–4.

132. Suffredini AF, Ognibene FP, Lack EE, et al. Non-specific interstitial penumonitis: a common cause of pulmonary disease in the acquired immunodeficiency syndrome. Ann Intern Med 1987;107:7–13.

133. Colclough AB. Interstitial pneumonia in human immunodeficiency virus infection: a report of a fatal case in childhood. Histopathology 1988;12:211–9.

134. Ognibene FP, Masur H, Rogers P, et al. Nonspecific interstitial pneumonitis without evidence of *Pneumocystis carinii* in asymptomatic patients infected with human immunodeficiency virus (HIV). Ann Intern Med 1988;109:874–9.

135. Travis WD, Fox CH, Devaney KO, et al. Lymphoid pneumonitis in 50 adult patients infected with the human immunodeficiency virus – lymphocytic interstitial pneumonitis versus nonspecific interstitial pneumonitis. Hum Pathol 1992;23:529–41.

136. Griffiths MH, Miller RF, Semple SJG. Interstitial pneumonitis in patients infected with the human immunodeficiency virus. Thorax 1995;50:1141–6.

137. Mankowski JL, Carter DL, Spelman JP, et al. Pathogenesis of simian immunodeficiency virus pneumonia: An immunopathological response to virus. Am J Pathol 1998;153:1123–30.

138. Fitzpatrick EA, Avdiushko M, Kaplan AM, et al. Role of virus replication in a murine model of AIDS-associated interstitial pneumonitis. Exp Lung Res 1999;25:647–61.

139. Fitzpatrick EA, Avdiushko M, Kaplan AM, et al. Role of T cell subsets in the development of AIDS-associated interstitial pneumonitis in mice. Exp Lung Res 1999;25:671–87.

140. Marchevsky A, Rosen MJ, Chrystal G, et al. Pulmonary complications of the acquired immunodeficiency syndrome: a clinicopathologic study of 70 cases. Hum Pathol 1985;16:659–70.

141. Stover DE, White DA, Romano PA, et al. Spectrum of pulmonary diseases associated with the acquired immune deficiency syndrome. Am J Med 1985;78: 429–37.

142. Klatt EC, Nichols L, Noguchi TT. Evolving trends revealed by autopsies of patients with the acquired immunodeficiency syndrome – 565 autopsies in adults with the acquired immunodeficiency syndrome, Los Angeles, Calif, 1992–1993. Arch Pathol Lab Med 1994;118:884–90.

143. Afessa B, Green W, Chiao J, et al. Pulmonary complications of HIV infection: Autopsy findings. Chest 1998;113:1225–9.

144. Wolff AJ, ODonnell AE. Pulmonary manifestations of HIV infection in the era of highly active antiretroviral therapy. Chest 2001;120:1888–93.

145. Joshi VV, Oleske JM, Minnefor AB, et al. Pathologic pulmonary findings in children with the acquired immunodeficiency syndrome: a study of ten cases. Hum Pathol 1985;16:241–6.

146. Joshi VV, Oleske JM. Pulmonary lesions in children with the acquired immunodeficiency syndrome. A reappraisal based on data in additional cases and follow-up study of previously reported cases. Hum Pathol 1986;17:641–2.

147. Joshi VV. Pathology of AIDS in children. Pathol Annu 1989;24:355–81.

148. Moran CA, Suster S, Pavlova Z, et al. The spectrum of pathological changes in the lung in children with the acquired immunodeficiency syndrome: an autopsy study of 36 cases. Hum Pathol 1994;25:877–82.

149. Yousem SA, Colby TV, Carrington CB. Follicular bronchitis/bronchiolitis. Hum Pathol 1985;16:700–6.

150. Itescu S, Brancato LJ, Winchester R. A sicca syndrome in HIV infection: association with HLA-DR5 and CD8 lymphocytosis. Lancet 1989;ii:466–8.

151. Carson PJ, Goldsmith JC. Atypical pulmonary diseases associated with AIDS. Chest 1991;100:675–7.

152. Murray JF, Mills J. Pulmonary infectious complications of human immunodeficiency virus infection. Am Rev Respir Dis 1990;1416:1356–72.

153. Harding CV. Blastomycosis and opportunistic infections in patients with acquired immunodeficiency syndrome – an autopsy study. Arch Pathol Lab Med 1991;115:1133–6.

154. Moore JA, Frenkel JK. Respiratory and enteric cryptosporidiosis in humans. Arch Pathol Lab Med 1991;115:1160–2.

155. Scaglia M, Sacchi L, Croppo GP, et al. Pulmonary microsporidiosis due to Encephalitozoon hellem in a patient with AIDS. J Infect 1997;34:119–26.

156. Nichols L, Balogh K, Silverman M. Bacterial infections in the acquired immune deficiency syndrome. Clinicopathologic correlations in a series of autopsy cases. Am J Clin Pathol 1989;92:787–90.

157. Hirschtick RE, Glassroth J, Jordan MC, et al. Bacterial pneumonia in persons infected with the human immunodeficiency virus. N Engl J Med 1995;333:845–51.

158. Diaz F, Collazos J, Martinez E, et al. Bronchiolitis obliterans in a patient with HIV infection. Respir Med 1997;91:171–3.

159. Valor RR, Polnitsky CA, Tanis DJ, et al. Bacterial tracheitis with upper airway obstruction in a patient with the acquired immunodeficiency syndrome. Am Rev Respir Dis 1992;146:1598–9.

160. Brudney K, Dobkin J. Resurgent tuberculosis in New York City – human immunodeficiency virus, homelessness, and the decline of tuberculosis control programs. Am Rev Respir Dis 1991;144:745–9.

161. Hill AR, Premkumar S, Brustein S, et al. Disseminated tuberculosis in the acquired immunodeficiency syndrome era. Am Rev Respir Dis 1991;144:1164–70.

162. Dolin PJ, Raviglione MC, Kochi A. Global tuberculosis incidence and mortality during 1990–2000. Bulletin of the World Health Organization 1994;72:213–20.

163. Rigsby MO, Curtis AM. Pulmonary disease from nontuberculous mycobacteria in patients with human immunodeficiency virus. Chest 1994;106:913–19.

164. Schwartz DA, Ogden PO, Blumberg HM, et al. Pulmonary malakoplakia in a patient with the acquired immunodeficiency syndrome – differential diagnostic considerations. Arch Pathol Lab Med 1990;114:1267–72.

165. Bishopric GA, d'Agay MF, Schlemmer B, et al. Pulmonary pseudotumor due to Corynebacterium equi in a patient with the acquired immunodeficiency syndrome. Thorax 1988;43:486–7.

166. Foltzer MA, Guiney WB, Wager GC, et al. Bronchopulmonary bacillary angiomatosis. Chest 1993;104:973–5.

167. Ruben FL, Talamo TS. Secondary pulmonary alveolar proteinosis occurring in two patients with acquired immune deficiency syndrome. Am J Med 1986;80:1187–90.

168. Sehonanda A, Choi YJ, Blum S. Changing patterns of autopsy findings among persons with acquired immunodeficiency syndrome in an inner-city population: a 12-year retrospective study. Arch Pathol Lab Med 1996;120:459–64.

169. Francis ND, Goldin RD, Forster SM, et al. Diagnosis of lung disease in acquired immune deficiency syndrome: biopsy or cytology and implications for management. J Clin Pathol 1987;40:1269–73.

170. del Rio C, Guarner J, Honig EG, et al. Sputum examination in the diagnosis of Pneumocystis carinii pneumonia in the acquired immunodeficiency syndrome. Arch Pathol Lab Med 1988;112:1229–32.

171. Coplan NL, Shimony RY, Ioachim HL, et al. Primary pulmonary hypertension associated with human immunodeficiency viral infection. Am J Med 1990;89:96–9.

172. Speich R, Jenni R, Opravil M, et al. Primary pulmonary hypertension in HIV infection. Chest 1991;100:1268–71.

173. Jacques C, Richmond G, Tierney L, et al. Primary pulmonary hypertension and human immunodeficiency virus infection in a non-hemophiliac man. Hum Pathol 1992;23:191–4.

174. Mette SA, Palevsky HI, Pietra GG, et al. Primary pulmonary hypertension in association with human immunodeficiency virus infection – a possible viral etiology for some forms of hypertensive pulmonary arteriopathy. Am Rev Respir Dis 1992;145:1196–200.

175. Cool CD, Kennedy D, Voelkel NF, et al. Pathogenesis and evolution of plexiform lesions in pulmonary hypertension associated with scleroderma and human immunodeficiency virus infection. Hum Pathol 1997;28:434–42.

176. Mehta NJ, Khan IA, Mehta RN, et al. HIV-Related pulmonary hypertension – analytic review of 131 cases. Chest 2000;118:1133–41.

177. Orenstein JM, Preble OT, Kind P, et al. The relationship of serum alpha-interferon and ultrastructural markers in HIV-seropositive individuals. Ultrastruct Pathol 1987;11:673–9.

178. Chetty R. Vasculitides associated with HIV infection. J Clin Pathol 2001;54:275–8.

179. Aaron SD, Warner E, Edelson JD. Bronchogenic carcinoma in patients seropositive for human immunodeficiency virus. Chest 1994;106:640–2.

180. Cadranel J, Naccache JM, Wislez M, et al. Pulmonary malignancies in the immunocompromised patient. Respiration 1999;66:289–309.

181. Cadranel J, Garfield D, Lavole A, et al. Lung cancer in HIV infected patients: facts, questions and challenges. Thorax 2006;61:1000–8.

182. Judson MA, Sahn SA. Endobronchial lesions in HIV-infected individuals. Chest 1994;105:1314–23.

183. Naccache JM, Antoine M, Wislez M, et al. Sarcoid-like pulmonary disorder in human immunodeficiency virus- infected patients receiving antiretroviral therapy. Am J Respir Crit Care Med 1999;159:2009–13.

184. Lassalle S, Selva E, Hofman V, et al. Sarcoid-like lesions associated with the immune restoration inflammatory syndrome in AIDS: absence of polymerase chain reaction detection of Mycobacterium tuberculosis in granulomas isolated by laser capture microdissection. Virchows Arch 2006;449:689–96.

185. Shelburne SA, III, Hamill RJ. The immune reconstitution inflammatory syndrome. AIDS Rev 2003;5:67–79.

186. Wang X, Chai H, Lin PH, et al. Roles and mechanisms of human immunodeficiency virus protease inhibitor ritonavir and other anti-human immunodeficiency virus drugs in endothelial dysfunction of porcine pulmonary arteries and human pulmonary artery endothelial cells. Am J Pathol 2009;174:771–81.

Chickenpox (varicella) and herpes zoster

187. Feldman S. Varicella-zoster virus pneumonitis. Chest 1994;106:S22–7.

188. Mohsen AH, McKendrick M. Varicella pneumonia in adults. Eur Resp J 2003;21:886–91.

189. Rice P, Banatvala J, Simmons K, et al. Near fatal chickenpox during prednisolone treatment. BMJ 1994;309:1069–70.

190. Raider L. Calcification in chickenpox pneumonia. Chest 1971;60:504–7.

191. Sargent EN, Carson MJ, Reilly ED. Roentgenographic manifestations of varicella pneumonia with postmortem correlation. Am J Roentgenol 1966;98:305–17.

192. Ellis ME, Neal KR, Webb AK. Is smoking a risk factor for pneumonia in adults with chickenpox? BMJ 1987;294:1002.

193. Pek S, Gikas PW. Pneumonia due to herpes zoster. Report of a case and review of the literature. Ann Intern Med 1965;62:350–8.

Hantavirus pulmonary syndrome

194. Duchin JS, Koster FT, Peters CJ, et al. Hantavirus pulmonary syndrome – a clinical description of 17 patients with a newly recognized disease. N Engl J Med 1994;330:949–55.

195. Butler JC, Peters CJ. Hantaviruses and hantavirus pulmonary syndrome. Clin Infect Dis 1994;19:387–95.

196. Foucar K, Nolte KB, Feddersen RM, et al. Outbreak of Hantavirus pulmonary syndrome in the southwestern United States. Response of pathologists and other laboratorians. Am J Clin Pathol 1994;101:S1–5.

197. Zaki SR, Khan AS, Goodman RA, et al. Retrospective diagnosis of Hantavirus pulmonary syndrome, 1978–1993: implications for emerging infectious diseases. Arch Pathol Lab Med 1996;120:134–9.

198. Wells RM, Sosa Estani S, Yadon ZE, et al. An unusual hantavirus outbreak in southern Argentina: person-to-person transmission? Hantavirus Pulmonary Syndrome Study Group for Patagonia. Emerg Infect Dis 1997;3:171–4.

199. Nolte KB, Feddersen RM, Foucar K, et al. Hantavirus pulmonary syndrome in the United States: a pathological description of a disease caused by a new agent. Hum Pathol 1995;26:110–20.

200. Zaki SR, Greer PW, Coffield LM, et al. Hantavirus pulmonary syndrome: pathogenesis of an emerging infectious disease. Am J Pathol 1995;146:552–79.

201. Colby TV, Zaki SR, Feddersen RM, et al. Hantavirus pulmonary syndrome is distinguishable from acute interstitial pneumonia. Arch Pathol Lab Med 2000;124:1463–6.

202. Nolte KB, Foucar K, Richmond JY. Hantaviral biosafety issues in the autopsy room and laboratory: concerns and recommendation. Hum Pathol 1996;27:1253–4.

Mycoplasmal pneumonia

203. British Thoracic Society Research Committee. Community acquired pneumonia in adults in British hospitals in 1982–83: a survey of aetiology, mortality, prognostic factors and outcome. Q J Med 1987;62:195–220.

204. Abele-Horn M, Busch U, Nitschko H, et al. Molecular approaches to diagnosis of pulmonary diseases due to *Mycoplasma pneumoniae*. J Clin Microbiol 1998;36:548–51.

205. Templeton KE, Scheltinga SA, Graffelman AW, et al. Comparison and evaluation of real-time PCR, real-time nucleic acid sequence-based amplification, conventional PCR, and serology for diagnosis of *Mycoplasma pneumoniae*. J Clin Microbiol 2003;41:4366–71.

206. Collier AM, Clyde WA. Relationships between *Mycoplasma pneumoniae* and human respiratory epithelium. Diag Radiology 1971;3:694–701.

207. Rosendal S, Vinther O. Experimental mycoplasmal pneumonia in dogs: electron microscopy of infected tissue. Acta Path Microbiol Scand Sect B 1977;85:462–5.

208. Rollins S, Colby T, Clayton F. Open lung biopsy in *Mycoplasma pneumoniae* pneumonia. Arch Pathol Lab Med 1986;110:34–4l.

209. Ebnother M, Schoenenberger RA, Perruchoud AP, et al. Severe bronchiolitis in acute *Mycoplasma pneumoniae* infection. Virchows Archiv 2001;439:818–22.

210. Donat WE, Shepard JAO, Mark EJ, et al. A 20-year-old man with diffuse pulmonary infiltrates and disseminated intravascular coagulation – mycoplasma pneumonia, with diffuse alveolar damage and disseminated intravascular coagulation. N Engl J Med 1992;326:324–36.

Rickettsial infection

211. Chayakul P, Panich V, Silpapojakul K. Scrub typhus pneumonitis: an entity which is frequently missed. Q J Med 1988;68:595–602.

212. Walker DH, Crawford CG, Cain BG. Rickettsial infection of the pulmonary microcirculation: the basis for interstitial pneumonitis in Rocky Mountain spotted fever. Human Pathology 1980;11:263–72.

213. Samuels MA, Newell KL, Trotman Dickenson B. A 43-year-old woman with rapidly changing pulmonary infiltrates and markedly increased intracranial pressure – Rocky Mountain spotted fever with meningoencephalomyelitis, vasculitis, and focal myocarditis. N Engl J Med 1997;337:1149–56.

Coxiella burnetti pneumonia (Q fever)

214. Spelman DW. Q fever. A study of 111 consecutive cases. Med J Aust 1959;1:547–53.

215. Marrie TJ. *Coxiella burnetii* pneumonia. Eur Resp J 2003;21:713–19.

216. Leone M, Honstettre A, Lepidi H, et al. Effect of sex on *Coxiella burnetii* infection: protective role of 17beta-estradiol. J Infect Dis 2004;189:339–45.

217. Janigan DJ, Marrie TJ. An inflammatory pseudotumor of the lung in Q fever pneumonia. N Engl J Med 1983;308:86–7.

218. deLlano LAP, Racamonde AV, Bande MJR, et al. Bronchiolitis obliterans with organizing pneumonia associated with acute *Coxiella burnetii* infection. Respiration 2001;68:425–7.

219. Kagawa FT, Wehner JH, Mohindra V. Q fever as a biological weapon. Semin Respir Infect 2003;18:183–95.

Bacillary angiomatosis

220. Walford N, Van der Wouw PA, Das PK, et al. Epithelioid angiomatosis in the acquired immunodeficiency syndrome: morphology and differential diagnosis. Histopathology 1990;16:83–8.

221. Stoler M, Bonfiglio T, Steigbigel R, et al. An atypical subcutaneous infection associated with acquired immune deficiency virus. Am J Clin Pathol 1993;80:714–18.

222. Slater LN, Min KW. Polypoid endobronchial lesions – a manifestation of bacillary angiomatosis. Chest 1992;102:972–4.

223. Finet JF, Abdalsamad I, Bakdach H, et al. Intrathoracic localization of bacillary angiomatosis. Histopathology 1996;28:183–5.

224. Koehler JE, Quinn FD, Berger TG, et al. Isolation of *Rochalimaea* species from cutaneous and osseous lesions of bacillary angiomatosis. N Engl J Med 1992;327:1625–31.

225. Leboit PE. In consultation – bacillary angiomatosis. Mod Pathol 1995;8:218–22.

226. Adal KA, Cockerell CJ, Petri WA. Cat scratch disease, bacillary angiomatosis, and other infections due to rochalimaea. N Engl J Med 1994;330:1509–15.

227. Kostianovsky M, Lamy Y, Greco MA. Immunohistochemical and electron microscopic profiles of cutaneous Kaposi's sarcoma and bacillary angiomatosis. Ultrastruct Pathol 1992;16:629–40.

5.2 Acute bacterial pneumonia

Acute bacterial infection of the lungs is still one of the commonest causes of death, especially in the young and the aged, but very often it is merely a terminal event secondary to some other debilitating process. Primary pneumonia is one that develops in a previously healthy individual. Whilst it is still possible to classify pneumonia on the classic basis of its lobar, bronchial (lobular) or interstitial distribution, an aetiological classification facilitates the choice of an appropriate antibiotic, and will be followed here as far as possible. Consideration of the clinical situation provides important clues to the likely bacterium responsible (Table 5.2.1), and so aids the initial treatment. Most bacterial pneumonia is endogenous, caused by microorganisms that make up the flora of the pharynx. Cultures taken at autopsy have identified similar bacterial species in lung and pharynx.[1–3]

Of outstanding importance is the Gram-positive diplococcus *Streptococcus pneumoniae*, which is generally known as the pneumococcus. This bacterium is responsible for almost all cases of lobar pneumonia and for most cases of bronchopneumonia. Other varieties of bacteria that may produce pneumonia, almost always in its bronchopneumonic form, include *Staphylococcus aureus*, *Streptococcus pyogenes*, *Haemophilus influenzae* (Pfeiffer's bacillus), *Klebsiella pneumoniae* (Friedlander's bacillus), and *Legionella pneumophila*.

Streptococcus pneumoniae is much the commonest cause of adult cases of community-acquired pneumonia requiring admission to hospital (Table 5.2.2).[4–10] However, the situation is very different in patients who develop pneumonia after admission to hospital (nosocomial pneumonia), in whom Gram-negative enteric bacilli such as *Pseudomonas aeruginosa* and members of the Enterobacteriaceae family (*Escherichia coli*, *Proteus* and *Klebsiella* species) are most commonly responsible.[11–15] This is largely due to the administration of wide-spectrum antibiotics. Soon after such antibacterial drugs are administered, the oral flora changes and the upper respiratory tract commonly becomes colonised by bowel organisms.[16,17] Acid suppressants also increase the risk of nosocomial pneumonia.[18] They act by countering an important natural defence mechanism against bacterial growth in the stomach and upper small intestine. The problem has been particularly seen in intensive care units where acid suppressants may be administered to minimise the risk of gastric stress ulceration.[12] Sometimes the lungs are infected by way of the blood stream and on rare occasions an exogenous source such as a contaminated ventilator or nebuliser has been identified.[19,20] The mechanisms involved in nosocomial pneumonia are summarised in Figure 5.2.1.

Bacteriological diagnosis is usually made from the direct examination or culture of expectorated sputum. Sputum is prone to be contaminated by upper respiratory tract commensals and bronchoscopic or transcutaneous tracheal aspirates free of this problem have much

Table 5.2.1 Acute pneumonia: inference of the bacterium responsible from the clinical situation

Clinical situation	Likely bacterium
Previously healthy individual	*Streptococcus pneumoniae*
Complication of viral infection	*Staphylococcus aureus* *Streptococcus pneumoniae*
Chronic bronchitis	*Streptococcus pneumoniae* *Haemophilus influenzae*
Cystic fibrosis	*Staphylococcus aureus* *Haemophilus influenzae* *Pseudomonas aeruginosa* *Burkholderia cepacia*
Immunosuppression	*Streptococcus pneumoniae* *Staphylococcus aureus* *Pseudomonas aeruginosa* *Klebsiella pneumoniae* Anaerobes
Hospital inpatient	*Pseudomonas aeruginosa* Enterobacteriaceae spp. *Staphylococcus aureus* (often methicillin-resistant)
Bronchial tumour	*Streptococcus pneumoniae* *Staphylococcus aureus* Anaerobes
Aspiration	Anaerobes
Alcoholism	*Streptococcus milleri* *Haemophilus influenzae* Anaerobes *Klebsiella pneumoniae*

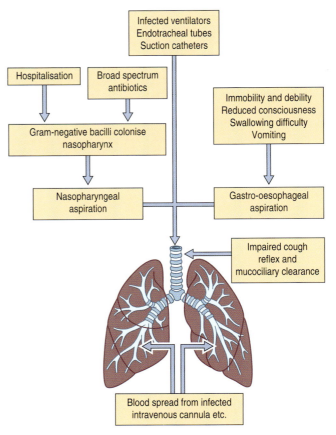

Figure 5.2.1 Mechanisms involved in the development of nosocomial pneumonia. Other risk factors include older age, underlying diseases such as cancer and diabetes mellitus, obesity and cigarette smoking.

Table 5.2.2 Microbial diagnoses (%) in adults admitted to hospital with community-acquired pneumonia

	UK[4]	New Zealand[5]	Spain[6]	Netherlands[7]	North America[a,8]	Chile[9]	Australia[10]
Streptococcus pneumoniae	34	27	39	20–60	11	24	5
Mycoplasma pneumoniae	18	6	16	1–6	4	2	9
Viruses	7	8	–	2–15	14	12	15
Haemophilus influenzae	6	8	11	3–10	0.4	3	5
Chlamydia	3	3	–	4–6	9	2	2
Legionella pneumophila	2	2	11	2–8	2	2	3
Staphylococcus aureus	1	–	–	3–5	–	1	1
Microbiologically negative	33	45	27	–	57	54	45

[a]Based on 15 separate reports.

to commend them. At autopsy, bacterial contamination is unavoidable and microbiological sampling of a consolidated area of lung should be through a surface sterilised by searing with a hot iron rod. A more elegant method entails the in situ culture of bacteria in the whole frozen organ using large Petri dishes.[21] By this method bacteria can be matched topographically to foci of consolidation, and contaminants recognised as being on the pleural surface of the lung.

BRONCHOPNEUMONIA

Although it has been resolved to follow an aetiological classification as far as possible, many bacteria cause a common morphological pattern of disease and this will be described before proceeding to specific aetiological agents. This pattern of pneumonia results from the successive infection of conductive airways and is therefore called bronchopneumonia.

Predisposing causes

Bronchopneumonia occurs most frequently in infants, debilitated young children and elderly people, and in such patients often proves fatal. The disease is particularly likely to complicate a condition that predisposes to infection by weakening either the local or general defence mechanisms. Local predisposing conditions include other acute infections of the respiratory tract, such as influenza, measles, pertussis and *Mycoplasma* infection, and chronic infective conditions such as chronic bronchitis and cystic fibrosis. Bronchopneumonia may also follow inhalation of irritant gases, aspiration of food or vomit, and obstruction of a bronchus by a foreign body or tumour.

Bronchopneumonia is also common after surgical operations. The pathogenesis of postoperative bronchopneumonia is complex. Tracheal intubation bypasses the nose, which normally warms and moistens the inspired air, whilst ether or other irritant vapours may further impair the ciliary defence mechanism of the bronchial tree. The unconscious patient may inhale infected material from the mouth or nose, and the temporary depression of the cough reflex may allow microorganisms to establish themselves in the lungs. Once the effect of the anaesthetic has worn off, the pain associated with movement, particularly of the abdominal wall, may restrict the normal aeration of the lower parts of the lungs. The haemorrhage and shock that may accompany any major surgical operation also result in some general depression of resistance to infection.

Other factors predisposing to bronchopneumonia include generalised metabolic disorders such as diabetes mellitus. Finally, bronchopneumonia is a very common terminal event in patients debilitated by cancer.

Clinical features

The onset of bronchopneumonia is insidious but once established it may have serious effects on respiratory function. The filling of many air spaces with exudate excludes air from much of the lungs and may lead to serious peripheral hypoxia. Healing is slow and the patient's temperature, which is seldom as high as in lobar pneumonia, subsides only gradually: resolution is said to be 'by lysis' rather than 'by crisis'.

Pathological features

Bronchopneumonia is characterised by widespread patchy areas of inflammation that begin as a widely dispersed bronchitis and bronchiolitis: focal areas of pneumonia then develop in the centres of the acini. The consolidated areas are generally larger and more

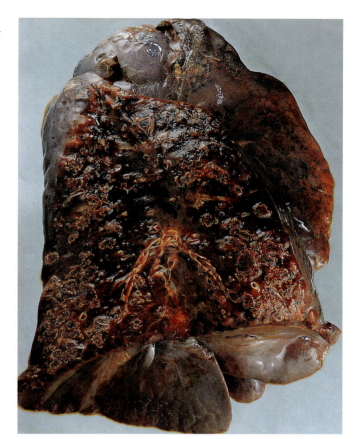

Figure 5.2.2 Bronchopneumonia. There are focal areas of pale consolidation surrounding small airways.

numerous in the lower lobes, where they may be several millimetres across. In the freshly cut lung they are commonly seen as pale, solid, centriacinar foci, often somewhat raised above the surface of the surrounding lung substance (Fig. 5.2.2). These consolidated areas can be felt as well as seen. Small beads of yellow mucopus can often be expressed from the bronchioles on the cut surface of the lung. In severe cases, the patches of consolidation may become confluent but even when this happens the affected area seldom presents the uniformity of texture and colour that is characteristic of lobar pneumonia, in which all parts of the lobe are involved almost simultaneously.

Once the organisms are established in the small bronchioles, they spread partly by the aspiration of pus and partly by penetrating the inflamed bronchiolar walls. When the bacteria reach the alveoli they excite an acute inflammation, with copious exudation of fluid and migration of neutrophils into the alveoli (Fig. 5.2.3). The air spaces nearest to the bronchioles show the most advanced degree of inflammation; those at a greater distance may be filled merely with fluid exudate.

The point at which neutrophils interact with the pulmonary vasculature is unusual. In contrast to other tissues where neutrophil migration takes place in postcapillary venules, in the lungs neutrophils leave the circulation through the thin walls of the alveolar capillaries, a difference that may serve to localise the inflammation to the alveoli.[22]

When recovery from bronchopneumonia takes place the exudate liquefies and is expectorated or absorbed and respiratory function is restored. However, healing by fibrosis rather than resolution is commoner in bronchopneumonia than in lobar pneumonia.

Figure 5.2.3 Bronchopneumonia. Pus fills a bronchiole (centre) and some of the adjacent alveoli.

Figure 5.2.4 Organising pneumonia. Micropolypoid buds of pale, myxoid, granulation tissue (Masson bodies) are seen in three alveoli.

Bronchopneumonia healing by fibrosis is the commonest cause of organising pneumonia. It takes the form of granulation tissue polyps, which are often known as 'Masson bodies', protruding into the alveoli and bronchioles (Fig. 5.2.4).

PNEUMOCOCCAL PNEUMONIA

In 1880 Sternberg and Pasteur independently recovered pneumococci from saliva of ill patients[23,24] and it was soon recognised that this bacterium was an important cause of lobar pneumonia. At least 90 types of pneumococcus are distinguished serologically on the basis of antigenic differences between their capsular polysaccharides.[25] Any serological type may be found from time to time in sputum from normal people and most, if not all, are capable of causing serious disease in humans. However, some types are more pathogenic than others. Type 3 is particularly pathogenic and is commonly isolated from patients with acute respiratory illness[26] and pneumococcal bacteraemia.[27] The distribution of the various serotypes differs from country to country and between different age groups but overall type 14 is the commonest, particularly in young children, followed by types 4, 1, 6 and 3.[25]

Host resistance is very dependent upon the development of opsonic anticapsular antibodies because the polysaccharide capsule of the pneumococcus impairs phagocytosis. The identification of the serological type of the pneumococcus responsible for each case of pneumonia was of great importance when effective treatment depended on the prompt administration of the appropriate type-specific antiserum but the introduction of sulphonamides and then antibiotics made serum therapy obsolete. Unfortunately, penicillin-resistant strains have now emerged. Serological typing is based on the Quellung reaction, an easily recognisable swelling of the bacterial capsule when the specific antiserum is applied.

Pathogenesis

The widespread distribution of all types of pneumococcus in the throats of healthy people is relevant to the pathogenesis of pneumococcal pneumonia, the development of which must be regarded as attributable to circumstances that sharply lower resistance to a potentially pathogenic strain of pneumococcus that has been carried in the nose or throat, perhaps over a long period. Pneumococcal pneumonia is, essentially, an endogenous infection, due to failure of the natural defences of the respiratory tract to prevent the spread of a potentially pathogenic strain of pneumococcus from the nasopharynx to the lungs, where it causes acute inflammation. Pneumococci may also cause bacteraemia and meningitis.

Although most cases of pneumococcal pneumonia occur sporadically, minor epidemics sometimes occur as a result of the spread of newly introduced pathogenic strains into a community, such as a school or military camp, where personal contacts are especially close.[28] Under these circumstances, a rise in the carrier rate for the responsible type generally precedes the outbreak.

In temperate climates, pneumococcal infections of the lungs, especially in infants and the elderly, are much commoner in winter than in summer. Low external temperature probably has the greatest bearing on the seasonal occurrence of pneumonia, partly by impairing the natural defences of the respiratory tract through cold air chilling its mucosa and partly indirectly, by aggravating the overcrowding that occurs in inclement weather. Both these mechanisms also promote viral infections of the respiratory tract that predispose to subsequent pneumococcal infection. The carrier rate for pneumococci in the general population also tends to rise considerably during the winter and thus to increase dispersal of the more pathogenic strains by droplet spread.

An absent or non-functioning spleen (perhaps removed because of trauma or destroyed by sickle cell disease) also predisposes to pneumococcal infection. Other contributory conditions include alcoholic binge-drinking, chronic chest disease, respiratory-depressant drugs, debilitating metabolic diseases such as diabetes mellitus, cirrhosis, the nephrotic syndrome, carcinomatosis, immunodeficiency or immunosuppression due to treatment or disease, including human immunodeficiency virus infection, and any condition, such as coma, that depresses the cough reflex and so impairs clearance of the respiratory tract.[27,29] Chronically high-risk individuals and elderly people in residential nursing homes benefit from a polyvalent vaccine containing purified capsular polysaccharide that is now available.[30]

Pneumococcal infection of the lungs may result in either lobar pneumonia or bronchopneumonia. These two forms of pneumonia differ greatly in their clinical and pathological features but the contributory conditions outlined above underlie both.[31] Whether the pneumonia has a lobar or bronchial distribution appears to depend more on the virulence of the particular serotype than on host defence. However, host factors involving hypersensitivity have been implicated in the development of lobar pneumonia, largely because of the

Figure 5.2.5 Temperature chart (Fahrenheit) of a patient spontaneously recovering from pneumococcal lobar pneumonia.

rapidity with which the disease spreads to involve a whole lobe. Bronchopneumonia is dealt with above and only lobar pneumonia will be considered here.

Clinical features

The onset of lobar pneumonia is typically abrupt. The patient feels ill, complains of a sharp pain in the side of the chest that is made worse by deep breathing, coughs up 'rusty' sputum, and quickly develops a fever of about 40°C. The respiration is shallow and its rate becomes fast, sometimes reaching 50 breaths/min or more: the ratio of pulse to respiration may fall from its usual 4 : 1 to 2 : 1. Cyanosis usually appears as the disease advances. A leukocytosis of 15–20 × 10⁹/l, mainly neutrophils, is frequently found. In many cases, pneumococci can be cultured from the blood during the height of the fever. The patient is delirious and before effective treatment became available the death rate was high. Before the days of chemotherapy, resolution generally began on about the eighth or ninth day of the illness, if the patient survived that long. Quite frequently, the fever fell suddenly, sweating was profuse, respiration became deeper and less rapid, the delirium abated and the temperature quickly returned to normal (Fig. 5.2.5). The healing was said to be 'by crisis', as opposed to the gradual abatement of symptoms seen in bronchopneumonia, which was described as healing 'by lysis'. This rapid recovery followed the appearance of specific antibodies against the pneumococcus responsible.

Structural changes in the lungs

As the name lobar pneumonia implies, it is usual for the typical changes to be uniform throughout the affected lobe. Sometimes two or even three lobes may be involved simultaneously or after brief intervals, in which case 2 or 3 days may separate the onset of involvement of the different lobes. The lower lobes are most commonly affected; there is no significant difference in the frequency of involvement of the two lungs. Before the introduction of effective treatment, the morphological alterations in the lungs generally followed a classic sequence which, following Laennec's original description, comprised four stages:

1. congestion
2. red hepatisation
3. grey hepatisation
4. resolution.

It should be realised that these terms apply to typical appearances, and that each stage shades into the next. Antibiotic treatment has curtailed and modified the natural course of lobar pneumonia, and reduced both its incidence and its mortality so that the classic morbid anatomical appearances are now rare.

Congestion

The stage of congestion generally lasts less than 24 hours. It is exceptional for patients to die so early in the disease, but when such cases are seen at necropsy, the affected lobe is more or less uniformly involved and appears disproportionately large in comparison with the other lobes, which collapse in the usual way when the pleural sacs are opened. The pneumonic lobe is heavy and congested with blood. A blood-stained, frothy fluid oozes freely from the cut surface.

Histological examination shows that alveolar capillaries are much dilated, and the air spaces are filled with pale eosinophilic fluid in which there are a few red cells and neutrophils. The uniformity of the appearances throughout the lobe is taken to indicate widespread, rapid dissemination of the bacteria through the pores of Kohn by a flood of oedema fluid. In Gram-stained sections, the paired, lanceolate pneumococci can often be seen, mainly free, in the alveolar fluid. At this stage, little fibrin has formed, and the affected lobe has not yet acquired the firm consistency typical of hepatisation.

Red hepatisation

The feature that led Laennec to popularise Morgagni's term 'hepatisation' is the consistency of the affected lobe, which resembles that of the liver. The cut surface of the lung is dry and there is a serofibrinous pleurisy. Small rough tags of fibrin cover much of the visceral pleura of the affected lobe. Congestion persists and the lung remains red.

The changes in the gross features of the affected lobe are readily explained by the histological changes that have taken place during the preceding few hours. The copious fluid exudate, which at the time of its formation contained abundant fibrinogen, has clotted in the alveolar spaces and interlacing strands of fibrin now occupy each air space and can often be seen connecting with those in neighbouring alveoli through the pores of Kohn. At the same time, more and more neutrophils have migrated from the congested capillaries into the fibrin meshwork. Usually, at this stage, the pneumococci are numerous, and many of them have been ingested by neutrophils.

Grey hepatisation

After 2–3 days, the affected lobe gradually loses its red colour and assumes the grey appearance that it retains for the next few days (Fig. 5.2.6). This change in colour, which starts at the hilum and spreads towards the periphery, is brought about by a lessening of the capillary

Figure 5.2.6 Lobar pneumonia in the stage of grey hepatisation. The lower lobe is uniformly consolidated.

Table 5.2.3 Pneumonia as a cause of septic shock

	Number of patients	Source of infection (%)			
		Lung	Abdomen	Urinary tract	Other
Warren et al. 2001[34]	2314	34	27	7	31
Abraham et al. 2003[35]	1754	51	28	13	8

congestion and by the migration of very large numbers of leukocytes, at first mainly neutrophils but later macrophages, into the fibrin in the alveoli. An almost complete shutdown of the vasculature of the affected lobe can be demonstrated in radiographs of the lungs after their injection at necropsy with radiopaque material. The temporary virtual cessation of blood flow through the unventilated lobe lessens the liability to systemic hypoxia that might otherwise develop, a good example of ventilation/perfusion matching (see p. 22).

The cut surface of the lung is now moist as the fibrin has contracted, expelling serum. Toward the end of the stage of grey hepatisation, pneumococci are less numerous and appear in degenerate forms, varying much in size, and often no longer Gram-positive.

Resolution

Resolution proceeds in a patchy yet progressive manner by liquefaction of the previously solid, fibrinous constituent of the exudate in the air spaces. Soon the affected lobe becomes more crepitant as the air spaces reopen. Liquefaction of the fibrin is thought to be due to a fibrinolytic enzyme liberated from senescent neutrophils. However, excessive neutrophil breakdown would probably damage the lung and an alternative form of cell death is also utilised, namely apoptosis:

apoptotic neutrophils are ingested by macrophages and excessive lysosomal enzyme release is thereby avoided.[32]

The now fluid contents of the alveoli are removed, partly by expectoration but mainly through the lymphatics, resulting in the hilar lymph nodes being soft, moist and swollen. By the end of the stage of resolution, completion of which is shown by chest radiographs to require several weeks, the lung has recovered its normal structure.

Complications

Lobar pneumonia may be complicated by dissemination of the pneumococci throughout the lungs and to other organs. In some patients acute pneumococcal bronchitis and foci of bronchopneumonia may be present in lobes other than that mainly involved. These accessory lesions, if severe, may exacerbate the disease by further impairing the respiratory exchange in the lungs. In many cases of lobar pneumonia there is a bacteraemia at the height of the infection. Acute endocarditis may then develop, and this is sometimes followed by the formation of an abscess in the brain after lodgement of an infected embolus. Pneumococcal meningitis, peritonitis and arthritis are rarer manifestations of the dissemination of the organisms by the blood but septicaemia with consequent septic shock are important complications in patients requiring hospital admission.[33] Pneumonia is the commonest cause of septic shock (Table 5.2.3).[34,35]

Although, in patients who recover, the area of lobar consolidation usually resolves completely, several complications may interfere with the healing process. Resolution may be delayed through incomplete digestion of the fibrin in the exudate within the alveoli, and organisation, followed by fibrosis ('carnification'), may develop. The fibrosis is essentially intraluminal, taking the form of micropolypoid buds of granulation tissue (Masson bodies) that largely fill alveoli and extend into alveolar ducts and respiratory bronchioles (organising pneumonia), as described above under bronchopneumonia (see Fig. 5.2.4). The contracting fibrous tissue may exert traction on the airways, leading to bronchiectasis, which may affect the whole or part of the lobe. Alternatively, part of the affected tissue may break down, especially in cases of infection by pneumococci of serotype 3, and a lung abscess may form.[36] On the pleural surface, the serofibrinous exudate may develop into empyema (see Fig. 13.6, p. 713) or be complicated by suppurative pericarditis.

STAPHYLOCOCCAL PNEUMONIA

Staphylococcus aureus pneumonia is a serious but relatively uncommon disease with a high case fatality rate. It often complicates influenza.

The special relationship of staphylococci and influenza virus has been dealt with on page 158. In children, staphylococcal pneumonia may follow measles or whooping cough. In infants a primary staphylococcal bronchopneumonia is known, with a case fatality rate as high as 80% in the pre-antibiotic era. The infection is generally endogenous, the bacteria frequently being derived from the patient's skin or nose and the infection air-borne. However, staphylococcal pneumonia or lung abscess sometimes follows bacteraemia or septicaemia,[37] particularly in drug addicts with right-sided bacterial endocarditis.

Although the mortality from most forms of pneumonia has been reduced by modern drugs, many strains of *Staphylococcus* now widely distributed in the population are resistant to the generally used antibiotics. Even relatively new antibiotics such as meticillin are inactive against some of these staphylococci, which have become known as meticillin-resistant *S. aureus* or MRSA. Such strains periodically become prevalent in hospitals,[15] carried in the nose by staff and patient, and fatalities from staphylococcal infection, often with pneumonia, have occurred among surgical patients who otherwise should have recovered from their operation. In addition, although MRSA is primarily viewed as the prototype of multiresistant nosocomial (hospital-acquired) infections, new lineages have emerged that cause community-acquired infections in individuals without risk factors, including rare cases of necrotising pneumonia.[38–40]

S. aureus owes its pathogenicity to a series of necrotising exotoxins that induce a marked neutrophil response resulting in suppurative tissue necrosis.[41] Particularly potent is a strain of meticillin-resistant *S. aureus* that secretes an exotoxin known as Panton–Valentine leukocidin. As well as complicating influenza,[42–44] this strain has resulted in fatal septic shock in previously healthy persons.[38]

At necropsy, the bronchi are acutely inflamed and the lungs contain many bright yellow centrilobular foci of suppuration (Fig. 5.2.7), which in the more advanced cases may have enlarged and coalesced to form abscesses 1 cm or more in diameter. Adjacent air spaces contain a purulent exudate. A superficial abscess may rupture into the pleura and cause empyema, which is a common complication of staphylococcal pneumonia. If the patient survives, there may be permanent damage to the lungs in the form of pulmonary fibrosis, bronchiectasis or large air-filled cysts known as pneumatoceles (Fig. 5.2.8).

Figure 5.2.7 Staphylococcal bronchopneumonia. The pneumonic foci show early suppuration.

STREPTOCOCCAL PNEUMONIA

In the pre-antibiotic era, up to 5% of all acute pneumonias were caused by group A β-haemolytic streptococci but *Streptococcus pyogenes* is now a rare cause of serious pulmonary infection; nevertheless, occasional cases of streptococcal pneumonia are still encountered,[45] and infective pulmonary embolism is recorded in streptococcal toxic shock.[46] Streptococcal pneumonia typically follows viral infections of the respiratory tract and is thought to have been a prominent bacterial superinfection during the 1919 influenza pandemic. Patients present with abrupt fever, dyspnoea and pleuritic chest pain. They often develop haemoptysis and cynosis. Death may take place within 2–3 days of the onset, in which case the lungs show haemorrhagic oedema and pneumonic consolidation is not well developed. In subacute cases there is bronchopneumonic consolidation, which is characteristically accompanied by early pleural involvement and effusion.

The anaerobic *Streptococus milleri* is now recognised to be an important cause of necrotising lung disease, causing lung abscess and empyema. Patients are often elderly men with periodontal disease, excessive alcohol consumption, malignant disease or recent thoracic surgery.[47]

Figure 5.2.8 Pneumatoceles in a child's lung, the consequence of staphylococcal pneumonia.

HAEMOPHILUS PNEUMONIA

The Gram-negative bacillus *Haemophilus influenzae* is a frequent isolate from the upper respiratory tract of healthy individuals and can often be cultured from the sputum of patients with pneumonia due to other organisms, the true pathogen being identified by lung aspiration or blood culture. It was first isolated in the 1889–90 influenza pandemic and so named because its discoverer, Pfeiffer, recovered it from a large proportion of cases and mistook it for the cause of influenza. Occasionally however *H. influenzae* is itself the cause of pneumonia.[48] Patients are often elderly or predisposed to pneumonia by alcoholism or chronic bronchitis. The consolidation may take the form of either lobar pneumonia or bronchopneumonia. The changes in the lung are similar to those in pneumococcal pneumonia (see above). Pleural effusion is a common feature.

MORAXELLA PNEUMONIA

The Gram-negative diplococcus *Moraxella catarrhalis*, previously known as *Branhamella catarrhalis* or *Neisseria catarrhalis*, is usually a harmless pharyngeal commensal but in the immunodeficient it can cause many serious infections, including pneumonia.[49–51] *M. catarrhalis* is one of the bacteria that colonise the bronchi in chronic bronchitis and are responsible for acute exacerbations of this disease.[52] Chronic bronchitis and lung cancer both predispose to *M. catarrhalis* pneumonia.[53–55] Other conditions predisposing to *M. catarrhalis* infection include old age, heart failure, diabetes mellitus and corticosteroid treatment. The incidence of *M. catarrhalis* colonisation and infection is highest in winter. The pathological appearances are those of acute bronchitis and bronchopneumonia.

Acinetobacter is another genus belonging to the family Moraxellaceae, one species of which (*A. baumannii*) has emerged as a potential cause of pneumonia in intensive care units. *Acinetobacter* are generally regarded as harmless soil-living commensals but they may colonise hospitals and cause serious respiratory illness in severely immunocompromised patients. *Acinetobacter* species are innately resistant to many classes of antibiotics.

LEGIONELLA PNEUMONIA (LEGIONNAIRE'S DISEASE)[56–58]

Aetiology and epidemiology

The legionellae were only discovered after prolonged investigations into the deaths of 34 of some 4500 members of the American Legion attending a convention in a Philadelphia hotel in 1976.[59,60] The investigations took so long because the responsible bacterium, subsequently named *Legionella pneumophila*, is resistant to conventional stains and fastidious in its culture requirements. Once identified, it was possible to recognise retrospectively from stored sera that *Legionella* had been responsible for pneumonia in the past. Sporadic cases were subsequently recognised.[61,62] These are commoner than those encountered in epidemic outbreaks but nevertheless only form a small proportion of community-acquired pneumonia (see Table 5.2.2). In addition to causing pneumonia (legionnaire's disease), *Legionella* is responsible for a less severe, non-pneumonic, acute febrile illness known as Pontiac fever. The term 'legionellosis' embraces both diseases.

Although *Legionella* pneumonia occurs in epidemics, the bacterium is seldom transmitted from person to person. Spread is usually due to atmospheric contamination. It is ironic that a bacterium so hard to grow in the laboratory can succeed so well in air-conditioning plants. These provide the necessary warm, moist conditions that the bacterium requires, drawing it in from the outside, fostering its growth and dispersing it around a building. The contaminated buildings are therefore generally modern, but with neglected engineering plants. Colonisation of the plant by certain free-living amoebae may also promote the growth and survival of legionellae for these bacteria are resistant to amoebic digestion and may survive exposure to disinfectants when the amoeba encysts.[63]

Passers-by as well as those within the building may be infected. In 1985, the 2-year-old Stafford General Hospital in the UK was the setting of one of the biggest outbreaks: 46 people died there of legionnaire's disease, mostly patients rather than staff. It is no coincidence that outbreaks affect hospitals or conventions of ex-servicemen, for the old, the infirm, heavy smokers and those who drink to excess are at particular risk. Hospital-acquired infection is particularly likely to affect immunocompromised patients, such as transplant recipients.[62] Also, mixed infections involving legionellae may be commoner than previously thought.[64]

Bacteriology

Legionellae are aerobic, 1–2-μm, Gram-negative bacilli that differ from other such bacilli in the fatty acid profile of their cell wall. They fail to grow on standard media and require buffered charcoal yeast extract, which is also useful for isolating *Nocardia*. The number of species has been continually increasing since the original isolation of *L. pneumophila* and now exceeds 50, of which about half are pathogenic to humans. In the USA *L. pneumophila* accounts for about 85% of *Legionella* infections, *L. micadadei* for about 8% and *L. longbeachae* for 1–3%. The legionellae are facultative intracellular organisms that are able to proliferate within phagocytic cells. They are also able to invade and proliferate within alveolar epithelial cells.[65]

Host defence

Humoral mechanisms of defence appear to be limited to opsonic enhancement of phagocytosis. The role of neutrophils is unclear: neutropenic patients are not particularly susceptible to legionnaire's disease. Macrophages activated by T-cell lymphokines appear to be more important.[66]

Clinical features

Legionnaire's disease is heralded by a vague prodromal illness that lasts about 5 days. Malaise and muscle pain are followed by rapidly rising fever, rigors, cough, chest pain and dyspnoea. There may also be confusion, diarrhoea and proteinuria. There is usually a moderate leukocytosis. Thus, the clinical features of legionnaire's disease are similar to those encountered in other bacterial pneumonias. The radiographic findings are similarly non-specific but detection of *Legionella* antigen in urine provides a reliable diagnostic test.[67] Macrolides, fluoroquinolones and rifampin (rifampicin) are the most widely used drugs in treatment.

Pathology[56,57,61,68–72]

The gross appearances of the lungs are those of a confluent or multifocal lobular pneumonia with a fibrinous pleurisy and a serosanguineous pleural effusion. If confluent, the boundaries of the consolidation generally fail to match the interlobar fissures (Fig. 5.2.9). There may be abscess formation[73] but this is not typical. A miliary distribution is another atypical manifestation.[74]

Microscopically, airways do not appear to be particularly involved in the inflammatory process, so the disease is not a bronchopneumonia. An acute, leukocytoclastic, fibrinopurulent pneumonia is characteristic (Fig. 5.2.10) but sometimes macrophages are more prominent than neutrophils. The legionellae resist digestion and multiply within the phagocytes, which they eventually destroy so that intense necrosis of the inflammatory cells is often observed. At low magnifications, alveolar walls may be difficult to recognise but even when there is extensive necrosis of the exudate, close inspection, perhaps aided by reticulin stains, shows that the alveolar architecture is generally intact. Occasionally however there are breaks in the alveolar walls or more widespread destruction may be seen. This may be due to vasculitis and thrombosis, which is sometimes evident in small blood vessels.

Demonstration of the organisms is difficult; the fickle and nonspecific Dieterle silver impregnation method is the best of the nonimmunological techniques used to stain the small coccobacilli. Fortunately the bacterial antigens withstand formalin fixation and routine processing, permitting immunostaining to be applied to paraffin sections.[75] Electron microscopy of the bacteria shows features that are indistinguishable from those of Gram-negative bacilli.[76] In practice, most cases are diagnosed without recourse to pathology.

The hilar lymph nodes are often infected and there is haematogenous dissemination to sites such as the spleen and bone marrow in 27% of cases.[61]

The process generally resolves completely but healing by organisation may be recognised in fatal cases as buds of connective tissue (Masson bodies) in the lumen of alveoli, alveolar ducts and respiratory bronchioles. Such postpneumonic fibrosis presumably accounts for the permanent impairment of lung function that has been noted in some patients.

KLEBSIELLA PNEUMONIA

Klebsiella pneumoniae (Friedlander's bacillus) is a rare cause of community-acquired pneumonia but accounts for a higher proportion of pneumonia acquired in hospital, where patients are more likely to be treated with antibiotics that permit this bacterium to dominate the pharyngeal flora.[77] *K. pneumoniae* is also a particularly common inhabitant of the oral cavity in those with poor dental hygiene and such persons are accordingly at increased risk of *Klebsiella* pneumonia. Alcoholics are also particularly susceptible to *Klebsiella* pneumonia, constituting about half the patients dying of *Klebsiella* infection.[78] Others at particular risk are the elderly and diabetics. The mortality of *Klebsiella* pneumonia is much higher than that of pneumococcal pneumonia: 21% in the general population and 64% in alcoholics.[78,79] Bacteraemia is a particularly adverse prognostic factor.[78]

Klebsiella pneumonia has a predilection for the upper lobes. There is often uniform diffuse consolidation but, with only part of the lobe involved, a sharply demarcated edge abutting interlobular septa rather than interlobar fissures: the part of the lobe affected by such consolidation enlarges by the progressive involvement of adjacent lobules (Fig. 5.2.11). The abundant mucoid coat of the klebsiellae gives the pneumonic lesions a distinctively slimy appearance and feel. This material is mucicarminophilic, a characteristic that is often helpful in identifying the infection in histological sections. *Klebsiella* pneumonia is particularly liable to suppurate and form lung abscesses (Fig. 5.2.12). These may progress to massive pulmonary gangrene.[80] Chronic *Klebsiella* pneumonia may mimic tuberculosis by presenting with cavitating upper-lobe disease.

Figure 5.2.9 Legionnaire's disease, represented by a confluent lobular pneumonia that does not show the uniform involvement of the affected lobe seen in lobar pneumonia.

PSEUDOMONAS PNEUMONIA

The species of *Pseudomonas* involved in lung infections is usually *Pseudomonas aeruginosa,* which is the commonest bacterium isolated in hospital-acquired pneumonia.[15] Infection may be inhalational or blood-borne. Infection via the airways generally follows colonisation of the pharynx, especially in patients on antibiotics that destroy the normal flora of the upper respiratory tract. As with many bacterial infections, prior viral injury promotes adhesion to the bronchial mucosa,[81,82] for it is difficult for *P. aeruginosa* to adhere to normal epithelial cells. Adhesion of the bacteria is dependent upon the transient expression of a sialoganglioside at the apex of the regenerating epithelial cells.[83] Inhalational *Pseudomonas* pneumonia has also developed in patients treated by tracheostomy and mechanical ventilation due to contamination and inadequate disinfection of the ventilators.[19] Several outbreaks in the USA were attributable to faulty bronchoscopes.[84,85]

Figure 5.2.10 Legionnaire's disease, showing widespread alveolar filling by fibrin and necrotic neutrophils.

Figure 5.2.11 Friedlander's (*Klebsiella*) pneumonia showing diffuse consolidation of the upper part of the upper lobe. The unaffected lower portion has collapsed on slicing but the consolidated, airless upper portion has retained its shape.

Figure 5.2.12 Abscess formation complicating Friedlander's (*Klebsiella*) pneumonia.

Pseudomonas pneumonia is often characterised by well-demarcated pale areas of necrosis, which histologically are composed of an amorphous coagulum containing many bacteria, the nuclear debris of necrotic neutrophils and small numbers of lymphocytes and macrophages.[86,87] *Pseudomonas* appears to be able not only to resist, but also to destroy neutrophils.[88] It is debatable whether the tissue necrosis is due to bacterial toxins or an immunological response.

Pseudomonas septicaemia may complicate *Pseudomonas* pneumonia[87] or abdominal infection. It results in further changes, notably prominent colonisation of blood vessels. So pronounced is this feature that the vessels exhibit a distinctive blue haze with haematoxylin, or a red one with a Gram stain.[89] The rod-like form of the bacteria is usually readily apparent at high magnification but the Sandiford modification of the Gram stain is especially useful for demonstrating Gram-negative bacteria in tissue sections (Fig. 5.2.13A).[90] The bacterial colonisation causes a vasculitis with resultant thrombosis and ischaemic necrosis (Fig. 5.2.13B). Such necrotising arteritis is not found in non-bacteraemic *Pseudomonas* pneumonia.[91] Meningitis, arthritis and jaundice are further manifestations of *Pseudomonas* septicaemia. There may also be striking skin lesions, including vesicles and sharply demarcated foci of cellulitis that enlarge rapidly and become haemorrhagic and necrotic.

BURKHOLDERIA INFECTION

Acute melioidosis

Melioidosis is a generalised infection caused by *Burkholderia* (formerly *Pseudomonas*) *pseudomallei*, a Gram-negative bacillus found in watery environments in certain tropical areas, notably south-eastern Asia and northern Australia.[92] However, isolated cases have been described in many other countries.[93,94] The route of infection is most often through the skin but may be through the respiratory tract, where cystic fibrosis appears to be a predisposing factor.[95] Early studies were made during the British occupation of Burma, whilst French and American servicemen were infected in Vietnam.[96] The prognosis was initially thought to be very poor but improved serological testing indicated that subclinical and mild forms of the disease are common in certain tropical areas.[96] The bacterium may lie dormant in an infected person for many years before causing disease and it is estimated on the basis of high antibody titres that many thousands of American veterans of the Vietnam war are at risk. Acute and chronic forms are recognised, and, in both, lesions are commonest in the lungs. Melioidosis is very similar clinically (but not epidemiologically) to the equine disease, glanders, which is caused by infection with *Malleomyces mallei*, with which *B. pseudomallei* shares certain antigenic determinants. Chronic melioidosis is described on page 213.

Acute melioidosis is characterised by the sudden onset of severe diarrhoea, overwhelming pneumonia and septicaemia, and if untreated is rapidly fatal. Numerous abscesses are found throughout the body. In chest radiographs these are seen as disseminated nodules.[97] The early lesions take the form of small foci of neutrophils surrounded by haemorrhagic zones. As the abscess enlarges, fibrin becomes more prominent and necrosis ensues. Cases with prominent pulmonary features are characterised by a confluent necrotising pneumonia which has a bronchitis element that is not evident when there are only discrete abscesses. Vasculitis, a feature of *P. aeruginosa* pneumonia, is not seen in melioidosis. Bacilli are generally quite numerous and often form distinct collections within multinucleate macrophages that are scattered amongst the numerous neutrophils.[98] They have been shown to survive and multiply within cells, including neutrophils.[99] The bacteria are most easily identified by the Giemsa stain, which can then be supplemented by a Gram preparation. Staining is strongest at the ends of the bacilli, which therefore have a bipolar appearance that has been likened to that of a closed safety pin.

Burkholderia cepacia pneumonia

Burkholderia cepacia (formerly *Pseudomonas cepacia*) is an important pathogen in cystic fibrosis[100] but is seldom isolated in the immunocompetent. The few pathological studies of *B. cepacia* pneumonia have shown necrotising granulomatous inflammation merging with areas of more conventional necrotising bronchopneumonia, occasionally with necrotising granulomas in the mediastinal lymph nodes.[101]

Figure 5.2.13 Blood-borne *Pseudomonas aeruginosa* pneumonia. (A) A Gram–Sandiford stain shows heavy colonisation of arterial walls by Gram-negative bacilli. (B) The consequent vasculitis has led to extensive infarction of the lower part of the lung.

PNEUMONIC PLAGUE

In humans, infection with the Gram-negative bacillus *Yersinia pestis* takes two main forms: bubonic plague, in which the bacillus is transmitted to humans by the bite of infected rat fleas, and pneumonic plague, in which the organism is usually spread from person to person by infected sputum droplets. Before the era of effective antibiotics both forms had a high case fatality rate: indeed, the plague bacillus has been the cause of some of the most widespread and devastating epidemics in human history.

In the pneumonic form the lungs show many areas of bronchopneumonia: these are sometimes confluent but the course of the untreated disease is generally too short for massive consolidation to develop. The pulmonary lesions are often haemorrhagic and they are usually accompanied by serofibrinous pleurisy and great enlargement of the hilar lymph nodes. Histologically the alveolar capillaries are engorged and the air spaces are full of fluid exudate containing few leukocytes but many bacilli. In successfully treated cases, progression to consolidation and rarely cavitation has been noted radiologically.[102]

TULARAEMIC PNEUMONIA

Tularaemia is caused by *Francisella* (formerly *Pasteurella*) *tularensis*, a Gram-negative coccobacillus that infects many wild animals in North America and, to a lesser extent, Scandinavia, Japan and elsewhere, including the UK.[103] The bacterium was named after Tulare county in California where human infection was first identified. The infected animals include rabbits, hares, muskrats and ground squirrels. Humans are infected when handling these animals or when bitten by ticks that act as vectors of the disease. Direct infection takes place through skin abrasions, mucous membranes, the conjunctivae, and, less commonly, the lungs. The bacterium is highly virulent and its handling poses an extreme hazard to microbiology staff. It is a facultative intracellular pathogen with its primary target being the macrophage.

Pulmonary involvement is usually by septicaemic spread from a lesion in the skin or eyes, via the local lymph nodes, but may be primary. Many patients show neither septicaemia nor pulmonary involvement but in fatal cases the incidence of pneumonia rises to 70%.

At necropsy, the lungs show necrotising bronchiolitis, bronchopneumonia, pleurisy and pleural effusions. The consolidation tends to become confluent and undergo necrosis.[104] The alveoli then contain abundant fibrin and necrotic macrophages, resembling the changes seen in *Legionella* pneumonia. Vasculitis and thrombosis may lead to necrosis of the alveolar walls. The bacteria are difficult to demonstrate in sections with conventional stains but can be identified by immunocytochemistry. Culture is important and the demonstration of a rising titre of antibodies is also helpful in establishing the diagnosis.

ANTHRAX PNEUMONIA (WOOLSORTER'S DISEASE)

Anthrax occurs in many species of domestic animals, especially herbivores. Spores of the causative organism, *Bacillus anthracis*, occasionally infect humans, most commonly by skin inoculation, where they cause a 'malignant pustule', least commonly by ingestion, or with devastating effect by inhalation, resulting in 'woolsorter's disease'.

Woolsorter's disease was formerly seen in the Yorkshire textile towns, where it was acquired by inhalation of dust from imported wool contaminated with anthrax spores. Others at risk include those exposed to infected hides, hair, bristle, bonemeal and animal carcasses. The spores are very resistant to drying but effective measures are now directed to their destruction by exposure of imported materials to antiseptics before they are handled; as a result anthrax is now very rare in Great Britain. In 1979 there was a major epidemic of anthrax resulting in over 60 deaths in a narrow corridor of land downwind of a military establishment near Sverdlovsk, Russia, which was suspected of conducting microbiological warfare research.[105,106] Anthrax spores were also used as a bioweapon by terrorists operating in the USA in 2001: of 11 people who were infected, 5 died. Screening procedures and plans to deal with the possibility of similar attacks have subsequently been put in place.[107–109]

If inhaled, the spores are rapidly transmitted to the mediastinal lymph nodes. It is here that the bacilli form and the disease starts. From the lymph nodes the bacilli reach the blood stream and are distributed in large numbers throughout the body. The septicaemia is often so severe that the organisms are recognisable in films of the circulating blood. Although the lungs may have provided the portal of entry, they are affected secondarily as part of a systemic blood-borne disease.[110,111]

The course of inhalational anthrax is dramatic. Non-specific influenza-like symptoms rapidly progress to cardiopulmonary failure and death within a few days.[112] Necropsy shows haemorrhagic necrosis of the infected tissues. The process is most advanced in the lymph nodes draining the site of primary infection.[106] Thus, in woolsorter's disease a haemorrhagic mediastinal mass is one of the principal findings at necropsy. Other changes commonly encountered at necropsy include a large, dark, soft spleen, haemorrhagic effusions, haemorrhagic intestinal ulceration, haemorrhagic meningitis (which is often limited to the top of the cerebral hemispheres in a so-called 'cardinal's cap'), haemorrhagic bronchitis and widespread, often confluent, areas of haemorrhagic pneumonia. As in other organs, the haemorrhagic inflammatory oedema that constitutes the exudate in the alveoli contains large numbers of the characteristic large Gram-positive bacilli, which are readily seen in haematoxylin and eosin preparations.[105,111,113] However, immunohistochemistry is proving more reliable than Gram staining in identifying the bacteria.[108,109]

LEPTOSPIRAL PNEUMONIA

Leptospirosis is a zoonosis of worldwide distribution with many wild and domestic animal reservoirs. Human infection occurs through direct contact with infected animals or, more commonly, through contact with water or soil contaminated with the urine of infected animals. Sewage workers, farmers, animal handlers and veterinarians are at particular risk. Pulmonary disease may be seen in cases of infection by leptospires of various serogroups: they are severest in cases of infection by *Leptospira icterohaemorrhagiae*, which is acquired from rats, but have been a conspicuous feature in a small proportion of cases of canicola fever (infection by *L. canicola*, acquired from dogs) and of infection by *L. bataviae*, which occurs in parts of south-eastern Asia. The spirochaetal leptospires can be demonstrated in the lesions by Levaditi's silver impregnation method, immunocytochemistry or in situ hybridisation.

Pulmonary involvement is manifest as cough and haemoptysis in association with patchy consolidation of the lungs.[114,115] Occasionally, severe pulmonary haemorrhage is the predominant or only manifestation of the infection.[116,117] but provided the disease is recognised, and treated early and efficiently, the case fatality rate is low.

The pulmonary lesions are foci of haemorrhagic pneumonia or, in some cases, of simple haemorrhage.[116] In the pneumonic foci there is a haemorrhagic fibrinous exudate that contains a few neutrophils and occasional macrophages; the exudate is most conspicuous within the alveoli but is seen also in the interalveolar septa, which are correspondingly thickened. Diffuse alveolar damage is occasionally observed. In cases of simple pulmonary haemorrhage, the bleeding is often associated with the profound thrombocytopenia that is an occasional accompaniment of leptospirosis but electron microscopy reveals that there is also profound capillary damage, culminating in endothelial necrosis[118]: a paucity of bacteria near the lesions supports the suggestion that they are due to toxins released elsewhere.[119]

CHLAMYDOPHILA PNEUMONIA (PSITTACOSIS, ORNITHOSIS)

The chlamydophilae, formerly known as the chlamydiae or bedsoniae and once considered to be viruses, are obligate, intracellular organisms, 0.25–0.50 μm in diameter, that are now classed as bacteria. The genus includes three species pathogenic for humans: *Chlamydophila psittaci*, *C. trachomatis* and *C. pneumoniae*.

C. psittaci pneumonia is contracted from infected birds, particularly parrots imported from South America, where the disease is enzootic. In contrast, *C. trachomatis* is almost exclusively confined to humans, causing trachoma, lymphogranuloma venereum and other genital diseases, and, in infants, pneumonia, which is usually accompanied by ocular infection.[120,121] *C. pneumoniae* was described as a separate pathogen in 1986 and in some communities is responsible for as many as 10% of pneumonia admissions to hospital,[122–125] although generally causing milder disease than *C. psittaci*.

Organisms similar to *C. psittaci* are found in many species of wild and domesticated birds in various parts of the world and at least some of these are pathogenic for humans. For this reason, the more generally applicable name, ornithosis, is more appropriate to this group of diseases rather than psittacosis (parrot's disease). Budgerigars are now the commonest source of ornithosis in the UK.[126] Outbreaks have also been associated with ducks, chickens and turkeys.[127,128]

Infected birds, which may show no signs of disease, excrete the organisms in droppings that eventually form a highly infected dust. It is usually through the inhalation of such dust while attending to the birds that individuals become infected, but the disease may also be contracted in poultry-processing plants or pillow-filling factories.[127] The infectivity of ornithosis is high and numerous instances have been recorded of nurses and relatives contracting the disease while caring for patients. The disease has also been acquired through exposure to the organism in the laboratory and in the performance of necropsies.

Clinical features

The clinical presentation of ornithosis varies from a mild influenza-like illness to fulminating pneumonia complicated by lesions in other systems. Fulminating cases carry a high mortality. Symptoms usually start within 1–2 weeks of exposure. The organism may be cultured from the patient's blood, but more usually the diagnosis is established by demonstrating a rising titre of complement-fixing antibodies. Cross-reactions with other organisms of the psittacosis–lymphogranuloma–trachoma group occur but should not be confusing in practice. Many patients with ornithosis give a positive skin reaction to Frei (lymphogranuloma venereum) antigen.

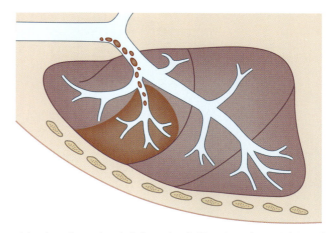

Figure 5.2.14 The effect of posture on the distribution of aspirated material. When the patient is fully supine (left) aspirated material is preferentially distributed by gravity to the apical segment of the lower lobe, whereas when tilted to one side (right) the lateral portions of the anterior and posterior basal segments of the upper lobe are affected. *(Reproduced from Brock et al. (1942)*[139] *courtesy of the Editor of* The Guy's Hospital Reports.*)*

Pathology

At necropsy, the lungs are bulky and patchily consolidated. The consolidated areas, which are usually haemorrhagic, are more numerous in the lower lobes than elsewhere. Where they abut the pleura there is local fibrinous pleurisy but pleural effusion is uncommon.

Microscopically, the changes are appropriate to a bacterial rather than to a viral pneumonia, for exudation within the alveoli is more marked than interstitial changes. However, the inflammatory cells are a mixture of those found in bacterial and viral pneumonia, macrophages predominating in the air spaces and a mixed lymphocytic and neutrophil infiltrate being seen in the interstitium. The changes are concentrated on the terminal bronchioles, from which they spread to involve adjacent alveoli and then the whole lobule, by which time there is often necrosis of the bronchiolar and bronchial epithelium.[129] There is engorgement and often thrombosis of capillaries that can result in foci of alveolar necrosis. Later, the alveoli develop a conspicuous lining of swollen epithelial cells. The chlamydophilae are just visible with the light microscope as cytoplasmic inclusion bodies (known as Levinthal–Coles–Lillie bodies, LCL bodies, or Levinthal bodies) that range from about 0.25 to 0.50 μm in diameter. They are to be seen in the cytoplasm of a variable proportion of the alveolar lining cells. They are basophilic and may most easily be found in preparations stained by the prolonged Giemsa method. As with many bacterial pneumonias, healing may be by repair rather than resolution, resulting in bronchiolitis obliterans organising pneumonia.[130]

C. pneumoniae pneumonia

C. pneumoniae is spread from person to person rather than from birds, infecting both upper and lower respiratory tracts and causing prolonged bronchitis and mild pneumonia of rather non-specific character, somewhat similar to that caused by *Mycoplasma pneumoniae*.[125] Retrospective studies of stored sera have shown that many patients diagnosed as having psittacosis on the basis of a positive serological test were actually infected with *C. pneumoniae*. Antibodies to *C. pneumoniae* have also been identified in many persons who give no history of respiratory disease.[131]

C. pneumoniae infection has a bimodal age distribution, affecting schoolchildren and the elderly. *C. pneumoniae* pneumonia is not fatal and there have consequently been few histopathological studies in humans. Experimental studies suggest that the bacterium causes a non-specific acute pneumonia.[125] *C. pneumoniae* has been linked to chronic obstructive lung disease[125,132,133] and an intriguing relationship between *C. pneumoniae* and atheroma has been identified.[124,134,135]

ASPIRATION PNEUMONIA[136]

Causes of aspiration pneumonia

Aspiration lesions include infective processes such as pneumonia and lung abscess, which are dealt with here, and non-infective processes such as exogenous lipid pneumonia and the chemical pneumonias or pulmonary fibrosis that result from the aspiration of gastric acid and other irritants. Aspiration is promoted by loss of consciousness and suppression of the cough reflex, particularly the latter.[137] It is therefore likely to complicate drunkenness, general anaesthesia, cerebrovascular accidents, drug overdosage or other causes of coma. Aspiration is also promoted by dysphagia, whether it be neurological or due to oesophageal diseases such as achalasia, stricture, diverticulum or involvement in systemic sclerosis.[138] Aspiration pneumonia and lung abscess are also promoted by poor oropharyngeal hygiene: they are rare in the edentulous.

Anatomical location

Aspiration lesions affect the dependent parts of the lungs so that their anatomical location is dictated by the position of the individual when aspiration occurs. Common sites of aspiration pneumonia include the apical segment of the lower lobe and the lateral parts of the basal segments of the upper lobe because gravity carries the aspirated material into these lung segments when the patient is in the prone and lateral positions respectively (Figs 5.2.14, 5.2.15).[139] Conversely, the right middle lobe is affected when gasoline is accidentally aspirated

Figure 5.2.15 Aspiration pneumonia showing necrotizing foci of consolidation in the apical segment of the lower lobe.

Figure 5.2.16 Aspiration pneumonia showing a bronchiole filled with pus in which there is a spicule of foreign material with attendant foreign-body giant cells.

Figure 5.2.17 Aspiration pneumonia characterised by florid foreign-body granulomas.

while it is being syphoned from a motor vehicle, a procedure that necessitates the person bending forward so that the right middle lobe and the lingula become the most dependent parts of the lungs.[140]

Pathological findings

Aspiration pneumonia is a bronchopneumonia in that the conductive air passages as well as the alveoli are filled with pus and the consolidation is peribronchiolar. The consolidation is particularly florid; individual foci are often much larger than those encountered in the more usual type of bronchopneumonia. The lesions also tend to undergo necrosis (see Fig. 5.2.15). Microscopically, particles of undigested food may sometimes be observed in the pus. These are generally attended by foreign-body giant cells (Fig. 5.2.16) and a florid granulomatous reaction may be provoked, sometimes termed 'pulse granuloma' (Fig. 5.2.17).[141–143] In such cases, the surgeon palpitating the lung at thoracotomy may suspect metastatic carcinoma but the pathologist is more likely to mistake the microscopic changes for a specific infective granulomatous disease, such as miliary tuberculosis, if the aspirated debris goes unrecognised. Less frequently, the granulomas may contain components of pharmaceutical tablets such as starch, talc, microcrystalline cellulose and crospovidone used as fillers, or kayexalate, which is a polystyrene sulphonate used in the treatment of hyperkalaemia.[143] The fillers may also gain access to the lungs via the blood stream in intra-

venous drug abusers and are described in the section on foreign-body emboli on page 411.

Clinical features

Fever, consolidation of the lung and leukocytosis may develop soon after the aspiration. Alternatively, the precipitating episode may not be recognised and the onset of the pneumonia may be insidious. Cavitation and the production of foul purulent sputum are common late manifestations of aspiration pneumonia.

Bacteriology

The bacteria responsible for aspiration pneumonia are the dominant components of the indigenous flora of the upper respiratory tract and mouth. Because of this, specimen contamination bedevils the interpretation of sputum samples. Cultures of blood, pleural fluid or transcutaneous tracheal aspirates are more informative. Facilities for anaerobic culture are essential as anaerobes outnumber aerobes by 10 to 1, as they do in the mouth and pharynx. Mixed infections are the rule, comprising either a variety of different anaerobes or mixed anaerobes and aerobes. The commonest isolates are *Bacteroides melaninogenicus, Fusobacterium necrophorum*, anaerobic or microaerophilic cocci and *Bacteroides fragilis*.[144] It is fortunate that all except the last of these are sensitive to penicillin. *B. fragilis* is sensitive to the cephamycin, cefoxitin. A predilection for opportunistic mycobacteria to infect lungs containing aspirated lipids, such as those in milk, is referred to on page 212.

LUNG ABSCESS

An abscess is a focus of suppuration consisting of a collection of pus that is walled off by chronic inflammatory granulation tissue and fibrous tissue. Although abscesses are very familiar lesions, in the lung they are often confused with other pus-filled cavities, particularly those of bronchiectasis. Similarly, when a lung abscess discharges into the air passages, as it is prone to do, the air-filled space that results is often confused with an empty bronchiectatic cavity. Lung abscess and bronchiectasis are fundamentally different diseases. The essential structural difference between them is that several airways communicate with an abscess cavity, whereas if multiple airways are ectatic, they only communicate at their normal branching points (see Fig. 3.34, page 119). This is because the formation of an abscess entails 'cross-country' destruction of lung tissue, something that is unique to an abscess, regardless of its aetiology.

Spontaneous rupture of an abscess into a bronchus is a likely event and if the patient survives this by coughing up the pus instead of disseminating it throughout the bronchial tree, a marked improvement in the patient's general condition can be expected. With time, the granulation tissue bordering the now empty cavity may become epithelialised. Also, the many airways cut across when the abscess formed may be sealed off by scar tissue. The cavity may then resemble a congenital cyst. A congenital bronchogenic cyst is distinguished by the presence of cartilage and glands in its wall, but a simple congenital cyst may be indistinguishable morphologically from a cavity that started as an abscess. Other congenital cysts (dealt with in Chapter 2) have their own special features (see Table 2.2, p. 56).

Sometimes the airways leading into a postinfective cavity only open in inspiration so that they act as check valves. The fibrous wall is then stretched progressively, resulting in a very thin-walled air sac that is often termed a pneumatocele. This process is seen particularly after staphylococcal infection (see Fig. 5.2.8). Pneumatoceles resemble emphysematous bullae but, although they are often multiple, the remainder of the lung tissue is generally free of emphysema, something that is unlikely with bullae.

Secondary lung abscess

Abscesses develop in the lungs as a complication of several conditions. Pneumococcal pneumonia was formerly a common cause but pneumonia due to staphylococci, klebsiellae (see Fig. 5.2.12) and anaerobic bacteria is now more important in this respect.[145] Local predisposing conditions include bronchial cancer and the presence of a foreign body. Septic embolism and multiple pyaemic abscesses of the lung were formerly common complications of such staphylococcal infections as osteomyelitis and carbuncle but antibiotics have rendered these rare. Still seen on occasion is necrobacillosis (Lemierre's disease), a severe septicaemic illness in which pharyngitis caused by the anaerobe *Fusobacterium necrophorum* is complicated by thrombophlebitis of the internal jugular vein and multiple metastatic abscesses, particularly in the lungs.[146–149]

Figure 5.2.18 Bilateral aspiration abscesses. High-resolution computed tomography scan shows bilateral consolidation and cavitation. Culture grew anaerobic bacteria.

Primary lung abscess: an aspiration lesion

The development of a secondary lung abscess is easily understood and clearly dependent upon some other underlying disease. On occasion, however, a lung abscess has no apparent cause and is therefore termed primary. The available evidence indicates that primary lung abscesses are nearly always a consequence of the aspiration of infected oropharyngeal secretions. First, there is usually some condition predisposing to aspiration or impairing the cough reflex, for example, alcoholic stupor, general anaesthesia, head injury or neurological disease causing loss of consciousness, dysphagia or primary oesophageal dysfunction. Second, dental hygiene is usually poor, and there is often periodontitis or gingivitis. Third, primary lung abscesses are usually found in the dependent parts of the lungs. They are commoner on the right, probably because the right main bronchus is a more direct continuation of the trachea than the left, and in the apical segment of the lower lobe and the lateral parts of the basal segments of the upper lobe, these being the most dependent parts in the prone and lateral positions respectively (Figs 5.2.14, 5.2.18 and 5.2.19).[139] Fourth, the bacteria responsible are usually the mixed anaerobes that predominate in the oropharynx, particularly in people with bad teeth (*Fusobacterium, Bacteroides* and *Peptostreptococcus* species), and aerobes such as *Streptococcus milleri*.[47,150,151] Thus, primary lung abscess has much in common with aspiration pneumonia and it is for this reason that it is dealt with here, rather than in Chapter 5.3, the chapter on chronic bacterial infection, which its indolent nature would justify. The bacteriology of empyema is similar to that of aspiration pneumonia and primary lung abscess but this condition is dealt with in Chapter 13, the chapter on pleural disease.

BOTRYOMYCOSIS

The term 'botryomycosis' is used to describe colonies of pyogenic bacteria growing within tissues such as the skin, muscle, bone and various viscera, including the lungs.[152–154] The colonies generally exist within pus-filled cavities and are often enclosed within sheaths of eosinophilic hyaline material (Splendore–Hoeppli reaction – see p. 214) (Fig. 5.2.20). They are indistinguishable from the granules of

Figure 5.2.19 Primary lung abscess straddling the fissure and involving the lateral parts of the basal segments of the upper lobe and the apical segment of the lower lobe.

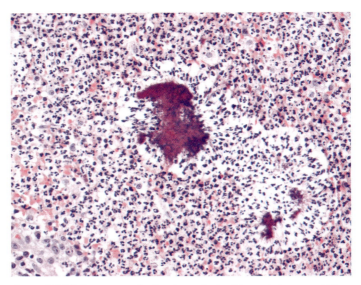

Figure 5.2.20 Botryomycosis. A colony of mixed bacteria is seen within a purulent exudate.

actinomycosis in sections stained by haematoxylin and eosin but Gram stains show cocci or bacilli rather than filamentous bacteria. The bacteria are viable but the growth of the colonies is slow and there is no invasion of the adjacent tissues: something approaching a state of balance exists between the body defences and the bacteria.

The size of the bacterial colonies varies. They may only be identifiable with the aid of a microscope or they may form visible flecks within the pus, similar to the sulphur granules of actinomycosis. Rarely the colonies are considerably larger; sometimes a single mass of bacteria may attain a size of 5 cm in diameter. One such colony simulated an aspergilloma and was called a 'botryomycoma'.[155]

The bacteria involved are often of mixed species but generally include anaerobes such as *Bacteroides* or peptostreptococci.[155] These are normal inhabitants of the pharynx and are generally found in aspiration pneumonia and primary lung abscess, thus relating botryomycosis to these aspiration lesions. Botryomycosis is also a complication of cystic fibrosis,[156] acquired immunodeficiency syndrome (AIDS)[157] and tracheopathia osteochondroplastica.[158]

REFERENCES

1. Smillie WG, Duerschner DR. The epidemiology of terminal bronchopneumonia II. The selectivity of nasopharyngeal bacteria in invasion of the lungs. Am J Hyg 1947;45:13–18.

2. Kneeland Y Jr, Price KM. Antibiotics and terminal pneumonia: a postmortem microbiological study. Am J Med 1960;29:967–79.

3. Knapp BE, Kent TH. Post-mortem lung cultures. Arch Pathol Lab Med 1968;85:200–3.

4. British Thoracic Society Research Committee. Community acquired pneumonia in adults in British hospitals in 1982–83: a survey of aetiology, mortality, prognostic factors and outcome. Q J Med 1987;62:195–220.

5. Neill AM, Martin IR, Weir R, et al. Community acquired pneumonia: aetiology and usefulness of severity criteria on admission. Thorax 1996;51:1010–16.

6. Almirall J, Bolibar I, Vidal J, et al. Epidemiology of community-acquired pneumonia in adults: a population-based study. Eur Resp J 2000;15:757–63.

7. Bohte R, Vanfurth R, Vandenbroek PJ. Aetiology of community-acquired pneumonia: a prospective study among adults requiring admission to hospital. Thorax 1995;50:543–7.

8. Bartlett JG, Mundy LM. Current concepts: community-acquired pneumonia. N Engl J Med 1995;333:1618–24.

9. Diaz A, Barria P, Niederman M, et al. Etiology of community-acquired pneumonia in hospitalized patients in Chile: the increasing prevalence of respiratory viruses among classic pathogens. Chest 2007;131:779–87.

10. Charles PG, Whitby M, Fuller AJ, et al. The etiology of community-acquired pneumonia in Australia: why penicillin plus doxycycline or a macrolide is the most appropriate therapy. Clin Infect Dis 2008;46:1513–21.

11. Heyland D, Mandell LA. Gastric colonization by Gram-negative bacilli and nosocomial pneumonia in the Intensive Care Unit patient – evidence for causation. Chest 1992;101:187–93.

12. Acourt C, Garrard CS. Nosocomial pneumonia in the Intensive Care Unit – mechanisms and significance .1. Thorax 1992;47:465–73.

13. Vincent JL, Bihari DJ, Suter PM, et al. The prevalence of nosocomial infection in intensive care units in Europe. Results of the European Prevalence of Infection in Intensive Care (EPIC) Study. EPIC International Advisory Committee. JAMA 1995;274:639–44.

14. Lynch JP. Hospital-acquired pneumonia – risk factors, microbiology, and treatment. Chest 2001;119:373S–84S.

15. Leroy O, Giradie P, Yazdanpanah Y, et al. Hospital-acquired pneumonia: microbiological data and potential adequacy of antimicrobial regimens. Eur Resp J 2002;20:432–9.

16. Johanson WG, Pierce AK, Sanford JP. Changing pharyngeal bacterial flora of

hospitalized patients. N Engl J Med 1969;281:1137–40.

17. Craven DE, Steger KA. Epidemiology of nosocomial pneumonia: new perspectives on an old disease. Chest 1995;108:S1–6.

18. Herzig SJ, Howell MD, Ngo LH, et al. Acid-suppressive medication use and the risk for hospital-acquired pneumonia. JAMA 2009;301:2120–8.

19. Phillips I. *Pseudomonas aeruginosa* respiratory tract infections in patients receiving mechanical ventilation. J Hyg 1967;65:229–35.

20. Estivariz CF, Bhatti LI, Pati R, et al. An outbreak of *Burkholderia cepacia* associated with contamination of albuterol and nasal spray. Chest 2006;130:1346–53.

21. Zanen-Lim OG, Zanen HC. Postmortem bacteriology of the lung by print culture of frozen tissue. A technique for in situ culture of microorganisms in whole frozen organs. J Clin Pathol 1980;33:474–80.

22. Lien DC, Henson PM, Capen RL, et al. Neutrophil kinetics in the pulmonary microcirculation during acute inflammation. Lab Invest 1991;65: 145–59.

Pneumococcal pneumonia

23. Sternberg GM. A fatal form of septicemia, produced by the injection of human saliva. An experimental research. Bull Nat Board Health USA 1881;2:781–3.

24. Pasteur L. Sur une maladie nouvelle, provoquée par la salive d'une enfant mort de la rage. Comptes rendus de l'Academie des Sciences 1881;92:159–65.

25. Kalin M. Pneumococcal serotypes and their clinical relevance. Thorax 1998;53:159–62.

26. Gould GA, Rhind GB, Morgan AD, et al. Pneumococcal serotypes in sputum isolates during acute respiratory illness in Edinburgh. Thorax 1987;42:589–92.

27. Gransden WR, Eykyn SJ, Phillips I. Pneumococcal bacteraemia: 325 episodes diagnosed at St Thomas's Hospital. BMJ 1985;290:505–8.

28. Gupta A, Khaw FM, Stokle EL, et al. Outbreak of *Streptococcus pneumoniae* serotype 1 pneumonia in a United Kingdom school. BMJ 2008;337:a2964.

29. de Roux A, Cavalcanti M, Marcos MA, et al. Impact of alcohol abuse in the etiology and severity of community-acquired pneumonia. Chest 2006;129:1219–25.

30. Whitney CG, Farley MM, Hadler J, et al. Decline in invasive pneumococcal disease after the introduction of protein-polysaccharide conjugate vaccine. N Engl J Med 2003;348:1737–46.

31. Ort S, Ryan JL, Barden G, et al. Pneumococcal pneumonia in hospitalized patients. Clinical and radiological presentations. JAMA 1983;249:214–8.

32. Haslett C. Resolution of acute inflammation and the role of apoptosis in the tissue fate of granulocytes. Clin Sci 1992;83:639–648.

33. Garcia-Vidal C, Ardanuy C, Tubau F, et al. Pneumococcal pneumonia presenting with septic shock: host- and pathogen-related factors and outcomes. Thorax 2010;65:77–81.

34. Warren BL, Eid A, Singer P, et al. Caring for the critically ill patient. High-dose antithrombin III in severe sepsis: a randomized controlled trial. JAMA 2001;286:1869–78.

35. Abraham E, Reinhart K, Opal S, et al. Efficacy and safety of tifacogin (recombinant tissue factor pathway inhibitor) in severe sepsis: a randomized controlled trial. JAMA 2003;290: 238–47.

36. Sawicki GS, Lu FL, Valim C, et al. Necrotising pneumonia is an increasingly detected complication of pneumonia in children. Eur Respir J 2008;31:1285–91.

Staphylococcal pneumonia

37. Naraqi S, McDonnell G. Hematogenous staphylococcal pneumonia secondary to soft tissue infection. Chest 1981;79: 173–5.

38. Vardakas KZ, Matthaiou DK, Falagas ME. Incidence, characteristics and outcomes of patients with severe community acquired-MRSA pneumonia. Eur Respir J 2009;34:1148–54.

39. Pantosti A, Venditti M. What is MRSA? Eur Respir J 2009;34:1190–6.

40. Defres S, Marwick C, Nathwani D. MRSA as a cause of lung infection including airway infection, community-acquired pneumonia and hospital-acquired pneumonia. Eur Respir J 2009;34:1470–6.

41. Hayashida A, Bartlett AH, Foster TJ, et al. *Staphylococcus aureus* beta-toxin induces lung injury through syndecan-1. Am J Pathol 2009;174:509–18.

42. Gillet Y, Issartel B, Vanhems P, et al. Association between *Staphylococcus aureus* strains carrying gene for Panton–Valentine leukocidin and highly lethal necrotising pneumonia in young immunocompetent patients. Lancet 2002;359:753–9.

43. Morgan M. *Staphylococcus aureus*, Panton–Valentine leukocidin, and necrotising pneumonia. BMJ 2005;331:793–4.

44. Micek ST, Dunne M, Kollef MH. Pleuropulmonary complications of Panton–Valentine leukocidin-positive community-acquired methicillin-resistant *Staphylococcus aureus*: importance of treatment with antimicrobials inhibiting exotoxin production. Chest 2005;128:2732–8.

Streptococcal pneumonia

45. McMurray JJ, Fraser DM, Brogan O. Fatal *Streptococcus pyogenes* pneumonia. J R Soc Med 1987;80:525–6.

46. Cramer SF, Tomkiewicz ZM. Septic pulmonary thrombosis in streptococcal toxic shock syndrome. Hum Pathol 1995;26:1157–60.

47. Wong CA, Donald F, Macfarlane JT. *Streptococcus milleri* pulmonary disease: a review and clinical description of 25 patients. Thorax 1995;50:1093–6.

Haemophilus pneumonia

48. Barnes DJ, Naraqi S, Igo JD. *Haemophilus influenzae* pneumonia in Melanesian adults: report of 15 cases. Thorax 1987;42:889–91.

Moraxella pneumonia

49. Diamond LA, Lorber B. *Branhamella catarrhalis* pneumonia and immunoglobulin abnormalities: A new association. Am Rev Respir Dis 1984;129:876–8.

50. Verghese A, Berk SL. *Branhamella catarrhalis*. A microbiologic and clinical update. Am J Med 1990;88:S1–56.

51. Murphy TF. *Branhamella catarrhalis*: epidemiological and clinical aspects of a human respiratory tract pathogen. Thorax 1998;53:124–8.

52. Mannion PT. Sputum microbiology in a district general hospital. The role of *Branhamella catarrhalis*. Br J Dis Chest 1987;81:391–6.

53. McLeod DT, Ahmad F, Capewell S, et al. Increase in bronchopulmonary infection due to *Branhamella catarrhalis*. BMJ 1986;292:1103–5.

54. Black AJ, Wilson TS. Immunoglobulin G (IgG) serological response to *Branhamella catarrhalis* in patients with acute bronchopulmonary infections. J Clin Pathol 1988;41:329–33.

55. Capewell S, McLeod DT, Croughan MJ, et al. Pneumonia due to *Branhamella catarrhalis*. Thorax 1988;43:929–30.

Legionella pneumonia

56. Winn WC, Myerowitz RL. The pathology of the legionella pneumonias. A review of 74 cases and the literature. Hum Pathol 1981;12:401–22.

57. Roig J, Domingo C, Morera J. Legionnaires' disease. Chest 1994;105:1817–25.

58. Stout JE, Yu VL. Current concepts: legionellosis. N Engl J Med 1997;337:682–7.

59. Fraser DW, Tsai TR, Orenstein W, et al. Legionnaires' disease. Description of an epidemic of pneumonia. N Engl J Med 1977;297:1189–97.

60. McDade JE, Shepard CC, Fraser DW, et al. Legionnaires' disease. Isolation of a bacterium and demonstration of its role in other respiratory disease. N Engl J Med 1977;297:1197–203.

61. Weisenberger DD, Helms CM, Renner ED. Sporadic legionnaires' disease. A pathologic study of 23 fatal cases. Arch Pathol Lab Med 1981;105:130–7.

62. England AC, Fraser DW, Plikaytis BD, et al. Sporadic legionellosis in the United States:

the first thousand cases. Ann Intern Med 1981;94:164–70.

63. Barker J, Brown MR, Collier PJ, et al. Relationship between *Legionella pneumophila* and *Acanthamoeba polyphaga*: physiological status and susceptibility to chemical inactivation. Appl Environ Microbiol 1992;58:2420–5.

64. Roig J, Sabria M, Pedro-Botet ML. *Legionella* spp.: community acquired and nosocomial infections. Curr Opin Infect Dis 2003;16:145–51.

65. Maruta K, Miyamoto H, Hamada T, et al. Entry and intracellular growth of *Legionella dumoffii* in alveolar epithelial cells. Am J Respir Crit Care Med 1998;157:1967–74.

66. Skerrett SJ, Martin TR. Alveolar macrophage activation in experimental legionellosis. J Immunol 1991;147:337–45.

67. Sabria M, Campins M. Legionnaires' disease: update on epidemiology and management options. Am J Respir Med 2003;2:235–43.

68. Blackmon JA, Chandler FW, Cherry WB, et al. Legionellosis. Am J Pathol 1981;103:429–65.

69. Winn WC, Glavin FL, Perl DP, et al. The pathology of legionnaires' disease. Fourteen fatal cases from the 1977 outbreak in Vermont. Arch Pathol Lab Med 1978;102:344–50.

70. Blackmon JA, Hicklin MD, Chandler FW. Legionnaires' disease. Pathological and historical aspects of a 'new' disease. Arch Pathol Lab Med 1978;102:337–43.

71. Lattimer GL, Rachman RA, Scarlato M. Legionnaires' disease pneumonia: histopathologic features and comparison with microbial and chemical pneumonias. Ann Clin Lab Sci 1979;9:353–61.

72. Hernandez FJ, Kirby BD, Stanley TM, et al. Legionnaires' disease. Postmortem pathologic findings of 20 cases. Am J Clin Pathol 1980;73:488–95.

73. Edwards D, Finlayson DM. Legionnaires' disease causing severe lung abscesses. CMA Journal 1980;123:524–6.

74. Cluroe AD. Legionnaire's disease mimicking pulmonary miliary tuberculosis in the immunocompromised. Histopathology 1993;22:73–5.

75. Theaker JM, Tobin OJ, Jones SEC, et al. Immunohistological detection of *Legionella pneumophila* in lung sections. J Clin Pathol 1987;40:143–6.

76. Chandler FW, Cole RM, Hicklin MD, et al. Ultrastructure of the legionnaires' disease bacterium. A study using transmission electron microscopy. Ann Intern Med 1979;90:642–7.

Klebsiella pneumonia

77. Garb JL, Brown RB, Garb JR, et al. Differences in etiology of pneumonia in nursing home and community patients. JAMA 1978;240:2169–72.

78. Jong GM, Hsiue TR, Chen CR, et al. Rapidly fatal outcome of bacteremic *Klebsiella pneumoniae* pneumonia in alcoholics. Chest 1995;107:214–7.

79. Dorff GJ, Rytel MW, Farmer SG, et al. Etiologies and characteristic features of pneumonias in a municipal hospital. Am J Med Sci 1973;266:349–58.

80. Schamaun M, von Buren U, Pirozynski W. Ausgedehnte Lungennekrose bei Klebsiellen-Pneumonie (sogenannte massive Gangran der Lunge). Schweiz Med Wochenschr 1980;110:223–5.

Pseudomonas pneumonia

81. Philippon S, Streckert HJ, Morgenroth K. Invitro study of the bronchial mucosa during *Pseudomonas aeruginosa* infection. Virchows Arch A Pathol Anat Histopathol 1993;423:39–43.

82. Tsang KWT, Rutman A, Kanthakumar K, et al. Interaction of *Pseudomonas aeruginosa* with human respiratory mucosa in vitro. Eur Respir J 1994;7:1746–53.

83. Debentzmann S, Roger P, Puchelle E. *Pseudomonas aeruginosa* adherence to remodelling respiratory epithelium. Eur Respir J 1996;9:2145–50.

84. Kirschke DL, Jones TF, Craig AS, et al. *Pseudomonas aeruginosa* and *Serratia marcescens* contamination associated with a manufacturing defect in bronchoscopes. N Engl J Med 2003;348:214–20.

85. Srinivasan A, Wolfenden LL, Song XY, et al. An outbreak of *Pseudomonas aeruginosa* infections associated with flexible bronchoscopes. N Engl J Med 2003;348:221–7.

86. Fetzer AE, Werner AS, Hagstrom JWC. Pathologic features of pseudomonal pneumonia. Am Rev Respir Dis 1967;96:1121–30.

87. Bonifacio SL, Kitterman JA, Ursell PC. *Pseudomonas* pneumonia in infants: An autopsy study. Hum Pathol 2003;34:929–38.

88. Teplitz C. Pathogenesis of *Pseudomonas* vasculitis and septic lesions. Arch Pathol 1965;80:297–307.

89. Barson AJ. Fatal *Pseudomonas aeruginosa* bronchopneumonia in a children's hospital. Arch Dis Child 1971;46:55–60.

90. Leaver RE, Evans BJ, Corrin B. Identification of Gram-negative bacteria in histological sections using Sandiford's counterstain. J Clin Pathol 1977;30:290–1.

91. Tillotson JR, Lerner AM. Characteristics of non-bacteremic *Pseudomonas* pneumonia. Ann Intern Med 1968;68:295–307.

Acute melioidosis

92. Currie BJ. Melioidosis: an important cause of pneumonia in residents of and travellers returned from endemic regions. Eur Resp J 2003;22:542–50.

93. Barnes PF, Appleman MD, Cosgrove MM. A case of melioidosis originating in North America. Am Rev Respir Dis 1986;134:170–1.

94. Ip M, Osterberg LG, Chau PY, et al. Pulmonary melioidosis. Chest 1995;108:1420–4.

95. OCarroll MR, Kidd TJ, Coulter C, et al. *Burkholderia pseudomallei*: another emerging pathogen in cystic fibrosis. Thorax 2003;58:1087–91.

96. Piggott JA, Hochholzer L. Human melioidosis. A histopathologic study of acute and chronic melioidosis. Arch Pathol 1970;90:101–11.

97. Dhiensiri T, Puapairoj S, Susaengrat W. Pulmonary melioidosis: clinical-radiologic correlation in 183 cases in northeastern Thailand. Radiology 1988;166:711–15.

98. Wong KT, Puthucheary SD, Vadivelu J. The histopathology of human melioidosis. Histopathology 1995;26:51–5.

99. Jones AL, Beveridge TJ, Woods DE. Intracellular survival of *Burkholderia pseudomallei*. Infect Immun 1996;64:782–90.

Burkholderia cepacia pneumonia

100. Stableforth DE, Smith DL. *Pseudomonas cepacia* in cystic fibrosis. Thorax 1994;49:629–30.

101. Belchis DA, Simpson E, Colby T. Histopathologic features of *Burkholderia cepacia* pneumonia in patients without cystic fibrosis. Modern Pathol 2000;13:369–72.

Pneumonic plague

102. Florman AL, Spencer RR, Sheward S. Multiple lung cavities in a 12-year-old girl with bubonic plague, sepsis, and secondary pneumonia. Am J Med 1986;80:1191–3.

Tularaemic pneumonia

103. Tarnvik A, Berglund L. Tularaemia. Eur Resp J 2003;21:361–373.

104. Shapiro DS, Mark EJ, Sabloff B, et al. A 60-year-old farm worker with bilateral pneumonia. Tularemic pneumonia. N Engl J Med 2000;342:1430–8.

Anthrax pneumonia (woolsorters' disease)

105. Abramova FA, Grinberg LM, Yampolskaya OV, et al. Pathology of inhalational anthrax in 42 cases from the Sverdlovsk outbreak of 1979. Proc Natl Acad Sci USA 1993;90:2291–4.

106. Grinberg LM, Abramova FA, Yampolskaya OV, et al. Quantitative pathology of inhalational anthrax I: Quantitative microscopic findings. Modern Pathol 2001;14:482–95.

107. Bush LM, Abrams BH, Beall A, et al. Index case of fatal inhalational anthrax due to

bioterrorism in the United States. N Engl J Med 2001;345:1607–10.

108. Guarner J, Jernigan JA, Shieh WJ, et al. Pathology and pathogenesis of bioterrorism-related inhalational anthrax. Am J Pathol 2003;163:701–9.

109. Hupert N, Bearman GM, Mushlin AI, et al. Accuracy of screening for inhalational anthrax after a bioterrorist attack. Ann Intern Med 2003;139:337–45.

110. Ross JM. The pathogenesis of anthrax following the administration of spores by the respiratory route. J Path Bact 1957;73:485–94.

111. Zaucha GM, Pitt MLM, Estep J, et al. The pathology of experimental anthrax in rabbits exposed by inhalation and subcutaneous inoculation. Arch Pathol Lab Med 1998;122:982–92.

112. Shafazand S, Doyle R, Ruoss S, et al. Inhalational anthrax – Epidemiology, diagnosis, and management. Chest 1999;116:1369–76.

113. Severn M. A fatal case of pulmonary anthrax. BMJ 1976;1:748.

Leptospiral pneumonia

114. Teglia OF, Battagliotti C, Villavicencio RL, et al. Leptospiral pneumonia. Chest 1995;108:874–5.

115. Tattevin P, Leveiller G, Flicoteaux R, et al. Respiratory manifestations of leptospirosis: a retrospective study. Lung 2005;183:283–9.

116. Zaki SR, Shieh WJ. Leptospirosis associated with outbreak of acute febrile illness and pulmonary haemorrhage, Nicaragua, 1995. The Epidemic Working Group at Ministry of Health in Nicaragua [letter] [see comments]. Lancet 1996;347:535–6.

117. Silva JJ, Dalston MO, Carvalho JE, et al. Clinicopathological and immunohistochemical features of the severe pulmonary form of leptospirosis. Rev Soc Bras Med Trop 2002;35:395–9.

118. Nicodemo AC, Duarte MI, Alves VA, et al. Lung lesions in human leptospirosis: microscopic, immunohistochemical, and ultrastructural features related to thrombocytopenia. Am J Trop Med Hyg 1997;56:181–7.

119. de Brito T, Bohm GM, Yasuda PH.. Vascular damage in acute experimental leptospirosis of the guinea pig. J Pathol 1979;128:177–82.

Chlamydophila pneumonia

120. Beem MO, Saxon EM. Respiratory tract colonization and a distinctive pneumonia syndrome in infants infected with Chlamydia trachomatis. N Engl J Med 1977;296:306–10.

121. Harrison HR, Enlish MG, Lee CK, et al. Chlamydia trachomatis infant pneumonitis. Comparison with matched controls and other infant pneumonitis. N Engl J Med 1978;298:702–8.

122. Grayston JT, Wang SP, Kuo CC, et al. Current knowledge on Chlamydia pneumoniae, strain TWAR: an important cause of pneumonia and other acute respiratory diseases. Eur J Clin Microbiol Infect Dis 1989;8:191–202.

123. Grayston IT, Campbell LA, Kuo C-C, et al. A new respiratory tract pathogen: Chlamydia pneumoniae strain TWAR. J Infect Dis 1990;161:618–25.

124. Marrie TJ. Chlamydia pneumoniae. Thorax 1993;48:1–4.

125. Hammerschlag MR. Chlamydia pneumoniae and the lung. Eur Resp J 2000;16:1001–7.

126. Grist NR, McLean C. Infections by organisms of psittacosis/lymphogranuloma venereum group in the west of Scotland. BMJ 1964;2:21–5.

127. Andrews BE, Major R, Palmer SR. Ornithosis in poultry workers. Lancet 1981;i:632–4.

128. Irons JV, Sullivan TD, Rowan J. Outbreak of psittacosis [ornithosis] from working with turkeys or chickens. Am J Public Health 1951;41:931–7.

129. Sax PE, TrotmanDickenson B, Klein RS, et al. Pneumonia and the acute respiratory distress syndrome in a 24-year-old man – psittacosis, causing the acute respiratory distress syndrome. N Engl J Med 1998;338:1527–35.

130. Diehl JL, Gisselbrecht M, Meyer G, et al. Bronchiolitis obliterans organizing pneumonia associated with chlamydial infection. Eur Respir J 1996;9:1320–2.

131. BenYaakov M, Eshel G, Zaksonski L, et al. Prevalence of antibodies to Chlamydia pneumoniae in an Israeli population without clinical evidence of respiratory infection. J Clin Pathol 2002;55:355–8.

132. Wu L, Skinner SJM, Lambie N, et al. Immunohistochemical staining for Chlamydia pneumoniae is increased in lung tissue from subjects with chronic obstructive pulmonary disease. Am J Respir Crit Care Med 2000;162:1148–51.

133. Webley WC, Tilahun Y, Lay K, et al. Occurrence of Chlamydia trachomatis and Chlamydia pneumoniae in paediatric respiratory infections. Eur Respir J 2009;33:360–7.

134. Jackson LA, Campbell LA, Schmidt RA, et al. Specificity of detection of Chlamydia pneumoniae in cardiovascular atheroma: Evaluation of the innocent bystander hypothesis. Am J Pathol 1997;150:1785–90.

135. Shor A, Phillips JI, Ong G, et al. Chlamydia pneumoniae in atheroma: consideration of criteria for causality. J Clin Pathol 1998;51:812–17.

Aspiration pneumonia and lung abscess

136. Marik PE. Primary care: Aspiration pneumonitis and aspiration pneumonia. N Engl J Med 2001;344:665–71.

137. Huxley EJ, Viroslav J, Gray WR, et al. Pharyngeal aspiration in normal adults and patients with depressed consciousness. Am J Med 1978;64:564–8.

138. Kennedy JH. 'Silent' gastroeosophageal reflux: an important but little known cause of pulmonary complications. Dis Chest 1962;42:42–5.

139. Brock RC, Hodgkiss F, Jones HO. Bronchial embolism and posture in relation to lung disease. Guy Hosp Rep 1942;91: 131–9.

140. Carlson DH. Right middle lobe aspiration pneumonia following gasoline siphonage. Chest 1981;80:246–7.

141. Crome L, Valentine JC. Lentil soup inhalation? J Clin Pathol 1962;15:21–5.

142. Matsuse T, Oka T, Kida K, et al. Importance of diffuse aspiration bronchiolitis caused by chronic occult aspiration in the elderly. Chest 1996;110:1289–93.

143. Mukhopadhyay S, Katzenstein A-LA. Pulmonary disease due to aspiration of food and other particulate matter: a clinicopathologic study of 59 cases diagnosed on biopsy or resection specimens. Am J Surg Pathol 2007;31:752–9.

144. Bartlett JG, Gorbach SL, Finegold SM. The bacteriology of aspiration pneumonia. Am J Med 1974;56:202–7.

145. Penner C, Maycher B, Long R. Pulmonary gangrene – a complication of bacterial pneumonia. Chest 1994;105: 567–73.

146. Lemierre A. On certain septicaemias due to anaerobic organisms. Lancet 1936;i: 701–3.

147. Moore-Gillon J, Lee TH, Eykyn SJ, et al. Necrobacillosis: a forgotten disease. BMJ 1984;288:1526–7.

148. Dykhuizen RS, Olson ES, Clive S, et al. Necrobacillosis (Lemierre's syndrome): a rare cause of necrotizing pneumonia. Eur Respir J 1994;7:2246–8.

149. Riordan T, Wilson M. Lemierre's syndrome: more than a historical curiosa. Postgrad Med J 2004;80:328–34.

150. Bartlett JG, Gorbach SL, Tally FP, et al. Bacteriology and treatment of primary lung abscess. Am Rev Respir Dis 1974;109:510–18.

151. Neild JE, Eykyn SJ, Phillips I. Lung abscess and empyema. Q J Med 1985;57: 875–82.

Botrymycosis

152. Multz AS, Cohen R, Azeuta V. Bacterial pseudomycosis: a rare cause of haemoptysis. Eur Respir J 1994;7: 1712–13.

153. Tuggey JM, Hosker HSR, DaCosta P. Primary pulmonary botryomycosis: a late complication of foreign body aspiration. Thorax 2000;55:1068–9.

154. Kathir K, Dennis C. Primary pulmonary botryomycosis: an important differential diagnosis for lung cancer. Respirology 2001;6:347–50.

155. Naidech H, Ruttenberg N, Axelrod R, et al. Pulmonary botryomycoma. Chest 1976;70:385–7.

156. Katznelsen D, Vawter GF, Foley GE, et al. Botryomycosis: a complication in cystic fibrosis. Report of 7 cases. J Pediatr 1964;65:525–39.

157. Katapadi K, Pujol F, Vuletin JC, et al. Pulmonary botryomycosis in a patient with AIDS. Chest 1996;109:276–8.

158. Shih JY, Hsueh PR, Chang YL, et al. Tracheal botryomycosis in a patient with tracheopathia osteochondroplastica. Thorax 1998;53:73–5.

Chapter | 5 |

5.3   Chronic bacterial infections

TUBERCULOSIS

Bacteriology

Tuberculosis is caused by certain mycobacteria. In the laboratory these microbes are difficult to stain and in the body they are difficult to kill. Their comparative resistance to the normal body defences is due to an ability to inhibit phagosome–lysosome fusion, permitting them to survive within the host's phagocytes.[1,2] Their resistance to ordinary stains is attributed to their cell walls being rich in mycolic acid waxes. This necessitates the use of hot concentrated carbol fuchsin for their demonstration, as in the Ziehl–Neelsen stain. Once stained in this way, they are difficult to decolorise, even with strong acids and alcohol, hence references to the acid- and alcohol-fast bacilli. Mycobacteria also show some resistance to formalin: of 138 tissue specimens from autopsy lungs fixed in formalin and showing histological evidence of acid-fast bacilli, 12 grew mycobacteria, including three *Mycobacterium tuberculosis* isolates.[3]

The bacilli are normally scanty in tuberculous tissue and their identification with the Ziehl–Neelsen stain may require tedious examination of many sections.[4] They are easier to identify in rhodamine-auramine-stained sections examined by fluorescence microscopy.[5–7] Tissue containing necrotising granulomas is most likely to give positive results whereas specimens showing only non-necrotising granulomas, poorly formed granulomas or acute inflammation are less likely to reveal acid-fast bacilli.[8,9] Culture is no more likely to identify the mycobacteria than the examination of tissue sections.[9,10] Failure to demonstrate them does not exclude a diagnosis of tuberculosis. The future lies in immunohistochemistry[11] or molecular techniques such as the polymerase chain reaction, which can be adapted for application to paraffin sections.[12–15a] The detection of mycobacterial RNA indicates that the bacilli are viable and is therefore preferable to tests for mycobacterial DNA. Molecular techniques are also useful in identifying drug resistance, distinguishing mycobacterial species and identifying specific strains of *M. tuberculosis*.[16–18]

The mycobacteria that cause tuberculosis in humans are sometimes listed as *M. tuberculosis*, *M. bovis*, *M. africanum* and *M. microti*, the so-called tuberculosis complex, although these four organisms are probably just variants of a single species. The first two correspond to the human and bovine tubercle bacilli while *M. africanum* includes a heterogeneous group of strains, with properties intermediate between the former two, isolated from humans in equatorial Africa and from African immigrants in Europe. The features and management of tuberculosis in humans caused by these three variants are very similar. *M. microti*, the vole tubercle bacillus, is of attenuated pathogenicity for humans and has been used as a vaccine.

M. tuberculosis is largely responsible for the disease and the infection is predominantly pulmonary, acquired through inhalation of this organism into the lungs. Formerly, intestinal tuberculosis, acquired by drinking milk infected with *M. bovis*, was much commoner, but the eradication of mycobacteriosis from cattle and the widespread pasteurisation of milk brought about a virtual disappearance of this form of disease in developed countries.

In addition to the human, bovine and vole types, the term 'tubercle bacillus' includes the avian and the 'cold-blooded' types. The avian tubercle bacillus is a distinct species, *M. avium*, while the 'cold-blooded' group includes the fish, turtle and frog tubercle bacilli, which are known as *M. marinum, M. chelonei* and *M. fortuitum* respectively. All these other 'tubercle bacilli' can cause opportunistic infections in humans and, together with a number of other opportunistic species, are often referred to as the atypical, anonymous or opportunistic mycobacteria. *M. intracellulare* is no longer distinguished from *M. avium*, and the collective *M. avium-intracellulare* is often used. Similarly, reference is sometimes made to *M. fortuitum-chelonei*. The opportunistic mycobacteria are dealt with separately later in this chapter (see p. 211).

Route of infection in pulmonary tuberculosis

In the past, there was much speculation about the possible routes of infection in tuberculosis. Today, there is little doubt that when the lesions are present in the lungs the infection has taken place as a result of inhalation of tubercle bacilli. That the respiratory tract should be the chief portal of entry is scarcely surprising in view of the great preponderance of the pulmonary form of chronic tuberculosis in humans and of the enormous numbers of tubercle bacilli that are eliminated daily in the sputum of most untreated active cases. Those in close contact with such patients are liable to inhale the bacilli and acquire the infection in their lungs. Although the smaller droplets of expectorated sputum, which may remain for many minutes suspended in the air after a cough, are probably the chief vehicle for the transmission of tubercle bacilli, it should be realised that the organisms are resistant to desiccation, and that in consequence, dried 'droplet nuclei', or the dust that they ultimately contaminate, may long remain as potential carriers of the infection. Tuberculosis transmission can be reduced however by hospitalising patients with positive sputa in isolation rooms equipped with ultraviolet light and exhaust ventilation.[19]

Other routes of infection which may have operated in pulmonary mycobacteriosis in the past include haematogenous dissemination from a primary focus of *M. bovis* infection in the intestine, acquired by drinking infected milk, and similar spread from a primary focus in the skin acquired by traumatic inoculation (a rare occupational hazard of pathologists and butchers, hence the old term 'butcher's wart'), but these have never been as important as droplet spread.

Epidemiology

In most developed countries there has been a considerable fall in the incidence of tuberculosis and its mortality over the last century (Fig. 5.3.1). This is attributable to a variety of factors that began to operate among the prosperous classes and subsequently extended to all strata of society. During almost the whole of this period an amelioration in social conditions took place in an almost uninterrupted, unspectacular manner and it is to these unspecific factors that for many years the progressive fall in mortality was essentially due, although it was aided by public health measures such as the eradication of tuberculous cattle and mass radiography screening. After 1950, the decline in mortality from tuberculosis was hastened by the introduction of effective antituberculosis drugs. By bringing about a great fall in the number – often even the complete disappearance – of bacilli in the sputum in cases of active respiratory tuberculosis, these drugs have much reduced the hazard of infection that was formerly incurred by those who inadvertently or by obligatory associations were brought into contact, at work or at home, with an infectious case of the disease.

The reduced incidence of the disease in developed countries led to changes in the ages of the affected patients. Whereas it was formerly a disease of the young, tuberculosis came to be largely limited to the elderly in these countries, the disease representing recrudescence of quiescent infection acquired in youth. Many of these elderly patients suffered from an insidiously progressive form of the disease and this is still the case today (see p. 210).

The situation remained very different elsewhere. Much of the world has still not shared the economic and health benefits enjoyed in the west and in many countries tuberculosis remains one of the most important specific communicable diseases. Furthermore, the considerable gains that have slowly been achieved are now in peril because of the acquired immunodeficiency syndrome (AIDS) and other factors.

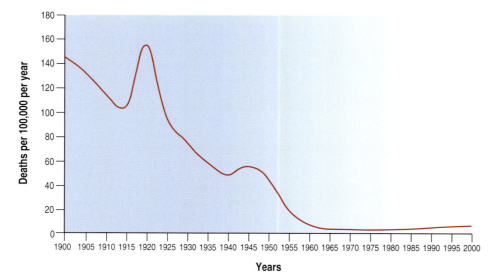

Figure 5.3.1 Deaths from tuberculosis in England and Wales in the twentieth century. The decline in mortality, temporarily checked by two world wars, was established well before specific chemotherapy became available, and is largely attributable to improved living standards.

There has been a resurgence of tuberculosis recently, even in groups where AIDS has yet to make a major impact, possibly due to new levels of urban deprivation and the influx of immigrants and refugees from countries with a high incidence of the disease.[20] In the UK, for example, immigrants from the Indian subcontinent have rates of tuberculosis about 25 times as high as that of the white population.[21] The decline in the incidence of tuberculosis in the UK slowed towards 1987 and has subsequently reversed: since that date case numbers have risen, particularly in inner London. The situation is similar in many other developed countries. Tuberculosis can therefore be regarded once more as a worldwide problem. It is estimated that about one-third of the world's population (approximately 2000 million people) have latent tuberculosis while the prevalence of active disease is put at more than 20 million worldwide. In 2006 there were 9.2 million new cases and 1.7 million deaths, which makes tuberculosis the largest cause of death from a single pathogen in the world.

Despite the prevalence of tuberculosis, the human response to infection is good. In the absence of immunosuppressive disorders such as human immunodeficiency virus (HIV) infection, only about 10% of those infected develop clinically evident disease. The basis of these patients' susceptibility is not well understood but tobacco smoking is a predisposing cause[22] and genetic factors appear to be involved.[23]

The impact of HIV infection

Following the advent of AIDS the downward trend in tuberculosis stabilised or was reversed.[24,25] An alarming resurgence of the disease is being witnessed, particularly in the poorer communities where drug abuse is prevalent (Table 5.3.1).[26–28] Furthermore, multidrug-resistant strains have emerged and now represent a global problem.[29–33] The mortality is high with such strains, even in patients who are not immunodeficient, but it is particularly high in AIDS.

It is estimated that worldwide more than 6 million people are dually infected with the tubercle bacillus and HIV, the majority in 10 sub-Saharan African countries. In 2007, there were an estimated 1.37 million new cases of tuberculosis among HIV-infected people and

456 000 deaths, one in four deaths from tuberculosis being HIV-related.[34] In sub-Saharan Africa, the AIDS epidemic is having a devastating effect on tuberculosis control programmes, with up to 100% increases in reported tuberculosis cases. The annual risk of active tuberculosis in those who are doubly infected is 10%, compared with a 10% lifetime risk in those who harbour the tubercle bacillus but are HIV-negative.[35] The situation in richer countries may not be so bad because HIV-infected persons tend to be young and those harbouring tuberculosis old, rendering recrudescence unlikely.[35] However, within HIV units, cross-infection is being reported.[31] Such nosocomial transmission has involved patients and hospital staff who are immunocompetent as well as other HIV-positive patients.[36]

The mechanism whereby HIV infection promotes tuberculosis is probably related to the pattern of cytokines produced by T-lymphocyte subsets. T-helper-1 lymphocytes produce interferon-γ and are central to antimycobacterial immune defence. However, when peripheral blood lymphocytes from HIV-infected patients with tuberculosis are exposed to tubercle bacilli in vitro they produce less interferon-γ than lymphocytes from HIV-negative patients with tuberculosis, suggesting that a reduced T-helper-1 response contributes to HIV-infected patients' susceptibility to tuberculosis.[37] It is also noteworthy that there is a reciprocal relationship between tuberculosis and HIV infection: tuberculosis appears to promote the course of HIV infection, probably by inducing macrophages to secrete cytokines that increase HIV replication.[38–40]

Not surprisingly in view of the interrelationship of HIV and the tubercle bacillus, the tuberculosis associated with HIV infection is particularly aggressive, being characterised by widespread dissemination throughout the body and a poor host response.[41] This nonreactive form of tuberculosis is similar to the insidious disease of elderly patients referred to above and described on page 210.

Primary and postprimary types of tuberculosis

Although the morbid anatomical changes that develop in tuberculosis assume a variety of forms, the great majority of cases fall into one or other of two distinctive types. The first type was formerly found mainly in children and became known as the 'childhood type' of tuberculosis. Further experience has shown that it is not so much the youth of these patients as the fact that they are infected for the first time that accounts for the distinctive structural features of their lesions. In consequence, this form of tuberculosis is now known as the 'primary type', and as the incidence of the disease in the general population has declined and the age of first infection has correspondingly risen, it is now met with increasing frequency in adults. The second morphological form – previously known as the 'adult type' of the disease – occurs in those patients who have been sensitised by an earlier exposure to tuberculosis: this type of disease is now generally termed 'postprimary tuberculosis'. Postprimary tuberculosis is due to either fresh infection or reactivation of a dormant primary lesion (Fig. 5.3.2). Reinfection is common in countries in which tuberculosis is prevalent but in the developed countries reactivation of infection acquired decades earlier is commoner. The various patterns of tuberculous infection are summarised in Box 5.3.1.

Primary tuberculosis

The very early stages of a tuberculous lesion in the human lung have seldom been seen, and our ideas on its pathogenesis have been derived almost wholly from study of lesions in experimental animals.[42] Initially, the presence of tubercle bacilli in an alveolus excites little immediate reaction, and for the first day or two the only change may

Table 5.3.1 The effect of human immunodeficiency virus (HIV) infection on the global toll of tuberculosis[27,28]

Region	People infected (millions)	New cases	Deaths	HIV-attributed
Western Pacific[a]	574	2 560 000	890 000	19 000
South-East Asia	426	2 480 000	940 000	66 000
Africa	171	1 400 000	660 000	194 000
Eastern Mediterranean	52	594 000	160 000	9000
The Americas[b]	117	560 000	220 000	20 000
The industrialized countries[c]	382	410 000	40 000	6000
Total	1722	8 004 000	2 910 000	315 000

[a]Excluding Japan, Australia and New Zealand.

[b]Excluding USA and Canada.

[c]Western Europe, USA, Canada, Japan, Australia and New Zealand.

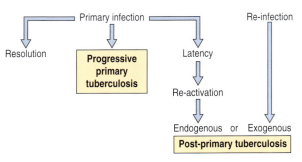

Figure 5.3.2 Possible events following infection by tubercle bacilli.

Box 5.3.1 **Summary of patterns of tuberculous infection of the lungs**

Primary tuberculosis[a]

Ghon focus + regional lymph node = primary complex

Reparative

Quiescent

Progressive

Pleural involvement

Airway dissemination (tuberculous bronchopneumonia, laryngeal lesions)

Epituberculosis (segmental tuberculosis)

Haematogenous (miliary tuberculosis, meningitis, solitary lesions in organs with a rich systemic blood supply and therefore a high oxygen tension, e.g. kidney. Also the lung apices because of their high ventilation/perfusion ratio)

Postprimary tuberculosis[a] (reactivation or reinfection)

Fibrocaseous apical cavitation (high oxygen tension)

Reparative

Quiescent

Progressive

Local extension

Pleural involvement

Airway dissemination (tuberculous bronchopneumonia)

Haematogenous (miliary tuberculosis)

Non-reactive tuberculosis (immunocompromised or elderly)

[a]Primary tuberculosis usually heals but if it progresses there is a greater chance of widespread dissemination than in postprimary disease, in which progression is more often local.

Figure 5.3.3 A tuberculous granuloma consisting of a central collection of epithelioid macrophages surrounded by lymphocytes. A Langhans giant cell is seen amongst the epithelioid cells.

are mixed with the epithelioid and giant cells and outside these, further lymphocytes form a dense outer mantle. This localised collection of epithelioid macrophages, Langhans giant cells and lymphocytes constitutes a tuberculous granuloma (Fig. 5.3.3). Immunocytochemistry shows that the lymphocytes in the inner zone of the granuloma are mainly T-helper (CD4) and memory (CD45RO) cells whereas the outer zone includes both CD4 and CD8 (T-suppressor) lymphocytes, while immediately adjacent to the outer zone and difficult to distinguish from it without immunocytochemistry there is a secondary centre composed of B lymphocytes and active (Ki-67+) antigen-presenting cells (Fig. 5.3.4).[45]

By the third week, the granuloma has usually grown sufficiently to be visible to the naked eye as a small, grey nodule, or tubercle, which gives the disease its name. As the tubercle enlarges, its centre turns yellow. Microscopical examination at this stage shows that the granuloma has undergone necrosis (Fig. 5.3.5). A ring of satellite tubercles then develops and as these undergo central necrosis they fuse together (Fig. 5.3.6). In this way the original granuloma gradually increases in size. The growth of a tuberculous lesion by the progressive development and subsequent incorporation of satellite tubercles is also seen in postprimary tuberculosis (see Fig. 5.3.19, p. 210).

It is characteristic of the classic active tuberculous lesions that the tubercle bacilli are scanty, probably reflecting a state of relatively strong immunity/hypersensitivity (see below). Also characteristic of tuberculosis is prolonged survival of the tubercle bacilli within the tissues, despite a vigorous host reaction. This is attributable to the tubercle bacillus inhibiting the fusion of macrophage lysosomes and phagosomes and so avoiding the bactericidal contents of the lysosomes.[1,2]

The type of necrosis found in a classic tuberculous lesion is distinctive, being dry, crumbling and cheesy (hence the term 'caseous' as a macroscopic description). It is of the coagulative rather than liquefactive type, probably because of the relative dearth of polymorphonuclear leukocytes. The necrosis is a hypersensitivity phenomenon; no

be a small amount of exudate and a few neutrophils round the organisms. Within the next few days, macrophages collect in increasing numbers, and ingest most of the bacilli.

Gradually, the macrophages, with living bacilli in their cytoplasm, aggregate to form microscopical nodules. The macrophages also develop an abundant eosinophilic cytoplasm and are described as 'epithelioid'. This represents a switch from their basic phagocytic function to a secretory one (see sarcoidosis, p. 286), modulated by lymphokines from T lymphocytes, notably interferon-γ.[23,43,44] This change promotes the antibacterial properties of the macrophage but also contributes to tissue necrosis, as outlined below. After about 2 weeks some of the more centrally placed macrophages fuse to form multinucleate cells of Langhans type. Small numbers of lymphocytes

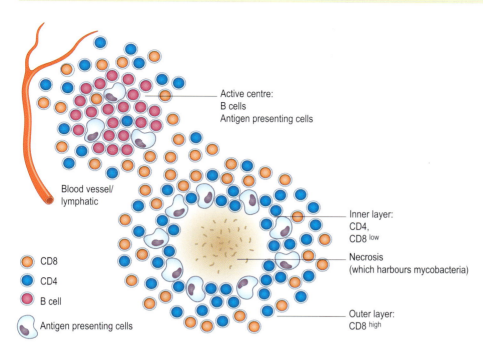

Figure 5.3.4 Diagrammatic representation of a tuberculous granuloma. The central necrosis, which harbours mycobacteria, is surrounded by an inner layer of antigen-presenting cells and CD4+ T lymphocytes, within which CD8+ cells are scarce. The outer lymphocyte infiltrate contains large numbers of CD8+ T cells and active (Ki-67+) centres with mycobacteria-containing antigen-presenting cells and B cells surrounded by both CD4+ and CD8+ T cells. *(Redrawn from Ulrichs et al.[45] by permission of the Journal of Pathology.)*

Active centre:
B cells
Antigen presenting cells

Blood vessel/
lymphatic

○ CD8
○ CD4
● B cell

○ Antigen presenting cells

Inner layer:
CD4,
CD8 low

Necrosis
(which harbours mycobacteria)

Outer layer:
CD8 high

Figure 5.3.5 A tuberculous granuloma showing central caseous necrosis.

Figure 5.3.6 Tuberculous granulomas clustered around more extensive areas of coagulative necrosis.

mycobacterial toxins have been identified. It represents apoptosis brought about by cytotoxic T cells and macrophages activated by subsets of T-helper cells. The epithelioid cells show strong immuno-expression of the proapoptotic proteins Bax and Fas, with the anti-apoptotic protein Bcl-2 being notably absent.[46,47]

The elastic tissue of the lung persists for a long time in necrotising tuberculous lesions. When stained appropriately, its distribution and pattern give information about the position of blood vessels and of alveolar walls within the necrotic centre that cannot be recognised clearly, if at all, in haematoxylin and eosin preparations. Ultimately, however, all trace of the lung's elastin framework is lost.

In the comparatively small number of human cases in which there is an opportunity to examine the lungs while the lesion of primary tuberculosis is still active, the latter – often known as the 'Ghon focus'[48] – is generally visible as a pale yellow, caseous nodule, a few millimetres to a centimetre or two in diameter. Characteristically, it is situated in the peripheral part of the lung underlying a localised area of chronic inflammation and thickening of the pleura. Usually, only one such focus is present, but if the lungs are searched carefully, preferably with the help of postmortem radiography, it will be found that there is more than one focus in a small proportion of cases. It is a point of importance in the distinction between primary and post-primary tuberculosis of the lungs that in the latter the lesions are almost invariably in the apical region of an upper lobe, whereas in the former they are found most frequently in the periphery of the lower lobes, where airflow is greatest.

Studies on primary tuberculosis in both humans and experimental animals show that within a few days of their deposition in subpleural alveoli some of the bacilli are carried centripetally in the lymphatics to establish infection in hilar lymph nodes. Thereafter, the granulomatous changes in the lung and lymph nodes, and the smaller foci that may have formed along the course of the intrapulmonary lymphatics, all develop at about the same rate but the caseating lesions in the lymph nodes tend to be larger than the primary focus in the lung. This combination of a peripheral Ghon focus with the corresponding focus of caseation in the regional lymph nodes is known as the primary complex of Ranke (Figs 5.3.6 and 5.3.7). The complex is the typical result of a primary tuberculous infection of the lungs.

Figure 5.3.7 Primary complex of tuberculosis with miliary spread. A small Ghon focus in the lower lobe of the lung is accompanied by prominent caseating tuberculous lymphadenitis. The infection has spread from one of the lymph nodes into a branch of a pulmonary artery, resulting in miliary haematogenous tuberculosis of the lower lobe. *(Courtesy of the Curator of the Pathology Museum, Charing Cross and Westminster Medical School, London, UK.)*

The primary complex may undergo a series of reparative changes, or it may continue to enlarge and in so doing implicate further structures and thus promote dissemination of the infection. The pathological features of healing and progressive primary complexes and the relative frequency of these processes will be considered next.

Reparative changes

The slow enlargement of the caseating primary complex is accompanied by the development of a fibrous capsule that impedes further centrifugal dispersal of the bacilli should any still remain alive. Later, there is often dystrophic calcification and even ossification, within which fatty and sometimes haemopoietic marrow may form. Diffuse racemose (dendriform) ossification (see p. 149) has also been reported in association with pulmonary tuberculosis.[49]

These old foci of caseous necrosis, walled off by fibrous tissue, may contain viable bacilli, despite an absence of inflammation. Such latent lesions, which are known as quiescent tuberculosis, are potential sites of recrudescence. Active disease is denoted by granulomatous inflammation.

Progressive changes

In a small proportion of cases of primary tuberculosis, the reparative changes fail to stem the progress of the disease. As the infected tissues undergo caseation, the bacilli tend to die in the central areas but to

Figure 5.3.8 Tuberculous empyema. The lung is compressed by a large cavity that was originally filled by caseous material, loculated collections of which persist at the apex. The walls of the cavity are formed by the thickened parietal and visceral layers of the pleura. *(Courtesy of the curator of the Gordon Museum, Guy's Hospital, London, UK.)*

survive and multiply in the surviving zone of granulation tissue that borders the lesion, leading to its peripheral extension. As a result of this, a caseous mass, several centimetres in diameter, may form either in the lung itself or in the now much enlarged and generally matted regional lymph nodes. If the lesion erodes into a bronchus, loss of the necrotic material through the airway leads to the creation of a cavity, often of a size little less than that of the parent caseous mass, and surrounded by a ragged lining of partly necrotic tuberculous granulation tissue. If the necrotic focus breaks through the pleura, the result is pleural effusion, pneumothorax, tuberculous empyema (Fig. 5.3.8) or pyopneumothorax. Sometimes this is the presenting manifestation of the disease, and occasionally the only clinical evidence of the disease. In tuberculous empyema the matter in the pleural sac is caseous and not purulent, despite the traditional terminology, unless there is a secondary infection by pyogenic organisms.

Figure 5.3.10 Dissemination of caseous material via the airways has led to widespread focal consolidation. *(Courtesy of Dr Max Millard, formerly of Florida, USA.)*

Figure 5.3.9 Primary complex of tuberculosis comprising a large caseating Ghon focus and marked enlargement of the infected mediastinal lymph nodes. A caseating lymph node to the right of the lower end of the trachea has become adherent to the latter, and the tuberculous process has extended through the tracheal wall to form a sinus. Aspiration of infective material from this sinus has led to the development of the tuberculous bronchopneumonia, represented by multiple small foci of consolidation scattered throughout the lung. *(Courtesy of the curator of the Gordon Museum, Guy's Hospital. London, UK.)*

Dissemination through the airways

Caseous material that enters the main respiratory passages is largely expectorated but some is dispersed to other parts of the lungs by the deep inspiration that usually accompanies coughing. Such dispersion of large numbers of organisms within the bronchial tree may lead to widespread tuberculous bronchopneumonia ('galloping consumption'), an often fatal condition (Figs 5.3.9–5.3.11). Smaller numbers of bacilli may infect the bronchial, tracheal or laryngeal mucosa, or, by being swallowed, the intestine. Infection of a bronchus causes ulceration, mucosal thickening or concentric scarring which may be complicated by collapse of the distal lung.

Caseous hilar nodes may compress a bronchus and lead to absorption collapse (see middle-lobe syndrome, p. 92).[50–52] Partial

Figure 5.3.11 Tuberculous bronchopneumonia. Almost the whole of the lung shows pale, confluent areas of caseation. *(Courtesy of the curator of the Gordon Museum, Guy's Hospital. London, UK.)*

obstruction may lead to air trapping and severe distension of a lobe, proper ventilation of which may be obtainable only by surgical evacuation of the caseous contents of the nodes responsible. Massive enlargement of paratracheal nodes, particularly those of the right side, may result in compression of the trachea, causing stridor and sometimes cyanosis.

A caseating hilar lymph node may also erupt into a bronchus. Very rarely, so much matter escapes suddenly that the patient, usually a child, is quickly asphyxiated. More often there is progressive change in the affected segment. This is the condition known as epituberculosis.

Epituberculosis (segmental tuberculosis)

This condition[53] is a fairly frequent radiological finding in cases of primary pulmonary tuberculosis. The radiographic picture is that of a segmental opacity. It is associated with little clinical disturbance and usually resolves completely over a period of months. It was once commonly assumed to represent absorption collapse due to compression of the segmental bronchus by the lymph node component of the primary complex, but this explanation is now recognised to be inadequate in many cases. The great majority of these lesions represent inflammatory consolidation caused by the lymph node component of the complex perforating into the segmental bronchus so that infected caseous material is disseminated throughout the distal air passages.

The affected segment is pale grey and the lobular markings are accentuated by thickening of the interlobular septa. There is exudation of both fluid and macrophages into the alveoli, and lymphocytic infiltration of the alveolar walls. That the lesion is not merely a non-specific obstructive pneumonitis is clear from the constant presence of numerous epithelioid cell granulomas. Initially the granulomas are non-necrotising but quite extensive caseation may develop. Tubercle bacilli are to be found in the caseous node but are usually very sparse in the consolidated lung.

The lesion can be reproduced experimentally by introducing either killed tubercle bacilli or the purified protein derivative of tuberculin into previously sensitised animals. The condition is therefore considered to represent a local hypersensitivity reaction to the aspiration of caseous material from the perforated hilar nodes. This is supported by the acceleration of the resolution that is achieved by adding corticosteroids to the usual specific antituberculous drugs, and by the dramatic reappearance of the disease if the corticosteroids are withdrawn.

The natural outcome of epituberculosis is variable. There may be complete resolution or patchy fibrosis with contracture and perhaps bronchiectasis. The perforation of the bronchus usually heals with only minor scarring, but occasionally it causes fibrous constriction of the bronchus similar to that caused by aerogenous spread to the bronchus from a lesion in the lung, as described above. A rare sequel, comparable in pathogenesis to the traction diverticula of the oesophagus, is the formation of a bronchial diverticulum.

Haematogenous dissemination

Tuberculous bacillaemia is a common early event in primary tuberculosis. Strom provided evidence of this when he used radiolabelled tubercle bacilli to induce the disease experimentally.[54,55] The bacilli are generally destroyed by phagocytes throughout the body but occasional organisms may escape this fate and – after their lodgement in a kidney, bone or joint, the central nervous system, an adrenal gland or some other organ favourable to their growth – set up an isolated focus of tuberculosis that may either remain latent for years or progress. The apices of the lungs are amongst the tissues that favour

the establishment of blood-borne tuberculosis. The reason for this is described below under 'Postprimary tuberculosis'.

When many bacilli enter the circulation simultaneously and a massive haematogenous dissemination ensues, generalised miliary tuberculosis develops. In this condition, as in all forms of bacteraemia, the organisms are removed from the circulating blood by phagocytic cells lining sinusoids in the liver, spleen, bone marrow and elsewhere. Although, to judge from experimental tuberculous bacillaemias, most of the circulating bacilli are promptly destroyed by the phagocytes, enough survive ingestion to set up innumerable small metastatic foci of infection.

The massive blood stream invasion by tubercle bacilli necessary to produce miliary tuberculosis is often brought about by a caseating tuberculous focus involving the wall of a neighbouring blood vessel. This is particularly likely to complicate the hilar lymph node component of a primary complex, for these caseous masses are not only larger than those in the lungs, but they develop in proximity to the large veins in the mediastinum (see Fig. 5.3.7). The wall of the affected blood vessel becomes replaced by tuberculous granulation tissue. In time, caseation develops, the lesion ulcerates through the intima and tubercle bacilli escape into the blood stream. In exceptional cases, the aorta may be eroded, with consequent rupture and rapidly fatal bleeding. However, it is not always possible to demonstrate vascular erosion and it seems likely that the organisms may on occasion reach the blood by way of the lymphatics.

Generalised miliary tuberculosis is usually fatal unless treated quickly and appropriately, particularly if the infection has involved the central nervous system and given rise to tuberculous meningitis. Necropsy in such cases shows enormous numbers of small, grey tubercles, a millimetre or less in diameter, most notably in the liver, spleen, bone marrow, lungs and meninges, and more sparsely in other organs (Fig. 5.3.12). The term 'miliary' derives from a supposed likeness of the tubercles to millet seeds. The preponderant distribution and typically uniform dispersal of tubercles in the parts affected may be ascribed partly to the particularly large number of phagocytic cells in the walls of the blood sinusoids of the tissues, and partly to the situation of the vessel invaded: if it is a systemic vein in the mediastinum, or the main thoracic duct, the bacilli are first carried to the lungs, where many are filtered out in the pulmonary capillaries to give origin to a preponderance of the miliary tubercles in the lungs; if it is a tributary of the pulmonary veins, they are carried to other organs in the systemic arterial circulation.

Histologically, miliary tubercles have a characteristic structure. A Langhans multinucleate giant cell commonly forms the centre and is enclosed by a zone of epithelioid macrophages and an outer shell of lymphocytes. If the patient survives for a month or more, the tubercles will be larger and their centres show early caseation. These more advanced lesions consist of small groups of satellite tubercles that have a general resemblance to the original one and surround the central caseous area that has taken its place.

Today, when many of those patients who develop generalised haematogenous dissemination of the infection are successfully treated, the progressive changes in the tubercles in the lungs can sometimes be followed in serial radiographs and the findings compared with those in histological preparations of the lungs of patients who died at the corresponding stage. Gradually, during the weeks following the institution of the treatment the finely dispersed opacities can be seen to regress until their presence is no longer detectable radiologically. At this stage, microscopical examination of the tubercle shows merely a minute scar composed almost wholly of hyaline collagen with no trace of the former distinctive cellular structure. If a cure follows at a more advanced stage of the disease, after caseation has occurred, the caseous material becomes calcified. This results in a fine mottling of the lung fields that may be seen radiologically for years after.

Figure 5.3.12 Miliary tuberculosis. The lung is studded with numerous tubercles, each the size of a millet seed. *(Courtesy of Dr M Kearney, Tromso, Norway.)*

Subclinical primary tuberculosis

The true prevalence of tuberculous infection in the general population is very much higher than overt clinical manifestations suggest. This inference is based on two main sources of evidence: first, identification of healed tuberculous lesions in necropsy studies on long series of consecutive cases of patients dying from all causes in large general hospitals; and second, immunological surveys on large samples of the population employing the tuberculin skin test as an indicator of previous infection.

The realisation that primary tuberculosis is followed by recovery in the great majority of those infected was the most important outcome of a pioneer study by Naegeli at the end of the nineteenth century in the postmortem room of the Zurich General Hospital. Employing acceptable anatomical criteria for the identification of healed and active tuberculous lesions, he reached two very significant conclusions: first, that practically all the adults who had died in that hospital from diseases of all kinds had, at some site in their body, recognisable tuberculous foci that, in the great majority, had healed; and second, that in only a minority of these patients could death be attributed to tuberculosis. Forty years later, a similar study was made at the same hospital, and again traces of a previous tuberculous infection were detected in the bodies of 80–90% of all adult patients.

The interest and surprise aroused by Naegeli's work stimulated numerous similar studies elsewhere: his general conclusions were fully confirmed and it was recognised that signs of past tuberculous infection, notably calcified mediastinal and mesenteric lymph nodes, were common in any population studied. Although in elderly people the frequency of evidence of such healed infections changed little over the ensuing half-century, in children and young adults it showed a decline that reflected the diminished incidence of clinical tuberculosis in western countries. A much larger fraction of the population than formerly became liable to reach adult life without a primary infection and, as a corollary, also without the valuable, if partial, immunity that results from an infection that has been overcome. Prophylactic immunisation in childhood was therefore instituted and is now widely practised.

The tuberculin skin test

As well as first identifying the tubercle bacillus in 1882, Robert Koch went on to develop a vaccine against the disease based upon the subcutaneous injection of a sterilised extract of the bacteria. It was not successful therapeutically but von Pirquet used Koch's 'old tuberculin' as a skin-testing agent after showing that reactivity to it indicates that a person has been infected by the tubercle bacillus. In the original test, a drop of old tuberculin was placed on the skin and a scratch was made through the drop, but reagents are now administered by intradermal injection (the Mantoux method) or by use of multiple-pronged devices (Heaf and tine tests). Old tuberculin has given way to purified protein derivative but the principle of the test remains unchanged and it provides a useful indication of the extent of transmission of tuberculosis in countries where tuberculin reactivity has not been artificially induced by bacillus Calmette–Guérin (BCG) vaccination (see below) or there is not heavy exposure to the opportunistic environmental mycobacteria. To circumvent the problem of opportunistic mycobacteria causing such spurious reactions, blood tests have been developed that measure T-cell interferon release in vitro in response to antigens unique to the tubercle bacillus.[56]

The tuberculin skin test becomes positive within a few weeks of tuberculous infection being acquired and remains so in the great majority for many years. Confidence in the reliability and specificity of the test is based mainly upon evidence from two sources. The first comes from surveys made on cattle just before slaughter: the result of the test correlated very closely with the presence or absence of tuberculous lesions in the carcass. The second is derived from tests on clinically tuberculous and clinically non-tuberculous children under 5 years of age: 94% of the former, and only 12% of the latter, were positive.

Tuberculin surveys have given incontestable support to the general conclusion drawn from necropsy studies that tuberculosis has been widespread in urban populations. In a tuberculin survey in London between the two world wars the percentage of positive reactors was found to rise progressively from well below 10 in children under 2 years to 90 in adults. Yet despite the great frequency of infection and the large number of deaths from the disease, the case fatality rate – the only numerical indicator of the probable outcome of an infection – is comparatively low. This is exemplified by the figures set out in Table 5.3.2, which shows that even in 1931 only one out of several thousand children who became infected actually died from the disease: a fatal outcome is even less frequent today.

The immunity and hypersensitivity that result from tuberculous infection

The frequency with which a primary tuberculous infection is overcome, usually without the patient being aware of its presence, roused interest in the possibility that in tuberculosis, as in many other infectious diseases, recovery from an attack might leave a heightened resistance to infection in the event of subsequent exposure to the same organism. Further, as some degree of immunity generally results from a natural infection, the question was raised whether similar protection could be conferred by some controllable prophylactic procedure. An affirmative answer has been given to both these questions.

The first study that disclosed convincingly that a primary infection conferred some protection was made by Heimbeck in Oslo. His conclusions were based on studying follow-up records of positive and negative tuberculin reactors among probationer nurses entering the municipal hospital in that city. Through a comparative study of the findings on enrolment and the subsequent medical history while nursing, it became apparent that, although all were equally exposed to the same general hospital environment and its hazards, the incidence of overt tuberculosis was significantly less in those girls who were positive reactors at the time of their entry.

Heimbeck's conclusions have since been scrutinised and confirmed in many studies elsewhere. The most extensive of these – the Prophit

Table 5.3.2 Comparison by age of positive tuberculin reactors in a sample London population with deaths from tuberculosis for England and Wales in 1931

Age group (years)	Positive reactors (%)	Deaths from tuberculosis (%)
0–5	12	0.076
6–10	30	0.026
11–20	61	0.060

Table 5.3.3 Incidence of clinical tuberculosis among positive and negative reactors to tuberculin in London, 1934–44[57]

Tuberculin reaction at outset	Number of people examined	Cases of tuberculosis recorded	Incidence (%)
Positive	7130	95	1.33
Negative	1745	69	3.95

Fund Tuberculosis Survey – was carried out on nearly 10 000 young people, mainly nurses and medical students, in London over the period from 1934 to 1944.[57] The results of this investigation are summarised in Table 5.3.3, which shows that there was about three times as high an incidence of clinical tuberculosis among young adults who were negative reactors at the start of the study as among similarly exposed positive reactors in London. This is almost the same as the average ratio derived from nearly 30 comparable surveys elsewhere in Europe and in America. It establishes the conclusion that, although a primary infection does not confer absolute immunity, it does give a valuable degree of protection against developing the disease in a clinical form after subsequent exposure to the same organism.

Specific prophylactic immunisation

Numerous efforts have been made to confer immunity to tuberculosis through prophylactic inoculation, many by veterinary surgeons who hoped to free cattle from the disease. The most significant conclusion from their work was that, unlike what had been found for many other infectious diseases, killed organisms were relatively impotent as immunising agents. Protection could be conferred only through an infection that had been overcome. In consequence of this, the search for an effective prophylactic agent became one for strains of the bacillus that were of such low natural virulence, or that had been so attenuated by appropriate methods of culture, that they could be inoculated safely while still alive. Such strains, it was hoped, would produce only a self-limiting infection. Of those that have been found, the organism now widely known, after those who developed it, as bacillus Calmette–Guérin or BCG has established itself as the agent of choice, and is now widely employed in antituberculosis schemes in many parts of the world. Yet, although the effectiveness of BCG has been demonstrated on many occasions (Table 5.3.4), in other studies it appears to have conferred no protection whatsoever.[58] The reason for these marked differences is poorly understood but may be connected with the fact that, since its introduction, numerous daughter strains of varying antigenicity have developed, which is not surprising as being a live bacterium it has had to be passaged in vitro over 1000 times.[59] Another possible reason is the variable prevalence of other mycobacteria in the

environment as these confer some protection against tuberculosis but also reduce the effectiveness of BCG.[59a] Table 5.3.4 shows that BCG is most effective when administered soon after birth, i.e. to the immunologically naïve.

In developing countries, where the prevalence of tuberculosis is high, BCG immunisation of the newborn is recommended to prevent the dangerous forms of childhood tuberculosis, but elsewhere it is only recommended for the Mantoux-negative members of certain high-risk groups – health workers, including mortuary and laboratory staff, veterinarians, case contacts, immigrants from countries with a high prevalence of tuberculosis together with their children and infants wherever born, and those intending to stay in Asia, Africa or Central or South America for longer than a month.

Although BCG inoculation is generally harmless, disastrous dissemination of the infection has been known to occur.[60] Impaired host immunity may be presumed to account for these rare instances as the dose and batch of the vaccine used in these exceptional cases have not differed from those used successfully in other children. Cases have been reported in the context of AIDS and inherited immunodeficiency states such as severe combined immunodeficiency and chronic granulomatous disease. However, in half the cases reported no well-defined inherited immunodeficiency state has been recognised. Some of these patients have been able to mount a good granulomatous response against the infection but others have developed disease similar to lepromatous leprosy, characterised by florid proliferation of the bacilli and an apparently ineffective non-granulomatous macrophage response.[61] It follows that any form of immunosuppression is a contraindication to BCG immunisation: this includes corticosteroid treatment and HIV infection.

BCG immunisation confers advantages other than protection against tuberculosis as it has heterologous effects on the immune response to many organisms and thereby exerts a beneficial influence on several human infections.[61a] It has also been suggested that children so immunised suffer less leukaemia and other malignancies but such claims are somewhat tenuous.[62] However, BCG has been injected into the pleural cavity or the bladder of patients with inoperable cancer of these regions in the hope that it would have a non-specific adjuvant effect on the immune reaction to the cancer and, as with its use in preventing tuberculosis, there are rare instances of the bacillus being disseminated widely throughout the body.[63,64]

The relationship of immunity to hypersensitivity in tuberculosis

The rapid translocation of tubercle bacilli to the regional lymph nodes, and perhaps beyond, on first infection, is less likely in post-primary tuberculosis, indicating some degree of acquired immunity, while the development of caseation at a time when cellular immune mechanisms may be expected to take effect suggests that hypersensitivity accompanies the immunity. Long ago, Rich showed that guinea pigs made allergic by the injection of non-virulent tubercle bacilli still retained resistance after gradual desensitisation with tuberculin, suggesting that hypersensitivity and immunity were distinct,[65] a proposition for which there is now considerable support.[66,67] Hypersensitivity and specific acquired immunity are both cell-mediated, but T-cell characterisation indicates that different T-cell subsets are involved.

Antigens are processed by specific cells, such as dendritic cells, and are presented in association with products of the major histocompatibility complex genes to T lymphocytes. Cytotoxic (CD8-positive) T cells are activated by products of the class I major histocompatibility genes (HLA-A and -B), which are expressed on the surface of antigen-presenting cells if microbial proliferation proceeds unchecked within phagocytes, the bacteria-containing phagocytes then being eliminated

Table 5.3.4 The protective effect of bacillus Calmette–Guérin (BCG) found in nine major studies[58]

Group studied	Date of commencement	Duration (years)	Age range	Protection (%)
Native North American	1935–38	9–11	0–20 years	80
Chicago, USA	1937–48	12–23	3 months	75
Georgia, USA	1947	20	6–17 years	0
Illinois, USA	1947–48	19–20	Young adults	0
Puerto Rico	1949–51	5–7.5	1–18 years	31
Georgia/Alabama, USA	1950	14	Over 5 years	14
Great Britain	1950–52	15	14–15 years	78
South India (Bangalore)	1950–55	9–14	All ages	30
South India (Madras)	1969–71	7.5[a]	All ages	0

[a]15-year follow-up has revealed some protection amongst those administered BCG as neonates.

by the T cells. On the other hand, effective processing of the bacteria results in the antigen-presenting cells expressing class II major histocompatibility genes (HLA-D), the products of which activate (CD4-positive) T-helper cells, so enhancing bacterial elimination.[68]

Two types of T-helper cells are recognised, one concerned mainly in immunity and the other with hypersensitivity. Type 1 T-helper lymphocytes (Th1) secrete interleukin-2 and the macrophage-activating cytokine interferon-γ, resulting in enhanced bacterial elimination; however, it also results in the secretion of tumour necrosis factor by the macrophage, which contributes to the hypersensitivity that derives from the activation of type 2 helper T cells (Th2).[69] Th2 cells secrete interleukins-4, -5, -6 and -10, which prime tissue cells to the necrotising action of tumour necrosis factor secreted by macrophages activated by Th1 cells. Thus, type 1 reactions are essentially protective but also contribute to the type 2 cell-mediated hypersensitivity (Fig. 5.3.13).[43,44,68,70] Many chronic infections are first characterised by a Th1 response which then shifts to a Th2 response, with detriment to the host. Animal models suggest that necrosis occurs in T-cell-dependent granulomas when Th2 involvement is superimposed on a Th1 reaction.[71]

Postprimary tuberculosis

In contrast to primary tuberculosis of the lungs, where the Ghon focus may develop in any lobe, the early lesions in the postprimary disease are almost invariably found near the apex of one of the upper lobes. Postprimary pulmonary tuberculosis obviously involves considerable spread of the infection. The dissemination is believed to be blood-borne. Using radiolabelled bacilli, Strom provided experimental evidence that tuberculous bacillaemia is a common and early event in primary tuberculosis.[54,55] In the great majority of people, both the primary complex and its haematogenous dissemination are quickly overcome, but in some the distant foci progress or remain latent. If tributaries of the pulmonary veins are involved in the spread of the infection, the bacilli pass out of the thorax, but if the blood stream is colonised via the lymphatics, the pulmonary capillaries are the first to be reached, and so the infection returns to the lungs.

Oxygen tension governs the predilection for blood-borne tuberculosis to favour the apical regions of the lungs and also sites such as the kidneys, meninges and metaphyses. These extrapulmonary sites are well vascularised and therefore have a relatively high oxygen tension. The tubercle bacillus is a strict aerobe and thrives in such organs. In the lung, more complex factors govern oxygen tension. The

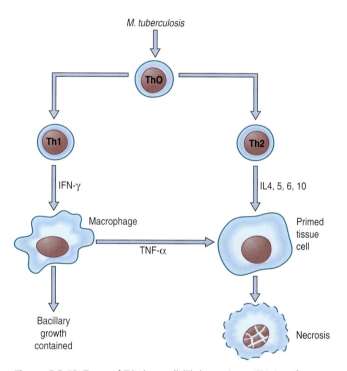

Figure 5.3.13 Types of T-helper cell (Th-) reactions. IFN, interferon-γ; IL, interleukin; TNF-α, tumour necrosis factor-α. (*Redrawn after Grange.*[68])

apices of the lungs are poorly perfused, but the pulmonary arteries bring deoxygenated blood. Ventilation on the other hand promotes oxygen tension, but the apices are also the most poorly ventilated parts of the lungs. The oxygen tension in the lungs is in fact dependent upon the ventilation/perfusion ratio. In the upright position, this declines from the apices to the bases of the lungs (Fig. 5.3.14),[72–75] and the oxygen tension is therefore highest at the top of the lungs, thus favouring the development of postprimary tuberculosis at the apices.

If the disease progresses, radiological opacities appear in the apex of one or both of the upper lobes. They may resolve or progressively enlarge and ultimately cavitate. Necropsy studies indicate that such lesions represent areas of caseating granulomatous inflammation that

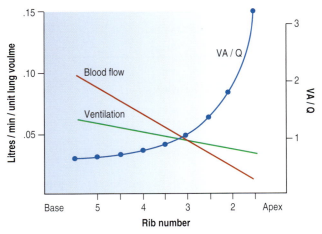

Figure 5.3.14 Regional differences in pulmonary blood flow, ventilation and ventilation/perfusion ratios (VA/Q), consequent upon gravitational forces. These result in a higher oxygen tension and poorer lymphatic drainage at the apices, thereby promoting the development of tuberculosis at this site. *(Redrawn after West.[74])*

ultimately develop large central areas of necrosis. It is through the expulsion of this dead tissue through the regional bronchi that the cavities so typical of the advanced lesions originate.

If the liquefying contents of a cavity escape into the bronchial tree, the bacilli become widely dispersed to other parts of both lungs, as in progressive primary tuberculosis. This diffuse bronchogenic infection gives rise to innumerable small areas of caseous pneumonia, mostly in the lower lobes, and occasionally, a rapidly developing confluent tuberculous bronchopneumonia involves almost the whole lower lobe. Microscopical examination may show tubercle bacilli and macrophages in very large numbers in the consolidated areas. Occasionally, such regions undergo caseation. They may become so confluent as to involve a whole lobe.

At necropsy, the lungs of a patient with long-standing, progressive, postprimary tuberculosis have a characteristic appearance. Large cavities may replace much of an upper lobe and one or more smaller, but otherwise similar, cavities may be present in the apical part of the lower lobe. The cavities may be filled with caseous material (Fig. 5.3.15) or the contents may have been evacuated through communicating bronchi (Figs 5.3.16–5.3.18). The cavities may be several centimetres in diameter, with walls formed by tuberculous granulation tissue in which the fibrotic remains of the larger bronchi and of branches of the pulmonary arteries form coarse, irregular bands. Usually the disease is bilateral, with similar, but often less advanced, changes in the opposite lung. As in progressive primary tuberculosis, satellite nodules are evident at the advancing edge (Fig. 5.3.19).

The hilar lymph nodes are less obviously involved in the postprimary form of tuberculosis than in the primary form of the disease but, on histological examination, tuberculous foci, often with small areas of caseation, can generally be seen in them.

Histological examination of the wall of a cavity usually discloses several zones, each grading into the next. The yellowish-grey lining is formed largely of granulation tissue that has undergone caseation but not yet liquefied. Acid-fast bacilli can generally be seen in this zone: their multiplication there and subsequent escape into the cavity largely account for the high infectivity of the sputum expectorated by patients with advanced pulmonary tuberculosis. Just deep to this is a zone of granulation tissue containing a profusion of macrophages and lymphocytes and occasional multinucleate giant cells. If the cavity has been infected secondarily by other organisms, as often happens, this

Figure 5.3.15 Postprimary tuberculosis. The upper lobe is consolidated and several large foci of caseous necrosis are evident. Smaller foci are also seen in the lower lobe. *(Courtesy of the Curator of the Gordon Museum, Guy's Hospital, London, UK.)*

zone may also contain many neutrophils. Outside this zone there is generally a mantle of satellite tubercles. Still deeper in the wall are traces of residual parenchyma, often with alveoli obliterated by compression and fibrosis. The cavities enlarge by incorporation of the satellite tubercles, more of which are constantly forming more peripherally (see Fig. 5.3.19). In this way tuberculous granulation tissue extends into the surrounding lung substance as its lining progressively caseates, liquefies and is expectorated. Eventually the process of cavitation may reach the pleura, but perforation into the sac hardly ever takes place, for the chronic pleurisy that accompanies the changes within the lungs results in the formation of firm adhesions between the visceral and parietal layers, with obliteration of the pleural sac.

Although the formation of a cavity is a serious development in the progress of a postprimary tuberculous infection of the lung, it does not represent an irreversible stage in the course of the disease. As long as it is small, a cavity may heal by scarring. Ultimately, such a lesion may only be recognisable as an area of fibrosis that stands out from the surrounding parenchyma because of its black pigmentation and the radiating pale strands of fibrous tissue that pucker the neighbouring lung substance. Alternatively, a balance may be achieved whereby the tubercle bacilli are not destroyed but their spread is halted and the process is held in check, typically by a fibrous capsule forming. Such an encapsulated mass of caseous material is sometimes termed a tuberculoma (Fig. 5.3.20). In such quiescent tuberculosis there is no

Figure 5.3.16 Postprimary tuberculosis. The caseous contents of this cavitating upper-lobe lesion have been partially evacuated through communicating airways. *(Courtesy of Dr M Kearney, Tromso, Norway.)*

Figure 5.3.17 Postprimary tuberculosis. The upper lobe is replaced by a large air-filled cavity, its caseous contents having emptied into the lobar bronchus with which the cavity communicates.

inflammation but viable bacilli may survive in the central caseation, ready to reactivate the disease should host defence weaken. Any granulomatous inflammation in the vicinity of such a lesion indicates active tuberculosis.

Local complications of postprimary pulmonary tuberculosis

Pulmonary tuberculosis is often attended by minor episodes of haemoptysis. That the involvement of blood vessels is not more frequently accompanied by haemoptysis is accounted for by the fact that the destructive process usually advances slowly, so that obliterative endarteritis leads to the closure of the lumen of the pulmonary and bronchial arteries before their walls have been penetrated. However, caseation sometimes advances too quickly for the artery to become completely blocked, and an aneurysm may form where the muscular and elastic coats are destroyed on the side nearer the cavity. It is through the rupture of such aneurysms (Rasmussen's aneurysms) that sudden and sometimes fatal haemorrhages occur.

Large tuberculous cavities may persist indefinitely once the tuberculous infection has been overcome. If the cavity is not able to drain freely into the bronchial tree, secretion may accumulate in it and predispose to secondary bacterial infection, sometimes with the formation of a lung abscess. Fungal colonisation may also take place, leading to the formation of an aspergilloma or other variety of intracavitary ball colony[76] (see p. 231).

In some cases the cavity acquires an epithelial lining: the epithelial lining may be of modified respiratory type or squamous. A squamous lining may be simple or stratified; sometimes keratinisation develops, and the lumen of the cavity may become filled by compressed desquamated cells, the appearances then being reminiscent of an epidermoid cyst. Squamous carcinoma occasionally arises from such areas of metaplasia.

Chronic tuberculosis of the lungs is usually accompanied by pleurisy. Although this begins in the neighbourhood of the most active lesions, in time it may extend to involve the whole surface of the lung. The condition advances slowly, generally without the formation of much exudate; by the time of necropsy the pleural lesions have usually undergone fibrosis. The damaged lung becomes firmly attached to the chest wall – indeed, the fibrosis may be so firm and extensive that the lung can be removed from the body only by dissection outside the parietal pleura. Occasionally, the entire lung may be enclosed by a dense white layer of hyaline connective tissue, several millimetres thick.

Extrapulmonary complications of postprimary respiratory tuberculosis

The proliferation of tubercle bacilli that takes place in the caseating lining of cavities in the lungs is often so great that it leads to heavy

Figure 5.3.18 Postprimary tuberculosis. Tuberculous bronchopneumonia is seen throughout the lower lobe, the result of aerogenous dissemination of infection from the cavitating focus at the apex of this lobe. A further focus of cavitating tuberculosis is seen in the midzone of the upper lobe.

Figure 5.3.19 Postprimary pulmonary tuberculosis progressing by the incorporation of satellite tubercles. Satellite tubercles are evident at the advancing edge of a chronic caseating focus of infection.

infection of the exudate and secretions, most of which are expelled by coughing, sometimes aided by the adoption of a posture that promotes gravitational drainage. These organisms form a potent reservoir for infection of the upper respiratory tract and of the alimentary canal.

In advanced cases of chronic respiratory tuberculosis small ulcers, each a few millimetres in diameter, often develop in the tracheobronchial mucosa,[77] as described above under the dissemination of primary

Figure 5.3.20 Quiescent tuberculosis forming a 'tuberculoma'. Growth of this apical focus of tuberculosis has been halted and its caseous contents walled off by a fibrous capsule. However, the infection has not necessarily been overcome as viable bacilli may persist in the caseous material and reactivate the disease if immunity wanes.

pulmonary tuberculosis via the airways. Occasionally it may mimic a neoplasm but generally there is just slight destruction of tissue and the ulceration amounts to little more than loss of epithelium; occasionally, it may extend more deeply and expose one or more rings of tracheal cartilage. Such tracheobronchial disease was identified in 42% of cases in the preantibiotic era.[77] Subsequently, it was rarely encountered, until AIDS appeared, since when there have been several reports of endobronchial tuberculosis.[78–81] Similar infection may involve the larynx, particularly the glottis and the aryepiglottic folds; the subsequent injury to the vocal cords leads both to hoarseness and to frequent stimulation of the cough reflex.

The passage through the mouth of sputum teeming with tubercle bacilli may also lead to infection of the oral mucous membrane. Most commonly, the lesions appear as ulcers on the margin of the tongue: these are probably initiated by some minor damage to the mucosa such as results from abrasion by a nearby carious tooth, the resulting breach in the epithelial surface giving access to the organisms. Once these ulcers form, they may penetrate deeply into the muscle. Sometimes, the organisms gain entry to the tonsils and there produce typical changes.

Unless trained not to do so, many patients with respiratory tuberculosis swallow much of their sputum and thus maintain a constant infection of the alimentary canal. Since tubercle bacilli are relatively resistant to acid in the concentrations found in gastric juice, they escape destruction in the stomach and enter the small intestine. The most typical lesions occur in the lowest 2 m of the ileum; these are chronic, circumferentially oriented ulcers that begin in, and finally destroy, Peyer's patches, and then extend towards the mesentery along the mucosal lymphatics.

Amyloidosis is prone to develop in many cases of slowly progressive pulmonary tuberculosis. Although many organs become infiltrated with the amyloid material, renal involvement is the commonest serious manifestation and the lungs are seldom involved. As in other forms of secondary amyloidosis, the amyloid is a polymer of the hepatic acute-phase protein A.

Tuberculosis in the elderly and immunodeficient: non-reactive tuberculosis

In developed countries, miliary tuberculosis is now a commoner cause of death in the elderly than the young.[82] It is thought to result from

Figure 5.3.21 Non-reactive tuberculosis in acquired immunodeficiency syndrome (AIDS). There is extensive necrosis but no granulomatous reaction. Such lesions teem with tubercle bacilli.

activation of old tuberculous foci, primary or postprimary, as a consequence of waning of the immunological defences. In many cases the disease takes a 'cryptic' form,[82–84] characterised by insidious onset and progression, and often lacking any evidence of miliary mottling in the chest radiograph. The diagnosis is usually not made until necropsy. Both cryptic and overt miliary tuberculosis in the elderly may be accompanied by changes in the blood, including pancytopenia and leukaemoid reactions: these may be the first manifestation of the illness, and their significance in such cases is sometimes overlooked. In the elderly, and especially in the immunodeficient, the disease may be non-reactive. Non-reactive tuberculosis differs from ordinary tuberculosis in lacking the usual giant cell granuloma formation.

At necropsy, disseminated miliary tuberculous lesions are found to be widespread. Microscopy shows that the lesions comprise foci of virtually structureless necrotic matter, sharply defined from the surrounding tissue, which shows little or no abnormality (Fig. 5.3.21). There is little or no granulomatous response. Appropriate staining shows that they teem with tubercle bacilli, and, unlike the caseation of classic tuberculosis, the necrotic material may contain much nuclear debris.[41,85,86] Neutrophil polymorphonuclear leukocytes are commonly seen.

Other forms of non-reactive tuberculosis include diffuse alveolar damage and vasculitis. In the former tubercle bacilli are generally demonstrable in the hyaline membranes[86] while in the latter they teem within the vessel walls.

Non-reactive tuberculosis is the result of a deficiency in the body's cellular defences. In some cases it develops as a complication of lymphoid neoplasia, particularly Hodgkin's disease and leukaemia. In other cases it has followed treatment with immunosuppressant drugs. More recently it has been seen in patients suffering from AIDS.[41,87] Often, however, no predisposing cause is found; such patients are generally elderly.

If the diagnosis of non-reactive tuberculosis is suspected during life, tubercle bacilli should be looked for in films of bone marrow. Biopsy may be helpful; any suggestion of a tuberculous reaction is potentially an important diagnostic guide. When any biopsy section includes unexplained areas of necrosis, particularly when there is little in the way of a related cellular reaction, it is imperative to look for tubercle bacilli.

It is to be remembered that the tissues in this form of tuberculosis are highly infective. Several cases of tuberculous infection in laboratory staff, including those working in mortuaries, have been traced to this source.

Postmortem recognition of pulmonary tuberculosis

It is estimated that many cases of active tuberculosis of the lungs go unrecognised until necropsy. This is particularly true of the elderly, whose resistance to the infection is lowered as an accompaniment of ageing: dormant lesions become active, and spread of the disease follows, often with little in the way of clinical manifestations to indicate the seriousness of the danger. Similarly, at any age, patients, whose resistance is lowered by conditions such as lymphoma and poorly controlled diabetes mellitus, are prone to reactivation of dormant tuberculosis and vulnerable to exogenous reinfection: often the presence of the infection is overlooked, even when it is the immediate cause of death, until disclosed in the postmortem room. Now that the necropsy rate is falling markedly in so many countries, many cases of active tuberculosis must go unrecognised. The danger that persists after the patient's death is that the infection may have been passed to relatives or associates without awareness of the need for treatment.

Treatment of tuberculosis

The treatment of tuberculosis is based on a combination of drugs (classically triple therapy) but is bedevilled by the emergence of drug-resistant strains, an inability of many countries to provide the drugs and poor compliance on the part of the patient.[88–91]

INFECTION BY OPPORTUNISTIC MYCOBACTERIA

Bacteriology

The organisms responsible for tuberculosis and leprosy are only two of about 40 species of mycobacteria, most of which live freely in the environment, particularly where water abounds, and seldom infect humans. Occasionally, however, especially when resistance is low, several of these environmental mycobacteria cause serious disease.[92,93] Their distinction from M. tuberculosis is important because they require special drug regimens; they do not respond to antituberculosis treatment. Formerly dismissed as 'atypical' or 'anonymous', these species are better described as the opportunistic mycobacteria. They include M. marinum and M. ulcerans, the causes of swimming-pool granuloma and Buruli ulcer respectively, and a group that causes disease that is very like tuberculosis. In infection by members of the latter group, as in tuberculosis itself, the lungs are the organs most often involved and there may be spread to lymph nodes, bone, meninges, kidneys and elsewhere, or massive dissemination throughout the body akin to miliary tuberculosis. The similarity to tuberculosis is also seen in that the gastrointestinal tract is another important portal of entry.[94]

The commonest opportunistic mycobacteria infecting the lungs are M. avium-intracellulare, M. kansasii and M. xenopi. Less frequent causes of tuberculosis-like disease are M. scrofulaceum, M. malmoense, M. szulgai, M. simiae, M. chelonei, M. fortuitum and M. gordonae. M. avium-intracellulare and M. scrofulaceum are often said to comprise the MAIS complex. They are all acid-fast but, unlike M. tuberculosis, many of them can also be demonstrated with periodic acid–Schiff and Grocott's stains. M. kansasii has a distinctive shape, being long, broad, beaded and bent.[95] Species-specific probes are available.[96,97]

Infection with these organisms comes from the environment, in contrast to tuberculosis, which is always transmitted from an infected individual. The infection rate of tuberculosis in the community bears a direct relation to the number of infectious cases but this is not the case with the opportunistic mycobacteria. The prevalence of opportunistic mycobacterial infection in a community is independent of that of tuberculosis and is not controlled by public health measures aimed at reducing the spread of tuberculosis.

Interpretation of cultured isolates

The interpretation of cultured isolates must always take account of the possibility that specimens may be contaminated with opportunistic mycobacteria from the environment. Whereas *M. tuberculosis* is an obligate parasite and its isolation indicates tuberculosis, the culture of opportunist mycobacteria does not necessarily indicate that they are the cause of the disease being investigated. Their isolation from granulomatous tissue strongly suggests that they have played a causative role, but sputum isolates need to be obtained consistently over a period of weeks, and other causes of granulomatous disease, especially tuberculosis, thoroughly excluded before a clinical diagnosis of opportunistic mycobacterial infection can be advanced with confidence.

Predisposing causes

Factors predisposing to opportunistic mycobacterial infection may be general or local.[98] General factors include any congenital or acquired immunodeficiency, but especially AIDS,[94,99,100] therapeutic immuno-suppression and autoimmune disease. Local factors include pneumo-coniosis, chronic bronchitis, cystic fibrosis, bronchiectasis and old tuberculosis. The virulence of mycobacteria is enhanced by lipid[101] and the growth of opportunistic mycobacteria, especially *M. fortuitum-chelonei*, appears to be promoted by lipid pneumonia.[102–104] The aspiration of milk may explain an observed association between achalasia and *M. fortuitum-chelonei* infection.[105,106]

Only rarely is no predisposing cause recognised.[107,108] Although some impairment of host defence is generally necessary for these bacteria to establish themselves in humans, heavy exposure may result in healthy individuals being infected. An example of this is the increasingly frequent presentation in affluent, non-immunocompro-mised individuals of diffuse lung disease due to the inhalation of aerosols from hot tubs and showers heavily infected by these bacteria. However, there are suggestions that this may represent extrinsic allergic alveolitis rather than infection.[96,109–114]

Despite the above, there appears to be an increasing incidence of infection by opportunistic mycobacteria in persons who are not obviously immunodeficient or heavily exposed. These individuals are often women and it has been suggested that their infection may be due to them suppressing their cough reflex for reasons of societal etiquette, an unlikely scenario but one that has nevertheless entered the medical argot as the Lady Windermere syndrome, a term taken from the fastidious character of the same name in Oscar Wilde's play *Lady Windermere's Fan*.[115] A survey of such patients found that they were taller and leaner than controls, had high rates of scoliosis, pectus excavatum, mitral valve prolapse and mutation of the cystic fibrosis transmembrane conductance regulator gene. This categorised the condition as one of women with a complex pre-existing morpho-type, suggesting that there was an underlying genetic defect.[116]

Pathological changes

The pathological changes produced by opportunistic mycobacteria are generally very similar, if not identical, to those of tuberculosis (Fig.

Figure 5.3.22 *Mycobacterium avium-intracellulare* infection. There is necrotising granulomatous inflammation similar to that seen in tuberculosis.

5.3.22), but there is more airway involvement leading to bronchiectasis[117–119] and a higher proportion of cases that lack the classic granulomatous response.[120] In one study, four histological features were identified that favoured non-tuberculous mycobacterial infection: the presence of microabscesses, the granulomas being ill defined, an absence of necrosis and a comparatively small number of giant cells,[121] but these are not absolute points of distinction.

Granulomatous disease indicates a strong immune response and the mycobacteria are then scanty, as in classic tuberculosis. However, in very severe immunodeficiency, as for example AIDS, the lesions may consist of numerous swollen macrophages, all of which contain large numbers of acid-fast bacilli (Fig. 5.3.23). Necrosis is not seen and granulomas are poorly formed or absent. The changes then resemble those of lepromatous leprosy[94] or, if the macrophages are spindle-shaped, inflammatory myofibroblastic tumour (see p. 620).[122–125] A leproma-like pattern has also been described in disseminated BCG infection but is unusual in non-reactive tuberculosis[126] which is characterised by sheets of necrosis unattended by the usual granulomas, the tubercle bacillus being more toxic to the macrophage than the opportunistic mycobacteria.[127]

Treatment

The treatment of opportunist mycobacteriosis is less well defined than for tuberculosis, there being few large clinical trials. However, the British Thoracic Society has published a set of guidelines.[97]

BRUCELLOSIS

Pneumonia is a rare form of brucellosis but has been reported in countries such as Kuwait and Arabia[128,129] where this zoonosis is endemic, and in farmers and meat packers in North America and Europe.[130,131] Cattle, sheep, goats and camels are common sources of infection, which is usually acquired by consuming unpasteurised milk or milk products. Close contact with infected animals or their carcasses may also be responsible for transmission of the disease to humans, either orally or, in the case of pneumonia, by inhalation.

Figure 5.3.23 *Mycobacterium avium-intracellulare/M. scrofulaceum* (MAIS complex) infection in a patient with acquired immunodeficiency syndrome (AIDS). Whereas the tissue reaction to opportunistic mycobacteria is usually identical to that seen in tuberculosis, in the immunodeficient it resembles the lepromatous form of leprosy, consisting of numerous macrophages with abundant pale cytoplasm (A); Ziehl–Neelsen staining demonstrates that this contains innumerable acid-fast bacilli (B). (C) Alternatively, the macrophages may be spindle-shaped and the cytoplasm eosinophilic, resulting in an appearance simulating inflammatory myofibroblastic tumour.

Patients with *Brucella* pneumonia develop a cough productive of mucopurulent sputum or present with fever of unknown cause.[132] Perihilar or peribronchial infiltrates, or less frequently coin lesions, are evident radiographically. Pleural effusion with a predominance of monocytic or lymphocytic infiltrates is also described.[133]

Histology shows necrotising epithelioid and giant cell granulomas, very similar to those of tuberculosis.[128,134,135] Diagnosis is dependent upon excluding tuberculosis and identifying brucellae by culture or brucellar DNA by polymerase chain reaction in blood or tissue.[135] Examination of sputum and bronchial washings is generally unrewarding.

CHRONIC MELIOIDOSIS

The general features and acute form of melioidosis have been described on page 186. Chronic melioidosis is acquired in the same way as the acute form and may represent persistence or recrudescence of acute disease or arise insidiously in someone unknown to have had acute disease. The disease progresses gradually over months or years. It takes the form of localised lesions that may affect any organ but most commonly involve the lungs, where chronic cavitatory melioidosis may closely mimic tuberculosis apart from relative sparing of the apices.[136-138] Pleural effusion and empyema are less common in chronic than acute disease. Before cavitation takes place, microscopy shows areas of necrosis surrounded by granulomatous inflammation. The central necrotic zones are often stellate, and may be suppurative or caseous. The surrounding granulomatous reaction consists of epithelioid and Langhans giant cells and is itself encompassed by a fibrous mantle. When necrosis is suppurative, the histological features mimic those of cat scratch disease or lymphogranuloma venereum, and, especially in the lungs, tularaemia (see p. 187) or sporotrichosis (see p. 244). When the necrosis is caseous, the histological picture is very similar to that of tuberculosis. In contrast to the acute form of the disease, the causative bacterium (*Burkholderia pseudomallei*) can be difficult to demonstrate in tissue sections (see p. 186 for staining methods). The diagnosis is then largely dependent upon serological techniques.

ACTINOMYCOSIS

Bacteriology

Actinomycetaceae (which include the genera *Actinomyces*, *Nocardia* and *Rhodococcus*) and Mycobacteriaceae (which include the genus *Mycobacterium*) are both families of the order Actinomycetales. Although Actinomycetales are classed as bacteria and mycobacterial diseases are invariably considered among bacterial infections, some of the pathogenic Actinomycetaceae are often mistakenly referred to as fungi and the diseases they cause are commonly grouped with those caused by the true fungi under the general heading of mycoses. It will be difficult to correct this misconception, particularly in view of such entrenched nosological nomenclature as actinomycosis, which by virtue of the ending '-mycosis' – its etymology is usually misinterpreted – is unlikely to be displaced from its common association with the true mycoses, in spite of other well-understood terminological paradoxes and pitfalls such as mycosis fungoides and mycotic aneurysm. However, as well as differing from fungi in size, structure and metabolism, the Actinomycetaceae are susceptible to antibacterial agents and resistant to specifically antifungal drugs.

Actinomyces israelii is by far the most frequent cause of actinomycosis in humans. *A. bovis*, the cause of actinomycosis in cattle, is an exceptionally rare cause of the disease in humans. Other species that occasionally cause actinomycosis in humans include *A. eriksonii*, *A. meyerii* and *A. naeslundii*. *A. propionicus* (*Arachnia proprionica*), an organism closely related to *Actinomyces israelii*, also causes disease indistinguishable from actinomycosis.

A. israelii is a strictly anaerobic, Gram-positive bacterium, formed of branching filaments 0.5–1.0 µm wide. The filaments readily break into bacillus-like fragments. They are not acid-fast. Like those of the nocardiae (see below), fragments of the *Actinomyces* may be mistaken for contaminant corynebacteria.

A. israelii is a common commensal or saprophyte in the human mouth and intestine and it is probable that most infections by this organism are endogenous. About 60% of cases of actinomycosis present with lesions in the region of the mouth, face or neck, the portal of entry being dental or tonsillar. About 25% of cases of actinomycosis involve the ileocaecal region and in the remaining 15% of cases the infection is in the lungs. It is presumed that pulmonary actinomycosis is the outcome of aspiration of infected matter from the tonsillar crypts or mouth, apart from the very small proportion of cases in which the disease has extended from known foci of infection in the abdomen. The diagnosis should therefore be particularly suspected in patients with dental caries or a history of unconsciousness with aspiration. The incidence of actinomycosis is in decline, probably due to a combination of improved dental hygiene and the early initiation of antibiotic therapy, the bacterium being highly sensitive to penicillin.

Most cases of actinomycosis are of mixed microbial aetiology, the pathogenicity of *Actinomyces* being enhanced by the synergistic action of other bacteria, notably microaerophilic streptococci, other anaerobes such as *Bacteroides* and *Fusobacterium*, and aerobic streptococci and staphylococci. *Actinobacillus actinomycetem comitans* is another constituent of the mouth flora – one that is seldom recovered in pure culture[139] but is often found in association with *Actinomyces israelii* in actinomycotic lesions. It secretes a powerful leukotoxin which probably contributes to the virulence of these mixed infections.

Clinical features

Pulmonary actinomycosis is promoted by poor dental hygiene, smoking and heavy drinking[140] and is recorded in AIDS.[141] It is usually a disease of adults, though may rarely occur in children.[142,143] It is characterised by fever and expectoration of mucopurulent sputum. Contrary to a common belief, 'sulphur granules' – the yellow colonial granules of the organisms – are not often to be found in the sputum. Haemoptysis is a significant complication and may require surgical treatment.[144] The diagnosis depends on recognition of the fine, Gram-positive, sometimes branching filaments in films, and isolation of the organism. It has to be remembered that the organism may be present in sputum only in short bacillary forms that are liable to be misinterpreted. The chest radiograph may show opacities of various sizes scattered through both lungs, particularly in the middle and lower zones. Alternatively, there may be a large pneumonic area, sometimes associated with an empyema: this type of disease may be accompanied by new bone formation on the inner aspects of several contiguous ribs due to elevation of the periosteum by the inflammatory infiltrate. Occasionally, infiltration of the chest wall suggests malignancy (Fig. 5.3.24). The presence of discharging sinuses on the chest wall is characteristic of advanced thoracic actinomycosis[145] but this stage is seldom encountered today.[146,147] It is in the pus discharging from these sinuses that the 'sulphur granules' referred to above are to be found. Recent series have been characterised by less specific features that have suggested tuberculosis or cancer.[140,141,148] The diagnosis has often been made only after lung tissue has been resected, but may be possible by biopsy, particularly when the process involves major airways.[141,149] It

Figure 5.3.24 Actinomycosis. (A) Computed tomography shows a mass in the right middle lobe extending through the chest wall and mimicking an invasive carcinoma. (B) The lobectomy specimen shows colonies of *Actinomyces* (arrow) within abscesses that extend into the fat of the chest wall.

should be confirmed by culture and, because *A. israelii* is a strict anaerobe and will die on exposure to atmospheric oxygen, prompt delivery to the laboratory for appropriate processing is imperative.

Pathological findings

Actinomycosis of the lungs typically affects the lower lobes but may involve any part. Characteristically, the affected tissue is riddled with chronic abscesses that range in diameter from a few millimetres to 3 cm. These lesions may communicate with one another, drain into the bronchial tree or extend to the pleural surface and open into the pleural sac. 'Sulphur granules' are often to be found within the abscesses. These colonies of *Actinomyces* consist of numerous radiating bacterial filaments that often terminate in a prominent cap of eosinophilic material that represents immune material, a reaction known as the Splendore–Hoeppli phenomenon (Fig. 5.3.25). Fibrosis surrounds the suppurative foci and extends more widely through the lungs, particularly involving the septa. The infection may spread to

Figure 5.3.25 Actinomycosis. Pus containing a colony of *Actinomyces* surrounded by an eosinophilic mantle of immune material. The eosinophilic mantle is known as the Splendore–Hoeppli phenomenon, although neither of these workers recognised its true nature. Splendore described the eosinophilic material around *Sporotrichum* in 1908 and erroneously assumed that it was a new species, while Hoeppli described the same material around schistosomes in 1932 and erroneously suggested that it was secreted by the parasite. The material is now considered to consist of immunoglobulin, complement and cellular debris. It is especially striking in actinomycosis, botryomycosis and various fungal infections, but may also be seen around parasites such as schistosomes and helminths, and even around foreign material.

the pleura and on into the spine and ribs, whether or not there is an actinomycotic empyema: the latter may be loculated or involve the entire pleural sac. Obliteration of the sac prevents empyema formation but does not present a barrier to the infection as it spreads outwards to involve not only the thoracic skeleton but also the soft tissues and skin of the chest wall, often with the establishment of the draining sinuses that are a classic, if rare, feature of the disease. Actinomycotic bacteraemia is uncommon but arises more frequently from pulmonary foci than from any other form of actinomycosis; it may give rise to metastatic abscesses in other viscera, the skeleton or soft tissues. Actinomycosis is occasionally complicated by amyloidosis.

NOCARDIOSIS

Bacteriology

Nocardiosis is caused by several genera of aerobic Actinomycetaceae. *Nocardia asteroides* is the usual cause: *N. brasiliensis* and *N. caviae* are less common human pathogens. None of these is part of the normal human flora. They are soil saprophytes that are often found in decaying organic matter and human infection is exogenous. *Nocardia* were first identified in cattle suffering from farcy in 1888.[150] Human disease was described shortly afterwards.[151,152]

In contrast to *A. israelii*, *N. asteroides* is an aerobic bacterium. It is formed of filaments measuring 0.5–1.0 μm in width, which are so highly branched that they have been likened to Chinese characters. They often break into bacillus-like fragments during preparation of films of infected exudate. They are Gram-positive but often weakly so, and although commonly acid-fast, they are seldom as strongly so as tubercle bacilli and they are not alcohol-fast; silver impregnation methods offer the best means of demonstrating this organism in tissue sections. In contrast to *A. israelii*, and to *N. brasiliensis* and *N. caviae*,

N. asteroides does not form macroscopically evident colonial granules in infected tissues.

Clinical features

Nocardiosis is typically acquired by inhalation but may extend beyond the respiratory tract. Infection may develop in a previously healthy person,[153] but in most cases there are predisposing factors, particularly those that compromise cellular immunity.[154–157] The disease is ordinarily chronic but may progress rapidly in the severely immunocompromised. Predisposing factors include diseases such as leukaemia and AIDS that interfere with resistance, therapeutic agents such as corticosteroids and cytotoxic drugs that similarly suppress immunity and underlying pulmonary diseases, including alveolar lipoproteinosis.[158,159] The overall incidence of nocardiosis appears to be rising, probably in the main because of the increasing use of the drugs that predispose to its occurrence. The disease is commoner in adults than children.

Pulmonary nocardiosis causes fever and cough productive of thick, sticky, purulent sputum that may be streaked with blood. The radiological findings vary from minor infiltrates to extensive consolidation, sometimes with abscess formation or empyema.[160,161] Less commonly, nocardiosis results in bronchial obstruction.[162–164]

Pathological findings

In general, the picture of nocardiosis is that of suppuration, with the development of multiple abscesses. The lesions have a notable tendency to confluence. Pulmonary nocardiosis may affect one or both lungs widely, with extensive consolidation round the suppurative foci: the exudate in the alveoli of these pneumonic foci initially contains much fibrinogen, and a fibrin coagulum forms, often with relatively little leukocytic involvement. The organisms are present in the exudate, and may be very numerous. Their number is often only inadequately disclosed by Gram or Ziehl–Neelsen stains: the Grocott–Gomori method is generally more reliable (Fig. 5.3.26).[165] Healing may result in extensive organising pneumonia.[166] Rarely, pulmonary nocardiosis may take the form of an intracavitary nocardioma[167] or invade contiguous vertebrae and compress the spinal cord.[168] *N. asteroides* has a particular affinity for the central nervous system; nocardial brain abscess and nocardial meningitis are frequent complications of pulmonary infection. Coexisting microbial agents are commonly identified. Treatment of nocardiosis is generally medical, typically employing sulphonamides or co-trimoxazole. Abscesses and empyema may require additional surgery.

RHODOCOCCUS PNEUMONIA

Rhodococcus equi (formerly *Corynybacterium equi*) is an aerobic, Gram-positive and acid-fast bacillus belonging to the order Actinomycetales, and is therefore closely related to the mycobacteria and *Nocardia*. Its natural habitat is the soil and its transmission is aerogenous. It is best known as a pathogen in foals, cattle, swine and sheep, where it is a lethal cause of suppurative granulomatous pneumonia, lymphadenitis, mediastinitis and pyometra. It has only recently been recognised as pathogenic to humans. Human infection often follows exposure to farm animals or to stockyards contaminated with animal excreta. Virtually all *Rhodococcus*-infected patients have been severely immunocompromised, typically suffering from AIDS, of which it is an infrequent complication.[169] The clinical presentation is often insidious, consisting of fatigue, fever and a non-productive cough.

Figure 5.3.26 Nocardiosis. Pus containing colonies of basophilic nocardia (A), which are better demonstrated by Grocott staining (B).

Figure 5.3.27 Malakoplakia. A mass lesion composed of histiocytes with abundant eosinophilic cytoplasm. Occasional Michaelis–Gutman bodies are evident (arrows).

R. equi infection causes pneumonic consolidation with abscesses. The disease typically affects the upper lobes and may simulate tuberculosis radiologically.[170–172] Spread to sites such as the brain and bone may occur. The inflammation is histiocytic in nature and may result in pulmonary malakoplakia.

Malakoplakia

Malakoplakia is a rare inflammatory disorder characterised by tumour-like accumulations of swollen macrophages. It usually affects immunocompromised persons and is due to a defect in macrophage function.[173] Bacteria are ingested normally but are not killed within the cell, suggesting that the fault lies in the lysosomes. Malakoplakia usually affects the lower genitourinary or gastrointestinal tracts and until recently few cases had been described with lung involvement. However, several cases of malakoplakia confined to the lungs have now been described, chiefly in the setting of AIDS but also associated with general debilitation, organ transplantation, haematopoietic malignancy and alcoholism.[170,171,174–183]

Bacteriology

Malakoplakia is associated with infection by various bacteria and fungi. In the urinary tract the organism is usually *Escherichia coli* but

in the lungs *Rhodococcus equi* (formerly *Corynebacterium equi*) is generally involved, although rare cases associated with other infections are described.[184] Rhodococci are Gram-positive coccobacilli that may be mistaken for commensal diphtheroids in sputum. They are sometimes acid-fast. *R. equi* has been recognised as an agent causing bronchopneumonia in horses and other domesticated animals since its first isolation from infected foals in 1923. Its habitat is the soil. Infection of both humans and beasts is thought to be acquired through the lungs. Human infection almost always involves patients who have defects in cell-mediated immunity. A history of exposure to animals is not invariably obtained.

Pathological and clinical features

Malakoplakia of the lungs may form solitary or multiple bilateral lesions, mimicking either primary or metastatic neoplasms radiologically. The gross appearances also mimic neoplastic disease. The lesions are well demarcated, firm and either solid or cavitating. Microscopically, the lung tissue is replaced by sheets of swollen macrophages with abundant eosinophilic, granular or vacuolated cytoplasm that stains well with periodic acid–Schiff reagents and is diastase-resistant. The appearances may suggest a granular cell tumour (see p. 640). A characteristic feature is the presence of Michaelis–Gutman bodies in the macrophage cytoplasm or free between the cells. These are faintly basophilic, round, target-like structures that measure up to 20 μm diameter (Fig. 5.3.27). They contain calcium and are therefore well shown by von Kossa's stain. The Michaelis–Gutman bodies represent mineralised bacteria-containing phagolysosomes.[183] Aggregates of bacteria can sometimes be demonstrated within macrophages by Gram stains.

SYPHILIS

Syphilitic lesions have never been particularly frequent in the lungs, and congenital pulmonary syphilis ('pneumonia alba') has probably always been the commonest manifestation. However, there has recently been an increase in syphilis and its protean manifestations should not be forgotten.[185,186]

Congenital pulmonary syphilis

The pallor and firmness of the lungs, which are larger than normal, account for this condition's old name, pneumonia alba. It is usually seen in stillborn syphilitic babies or those who die within a few hours of birth: in the latter, the aerated lobules stand out above the indurated parts. Microscopically, there is widespread thickening of the alveolar walls by fibroblastic connective tissue accompanied by an accumulation of plasma cells with some lymphocytes. In places there are microscopical foci of necrosis, maybe with histiocytic proliferation round them, as well as some accumulation of neutrophils: these lesions occasionally merge to form gummatous foci that may be evident macroscopically. Usually there is a conspicuous lining of cuboidal type II alveolar epithelial cells and many alveoli may be filled with macrophages. Silver impregnation methods show the presence of great numbers of treponemes in the tissues. The bacteria may also be demonstrated immunohistochemically.[187] Imaging may show diffuse pulmonary infiltrates, which persist long after adequate antibiotic treatment.[188]

Somewhat similar macroscopical and microscopical changes may result from viral infections in the neonatal period. Also, *Pneumocystis* pneumonia may be mistaken for syphilitic pneumonia in those cases in which interstitial accumulation of plasma cells is particularly marked (see p. 226).

Acquired pulmonary syphilis

Gummas and interstitial fibrosis are the manifestations of acquired syphilis in the lungs. The gummas may be solitary or multiple, and small or large. They may occur in the trachea and bronchi as ulcerative lesions, with a tendency to destroy the cartilage of the wall. These cause cough and haemorrhage whereas gummas in the lung substance may be clinically silent.

Bronchopulmonary gummas have the structure that is common to these lesions wherever they occur in the body. They consist of a necrotic core surrounded by granulation tissue that is heavily infiltrated by plasma cells and lymphocytes with scanty giant cells. Satellite lesions, as seen in tuberculosis, are not a feature. As elsewhere, gummas tend ultimately to produce dense scars that contract and produce deep cicatricial fissures in the surface of the lungs, an appearance comparable to that of the classic hepar lobatum of tertiary syphilis.

It is very important to consider and exclude other types of infection, particularly mycobacterioses and mycoses, before a diagnosis of gumma can be sustained, even when the patient's serological tests indicate the presence of syphilis. Moreover, primary and secondary tumours are commoner causes of discrete shadows in chest radiographs than gummas, even in patients with syphilis. The necrotic pulmonary lesions of Wegener's granulomatosis and even pulmonary infarcts are among other conditions to be considered in the differential diagnosis.

Other thoracic manifestations of acquired syphilis include diffuse pulmonary fibrosis of non-specific character, hilar lymphadenopathy and pleural fibrosis.[185,186]

REFERENCES

Tuberculosis

1. Armstrong JA, D'Arcy Hart P. Response of cultured macrophages to *Mycobacterium tuberculosis* with observations on fusion of lysosomes and phagosomes. J Exp Med 1971;134:713–40.

2. Lowrie DB, Andrew PW. Macrophage antimycobacterial mechanisms. Br Med Bull 1988;44:624–34.

3. Gerston KF, Blumberg L, Tshabalala VA, et al. Viability of mycobacteria in formalin-fixed lungs. Human Pathology 2004;35:571–5.

4. Fukunaga H, Murakami T, Gondo T, et al. Sensitivity of acid-fast staining for *Mycobacterium tuberculosis* in formalin-fixed tissue. Am J Respir Crit Care Med 2002;166:994–7.

5. Cserni G. Auramine fluorescence for acid-fast bacilli in formalin-fixed paraffin-embedded tissues. Am J Clin Pathol 1995;103:114.

6. Popper HH. Auramine fluorescence for acid-fast bacilli in formalin-fixed paraffin-embedded tissues – reply. Am J Clin Pathol 1995;103:114.

7. Wockel W. Auramine fluorescence for acid-fast bacilli in formalin-fixed, paraffin-embedded tissues. Am J Clin Pathol 1995;103:667–8.

8. Ulbright TM, Katzenstein ALA. Solitary necrotizing granulomas of the lung. Am J Surg Pathol 1980;4:13–28.

9. Tang YW, Procop GW, Zheng XT, et al. Histologic parameters predictive of mycobacterial infection. Am J Clin Pathol 1998;109:331–4.

10. Chitkara YK. Evaluation of cultures of percutaneous core needle biopsy specimens in the diagnosis of pulmonary nodules. Am J Clin Pathol 1997;107:224–8.

11. Ulrichs T, Lefmann M, Reich M, et al. Modified immunohistological staining allows detection of Ziehl–Neelsen-negative *Mycobacterium tuberculosis* organisms and their precise localization in human tissue. J Pathol 2005;205:633–40.

12. Mustafa T, Wiker HG, Mfinanga SGM, et al. Immunohistochemistry using a *Mycobacterium tuberculosis* complex specific antibody for improved diagnosis of tuberculous lymphadenitis. Mod Pathol 2006;19:1606–14.

13. Cheng VCC, Yam WC, Hung IFN, et al. Clinical evaluation of the polymerase chain reaction for the rapid diagnosis of tuberculosis. J Clin Pathol 2004;57:281–5.

14. Selva E, Hofman V, Berto F, et al. The value of polymerase chain reaction detection of *Mycobacterium tuberculosis* in granulomas isolated by laser capture microdissection. Pathology 2004;36:77–81.

15. Nopvichai C, Sanpavat A, Sawatdee R, et al. PCR detection of *Mycobacterium tuberculosis* in necrotising non-granulomatous lymphadenitis using formalin-fixed paraffin-embedded tissue: a study in Thai patients. J Clin Pathol 2009;62:812–15.

15a. Park JS, Kang YA, Kwon SY, et al. Nested PCR in lung tissue for diagnosis of pulmonary tuberculosis. Eur Respir J 2010;35:851–7.

16. Schulz S, Cabras AD, Kremer M, et al. Species identification of mycobacteria in paraffin-embedded tissues: frequent detection of nontuberculous mycobacteria. Mod Pathol 2005;18:274–82.

17. Schewe C, Goldmann T, Grosser M, et al. Inter-laboratory validation of PCR-based detection of *Mycobacterium tuberculosis* in formalin-fixed, paraffin-embedded tissues. Virchows Arch 2005;447:573–85.

18. Greco S, Girardi E, Navarra A, et al. Current evidence on diagnostic accuracy of commercially based nucleic acid amplification tests for the diagnosis of pulmonary tuberculosis. Thorax 2006;61:783–90.

19. Escombe AR, Moore DA, Gilman RH, et al. Upper-room ultraviolet light and negative air ionization to prevent tuberculosis transmission. PLoS Med 2009;6:e43.

20. Callister ME, Barringer J, Thanabalasingam ST, et al. Pulmonary tuberculosis among political asylum seekers screened at

Heathrow Airport, London, 1995–9. Thorax 2002;57:152–6.

21. Meredith SK, Nunn AJ, Byfield SP, et al. National survey of notifications of tuberculosis in England and Wales in 1988. Thorax 1992;47:770–5.

22. Kolappan C, Gopi PG. Tobacco smoking and pulmonary tuberculosis. Thorax 2002;57:964–6.

23. Levin M, Newport M. Unravelling the genetic basis of susceptibility to mycobacterial infection. J Pathol 1997;181:5–7.

24. Murray JF. Cursed duet: HIV infection and tuberculosis. Respiration 1990;57:210–20.

25. Heckbert SR, Elarth A, Nolan CM. The impact of human immunodeficiency virus infection on tuberculosis in young men in Seattle-King county, Washington. Chest 1992;102:433–7.

26. Brudney K, Dobkin J. Resurgent tuberculosis in New York City – human immunodeficiency virus, homelessness, and the decline of tuberculosis control programs. Am Rev Respir Dis 1991;144:745–9.

27. Kochi A. The global tuberculosis situation and the new control strategy of the World Health Organization. Tubercle 1991;72:1–6.

28. Dolin PJ, Raviglione MC, Kochi A. Global tuberculosis incidence and mortality during 1990–2000. Bulletin of the World Health Organization 1994;72:213–20.

29. Busillo CP, Lessnau KD, Sanjana V, et al. Multidrug resistant *Mycobacterium tuberculosis* in patients with human immunodeficiency virus infection. Chest 1992;102:797–801.

30. Chawla PK, Klapper PJ, Kamholz SL, et al. Drug-resistant tuberculosis in an urban population including patients at risk for human immunodeficiency virus infection. Am Rev Respir Dis 1992;146:280–4.

31. Edlin BR, Tokars JI, Grieco MH, et al. An outbreak of multidrug-resistant tuberculosis among hospitalized patients with the acquired immunodeficiency syndrome. N Engl J Med 1992;326:1514–21.

32. PablosMendez A, Raviglione MC, Laszlo A, et al. Global surveillance for antituberculosis-drug resistance, 1994–1997. N Engl J Med 1998;338:1641–9.

33. Kruijshaar ME, Watson JM, Drobniewski F, et al. Increasing antituberculosis drug resistance in the United Kingdom: analysis of National Surveillance Data. BMJ 2008;336:1231–4.

34. World Health Organization. Global TB Control Report. 2009. Available online at: www.who.int/tb.

35. Selwyn PA, Hartel D, Lewis VA, et al. A prospective study of the risk of tuberculosis among intravenous drug users with human immunodeficiency virus infection. N Engl J Med 1989;320:545–50.

36. Centers for Disease Control. Nosocomial transmission of mutlidrug-resistant tuberculosis to health-care workers and HIV-infected patients in an urban hospital – Florida. Mortality and Morbidity Weekly Reports 1990;39:718–22.

37. Havlir DV, Barnes PF. Tuberculosis in patients with human immunodeficiency virus infection. N Engl J Med 1999;340:367–73.

38. Goletti D, Weissman D, Jackson RW, et al. Effect of *Mycobacterium tuberculosis* on HIV replication. Role of immune activation. J Immunol 1996;157:1271–8.

39. Toossi Z, Nicolacakis K, Xia L, et al. Activation of latent HIV-1 by *Mycobacterium tuberculosis* and its purified protein derivative in alveolar macrophages from HIV-infected individuals in vitro. J Acquir Immune Defic Syndr Hum Retrovirol 1997;15:325–31.

40. Garrait V, Cadranel J, Esvant H, et al. Tuberculosis generates a microenvironment enhancing the productive infection of local lymphocytes by HIV. J Immunol 1997;159:2824–30.

41. Hill AR, Premkumar S, Brustein S, et al. Disseminated tuberculosis in the acquired immunodeficiency syndrome era. Am Rev Respir Dis 1991;144:1164–70.

42. Medlar EM. The behavior of pulmonary tuberculosis lesions: a pathological study. Am Rev Tuberc 1955;71:1–244.

43. Rook GAW, Al Attiyah R. Cytokines and the Koch phenomenon. Tubercle 1991;72:13–20.

44. Chensue SW, Warmington K, Ruth J, et al. Cytokine responses during mycobacterial and schistosomal antigen-induced pulmonary granuloma formation – production of Th1 and Th2 cytokines and relative contribution of tumor necrosis factor. Am J Pathol 1994;145:1105–13.

45. Ulrichs T, Kosmiadi GA, Trusov V, et al. Human tuberculous granulomas induce peripheral lymphoid follicle-like structures to orchestrate local host defence in the lung. J Pathol 2004;204:217–28.

46. Leong ASY, Wannakrairot P, Leong TYM. Apoptosis is a major cause of so-called 'caseous necrosis' in mycobacterial granulomas in HIV-infected patients. J Clin Pathol 2008;61:366–72.

47. Mustafa T, Wiker H, Morkve O, et al. Differential expression of mycobacterial antigen MPT64, apoptosis and inflammatory markers in multinucleated giant cells and epithelioid cells in granulomas caused by *Mycobacterium tuberculosis*. Virchows Archiv 2008;452:449–56.

48. Ober WB. Ghon but not forgotten: Anton Ghon and his complex. Pathol Annu 1983;18:79–85.

49. Chow LTC, Shum BSF, Chow WH, et al. Diffuse pulmonary ossification – a rare complication of tuberculosis. Histopathology 1992;20:435–7.

50. Brock RC, Cann RJ, Dickinson JR. Tuberculous mediastinal lymphadenitis in childhood; secondary effects on the lungs. Guy Hosp Rep 1937;87:295–317.

51. MacPherson AMC, Zorab PA, Reid L. Collapse of the lung associated with primary tuberculosis: a review of 51 cases. Thorax 1960;15:346–54.

52. Husson RN, Bramson RT, Newton AW, et al. A 10-month-old girl with fever, upper-lobe pneumonia, and a pleural effusion – Pulmonary tuberculosis, infantile. N Engl J Med 1999;341:353–60.

53. Seal RME. The pathology of tuberculosis. Br J Hosp Med 1971;5:783–90.

54. Strom L. Experiments with radioactive Calmette (BCG) vaccine. Acta Paed 1950;39:453–4.

55. Strom L, Rudback L. On labelling tubercle bacteria with radioactive phosphorus. Acta tuberculosea Scandinavica 1949;98–101.

56. Lalvani A. Diagnosing tuberculosis infection in the 21st century: new tools to tackle an old enemy. Chest 2007;131:1898–906.

57. Daniels M, Ridehalgh F, Springett VH, et al. Tuberculosis in young adults. Report on the Prophit tuberculosis survey 1935–1944. London: HK Lewis; 1948.

58. Grange JM. Mycobacteria and Human Disease. London: Edward Arnold; 1988. 88.

59. Behr MA, Wilson MA, Gill WP, et al. Comparative genomics of BCG vaccines by whole-genome DNA microarray [see comments]. Science 1999;284:1520–3.

59a. Fine PE. Variation in protection by BCG: implications of and for heterologous immunity. Lancet 1995;346:1339–45.

60. Abramowsky C, Gonzalez B, Sorensen RU. Disseminated bacillus Calmette-Guerin infections in patients with primary immunodeficiences. Am J Clin Pathol 1993;100:52.

61. Emile J-F, Patey N, Altare F, et al. Correlation of granuloma structure with clinical outcome defines two types of idiopathic disseminated BCG infection. J Pathol 1997;181:25–30.

61a. Clark IA. Heterologous immunity revisited. Parasitology 2001;122:S51–9.

62. Grange JM, Stanford JL. BCG vaccination and cancer. Tubercle 1990;71:61–4.

63. Bakker W, Nijhuis-Heddes JM. Post-operative intrapleural BCG in lung cancer: a 5-year follow-up report. Cancer Immunol Immunother 1986;22:155–9.

64. Tan L, Testa G, Yung T. Diffuse alveolar damage in BCGosis: A rare complication of intravesical bacillus Calmette-Guerin therapy for transitional cell carcinoma. Pathology 1999;31:55–6.

65. Rich AR. The pathogenesis of tuberculosis. 2nd ed. Springfield, Ill.: Charles C Thomas; 1951. 500–60.

66. Youmans GP. Mechanisms of immunity in tuberculosis. In: Ioachim HL, editor. Pathology Annual Vol. 9. New York: Raven Press; 1979. p. 137–57.

67. Bothamley GH, Grange JM. The Koch phenomenon and delayed hypersensitivity: 1891–1991. Tubercle 1991;72:7–11.

68. Grange JM. The immunophysiology and immunopathology of tuberculosis. In: Davies PDO, editor. Tuberculosis. 2nd ed. London: Chapman and Hall; 1998.

69. Schluger NW. Recent advances in our understanding of human host responses to tuberculosis. Respir Res 2001;2:157–63.

70. Myatt N, Coghill G, Morrison K, et al. Detection of tumour necrosis factor alpha in sarcoidosis and tuberculosis granulomas using in situ hybridisation. J Clin Pathol 1994;47:423–6.

71. Grange JM, Stanford JL, Rook G, et al. Tuberculosis and HIV: light after darkness. Thorax 1994;49:537–9.

72. Dock W. Apical localization of phthisis. Am Rev Tuberc 1946;53:297–305.

73. West JB, Dollery CT. Distribution of blood flow and ventilation perfusion ratio in the lung, measured with radioactive CO_2. J Appl Physiol 1960;15:405–10.

74. West JB. Ventilation/Blood Flow and Gas Exchange. 3rd ed. Oxford: Blackwell; 1977. 30.

75. Goodwin RA, Des Prez RM. Apical localization of pulmonary tuberculosis, chronic pulmonary histoplasmosis, and progressive massive fibrosis of the lung. Chest 1983;83:801–5.

76. British Thoracic and Tuberculosis Association. Aspergilloma and residual tuberculous cavities – the results of a resurvey. Tubercle 1970;51:227–45.

77. Auerbach O. Tuberculosis of the trachea and major bronchi. Am Rev Tuberc 1949;60:604–20.

78. Vandenbrande P, Lambrechts M, Tack J, et al. Endobronchial tuberculosis mimicking lung cancer in elderly patients. Respir Med 1991;85:107–9.

79. Wasser LS, Shaw GW, Talavera W. Endobronchial tuberculosis in the acquired immunodeficiency syndrome. Chest 1988;94:1240–4.

80. Lee JH, Park SS, Lee DH, et al. Endobronchial tuberculosis – clinical and bronchoscopic features in 121 cases. Chest 1992;102:990–4.

81. Hoheisel G, Chan BKM, Chan CHS, et al. Endobronchial tuberculosis: diagnostic features and therapeutic outcome. Respir Med 1994;88:593–7.

82. King D, Davies PDO. Disseminated tuberculosis in the elderly: still a diagnosis overlooked. J R Soc Med 1992;85:48–50.

83. Proudfoot AT. Cryptic disseminated tuberculosis. Br J Hosp Med 1971;5:773–80.

84. Morris CDW. Pulmonary tuberculosis in the elderly – a different disease. Thorax 1990;45:912–13.

85. Singh R, Joshi RC, Christie J. Generalised non-reactive tuberculosis: a clinicopathological study of four patients. Thorax 1989;44:952–5.

86. Benatar SR, Mark EJ, McLoud TC, et al. A 44-year-old woman with pulmonary infiltrates, respiratory failure, and pancytopenia – pulmonary tuberculosis, nonreactive and miliary, with diffuse alveolar damage (adult respiratory distress syndrome), with miliary tuberculosis in the liver, spleen, adrenal glands, bone marrow, and kidneys. Kaposi's sarcoma of the jejunum. N Engl J Med 1995;333:241–8.

87. Nambuya A, Sewankambo N, Mugerwa J, et al. Tuberculous lymphadenitis associated with human immunodeficiency virus (HIV) in Uganda. J Clin Pathol 1988;41:91–6.

88. Iseman MD. Tuberculosis therapy: past, present and future. Eur Respir J Suppl 2002;36:87s–94s.

89. Loddenkemper R, Sagebiel D, Brendel A. Strategies against multidrug-resistant tuberculosis. Eur Respir J Suppl 2002;36:66s–77s.

90. Blumberg HM, Burman WJ, Chaisson RE, et al. American Thoracic Society/Centers for Disease Control and Prevention/Infectious Diseases Society of America: treatment of tuberculosis. Am J Respir Crit Care Med 2003;167:603–62.

91. Caminero JA, de March P. Statements of ATS, CDC, and IDSA on treatment of tuberculosis. Am J Respir Crit Care Med 2004;169:316–17.

Opportunistic mycobacteria

92. Chester AC, Winn WC. Unusual and newly recognized patterns of nontuberculous mycobacterial infection with emphasis on the immunocompromised host. Pathol Annu 1986;21:251–70.

93. Grange JM, Yates MD. Infections caused by opportunist mycobacteria: a review. J R Soc Med 1986;79:226–9.

94. Wallace JM, Hannah JB. Mycobacterium avium complex infection in patients with the acquired immunodeficiency syndrome. A clinicopathologic study. Chest 1988;93:926–32.

95. Smith MB, Molina CP, Schnadig VJ, et al. Pathologic features of Mycobacterium kansasii infection in patients with acquired immunodeficiency syndrome. Arch Pathol Lab Med 2003;127:554–60.

96. Kahana LM, Kay JM, Yakrus MA, et al. Mycobacterium avium complex infection in an immunocompetent young adult related to hot tub exposure. Chest 1997;111:242–5.

97. Management of opportunist mycobacterial infections: Joint Tuberculosis Committee Guidelines 1999. Subcommittee of the Joint Tuberculosis Committee of the British Thoracic Society. Thorax 2000;55:210–18.

98. Sexton P, Harrison AC. Susceptibility to nontuberculous mycobacterial lung disease. Eur Respir J 2008;31: 1322–33.

99. Rigsby MO, Curtis AM. Pulmonary disease from nontuberculous mycobacteria in patients with human immunodeficiency virus. Chest 1994;106:913–19.

100. Nash G, Said JW, Nash SV, et al. The pathology of AIDS – intestinal Mycobacterium avium complex (MAC) infection in AIDS. Mod Pathol 1995;8:209–11.

101. Laporte R. A l'études des bacillus paratuberculeux. I Propriétés pathogènes II. Histo-cytologie des lésions paratuberculeuses. Ann Inst Pasteur 1940;65:415–34.

102. Guest JL, Arean VM, Brenner HA. Group IV atypical mycobacterium infection occurring in association with mineral oil granuloma of lungs. Am Rev Respir Dis 1967;95:656–62.

103. Greenberger PA, Katzenstein ALA. Lipid pneumonia with atypical mycobacterial colonization. Association with allergic bronchopulmonary aspergillosis. Arch Intern Med 1983;143:2003–5.

104. Jouannic I, Desrues B, Lena H, et al. Exogenous lipoid pneumonia complicated by Mycobacterium fortuitum and Aspergillus fumigatus infections. Eur Respir J 1996;9:172–4.

105. Gibson JB. Infection of the lungs by 'saprophytic' mycobacteria in achalasia of the cardia, with report of a fatal case showing lipoid pneumonia due to milk. J Pathol Bacteriol 1953;65:239–51.

106. Burke DS, Ullian RB. Megaesophagus and pneumonia associated with Mycobacterium chelonei A case report and a literature review. Am Rev Respir Dis 1977;116:1101–7.

107. Levin M, Newport M, D'Souza S, et al. Familial disseminated atypical mycobacterial infection in childhood: a human mycobacterial susceptibility gene? Lancet 1995;345:79–83.

108. Asano T, Itoh G, Itoh M. Disseminated Mycobacterium intracellulare infection in an HIV-negative, nonimmunosuppressed patient with multiple endobronchial polyps. Respiration 2002;69:175–7.

109. Khoor A, Leslie KO, Tazelaar HD, et al. Diffuse pulmonary disease caused by nontuberculous mycobacteria in immunocompetent people (hot tub lung). Am J Pathol 2001;115:755–62.

110. Kahana LM, Kay JM. Pneumonitis due to Mycobacterium avium complex in hot tub water: infection or hypersensitivity? Chest 1997;112:1713–4.

111. Marras TK, Wallace RJ, Jr., Koth LL, et al. Hypersensitivity pneumonitis reaction to Mycobacterium avium in household water. Chest 2005;127:664–71.

112. Cappelluti E, Fraire AE, Schaefer OP. A case of 'hot tub lung' due to Mycobacterium

avium complex in an immunocompetent host. Arch Intern Med 2003;163:845–8.

113. Hanak V, Kalra S, Aksamit TR, et al. Hot tub lung: presenting features and clinical course of 21 patients. Respir Med 2006;100:610–5.

114. Zota V, Angelis SM, Fraire AE, et al. Lessons from *Mycobacterium avium* complex-associated pneumonitis: a case report. J Med Case Reports 2008;2:152.

115. Reich JM, Johnson RE. *Mycobacterium avium* complex pulmonary disease presenting as an isolated lingular or middle lobe pattern. The Lady Windermere syndrome. Chest 1992;101:1605–9.

116. Kim RD, Greenberg DE, Ehrmantraut ME, et al. Pulmonary Nontuberculous Mycobacterial Disease: Prospective Study of a Distinct Preexisting Syndrome. Am J Respir Crit Care Med 2008;178:1066–74.

117. Fujita J, Ohtsuki Y, Suemitsu I, et al. Pathological and radiological changes in resected lung specimens in *Mycobacterium avium intracellulare* complex disease. Eur Resp J 1999;13:535–40.

118. Fujita J, Ohtsuki Y, Shigeto E, et al. Pathological findings of bronchiectases caused by *Mycobacterium avium intracellulare* complex. Resp Med 2003;97:933–8.

119. Fukuoka K, Nakano Y, Nakajima A, et al. Endobronchial lesions involved in *Mycobacterium avium* infection. Resp Med 2003;97:1261–4.

120. Christianson LC, Dewlett HJ. Pulmonary disease in adults associated with unclassified mycobacteria. Am J Med 1960;29:980–91.

121. Kraus M, Benharroch D, Kaplan D, et al. Mycobacterial cervical lymphadenitis: the histological features of non-tuberculous mycobacterial infection. Histopathology 1999;35:534–8.

122. Loo KT, Seneviratne S, Chan JKC. Mycobacterial infection mimicking inflammatory 'pseudotumour' of the lung. Histopathology 1989;14:217–19.

123. Umlas J, Federman M, Crawford C, et al. Spindle cell pseudotumor due to *Mycobacterium-avium-intracellulare* in patients with acquired immunodeficiency syndrome (AIDS) – positive staining of mycobacteria for cytoskeleton filaments. Am J Surg Pathol 1991;15:1181–7.

124. Chen KTK. Mycobacterial spindle cell pseudotumor of lymph nodes. Am J Surg Pathol 1992;16:276–81.

125. Suster S, Moran CA, Blanco M. Mycobacterial spindle-cell pseudotumor of the spleen. Am J Clin Pathol 1994;101:539–42.

126. Sekosan M, Cleto M, Senseng C, et al. Spindle cell pseudotumors in the lungs due to *Mycobacterium tuberculosis* in a transplant patient. Am J Surg Pathol 1994;18:1065–8.

127. Lucas SB. Mycobacteria and the tissues of man. In: Ratledge C, Stanford JL, Grange JM, editors. Biology of Mycobacteria, Vol. 3. London: Academic Press; 1989. p. 107–76.

Brucellosis

128. Lubani MM, Lulu AR, Araj GF, et al. Pulmonary brucellosis. Q J Med 1989;71:319–24.

129. Al-Jam'a AH, Elbashier AM, Al-Faris SS. *Brucella* pneumonia: a case report. Ann Saudi Med 1993;13:74–7.

130. Greer AE. Pulmonary brucellosis. Dis Chest 1956;29:508–19.

131. Hunt AC, Bothwell PW. Histological findings in human brucellosis. J Clin Pathol 1967;20:267–72.

132. Saltoglu N, Tasova Y, Midikli D, et al. Fever of unknown origin in Turkey: evaluation of 87 cases during a nine-year-period of study. J Infect 2004;48:81–5.

133. Pappas G, Bosilkovski M, Akritidis N, et al. Brucellosis and the respiratory system. Clin Infect Dis 2003;37:e95–9.

134. Weed LA, Sloss PT, Clagett OT. Chronic localised pulmonary brucellosis. JAMA 1956;161:1044–7.

135. Theegarten D, Albrecht S, T+Åtsch M, Teschler H, Neubauer H, Al Dahouk S. Brucellosis of the lung: case report and review of the literature. Virchows Archiv 2008;452:97–101.

Chronic melioidosis

136. Piggott JA, Hochholzer L. Human melioidosis. A histopathologic study of acute and chronic melioidosis. Arch Pathol 1970;90:101–11.

137. Wong KT, Puthucheary SD, Vadivelu J. The histopathology of human melioidosis. Histopathology 1995;26:51–5.

138. Dhiensiri T, Puapairoj S, Susaengrat W. Pulmonary melioidosis: clinical-radiologic correlation in 183 cases in northeastern Thailand. Radiology 1988;166:711–15.

Actinomycosis

139. Bowker CM, Connellan SJ, Freeth MG. A case of thoracic *Actinobacillus* infection. Respir Med 1992;86:53–4.

140. Hsieh MJ, Liu HP, Chang JP, et al. Thoracic actinomycosis. Chest 1993;104:366–70.

141. Cendan I, Klapholz A, Talavera W. Pulmonary actinomycosis – a cause of endobronchial disease in a patient with AIDS. Chest 1993;103:1886–7.

142. Lee JP, Rudoy R. Pediatric thoracic actinomycosis. Hawaii Med J 2003;62:30–2.

143. Mabeza GF, Macfarlane J. Pulmonary actinomycosis. Eur Respir J 2003;21:545–51.

144. Lu MS, Liu HP, Yeh CH, et al. The role of surgery in hemoptysis caused by thoracic actinomycosis; a forgotten disease. Eur J Cardiothorac Surg 2003;24:694–8.

145. Bates M, Cruickshank G. Thoracic actinomycosis. Thorax 1957;12:99–124.

146. Brown JR. Human actinomycosis. A study of 181 subjects. Hum Pathol 1973;4:319–30.

147. Slade PR, Slesser BV, Southgate J. Thoracic actinomycosis. Thorax 1973;28:73–85.

148. Dalhoff K, Wallner S, Finck C, et al. Endobronchial actinomycosis. Eur Respir J 1994;7:1189–91.

149. Ariel I, Breuer R, Kamal NS, et al. Endobronchial actinomycosis simulating bronchogenic carcinoma. Diagnosis by bronchial biopsy. Chest 1991;99:493–5.

Nocardiosis

150. Nocard ME. Note sur la maladie des boeufs de la Guadeloupe connue sous le nom de farcin. Ann Inst Pasteur 1888;2:293–302.

151. Eppinger H. Ueber eine neue pathogene Cladothrix und eine durch sie hervorgerufene Pseudotuberculose. Wien Klin Wschr 1890;3:321.

152. Eppinger H. Uber eine neue, pathogene Cladothrix und eine durch sie hervorgerufene Pseudotuberculosis (cladothrichica). Beitr Pathol Anat 1891;9:287–328.

153. Brechot JM, Capron F, Prudent J, et al. Unexpected pulmonary nocardiosis in a non-immunocompromised patient. Thorax 1987;42:479–40.

154. Saltzman HA, Chick EW, Conant NF. Nocardiosis as a complication of other diseases. Lab Invest 1962;11:1110–7.

155. Uttamchandani RB, Daikos GL, Reyes RR, et al. Nocardiosis in 30 patients with advanced human immunodeficiency virus infection: clinical features and outcome. Clin Infect Dis 1994;18:348–53.

156. Menendez R, Cordero PJ, Santos M, et al. Pulmonary infection with Nocardia species: a report of 10 cases and review. Eur Respir J 1997;10:1542–6.

157. Hui CH, Au VWK, Rowland K, et al. Pulmonary nocardiosis re-visited: experience of 35 patients at diagnosis. Resp Med 2003;97:709–17.

158. Burbank B, Morrione TG, Cutler SS. Pulmonary alveolar proteinosis and nocardiosis. Am J Med 1960;28:1002–7.

159. Summers JE. Pulmonary alveolar proteinosis. Review of the literature with follow-up studies and report of two new cases. Calif Med 1966;104:428–36.

160. Frazier AR, Rosenow ECI, Roberts GD. Nocardiosis: a review of 25 cases occurring during 24 months. Mayo Clin Proc 1975;50:657–63.

161. Wada R, Itabashi C, Nakayama Y, et al. Chronic granulomatous pleuritis caused by nocardia: PCR based diagnosis by nocardial 16S rDNA in pathological specimens. J Clin Path 2003;56:966–9.

162. McNeil KD, Johnson DW, Oliver WA. Endobronchial nocardial infection. Thorax 1993;48:1281–2.

163. Fielding DI, Oliver WA. Endobronchial nocardial infection. Thorax 1994;49: 385.

164. Casty FE, Wencel M. Endobronchial nocardiosis. Eur Respir J 1994;7: 1903–5.

165. Robboy SJ, Vickery AL Jr. Tinctorial and morphologic properties distinguishing actinomycosis and nocardiosis. N Engl J Med 1970;282:593–6.

166. Camp M, Mehta JB, Whitson M. Bronchiolitis obliterans and *Nocardia asteroides* infection of the lung. Chest 1987;92:1107–8.

167. Murray JF, Finegold SM, Froman S, et al. The changing spectrum of nocardiosis. A review and presentation of nine cases. Am Rev Respir Dis 1961;83:315–30.

168. Petersen JM, Awad I, Ahmad M, et al. Nocardia osteomyelitis and epidural abscess in the nonimmunosuppressed host. Cleve Clin Q 1983;50: 453–9.

Rhodococcus infection and malakoplakia

169. TorresTortosa M, Arrizabalaga J, Villanueva JL, et al. Prognosis and clinical evaluation of infection caused by *Rhodococcus equi* in HIV-infected patients – A multicenter study of 67 cases. Chest 2003;123: 1970–6.

170. Kwon KY, Colby TV. *Rhodococcus equi* pneumonia and pulmonary malakoplakia in acquired immunodeficiency syndrome – pathologic features. Arch Pathol Lab Med 1994;118:744–8.

171. Scott MA, Graham BS, Verrall R, et al. *Rhodococcus equi* – an increasingly recognized opportunistic pathogen: report of 12 cases and review of 65 cases in the literature. Am J Clin Pathol 1995;103:649–55.

172. Hamrock D, Azmi FH, ODonnell E, et al. Infection by *Rhodococcus equi* in a patient with AIDS: histological appearance mimicking Whipple's disease and *Mycobacterium avium-intracellulare* infection. J Clin Pathol 1999;52:68–71.

173. Biggar WD, Keating A, Bear RA. Malakoplakia: evidence for an acquired disease secondary to immunosuppression. Transplantation 1981;31:109–12.

174. Gupta RK, Schuster RA, Christian WD. Autopsy findings in a unique case of malacoplakia. A cytoimmunohistochemical study of Michaelis–Gutmann bodies. Arch Pathol Lab Med 1972;93:42–8.

175. Colby TV, Hunt S, Pelzmann K, et al. Malakoplakia of the lung. A report of two cases. Respiration 1980;39:295–9.

176. Hodder RV, St George-Hyslop P, Chalvardjian A, et al. Pulmonary malakoplakia. Thorax 1984;39:70–1.

177. Crouch E, Wright J, White V, et al. Malakoplakia mimicking carcinoma metastatic to lung. Am J Surg Pathol 1984;8:151–6.

178. Byard RW, Thorner PS, Edwards V, et al. Pulmonary malacoplakia in a child. Pediatr Pathol 1990;10:417–24.

179. Scannel KA, Portoni EJ, Finkel HI, et al. Pulmonary malakoplakia and *Rhodococcus equi* infection in a patient with AIDS. Chest 1990;97:1000–1.

180. Schwartz DA, Ogden PO, Blumberg HM, et al. Pulmonary malakoplakia in a patient with the acquired immunodeficiency syndrome – differential diagnostic considerations. Arch Pathol Lab Med 1990;114:1267–72.

181. Mollo JL, Groussard O, Baldeyrou P, et al. Tracheal malacoplakia. Chest 1994;105:608–10.

182. Deperalta-Venturina MN, Clubb FJ, Kielhofner MA. Pulmonary malacoplakia associated with *Rhodococcus equi* infection in a patient with acquired immunodeficiency syndrome. Am J Clin Pathol 1994;102:459–63.

183. Yuoh G, Hove MGM, Wen J, et al. Pulmonary malakoplakia in acquired immunodeficiency syndrome: an ultrastructural study of morphogenesis of Michaelis–Gutmann bodies. Mod Pathol 1996;9:476–83.

184. Bastas A, Markou N, Botsi C, et al. Malakoplakia of the lung caused by *Pasteurella multocida* in a patient with AIDS. Scand J Infect Dis 2002;34: 536–8.

Syphilis

185. Edmonds LC, Stubbs SE, Ryu JH. Syphilis – a disease to exclude in diagnosing sarcoidosis. Mayo Clin Proc 1992;67:37–41.

186. Dooley DP, Tomski S. Syphilitic pneumonitis in an HIV-infected patient. Chest 1994;105:629–31.

187. Guarner J, Greer PW, Bartlett T, et al. Congenital syphilis in a newborn: An immunopathologic study. Modern Pathol 1999;12:82–7.

188. Austin R, Melhem RE. Pulmonary changes in congenital syphilis. Pediatr Radiol 1991;21:404–5.

Chapter | 5 |

5.4 Fungal infections

In certain regions of the world, environmental soil conditions support the saprophytic phase of pathogenic fungi such as *Histoplasma capsulatum*, *Blastomyces dermatitidis*, *Coccidioides immitis* and *Paracoccidioides brasiliensis* that are able to cause disease in previously healthy people. Other fungi invade the tissues only because of lowering of the patient's resistance by some other disease or as a side-effect of treatment. Some of the fungi that cause these so-called opportunistic infections are seldom, if ever, responsible for illness in healthy individuals: this is particularly so of mucormycetes. Others cause disease in healthy individuals of a type very different from the progressive, destructive, disseminated infection that they set up in those whose resistance has been reduced: asthma from sensitisation to aspergilli and saprophytic growth in previously formed cavities are examples of such disease.

Many fungi that infect humans are dimorphic – that is, they grow as yeast-like organisms at certain temperatures and in mycelial form at others. Sporulating conidiophores (or 'fruiting heads') form on the mycelial hyphae when oxygen is plentiful and release spores into the atmosphere. The spores are particularly likely to be inhaled and germinate into hyphae in the lungs. The size and shape of the fungus in its various forms often enable the histopathologist to identify the genus (Box 5.4.1) but speciation generally requires culture.

The ease and frequency of international travel make many hitherto 'exotic' diseases the immediate practical concern of doctors who have no personal experience in their recognition and management. The fact that fungi which are frequently the cause of disease in other parts of the world are not indigenous where the doctor is in practice is no longer an excuse for not considering the possibility that a patient may have acquired infection while visting another country or through exposure to contaminated, imported materials. Neither histoplasmosis nor coccidioidomycosis, for instance, occurs naturally in western Europe, yet every year in countries such as the UK patients are seen whose symptoms are due to these diseases: the cardinal importance of the patient's geographical history, and of the doctor's knowledge of geographical medicine, is self-evident.

PNEUMOCYSTOSIS[1,2]

Microbiology

Pneumocystosis is caused by organisms discovered in the early twentieth century by Chagas and soon after by Carini. They both thought the organism to be a stage in the life cycle of trypanosomes as they found it in the lungs of rats experimentally infected with trypanosomiasis. The Delanoës recognised that it was a distinct species, *Pneumocystis carinii*. *Pneumocystis* organisms were first identified as a cause of human disease in 1942, in Belgium, in association with cases of the condition, previously of unknown causation, that had been described in 1937 as interstitial plasma cell pneumonia. Outbreaks of the latter occurred during the Second World War, and for some years after, in orphanages and other institutions that housed malnourished children, particularly in eastern Europe and the Middle East.[3] The causative role of the *Pneumocystis* in this type of pneumonia in young children was generally recognised following work of Jirovec in

Czechoslovakia in the years immediately after the war.[4,5] Subsequently it has been recognised that the human pathogen is a separate species, *P. jirovecii*. Although pneumocysts were long thought to be protozoal, they are now regarded as a primitive fungus in which the mycelium is reduced to a unicellular state but is still able to sporulate.[6–8] Despite this, various forms of the fungus are still referred to as sporozoa or trophozoites, as if it was a protozoa.

Electron microscopy[6,9–12] provides an insight into the structure of the organism and the pathogenesis of *Pneumocystis* pneumonia. It shows that the organism forms cysts measuring 3–6 μm in diameter, which have a thick wall or pellicle (Fig. 5.4.1). The pellicle is particularly thick at one point, a feature that is evident by light microscopy in silver-stained preparations as a peripheral dot on the cyst wall. The pellicle is triple-layered, consisting of an outer electron-dense zone about 75 nm thick, an electron-lucent intermediate zone 250 nm thick and an inner 7-nm membrane. Numerous small tubular structures are associated with the inner layer. Up to eight nucleated intracystic bodies or sporozoa are also probably derived from this membrane. These are released when the cyst ruptures (Fig. 5.4.2). Collapsed cysts are largely empty and the innermost membrane of the wall is either detached or absent. The released sporozoa grow from about 1.5 to 6 μm, have a thin pellicle and are highly irregular in shape (Fig. 5.4.3). They are now known as trophozoites and possibly undergo binary fission before entering a precyst stage in which their pellicles thicken (Fig. 5.4.4).

Cysts tend to be sparse near the alveolar walls, which are bordered chiefly by trophozoites, suggesting that limitation of some nutritional factor promotes cyst formation. In successfully treated cases only empty cysts are found, indicating that all viable forms of the parasite, whether free-living or encysted, are vulnerable to chemotherapy. Although there is not a heavy cellular reaction within the alveoli, cysts and trophozoites may fill these air spaces.

Electron microscopy also shows that the trophozoites attach to type I alveolar epithelial cells, eventually causing these cells to slough away from the alveolar walls.[13] Tracer studies show that there is increased permeability in the lung, even before epithelial cells are lost.[14] In severe cases, trophozoites are observed within the alveolar interstitium. From here they may gain access to the blood stream and disseminate widely.[15]

Epidemiology

The epidemic *Pneumocystis* pneumonia mentioned above as a feature of malnourished children is no longer seen in Europe but is still encountered in parts of the world where poverty and malnutrition are rife. *Pneumocystis* pneumonia is also recognised as a complication of immunodeficiency states, both congenital and acquired. Until the appearance of the acquired immune deficiency syndrome (AIDS), such immunodeficiency was generally due to lymphoproliferative disease or immunosuppressive therapy but interest now centres on *Pneumocystis* pneumonia as being by far the commonest opportunistic infection in AIDS (see Table 5.1.1, p. 167). *P. jirovecii* is kept in check by T lymphocytes and suppression of these cells, as in AIDS, allows the parasite to proliferate and cause pneumonia. In very severe T-lymphocyte depletion extrapulmonary dissemination is found (see below). Patients who have undergone heart/lung transplantation are also at risk of developing *Pneumocystis* pneumonia,[16] as are those with cancer.[17] Whatever the cause of the immunoparesis, *Pneumocystis* pneumonia in immunodeficient individuals lacks the intense plasma cell infiltration seen in malnourished children.

Antibodies to *P. jirovecii* can be detected in most of the population by the age of 4 years[18] but the absence of the organism from normal lungs suggests that the pneumonia represents reinfection rather than

Figure 5.4.1 *Pneumocystis jirovecii*. Cyst form. The cyst wall has three layers: an outer electron-dense zone about 75 nm thick, an electron-lucent intermediate zone 250 nm thick and an inner 7-nm membrane. Numerous small tubular structures are associated with the inner layer, which also spawns up to eight intracystic bodies or sporozoites, one of which is visible here. Electron micrograph. *(Reproduced from Corrin & Dewar (1992).[12])*

Figure 5.4.3 *Pneumocystis jirovecii*. Trophozoites. These are irregular in shape and have a thin unit membrane wall. Electron micrograph. *(Reproduced from Corrin & Dewar 1992.[12])*

Figure 5.4.2 *Pneumocystis jirovecii*. Collapsed cyst releasing its contents. Electron micrograph *(Reproduced from Corrin & Dewar (1992).[12])*

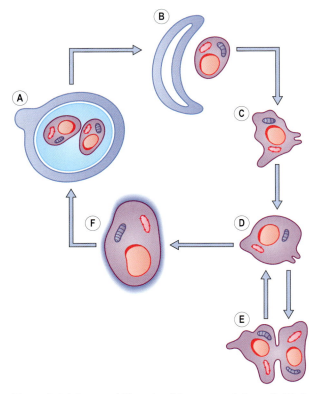

Figure 5.4.4 Proposed life cycle of *Pneumocystis jirovecii*. (A) Cystic form containing two intracystic bodies. Note the focal thickening of the pellicle. (B) Discharge of cyst contents and collapse of the cyst. (C–E) Trophozoites, which possibly undergo binary fission. (F) Trophozoite in precystic stage.

reactivation.[8,19,20] Infection is presumed to be by inhalation from an as yet poorly characterised environmental source. Although *P. jirovecii* has been found in a wide range of animals it shows host specificity and is the species prevalent in humans.

Autopsy in cases of *Pneumocystis* pneumonia presents no danger except in AIDS where there is a possibility of mortuary staff being infected by the HIV virus.

Clinical features

Pneumocystis pneumonia is characterised by breathlessness, cough and fever, generally of insidious onset. Untreated, the disease progresses with mounting tachypnnoea, hypoxaemia and cyanosis. Radiographs typically show widespread bilateral opacification. Late features include calcification, cavitation and pneumothorax. Diagnosis requires demonstration of the organisms, for which sputum production is generally induced by the inhalation of a saline aerosol or bronchoalveolar

Figure 5.4.5 *Pneumocystis jirovecii* pneumonia. The lung shows diffuse consolidation. *(Courtesy of the late Dr AA Liebow, San Diego, USA and Dr T Jelihovsky, Sydney, Australia.)*

Figure 5.4.6 *Pneumocystis jirovecii* pneumonia. The alveoli are filled by a foamy exudate and the alveolar walls are thickened by a lymphoid infiltrate.

Figure 5.4.7 *Pneumocystis jirovecii* demonstrated by Grocott's methenamine silver stain. The smaller group includes crescentic forms representing collapsed cysts and other cysts that show a characteristic dot representing focal thickening of the cyst wall.

lavage is undertaken.[21] The organisms may be demonstrated with toluidine blue, Giemsa stain, Grocott's methenamine silver stain or by immunofluorescence, but detection of *Pneumocystis* DNA by the polymerase chain reaction is much more sensitive.[22–28]

Morbid anatomy

Fatal *Pneumocystis* pneumonia is generally characterised by widespread bilateral consolidation with relative sparing of the bases and apices of the lungs (Fig. 5.4.5). Rarely, the disease takes the form of solid or cavitating pulmonary nodules.[29,30]

Histological appearances

Microscopically, the alveoli are filled by a foamy, pale, eosinophilic exudate (Fig. 5.4.6). The parasite is unstained in haematoxylin and eosin preparations but with Grocott's methenamine silver stain the alveoli are seen to contain numerous round cysts that measure about 5 µm across. Crescent-shaped forms (Fig. 5.4.7) represent collapsed cysts and their presence is helpful if there is concern that erythrocytes

have not been successfully differentiated in the staining procedure, especially if bronchial washings or bronchoalveolar lavage fluids are being examined and the topographical features provided by a biopsy cannot be studied. Another helpful feature is a dot, generally seen on the edge of the cyst (see Fig. 5.4.7); this represents a focal thickening of cyst wall.[31] Various quick modifications of fixation and processing and of the Grocott stain have been introduced to speed the diagnosis,[32–34] but the importance of fixation in killing any concomitant human immunodeficiency virus (HIV) should not be overlooked. Other special stains that find favour include the Gram Weigert and Giemsa methods[35,36] and those using monoclonal antibodies (Fig. 5.4.8).[22] The last two methods stain the trophozoite as well as the encysted form of the parasite, but as the cysts are invariably present in *Pneumocystis* pneumonia (and are shown by Grocott's stain), this is a dubious advantage: the Grocott stain is clearer and has the advantage of staining any other fungi that may also be present.[37] However, in sputa and other cytological specimens where the pneumocysts may be sparse the greater sensitivity of immunochemical stains and molecular techniques is advantageous.[23–27] In situ hybridisation has also been used to demonstrate pneumocysts in tissue sections.[38]

Figure 5.4.8 Immunocytochemical staining of *Pneumocystis jirovecii* demonstrates the trophozoites as well as the cysts.

Table 5.4.1 *Pneumocystis jirovecii* pneumonia: atypical histological features[43]

	No. of cases	%
Fibrosis	77	63
Interstitial	44	36
Intraluminal	23	19
Absence of typical exudates	11	9
Numerous alveolar macrophages	6	5
Granulomatous inflammation	5	4
Hyaline membranes	4	3
Marked interstitial pneumonitis	3	2
Parenchymal cavities	3	2
Interstitial microcalfication	2	2
Minimal histological reaction	1	1
Vascular permeation	1	1

The alveolar exudate in which the parasites are found is virtually free of host cells except for a mild increase in the number of alveolar macrophages. The reaction to the parasite is largely an interstitial infiltrate of lymphocytes and plasma cells (see Fig. 5.4.6). In most immunodeficient patients the infiltrate is generally mild but in malnourished children it is intense, warranting the original descriptive term interstitial plasma cell pneumonia.

Changes other than the classic one of foamy alveolar exudates may be found in *Pneumocystis* pneumonia, particularly in AIDS (Table 5.4.1 and Fig. 5.4.9),[29,30,39-46] demonstrating that pathological changes in infective disorders are dependent on host factors as well as the parasite. In addition to the cavitating nodules mentioned above,[29,30] necrotising granulomatous inflammation,[26,39,42-44,47] diffuse alveolar damage,[41] calcification,[40,45,48] lymphoid interstitial pneumonia (particularly in children)[49-51] and interstitial[52,53] and vascular invasion have been described, the latter sometimes resulting in a necrotising vascu-

litis.[30] The invasion of the interstitium and pulmonary blood vessels probably causes the necrosis that underlies the cavitating nodules.[30,53,54] The cavities develop into air cysts, which are prone to rupture into the pleural cavities, resulting in both pneumothorax and *Pneumocystis* infection of the pleura.[55,56] Alternatively, there may be interstitial spread and infection of the pleural cavities in the absence of any direct fistulous communication.[52]

In view of the vascular invasion it is not surprising that widespread blood-borne dissemination is also reported, particularly in AIDS.[15,39,57-61] The fact that this sometimes develops in the absence of obvious pneumonia has been attributed to the prophylactic use of inhaled pentamidine which reduces the risk of *Pneumocystis* pneumonia but does not prevent the organism spreading to other organs. Restitution of the immune response following effective antiviral therapy is sometimes accompanied by an 'immune reaction inflammation syndrome' (IRIS)[62] and this may ultimately result in widespread interstitial pulmonary fibrosis.

Although opportunistic infections are often multiple, there appears to be a special relationship between *P. jirovecii* and cytomegalovirus because these two organisms coexist particularly frequently in the infected lung (Fig. 5.4.10). It has been suggested that *P. jirovecii* acts as an intermediate host for cytomegalovirus.[63]

Differential diagnosis

The differential diagnosis of classic *Pneumocystis* pneumonia is from pulmonary oedema and alveolar lipoproteinosis. These three conditions are all characterised by the alveoli being filled by a largely acellular material, but whereas in oedema the material is amorphous, in lipoproteinosis it is granular and in *Pneumocystis* pneumonia it has a foamy appearance. Alveolar lipoproteinosls is further distinguished from *Pneumocystis* pneumonia by the presence of cholesterol crystal clefts and a few foamy fat-filled macrophages in the alveolar deposit and by the strong periodic acid–Schiff-positivity of the deposit (compare Fig. 5.4.6 with Fig. 6.2.18A, p. 319).

ASPERGILLOSIS

Mycology

Aspergilli are common saprophytes found throughout the world in decaying organic matter where their spores may be so numerous that they can be seen as a dense dust cloud when piles of such material are disturbed. Several species have been identified as causes of human disease but *Aspergillus fumigatus* is by far the most frequent, particularly in European cases of pulmonary disease and septicaemia. Other species responsible for disease in humans include *A. flavus* and *A. niger*, the latter more common in the USA.

Definitive diagnosis requires culture but this is not always successful. In histological preparations an aspergillus has a characteristic appearance and can be generically identified by the morphology of its hyphae (Fig. 5.4.11). *Aspergillus* hyphae are usually visible in haematoxylin and eosin preparations, and sometimes are so intensely haematoxyphil that they are immediately evident at low magnifications. Although the periodic acid–Schiff stain and the Gridley stain for fungi facilitate their recognition, the Grocott–Gomori methenamine silver nitrate method is very much more reliable. The hyphae are septate and their hyphal diameter, which varies from 3 to 6 μm, is fairly regular. Typically, the hyphae branch dichotomously at relatively narrow angles (35–45°), the branches then tending to orient themselves parallel to each other. Rare fungi of similar morphology, such as

Figure 5.4.9 Atypical reactions to *Pneumocystis jirovecii* in severely immunodeficient patients. (A, B) Necrotising, granulomatous inflammation. (C) Necrosis, cavitation and dystrophic calcification. (D) Invasion of the interstitium, evident from the foamy exudate expanding alveolar walls as well as occupying alveoli. *(Courtesy of Dr R Steele, Brisbane, Australia; and Professor F Capron and Dr I Abdalsamad, Paris, France.)*

Figure 5.4.10 *Pneumocystis jirovecii* and cytomegalovirus pneumonia. As well as the foamy exudate of *Pneumocystis* pneumonia there are prominent viral inclusions (centre).

Chaetomium globosum, can be distinguished by immunocytochemistry, culture or molecular methods.[64–67]

The conidiophores (or fruiting heads), that are so striking a feature of aspergilli when growing as saprophytes, are seen in infected tissues only when the fungus is exposed to air: they are never found within the solid structure of colonised organs and tissues, but may occasionally be seen in the lung if the lesion communicates with a bronchus (Fig. 5.4.12). Species identification is based on colonial characteristics and on the structure of the conidiophores, which is best studied in culture (Figs 5.4.13 and 5.4.14).

Oxalate crystal deposition

Crystals of calcium oxalate have been identified in tissues infected by aspergilli, particularly *A. niger*, of which oxalic acid is a fermentation product. In some cases local tissue injury and even generalised acute oxalosis and renal failure have resulted from the production of oxalic acid by the fungus.[68,69] Its widespread deposition as insoluble calcium oxalate may be accompanied by sudden hypocalcaemia.[70] Tissue toxicity is attributed to calcium oxalate complexing with iron, resulting in the production of free oxidants.[71] Oxalosis is commonest with saprophytic aspergillosis but is also recorded with the allergic and

Figure 5.4.11 *Aspergillus* hyphae are septate, of fairly uniform thickness (3-6 μm diameter) and branch dichotomously. Grocott's methenamine silver stain.

invasive varieties of the infection (described below). The demonstration of oxalate crystals in biopsy and cytology specimens can be a useful aid in the diagnosis of pulmonary aspergillosis.[72–74] The crystals are birefringent (Fig. 5.4.15), stain with alizirin red[75] and can be confirmed as oxalate by crystallography and X-ray diffraction.[76]

Predisposing causes and types of pulmonary aspergillosis[77,78]

Although exposure to *Aspergillus* spores is common, the fungus is not a frequent pathogen. Only if the individual is atopic, or the lungs have been previously damaged, or general resistance is lowered by other conditions are ill-effects likely to occur. Bronchopulmonary disease caused by aspergilli may accordingly be classified respectively as allergic, saprophytic and invasive.[77,79] Rarely, different forms of pulmonary aspergillosis occur in the same patient. For example, an aspergilloma may be complicated by allergic aspergillosis,[80,81] even in a non-atopic patient, whilst an aspergilloma may develop within the bronchiectasis resulting from allergic aspergillosis.[82,83]

Allergic bronchopulmonary aspergillosis

Persons suffering from this form of aspergillosis are generally atopic and give a history of asthma.[84–87] There is also an increased incidence of allergic aspergillosis in patients with cystic fibrosis, but nearly half those so affected are also atopic.[88] It is important to reiterate that this form of aspergillosis is not characterised by invasion of the tissues by the fungus: it is an allergic response to *Aspergillus* that remains confined to the airways. Furthermore, as the disease is a hypersensitivity phenomenon, hyphae are very sparse and have to be searched for diligently, in contrast to both the other main forms of aspergillosis (saprophytic and invasive) in which hyphae are numerous.

The allergic reaction in the lung is frequently reflected in a raised blood eosinophil count: eosinophilia is also seen in lung tissue and sputum. Circulating precipitating antibodies to *Aspergillus* antigens may be demonstrable and immunoglobulin E, both total and specific, is generally raised; indeed, these immunological tests, together with the demonstration of immediate (and late) skin reactions to *Aspergillus* antigens, are now the main means of confirming the clinical diagnosis of allergic aspergillosis. There is, however, a wide range of specific antibodies to various antigenic components of the fungus, and con-

Figure 5.4.12 The fruiting heads or conidiophores of *Aspergillus* in a pulmonary cavity that communicated with the bronchi, so affording the fungus the oxygen that stimulates this form of reproduction. (A) Grocott's methenamine silver stain; (B) lactophenol cotton blue stain.

centration of the serum may be necessary to detect them for they are often not present in the high concentrations found in association with an aspergilloma. Poor antigens may give false-negative results and corticosteroids may depress the antibody response and thus both skin and serological reactions. Culture of the sputum is not always positive and on occasion the diagnosis of allergic bronchopulmonary aspergillosis is first made by the histopathologist after surgery has been undertaken for a suspected malignancy (Fig. 5.4.16 and see Fig. 9.8, p. 464).[89]

The term 'allergic bronchopulmonary aspergillosis' is generally limited to a syndrome that is chiefly characterised by the expectoration of mucous plugs or the impaction of such plugs and the consequent development of bronchiectasis. However, allergy to *Aspergillus* may have further bronchopulmonary consequences, notably bronchocentric granulomatosis and eosinophilic pneumonia, both of which are dealt with elsewhere (see pp. 461 and 464). Attention here will be limited to mucoid impaction.

Mucoid impaction

In some asthmatic individuals particularly large mucous plugs develop, typically 1–2 cm thick and 2–5 cm long. They generally form in proximal bronchi (see Fig. 5.4.16) and can be clearly seen in plain

Figure 5.4.13 *Aspergillus* colonies in culture. The hyphal mycelium is white in all species but the conidiophores' colour is distinctive. (A) *A. fumigatus*; (B) *A. niger*.

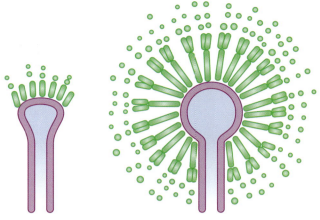

Figure 5.4.14 *Aspergillus* conidiophores. The structure of the conidiophores shows marked species variation. (A) Diagrammatic appearances of *A. fumigatus* on the left and *A. flavus* on the right. (B) A conidiophore in culture.

Figure 5.4.15 Calcium oxalate crystal deposition in the tissues bordering an aspergilloma viewed with (A) non-polarised and (B) polarised light. As is usually the case, much of the fungal colony is dead but here the adjacent host tissue is also necrotic; this change is attributable to oxalic acid secretion by the fungus. The oxalic acid combines with free calcium ions in the tissues to precipitate as insoluble, birefringent crystals.

radiographs as finger-like opacities near the hilum of the lung. They are frequently expectorated spontaneously (Fig. 5.4.17). The airway involved is dilated and its wall shows non-specific chronic inflammatory changes which vary from a mild infiltrate to a severe reaction that includes many eosinophils. The affected airway may be merely distended and therefore returns to normal after the plug is expectorated, or its wall may be largely destroyed by the inflammation so that there is permanent bronchiectasis (Fig. 5.4.18). The proximal distribution of this form of bronchiectasis contrasts with that of the postinfective form, which generally affects the bases.

Figure 5.4.16 Allergic bronchopulmonary aspergillosis identified as the cause of a pulmonary opacity thought to be neoplastic. (A) Several bronchi are distended by plugs of viscous mucus. (B, C) Microscopy shows alternating eosinophilic bands, the pink ones representing mucus and the red conglomerations of eosinophils. In (C) the walls of the bronchi also show chronic inflammation, which weakens them and leads to proximal bronchiectasis. *(Courtesy of Professor DH Wright, Southampton, UK.)*

Figure 5.4.17 A mucous plug spontaneously expectorated by a patient with allergic bronchopulmonary apergillosis. Such plugs are short and stubby, very different from the long, many-tailed plugs expectorated in plastic bronchitis (compare with Fig. 3.20, p. 109). *(Courtesy of Dr T Jelihovsky, Sydney, Australia.)*

The mucous plugs undergo inspissation and often have the consistency of hard rubber. Although they may form casts of several generations of bronchi, they tend to be shorter and stubbier than the long stringy casts expectorated in plastic bronchitis (see p. 109). The microscopic appearances also differ. Mucous plugs characteristically consist of bands of agglutinated eosinophils alternating with layers of mucus (see Fig. 5.4.16). The bands of eosinophils are arranged parallel to the airway wall and frequently diminish in length towards the centre of the lumen so that wedges of alternating cellular and mucous bands point inwards, presenting an appearance that has been likened to fir trees.[90] Sparse *Aspergillus* hyphae are generally to be found in the mucous plugs.

In exceptional cases other fungi are responsible for similar changes, resulting in reports of allergic bronchopulmonary stemphyliosis, curvulariosis, drechsleriasis, candidosis, helminthosporiosis, penicilliosis, torulopsosis, fusariosis and pseudallescheriosis.[91–96] and the term 'allergic bronchopulmonary fungal disease' is therefore sometimes preferred.[97]

Extrinsic allergic alveolitis

Extrinsic allergic alveolitis may also be a manifestation of allergy to *Aspergillus*, but here it is heavily exposed non-atopic individuals who are affected. One example is 'malt worker's lung', which occurs in

Figure 5.4.18 Allergic bronchopulmonary aspergillosis. The proximal bronchi (top) are dilated and some contain mucous plugs. More peripherally there is coagulative necrosis representing bronchocentric granulomatosis and beyond that pale foci of eosinophilic pneumonia are seen. *(Courtesy of the late Dr AA Liebow, San Diego, USA.)*

Figure 5.4.19 Aspergilloma. Computed tomography shows a cavity in the apical segment of the right lower lobe, containing an intracavitary body consistent with an aspergilloma, which was confirmed following lobectomy.

brewery staff working with mouldy barley; the species of *Aspergillus* involved here is usually *A. clavatus*. Extrinsic allergic alveolitis may also develop in patients harbouring an aspergilloma.[81] These forms of allergy to *Aspergillus* are similar, both clinically and pathologically, to the extrinsic allergic alveolitis that develops in response to other allergens (see p. 279).

SAPROPHYTIC ASPERGILLOSIS

Aspergilli may grow saprophytically within stagnant secretions in the bronchi in cases of chronic bronchitis and, less often, bronchiectasis. In certain circumstances this may be very marked, resulting in obstructive aspergillosis (see below). Other varieties of saprophytic aspergillosis include the colonisation of an infarct,[98] a tumour,[99] the bronchial anastomosis following transplantation[100,101] and a preformed cavity, resulting in the last case in the formation of an aspergilloma (intracavitary *Aspergillus* ball colony).[102]

Aspergilloma

In an aspergilloma the fungus grows in the lumen of a cavity in the lung without invading the tissues to any appreciable extent, drawing its nutriment from such exudate as may be present. The ball usually forms in an existing cavity, particularly an old tuberculous cavity,[102] but sometimes in a cavity resulting from conditions such as sarcoidosis (see Fig. 6.1.37, p. 289), bronchiectasis, abscess or emphysema, or in a congenital cyst. Aspergilloma formation has been observed both in the bronchiectatic lung distal to an obstructing carcinoma and within the cavity resulting from necrosis at the centre of a peripheral carcinoma.[103] Although usually single, aspergillomas may be present in cavities in both lungs, and in some cases there are several such lesions.

The term 'mycetoma' is frequently misapplied to intracavitary fungal balls, such as aspergillomas. The term is correctly limited to a type of fungal granuloma that is characterised by the formation of multiple sinuses and is usually the outcome of penetration of the soft tissues by a thorn, or the like, contaminated by the causative organism. Such lesions are most frequent on the extremities and 'Madura foot' is the type example. In this sense a mycetoma represents a lesion caused by invasion of the tissues by the organism concerned, in contrast to an intracavitary fungal ball, which is essentially outside the tissues and does not, except in unusual circumstances, lead to extension of the infection into the wall of the cavity itself. Many varieties of fungus cause mycetomas: most of them seldom, if ever, cause other disease.

While most intracavitary fungal ball colonies are formed by *A. fumigatus*, other species of *Aspergillus* have been identified in some cases and, exceptionally, fungi such as *Pseudallescheria (Petriellidium) boydii*,[104] *Cladosporium cladosporidioides*[105] and species of *Penicillium*, *Candida* or *Syncephalastrum*[106] have been responsible. Also, ball colonies similar to an aspergilloma may on rare occasions consist solely of bacteria (see nocardioma on p. 215 and botryomycoma on p. 192).

Radiology

The radiological appearances of an aspergilloma are often characteristic. The fungal ball appears as a sharply demarcated radiopaque spheroid that rests on the wall of the dependent part of the cavity and is separated from it elsewhere by a crescent of air (Fig. 5.4.19). In cases of long standing the colony may fill the cavity completely but the fungal ball is often able to move within the cavity in accordance with the patient's posture. However, although these features are characteristic of an aspergilloma, they may also be given by an indolent necrotising form of invasive aspergillosis which is considered below. A true aspergilloma is often demonstrated in radiographs over a period of several years, sometimes with little or no detectable change in its

Figure 5.4.20 An *Aspergillus* fungal ball (an aspergilloma) filling an apical cavity. In its fresh state the fungal ball forms a soft, brown, pultaceous mass but as seen here after fixation, it is more friable.

Figure 5.4.21 Aspergilloma. (A) The centre of the fungus ball consists of a dense feltwork of dead fungal hyphae. Only at the periphery is the fungus viable. (B) The edge of the fungus ball is coated by a layer of eosinophilic immune material (Splendore–Hoeppli phenomenon).

appearance, sometimes with appreciable phases of shrinkage and enlargement.

Antibody production

Most patients with an aspergilloma have strong serum precipitins against *Aspergillus* antigens but, unless allergy with asthma has developed, skin tests against extracts of the fungus are negative. Occasionally the circulating precipitins combine with fungal antigen disseminated via the airways to produce the changes of extrinsic allergic alveolitis elsewhere in the lung or there may be immune complex-mediated vasculitis elsewhere in the body.

Morbid anatomy

The fungal colony appears macroscopically as a grey or reddish brown, rarely white or green-tinged mass, sometimes firm or rubbery in consistency but often friable or pultaceous (Fig. 5.4.20). Old colonies may have a gritty feel, from deposition of calcium salts, and exceptionally

there may be so much calcification that the ball becomes stony and may be classified among the so-called 'pneumonoliths'.

Histological appearances

Microscopically, an aspergilloma consists of a dense feltwork of hyphae, most of which are dead. Only the hyphae at the surface are well preserved. The tips of these may be abundantly coated with hyaline eosinophilic material of probable immune origin (Splendore–Hoeppli phenomenon; see Fig. 5.3.25, p. 215), giving the edge of the aspergilloma a distinctive appearance (Fig. 5.4.21). The lining of the cavity that contains an aspergilloma varies according to the nature of the condition that has given rise to it. The wall of an old tuberculous cavity may consist of dense, hyaline fibrous tissue, sometimes devoid of an epithelial covering; in other cases there may be a lining zone of chronic inflammatory granulation tissue, which usually is without specific features of tuberculosis or other former disease. When present, an epithelial lining may be of either respiratory or squamous type.

Chronic inflammatory changes in the lining of the cavity that are attributable to the fungal ball are variable but their presence underlies any enlargement of the cavity. It is mentioned above that numerous calcium oxalate crystals are occasionally present. These are found in the cavity lining, particularly near the surface and in relation to the sides of blood vessels that face the fungus ball (see Fig. 5.4.15). The toxic nature of oxalic acid contributes to the progressive enlargement of the cavity but proteinases secreted by the fungus are probably more important in this respect.[107] Sometimes non-specific chronic inflammation is due to secondary bacterial infection.

It is exceptional for the fungus to invade the tissues, although this has been observed. Such a change from saprophytosis to invasive growth is more likely to occur when the patient's resistance is lowered, particularly by immunosuppressant and cytotoxic therapy and less often by administration of corticosteroids.

Haemorrhage

Haemoptysis is a common feature of aspergilloma. Usually it causes no more than anaemia, but in some cases it has been massive and death has resulted. It often accompanies the development of further excavation of the lung tissue round the colonised lesion. The rich capillary bed of a granulation tissue lining is generally the source of the haemorrhage,[108] but larger vessels are occasionally involved; the endarteritis obliterans usually found in chronic inflammation fails to seal them completely. The blood supply to the wall of an aspergilloma cavity ultimately derives from the bronchial circulation and the haemoptysis can sometimes be controlled by cannulation of the bronchial arteries concerned under radiographic control and the introduction of occlusive synthetic emboli (see Fig. 8.1.15, p. 412).

Obstructive aspergillosis

This form of aspergillosis was first described in patients with AIDS[109] and subsequently in the recipients of organ transplants.[110] It is characterised by a progressive cough, which is sometimes productive of bronchial casts composed entirely of *Aspergillus* hyphae, in contrast to the mucous plugs of allergic bronchopulmonary aspergillosis in which hyphae are scanty. There is no wheezing or eosinophilia but the patient rapidly develops hypoxaemia. Chest radiographs show areas of collapse and at bronchoscopy some airways are found to be completely obstructed by fungal casts. When these are removed the bronchial mucosa appears normal. The condition therefore represents saprophytic infection. Nevertheless, it is probably a precursor of the locally invasive pseudomembranous *Aspergillus* tracheobronchitis, described below.

INVASIVE AND SEPTICAEMIC ASPERGILLOSIS

Excluding saprophytic colonisation of pulmonary infarcts and superficial invasion round an aspergilloma – each a relatively rare occurrence – most instances of *Aspergillus* pneumonia are due to the patient's resistance being undermined by factors that cause prolonged granulocytopenia, such as lymphoproliferative disease, leukaemia and corticosteroid therapy.[111–115] Less often, invasive pulmonary aspergillosis complicates influenza or other viral infection[116,117] or chronic obstructive pulmonary disease.[117a,118] AIDS is another predisposing cause[119–121] but the incidence of invasive aspergillosis is nevertheless lower than that of many other opportunistic infections in this group of patients,[109,122,123] probably because the HIV attacks lymphocytes rather than granulocytes. Rarely, the patient is apparently immunocompetent.[124] In severely immunodeficient patients the infection spreads quickly and often disseminates via the blood stream, whereas in less debilitated patients infection results in more indolent localised lesions.

Figure 5.4.22 Invasive aspergillosis. The fungal hyphae grow through all constituents of the lung tissue, including blood vessels, which thrombose, resulting in infarction.

Invasive aspergillosis

In neutropenic patients invasive aspergillosis is characterised by star-like clusters of radiating hyphae that extend widely throughout the lung tissue (Fig. 5.4.22). There is vascular invasion leading to thrombosis, infarction and generalisation of the infection through the body. Non-neutropenic patients are more likely to show neutrophilic and monocytic exudates and inflammatory necrosis.[125]

Septicaemic aspergillosis

Septicaemic aspergillosis is commonly first recognised at necropsy, and often not until the tissues are examined with the microscope. In many cases the portal of invasion of the blood stream by the fungus is not apparent. In others it is a recognisable local infection such as *Aspergillus* pneumonia. There may be a rapidly overwhelming septicaemia, with little to show in the way of focal lesions, or there may be many large foci of necrosis, most frequently in the brain, heart and kidneys. The lesions are often so heavily colonised by the *Aspergillus* that, very soon after exposure to the air at necropsy, condiophores develop and colour the necrotic tissue – green in the case of *A. fumigatus* and *A. flavus* and black if the fungus is *A. niger*. There may even be an obvious growth of the pigmented mould on the surface. Microscopical examination often shows that the hyphae of the invading fungus are surrounded by a spreading zone of necrosis in advance of their progress through the tissues: this is probably a result of diffusion from the infected part of toxins and degradative enzymes produced by the *Aspergillus*.[68,107] Occasionally, the lesions are suppurative. Infection by other fungi may be present at the same time.

Chronic necrotising *Aspergillus* pneumonia (acute cavitary pulmonary aspergillosis)

This is a localised form of invasive aspergillosis in which the necrotic lung tissue may separate away as a sequestrum and mimic an aspergilloma both radiographically and macroscopically (Fig. 5.4.23)[126–134]; microscopically, however, infected lung tissue is easily distinguishable from an intraluminal ball colony of fungus, even though both are largely necrotic.

Figure 5.4.23 Chronic necrotising *Aspergillus* pneumonia. The lung contains a cavity partly lined by a plaque of *Aspergillus nigra*. The appearances simulate those of an aspergilloma but the cavity is newly formed and its contents consist of necrotic lung tissue heavily infiltrated by the fungus. Compare the colour of this non-sporing mycelium with the cultured colony of the same species, which is exposed to oxygen and is therefore producing black conidiophores (Fig. 5.4.13b). *(Reproduced from Wiggins et al. (1989) by permission of the editor of* Thorax.[130])

Pseudomembranous *Aspergillus* tracheobronchitis

Pseudomembranous *Aspergillus* tracheobronchitis involves only a narrow zone of tissue bordering the major airways; the intervening lung parenchyma is spared.[135-140] In this form of invasive aspergillosis the airways are occluded by a mixture of necrotic debris and fungal hyphae (Fig. 5.4.24). It may be preceded by the obstructive form of saprophytic aspergillosis, described above. A granulomatous response to the fungus may develop, mimicking bronchocentric granulomatosis.[141,142]

MUCORMYCOSIS

Mycology

Mucormycosis (formerly zygomycosis or phycomycosis) is the name most widely familiar for any infection caused by a fungus that is a member of the class Zygomycetes (formerly Phycomycetes). This class includes the orders Mucorales and Entomophthorales. They are found in soil, dung and dust throughout the world and are common causes of food spoilage. The classic form of mucormycosis is rhinocerebral, where the fungi grow from an infected ulcer in the nasal space to invade the cranial cavity, cerebral blood vessels and the contents of one or both orbits.[143,144] Some of the mucormycoses are primary subcutaneous or orificial mucosal infections, occurring without predisposing disease. Very rarely, dissemination of the fungus from these primary sites results in visceral infection, including pulmonary mucormycosis due to the Entomophthorales *Basidiobolus haptosporus* (*B. meristosporus*) and *Conidiobolus coronatus* (*Entomophthora coronata*). Much more commonly, pulmonary mucormycosis is direct and attributable to lowering of resistance to invasion of the tissues by Mucorales of the species *Absidia*, *Mucor* and *Rhizopus* which ordinarily are sapro-

Figure 5.4.24 Pseudomembranous *Aspergillus* bronchitis. Many airways are plugged by fungal hyphae and necrotic debris. Invasion is generally limited but in this patient the process has already affected the adjacent pulmonary artery. (A) Gross appearances; (B) microscopy.

phytes on decaying organic matter. It is quite exceptional for one of these moulds to set up progressive infection in a patient who is otherwise in good health.[145]

The Mucorales that cause pulmonary infection are recognisable as such in histological sections by their characteristic morphology (Fig. 5.4.25A) but this does not allow identification of genus or species, which requires immunohistochemistry.[66] The hyphae are characteristically of variable but generally broad diameter, ranging from 3 to 20 μm. They tend to branch perpendicularly, and septation of the hyphae is absent or at most very infrequent. A false impression of septum formation may be given by folds that result from shrinkage. Because of their irregular appearance and the sometimes striking effects of shrinkage during histological processing the hyphae have been likened to lengths of crushed ribbon. Although visible in haematoxylin and eosin preparations, the mucoraceous fungi are best shown by special methods: the methenamine silver stain is often useful, but better results may be obtained by the silver impregnation methods used in the demonstration of reticulin fibres. As in the case of aspergilli, such morphologically specific structures as sporangiophores develop only when the mould is growing in air: they are seldom, if ever, seen in pulmonary lesions in the fresh state, but they may form if a specimen has inadvertently been left exposed before being placed in fixative solution. Culture often fails and

Figure 5.4.25 Mucor. (A) Mucor hyphae have few septa and are irregular in outline. The rounded structures that resemble spores are hyphae cut transversely. (B) Mucormycosis in a lung excised because of massive haemoptysis. Haemorrhage surrounds a partially thrombosed ruptured blood vessel. (C) The wall of the ruptured vessel shows necrotising granulomatous angiitis.

histology may then be the first means of identification, supplemented if required by molecular techniques.[67] The distinction from aspergilli is important because the treatment differs.

Predisposing causes

Conditions predisposing to visceral mucormycosis include AIDS, leukaemia, pancytopenia, myelomatosis, diabetes mellitus and immunosuppression to prevent graft rejection.[142,146,147] Certain therapeutic measures also predispose to these infections, particularly desferrioxamine and the administration of cytotoxic and immunosuppressant drugs, including corticosteroids. Cannulation of blood vessels, when long continued, is a further occasional factor, being a potential portal of infection. Burns, too, have repeatedly become not merely a site of superficial infection but the source of haematogenous dissemination. The predisposing factors to some extent determine the site of predominant infection. For instance, the syndrome of naso-orbitomeningingocerebral mucormycosis occurs usually as a complication of diabetes mellitus or renal failure: these metabolic disorders are comparatively seldom responsible for the development of pulmonary or primarily septicaemic mucormycosis, which in most cases occur as complications of severe blood disease or of the resistance-lowering side-effects of drugs. Similarly, severe malnutrition predisposes to mucormycosis of the stomach or intestine.

Pathological findings

Mucormycotic lesions in the lungs vary greatly in size and number. Multiple lesions are usually the result of haematogenous dissemination, as may occur in cases of naso-orbitocerebral mucormycosis, whereas lesions that are single or few may be the result of direct infection of the lungs by way of the airways. The lesions are firm, hyperaemic or haemorrhagic, and often necrotic. If they extend to the pleura, a fibrinous exudate is found over them and there are often petechial or larger foci of bleeding. Central lesions tend to be spherical and peripheral ones wedge-shaped,[148] the former resembling chronic necrotising pulmonary aspergillosis (see above) and the latter representing infarcts.

Microscopically, the most significant finding is fungal invasion of blood vessels of all sizes, with thrombosis and colonisation of the thrombus by the fungus, and infarction (Fig. 5.4.25B, C). It is clear that many strains of these fungi are thrombogenic, and staining the lesions with phosphotungstic acid haematoxylin or by other appropriate methods clearly demonstrates the formation of fine radiating threads of fibrin on the surface of the hyphae within the blood vessels. Perineural invasion is also commonly seen.[144] The hyphae may be present in great number, not only in the thrombi but throughout the resulting infarcts. The latter soon liquefy, and there may be secondary bacterial infection. Calcium oxalate crystal deposition, as described in aspergillosis (see above), is rarely reported in mucormycosis.[149]

As with other fungal infections occurring as a consequence of predisposing illnesses and drug-induced failure of resistance, mucormycosis is often accompanied by one or more other opportunistic infections, even of the same part. Frequent associations are of mucormycosis with aspergillosis or candidosis but bacterial, viral and protozoal infections may also be present.

CANDIDOSIS (MONILIASIS)

Candida is a yeast-like fungus that forms round or oval budding cells (blastospores), septate hyphae and intermediate structures called pseudohyphae (Fig. 5.4.26). Candidosis generally represents infection

Figure 5.4.26 'Mycotic' candidal aneurysm of a pulmonary artery complicating surgery for complex congenital heart disease. (A) Severe inflammation of the artery has led to mural necrosis (below) and thrombosis. (B) Grocott staining reveals *Candida* spores and hyphae within the thrombosed vessel. Note: the term 'mycotic' is applied to any aneurysm caused by infected emboli regardless of whether the infection is fungal or bacterial.

by *Candida albicans* (formerly known as *Monilia albicans*) but other species may be involved.[150] Speciation requires culture as the species are morphologically identical. *C. (Torulopsis) glabrata* is dealt with separately (see p. 244).

The commonest form of candidosis is oral thrush, but the organism can attack any mucous or moist cutaneous surface. The fungus is often found in the sputum but its presence there generally represents no more than saprophytic growth. The diagnosis of bronchopulmonary candidosis therefore often depends on finding the organism histologically. It is found as a secondary invader of the lower respiratory tract in cases of chronic bronchitis, bronchiectasis and bronchial carcinoma, and in severely ill patients with immunosuppression, including

AIDS.[119] In sections, *Candida* may be seen within a pseudomembrane consisting of purulent exudate on the surface of a bronchus, or very rarely in lung tissue as a cause of pneumonia or even lung abscess. In agranulocytic patients there is necrosis with minimal inflammation. *Candida* pneumonia may represent a peripheral extension of *Candida* bronchitis or result from haematogenous dissemination complicating diseases or therapeutic measures that lower resistance. Pulmonary vascular candidosis may complicate endocarditis or infection of central venous catheters inserted for prolonged parenteral feeding (see Fig. 5.4.26).[151,152] Features that distinguish *Candida* from *P. jirovecii* and other yeast-forming fungi such as *Histoplasma* include the mixture of budding yeast cells with pseudohyphae and the pyogenic or necrotising host reaction. The invariable presence of yeasts distinguishes candidosis from aspergillosis and mucormycosis.

CRYPTOCOCCOSIS

Mycology

Cryptococcosis, a disease of worldwide distribution, is caused by the monomorphic yeast-like fungus, *Cryptococcus neoformans*. This organism was formerly known as *Torula histolytica*, and the disease as torulosis. Because it was first recognised in Europe, and is caused by a fungus the cells of which reproduce by budding, cryptococcosis was also sometimes known as European blastomycosis, in contrast to the so-called North and South American blastomycoses (now blastomycosis and paracoccidioidomycosis respectively).

Although perhaps most familiar as a complication of leukaemia or lymphoma, in which the infection typically presents as a progressive meningoencephalitis, cryptococcosis is also known as a primary disease of the lungs without predisposing conditions, particularly when *Cryptococcus neoformans* var. *gattii* is involved.[153,154] The lung is the principal portal of entry and infection of the lungs is probably much commoner than at present recognised. The primary pulmonary lesion of cryptococcosis is comparable to the initial lesion of histoplasmosis and coccidioidomycosis and to the Ghon focus of tuberculosis. Other diseases predisposing to secondary pulmonary cryptococcosis include alveolar lipoproteinosis and AIDS.[119,155,156] Cryptococcal inflammatory pseudotumours are recorded in HIV-positive patients.[157]

C. neoformans is a spheroidal or ovoid organism (Fig. 5.4.27). A characteristic feature is variability in size, the cell body measuring from 3 to 20 µm in diameter, although in many instances it is within the range of 6–9 µm. Another prominent feature is single, narrow-based budding, as opposed to the single, broad-based budding of *Blastomyces dermatitidis* and the multiple narrow-based budding of *Paracoccidioides brasiliensis* (Fig. 5.4.27A). The organism has a mucoid capsule that usually stains with mucicarmine, a reaction that is not given by any other pathogenic yeast-like fungus. Cryptococci can be seen in haematoxylin and eosin preparations because they are refractile and, in polarised light, birefringent. They can also be demonstrated by any of the special methods for staining fungi (Fig. 5.4.27B). The capsule is sometimes deficient, in which case the fungus is not mucicarminophilic.[158] However, in most cases of capsule-deficient cryptococcosis some carminophilic capsular material can be identified around a few yeasts. A Masson–Fontana stain can also help in the recognition of capsule-deficient cryptococci because, unlike other yeasts, cryptococci produce a melanin-like pigment.[159] Alternatively, capsule-deficient strains may be identified by immunohistochemistry.

The cryptococci may be found in the sputum in cases of pulmonary involvement. They may be seen on microscopical examination of wet films, particularly when the sputum has been mixed with India ink or

Figure 5.4.27 Cryptococcosis. (A) A single *Cryptococcus* exhibiting single narrow-based budding (haematoxylin and eosin stain). *(Courtesy of Dr A Paiva-Correia, formerly of Oporto, Portugal.)* (B) Cryptococci demonstrated by periodic acid–Schiff staining. (C) A necrotising 4-cm cryptococcoma excised after its chance radiographic discovery. *(Courtesy of Dr M Jagusch, formerly of Auckland, New Zealand).* (D) Fungal spores (arrows) are seen amongst neutrophils in an immunosuppressed patient with disseminated disease. *(B and D courtesy of Dr PM Cury, Rio Preto, Brazil.)*

nigrosin to display the capsule. In dry films the fungal cells disintegrate or become smudged and usually cannot be recognised, although sometimes staining with mucicarmine is conclusive. Cultures are generally the preferred means of confirming the diagnosis, but some strains of the cryptococcus do not grow well and several attempts may have to be made before the organism is isolated. It is notable that the cryptococcus is only exceptionally, if ever, found in sputum in the absence of infection, in spite of its near ubiquity in our environment.

The fungus is often found in the dried droppings of birds, particularly pigeons and starlings; these provide a good culture medium and pathogenic cryptococci can often be isolated from buildings on which these birds roost.[160] Isolation from soil is less frequent, probably because of the avidity with which cryptococci are phagocytosed by soil amoebae. As in the case of histoplasmosis, cryptococcosis has been known to develop in people who have worked in bird-infested build-ings, particularly during demolition. The infection in such patients is slow to appear, in contrast to the acute pneumonic form of histoplasmosis. It is clear that exposure to cryptococci must occur very frequently: equally, the great majority of people must have a high immunity, for cryptococcosis is rare in any population.

It is important to remember that any patient with active cryptococcosis is at risk of developing infection of the central nervous system because of the peculiar affinity of the organism for the brain and meninges and the frequency of its dissemination in the blood.

Clinical features

Clinical features range from asymptomatic pulmonary involvement to life-threatening meningitis and overwhelming cryptococcaemia. Imaging shows single or multiple well-circumscribed masses, poorly demarcated opacities or segmental consolidation.

Morbid anatomy

Pulmonary cryptococcosis takes several forms: primary, crypto-coccoma, cavitary, pneumonic, miliary and inflammatory pseudo-tumour.[153,155–157,161–163] Isolated, discrete, encapsulated, subpleural granulomas are occasionally seen at necropsy: these are healed or healing lesions, and the implication of their presence is that they are a manifestation of a primary and non-progressive infection. Less rarely, there are one or more focal lesions in the lungs, up to several centimetres in diameter, that prove to be foci of progressive crypto-coccal infection. These are known as cryptococcomas (formerly toru-lomas) (Fig. 5.4.27C). They are firm, pale tan and rather sharply defined but are encapsulated only when healing. Their cut surface may be dry or gelatinous: the latter is the case when there is less inflam-matory reaction to the organisms, which, packed closely in great numbers, account for the mucoid appearance and consistence of such lesions. Cryptococcal inflammatory pseudotumours are solid, firm and grey. Progressive cavitary disease occurs in about 10% of cases. Confluence and continuing enlargement of multiple foci may produce a gelatinous pneumonia involving a segment or the greater part of one or more lobes. In cases of generalised haematogenous dissemina-tion of cryptococcosis both lungs may be studded with miliary or larger foci: close inspection of these discloses their gelatinous nature; they tend to be sharper in outline than miliary tubercles or pyaemic abscesses. The gelatinous collection of cryptococci at the centre of the lesion may be washed out during examination of the tissue, leaving a minute cavity.

Histological appearances

Microscopically, the lesions may be composed largely of the crypto-cocci themselves, with little cellular reaction: the alveoli and intersti-tial tissue contain the closely packed organisms, their cell bodies separated by the variable extent of their mucoid capsule. In other cases, particularly those involving capsule-deficient strains, there may be a tuberculoid reaction, the fungal cells being found within the cytoplasm of multinucleate giant cells and of mononuclear macro-phages as well as free in the tissue spaces. In lesions of long standing, lymphocytes and plasma cells may be present in large numbers, and fibrosis may be a feature, although not often conspicuous. Occasionally, neutrophils accumulate in considerable numbers (Fig. 5.4.27D), par-ticularly in miliary haematogenous lesions, but in the absence of bacterial infection frank suppuration is not found. Caseation is a rare development, and has to be distinguished from the somewhat similar appearance that may result when large numbers of cryptococci have died and disintegrated into an amorphous, finely granular, eosinophile mass. Cryptococcal inflammatory pseudotumours are composed of plump spindle cells mixed with lymphocytes, plasma cells and the yeast forms of the fungus.

HISTOPLASMOSIS

The first report of *Histoplasma* infection was in 1905 by Samuel Darling, a US Army pathologist stationed in Panama around the time of the building of the canal. Darling observed the organisms in histio-cytes (hence the prefix 'histo'), likened them to plasmodia (hence 'plasma') and incorrectly assumed that an artefactual clear space around each organism was a capsule (hence 'capsulatum').

Mycology

Two species of *Histoplasma* are pathogenic in humans, *H. capsulatum* and *H. duboisii*. The latter is found exclusively in tropical Africa and the disease that it causes differs significantly from that caused by *H. capsulatum*, an organism that is geographically far more widespread. In general, when the word histoplasmosis is used without elaboration it refers to disease caused by *H. capsulatum*.

The histoplasmas are dimorphic fungi, growing as ovoid, yeast-like organisms in cultures at 37°C and in infected tissues (parasitic phase), and in mycelial form, producing characteristic tuberculate macroco-nidia, in cultures at laboratory temperature (about 18°C) and in their free-living state in the soil (saprophytic phase). Spores released by the macroconidia are inhaled and at body temperature germinate into yeasts that grow by binary fission.

Histoplasmas can rarely be demonstrated in sputum, even by culture, but complement fixation and precipitin tests may be helpful. However, on occasion, biopsy may be necessary. When this is under-taken, the opportunity to set up cultures must not be lost, although histology is more sensitive than culture.[164] The fungi may be quite focal in their distribution, and therefore difficult to find, but within these foci the spores are usually present in large numbers within the cytoplasm of macrophages or in areas of necrosis. They are readily seen in haematoxylin and eosin preparations, but only if recently viable. They measure $1{-}3 \times 3{-}5 \ \mu m$ and may contain a distinct nucleus. Histoplasmas that have been dead for some time may escape detection in such preparations, although sometimes birefringence, induced by histological processing, may make a proportion of them visible in polarised light. Fortunately, the methenamine silver stain commonly demonstrates histoplasmas very clearly, even when they have long been dead. Unfortunately, they are difficult to distinguish from other budding yeasts but a granulomatous reaction, their intra-cellular location and an absence of pseudohyphae help separate them from *Candida* species and *P. jirovecii*.

Epidemiology

H. capsulatum is a soil-inhabiting fungus that requires organic nitrates for growth. These are generally provided by bird droppings. Histo-plasmosis results from inhalation of infective spores and the geo-graphical distribution of the disease is determined by environmental conditions. In regions where the fungus cannot survive to complete its saprophytic phase in soil or other organic debris, histoplasmosis does not occur naturally – infection does not ordinarily take place from person to person, the tissue form of the fungus being in general unable to convey the disease. In those parts of the world where the soil or the climate is unsuitable for the saprophytic phase of *H. cap-sulatum*, the disease is found only among those who have acquired the infection in lands where the fungus is present in the environment, or, much more rarely, as a result of exposure to imported materials contaminated by the infective spores[165] or to laboratory cultures of the saprophytic phase, which develops when the tissue form is grown at laboratory temperature.

Histoplasmosis is endemic in many parts of North, Central and South America, Asia and Africa. In North America, infection is particu-larly common in the basin of the Ohio and Mississippi river valleys, where as many as 90% of the population give a positive reaction to the histoplasmin skin test. The histoplasmin test has the same signifi-cance in relation to histoplasmosis as the tuberculin test in relation to infection by *Mycobacterium tuberculosis*. In Africa, infection by *H. capsulatum* is endemic over an area far greater than that in which infec-tion by the 'African histoplasma', *H. duboisii*, occurs. Histoplasmosis is also endemic in India and South-east Asia but it has not been recognised as an indigenous infection in Australia. Its occurrence in Europe, other than as a result of travel to an endemic area or accidental exposure to the fungus, is exceptionally rare.

Most people who acquire histoplasmosis have no more than a subclinical infection. It has been estimated that clinical manifestations

Figure 5.4.29 Histoplasmoma representing quiescent disease.

Figure 5.4.28 Histoplasmosis. A chest radiograph shows multiple bilateral calcific nodules in a patient with quiescent histoplasmosis.

occur in only about 1% of cases and that few of these patients develop serious illness. Histoplasmosis is seen in rural communities exposed to bird droppings and in urban dwellers exposed to demolition and building sites. Bat guano is rich in organic phosphates and histoplasmas and the likely cause of an acute illness of cave explorers. Several forms of histoplasmosis are desribed, which will now be considered.

Primary pulmonary histoplasmosis

The primary focus of histoplasmosis resembles that of tuberculosis. As with mycobacteria, the main line of host defence is the macrophage. Specific T-cell immunity appears about 10–14 days after infection and macrophages so activated usually terminate the infection. If not, the organisms continue to grow within the macrophage cytoplasm. The disease is spread during its primary stage by infected macrophages migrating to the regional lymph nodes and beyond to disseminate by the blood stream to all organs, but being filtered out particularly well by those rich in reticuloendothelial cells so that the liver and spleen are commonly involved.

The primary lesion may be solitary or there may be two or more, sometimes many, primary lesions in the lungs, the number depending on the heaviness of the exposure to the infecting spores. Primary lesions may occur in any part of the lungs. Generally, and especially when solitary, it is larger than the corresponding lesion of primary tuberculosis but otherwise similar, showing epithelioid and giant cell granulomatous inflammation. Caseation develops within a few weeks of infection and its appearance is believed to coincide with the development of skin reactivity to histoplasmin, an observation comparable to the corresponding events in tuberculosis. Early calcification and the formation of a fibrous capsule are common (Fig. 5.4.28). As in tuber-

culosis, there is spread of the infection to the hilar lymph nodes, which undergo comparable changes. It is a characteristic of calcified lesions of histoplasmosis that they have a massively chalky appearance and often show a peculiar stippled pattern in radiographs, particularly lesions in lymph nodes. Occasionally, the calcified foci in the lungs have a target-like radiographic shadow because of concentric zones of greater and lesser transradiancy.

Histoplasmoma

The name histoplasmoma is given to any circumscribed, persistent focus of *Histoplasma* infection in a lung. The lesion is an outcome of a primary focus, akin to a tuberculoma rather than an aspergilloma. It occurs typically just under the pleura, and is roughly spherical and from 1 to 4 cm, sometimes more, in diameter (Fig. 5.4.29). Both in radiographs and when examined with the naked eye it has a characteristically concentric pattern of closely set laminae, which may contain appreciable amounts of calcium salts, although by no means invariably. This laminar structure is so characteristic of chronic caseous granulomas of fungal origin that in some centres it is regarded as proof of the non-neoplastic nature of 'coin shadows': this is not necessarily justified, for it has been known for carcinoma to arise in the fibrotic capsular zone round such a long-standing mycotic lesion. In general, histoplasmomas are altogether benign in outlook, and may be left in situ with little chance that the infection will be activated and progress; they may become more heavily calcified as the years pass. If resected, they usually prove to be sterile on culture. The causative organism may then be demonstrated most reliably by the methenamine silver stain, even though it is no longer viable.

Cavitary histoplasmosis

Histoplasmosis may closely reproduce the clinical and radiological picture of cavitating pulmonary tuberculosis. Moreover, if such patients are exposed to a substantial risk of infection by *Mycobacterium tuberculosis*, as may occur if they are nursed in company with tuberculous patients, tuberculosis may be superimposed on the histoplasmic lesions, with detriment to the chances of successfully treating either infection. In general, cavitary histoplasmosis is seen most frequently in older patients, particularly men with emphysema or other chronic lung disease.[166] It is attributed to a local breakdown in immunity at the site of dormant subapical histoplasmic granulomas. In some cases it is possible that the condition is due to reinfection, thus adding to the similarities between histoplasmosis and tuberculosis. Like the cavities of chronic pulmonary tuberculosis, the lesion of cavitary histoplasmosis may become the site of an aspergilloma. Tuberculoid granulomatous tissue in the lining and vicinity of the cavities contains typical intracellular histoplasmas.

Acute ('epidemic') pulmonary histoplasmosis

The condition that has been described as 'epidemic' pulmonary histoplasmosis is a form of acute histoplasmosis characterised by a severe influenza-like illness that occurs as a result of a particularly heavy inhalational infection in an unprotected individual.[167] The epithet 'epidemic' has been applied because such cases are commonly seen in several patients simultaneously, all of them exposed on the same occasion to a massive contamination of the air by infective spores. It is an unfortunate name, for such cases may occur singly when individuals are so unfortunate as to stir up large numbers of spores when working alone in a contaminated environment. These outbreaks have occurred when infected dust is disturbed in the course of cleaning or demolishing buildings, ranging from hen houses to city halls, that have harboured birds that over years have left the droppings that so perfectly favour the growth of the saprophytic phase of *H. capsulatum*. Similarly, those who enter caves where bat and bird droppings have encouraged the *Histoplasma* to proliferate may suffer comparable group outbreaks of acute histoplasmic pneumonia. The multiple foci of histoplasmosis that form in the lungs of heavily infected patients have the same structure and run the same course as the solitary primary foci described above. However, in some cases the infection is so heavy, and the resulting changes in the lungs are so widespread, that death occurs. Those who have not previously had a histoplasmic infection tend to suffer the severest illness in these outbreaks, but even those already known to have had a primary infection may develop fatal pneumonic lesions under such conditions of massive reinfection. Fatal opportunistic *Histoplasma* pneumonia is recorded[168] but immunosuppression is by no means necessary.

Progressive disseminated histoplasmosis

Mention has been made above of haematogenous dissemination of the infection during its primary stage. In most such cases the widespread lesions heal without ill effects. However, there is another form of disseminated histoplasmosis in which the disease progresses and eventually kills the patient. In some cases of this sort there are no obvious predisposing causes but in most the patient's resistance is lowered by the presence of serious underlying disease leading to defective T-cell function.[169] AIDS is now an important cause of such progressive disease (Fig. 5.4.30).[170,171]

Fatal disseminated histoplasmosis is characterised by heavy parasitisation of the reticuloendothelial cells resulting in hepatosplenomegaly and leukoerythroblastic anaemia. Painful ulcers develop at mucocutaneous junction zones or within the orifices of the body or in the pharynx and larynx. Organising pneumonic exudates and thin-walled cavities may be found in the lungs. Well-formed granulomas are not usually found. Fatal adrenal cortical insufficiency is another important manifestation.

Figure 5.4.30 Progessive disseminated histoplasmosis in a patient dying of acquired immunodeficiency syndrome (AIDS). (A) A pulmonary vessel shows only slight granulomatous inflammation but (B) Grocott staining shows extensive infiltration of the vessel by histoplasmas. *(Courtesy of Dr PM Cury, Rio Preto, Brazil.)*

Fibrosing mediastinitis

In those countries where histoplasmosis is prevalent mediastinal fibrosis with obstruction of some, or all, of the mediastinal contents is recorded as a complication of such infection.[172]

African histoplasmosis

Histoplasma duboisii, an organism larger than *H. capsulatum*, has been recognised as a cause of disease throughout much of Africa between the Sahara and the Zambesi. Its distribution overlaps that of *H. capsulatum*, which, however, is much more widespread on the continent. The source of the infection and the portal of entry of the fungus remain debatable. There is growing evidence that the organism has a saprophytic phase, probably in soil, and that it may enter the body either through the lungs or, in certain cases, by inoculation into the skin. Pulmonary disease as one of its manifestations has attracted less attention than cutaneous and skeletal involvement, but it is possible that in many cases the lesions in the skin, like those in bones, are the result of dissemination in the blood from inapparent pulmonary foci.

A feature typical of African histoplasmosis is that the fungal cells provoke a foreign-body giant cell reaction, not a simple histiocytosis with or without tuberculoid metamorphosis, as occurs in cases of infection by *H. capsulatum*. The organism is ovoid, has a distinct cell wall and some internal structure, and measures 5–12 μm in its longer dimension. It stains well with all the fungal stains, but is unlikely to be overlooked by the careful microscopist in haematoxylin and eosin preparations.

COCCIDIOIDOMYCOSIS[173–175]

Epidemiology

This disease is endemic in certain parts of North and South America, occurring especially in hot semiarid regions such as Arizona and the San Joaquin valley of California, but also in other such areas of the Americas down to Argentina. It is caused by the fungus *Coccidioides immitis*, the saprophytic, free-living form of which requires special environmental conditions of soil and climate for its survival: these determine its geographical distribution. *C. immitis* grows best in soils free of competing microflora, losing out to competitors when the soil is irrigated. Upsurges of infection may follow dust storms that release the fungus into the air. The fungus may also be transported on inanimate objects such as crops or native artefacts and infect persons outside endemic areas, and of course patients may travel to non-endemic regions while incubating the disease.[176] For example, the 2001 model airplane-flying world championship was held in an endemic region of California and several of those attending from other areas were found to have contracted coccidioidomycosis when they returned home.[177]

Mycology

C. immitis is a dimorphic fungus. Saprophytically, it grows as a mould that produces highly infective arthroconidia: these, inhaled in soil dust, establish the disease. As a parasite, the organism is found almost exclusively in the form of spherules: hyphae develop occasionally in the wall of coccidioidal cavities when air is admitted by them communicating with an airway, but this is exceptional: only spherules and their released spores are usually present, even when air is admitted (Figs 5.4.31 and 5.4.32).

Coccidioides is one of the most dangerous of all organisms in terms of risk of accidental infection of laboratory personnel. It is imperative that clinicians communicate to the laboratory any suspicion that a specimen may contain *C. immitis*. Laboratories dealing with coccidioidal cultures must operate with stringent precautions, including the exclusion of staff not known to have acquired some natural immunity through previous infection. The coccidioidin skin reaction is an invaluable screening test.

Once in the lungs, the arthroconidia develop into endosporulating spherules. These range from 30 to 60 μm or more in diameter and contain from scores to hundreds of endospores (see Fig. 5.4.32). The maturing spherule is usually accompanied by a histiocytic reaction, with the formation of many multinucleate giant cells: the parasite may be enclosed by the latter or lie free in the tissues. The mature spherule attracts neutrophils, which collect to form microabscesses at the centre of the histiocytic granulomatous foci. When the spherule ruptures, the freshly released spores, which range from 5 to 10 μm in diameter, at first lie free in the purulent exudate but soon are engulfed by mononucleate or multinucleate macrophages. They grow, and eventually

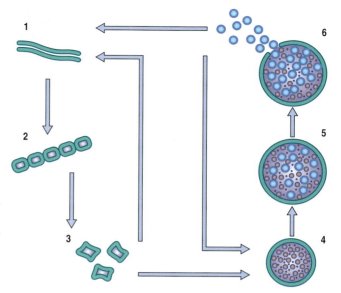

Figure 5.4.31 Life cycle of *Coccidioides immitis*. 1–3: Saprophytic phase in soil; 4–6: parasitic phase in lungs. Mycelial strands (1) growing in soil mature into chains of barrel-shaped arthroconidia (2), which disarticulate (3), become air-borne, and are returned to the soil or are inhaled. The parasitic phase in the lungs begins with the enlargement of the inhaled arthroconidia and their development into thick-walled spherules (4), within which endospores form (5). Released spores (6) can initiate the development of a new spherule in the lungs or if infected material returns to the soil, mycelia (1), so completing the cycle.

Figure 5.4.32 Coccidioidomycosis. Spherules discharging their spores within lung tissue. Grocott methenamine silver stain. (*Courtesy of Dr JT Gmelich, formerly of Pasadena, USA.*)

become transformed into further spherules, thus repeating the cycle and leading to extension of the infection.

The fungal cells are usually well seen in haematoxylin and eosin preparations, except in the early stages when only a few, newly released spores are present, which may be so inconspicuous as to escape detection. The methenamine silver and other stains for fungi demonstrate all forms of the organism very clearly. Whilst the mature or even ruptured spherule is diagnostic, immature spherules or free spores are not: the former may be confused with *Blastomyces* or *Paracoccidioides* and the latter with cryptococci or histoplasmas.

Figure 5.4.33 Coccidioidomycoma representing quiescent disease.

Figure 5.4.34 Blastomycosis. There is a neutrophil and giant cell reaction to *Blastomyces dermatitidis* yeasts, several of which have been ingested by giant cells. (A) Haematoxylin and eosin; (B) Grocott stain.

Clinical features

The initial coccidioidal infection is symptomless in about 60% of persons.[178] When disease develops, there is usually an influenza-like fever, which characteristically may be accompanied by erythema nodosum – hence its popular name of 'the bumps' in the San Joaquin valley, where it is also called 'valley fever'. In most cases there is spontaneous recovery from the primary infection. When the disease is more severe, which is likelier to be the case in patients of African or Asian ethnic origin, it may mimic tuberculosis in any of its manifestations. In severe infections generalisation through the blood is a frequent and particularly grave complication. Meningitis is another common complication. Many patients are left with quiescent pulmonary foci.

Pathological findings

At necropsy, the lungs may show focal consolidation, necrotic haemorrhagic areas or extensive necrotic excavating granulomatous nodules. Histologically, there may be a suppurative exudate in the alveoli, or necrotic haemorrhagic and fibrinous lesions, or a tuberculoid granulomatous reaction. Granulomatous inflammation is in general associated with good resistance, and purulent inflammation with poor resistance. However, when a spherule ruptures to release its spores (see Fig. 5.4.32), there may be a transient neutrophil response whatever the underlying pattern of inflammation. Also, the type of reaction is partly determined by the maturity of the developing fungal cells. Patients whose resistance is lowered by other diseases may develop generalised haematogenous coccidioidomycosis as a consequence of activation of a dormant pulmonary focus. The lesion of quiescent pulmonary coccidioidomycosis is typically a fibrocaseous nodule containing a few viable organisms (Fig. 5.4.33).

BLASTOMYCOSIS ('NORTH AMERICAN' BLASTOMYCOSIS)

Epidemiology

It is now recognised that infection with *Blastomyces dermatitidis* occurs very widely throughout Africa and that the geographical designation 'North American', intended to distinguish this disease from 'European blastomycosis' (cryptococcosis) and 'South American blastomycosis' (paracoccidioidomycosis), is inappropriate.

In North America, the greatest prevalence is in the south-eastern and north central USA, the area drained by the Mississippi, Missouri and Ohio rivers, the Great Lakes region and the eastern provinces of Canada.[179,180] The natural habitat of the fungus is soil, particularly that subjected to flooding. Infection is believed to occur by inhalation.

In Africa, lung disease is not so predominant. Many patients present with bone lesions or skin disease. Also, the antigenic make-up of the fungus differs from that encountered in North America, suggesting that there are at least two variants of blastomycosis, one seen in North America and in scattered foci in other countries (Mexico, Lebanon, Israel, Saudi Arabia and India), the other restricted to Africa.

Mycology

Like the histoplasmas, *B. dermatitidis* is a diphasic fungus.[181] In tissues and in cultures at 37°C it grows as a yeast whereas in cultures at laboratory temperature, and presumably in nature, it grows as a mycelium from which project special slender hyphae known as conidiophores which bear conidia, the infective agents. The yeasts are rounded and usually within the range of 7–15 μm in diameter, although some cells may be as much as 30 μm across (Fig. 5.4.34). They have a thick wall, which may give them a double-contoured appearance, but they differ from the spores of *Cryptococcus neoformans*, which they otherwise resemble, in lacking a capsule and therefore failing to stain with mucicarmine. It is a special feature of *B. dermatitidis* that it reproduces in tissues by the formation of a single broad-necked bud that protrudes from the surface of the parent cell, enlarging even until it has reached as much as half the diameter of the latter, or more, before the two separate.

Clinical features

As with several other fungi, *Blastomyces* causes a variety of clinical syndromes, including primary, progressive and disseminated disease. Asymptomatic disease is rarely documented, probably because there are no reliable skin or serological tests of infection. The disease is generally first identified on cytology or histology with subsequent positive culture.[181,182] Most patients are immunocompetent.

Primary blastomycosis is characterised by the abrupt onset of chills and cough accompanied by patchy radiographic opacities. Such illness may be self-limiting or followed by progressive disease, which is sometimes first manifest many months or years later, affecting either the lung or extrapulmonary sites. Some patients who have no history of pulmonary involvement develop blastomycosis in tissues such as the skin, the fungus probably having spread there during the course of asymptomatic primary lung infection.

Pathological features

The lungs are the usual portal of entry and within the lungs the upper lobes are predominantly involved.[183] The histological reaction to the fungus is characterised by necrotising granulomas that are typically suppurative, the fungal cells either lying free in the purulent exudate or engulfed by phagocytes. Although neutrophils are generally conspicuous, tuberculoid granulomas also form. A characteristic feature is the so-called 'suppurating pseudotubercle', in which a central microabscess is enclosed within a complex of epithelioid histiocytes and multinucleate giant cells (see Fig. 5.4.34). Alternatively, an overwhelming infection may cause diffuse alveolar damage.[184,185] The infection is usually confined to the lungs and hilar lymph nodes but dissemination by the blood stream may occur, particularly if immunity is impaired.[186] However, blastomycosis is not a common manifestation of AIDS.

PARACOCCIDIOIDOMYCOSIS ('SOUTH AMERICAN BLASTOMYCOSIS')[187,188]

Epidemiology

Infection with *Paracoccidioides brasiliensis* is limited to Latin American countries from Mexico to Argentina but does not occur in all countries in this area. The endemic regions are the tropical and subtropical forests, particularly those of Brazil, Venezuela and Colombia. Paracoccidioidomycosis has not been proved to occur in any other part of the world. Cases reported from North America[189] and England[190] had all lived in South or Central America. The fungus is thought to live in the soil but its exact ecological niche is still unknown. Humans are the only known naturally infected animal host. Person-to-person transmission is of little importance in the epidemiology of the disease, which is thought to be acquired by inhalation.

Mycology

P. brasiliensis is a dimorphic fungus that grows as a mould at ambient temperatures and as a yeast at 37°C. Infection is acquired by inhalation of conidia produced in the mycelial phase. The spores that form its tissue form are round or ovoid and vary in size from 5 to 30 μm.

Figure 5.4.35 *Paracoccidioides brasiliensis.* The larger of the organisms illustrated is forming multiple buds. Grocott's methenamine silver stain. *(Courtesy of Dr PM Cury, Rio Preto, Brazil.)*

A characteristic feature is that they reproduce by the development of multiple buds over the surface of the parent cell. The buds have been likened to the handles of a ship's wheel or Mickey Mouse's ears (Fig. 5.4.35). The presence of buds distinguishes *Paracoccidioides* from *Coccidioides* and their multiplicity from *Blastomyces*.

Clinicopathological features

Both pulmonary and disseminated forms of the disease are described.[187] After the establishment of a primary complex in the lung and hilar lymph nodes there may be haematogenous dissemination. Primary infection occurs in childhood and generally heals spontaneously. The sexes are affected equally in childhood but the development of the yeasts is inhibited by oestrogens and in adults the disease is largely limited to male agricultural workers. It is also described in patients with AIDS.[191] Disseminated disease tends to be acute and generalised in children and chronic and localised in adults. Chronic disseminated disease may take the form of lymphadenopathy, painful oropharyngeal ulceration or destruction of tissues such as the adrenal glands. Progressive pulmonary paracoccidioidomycosis is characterised by multiple cavities that mimic tuberculosis, or by progressive fibrosis of the lower lobes with traction bronchiectasis and paracicatricial emphysema in a bilaterally symmetrical distribution.[192] The tissue response is generally granulomatous but may be purulent (Fig. 5.4.36). Calcification is not a prominent feature. The diagnosis is established by recognising the spores in smears or culture of sputum or pus, or in tissue sections, or by serology. Biopsy is an excellent diagnostic procedure. The spores are best recognised with silver stains.

RARE PULMONARY MYCOSES

Fungi responsible for extrinsic allergic alveolitis are listed in Table 6.1.4 (p. 279) and the occurrence of intracavitary colonies of various fungi is mentioned on page 231. Allergic bronchopulmonary candidosis, helminthosporiosis, penicilliosis and curvulariosis, similar to the more familiar allergic aspergillosis, have all been described on rare occasions.[97]

Figure 5.4.36 Paracoccidioidomycosis. There is a giant cell and neutrophil reaction to numerous spores of *Paracoccidioides brasiliensis*.

Pulmonary mycoses not dealt with above are rare and ordinarily occur as a result of lowering of the body's resistance by other diseases or their treatment.[193] Some examples are dealt with below. Others include infection by the common saprophytic mould *Geotrichum candidum*, *Trichosporon cutaneum*, the organism of white piedra (tinea alba),[194,195] *Chaetomium globosum*,[65] *Paecilomyces lilacinus*,[196] *Dactylaria gallopava*[197] and *Ochroconis galloparvum*.[198] Chromomycosis (caused by species of *Phialophora* or *Cladosporium*) and rhinosporidiosis (caused by *Rhinosporidium seeberi*) are very occasionally found as infections of the lungs; in most cases such infection has spread, by the airways or in the blood, from a site elsewhere in the body.

Torulopsosis

Torulopsis glabrata, also known as *Candida glabrata*, is a common yeast on the body surface, and is frequently isolated as a contaminant of urine cultures. Human infection is usually opportunistic, taking the form of pneumonia, septicaemia, pyelonephritis or endocarditis in debilitated or immunocompromised patients, particularly those with AIDS or advanced cancer or being treated with wide-spectrum antibiotics.[199,200] Pulmonary infection is often by aspiration. Unlike *Candida albicans* it does not form hyphae. Its cells are nearly invisible in haematoxylin and eosin sections but are easily seen in Grocott preparations. They are difficult to distinguish from those of *Histoplasma capsulatum* but are rounded rather than ovoid.

Sporotrichosis

Sporotrichosis is usually seen as an indurated ulcer of the finger acquired from the prick of a thorn. Pulmonary involvement is rare and when present is generally secondary to disseminated lymphocutaneous sporotrichosis. Primary pulmonary sporotrichosis (involvement of the lung in the absence of cutaneous disease) is distinctly unusual.[201–203] However, because it mimics tuberculosis, its incidence may be greater than is generally recognised. The causative agent, *Sporothrix schenckii*, is a yeast-like fungus that occurs worldwide on decaying vegetation, contaminated soil and living plants, especially roses. Primary pulmonary sporotrichosis is acquired by inhalation of the spores and usually presents as a chronic, cavitary, bilateral, apical disease, most often in a clinical setting of alcoholism and chronic obstructive airway disease: less often it forms a solitary, necrotising, peripheral pulmonary nodule.[202] Fungal stains demonstrate many

round or ovoid budding yeast forms, 2–4 μm in size, in the areas of necrosis. Hyphae bearing sessile budding yeasts are found infrequently.

Adiaspiromycosis[204–212]

Adiaspiromycosis is caused by a remarkable fungus, *Emmonsia* (also known as *Chrysosporium*), which is a dimorphic filamentaous soil saprophyte of worldwide distribution. Its principal species are *E. crescens* and *E. parva*. The term 'adiaspiromycosis' derives from the conidia of this fungus, which are quite small but at 37 °C exhibit the unique property of progressive enlargement, perhaps a million-fold in volume, without replication, when they are known as adiaspores.

The disease is ordinarily limited to wild rodents but has been seen exceptionally in humans. It is characterised by the formation of tuberculoid granulomas around the inhaled adiaspores, which are usually solitary. The adiaspores have a prominent yellowish wall, up to about 8 μm in thickness, surrounding a central mass of amorphous cytoplasm in which there is a single nucleus. The adiaspores are remarkable for the great size that they may reach – as much as 600 μm in diameter. They are too large to be effectively mobilised by the host cells and the granulomatous response usually maintains a bronchiolocentric distribution indicative of inhalational infection. Dissemination is unusual but is recorded in AIDS.[210] Diagnosis relies on recognition of the fungus in tissue sections, as serology and culture are unreliable.

Light infection may result in a solitary adiaspiromycotic granuloma which would only be found incidentally in an asymptomatic individual. Widespread adiaspiromycotic granulomas are indicative of heavy infection and patients so affected may complain of fever, cough and dyspnoea and show a diffuse, micronodular pattern on chest radiographs.[207] Death is very unusual.[208] Healing is by progressive fibrosis and calcification.

Malasseziosis

Malassezia furfur, the causative organism of tinea versicolor (pityriasis versicolor), is dependent for its growth on high concentrations of fatty acids and is normally limited to the skin. Systemic infection has however complicated prolonged lipid infusions through central venous catheters, in which circumstances the small yeast-like organisms have been noted infiltrating the walls of pulmonary arteries and in small pulmonary thromboemboli.[213,214] As is so often the case with fungi, identification of the species depends upon cultural characteristics.

Pseudallescheriosis (monosporiosis)

Pseudallerscheria boydii (syn. *Petriellidium boydii*, *Allescheria boydii*) is a fungus of worldwide distribution in soils, and is of low pathogenicity. It is the commonest cause of mycetoma in Europe and North America, gaining access to the subcutaneous tissues through cuts and abrasions in the skin. Pulmonary involvement may occur through the inhalation of airborne spores, taking the form of an intracavitary fungal ball, comparable to an aspergilloma, or in conditions such as leukaemia it may be invasive and disseminate widely.[104,215–218] Allergic bronchopulmonary pseudallescheriosis is also described.[96]

Pseudallerscheria boydii usually grows in hyphal form within the body but within air-filled cavities conidia may develop. The conidial state is known as *Monosporium* (syn. *Scedosporium*) *apiospermum* and infection showing such growth may be termed monosporiosis. The hyphae are slender, thin-walled and of fairly constant diameter with numerous septa and branching points. The hyphae are slightly indented at the septa. They are more slender and their branches less clearly dichotomous than those of aspergilli but the differences are insufficient to discriminate between them with confidence morphologically. This requires immunohistochemistry.[66] The distinction of these two fungi is important because their drug sensitivities differ.[217]

Penicillium marneffei infection

Penicillium marneffei is a dimorphic fungus endemic in South-east Asia.[219] At room temperature it grows as a mould with red to black conidia whereas in tissue it forms a 3–5-μm yeast-like cell that divides by binary fission. The yeasts therefore display clear central septation, unlike H. capsulatum and other fungi that divide by budding. Infection, which is highest after the rainy season, is by inhalation but the pulmonary changes are usually overshadowed by systemic features such as hepatosplenomegaly, skin lesions and bone marrow involvement. However, there may be diffuse infiltration, mass lesions or cavities in the lungs. While it can affect the immunocompetent, infection is mainly associated with AIDS, for which it is a clinical marker in the endemic areas.[220]

Microsporidiosis

Microsporidia, once thought to be protozoa, are now regarded as extremely reduced fungi. They are obligate intracellular parasites that infect many animals and have emerged as important opportunistic pathogens in AIDS.[221,222] They are also being increasingly recognised in HIV-negative individuals.[223] Four microsporidian genera, Enterocytozoon, Encephalitozoon, Pleistophora and Nosema, have been reported to infect humans. Infection generally involves the gastro-intestinal tract but may become generalised.[223,224] Pulmonary involvement is unusual but heavy infestation of the tracheobronchial mucosa is recorded.[225–229] The infected respiratory epithelium may show focal proliferation with little inflammation or there may be a lymphocytic infiltrate of the airway epithelium similar to that seen in the bowel; heavy infestations cause sloughing and ulceration of the tracheobronchial mucosa and severe subacute inflammation. In haematoxylin and eosin-stained sections the parasite appears as a supranuclear 'blue body' but the staining is weak and it is easily overlooked, even when infestation is heavy. It is ovoid or spherical, and measures approximately 2 μm in length, and is Gram-positive. Microsporidia differ from cryptosporidia, which attach to the outer surface of infected epithelial cells, in being obligate intracellular parasites. Immunocytochemistry, electron microscopy and in situ hybridisation are useful for confirming the diagnosis.[230] Antiretroviral therapy has been shown to improve gastrointestinal symptoms, presumably through restoring immunity,[231] and albendazole has also been effective in some patients.

REFERENCES

Pneumocystosis

1. Watts JC, Chandler FW. Evolving concepts of infection by Pneumocystis carinii. Pathol Annu 1991;26:93–138.

2. Miller R, Huang L. Pneumocystis jirovecii infection. Thorax 2004;59:731–3.

3. Dutz W, Jennings-Khodadad E, Post C, et al. Marasmus and Pneumocystis carinii pneumonia in institutionalised infants. Observations during an endemic. Z Kinderheilk 1974;117:241–58.

4. Vanek J, Jivorec O, Luckes J. Interstitial plasma cell pneumonia in infants. Ann Pediatr 1953;180:1–21.

5. Lunseth JH, Kirmse TW, Prezyna AP, et al. Interstitial plasma cell pneumonia. J Pediatr 1955;46:137–45.

6. Haque A, Plattner SB, Cook RT, et al. Pneumocystis carinii. Taxonomy as viewed by electron microscopy. Am J Clin Pathol 1987;87:504–10.

7. Edman JC, Kovacs JA, Masur H, et al. Ribosomal RNA sequence shows Pneumocystis carinii to be a member of the fungi. Nature 1988;334:519–22.

8. Sidhu GS, Cassa ND, Pei ZH. Pneumocystis carinii: An update. Ultrastruct Pathol 2003;27:115–22.

9. Ham EK, Greenberg SD, Reynolds RC, et al. Ultrastructure of Pneumocystis carinii. Exp Mol Pathol 1971;14:362–72.

10. Campbell WG. Ultrastructure of Pneumocystis in human lung. Arch Pathol 1972;93:312–24.

11. Sueishi K, Hisano S, Sumiyoshi A, et al. Scanning and transmission electron microscopic study of human pulmonary pneumocystosis. Chest 1977;72:213–16.

12. Corrin B, Dewar A. Respiratory diseases. In: Papadimitriou JM, Henderson DW, Spagnolo DV, editors. Diagnostic Ultrastructure of Non-Neoplastic Diseases. Edinburgh: Churchill Livingstone; 1992. p. 264–86.

13. Lanken PN, Minda M, Pietra GG, et al. Alveolar response to experimental Pneumocystis carinii pneumonia in the rat. Am J Pathol 1980;99:561–88.

14. Yoneda K, Walzer PD. Mechanism of pulmonary alveolar injury in experimental Pneumocystis carinii pneumonia in the rat. Br J Exp Pathol 1981;62:339–46.

15. Coker RJ, Clark D, Claydon EL, et al. Disseminated Pneumocystis carinii infection in AIDS. J Clin Pathol 1991;44:820–3.

16. Gryzan S, Paradis IL, Zeevi A, et al. Unexpectedly high incidence of Pneumocystis carinii infection after heart–lung transplantation. Implications for lung defense and allograft survival. Am Rev Respir Dis 1988;137:1268–74.

17. Varthalitis I, Aoun M, Daneau D, et al. Pneumocystis carinii pneumonia in patients with cancer – an increasing incidence. Cancer 1993;71:481–5.

18. Pifer LL, Hughes WT, Stagno S, et al. Pneumocystis carinii infection: evidence for high prevalence in normal and immunosuppressed children. Pediatrics 1978;61:35–41.

19. Peters SE, Wakefield AE, Sinclair K, et al. A search for latent Pneumocystis carinii infection in post-mortem lungs by DNA amplification. J Pathol 1991;166:195–8.

20. Miller RF, Mitchell DM. AIDS and the lung – Update 1992 .1. Pneumocystis carinii pneumonia. Thorax 1992;47:305–14.

21. Young JA, Stone JW, McGonigle RJS, et al. Diagnosing Pneumocystis carinii pneumonia by cytological examination of bronchoalveolar lavage fluid: report of 15 cases. J Clin Pathol 1986;39:945–9.

22. Elvin KM, Bjorkman A, Linder E, et al. Pneumocystis carinii pneumonia: detection of parasites in sputum and bronchoalveolar lavage fluid by monoclonal antibodies. BMJ 1988;297:381–4.

23. Wakefield AE, Pixley FJ, Banerji S, et al. Detection of Pneumocystis carinii with DNA amplification. Lancet 1990;336:451–3.

24. Lipschik GY, Gill VJ, Lundgren JD, et al. Improved diagnosis of Pneumocystis carinii infection by polymerase chain reaction on induced sputum and blood. Lancet 1992;340:203–6.

25. Leigh TR, Gazzard BG, Rowbottom A, et al. Quantitative and qualitative comparison of DNA amplification by PCR with immunofluorescence staining for diagnosis of Pneumocystis carinii pneumonia. J Clin Pathol 1993;46:140–4.

26. Wakefield AE, Miller RF, Guiver LA, et al. Granulomatous Pneumocystis carinii pneumonia: DNA amplification studies on bronchoscopic alveolar lavage samples. J Clin Pathol 1994;47:664–6.

27. Eisen D, Ross BC, Fairbairn J, et al. Comparison of *Pneumocystis carinii* detection by toluidine blue O staining, direct immunofluorescence and DNA amplification in sputum specimens from HIV positive patients. Pathology 1994;26:198–200.

28. Armbuster CH, Pokieser L, Hassl A. Diagnosis of *Pneumocystis carinii* pneumonia by bronchoalveolar lavage in AIDS patients. Comparison of Diff-Quik, Fungifluor stain, direct immunofluorescence test and polymerase chain reaction. Acta Cytol 1995;39:1089–93.

29. Barrio JL, Suarez M, Rodriguez JL, et al. *Pneumocystis carinii* pneumonia presenting as cavitating and noncavitating solitary pulmonary nodules in patients with the acquired immunodeficiency syndrome. Am Rev Respir Dis 1986;134:1094–6.

30. Liu YC, Tomashefski JF, Tomford JW, et al. Necrotizing *Pneumocystis carinii* vasculitis associated with lung necrosis and cavitation in a patient with acquired immunodeficiency syndrome. Arch Pathol Lab Med 1989;113:494–7.

31. Watts JC, Chandler FW. *Pneumocystis carinii* pneumonitis. The nature and diagnostic significance of the methenamine silver-positive 'intracystic bodies'. Am J Surg Pathol 1985;9:744–51.

32. Mahan CT, Sale GE. Rapid methenamine silver stain for *Pneumocystis* and fungi. Arch Pathol 1978;102:351–2.

33. Musto L, Flanigan M, Elbadawi A. Ten-minute silver stain for *Pneumocystis carinii* and fungi in tissue sections. Arch Pathol 1982;106:292–4.

34. Shimono LH, Hartman B. A simple and reliable rapid methenamine silver stain for *Pneumocystis carinii* and fungi. Arch Pathol Lab Med 1986;110:855–6.

35. Kim H-K, Hughes WT. Comparison of methods for identification of *Pneumocystis carinii* in pulmonary aspirates. Am J Clin Pathol 1973;60:462–6.

36. Cameron RB, Watts JC, Kasten BL. *Pneumocystis carinii* pneumonia: an approach to rapid laboratory diagnosis. Am J Clin Pathol 1979;72:90–3.

37. Amin MB, Mezger E, Zarbo RJ. Detection of *Pneumocystis carinii* – comparative study of monoclonal antibody and silver staining. Am J Clin Pathol 1992;98:13–18.

38. Kobayashi M, Urata T, Ikezoe T, et al. Simple detection of the 5S ribosomal RNA of *Pneumocystis carinii* using in situ hybridisation. J Clin Pathol 1996;49:712–6.

39. LeGolvan DP, Heidelberger KP. Disseminated, granulomatous *Pneumocystis carinii* pneumonia. Arch Pathol 1973;95:344–18.

40. Weber WR, Askin FB, Dehner LP. Lung biopsy in *Pneumocystis carinii* pneumonia. A histopathologic study of typical and atypical features. Am J Clin Pathol 1977;67:11–19.

41. Askin FB, Katzenstein AA. *Pneumocystis* infection masquerading as diffuse alveolar damage. A potential source of diagnostic error. Chest 1981;79:420–2.

42. Cupples JB, Blackie SP, Road JD. Granulomatous *Pneumocystis carinii* pneumonia mimicking tuberculosis. Arch Pathol Lab Med 1989;113:1281–4.

43. Travis WD, Pittaluga S, Lipschik GY, et al. Atypical pathologic manifestations of *Pneumocystis carinii* pneumonia in the acquired immune deficiency syndrome. Review of 123 lung biopsies from 76 patients with emphasis on cysts, vascular invasion, vasculitis, and granulomas. Am J Surg Pathol 1990;14:615–24.

44. Birley HDL, Buscombe JR, Griffiths MH, et al. Granulomatous *Pneumocystis carinii* pneumonia in a patient with the acquired immunodeficiency syndrome. Thorax 1990;45:769–71.

45. Lee MM, Schinella RA. Pulmonary calcification caused by *Pneumocystis carinii* pneumonia – a clinicopathological study of 13 cases in acquired immune deficiency syndrome patients. Am J Surg Pathol 1991;15:376–80.

46. Foley NM, Griffiths MH, Miller RF. Histologically atypical *Pneumocystis carinii* pneumonia. Thorax 1993;48:996–1001.

47. Blumenfeld W, Basgoz N, Owen WF, et al. Granulomatous pulmonary lesions in patients with the acquired immunodeficiency syndrome (AIDS) and *Pneumocystis carinii* infection. Ann Intern Med 1988;109:505–7.

48. Nash G, Said JW, Nash SV, et al. The pathology of AIDS – bronchiectasis, pulmonary fibrosis with honeycombing, necrotizing bacterial pneumonia, invasive fungal infection consistent with aspergillosis, cytomegalovirus pneumonia, and healed pneumocystis pneumonia with pulmonary calcification. Mod Pathol 1995;8:203–5.

49. Travis WD, Fox CH, Devaney KO, et al. Lymphoid pneumonitis in 50 adult patients infected with the human immunodeficiency virus – lymphocytic interstitial pneumonitis versus nonspecific interstitial pneumonitis. Hum Pathol 1992;23:529–41.

50. Moran CA, Suster S, Pavlova Z, et al. The spectrum of pathological changes in the lung in children with the acquired immunodeficiency syndrome: an autopsy study of 36 cases. Hum Pathol 1994;25:877–82.

51. Saldana MJ, Mones JM. Pulmonary pathology in AIDS: atypical *Pneumocystis carinii* infection and lymphoid interstitial pneumonia. Thorax 1994;49:S46–55.

52. Mariuz P, Raviglione MC, Gould IA, et al. Pleural *Pneumocystis carinii* infection. Chest 1991;99:774–6.

53. Murry CE, Schmidt RA. Tissue invasion by *Pneumocystis carinii* – a possible cause of cavitary pneumonia and pneumothorax. Hum Pathol 1992;23:1380–7.

54. Ferre C, Baguena F, Podzamczer D, et al. Lung cavitation associated with *Pneumocystis carinii* infection in the acquired immunodeficiency syndrome – a report of six cases and review of the literature. Eur Respir J 1994;7:134–9.

55. Lazard T, Guidet B, Meynard JL, et al. Generalized air cysts complicated by fatal bilateral pneumothoraces in a patient with AIDS-related *Pneumocystis carinii* pneumonia. Chest 1994;106:1271–2.

56. Light RW, Hamm H. Pleural disease and acquired immune deficiency syndrome. Eur Resp J 1997;10:2638–43.

57. Grimes MM, LaPook JD, Bar MH, et al. Disseminated *Pneumocystis carinii* infection in a patient with acquired immunodeficiency syndrome. Hum Pathol 1987;18:307–8.

58. Ragni MV, Dekker A, Derubertis FR, et al. *Pneumocystis carinii* infection presenting as necrotizing thyroiditis and hypothyroidism. Am J Clin Pathol 1991;95:489–93.

59. Matsuda S, Urata Y, Shiota T, et al. Disseminated infection of *Pneumocystis carinii* in a patient with the acquired immunodeficiency syndrome. Virchows Arch A Pathol Anat Histopathol 1989;414:523–7.

60. Deroux SJ, Adsay NV, Ioachim HL. Disseminated pneumocystosis without pulmonary involvement during prophylactic aerosolized pentamidine therapy in a patient with the acquired immunodeficiency syndrome. Arch Pathol Lab Med 1991;115:1137–40.

61. Fishman JA, Mattia AR, Lee MJ, et al. A 29-year-old man with AIDS and multiple splenic abscesses – disseminated *Pneumocystis carinii* infection and *Mycobacterium avium* complex infection involving the spleen and liver. N Engl J Med 1995;332:249–57.

62. Shelburne SA, III, Hamill RJ. The immune reconstitution inflammatory syndrome. AIDS Rev 2003;5:67–79.

63. Wang N-S, Huang S-N, Thurlbeck WM. Combined *Pneumocystis carinii* and cytomegalovirus infection. Arch Pathol 1970;90:529–35.

Aspergillosis

64. Verweij PE, Smedts F, Poot T, et al. Immunoperoxidase staining for identification of *Aspergillus* species in routinely processed tissue sections. J Clin Pathol 1996;49:798–801.

65. Yeghen T, Fenelon L, Campbell CK, et al. Chaetomium pneumonia in a patient with acute myeloid leukaemia. J Clin Pathol 1996;49:184–6.

66. Jensen HE, Salonen J, Ekfors TO. The use of immunohistochemistry to improve

sensitivity and specificity in the diagnosis of systemic mycoses in patients with haematological malignancies. J Pathol 1997;181:100–5.

67. Bialek R, Konrad F, Kern J, et al. PCR based identification and discrimination of agents of mucormycosis and aspergillosis in paraffin wax embedded tissue. J Clin Pathol 2005;58:1180–4.

68. Nime FA, Hutchins GM. Oxalosis caused by *Aspergillus* infection. Johns Hopkins Med J 1973;133:183–94.

69. Roehrl M, Croft W, Liao Q, et al. Hemorrhagic pulmonary oxalosis secondary to a noninvasive *Aspergillus niger* fungus ball. Virchows Archiv 2007;451:1067–73.

70. Bryan RL, Hubscher SG. Aspergillosis associated with calcinosis and hypocalcaemia following liver transplantation. J Pathol 1988;155:353A.

71. Ghio AJ, Peterseim DS, Roggli VL, et al. Pulmonary oxalate deposition associated with *Aspergillus niger* infection – an oxidant hypothesis of toxicity. Am Rev Respir Dis 1992;145:1499–502.

72. Lee SH, Barnes WG, Schaetzel WP. Pulmonary aspergillosis and the importance of oxalate crystal recognition in cytology specimens. Arch Pathol Lab Med 1986;110:1176–9.

73. Benoit G, de Chauvin MF, Cordonnier C, et al. Oxalic acid level in bronchoalveolar lavage fluid from patients with invasive pulmonary aspergillosis. Am Rev Respir Dis 1985;132:748–51.

74. Nakajima M, Niki Y, Manabe T. False-positive antineutrophil cytoplasmic antibody in aspergillosis with oxalosis. Arch Pathol Lab Med 1996;120:425–6.

75. Proia AD, Brinn NT. Identification of calcium oxalate crystals using alizarin red S stain. Arch Pathol Lab Med 1985;109:186–9.

76. Kurrein F, Green GH, Rowles SL. Localized deposition of calcium oxalate around a pulmonary *Aspergillus niger* fungus ball. Am J Clin Pathol 1975;64:556–63.

77. Soubani AO, Chandrasekar PH. The clinical spectrum of pulmonary aspergillosis. Chest 2002;121:1988–99.

78. Kradin RL, Mark EJ. The pathology of pulmonary disorders due to *Aspergillus* spp. Arch Pathol Lab Med 2008;132:606–14.

79. Barth PJ, Rossberg C, Koch S, et al. Pulmonary aspergillosis in an unselected autopsy series. Pathol Res Pract 2000;196:73–80.

80. Makker H, McConnochie K, Gibbs AR. Postirradiation pulmonary fibrosis complicated by aspergilloma and bronchocentric granulomatosis. Thorax 1989;44:676–7.

81. Ein ME, Wallace Jr RJ, Williams Jr TW. Allergic bronchopulmonary aspergillosis-like syndrome consequent to aspergilloma. Am Rev Respir Dis 1979;119:811–20.

82. McCarthy DS, Pepys J. Allergic bronchopulmonary aspergillosis. Clinical immunology: (1) Clinical features. Clin Allergy 1971;1:261–86.

83. Reich JM. Pneumothorax due to pleural perforation of a pseudocavity containing aspergillomas in a patient with allergic bronchopulmonary aspergillosis. Chest 1992;102:652–3.

84. Hinson KFW, Moon AJ, Plummer NS. Broncho-pulmonary aspergillosis: a review and report of eight cases. Thorax 1952;7:317–33.

85. Sanerkin NG, Seal RME, Leopold JG. Plastic bronchitis, mucoid impaction of the bronchi and allergic broncho-pulmonary aspergillosis, and their relationship to bronchial asthma. Ann Allergy 1966;24:586–94.

86. Bosken CH, Myers JL, Greenberger PA, et al. Pathologic features of allergic bronchopulmonary aspergillosis. Am J Surg Pathol 1988;12:216–22.

87. Zander DS. Allergic bronchopulmonary aspergillosis: an overview. Arch Pathol Lab Med 2005;129:924–8.

88. Nelson LA, Callerame ML, Schwartz RH. Aspergillosis and atopy in cystic fibrosis. Am Rev Respir Dis 1979;120:863–73.

89. Aubry MC, Fraser R. The role of bronchial biopsy and washing in the diagnosis of allergic bronchopulmonary aspergillosis. Modern Pathol 1998;11:607–11.

90. Jelihovsky T. The structure of bronchial plugs in mucoid impaction, bronchocentric granulomatosis and asthma. Histopathology 1983;7:153–67.

91. Benatar S, Allan B, Hewitson R, et al. Allergic broncho-pulmonary stemphyliosis. Thorax 1980;35:515–18.

92. Glancy JJ, Elder JL, McAleer R. Allergic bronchopulmonary fungal disease without clinical asthma. Thorax 1981;36:345–9.

93. McAleer R, Kroenert D, Elder J, et al. Allergic bronchopulmonary disease caused by *Curvularia lunata* and *Drechslera hawaiiensis*. Thorax 1981;36:338–44.

94. Halwig JM, Brueske DA, Greenberger PA, et al. Allergic bronchopulmonary curvulariosis. Am Rev Respir Dis 1985;132:186–9.

95. Backman KS, Roberts M, Patterson R. Allergic bronchopulmonary mycosis caused by *Fusarium vasinfectum*. Am J Respir Crit Care Med 1995;152:1379–81.

96. Miller MA, Greenberger PA, Amerian R, et al. Allergic bronchopulmonary mycosis caused by *Pseudallescheria boydii*. Am Rev Respir Dis 1993;148:810–2.

97. Travis WD, Kwonchung KJ, Kleiner DE, et al. Unusual aspects of allergic bronchopulmonary fungal disease – report of two cases due to *Curvularia* organisms associated with allergic fungal sinusitis. Hum Pathol 1991;22:1240–8.

98. Buchanan DR, Lamb D. Saprophytic invasion of infarcted pulmonary tissue by *Aspergillus* species. Thorax 1982;37:693–8.

99. Smith FB, Beneck D. Localized *Aspergillus* infestation in primary lung carcinoma – clinical and pathological contrasts with post-tuberculous intracavitary aspergilloma. Chest 1991;100:554–6.

100. Mehrad B, Paciocco G, Martinez FJ, et al. Spectrum of aspergillus infection in lung transplant recipients – Case series and review of the literature. Chest 2001;119:169–75.

101. Nunley DR, Gal AA, Vega JD, et al. Saprophytic fungal infections and complications involving the bronchial anastomosis following human lung transplantation. Chest 2002;122:1185–91.

102. British Thoracic and Tuberculosis Association. Aspergilloma and residual tuberculous cavities – the results of a resurvey. Tubercle 1970;51:227–45.

103. McGregor DH, Papasian CJ, Pierce PD. Aspergilloma within cavitating pulmonary adenocarcinoma. Am J Clin Pathol 1989;91:100–3.

104. McCarthy DS, Longbottom JL, Riddell RW, et al. Pulmonary mycetoma due to *Allescheria boydii*. Am Rev Respir Dis 1969;100:213–6.

105. Kwon-Chung KJ, Schwartz IS, Rybak BJ. A pulmonary fungus ball produced by *Cladosporium cladosporioides*. Am J Clin Pathol 1975;64:564–8.

106. Kirkpatrick MB, Pollock HM, Wimberley NE, et al. An intracavitary fungus ball composed of *Syncephalastrum*. Am Rev Respir Dis 1979;120:943–7.

107. Iadarola P, Lungarella G, Martorana PA, et al. Lung injury and degradation of extracellular matrix components by *Aspergillus fumigatus* serine proteinase. Exp Lung Res 1998;24:233–51.

108. Awe RJ, Greenberg SD, Mattox KL. The source of bleeding in pulmonary aspergillomas. Texas Medicine 1984;80:58–61.

109. Denning DW, Follansbee SE, Scolaro M, et al. Pulmonary aspergillosis in the acquired immunodeficiency syndrome. N Engl J Med 1991;324:654–62.

110. Hummel M, Schuler S, Hempel S, et al. Obstructive bronchial aspergillosis after heart transplantation. Mycoses 1993;36:425–8.

111. Williams AJ, Zardawi I, Walls J. Disseminated aspergillosis in high dose steroid therapy. Lancet 1983;i:1222.

112. Lake KB, Browne PM, Van Dyke JJ, et al. Fatal disseminated aspergillosis in an asthmatic patient treated with corticosteroids. Chest 1983;83:138–9.

113. Karam GH, Griffin FM. Invasive pulmonary aspergillosis in non immunocomprised non neutropenic hosts. Rev Infect Dis 1986;8:357–63.

114. Gerson SL, Talbot GH, Hurwitz S, et al. Prolonged granulocytopenia: the major risk factor for invasive pulmonary aspergillosis in patients with acute leukemia. Ann Intern Med 1984;100:345–51.

115. Vaideeswar P, Prasad S, Deshpande JR, et al. Invasive pulmonary aspergillosis: A study of 39 cases at autopsy. J Postgrad Med 2004;50:21–6.

116. Variwalla AG, Smith AP, Melville-Jones G. Necrotising aspergillosis complicating fulminating viral pneumonia. Thorax 1980;35:215–16.

117. Lewis M, Kallenbach J, Ruff P, Zaltzman M, et al. Invasive pulmonary aspergillosis complicating influenza A pneumonia in a previously healthy patient. Chest 1985;87:691–3.

117a. Rello J, Esandi ME, Mariscal D, Gallego M, Domingo C, Valles J. Invasive pulmonary aspergillosis in patients with chronic obstructive pulmonary disease: report of eight cases and review. Clin Infect Dis 1998;256:1473–5.

118. Ali ZA, Ali AA, Tempest ME, et al. Invasive pulmonary aspergillosis complicating chronic obstructive pulmonary disease in an immunocompetent patient. J Postgrad Med 2003;49:78–80.

119. Marchevsky A, Rosen MJ, Chrystal G, et al. Pulmonary complications of the acquired immunodeficiency syndrome: a clinicopathologic study of 70 cases. Hum Pathol 1985;16:659–70.

120. Nash G, Irvine R, Kerschmann RL, et al. Pulmonary aspergillosis in acquired immune deficiency syndrome: Autopsy study of an emerging pulmonary complication of human immunodeficiency virus infection. Hum Pathol 1997;28:1268–75.

121. Mylonakis E, Barlam TF, Flanigan T, et al. Pulmonary aspergillosis and invasive disease in AIDS: Review of 342 cases. Chest 1998;114:251–62.

122. Klapholz A, Salomon N, Perlman DC, et al. Aspergillosis in the acquired immunodeficiency syndrome. Chest 1991;100:1614–18.

123. Miller WT, Sais GJ, Frank I, et al. Pulmonary aspergillosis in patients with AIDS – clinical and radiographic correlations. Chest 1994;105:37–44.

124. Cornet M, Mallat H, Somme D, et al. Fulminant invasive pulmonary aspergillosis in immunocompetent patients – a two-case report. Clin Microbiol Infect 2003;9:1224–7.

125. Stergiopoulou T, Meletiadis J, Roilides E, et al. Host-dependent patterns of tissue injury in invasive pulmonary aspergillosis. Am J Clin Pathol 2007;127:349–55.

126. Gefter W, Weingrad T, Ochs RH, et al. 'Semi-invasive' pulmonary aspergillosis. A new look at the spectrum of Aspergillus infections of the lung. Radiology 1981;140:313–21.

127. Binder RE, Faling LJ, Pugatch RD, et al. Chronic necrotizing pulmonary aspergillosis: a discrete clinical entity. Medicine (Baltimore) 1982;61:109–24.

128. Slevin ML, Knowles GK, Phillips MJ, et al. The air crescent sign of invasive pulmonary aspergillosis in acute leukaemia. Thorax 1982;37:554–5.

129. Kibbler CC, Milkins SR, Bhamra A, et al. Apparent pulmonary mycetoma following invasive aspergillosis in neutropenic patients. Thorax 1988;43:108–12.

130. Wiggins J, Clark TJH, Corrin B. Chronic necrotising pneumonia caused by Aspergillus niger. Thorax 1989;44:440–1.

131. Yamaguchi M, Nishiya H, Mano K, et al. Chronic necrotising pulmonary aspergillosis caused by Aspergillus niger in a mildly immunocompromised host. Thorax 1992;47:570–1.

132. Yousem SA. The histological spectrum of chronic necrotizing forms of pulmonary aspergillosis. Hum Pathol 1997;28:650–6.

133. Kradin RL, Drucker EA, Malhotra A, et al. An 83-year-old woman with long-standing asthma and rapidly progressing pneumonia – Chronic necrotizing pulmonary aspergillosis (Aspergillus fumigatus), with elements of bronchocentric granulomatosis. N Engl J Med 1998;339:1228–36.

134. Hiltermann TJ, Bredius RG, Gesink-vd Veer BJ, et al. Bilateral cavitary pulmonary consolidations in a patient undergoing allogeneic bone marrow transplantation for acute leukemia. Chest 2003;123:929–34.

135. Pervez NK, Kleinerman J, Kattan M, et al. Pseudomembranous necrotizing bronchial aspergillosis. A variant of invasive aspergillosis in a patient with haemophilia and acquired immune deficiency syndrome. Am Rev Respir Dis 1985;131:961–3.

136. Hines DW, Haber MH, Yaremko L, et al. Pseudomembranous-tracheobronchitis caused by Aspergillus. Am Rev Respir Dis 1991;143:1408–11.

137. Niimi T, Kajita M, Saito H. Necrotizing bronchial aspergillosis in a patient receiving neoadjuvant chemotherapy for non-small-cell lung carcinoma. Chest 1991;100:277–9.

138. Kramer MR, Denning DW, Marshall SE, et al. Ulcerative tracheobronchitis after lung transplantation – a new form of invasive aspergillosis. Am Rev Respir Dis 1991;144:552–6.

139. Tait RC, O'Driscoll BR, Denning DW. Unilateral wheeze caused by pseudomembranous Aspergillus tracheobronchitis in the immunocompromised patient. Thorax 1993;48:1285–7.

140. Nicholson AG, Sim KM, Keogh BF, et al. Pseudomembranous necrotising bronchial aspergillosis complicating chronic airways limitation. Thorax 1995;50:807–8.

141. Tron V, Churg A. Chronic necrotizing pulmonary aspergillosis mimicking bronchocentric granulomatosis. Pathol Res Pract 1986;181:621–6.

142. Tazelaar HD, Baird AM, Mill M, et al. Bronchocentric mycosis occurring in transplant recipients. Chest 1989;96:92–5.

Mucormycosis

143. Brown RB, Lau SK, Gonzalez RG, et al. A 59-year-old diabetic man with unilateral visual loss and oculomotor-nerve palsy – Invasive fungal sinusitis and osteomyelitis due to mucormycosis. (Diabetes mellitus.). N Engl J Med 2001;344:286–93.

144. Frater JL, Hall GS, Procop GW. Histologic features of zygomycosis – Emphasis on perineural invasion and fungal morphology. Arch Pathol Lab Med 2001;125:375–8.

145. Matsushima T, Soejima R, Nakashima T. Solitary pulmonary nodule caused by phycomycosis in a patient without obvious predisposing factors. Thorax 1980;35:877–8.

146. Murray HW. Pulmonary mucormycosis: one hundred years later. Chest 1977;72:1–3.

147. Bigby TD, Serota ML, Tierney LM, et al. Clinical spectrum of pulmonary mucormycosis. Chest 1986;89:435–9.

148. Harada M, Manabe T, Yamashita K, et al. Pulmonary mucormycosis with fatal massive hemoptysis. Acta Pathol Jpn 1992;42:49–55.

149. Rassaei N, Shilo K, Lewin-Smith MR, et al. Deposition of calcium salts in a case of pulmonary zygomycosis: histopathologic and chemical findings. Human Pathology 2009;40:1353–7.

Candidosis (moniliasis)

150. Hopfer RL, Fainstein V, Luna MP, et al. Disseminated candidiasis caused by four different Candida species. Arch Pathol Lab Med 1981;105:454–5.

151. Knox WF, Hooton VN, Barson AJ. Pulmonary vascular candidiasis and use of central venous catheters in neonates. J Clin Pathol 1987;40:559–65.

152. O'Driscoll BRC, Cooke RDP, Mamtora H, et al. Candida lung abscesses complicating parenteral nutrition. Thorax 1988;43:418–19.

Cryptococcosis

153. Campbell GD. Primary pulmonary cryptococcosis. Am Rev Respir Dis 1965;94:236–43.

154. Torda A, Kumar RK, Jones PD. The pathology of human and murine pulmonary infection with Cryptococcus neoformans var. gattii. Pathology 2001;33:475–8.

155. Douketis JD, Kesten S. Miliary pulmonary cryptococcosis in a patient with the acquired immunodeficiency syndrome. Thorax 1993;48:402–3.

156. Nash G, Said JW, Nash SV, Degirolami U. The pathology of AIDS – pulmonary cryptococcosis. Mod Pathol 1995;8:202–3.
157. Sing Y, Ramdial PK. Cryptococcal inflammatory pseudotumors. Am J Surg Pathol 2007;31:1521–7.
158. Harding SA, Scheld WM, Feldman PS, et al. Pulmonary infection with capsule-deficient *Cryptococcus neoformans*. Virchows Arch A Pathol Anat Histopathol 1979;382:113–18.
159. Lazcano O, Speights VO, Strickler JG, et al. Combined histochemical stains in the differential diagnosis of *Cryptococcus neoformans*. Mod Pathol 1993;6: 80–4.
160. Levitz SM. The ecology of *Cryptococcus neoformans* and the epidemiology of cryptococcosis. Rev Infect Dis 1991;13:1163–9.
161. Baker RD. The primary pulmonary lymph node complex of crytptococcosis. Am J Clin Pathol 1976;65:83–92.
162. Haugen RK, Baker RD. The pulmonary lesions in cryptococcosis with special reference to subpleural nodules. Am J Clin Pathol 1954;24:1381–90.
163. McDonnell JM, Hutchins GM. Pulmonary cryptococcosis. Hum Pathol 1985;16:121–8.

Histoplasmosis

164. Weydert JA, Van Natta TL, Deyoung BR. Comparison of fungal culture versus surgical pathology examination in the detection of *Histoplasma* in surgically excised pulmonary granulomas. Arch Pathol Lab Med 2007;131:780–3.
165. Symmers WStC. Histoplasmosis contracted in Britain: a case of histoplasmic lymphadenitis following clinical recovery from sarcoidosis. BMJ 1956;2:786–9.
166. Goodwin RA, Loyd JE, Des Prez RM. Histoplasmosis in normal hosts. Medicine (Baltimore) 1981;60:231–66.
167. Lehan PH, Furculow ML. Epidemic histoplasmosis. J Chronic Dis 1957;5:489–503.
168. Peterson MW, Pratt AD, Nugent KM. Pneumonia due to *Histoplasma capsulatum* in a bone marrow transplant recipient. Thorax 1987;42:698–9.
169. Sathapatayavongs B, Batteiger BE, Wheat J, et al. Clinical and laboratory features of disseminated histoplasmosis during two large urban outbreaks. Medicine 1983;62:263–70.
170. Wheat LJ, Conolly-Stringfield PA, Baker RL, et al. Disseminated histoplasmosis in the acquired immune deficiency syndrome: clinical findings, diagnosis and treatment, and review of the literature. Medicine 1990;69:361–74.
171. Levitz SM, Mark EJ, Ko JP, et al. A 19-year-old man with the acquired immunodeficiency syndrome and persistent fever – Disseminated histoplasmosis. Acquired immunodeficiency syndrome. N Engl J Med 1998;339:1835–43.
172. Godwin RA, Nickell JA, Des Prez AM. Mediastinal fibrosis complicating healed primary histoplasmosis and tuberculosis. Medicine 1972;51:227–46.

Coccidioidomycosis

173. Bayer AS. Fungal pneumonias; pulmonary coccidioidal syndromes (part 1). Chest 1981;79:575–83.
174. Bayer AS. Fungal pneumonias: pulmonary coccidioidal syndromes (part 2). Chest 1981;79:686–91.
175. Feldman BS, Snyder LS. Primary pulmonary coccidioidomycosis. Semin Respir Infect 2001;16:231–7.
176. Panackal AA, Hajjeh RA, Cetron MS, et al. Fungal infections among returning travelers. Clin Infect Dis 2002;35:1088–95.
177. Centers for Disease Control and Preventation. Coccidioidomycosis among persons attending the world championship of model airplane flying – Kern County, California, October 2001. JAMA 2002;287:312.
178. Kirkland TN, Fierer J. Coccidioidomycosis: a reemerging infectious disease. Emerg Infect Dis 1996;2:192–9.

Blastomycosis

179. Sarosi GA, Davies SF. Blastomycosis. Am Rev Respir Dis 1979;120:911–38.
180. Bradsher RW, Chapman SW, Pappas PG. Blastomycosis. Infect Dis Clin North Am 2003;17:21–40, vii.
181. Taxy JB. Blastomycosis: contributions of morphology to diagnosis: a surgical pathology, cytopathology, and autopsy pathology study. Am J Surg Pathol 2007;31:615–23.
182. Lemos LB, Guo M, Baliga M. Blastomycosis: organ involvement and etiologic diagnosis. A review of 123 patients from Mississippi. Ann Diagn Pathol 2000;4:391–406.
183. Patel RG, Patel B, Petrini MF, et al. Clinical presentation, radiographic findings, and diagnostic methods of pulmonary blastomycosis: a review of 100 consecutive cases. South Med J 1999;92:289–95.
184. Meyer KC, McManus EJ, Maki DG. Overwhelming pulmonary blastomycosis associated with the adult respiratory distress syndrome. N Engl J Med 1993;329:1231–6.
185. Lemos LB, Baliga M, Guo M. Acute respiratory distress syndrome and blastomycosis: presentation of nine cases and review of the literature. Ann Diagn Pathol 2001;5:1–9.
186. Guccion JG, Rohatgi PK, Saini NB, et al. Disseminated blastomycosis and acquired immunodeficiency syndrome: a case report and ultrastructural study. Ultrastruct Pathol 1996;20:429–35.

Paracoccidioidomycosis

187. Londero AT, Ramos CD. Paracoccidioidomycosis: a clinical and mycologic study of forty-one cases observed in Santa Maria, RS, Brazil. Am J Med 1972;52:771–775.
188. Bethlem EP, Capone D, Maranhao B, et al. Paracoccidioidomycosis. Curr Opin Pulm Med 1999;5:319–25.
189. Murray HW, Littman ML, Roberts RB. Disseminated paracoccidioidomycosis (South American blastomycosis) in the United States. Am J Med 1974;56: 209–20.
190. Bowler S, Woodcock A, Da Costa P, et al. Chronic pulmonary paracoccidioidomycosis masquerading as lymphangitis carcinomatosa. Thorax 1986;41:72–3.
191. Goldani LZ, Martinez R, Landell GAM, et al. Paracoccidioidomycosis in a patient with acquired immunodeficiency syndrome. Mycopathologia 1989;105:71–4.
192. Funari M, Kavakama J, Shikanai-Yasuda MA, et al. Chronic pulmonary paracoccidioidomycosis (South American blastomycosis): high-resolution CT findings in 41 patients. AJR Am J Roentgenol 1999;173:59–64.

Rare pulmonary mycoses

193. Huang S-N, Harris LS. Acute disseminated penicilliosis. Report of a case and review of pertinent literature. Am J Clin Pathol 1963;39:167–74.
194. Saul SH, Khachatoorian T, Poorsattar A, et al. Opportunistic *Trichosporon* pneumonia. Arch Pathol Lab Med 1981;105:456–9.
195. Ito T, Ishikawa Y, Fujii R, et al. Disseminated *Trichosporon capitatum* infection in a patient with acute leukaemia. Cancer 1988;61:585–8.
196. Ono N, Sato K, Yokomise H, et al. Lung abscess caused by *Paecilomyces lilacinus*. Respiration 1999;66:85–7.
197. Mazur JE, Judson MA. A case report of a dactylaria fungal infection in a lung transplant patient. Chest 2001;119: 651–3.
198. Odell JA, Alvarez S, Cvitkovich DG, et al. Multiple lung abscesses due to *Ochroconis gallopavum*, a dematiaceous fungus, in a nonimmunocompromised wood pulp worker. Chest 2000;118:1503–5.
199. Aisner J, Schimpff SC, Sutherland JC, et al. *Torulopsis glabrata* infections in patients with cancer. Increasing incidence and relationship to colonisation. Am J Med 1976;61:23–8.
200. Srivastava S, Kleinman G, Manthous CA. *Torulopsis* pneumonia – a case report and review of the literature. Chest 1996;110:858–861.
201. Beland JE, Mankiewicz E, MacIntosh DJ. Primary pulmonary sporotrichosis. Can Med Assoc J 1968;99:813–16.

202. England DM, Hochholzer L. Primary pulmonary sporotrichosis. Am J Surg Pathol 1985;9:193–204.

203. England DM, Hochholzer L. *Sporothrix* infection of the lung without cutaneous disease. Primary pulmonary sporotrichosis. Arch Pathol Lab Med 1987;111:298–300.

204. Watts JC, Callaway CS, Chandler FW, et al. Human pulmonary adiaspiromycosis. Arch Pathol 1975;99:11–5.

205. Schwarz J. Adiaspiromycosis. Pathol Annu 1978;13:41–53.

206. Rippon JW. Medical Mycology: The Pathogenic Fungi and the Pathogenic Actinomycetes. 3rd ed. Philadelphia: W.B. Saunders; 1988. p. 718–21.

207. Filho JVB, Amato MBP, Deheinzelin D, et al. Respiratory failure caused by adiaspiromycosis. Chest 1990;97:1171–5.

208. Peres LC, Figueiredo F, Peinado M, et al. Fulminant disseminated pulmonary adiaspiromycosis in humans. Am J Trop Med Hyg 1992;46:146–50.

209. England DM, Hochholzer L. Adiaspiromycosis – an unusual fungal infection of the lung – report of 11 cases. Am J Surg Pathol 1993;17:876–86.

210. Echavarria E, Cano EL, Restrepo A. Disseminated adiaspiromycosis in a patient with AIDS. J Med Vet Mycol 1993;31:91–7.

211. Nuorva K, Pitkanen R, Issakainen J, et al. Pulmonary adiaspiromycosis in a two year old girl. J Clin Pathol 1997;50:82–5.

212. Denson JL, Keen CE, Froeschle PO, et al. Adiaspiromycosis mimicking widespread malignancy in a patient with pulmonary adenocarcinoma. J Clin Pathol 2009;62:837–9.

213. Redline RW, Redline SS, Boxerbaum B, et al. Systemic *Malassezia furfur* infections in patients receiving intralipid therapy. Hum Pathol 1988;16:852–4.

214. Shek YH, Tucker MC, Viciana AL, et al. *Malassezia furfur* – Disseminated infection in premature infants. Am J Clin Pathol 1989;92:595–603.

215. Tadros TS, Workowski KA, Siegel RJ, et al. Pathology of hyalohyphomycosis caused by *Scedosporium apiospermum* (*Pseudallescheria boydii*): An emerging mycosis. Hum Pathol 1998;29:1266–72.

216. Nonaka D, Yfantis H, Southall P, et al. Pseudallescheriasis as an aggressive opportunistic infection in a bone marrow transplant recipient. Arch Pathol Lab Med 2002;126:207–9.

217. Raj R, Frost AE. *Scedosporium apiospermum* fungemia in a lung transplant recipient. Chest 2002;121:1714–16.

218. Jayamohan Y, Ribes JA. Pseudallescheriasis: a summary of patients from 1980–2003 in a tertiary care center. Arch Pathol Lab Med 2006;130:1843–6.

219. Deng Z, Ribas JL, Gibson DW, et al. Infections caused by *Penicillium marneffei* in China and Southeast Asia: review of eighteen published cases and report of four more Chinese cases. Rev Infect Dis 1988;10:640–52.

220. McShane H, Tang CM, Conlon CP. Disseminated *Penicillium marneffei* infection presenting as a right upper lobe mass in an HIV positive patient. Thorax 1998;53:905–6.

221. Shadduck JA, Orenstein JM. Comparative pathology of microsporidiosis. Arch Pathol Lab Med 1993;117:1215–19.

222. Schwartz DA, Sobottka I, Leitch GJ, et al. Pathology of microsporidiosis: emerging parasitic infections in patients with acquired immunodeficiency syndrome. Arch Pathol Lab Med 1996;120:173–88.

223. Orenstein JM. Diagnostic pathology of microsporidiosis. Ultrastruct Pathol 2003;27:141–9.

224. Tosoni A, Nebuloni M, Ferri A, et al. Disseminated microsporidiosis caused by *Encephalitozoon cuniculi* III (Dog type) in an Italian AIDS patient: a retrospective study. Modern Pathol 2002;15:577–83.

225. Schwartz DA, Bryan RT, Hewanlowe KO, et al. Disseminated microsporidiosis (*Encephalitozoon hellem*) and acquired immunodeficiency syndrome – autopsy evidence for respiratory acquisition. Arch Pathol Lab Med 1992;116:660–8.

226. Weber R, Kuster H, Keller R, et al. Pulmonary and intestinal microsporidiosis in a patient with the acquired immunodeficiency syndrome. Am Rev Respir Dis 1992;146:1603–5.

227. Schwartz DA, Visvesvara GS, Leitch GJ, et al. Pathology of symptomatic microsporidial (*Encephalitozoon hellem*) bronchiolitis in the acquired immunodeficiency syndrome – a new respiratory pathogen diagnosed from lung biopsy, bronchoalveolar lavage, sputum, and tissue culture. Hum Pathol 1993;24:937–43.

228. Cowley GP, Miller RF, Papadaki L, et al. Disseminated microsporidiosis in a patient with acquired immunodeficiency syndrome. Histopathology 1997;30:386–9.

229. Scaglia M, Sacchi L, Croppo GP, et al. Pulmonary microsporidiosis due to *Encephalitozoon hellem* in a patient with AIDS. J Infect 1997;34:119–26.

230. Velasquez JN, Carnevale S, Labbe JH, et al. In situ hybridization: A molecular approach for the diagnosis of the microsporidian parasite *Enterocytozoon bieneusi*. Hum Pathol 1999;30:54–8.

231. Maggi P, laRocca AM, Quarto M, et al. Effect of antiretroviral therapy on cryptosporidiosis and microsporidiosis in patients infected with human immunodeficiency virus type 1. Eur J Clin Microbiol Infect Dis 2000;19:213–17.

5.5 Parasitic infestations

This chapter describes infestation of the lungs by certain parasitic protozoa, helminths and arthropods, of which man may be either the natural or the accidental host.

Protozoal diseases of the lungs include toxoplasmosis, leishmaniasis and amoebic abscess while severe malaria may be complicated by acute respiratory failure. Also, parasites usually confined to other organs may be identified in the lungs, for example cryptosporidia in AIDS and trichomonas in aspiration lesions.

Helminths of all three major classes may infest the lung. Trematodes include the blood flukes (genus *Schistosoma*), the lung flukes (genus *Paragonimus*) and certain liver flukes (genus *Opisthorchis*). The cestodes are represented by the larval forms of *Echinococcus* and *Taenia*, which

are responsible for hydatid disease and cysticercosis respectively, whilst nematodes found in the lung include immature forms of *Ascaris, Strongyloides, Ancylostoma, Necator, Wuchereria* and *Brugia* and the adult forms of heartworm (*Dirofilaria*) and gapeworm (*Syngamus*).

Arthropods include the ticks and mites (arachnids), adult forms of which may cause pulmonary acariasis. Pulmonary pentastomiasis is a manifestation of infestation by larvae of *Linguatula* or of *Armillifer*.

The mode of transmission is variable. Some of these parasites are transmitted by an insect bite e.g. those causing tropical pulmonary eosinophilia, dirofilariasis and malaria, while some penetrate the skin directly e.g. *Strongyloides*, hookworms and schistosomes, and others are ingested e.g. *Paragonimus, Entamoeba* and *Echinococcus*.

The human lungs may be involved in the life-cycle of these parasites in various ways:

1. The lungs may be the natural location of the parasite, for example *Paragonimus* and *Syngamus*.
2. The larval form of the parasite may encyst in the lungs, for example *Echinococcus*.
3. The lung may be a migratory route for the larvae of the parasite: this includes most of the nematodes listed above and the larvae responsible for pentastomiasis.
4. The parasite may reach the lungs as an embolus: most schistosomal ova and the dead adult canine heartworm, *Dirofilaria*, are examples of this.
5. The parasite may invade the lung through the diaphragm from the liver, for example *Entamoeba histolytica* and the liver fluke *Opisthorchis*.
6. The lungs may be involved in disseminated parasitosis, for example microsporidiosis in the acquired immune deficiency syndrome.

Although immunodeficient patients are particularly prone to parasitic infestation, most of these pulmonary parasites are capable of infecting and causing disease in the immunocompetent; only a few are opportunists (e.g. Cryptosporidium spp.). Many of them have a characteristic distribution, often in tropical or subtropical countries. In the developed world parasitic diseases of the lung mainly affect immigrants and tourists.

PROTOZOA

Protozoa are unicellular eukaryotic microbes that reproduce vegetatively (as trophozoites) but encyst when conditions are unfavourable. Some are parasitic to man. A comprehensive review of those that affect the human lungs, including their taxonomy and treatment, has recently been provided.[1]

Toxoplasmosis

Toxoplasmosis represents infection with the coccidian parasite *Toxoplasma gondii*, this name deriving from the crescentic bow shape of the parasite's tachyzoites and its discovery in the gondi, a North African rodent used as a laboratory animal. The domestic cat is the usual definitive host from which man is infected but the disease occurs in many species of wild and domestic birds and mammals, all of which provide a ready source of human infection. Ingestion of infected animal material is the usual route of infection of adults but neonatal disease generally reflects placental transmission. Toxoplasmosis is one of the most prevalent protozoal infections of man but the parasite rarely harms its host and the vast majority of human infections remain occult throughout life, causing damage only when cellular immunity is impaired. Gametogenesis and oocyst formation take place in the intestine of animals such as cats; outside the body, sporozoites are liberated which can infect other species, including man. Only asexual cysts containing dormant bradyzoites are formed in normal accidental hosts but if immunity fails the cysts liberate motile tachyzoites and it is these that swarm through the host tissues causing cell damage and inflammation.

Pulmonary toxoplasmosis is rare and most cases have been in patients suffering from generalised disease attributable to immunodeficiency from diseases such as lymphoma and AIDS. Transplant recipients are also liable to develop toxoplasmosis. Because many of these patients undergo toxoplasma sero-conversion after they receive new organs, it is likely that the parasite is introduced in the donor tissues in which it presumably lay dormant. In lung transplant patients, recognition of the parasites in transbronchial biopsies is important in distinguishing infection from the changes of graft rejection. Because of the size of the parasite relative to the thickness of tissue sections, many laboratories involved in transplantation work cut serial sections through these small biopsies.

Pulmonary infection is initially non-specific. There is an interstitial infiltrate of lymphocytes, and alveolar macrophages are increased. Hyaline membranes may develop, indicating necrosis of the alveolar epithelium, and the changes are then those of diffuse alveolar damage. Alveoli adjacent to those lined by hyaline membranes show type II pneumocyte hyperplasia. Up to this stage the parasites are scanty but if immunity is sufficiently impaired, enormous numbers of tachyzoites develop. These cause necrosis on a major scale. Air spaces may be filled with necrotic debris or broad tracts of the lung undergo coagulative necrosis.[2–7] In one case macrophages filled with toxoplasma trophozoites formed a mass lesion.[8]

Individual tachyzoites are very difficult to recognise in histological sections but their identification is facilitated by immunocytochemistry,[6,7] which is superior to the Giemsa stain formerly used. The tachyzoites are crescentic in shape and measure within the range 4–7 × 2–3 μm with a prominent central nucleus.[9] The intracystic bradyzoites tend to be shorter and more rounded. The cysts, which represent the latent form of the parasite, lie free in the intercellular tissues and provoke no inflammatory response (Fig. 5.5.1). They vary considerably in size but are commonly of the order of 60 μm in diameter. Single tachyzoites are difficult to identify but they invade

Figure 5.5.1 A *Toxoplasma* cyst exciting little inflammatory reaction in the surrounding lung.

and proliferate within host cells to form distinctive collections known as pseudocysts. These resemble true cysts in size and appearance but are intracellular and lack an outer membrane. Cysts and pseudocysts are easier to recognise than individual tachyzoites but both are generally very rare.

Treatment with pyrimethamine and sulfonamides is effective if initiated promptly.[10] The mortality for toxoplasma pneumonia is 55%, although survival is much better in the immunocompetent.[11]

Amoebiasis

Entamoeba histolytica, the causative organism of amoebic dysentery, is a protozoon with a trophozoite and a cystic stage that is endemic in much of sub-Saharan Africa, South America and southern Asia. Infection is acquired by the ingestion of food or water contaminated by amoebic cysts. Trophozoites develop in the small intestine and are carried to the large bowel, which they ulcerate. From there they may spread in the blood, giving rise to metastatic foci of infection. These are found most frequently in the liver, lungs and brain, in that order. Although the lesions in these organs are conventionally described as abscesses, they are not accompanied by suppuration unless there is secondary bacterial infection.

If there is amoebic ulceration of the lower part of the rectum, amoebae may reach the rectal venous plexus and, bypassing the liver, make their way directly in the systemic circulation to the lungs. More often, amoebic pulmonary abscesses are secondary to those in the liver: the amoebae pass though the diaphragm to infect the lungs and are therefore commoner in the right lung. Whether the pleural cavity becomes infected in the course of this extension of the disease from liver to lung depends on whether adhesions have formed that bind the apposed pleural surfaces sufficiently to protect the cavity from invasion. Pleuropulmonary complications develop in less than 5% of patients with intestinal amoebiasis but in 50% of those with liver abscesses. They may include bronchohepatic fistulas.[12]

An amoebic abscess in the lung, like one in the liver, is essentially a focus of localised destruction in which part of the lung is converted into a cavity filled with reddish-brown, viscous fluid. There is little inflammatory reaction in the surrounding tissues but amoebae with their characteristic ingested erythrocytes may be seen in the zone bordering the cavity or on aspiration cytology.[13] Often the area of destruction extends to involve one of the bronchi, and much of the contents, often blood-stained, may then be expectorated. Should this happen, there may be secondary bacterial infection of the cavity. Metronidazole is the treatment of choice.[12]

In addition to *E.histolytica*, certain free-living amoebae have occasionally caused disease in man, of which two, Acanthamoeba spp. and *Balamuthia mandrillaris* have been responsible for pulmonary disease.[14]

Malaria

Severe *Plasmodium falciparum* malaria may be complicated by acute respiratory failure.[15–17] This is usually due to non-cardiogenic oedema, reflecting increased permeability of the alveolar capillaries.[18] Alternatively, patients may display the acute respiratory distress syndrome, which as usual has diffuse alveolar damage as its pathological basis.

It is suggested that the various cytokines that have been identified in the general circulation in complicated forms of malaria[19–21] may be more important than the ischaemia occasioned by heavy erythrocyte parasite burdens rendering the red blood cells less deformable and so inclined to occlude capillaries. However, blood sludging undoubtedly takes place in the lungs as well as the brain and elsewhere. The pulmonary capillaries are engorged with parasitised erythrocytes, pigment-laden macrophages and neutrophils. This is contributed to by endothelial activation and increased expression of intercellular adhesion molecule-1[22] as well as the non-deformability of the parasitised cells. The alveoli are filled with protein-rich or haemorrhagic oedema fluid, often containing pigment-laden macrophages, or show the hyaline membranes of diffuse alveolar damage.

The parasites in the lung are largely early trophozoites or ring forms rather than the later schizonts that predominate in cerebral vessels, possibly because the higher oxygen levels in the lung inhibit plasmodium maturation.[23] Therapeutic measures resulting in fluid overload and oxygen toxicity may aggravate the respiratory distress. Even after treatment, altered pulmonary function in malaria is common, with airflow obstruction, impaired ventilation, impaired gas transfer, and increased pulmonary phagocytic activity. This occurs in both vivax and falciparum malaria suggesting common underlying inflammatory mechanisms.[24]

Leishmaniasis

Visceral leishmaniasis, which is contracted by the bite of an infected sandfly, is characterised by fever, weight loss, splenomegaly and hepatomegaly. Most patients also complain of cough but there are few reports of pulmonary involvement. As in the spleen and liver, the leishmania are contained within macrophages (Fig. 5.5.2) but are difficult to find. One study identified chronic interstitial pneumonitis in 10 of 13 cases of visceral leishmaniasis, accompanied in 7 by focal interstitial fibrosis.[25] *Leishmania donovani* were identified in only 3 cases but leishmanial antigenic material was recognised immunocytochemically in all cases showing pneumonitis and in none of the others.

Cryptosporidiosis

Cryptosporidia species cause diarrhoea in many species.[26] In man, enteric cryptosporidiosis was first recognised in an immunodeficient patient and the disease has now become a serious problem in AIDS.[27] It also affects the immunocompetent and is a common cause of short-term diarrhoea in day nurseries and in travellers. Infection is by

Figure 5.5.2 Pulmonary involvement in disseminated leishmaniasis. The protozoa are seen within macrophages in alveoli and capillaries. *(Courtesy of Dr J DeGaetano, Malta.)*

Figure 5.5.3 Cryptosporidia (arrows) are seen in the bronchial lumen of a patient suffering from acquired immunodeficiency syndrome (AIDS). *(Courtesy of Dr M Antoine, Paris, France.)*

faecal–oral transmission of an encysted form and generally involves drinking contaminated water. A small number of immunocompromised patients show respiratory as well as enteric infection, complaining of cough and chest pain (Fig. 5.5.3).[28–31]

Cryptosporidia are extracellular protozoan parasites which adhere to the surface of lining epithelia. They are seen as faintly haematoxyphil dots measuring up to 5 μm arrayed along the mucosal surface. In the respiratory tract they have been identified on the surface and glandular epithelium of the trachea and bronchi and in the lung parenchyma, associated with extensive squamous metaplasia of the conductive airways.[29] The superficial location of cryptosporidia helps distinguish them from microsporidia, which are found within the cytoplasm of epithelial cells. Electron microscopy shows that cryptosporidia occupy a vacuole that communicates with the cell surface: they lie just beneath the level of cell membrane but are nevertheless extracellular.

Treatment may require immune reconstitution as well as the administration of drugs such as paromomycin, azithromycin and nitazoxanide, for which varying success is reported.[26,32,33]

Trichomoniasis

The finding of trichomonads in human lungs is rare. *Trichomonas hominis*, the intestinal trichomonas, has spread to the pleura via an enteropleural fistula, and *T.vaginalis* has been isolated from the respiratory tracts of newborn babies, but pulmonary trichomoniasis is usually caused by aspirated *T.tenax*.[34–36] Trichomonads cannot persist without associated bacterial infection and *T.tenax* is generally found as a harmless commensal in patients with poor oral hygiene, surviving in carious teeth where it feeds on the bacteria responsible for the dental decay. Pulmonary trichomoniasis is usually found as part of a mixed infection in adult men with chronic purulent or necrotic lung disease such as lung abscess or bronchiectasis. The flagellated protozoan may be identified by microscopic examination of wet-smear, Gram-stained or Papanicolaou-stained preparations but cultural identification is reputed to be superior to these methods.[34] Aspirated pulmonary trichomoniasis is an opportunistic infection of dubious pathogenicity, but it seems advisable that it be treated appropriately (with metronidazole).

HELMINTHS

Trematodes

Schistosomiasis

Pulmonary schistosomiasis (bilharziasis) may be due to any of the three most important species of human blood fluke, *Schistosoma haematobium*, *S.mansoni* and *S.japonicum*. Although involvement of the lung is relatively infrequent as a cause of clinical disease in comparison with the major locations of schistosomal infestation, it is recognised wherever schistosomiasis is endemic. However, with increased international travel, it seems that the non-endemic population has a higher incidence of pulmonary involvement once infected.[37,38] Specific changes are found in the lungs in a third of cases of clinically evident schistosomiasis in Egypt but contribute to death in only about 2% of these patients.[39,40] The frequency of pulmonary involvement is least in the Far East where schistosomiasis is due to *S.japonicum*.

The schistosomal cercariae thrive in fresh water and penetrate the skin to to transform into immature adults, which are transported in the blood to mature in venous plexuses around the bladder or rectum, where they reproduce. Pulmonary infestation generally comes from ova being carried to the lungs in the blood, either bypassing the portal venous circulation or having been produced by flukes inhabiting plexuses that drain directly into the inferior vena cava. Alternatively, if adult parasites are present within the pulmonary vasculature itself, ova are produced locally.

The ova, which measure from 70 to 170 μm in length by 50 to 70 μm in breadth, according to the species, are bound by their dimensions to lodge in blood vessels of corresponding calibre; local thrombosis and organisation result, with the formation of a characteristic tuberculoid granuloma round the egg itself (Figs 5.5.4 and 5.5.5).[39] Medial hypertrophy, intimal fibrosis, thrombosis, necrotising angiitis and angiomatoid lesions (see p. 422) develop in the obstructed arteries.[39,41] Eosinophils may be conspicuously numerous in the vicinity of the ova. It is uncertain whether the necrotising arteritis and

Figure 5.5.4 Schistosomiasis. Schistosomal ova are evident (centre) within the alveolar interstitium, which also shows a lymphocytic infiltrate.

Figure 5.5.5 Schistosomiasis. Lodgement of the schistosomal eggs in the pulmonary microcirculation has provoked a vigorous granulomatous response.

consequent angiomatoid lesions are attributable to vascular obstruction by the ova, to an allergic response to the parasite, or to the 'pipestem' hepatic fibrosis that is commonly found in schistosomiasis permitting vasoconstrictive substances that normally are metabolised in the liver to reach the pulmonary arteries.[41] Cor pulmonale may complicate pulmonary schistosomiasis and aneurysmal dilatation of the pulmonary trunk has been observed in long standing cases.

The ova also pass through the walls of the pulmonary vessels and initiate parenchymal lesions characterised by a similar granulomatous reaction and more widespread lymphocytic infiltrate and interstitial fibrosis. Although the ova may be much distorted during tissue processing, they are readily seen and recognised, particularly if they were viable at the time when the specimen was obtained (see Fig.

5.5.4). Dead ova often become heavily calcified but may long retain identifiable traces of the contained embryo. Eosinophilic infiltration and necrotising angiitis are only seen in the presence of viable ova. The presence of eggs, viable or dead, is generally the clue to the diagnosis, but in some cases pulmonary arterial lesions, including thrombosis and arteritis, develop where no ova are demonstrable.

Occasionally, ova reach the respiratory bronchioles and cause ·a local tuberculoid bronchiolitis. Sometimes a tumour-like mass forms in the lungs, abutting and obstructing a bronchus: this proves to be a confluent growth of granulomatous tissue and scarring around great numbers of schistosome ova.

When adult flukes reach the lungs they appear to cause no reaction while alive, any associated lesions being caused by the presence of their ova. However, when the flukes die, thrombosis and arteritis result, and there is commonly an accompanying focal consolidation of the adjacent parenchyma. This gives rise to nodules up to 1 cm and more in diameter that show as small 'coin' shadows in chest radiographs.

Katayama fever

As well as the classic chronic form of schistosomiasis described above, pulmonary symptoms such as cough feature in the severe form of acute schistosomiasis known as Katayama disease.[15] This systemic illness signifies seroconversion and develops about 3–6 weeks after penetration of the skin by water-borne cercariae. It is almost exclusively a disease of non-immune visitors to endemic areas and has been reported in several groups of tourists returning from such areas, especially those participating in water sports. The disease is self-limiting but recognition and treatment are important to avoid the sequelae of chronic infection.

Paragonimiasis

Infestation by lung flukes is endemic in the Far East, and to a lesser extent in central Africa and parts of the Americas. [42–44] In its early stages the disease is characterised by chest pain or discomfort. Later, when it has become chronic, there is persistent cough and recurrent haemoptysis. Characteristic operculate eggs can then be found in the sputum; they are golden-brown and measure about 90 μm in length. In some cases the presence of the parasite is borne well; in others it leads to anorexia and debility. As long as the flukes remain in the lungs the disease is rarely fatal, but should they reach the brain, as happens in a minority of cases, the prognosis is grave. Occasionally the disease mimics lung cancer.[45] Rapid and reliable immunodiagnostic methods are now available, and there are PCR techniques that distinguish individual species.[46,47]

The species most frequently responsible are *Paragonimus westermani* in the Far East and *P.kellicotti* in the Americas.[44] Morphologically these differ from each other only slightly. The adults infest the lungs of many predatory animals: *P westermani* in the dog, cat and pig, and *P.kellicotti* in the mink. Small groups of them become sexually mature within the lung tissue, where necrosis and the formation of a fibrous capsule produce characteristic 'worm cysts' (abscess cavities) that eventually enlarge and break into the bronchial lumen (Fig. 5.5.6). The ova that thus escape pass up the respiratory tract and are either expectorated or swallowed, to be eventually excreted in the stools. The life cycle of the fluke is a complex one: after several weeks in water or moist earth, the ovum hatches into a miracidium, a free-swimming form that eventually enters and parasitises water snails of the genus *Melania*. After its larval life in the snail, the fluke emerges as a cercaria, which in turn parasitises small fresh-water crabs and crayfish. It is through the consumption of these crustaceans, raw or insufficiently

Figure 5.5.6 Paragonimiasis. (A) A 'worm cyst' including several *Paragonimus* eggs in the chronic inflammatory granulation tissue that borders the central necrosis. (B) *Paragonimus* eggs removed from the lung (scale divisions = 10 μm).

cooked, that man becomes infested. Pickling the crabs does not destroy the parasite. The disease may also be acquired by eating the flesh of another host, such as a pig, that has eaten infected crabs or crayfish. On reaching the duodenum of the human host, the parasite penetrates the gut wall and thence passes by way of the peritoneal cavity and diaphragm to the pleura and the lungs. It grows to a length of 12 mm and attains maturity about five weeks after reaching the lungs and so completing its life cycle.

In man the flukes often lie singly in the connective tissue 'worm cysts', the number of which rarely exceeds ten, each about 1 to 2 cm across. They may excite an eosinophilic pneumonia, give rise to a pleural effusion or cause pneumothorax.[48] Sometimes the young worms go astray and reach the liver, spleen, kidneys or brain. Occasionally dead worms in the lungs are associated with distant tissue reactions that probably have a hypersensitivity basis. The diagnosis is based on the demonstration of the eggs in bronchial secretions, pleural fluid or faeces.

Opisthorchiasis

Liver flukes generally remain within the hepatic bile ducts but in Thailand *Opisthorchis viverrini* has on rare occasions made its way from the liver through the diaphragm to the right lung.[49]

Figure 5.5.7 Hydatid cyst, the encysted larval form of the *Echinococcus granulosus* tapeworm, filled with numerous 'daughter' cysts.

Figure 5.5.8 Hydatid cyst. The encysted larva of the *Echinococcus granulosus* tapeworm has died and the parasite's capsule has collapsed away from the fibrous capsule formed by its human host.

Figure 5.5.9 Hydatid cyst. The convoluted chitinous layer of a collapsed dead hydatid cyst.

Cestodes

Hydatid disease (larval echinococcosis)

This disease has long been endemic in sheep-raising countries, notably Australia, New Zealand, Wales, parts of South Africa and South America, and the Middle East.[50] Control measures are steadily lessening its incidence. The dog is the usual host of the mature tapeworm, *Echinococcus granulosus*, and sheep the commonest host of its larval stage. The ova in the faeces of the dog reach sheep or man in contaminated food or water and, after hatching in the small intestine, larvae penetrate the gut wall and enter the portal circulation. Most are retained in the liver, but some negotiate the hepatic barrier to reach the systemic venous circulation and the lungs. The larval forms of this helminth thus tend to occur most frequently in the liver and the lungs. They take the form of hydatid cysts (Fig. 5.5.7). If a hydatid cyst is demonstrated in the lung, others are almost always present in the liver. Pulmonary hydatid cysts are usually solitary but bilateral instances are recorded.[50–52]

The wall of a hydatid cyst is formed of a semipermeable laminated capsule, which is composed of chitin, and an inner germinal layer. Outside these is the pericyst, formed of a layer of chronic inflammatory granulation tissue or a fibrous capsule, these representing the host reaction to the parasite (Figs 5.5.8 and 5.5.9). The germinal layer gives rise to brood capsules and from the germinal layer of these arise scolices. Free brood capsules and scolices form the hydatid 'sand' that can be seen as minute white grains in the otherwise clear cyst fluid (Fig. 5.5.10). When sheep tissues containing hydatid cysts are eaten by a dog, the scolices attach to the intestinal mucosa and develop into the adult worms, thus completing the life cycle. Scolices also have the

potential to develop into secondary cysts if released by cyst rupture. They also form daughter cysts within the mother cyst, each daughter cyst being an exact true replica of the mother cyst. The daughter cysts may be packed together in the mother cyst or float freely in the mother cyst cavity. In older cysts, the contents degenerate into gelatinous material known as the matrix, which may be mistaken for pus. The cysts are usually bacteriologically sterile but they may become infected, resulting in true suppuration. Calcification commonly develops in the pericyst without affecting the viability of the parasite but calcification of the endocyst indicates that it is dead.

Because the parasite has evolved mechanisms to avoid host immunity, the infection is often asymptomatic until a mechanical complication occurs.[53] Thus, most cases of pulmonary hydatid disease are discovered on routine chest radiography. Symptoms stem from compression, infection or rupture into a bronchus. The sudden escape of a large amount of its fluid contents may give rise to a grave, even fatal,

Figure 5.5.10 Hydatid cyst. An echinococcal scolex from a ruptured hydatid cyst is surrounded by pus.

anaphylactic reaction. Rupture of a hydatid cyst into a bronchus may also cause bronchocentric granulomatosis[54] or lymphoid hyperplasia. Aspiration of the cyst contents should not be undertaken because of the risk of spillage and a consequent hypersensitivity reaction. The treatment of choice for compressive cysts is surgical resection, with particular care being exercised to avoid rupture of the cyst, and post-operative drug therapy using albendazole.[55–57]

Cysticercosis (larval taeniasis)

Cysticercosis occurs when man becomes the intermediate host of the porcine tapeworm, *Taenium solium*, through the ingestion of the worm's eggs present in faecally contaminated water or food or on soiled hands, or by the eggs hatching within the intestine of those harbouring the adult worm.[58,59] The disease is common in Africa, China, south east Asia and South America. Once hatched, the embryo penetrates the intestinal wall and is disseminated by the blood stream, giving rise to an encysted larva. Such cysticerci may form anywhere but the brain is particularly vulnerable. The lungs are seldom affected but may be the seat of either solitary or multiple lesions, the latter generally as part of disseminated disease, which probably reflects immune impairment. The larva has an inverted scolex and lies within clear fluid bounded by a thin fibrous capsule. Little inflammation is induced while the larvae are alive but after their death a variable response is seen, often culminating in calcification.

Nematodes

Ascariasis and toxocariasis ('visceral larva migrans')

Although essentially an intestinal parasite, the large roundworm *Ascaris lumbricoides* passes through the lungs during one phase of its complex life cycle. Infection is endemic in much of Africa, Asia and South America. The infestation is acquired by ingesting food or water contaminated with ova passed in the faeces of an earlier host. The ova hatch in the small intestine, where the larvae quickly penetrate the mucosa and are carried either to the liver in the portal bloodstream or in lymph to the systemic veins, reaching the lungs about five or six days after ingestion of the eggs. In the lungs, the larvae pierce the alveolar wall to reach the air space, whence they are cleared to the pharynx to be swallowed. Maturation, copulation and ovulation occur in the small intestine.

Toxocara canii and *cati* are respectively the corresponding round-worms of dogs and cats, human infection by which is acquired through close contact with these animals or with soil contaminated by their faeces. Toxocarae do not complete their life-cycle in man but dissemination of their larvae simulates visceral ascariasis, resulting in what is known as visceral larva migrans.

Migration of these worms through the lungs may cause self-limiting pulmonary eosinophilia (Löffler's syndrome, see p. 460) during which eosinophils and Charcot–Leyden crystals are often conspicuous in the sputum, although the larvae themselves are rarely seen. The illness is usually over within three weeks but in exceptional cases respiratory distress becomes so severe that the patient may die.[60]

Microscopical studies of the pulmonary lesions have been infrequent except in the rare fatal cases, or when the parasites are present by chance in lungs examined as a result of other disease. The larvae may be found in capillaries, the interstitial tissues, or air spaces, accompanied by eosinophils and neutrophils. When a larva dies, an intense reaction may develop, with dense local accumulation of eosinophils, lesser numbers of macrophages and neutrophils, and fibrin. Identifiable remnants of larvae may be seen, sometimes in multinucleate giant cells. There may be local haemorrhage.

The larvae of *A.lumbricoides*, the ascarid parasite of man, are difficult to distinguish from those of other ascarids, such as species of *Toxocara*, that may also be found in human lung tissue or pleural fluid.[61] Morphological differentiation of these larvae in histological preparations is commonly beyond the ability even of professional parasitologists but investigation by means of specific immuno-cytochemical staining may be decisive. The larvae of the toxocarae have a greater tendency than those of *A.lumbricoides* to die in the lungs when they infest man: they then cause pulmonary eosinophilia and tuberculoid granulomas that eventually lead to fibrous encapsulation of the remains of the parasites.

Strongyloidiasis

Strongyloides stercoralis is another intestinal parasite that at one stage in its development passes through the lungs. Infection is endemic in much of the tropics and subtropical regions. The filariform larvae of strongyloides, like those of hookworms and schistosomal cercariae, have the ability to penetrate intact human skin, following which they are carried to the lungs where they penetrate the alveoli and migrate via the airways and upper gastrointestinal tract to the small intestine. Here they mature into parthenogenetic adult females, the eggs of which release rhabditiform larvae within the intestine, unlike the eggs of other intestinal helminths which are passed intact in the faeces to embryonate in the soil. The rhabditiform larvae of *Strongyloides* may pass with the faeces to complete a free-living sexual cycle in the soil or differentiate within the intestine into filariform larvae, which are capable of penetrating the bowel wall or the perianal skin to repeat their parasitic asexual cycle, an endogenous process known as auto-infection. This difference between *Strongyloides* and other intestinal helminths is important in maintaining the infection and, in immuno-compromised hosts, leading to potentially fatal hyperinfestation.

Chronic strongyloidiasis has been well described among individuals who were prisoners of the Japanese during the second world war: decades later, it affected a fifth of the survivors of those who worked on the notorious Burma railway.[62,63] Most infestations cause at most a creeping skin eruption (larva migrans) or chronic diarrhoea but there is a real danger of fatal hyperinfestation if the individual becomes immunosuppressed. This may happen when corticosteroid drugs are

Figure 5.5.11 *Strongyloides stercoralis* filaria in the lung in a case of strongyloides superinfection. *(Courtesy of the late Professor BE Heard, Brompton, UK.)*

Filariasis: tropical eosinophilia

Filariasis is endemic in the tropics. The adult nematodes, *Wuchereria bancrofti, Brugia malayi, Brugia pahangi* and *Onchocerca volvulus* inhabit lymphatics where they produce eggs from which are released embryos known as microfilariae. These circulate in the blood and disseminate widely in the tissues, to be transmitted to others by mosquitoes.

Some of those infected present with 'tropical eosinophilia', a name that was given to a condition that was initially described from the coast of southern India but is now known to have a far wider distribution in the tropics.[72] The clinical signs are fever, loss of weight, dyspnoea and asthmatic attacks; there is marked blood eosinophilia and radiographs show nodular shadows in the lungs. The condition is benign and little is known of the changes in the lungs. Such reports as have been published describe whitish nodules 3 to 5 mm in diameter, scattered irregularly throughout the lungs. Histologically, the nodules are composed of groups of alveoli consolidated by eosinophils enmeshed in fibrin. In the centre of some of the nodules, the alveolar walls are destroyed and the area becomes an 'eosinophil abscess'. In others, a central collection of epithelioid cells becomes arranged in a palisade manner round deeply eosinophilic hyaline material that probably represents inspissated granules of eosinophil leukocytes. Giant cells and fibrosis are seen in some lesions and microfilariae are sometimes observed.[73,74] The condition is thought to represent an immunopathological response to the parasite rather than direct damage by the microfilariae because it is confined to those individuals who are highly sensitised to filarial antigens.

Tropical eosinophilia is readily distinguished from other forms of eosinophilia (which are described in Chapter 9) by the patient's history of residence in the tropics, by the presence of extraordinarily high levels of both serum IgE and antifilarial antibodies, and by a dramatic therapeutic response to the filaricide diethylcarbamazine.

Dirofilariasis (heartworm infestation)

Pulmonary dirofilariasis occurs when man becomes an alternative host of the canine heartworm, *Dirofilaria immitis*, after being bitten by a mosquito or sandfly infested with the microfilariae. Early development occurs in a subcutaneous nodule, whence after a few weeks' development the young adult worm migrates to the right side of the heart and the pulmonary arteries. In man, the adult worm typically dies while it is immature and is carried from the heart to the lungs as a parasitic embolus to occlude a small pulmonary artery. This generally causes no symptoms. A necrotising granuloma forms about the dead worm and this is seen as an incidental 'coin' lesion in chest radiographs,[75] often prompting a needless thoracotomy as carcinoma is the principal differential diagnosis. The diagnosis is almost always made only when resected tissue is submitted to microscopy. The granuloma is rounded rather than wedge-shaped and is not haemorrhagic, appearances favouring an immune reaction to the worm rather than infarction. The young adult worm in the centre of the granuloma is about 3cm in length but the mature female measures up to 30cm x 2mm with the male about 20cm x 2mm. Very rarely an embolic tangle of worms results in major pulmonary infarction (Fig. 5.5.12A).

Heartworm is enzootic in the Gulf states of America but since the first report of human infestation in 1961 it has become recognised in dogs throughout the United States and in southern parts of Canada. Human cases have now been reported also from Japan, Australia, Brazil and various other countries.[76–81] The smaller *D.repens*, which is common in Italy, may result in a similar pulmonary nodule but the lung is a relatively rare locus for this species.[82–84]

The lesions in man are usually solitary, peripheral and lower lobar in distribution (Fig. 5.5.12B), but multiple bilateral nodules have been reported. They range in size from 1 to 4 cm. Most patients are

administered, particularly in the treatment of unrelated conditions but also because of resistant asthma caused by unrecognised strongyloidiasis. In cases of such asthma the dose of corticosteroids may be progressively increased when the patient would have been better treated with anti-helminthic drugs.[64] Worsening asthma as the steroid dosage is increased should alert the clinician to the possibility of hyperinfestation. Heavy infestation is often associated with blood eosinophilia and fleeting pulmonary opacities that represent eosinophilic pneumonia but these features may be absent in those who are immunosuppressed. Other risk factors include advanced age, chronic lung disease and altered cellular immunity, particularly that found in adult T-cell leukaemia complicating human T-lymphotropic retrovirus (HTLV-1) infection.[65–68]

The respiratory features in hyperinfestation may be those of the acute respiratory distress syndrome. At necropsy in such cases, the larvae are seen in huge numbers within the lumen and walls of airways of all sizes down to the alveoli and within interlobular septa (Fig. 5.5.11). They excite an inflammatory response, chiefly of plasma cells with smaller numbers of lymphocytes and eosinophils. Diffuse alveolar haemorrhage may be seen.[69] More chronic infestation may result in restrictive lung disease due to interlobular septal fibrosis[70] or a mass lesion.[71]

Hookworm infestation

The larval forms of the hookworms *Ancylostoma duodenale* and *Necator americanus*, like those of *Ascaris lumbricoides* and *Strongyloides stercoralis*, migrate through the heart, lungs and trachea to reach the intestine where they mature. On their way through the lungs, they may similarly cause fleeting eosinophilic pneumonia.

Figure 5.5.12 *Dirofilaria immitis*, the dog heart worm. (A) A tangle of *Dirofilaria* worms that was removed surgically from the pulmonary artery of a merchant seaman. Magnification ×1.8. *(Courtesy of Professor F Ho, Hong Kong.)* (B–D) *Dirofilaria immitis* causing a 3-cm, rounded, necrotising nodule in the lung of a man who had lived rough in tropical countries. (B) Gross appearances; (C) microscopy; (D) elastin stain showing the worm situated within a pulmonary artery. *(B–D courtesy of Dr M Jagusch, Auckland, New Zealand.)*

asymptomatic but some complain of cough, chest pain, haemoptysis and fever, with up to 20% showing eosinophilia. Microscopically, a large central area of coagulative necrosis is surrounded by a thin band of chronic inflammatory granulomatous tissue containing occasional giant cells (Fig. 5.5.12C).[83,85,86] Eosinophils may be numerous but are often absent. The diagnosis is made by identifying the dead worm within a thrombosed artery in the central area of necrosis (Fig. 5.5.12D). This may require step sections, which are therefore advisable when examining any necrobiotic nodule of obscure aetiology. Methenamine silver and elastin stains aid the identification and localisation of the parasite (Fig. 5.5.12D), which has a thick cuticle and in man seldom measures more than 300 μm in diameter.

Syngamiasis (gapeworm infestation)

Gapeworms of the Syngamidae family infest domestic mammals, rodents and birds, producing in domestic fowl a disease known as 'the gapes', which is characterised by dyspnoea and an asphyxial death due to the worms obstructing the bird's trachea and bronchi. Human infection is rare but isolated cases have been reported from the West Indies, Brazil, the Philippines and Korea.[87–90] Affected patients complain of dyspnoea, cough, wheeze and pain or a feeling of tightness in the chest. Ova and adult worms may be found in the sputum or on bronchoscopy. The adults live off the host's blood and are therefore bright red. The female measures up to 2 cm and the male a quarter of this. They live in permanent copulation and since the vulva opens in the mid region of the female's body, each pair forms a characteristic Y shape. It must be disconcerting to see the paired worms wriggling away from the bronchoscopy forceps.[87]

ARTHROPODS

Pulmonary acariasis

Adult ticks and mites are occasionally found in the sputum of those exposed to organic dust in tropical climates, probably representing bronchial saprophytes. This is known as pulmonary acariasis. Mites were found in the sputum of 5% of Chinese grain workers.[91]

Pentastomiasis

The upper or lower respiratory passages of some dogs, birds and snakes are inhabited by certain arthropods of debatable taxonomic standing, the so-called 'tongueworms' or pentastomes, which include *Linguatula* and *Armillifer*.[92,93] The eggs of *Armillifer* may be transmitted to snake handlers in Africa and the Far East and those of *Linguatula* are transmitted to dog handlers worldwide. Larvae develop in the human intestine and penetrate the wall to reach many viscera, including the lungs, where in their natural host they mature to adults but where in man they die. A recognisable larva is occasionally encountered in human lungs but more often, barely recognisable parasitic remnants are observed within encapsulated, partly calcified, necrotic debris. Their identification from other metazoal remnants may be impossible, even for professional parasitologists.

Myiasis

Myiasis is caused by parasitic dipterous fly larvae feeding on the host's necrotic or living tissue. The disease is a serious problem in the livestock industry and is fairly common in rural human populations in tropical and subtropical regions. The insect that attacks man is *Dermatobia hominis*, the human bot-fly. The infestation is usually cutaneous but many other parts of the body may be affected, including the respiratory tract on rare occasions. Respiratory involvement is usually identified when a patient complaining of cough or haemoptysis coughs up a recognisable maggot.

REFERENCES

1. Martinez-Giron R, Esteban JG, Ribas A, et al. Protozoa in respiratory pathology: a review. Eur Respir J 2008;32:1354–70.

Toxoplasmosis

2. Marchevsky A, Rosen MJ, Chrystal G, et al. Pulmonary complications of the acquired immunodeficiency syndrome: a clinicopathologic study of 70 cases. Hum Pathol 1985;16:659–70.
3. Tschirart D, Klatt EC. Disseminated toxoplasmosis in the acquired immunodeficiency syndrome. Arch Pathol Lab Med 1988;112:1237–41.
4. Bergin C, Murphy M, Lyons D, et al. Toxoplasma pneumonitis – fatal presentation of disseminated toxoplasmosis in a patient with AIDS. Eur Respir J 1992;5:1018–20.
5. Artigas J, Grosse G, Niedobitek F. Anergic disseminated toxoplasmosis in a patient with the acquired immunodeficiency syndrome. Arch Pathol Lab Med 1993;117:540–1.
6. Schurmann D, Ruf B. Extracerebral toxoplasmosis in AIDS – Histological and immunohistological findings based on 80 autopsy cases. Pathol Res Pract 1993;189:428–36.
7. Nash G, Kerschmann RL, Herndier B, et al. The pathological manifestations of pulmonary toxoplasmosis in the acquired immunodeficiency syndrome. Hum Pathol 1994;25:652–8.
8. Monso E, Vidal R, de Gracia X, et al. Pulmonary toxoplasmoma presenting as obstructive pneumonia. Thorax 1986;41:489–90.
9. Dubey JP, Lindsay DS, Speer CA. Structures of *Toxoplasma gondii* tachyzoites, bradyzoites, and sporozoites and biology and development of tissue cysts. Clin Microbiol Rev 1998;11:267–99.
10. Mariuz P, Bosler EM, Luft BJ. *Toxoplasma* pneumonia. Semin Respir Infect 1997;12:40–3.

11. Pomeroy C, Filice GA. Pulmonary toxoplasmosis: a review. Clin Infect Dis 1992;14:863–70.

Amoebiasis

12. Lyche KD, Jensen WA. Pleuropulmonary amebiasis. Semin Respir Infect 1997;12:106–12.
13. Bhambhani S, Kashyap V. Amoebiasis: diagnosis by aspiration and exfoliative cytology. Cytopathology 2001;12:329–33.
14. Visvesvara GS. Pathogenic and opportunistic free-living amoebae: *Acanthamoeba* spp., *Balamuthia mandrillaris*, *Naegleria fowleri*, and *Sappinia diploidea*. FEMS immunology and medical microbiology 2007;50:1–26.

Malaria

15. Johnson S, Wilkinson R, Davidson RN. Acute tropical infections and the lung. Thorax 1994;49:714–18.
16. Torres JR, Perez H, Postigo MM, et al. Acute non-cardiogenic lung injury in benign tertian malaria. Lancet 1997;350:31–2.
17. Taylor WR, White NJ. Malaria and the lung. Clin Chest Med 2002;23:457–68.
18. Taylor WR. Pulmonary manifestations of malaria: recognition and management. Treatments in respiratory medicine 2006;5:419–28.
19. Kern P, Hemmer JC, Van Damme J, et al. Elevated tumour necrosis factor alpha and interleukin-6 serum levels as markers for complicated *Plasmodium falciparum* malaria. Am J Med 1989;87:139–43.
20. Kwiatkowski D, Hill AVS, Sambou I, et al. Tumour necrosis factor concentration in fatal cerebral, non-fatal cerebral, and uncomplicated *Plasmodium falciparum* malaria. Lancet 1990;336:1201–4.
21. Davis TME, Sturm M, Yue-Rong Z, et al. Platelet-activating factor and lipid metabolism in acute malaria. J Infect 1993;26:279–85.

22. Turner GDH, Morrison H, Jones M, et al. An immunohistochemical study of the pathology of fatal malaria – evidence for widespread endothelial activation and a potential role for intercellular adhesion molecule-1 in cerebral sequestration. Am J Pathol 1994;145:1057–69.
23. Macpherson GG, Warrell MJ, White NJ, et al. Human cerebral malaria, a quantitative ultrastructural analysis of parasitised erythrocyte sequestration. Am J Pathol 1985;119:385–401.
24. Anstey NM, Jacups SP, Cain T, et al. Pulmonary manifestations of uncomplicated falciparum and vivax malaria: cough, small airways obstruction, impaired gas transfer, and increased pulmonary phagocytic activity. J Infect Dis 2002;185:1326–34.

Leishmaniasis

25. Duarte MI, da Matta VLR, Corbett CEP, et al. Interstitial pneumonitis in human visceral leishmaniasis. Trans Roy Soc Trop Med Hyg 1989;83:73–6.

Cryptosporidiosis

26. Davies AP, Chalmers RM. Cryptosporidiosis. BMJ 2009;339:b4168.
27. Chen XM, Keithly JS, Paya CV, et al. Current concepts: Cryptosporidiosis. N Engl J Med 2002;346:1723–31.
28. Travis WD, Schmidt K, MacLowry JD, et al. Respiratory cryptosporidiosis in a patient with malignant lymphoma. Report of a case and review of the literature. Arch Pathol Lab Med 1990;114:519–22.
29. Moore JA, Frenkel JK. Respiratory and enteric cryptosporidiosis in humans. Arch Pathol Lab Med 1991;115:1160–2.
30. Meynard JL, Meyohas MC, Binet D, et al. Pulmonary cryptosporidiosis in the acquired immunodeficiency syndrome. Infection 1996;24:328–31.
31. Clavel A, Arnal AC, Sanchez EC, et al. Respiratory cryptosporidiosis: case series

and review of the literature. Infection 1996;24:341–6.

32. Maggi P, laRocca AM, Quarto M, et al. Effect of antiretroviral therapy on cryptosporidiosis and microsporidiosis in patients infected with human immunodeficiency virus type 1. Eur J Clin Microbiol Infect Dis 2000;19:213–17.

33. Palmieri F, Cicalini S, Froio N, et al. Pulmonary cryptosporidiosis in an AIDS patient: successful treatment with paromomycin plus azithromycin. Int J STD AIDS 2005;16:515–17.

Trichomoniasis

34. Hersh SM. Pulmonary trichomoniasis and Trichomonas tenax. J Med Microbiol 1985;20:1–10.

35. McLaren LC, Davis LE, Healy GR, et al. Isolation of Trichomonas vaginalis from the respiratory tract of infants with respiratory disease. Pediatrics 1983;71:888–90.

36. Radosavljevicasic G, Jovanovic D, Radovanovic D, et al. Trichomonas in pleural effusion. Eur Respir J 1994;7:1906–8.

Schistosomiasis

37. Schwartz E, Rozenman J, Perelman M. Pulmonary manifestations of early schistosome infection among nonimmune travelers. Am J Med 2000;109:718–22.

38. Schwartz E. Pulmonary schistosomiasis. Clin Chest Med 2002;23:433–43.

39. Shaw AFB, Ghareeb AA. The pathogenesis of pulmonary schistosomiasis in Egypt with special reference to Ayerza's disease. J Pathol Bacteriol 1938;46:401–23.

40. Cheever AW, Kamel IA, Elwi AM, et al. Schistosoma mansoni and S. haematobium infections in Egypt. Am J Trop Med Hyg 1978;27:55–75.

41. Harris P, Heath D. The Human Pulmonary Circulation. Its Form and Function in Health and Disease. 3rd ed. Edinburgh: Churchill Livingstone; 1986.

Paragonimiasis

42. Mukae H, Taniguchi H, Matsumoto L, et al. Clinicoradiologic features of pleuropulmonary Paragonimus westermani on Kyusyu Island, Japan. Chest 2001;120:514–20.

43. DeFrain M, Hooker R. North American paragonimiasis – Case report of a severe clinical infection. Chest 2002;121:1368–72.

44. Castilla EA, Jessen R, Sheck DN, et al. Cavitary mass lesion and recurrent pneumothoraces due to Paragonimus kellicotti infection – North American paragonimiasis. Amer J Surg Pathol 2003;27:1157–60.

45. Watanabe S, Nakamura Y, Kariatsumari K, et al. Pulmonary paragonimiasis mimicking lung cancer on FDG-PET imaging. Anticancer Res 2003;23:3437–40.

46. Sugiyama H, Morishima Y, Kameoka Y, et al. Polymerase chain reaction (PCR)-based molecular discrimination between Paragonimus westermani and P. miyazakii at the metacercarial stage. Mol Cell Probes 2002;16:231–6.

47. Nakamura-Uchiyama F, Mukae H, Nawa Y. Paragonimiasis: a Japanese perspective. Clin Chest Med 2002;23:409–20.

48. Al Mohaya SA, Al Sohaibani M, Bukhari H, et al. Pulmonary paragonimiasis presenting as a hemorrhagic pleural effusion. Eur J Respir Dis 1987;71:314–6.

Opisthorchiasis

49. Prijyanonda B, Tandhanand S. Opisthorchiasis with pulmonary involvement. Ann Intern Med 1961;54:795–9.

Hydatid disease (larval echinococcosis)

50. Tor M, Atasalihi A, Altuntas N, et al. Review of cases with cystic hydatid lung disease in a tertiary referral hospital located in an endemic region: A 10 years' experience. Respiration 2000;67:539–42.

51. Scully RE, Mark EJ, McNeely WF, et al. A 34-year-old woman with one cystic lesion in each lung – Bilateral pulmonary echinococcal cysts. N Engl J Med 1999;341:974–82.

52. Eroglu A, Kurkcuoglu C, Karaoglanoglu N. Bilateral multiple pulmonary hydatid cysts. Eur J Cardiothorac Surg 2003;23:1053.

53. Baden LR, Elliott DD, Miseljic S, et al. Case 4–2003: A 42-year-old woman with cough, fever, and abnormalities on thoracoabdominal computed tomography – Echinococcus granulosus infection. N Engl J Med 2003;348:447–55.

54. Den Hertog RW, Wagenaar SjSc, Westermann CJJ. Bronchocentric granulomatosis and pulmonary echinococcosis. Am Rev Respir Dis 1982;126:344–347.

55. Dakak M, Genc O, Gurkok S, et al. Surgical treatment for pulmonary hydatidosis (a review of 422 cases). J R Coll Surg Edinb 2002;47:689–92.

56. Kabiri e, Caidi M, al Aziz S, et al. Surgical treatment of hydatidothorax. Series of 79 cases. Acta Chir Belg 2003;103:401–4.

57. Ayed AK, Alshawaf E. Surgical treatment and follow-up of pulmonary hydatid cyst. Med Princ Pract 2003;12:112–16.

Cysticercosis (larval taeniasis)

58. Walts AE, Nivatpumin T, Epstein A. Pulmonary cysticercus. Mod Pathol 1995;8:299–302.

59. Mauad T, Battlehner CN, Bedrikow CL, et al. Case report: massive cardiopulmonary cysticercosis in a leukemic patient. Pathol Res Pract 1997;193:527–9.

Ascariasis and toxocariasis ('visceral larva migrans')

60. Heggers JP, Muller MJ, Elwood E, et al. Ascariasis pneumonitis: a potentially fatal complication in smoke inhalation injury. Burns 1995;21:149–51.

61. Jeanfaivre T, Cimon B, Tolstuchow N, et al. Pleural effusion and toxocariasis. Thorax 1996;51:106–7.

Strongyloidiasis

62. Gill V, Bell DR. Strongyloidiasis in ex-prisoners of war in south-east Asia. BMJ 1982;280:1319.

63. Gill GV, Bell DR. Strongyloides stercoralis infection in Burma Star veterans. BMJ 1987;294:1003–4.

64. Higenbottam TW, Heard BE. Opportunistic pulmonary strongyloidiasis complicating asthma treated with steroids. Thorax 1976;31:226–32.

65. Ting YM. Pulmonary strongyloidiasis – case report of 2 cases. Kaohsiung J Med Sci 200016:269–74.

66. O'Doherty MJ, Van de Pette JE, Nunan TO, et al. Recurrent Strongyloides stercoralis infection in a patient with T-cell lymphoma-leukaemia. Lancet 1984;1:858.

67. Newton RC, Limpuangthip P, Greenberg S, et al. Strongyloides stercoralis hyperinfection in a carrier of HTLV-I virus with evidence of selective immunosuppression. Am J Med 1992;92:202–8.

68. Robinson RD, Lindo JF, Neva FA, et al. Immunoepidemiologic studies of Strongyloides stercoralis and human T lymphotropic virus type I infections in Jamaica. J Infect Dis 1994;169:692–6.

69. Kinjo T, Tsuhako K, Nakazato I, et al. Extensive intra-alveolar haemorrhage caused by disseminated strongyloidiasis. Int J Parasitol 1998;28:323–30.

70. Lin AL, Kessimian N, Benditt JO. Restrictive pulmonary disease due to interlobular septal fibrosis associated with disseminated infection by Strongyloides stercoralis. Am J Respir Crit Care Med 1995;151:205–9.

71. Mayayo E, Gomez-Aracil V, Azua-Blanco J, et al. Strongyloides stercolaris infection mimicking a malignant tumour in a non-immunocompromised patient. Diagnosis by bronchoalveolar cytology. J Clin Pathol 2005;58:420–2.

Filariasis: tropical eosinophilia

72. Udwadia FE. Tropical eosinophilia – a review. Respir Med 1993;87:17–21.

73. Webb JGK, Job CK, Gault EW. Tropical eosinophilia : demonstration of microfilariae in lung, liver, and lymph nodes. Lancet 1960;1:835–42.

74. Danaraj TJ, Pacheco G, Shanmugaratnam K, et al. The etiology and pathology of eosinophilic lung (tropical eosinophilia). Am J Trop Med Hyg 1966;15:183–9.

Dirofilariasis (heartworm infestation)

75. Kido A, Ishida T, Oka T, et al. Pulmonary dirofilariasis causing a solitary lung mass and pleural effusion. Thorax 1991;46:608–9.

76. Awe RJ, Mattox KL, Alvarez BA, et al. Solitary and bilateral pulmonary nodules due to *Dirofilaria immitis*. Am Rev Respir Dis 1975;112:445–9.

77. Merrill JD, Otis J, Logan WD, et al. The dog heartworm (*Dirofilaria immitis*) in man. An epidemic pending or in progress? JAMA 1980;243:1066–8.

78. Tsukayama C, Manabe T, Miura Y. Dirofilarial infection in human lungs. Acta Pathol Jpn 1982;32:157–62.

79. Chesney TM, Martinez LC, Painter MW. Human pulmonary dirofilarial granuloma. Ann Thorac Surg 1983;36:214–17.

80. Nicholson CP, Allen MS, Trastek VF, et al. *Dirofilaria immitis* – a rare, increasing cause of pulmonary nodules. Mayo Clin Proc 1992;67:646–50.

81. deCampos JRM, Barbas CSV, Filomeno LTB, et al. Human pulmonary dirofilariasis: Analysis of 24 cases from São Paulo, Brazil. Chest 1997;112:729–33.

82. Pampiglione S, Rivasi F, Paolino S. Human pulmonary dirofilariasis. Histopathology 1996;29:69–72.

83. Pampiglione S, Rivasi F, Angeli G, et al. Dirofilariasis due to *Dirofilaria repens* in Italy, an emergent zoonosis: report of 60 new cases. Histopathology 2001;38:344–54.

84. Pampiglione S, Rivasi F, Gustinelli A. Dirofilarial cases in the Old World, attributed to *Dirofilaria immitis*: a critical appraisal. Histopathology 2009;54:192–204.

85. Flieder DB, Moran CA. Pulmonary dirofilariasis: A clinicopathologic study of 41 lesions in 39 patients. Hum Pathol 1999;30:251–6.

86. Hiroshima K, Iyoda A, Toyozaki T, et al. Human pulmonary dirofilariasis: report of six cases. Tohoku J Exp Med 1999;189:307–14.

Syngamiasis (gapeworm infestation)

87. Basden RDE, Jackson JW, Jones EI. Gapeworm infestation in man. Br J Dis Chest 1974;68:207–9.

88. Grell GAC, Watty EI, Muller RL. Syngamus in a West Indian. BMJ 1978;2:1464.

89. Delara TDC, Barbosa MA, Deoliveira MR, et al. Human syngamosis – two cases of chronic cough caused by *Mammomonogamus laryngeus*. Chest 1993;103:264–5.

90. Kim HY, Lee SM, Joo JE, et al. Human syngamosis: the first case in Korea. Thorax 1998;53:717–18.

Acariasis

91. Li C, Li L. Human pulmonary acariasis in Anhui Province: an epidemiological survey. Zhongguo Ji. Sheng Chong. Xue Yu Ji. Sheng Chong. Bing. Za Zhi 1990;8:41–4.

Pentastomiasis

92. Guardia SN, Sepp H, Scholten T, et al. Pentastomiasis in Canada. Arch Pathol Lab Med 1991;115:515–17.

93. Morsy TA, El Sharkawy IM, Lashin AH. Human nasopharyngeal linguatuliasis (Pentasomida) caused by *Linguatula serrata*. J Egypt Soc Parasitol 1999;29:787–90.

Chapter | 6 |

Diffuse parenchymal disease of the lung

Some diseases that affect the periphery of the lung largely involve the alveolar interstitium whereas others encroach upon, or preponderate within, the alveolar lumen. Until the advent of modern imaging techniques this distinction was not fully appreciated by clinicians, with the result that many diseases have been termed interstitial, irrespective of the lung compartment predominantly involved. A classification formulated by a joint committee of the American Thoracic Society and the European Respiratory Society in 2002 (the ATS/ERS classification) corrects this anomaly by referring to them as the diffuse parenchymal lung diseases.[1]

The parenchyma of an organ is the part concerned with function. In most viscera, function resides in the epithelium, and the interstitial connective tissue merely acts in a supporting role. This is not the case in the lungs. The function of the lungs is of course gas exchange, which takes place in the alveoli. It is unlikely that gas exchange could take place if any component of the alveolus or its wall was lacking. The lung parenchyma is therefore to be regarded as all the tissue of the gas-exchanging region, which is that portion beyond the terminal bronchiole – the pulmonary acinus (see p. 4 and Fig. 1.4, p. 5). An earlier term synonymous with diffuse parenchymal lung disease is acinar lung disease.[2] The lung acinus includes the alveolar interstitium and endothelium as well as its epithelium and air space. Thus the term 'diffuse parenchymal (or acinar) lung disease' is highly appropriate for a group of diseases that includes some which are truly interstitial and others that represent alveolar filling defects.

The idiopathic interstitial pneumonias form a major subgroup of the diffuse parenchymal lung diseases, and represent one in which there have been several recent advances. Of particular importance is the recognition that ongoing fibrosis is a better prognostic indicator than inflammation. Histopathological patterns such as usual interstitial pneumonia (UIP) have therefore been defined more precisely and separated from less specific patterns, leading to the introduction of terms such as non-specific interstitial pneumonia (NSIP). Considerable work has gone into correlating histopathological patterns with clinical course and radiological detail, as revealed by modern imaging techniques. The result has been an intensification in clinicopathological correlation and a better appreciation of the likely clinical outcome.

The ATS/ERS classification concentrates upon the idiopathic interstitial pneumonias and in this area seeks to match disease diagnosis with predominant histological pattern so that there is often dual terminology (Table 6.1).[1] It brings together clinical, imaging and histological criteria and is of undoubted prognostic and therapeutic value. However, it is not above criticism, particularly in its retention of terms such as 'interstitial pneumonia' for a group of parenchymal diseases that may be either interstitial or intra-alveolar. The term 'desquamative interstitial pneumonia' (DIP) is retained, although it is now well established that this process is not desquamative but exudative and has only a minor interstitial component. Cryptogenic organising pneumonia is a further condition listed under the idiopathic interstitial pneumonias despite it affecting the alveolar space rather than the interstitium. Furthermore, DIP and respiratory bronchiolitis are largely caused by smoking and are therefore not strictly idiopathic. Similarly, lymphoid interstitial pneumonia (LIP) is virtually never idiopathic and it is questionable whether it should be regarded as an interstitial pneumonia or a lymphoproliferative disease.

The prime reason for assembling the seven disparate entities listed in Table 6.1 under the heading idiopathic interstitial pneumonias is that, although they differ in their prognosis and treatment, they may enter the differential diagnosis of idiopathic pulmonary fibrosis (IPF) at initial presentation. These patterns are also of considerable prognostic value.[1,3–8] The ATS/ERS classification provides pathological criteria that allow these patterns to be distinguished in a fairly reproducible manner.[9] However, pathologists should be aware that they are only identifying a particular histological pattern, not a specific disease, subsequent correlation with clinical and imaging data being required to reach a final diagnosis.[1] Mixed patterns may be encountered. For example, diffuse alveolar damage, the pathological basis of acute interstitial pneumonia (AIP), may be superimposed on UIP in acute exacerbations of IPF,[10] different lobes may concurrently show different histological patterns in the same patient[11] and different histological patterns may be seen in successive samples of the same lung.[12] However, there is nothing to stop pathologists reviewing all the data and coming to a final diagnosis themselves.[13]

It is also worth noting that, whereas a UIP pattern is typical of IPF, conditions other than IPF may show UIP on occasion, while diffuse alveolar damage has many recognisable causes besides being the basis of AIP (see Box 4.2, p. 143) and NSIP is seen in a variety of unrelated conditions.[3] One review estimated that 68% of cases showing NSIP

DOI: 10.1016/B978-0-7020-3369-8.00006-9

Table 6.1 Classification of diffuse parenchymal lung disease[1]

1. Of known cause, e.g. drugs (Chapter 7.3) or of known association, e.g. collagen vascular disease (Chapter 10)
2. Idiopathic interstitial pneumonias

Diagnosis	Predominant histological pattern
Idiopathic pulmonary fibrosis (cryptogenic fibrosing alveolitis)	Usual interstitial pneumonia
Non-specific interstitial pneumonia (provisional)[a]	Non-specific interstitial pneumonia
Desquamative interstitial pneumonia	Desquamative interstitial pneumonia
Respiratory bronchiolitis-associated interstitial lung disease	Respiratory bronchiolitis
Acute interstitial pneumonia	Diffuse alveolar damage
Cryptogenic organising pneumonia[b]	Organising pneumonia
Lymphoid interstitial pneumonia	Lymphoid interstitial pneumonia

3. Granulomatous, e.g. sarcoidosis
4. Environmental or occupational (Chapters 7.1 and 7.2)
5. Others, e.g. lymphangioleiomyomatosis, Langerhans cell histiocytosis

[a]A heterogeneous group of diseases with poorly characterised clinical and radiological features that need further study.
[b]Synonymous with idiopathic bronchiolitis obliterans organising pneumonia.

were idiopathic, 22% were associated with connective tissue disease, 8% represented atypical cases of extrinsic allergic alveolitis and 2% followed the acute respiratory distress syndrome.[14] Another group estimated that 88% of patients classified as idiopathic NSIP had what they termed unclassified connective tissue disease.[15]

The terms 'acute interstitial pneumonia' (AIP) and NSIP are relatively new and when the adjective 'usual' was originally introduced it was to contrast UIP with four other patterns of idiopathic interstitial pneumonia, namely DIP, LIP, a pattern occurring in association with bronchiolitis obliterans (BIP) and one marked by the presence of giant cells (GIP).[16] It was hoped that this histopathological classification would facilitate a better understanding of aetiology, pathogenesis and clinical features. This hope has been partly realised in that many cases of GIP are now known to be caused by hard-metal alloys. The term BIP is no longer used, having been superseded initially by idiopathic bronchiolitis obliterans organising pneumonia and now by cryptogenic organising pneumonia.

A further pattern, described since the ATS/ERS classification was formulated, is one that has been termed bronchiolocentric interstitial pneumonia.[17–20] This lacks any specific features and is of unknown cause but before using the term bronchiolocentric interstitial pneu-

monia, the pathologist should consider the possibility that the changes may represent inactive forms of such centriacinar diseases as extrinsic allergic alveolitis. Having done so, one group suggested that the changes were the result of gastric aspiration.[18]

The term cryptogenic fibrosing alveolitis (CFA) was introduced in the 1960s to link IPF to the pulmonary fibrosis that is occasionally seen in association with the collagen vascular disorders, the prefixes 'lone' and 'system' being used to distinguish the two.[21–23] However, the prefixes are now seldom used and the unqualified term CFA has become an unnecessary synonym for IPF[1] or is used as a general umbrella term for pulmonary fibrosis of uncertain aetiology.[24]

Antedating all these terms but now largely abandoned are those applied by nineteenth-century morbid anatomists who were evidently familiar with the pathological changes seen in IPF and applied graphic descriptive terms such as muscular cirrhosis of the lung[25] and cirrhosis cystica pulmonum.[26]

DIFFUSE PARENCHYMAL LUNG DISEASE IN CHILDHOOD

Diffuse parenchymal lung disease in children is very different from that seen in adults. IPF with its characteristic pattern of UIP is virtually unknown in children,[27,28] most reports antedating the ATS/ERS consensus classification. When the criteria recommended in this classification are applied to the paediatric cases it is found that patterns other than UIP are more common. AIP is also very rare in children, although its histological pattern of diffuse alveolar damage was first recognised in premature babies dying of the infantile respiratory distress syndrome. On the other hand, LIP is common in childhood, where it is nearly always associated with either connective tissue disease or immunodeficiency, both congenital and acquired.[27,28] It is a well-described complication of paediatric acquired immunodeficiency syndrome (AIDS), occurring in over 30% of children infected perinatally by human immunodeficiency virus (HIV). NSIP is also increasingly recognised in children and some cases are a result of surfactant gene mutations. DIP is rare and its outcome is worse in children compared to adults. Some childhood cases of DIP represent inborn errors of metabolism such as surfactant B deficiency and lipid storage diseases.[29–31] Cryptogenic organising pneumonia is exceptionally rare in children and respiratory bronchiolitis has not been reported. Disorders such as extrinsic allergic alveolitis and eosinophilic pneumonia are uncommon in children but have to be considered in the differential diagnosis, as do infections and their sequelae, which tend to be diffuse in this age group. Langerhans cell histiocytosis is seen in children with the systemic forms of the disease, especially Letterer–Siwe disease, but the type confined to the lung is largely a disease of cigarette smokers. After all these conditions have been considered there remain diffuse parenchymal diseases that feature in the perinatal period: these are considered in Chapter 2 (see Table 2.2, p. 51).[32,33]

REFERENCES

1. American Thoracic Society/European Respiratory. Society international multidisciplinary consensus classification of the idiopathic interstitial pneumonias. Am J Respir Crit Care Med 2002;165: 277–304.
2. Scadding JG. Talking clearly about diseases of the pulmonary acini. Br J Dis Chest 1978;72:1–12.
3. Katzenstein ALA, Fiorelli RF. Nonspecific interstitial pneumonia/fibrosis – histologic features and clinical significance. Am J Surg Pathol 1994;18:136–47.

4. Bjoraker JA, Ryu JH, Edwin MK, et al. Prognostic significance of histopathologic subsets in idiopathic pulmonary fibrosis. Am J Respir Crit Care Med 1998;157:199–203.

5. Katzenstein ALA, Myers JL. Idiopathic pulmonary fibrosis: Clinical relevance of pathologic classification. Am J Respir Crit Care Med 1998;157:1301–15.

6. Nicholson AC, Colby TV, Dubois RM, et al. The prognostic significance of the histologic pattern of interstitial pneumonia in patients presenting with the clinical entity of cryptogenic fibrosing alveolitis. Am J Respir Crit Care Med 2000;162:2213–17.

7. King TE, Schwarz MI, Brown K, et al. Idiopathic pulmonary fibrosis – Relationship between histopathologic features and mortality. Am J Respir Crit Care Med 2001;164:1025–32.

8. Flaherty KR, Toews GB, Travis WD, et al. Clinical significance of histological classification of idiopathic interstitial pneumonia. Eur Resp J 2002;19:275–83.

9. Nicholson AG, Addis BJ, Bharucha H, et al. Inter-observer variation between pathologists in diffuse parenchymal lung disease. Thorax 2004;59:500–5.

10. Kondoh Y, Taniguchi H, Kawabata Y, et al. Acute exacerbation in idiopathic pulmonary fibrosis – analysis of clinical and pathologic findings in three cases. Chest 1993;103:1808–12.

11. Flaherty KR, Travis WD, Colby TV, et al. Histopathologic variability in usual and nonspecific interstitial pneumonias. Am J Respir Crit Care Med 2001;164:1722–7.

12. Katzenstein ALA, Zisman DA, Litzky LA, et al. Usual interstitial pneumonia – Histologic study of biopsy and explant specimens. Am J Surg Pathol 2002;26:1567–77.

13. Myers JL, Katzenstein ALA. Beyond a consensus classification for idiopathic interstitial pneumonias: progress and controversies. Histopathology 2009;54:90–103.

14. Cottin V, Loire R, Chalabreyesse L, et al. Pneumopathie interstitielle non specifique: une nouvelle entité anatomoclinique au sein des pneumopathies interstitielles diffuses idiopathiques. Rev Mal Respir 2001;18:25–33.

15. Kinder BW, Collard HR, Koth L, et al. Idiopathic nonspecific interstitial pneumonia: lung manifestation of undifferentiated connective tissue disease? Am J Respir Crit Care Med 2007;176:691–7.

16. Liebow AA. New concepts and entities in pulmonary disease. In: International Academy of Pathology monograph No. 8. The Lung. Baltimore: Williams & Wilkins; 1967. p. 332–65.

17. Yousem SA, Dacic S. Idiopathic bronchiolocentric interstitial pneumonia. Modern Pathol 2002;15:1148–53.

18. deCarvalho MEP, Kairalla RA, Capelozzi VL, et al. Centrilobular fibrosis: A novel histological pattern of idiopathic interstitial pneumonia. Pathol Res Pract 2002;198:577–83.

19. Churg A, Myers J, Suarez T, et al. Airway-centered interstitial fibrosis – A distinct form of aggressive diffuse lung disease. Am J Surg Pathol 2004;28:62–8.

20. Fukuoka J, Franks TJ, Colby TV, et al. Peribronchiolar metaplasia: a common histologic lesion in diffuse lung disease and a rare cause of interstitial lung disease: clinicopathologic features of 15 cases. Am J Surg Pathol 2005;29:948–54.

21. Scadding JG. Fibrosing alveolitis. BMJ 1964;2:686.

22. Scadding JG, Hinson KFW. Diffuse fibrosing alveolitis (diffuse interstitial fibrosis of the lungs): correlation of histology at biopsy with prognosis. Thorax 1967;22:291–304.

23. Scadding JG. Diffuse pulmonary alveolar fibrosis. Thorax 1974;29:271–81.

24. Wells AU, Hansell DM, Nicholson AG. What is this thing called CFA? Thorax 2007;62:3–4.

25. Buhl VL. Muscular Zirrhose der Lungen. Lungenentzundung, Tuberkulose und Schwindsucht. Munich: R. Olderburg; 1873. p. 169.

26. Rindfleisch GE. Ueber Cirrhosis Cystica Pulmonum. Zentralbl Pathol 1897;8:864–5.

Diffuse parenchymal lung disease in childhood

27. Fan LL, Kozinetz CA, Wojtczak HA, et al. Diagnostic value of transbronchial, thoracoscopic, and open lung biopsy in immunocompetent children with chronic interstitial lung disease. J Pediatr 1997;131:565–9.

28. Nicholson AG, Kim H, Corrin B, et al. The value of classifying interstitial pneumonitis in childhood according to defined histological patterns. Histopathology 1998;33:203–11.

29. Amir G, Ron N. Pulmonary pathology in Gaucher's disease. Hum Pathol 1999;30:666–70.

30. Stillwell PC, Norris DG, O'Connell EJ, et al. Desquamative interstitial pneumonitis in children. Chest 1980;77:165–71.

31. Tal A, Maor E, Bar-Ziv J, et al. Fatal desquamative interstitial pneumonia in three infants siblings. J Pediatr 1984;104:873–6.

32. Deutsch GH, Young LR, Deterding RR, et al. Diffuse Lung Disease in Young Children: Application of a Novel Classification Scheme. Am J Respir Crit Care Med 2007;176:1120–8.

33. McFetridge L, McMorrow A, Morrison PJ, et al. Surfactant metabolism dysfunction and childhood interstitial lung disease (chILD). Ulster Med J 2009;78:7–9.

Chapter | 6 |

6.1 Interstitial lung disease

The diseases described in this section predominantly involve the alveolar interstitium, which constitutes the connective tissue framework of the alveolar walls. Its boundaries are the epithelial and endothelial basement membranes (see Fig. 1.28, p. 17). Many of the diseases considered here involve the interstitial fibroblasts and progress to interstitial fibrosis and ultimately 'honeycombing' (see p. 149). They represent examples of restrictive lung disease, the other major cause of which is interstitial oedema, which is dealt with in Chapter 8.1 (p. 401). Lymphangioleiomyomatosis is an exception in that it progresses to severe cystic change without any appreciable degree of fibrosis.

USUAL INTERSTITIAL PNEUMONIA AND IDIOPATHIC PULMONARY FIBROSIS

Usual interstitial pneumonia (UIP) is the commonest histological pattern seen in idiopathic interstitial pneumonia. It generally corre-lates clinically with idiopathic pulmonary fibrosis (IPF). However, it may also, on rare occasions, be encountered in drug reactions, collagen vascular diseases and hypersensitivity pneumonia, and IPF can only be diagnosed when these possibilities have been excluded.[1-3] Some regard UIP as the only acceptable pattern in IPF,[1] but others report fibrotic non-specific interstitial pneumonia (NSIP) in a minority of patients with this disease.[4-7] Occasionally, UIP is observed in one lobe and NSIP in another, in which case the prognosis is that of UIP.[4,7] Although abundant macrophages may accompany UIP, desquamative interstitial pneumonia (DIP) is now considered to represent a separate process, which is dealt with on page 311.[5,8-11]

Epidemiology

IPF shows a wide age spectrum. The mean age at presentation is 71 years,[12] somewhat older than earlier studies that possibly included patients with DIP.[13,14] The disease affects twice as many men as women and there is a strong association with smoking.[14-16] Prevalence is between 1 and 5 per 100 000 population.[17] In the UK the reported incidence doubled between 1990 and 2003 while in the USA age-adjusted death rates over a similar period increased 28% in men and 41% in women.[12,18] There is no predilection for specific countries, ethnic groups or urban/rural locations.[1] Occasionally, several members of a family are affected.[19,20]

Clinical features

Most patients with IPF complain of breathlessness on exertion, dry cough and loss of weight.[16] Bilateral basal crackles are heard on inspiration and digital clubbing is commonly found. Functional studies show a restrictive respiratory defect, the lungs being small and stiff. Chest X-rays may show a 'ground-glass' pattern or fine linear mottling, predominantly affecting the subpleural region of the lung bases. Progressive elevation of the diaphragm and 'honeycombing' accompany the shrinkage of the fibrotic lung tissue (Fig. 6.1.1A). On high-resolution computed tomography (HRCT), the dominant pattern comprises irregular lines forming a reticular pattern, mainly involving the bases of the lungs. As the disease progresses, the reticular pattern becomes coarser and 'honeycombing' and 'traction bronchiectasis' develop (Fig. 6.1.1B). Serological abnormalities and changes detect-

Figure 6.1.1 (A) Chest radiograph of a patient with idiopathic pulmonary fibrosis. Note the predominantly basal distribution with involvement of the costophrenic angles, which is characteristic of this disease. (B) High-resolution computed tomography scan of usual interstitial pneumonia. The lung bases show subpleural honeycombing. *(Courtesy of Dr I Kerr and Professor DM Hansell, Brompton, UK.)*

able on bronchoalveolar lavage (outlined below under pathogenesis) contribute to a distinctive clinical picture.

The disease is generally diagnosed on the above clinical and imaging features; indeed, the diagnostic accuracy of HRCT in identifying patients with a UIP pattern and hence IPF is now such that many patients do not have a biopsy.[1,21] In the UK only 40% of patients with IPF undergo any form of biopsy: 28% have a transbronchial biopsy and 12% a surgical lung biopsy.[16] Transbronchial biopsy may establish an alternative diagnosis, but a surgical biopsy is nearly always required to determine the pattern of interstitial pneumonia, and is now usually obtained at video-assisted thoracoscopy. In these instances, it is the presence of UIP that establishes the diagnosis (of IPF) and dictates prognosis.[22]

Course of the disease

Early studies showed a mean survival of about 4 years[14] but in later series limited to patients with UIP this figure was reduced to about 2 years (Fig. 6.1.2).[1,5,8,22,23] The later stages of the disease are characterised by cyanosis and dyspnoea at rest. These features presage death from respiratory failure, cor pulmonale or lung cancer, this last being an important complication that is dealt with below. Although IPF is typically characterised by a steady, predictable decline, some patients experience more rapid deterioration, either episodically or as a terminal event.[3,24–32] These acute exacerbations are defined as clinically significant deteriorations in patients with underlying IPF, characterised by subjective worsening over 30 days or less, new bilateral radiographic opacities and the absence of infection or another identifiable aetiology.[31]

Until recently, treatment was largely based on immunosuppression but this has seldom proved effective[23,33] and in the last decade several other drugs have either been or are being assessed.[3] These include interferon-γ, which initially showed promise[34] but has since shown no advantage.[35] In recent trials neither etanercept (a tumour necrosis factor-α antagonist) nor imatinib (a tyrosine kinase inhibitor) influenced the primary study endpoint, although both showed some evidence of decreasing disease progression.[36,37] More promising was a study with N-acetyl cysteine in combination with steroids and azathioprine that achieved its primary endpoint in showing a significant slowing of disease progression,[38] and initial trials of both bosentan (an endothelin-1 receptor antagonist)[39] and pirfenidone[40,41] have suggested a positive effect. Another agent to show a positive treatment effect, notably a reduction in mortality, has been warfarin.[42] The introduction of these drugs reflects advances in our understanding of the pathogenesis of IPF that have in part arisen from the more precise definition of the disease within the consensus classification.[43–47] Currently however, the only treatments that can be recommended outside a drug trial are oxygen therapy and transplantation.[3]

Morbid anatomy

In a typical case, the lungs are shrunken and firm when removed at autopsy or in preparation for transplantation. The lower lobes are most severely affected, with the pleura having a finely nodular 'cobblestone' pattern, resembling that of a cirrhotic liver (Fig. 6.1.3). Pleural fibrosis is uncommon, in contrast to asbestosis which IPF otherwise resembles macroscopically. The cut surface of the lung shows fibrosis and a variable degree of 'honeycombing', which is most marked beneath the pleura (Figs 6.1.4 and 6.1.5). The posterior basal segment is maximally affected and from here the process extends upwards, involving particularly the subpleural lung tissue. This rind of contracted fibrous tissue prevents the lungs from expanding and is an important factor contributing to the restrictive respiratory defect.

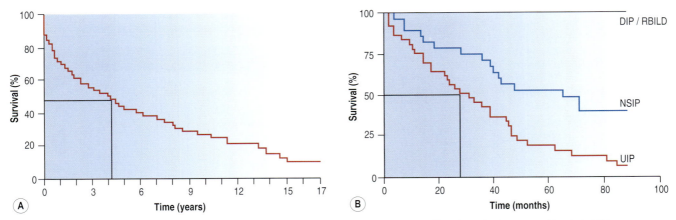

Figure 6.1.2 The survival curve of two groups of patients treated for idiopathic pulmonary fibrosis at the Brompton Hospital. (A) In a group antedating the distinction of usual interstitial pneumonia (UIP) and non-specific interstitial pneumonia (NSIP) the median survival was about 4 years from the onset of symptoms whereas in a later group (B) categorised according to their histological pattern, those with a UIP pattern had a median survival nearer to 2 years. DIP, desquamative interstitial pneumonia; RBILD, respiratory bronchiolitis-associated interstitial lung disease.

Figure 6.1.3 Idiopathic pulmonary fibrosis. The visceral pleura shows a 'cobblestone' pattern, reflecting changes in the underlying lung parenchyma. The pleura itself is not affected by the fibrotic process. *(Courtesy of Dr RVP Dissanayake, Ilford, UK.)*

Figure 6.1.4 Idiopathic pulmonary fibrosis. The lung shows basal subpleural 'honeycombing'.

Figure 6.1.5 Idiopathic pulmonary fibrosis. Paper-mounted whole-lung section. Note the predominance of the disease in the basal parts of the lung.

Histological changes

The cardinal features of UIP[2] are:

- subpleural and paraseptal predominance
- patchy parenchymal involvement
- established (i.e. collagenous) fibrosis leading to loss of architecture ('honeycombing')
- fibroblastic foci adjacent to the established fibrosis, indicative of progressive disease
- only mild to moderate chronic interstitial inflammation
- an absence of any causal feature such as inorganic dust, granulomas or accumulations of Langerhans cells.

As noted above, the disease is most marked immediately beneath the pleura and characteristic low-power feature is that the changes are patchy. Areas of chronic interstitial inflammation and fibrosis alternate with foci of relatively normal lung (Fig. 6.1.6). Much of the fibrosis is well established, consisting of poorly cellular hyaline collagen, but lying immediately adjacent to this older fibrous tissue are localised areas of granulation tissue consisting of plump fibroblasts set in a slightly haematoxyphilic myxoid stroma (Fig. 6.1.7). This variation in the age of the fibrosis is sometimes described as evidence of 'temporal heterogeneity'. The foci of immature fibrous tissue,

termed 'fibroblastic foci', can be highlighted by staining the abundant acidic proteoglycans present in such granulation tissue with alcian blue or Movat's stain (see Fig. 6.1.7C). They are thought to represent the sites of repeated lung damage.[13] Their progression is characterised by weakening alcianophilia and increasing collagenisation.[48] Most studies suggest that a profusion of these foci predicts poor survival whereas the more traditional feature of disease activity, interstitial mononuclear cell infiltration, is of only limited prognostic value.[49–52] Despite the term 'interstitial pneumonia', chronic inflammatory cell infiltration is generally only mild to moderate in intensity. Lymphoid follicles are not usually prominent in idiopathic disease and when present suggest collagen vascular disease.[53] As the process becomes more advanced, there is increased loss of alveolar architecture with remodelling and eventual formation of cysts separated by bands of fibrosis, so-called honeycombing.

This full constellation of histological features permits the pathologist to recognise a UIP pattern with confidence but in some cases only some of these features are evident, in which case only an opinion of probable or possible UIP can be offered. However, histological assessment is also of value in that it sometimes permits the confident exclusion of UIP (Table 6.1.1, p. 272).[3]

Although widespread 'honeycombing' usually represents advanced IPF, attempts to differentiate end-stage UIP from end-stage NSIP have shown poor reproducibility[5] and it is preferable to classify these changes merely as end-stage lung rather than assign a particular histological pattern.[5,54] Such areas can often be avoided if the surgeon discusses the cases with radiologist and pulmonologist before taking the biopsy to ascertain the probable sites of active disease.[2] Many centres now biopsy two sites to reduce the possibility of sampling error.[4,7]

A variety of secondary changes that are not specific to UIP and are of limited diagnostic value may also be observed:

- The residual air spaces are often lined by hyperplastic bronchiolar or cuboidal alveolar epithelium (Fig. 6.1.8A), sometimes showing squamous metaplasia (Fig. 6.1.8B) or goblet cell proliferation. Dysplasia and neoplasia may also develop (see below).
- The distorted air spaces often contain mucin, cellular debris, cholesterol crystal clefts, macrophages and other inflammatory cells.
- Blood vessel walls are usually thickened by intimal fibrosis in the affected areas but are normal elsewhere, unless there is secondary pulmonary hypertension.
- Reactive smooth-muscle hyperplasia is often very marked (Fig. 6.1.8C), contributing to the archaic term 'muscular cirrhosis of the lung'. The hyperplastic muscle is probably derived from bronchioles and small blood vessels rather than the myofibroblasts of young fibrous tissue, but its origin is seldom evident.
- Occasionally, eosinophilic pneumonia-like areas may be seen.[55]
- Other non-specific features include focal alveolar macrophage accumulation (sometimes mimicking DIP), mild pleuritis and pleural fibrosis, subpleural fatty metaplasia, dilated lymphatics, neutrophil accumulation (especially within areas of honeycomb change), osseous metaplasia, focal alveolar fibrin, and hyaline cytoplasmic inclusions in pneumocytes.[2]

Patients with IPF frequently smoke and it is therefore not surprising that a variety of further changes commonly found in smokers may be seen in addition to UIP, namely centriacinar emphysema, respiratory bronchiolitis, DIP-like changes and what has been termed air space enlargement with fibrosis.[56]

Figure 6.1.6 Usual interstitial pneumonia. Patchy subpleural and paraseptal fibrosis is characteristic of this pattern of interstitial pneumonia. In all cases, the fibrosis is interspersed with unaffected normal lung. Arrows pleura.

Figure 6.1.7 Usual interstitial pneumonia. (A) A fibroblastic focus consisting of granulation tissue adjacent to more collagenous interstitial fibrosis. (B) A fibroblastic focus showing a greater degree of collagenisation and overlying epithelialisation as it becomes incorporated in the interstitium. (C) Granulation tissue rich in alcianophilic proteoglycans (top) covers older, more mature fibrous tissue (Alcian blue stain).

Figure 6.1.8 Secondary changes commonly associated with usual interstitial pneumonia but not essential to its recognition. (A) Type II cell hyperplasia. (B) The regenerating alveolar epithelium has undergone marked squamous metaplasia. (C) An area of advanced interstitial fibrosis shows marked smooth-muscle hyperplasia and hypertrophy.

Table 6.1.1 Histopathological criteria for usual interstitial pneumonia (UIP)[3]

UIP (all four criteria present)	Probable UIP	Possible UIP (all three criteria present)	Not UIP (any of the six criteria present)
Marked fibrosis with architectural distortion in a predominantly subpleural and paraseptal distribution Patchy involvement Fibroblast foci Absence of features suggesting an alternative diagnosis (see fourth column)	Marked fibrosis with architectural distortion in a predominantly subpleural and paraseptal distribution Absence of either patchy involvement or fibroblastic foci, but not both Absence of features suggesting an alternative diagnosis (see fourth column) or Honeycomb changes only[c]	Patchy or diffuse parenchymal fibrosis, with or without interstitial inflammation Absence of other criteria for UIP (see UIP pattern column) Absence of features suggesting an alternative diagnosis (see fourth column)	Hyaline membranes[a] Organising pneumonia[b] Granulomas[b] Marked interstitial inflammatory cell infiltrate away from honeycombing Predominance of airway-centred changes Other features suggestive of an alternative diagnosis

[a]Can be superimposed upon UIP in acute exacerbations of idiopathic pulmonary fibrosis.
[b]An isolated or occasional granuloma or a little organising pneumonia may rarely coexist with UIP.
[c]End-stage fibrotic lung disease, which is usually evident on high-resolution computed tomography (HRCT) and can be avoided by preoperative HRCT targeting of biopsy sites away from these areas.

Electron microscopy

Ultrastructural studies support the view that the alveolar epithelium is the target tissue, identifying foci of bare epithelial basement membrane as an early feature of the disease (Fig. 6.1.9).[57–59]

Differential diagnosis

IPF was formerly categorised as either 'cellular' or 'fibrotic' and, although this was of prognostic value,[14,60,61] the 'cellular' cases would now be recognised as having a different histological pattern, such as cellular NSIP, DIP or respiratory bronchiolitis. It is important to distinguish UIP from these other patterns of interstitial pneumonia because IPF differs radically from the other interstitial lung disease in its prognosis and treatment (see Fig. 6.1.2). The most problematic area is the distinction of UIP from fibrotic NSIP.[62] The key features in this are a relatively diffuse pattern of interstitial fibrosis and an absence or dearth of fibroblastic foci (lack of temporal heterogeneity) in NSIP.[2] In reality, this can be very difficult and diagnostic confidence is often low,[62] not helped by the fact that, as well as areas showing UIP and normal lung, foci indistinguishable from NSIP are often seen.[6] In these difficult cases, consideration of the clinical and imaging features may be of great help.[62a]

Sometimes there are abundant macrophages, resulting in a DIP-like pattern, but attention to the alveolar walls reveals the characteristic fibroblastic foci and patchy subpleural distribution of UIP.[2,63,64] Any fibrosis found in DIP is mild, diffuse and non-fibroblastic.

Diffuse alveolar damage (DAD) is easily distinguished by its characteristic hyaline membranes but may be superimposed upon UIP in acute exacerbations of IPF (Fig. 6.1.10).[25,27–31]

Organising pneumonia may progress to interstitial fibrosis and when the polypoid foci of granulation tissue are closely applied to the alveolar wall they may resemble the fibroblastic foci of UIP, but the subpleural distribution of UIP is not seen and the intra-alveolar tufts of granulation tissue are generally evident elsewhere in the biopsy. In such cases, previous scans will usually show features more characteristic of organising pneumonia progressing to fibrosis. Clinical review also helps exclude an acute exacerbation of IPF.

UIP differs from asbestosis by the absence of asbestos bodies, from granulomatous diseases such as Langerhans cell histiocytosis and sarcoidosis by the absence of granulomas, and from lymphangioleio-myomatosis by the different nature of the smooth muscle, which is atypical and differs markedly from that seen as reactive hyperplasia in IPF (compare Figs 6.1.8C and 6.1.48).

Extrinsic allergic alveolitis can also usually be excluded by the presence of granulomas, but chronic cases may be difficult to distinguish from UIP.[65,66] This again emphasises the need to correlate the biopsy findings with clinical and imaging data.[67]

If the vascular changes are so severe that primary pulmonary hypertension enters the differential diagnosis, attention should be paid to the vessels in the comparatively normal areas of the biopsy, when it will generally be appreciated that the abnormal blood vessels are limited to areas of diseased parenchyma, unlike the generalised vascular hypertrophy seen in primary pulmonary hypertension. Pulmonary hypertension can of course complicate IPF, when it is an adverse prognostic indicator.[68]

Occasionally, lung biopsy reveals fibrosis that does not conform to the pattern of either UIP or any other idiopathic interstitial pneumonia and for these cases the term 'non-classifiable fibrosis' is recommended.[3] Table 6.1.2 summarises the pertinent features of UIP and the other interstitial lung diseases and may be used as part of a diagnostic algorithm.

Aetiology and pathogenesis[69,70]

The histological features of IPF suggest that the disease results from repeated episodes of focal damage to the alveolar epithelium but provide no clue to the nature of the injurious agent. However, IPF has many features in common with the so-called collagen vascular diseases and the concept of lone versus systemic cryptogenic fibrosing alveolitis (CFA) links the two (see p. 264).[71] Hyperglobulinaemia is common and circulating non-organ-specific autoantibodies such as rheumatoid factor and antinuclear factor are often present in IPF.[61,72] In a national British survey of patients with 'lone CFA', rheumatoid factor was positive in 19% and antinuclear factor in 26%.[16] Antibodies directed against the alveolar epithelium have also been identified.[73,74] Immune complexes have been demonstrated in the serum[75] and occasionally in the wall of pulmonary capillaries, particularly in early cases.[76,77] It seems likely therefore that IPF has in part an autoimmune basis, with the alveolar epithelium being the target tissue (see Fig. 6.1.9). The initiating cause remains unknown although environmental and occupational pollutants,[15,16,78,79] gastric reflux,[80] viruses[81–86] and

Figure 6.1.9 Idiopathic pulmonary fibrosis. Electron microscopy shows patchy loss of the alveolar epithelium (bottom right), remnants of which are shrunken and electron-dense (upper right). Between these cytoplasmic remnants, denuded epithelial basement membrane is exposed to alveolar air. *(Reproduced from Corrin et al.[58] by permission of the editor of the* Journal of Pathology.*)*

Table 6.1.2 A diagnostic algorithm for usual interstitial pneumonia and the other interstitial lung diseases

Collagenous or inflammatory?	Histology	Diagnosis
A predominance of collagen	Patchy subpleural and paraseptal distribution, loss of architecture, and presence of fibroblastic foci	Usual interstitial pneumonia (idiopathic pulmonary fibrosis in most cases)
	With chronic peribronchiolar inflammation and possibly granulomas or isolated giant cells	Chronic extrinsic allergic alveolitis
	Stellate peribronchiolar scars (often masked by excess macrophages)	Burnt-out Langerhans cell histiocytosis
	No significant architectural disruption or consistent zonal distribution	Fibrotic non-specific interstitial pneumonia
	None of the above	Unclassified fibrosis
A predominance of inflammation	Peribronchiolar with granulomas	Extrinsic allergic alveolitis
	Peribronchiolar with eosinophils and Langerhans cells	Langerhans cell histiocytosis
	Peribronchiolar with intraluminal pigmented macrophages	Respiratory bronchiolitis
	Diffuse with hyaline membranes and fibroblast proliferation	Diffuse alveolar damage
	No consistent zonal distribution – mild intensity	Cellular non-specific interstitial pneumonia
	No consistent zonal distribution – marked intensity	Lymphoid interstitial pneumonia
	Non-necrotising granulomas in a lymphatic distribution	Sarcoidosis

drugs[87] have all been incriminated from time to time. However, there is no firm evidence that any of these plays a causative role.[88]

Against IPF having an immune basis is the ineffectiveness of therapeutic immunosuppression[3,23,33] and the accelerated rate of progression of the disease seen in the native lung of patients who have undergone single-lung transplantation despite the profound immunosuppression necessary to prevent rejection of the donor lung.[89]

The fact that the disease is occasionally familial[19,20,90] suggests that genetic susceptibility may be important. There is evidence that in some families, susceptibility to the disease is inherited in an autosomal-dominant manner.[90,91] One gene that is potentially responsible for such susceptibility is situated on chromosome 14q32, close to the alleles responsible for α_1-antitrypsin deficiency.[92] Rarely, several family members suffer from either IPF or α_1-antitrypsin deficiency.[93]

Other genes identified include ones encoding for surfactant protein C and telomerase.[94,95] HRCT of the asymptomatic relatives of patients with familial IPF identified abnormalities in 22%, with diverse patterns being found on lung biopsy.[96] Several subtypes of idiopathic interstitial pneumonia may occur within the same family,[90] which suggests that there may be an interaction between a specific environmental exposure and a predisposing gene (or genes) such that the insult predicates the pattern of fibrosing lung disease rather than the gene itself.

Following recognition of the alveolar epithelium as the site of initial injury, from which dysregulated repair and eventual fibrosis ensue, considerable attention has been paid to the cytokines associated with the regenerating epithelial cells. These cells express numerous profibrotic cytokines, including transforming growth factor-β

Figure 6.1.10 Terminal acute exacerbation of idiopathic pulmonary fibrosis in which diffuse alveolar damage is superimposed upon a background of usual interstitial pneumonia. (A) Extensive honeycombing affects the peripheral parts of the lung while the non-fibrotic central part is deeply congested. (B) Microscopically, the hyaline membranes that characterise diffuse alveolar damage are evident, superimposed upon the interstitial fibrosis.

(Fig. 6.1.11),[97–99] interleukin (IL)-10,[99] endothelin,[100] tumour necrosis factor-α,[101] insulin-like growth factor-1,[102] transcription factor GATA-3,[103] gremlin[104] and connective tissue growth factor.[105] Receptors for these profibrotic cytokines such as CCR7 have been localised to the interstitial compartment in UIP.[106] Other factors identified in the regenerating epithelium include proteinases,[107] tenascin[98] and cytokines that inhibit cell migration and further re-epithelialisation, which may be important in the delayed or defective re-epithelialisation that has been held responsible for fibroblast recruitment, activation and sustained proliferation.[108] Poor re-epithelialisation may be due in part to increased pneumocyte apoptosis, promoted by some of the above cytokines, for example, transforming growth factor-β.

Epithelial loss with resultant surfactant deficiency would also explain the focal collapse with apposition of bare basement membranes that has been described by electron microscopists, a change that is rendered permanent by regenerating epithelial cells bridging the mouths of collapsed alveoli (atelectatic induration).[59,109] This is at its most extreme in relation to acute exacerbations when hyaline membranes are seen (see Fig. 6.1.10).[29,110–113]

The fibrosis that follows the epithelial injury is initially fibroblastic and in advanced disease the most recent injury is recognisable as foci of granulation tissue rich in these cells. The number of these fibroblastic foci correlates with the rate of disease progression and mortality.[49,114,115] The fibroblasts show an altered phenotype, typically myofibroblastic, that reflects activation and the production of extracellular matrix proteins. This is part of normal tissue repair but the persistence of an activated fibroblast phenotype probably contributes to the chronic progression to fibrosis and remodelling. This is enhanced by a reduced capacity for degradation of extracellular matrix proteins, through imbalances between matrix metalloproteinases and their tissue inhibitors. Myofibroblasts also produce cytokines that induce epithelial cell apoptosis, thereby contributing to reduced re-lymphocyte is the predominant interstitial inflammatory cell. Focal collections of B lymphocytes cluster about the airways while the diffuse infiltrate largely comprises T lymphocytes, particularly of the suppressor/cytotoxic (T8) variety.[122,123] The alveolar epithelial cells show aberrant expression of HLA-DR antigen, suggesting that the epithelium may be recognised as autoantigenic by the cytotoxic T8 cells.[124,125] However T4 (helper) lymphocytes are also found and a shift from their type I to type II cytokine profile may be important in the progression of inflammation to fibrosis, type II cytokine (IL-4 and IL-13) receptors being overexpressed in IPF[126] and type I cytokines, particularly interferon-γ, being antifibrotic.[108]

Other inflammatory cells that may contribute to disease activity include macrophages and neutrophils, both of which are increased in lavage fluid in IPF (see Table A2, p. 759).[127] Suitably stimulated, these cells secrete a variety of proteases and toxic oxygen and hydroxyl radicals.[128–130] Proteases may so disturb the healing process as to perpetuate it, whilst the toxic radicals may be responsible for damage to the capillary endothelium and alveolar epithelium[128–130] that is evident on electron microscopy (see Fig. 6.1.9).[57–59]

Bronchoalveolar lavage also highlights a potential role for mast cells in IPF[131] and when mast cells are sought by appropriate staining in tissue sections they are seen to be numerous in the interstitial tissues of the lungs in this disease, and undergoing degranulation.[132] Electron microscopy demonstrates that they are frequently in close apposition to fibroblasts.[133] A variety of cytokines, including those that stimulate fibroblasts, are known to be released by mast cells and immunophenotyping indicates that these cells are highly activated in a variety of interstitial lung diseases.[134–136]

Endothelial damage and interstitial oedema, which are evident on electron microscopy,[58] are probably also important since it is known that chronic interstitial oedema contributes to interstitial fibrosis in other circumstances, e.g. the 'brown induration' of the lungs seen in long-standing mitral stenosis (see p. 403).[137] Various mechanisms contributing to microvascular injury have been identified.[138] However, although likely to play a role in the development of pulmonary fibrosis in IPF, the exact role and relative importance of angiogenesis and vascular remodelling remain uncertain at present.[139]

In conclusion, a combination of environmental and genetic factors, age and other unknown agents appear to cause an initial injury to the alveolar epithelium that progresses to a state of persistent dysregulated repair, eventually leading to irreversible architectural remodelling. The mechanisms involved in this process are represented diagrammatically in Figure 6.1.12.[108]

Figure 6.1.11 Usual interstitial pneumonia. (A) Immunocytochemistry demonstrates the intracellular form of transforming growth factor-β within the hyperplastic alveolar epithelium. *(Reproduced from Corrin et al.[97] with permission of the editor of* Histopathology.*)* (B) The extracellular form of transforming growth factor-β is seen within the alveolar interstitium immediately beneath the alveolar epithelium, compatible with it having been secreted by these cells.

epithelialisation.[108] Direct signalling between epithelial cells and fibroblasts may also be possible in view of the contacts that have been described between these cells through gaps in the epithelial basement membrane.[116,117] A further role for the epithelium involves a direct contribution to the fibrosis in a process of epithelial–mesenchymal transition.[118,119]

Eicosanoids, which are lipid metabolites that play a role in many inflammatory processes, have also been suggested as playing a role in patients with IPF, with an imbalance of molecules leading to increased profibrotic leukotrienes and a decrease of the antifibrotic prostaglandin PGE₂.[108]

It is noticeable from the above that the emphasis on pathogenesis has shifted away from a process driven primarily by inflammation to one initiated by epithelial cell injury coupled with aberrant wound healing.[120] This view gains support from genetic profiling, IPF being characterised by genes concerned with tissue remodelling rather than inflammation.[121] Nevertheless, it is likely that inflammatory cells play a contributory role. Histological studies show that the severity of the interstitial inflammation correlates with disease progression.[49] The

Cancer in IPF

A notable complication of IPF is the development of lung cancer, which has been reported in up to 13% of fatal cases.[140,141] In an early study, in which the patients were matched for age and smoking habit, it was claimed that IPF contributed a 14-fold increased risk of lung cancer.[142] However, although a later study confirmed the association the authors were not convinced that the association was causal.[143]

The tumour may be of any histological type. Reports on the relative prevalence of the various histological types vary but overall their distribution does not appear to depart significantly from that found in the general population. The epithelial hyperplasia–metaplasia–dysplasia sequence found in IPF (see Fig. 6.1.8B) is thought to represent the starting point of the cancer. Mutations of the *p53* oncogene have been demonstrated therein[144] and a high proportion of the cancers arise in the periphery of the lower lobes where the fibrosis and dysplasia are most severe.[141] Non-small cell carcinoma complicating IPF may be resectable but operative mortality is high.[145] A few cases

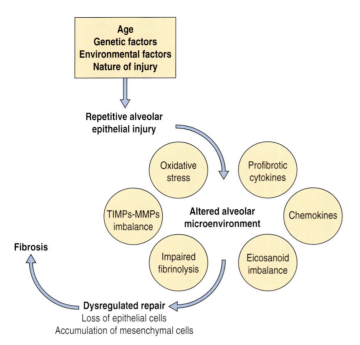

Figure 6.1.12 Pathogenesis of idiopathic pulmonary fibrosis. Progressive pulmonary fibrosis results from dynamic alterations in the alveolar microenvironment that eventually promote loss of alveolar epithelial cells and accumulation of activated fibroblasts/myofibroblasts. TIMPs, tissue inhibitors of matrix metalloproteinases; MMPs, matrix metalloproteinases. *(Redrawn from Thannickal et al.*[108] *with permission of* The Annual Review of Medicine.*)*

Figure 6.1.13 Non-specific interstitial pneumonia. High-resolution computed tomography shows ground-glass and faint reticular opacities.

of IPF have been complicated by the development of pulmonary lymphoma.[146]

NON-SPECIFIC INTERSTITIAL PNEUMONIA

The term NSIP was first used in the context of human immunodeficiency virus (HIV) infection[147] and only later applied to a pattern of supposedly idiopathic interstitial pneumonia that lacked specific features and could not be classified as one of the better-defined subsets.[148] The cause was unclear but clinical correlation suggested that it was multifactorial, some cases showing evidence of connective tissue disease, exposure to environmental allergens or previous acute lung injury. This uncertainty is reflected in the American Thoracic Society and European Respiratory Society classification in that the diagnosis allocated to a histological pattern of NSIP is merely given as NSIP (provisional). However, the term is of value in that patients with a histological pattern of NSIP have consistently been shown to respond better to treatment and have a more favourable prognosis than patients with UIP (see Fig. 6.1.2).[2,4,5,8,9,148–150]

Subsequent studies have provided further support for the multifactorial nature of NSIP and shown that only a minority of cases are idiopathic.[151,152] An NSIP pattern has been reported in further cases of extrinsic allergic alveolitis[66,67,153] and it is now realised that some drug reactions result in a pattern of NSIP.[154] Similarly, it is now clear that organising pneumonia and DAD may progress to NSIP.[148,155] Foci of NSIP may also be seen in IPF, with the classic UIP pattern evident elsewhere in the lung.[4–6,156]

Imaging provides further support that NSIP is multifactorial. HRCT scans of NSIP are sometimes suggestive of organising pneumonia,

sometimes of extrinsic allergic alveolitis and occasionally of IPF.[157] Genetic profiling also supports a multifactorial aetiology, some cases of NSIP expressing genes associated with IPF (such as those concerned with remodelling), some with extrinsic allergic alveolitis (such as inflammation and immune processes) and yet others that defy characterisation.[121]

NSIP may also represent connective tissue disorders that as yet lack systemic features, it being a common histological pattern in fully developed cases of systemic sclerosis, polymyositis, Sjögren's syndrome and, to a lesser extent, rheumatoid disease.[155,158–161] One group reported that 10% of patients originally diagnosed as having idiopathic NSIP subsequently developed collagen vascular disease.[152] Patients with such early connective tissue disease tend to be young, female non-smokers and in one centre constituted 88% of cases with NSIP.[162] There is also indirect evidence that some cases of fibrotic NSIP may be smoking-related.[163]

A histological pattern of NSIP should therefore be viewed as no more than a category from which the clinician can return to the patient to look for these potential associations, rather than a 'waste-basket' diagnosis.[156] Thus, the clinical disease 'idiopathic NSIP' should only be diagnosed after all these possible associations have been excluded.[151]

Clinical features

In patients with idiopathic disease, symptoms and signs are similar to those seen in IPF. The patients complain of breathlessness, cough and fever and are found to have crackles on auscultation. Clubbing is frequently evident. Some bronchoalveolar lavage studies record increased numbers of lymphocytes,[164] but others have shown no difference from UIP in this respect.[165] Functional studies generally show restrictive impairment.[151] HRCT shows varying patterns but a common one is of ground-glass opacities and reticular changes which may be diffuse but mainly involve the lower lobes (Fig. 6.1.13).[151,157,162,166,167] Volume loss and traction bronchiectasis may also be seen.[151] Honeycombing is less prevalent than in UIP but may be encountered.[166,167]

Histopathology

NSIP is characterised by expansion of the interstitium by variable amounts of chronic inflammation and fibrosis, the distribution of

Figure 6.1.15 Non-specific interstitial pneumonia. The interstitium is infiltrated by lymphocytes, histiocytes and plasma cells, whilst the fibrosis is collagenous and lacks the fibroblastic foci of usual interstitial pneumonia.

Figure 6.1.14 Non-specific interstitial pneumonia. (A) The changes are more diffuse than in usual interstitial pneumonia. (B) The cellular variant shows mild uniform expansion of the interstitium by a non-specific chronic inflammatory cell infiltrate.

Table 6.1.3 Major histological features of cellular and fibrotic forms of non-specific interstitial pneumonia

Cellular	Fibrotic
Diffuse involvement of affected parenchyma	Diffuse involvement of affected parenchyma
Moderate chronic interstitial inflammation	Mild to moderate chronic interstitial inflammation
Little or no fibrosis	Variable degree of interstitial fibrosis
Preservation of alveolar architecture	Little loss of alveolar architecture (no honeycombing)

Any features that suggest a specific aetiology, such as inorganic dust, granulomas, eosinophils and Langerhans cells, exclude non-specific interstitial pneumonia.

which is diffuse and usually lacks evidence of being either centriacinar or subpleural/paraseptal (Fig. 6.1.14). Foci of organising pneumonia may be seen but they are not the dominant component. At high power, the inflammatory cell infiltrate is seen to comprise small lymphocytes with occasional plasma cells, whilst the fibrosis may be predominantly collagenous or fibroblastic in nature (Figs 6.1.15 and 6.1.16). However, the fibrotic process is all of the same age (i.e. temporally homogeneous) with fibroblastic foci being absent or, at most, scanty.[2]

NSIP was initially divided into inflammatory, mixed and fibrotic types (grades 1–3) but subsequent studies showed that the survival for the mixed and fibrotic patterns is similar.[5,9] NSIP is therefore now divided only into cellular and fibrotic, the latter having the worse prognosis. Table 6.1.3 summarises the histological features of NSIP.

Differential diagnosis

The principal differential diagnosis is between fibrotic NSIP and UIP, the key features of which are described on page 269 and in Table 6.1.2.

The separation of cellular NSIP from DIP is facilitated by the relative dearth of alveolar macrophages in NSIP but rare cases of DIP may show mild to moderate fibrosis and overlap histologically with fibrotic NSIP.

The exudative and organising phases of DAD are easily distinguishable from NSIP as neither hyaline membranes nor diffuse organising pneumonia is present, but in long-term survivors of DAD the histological features may be indistinguishable,[148] again emphasising the importance of clinical correlation.

Extrinsic allergic alveolitis may also simulate fibrotic NSIP, in which case the presence of even a single granuloma or a suggestion of bronchiolocentricity should raise the suspicion of hypersensitivity.

The distinction of cellular NSIP from lymphoid interstitial pneumonia (LIP – see p. 655) is subjective, being primarily based upon the intensity of the interstitial chronic inflammatory cell infiltrate, which is much more marked in LIP than in NSIP. Again imaging is of value as LIP more frequently shows cystic changes superimposed on the ground-glass opacities. From a clinical perspective, the distinction between LIP and cellular NSIP is not particularly important as their prognoses are similar.

Figure 6.1.16 Cellular and fibrotic non-specific interstitial pneumonia. (A) Cellular non-specific interstitial pneumonia (NSIP) shows mild interstitial chronic inflammation without fibrosis. (B) Fibrotic NSIP shows variably intense interstitial chronic inflammation in association with established fibrosis.

IgG$_4$-related systemic sclerosing disease is a further condition that may be confused with cellular NSIP. It is characterised by a heavy infiltrate of IgG$_4$-bearing plasma cells, the recognition of which is key to the diagnosis (see p. 485).

Mixed patterns should alert one to the possibility of an adverse drug reaction or a collagen vascular disease.

Prognosis

Patients with cellular NSIP show a good response to steroid therapy and have an excellent prognosis, their 5-year survival being close to 100%.[5,9,150] Data on fibrotic NSIP are less consistent but it is universally reported that the 5-year survival is better than with

UIP,[2,4,5,8,9,148–150] 82% in one study and 74% in another.[151,152] Rare patients experience acute exacerbations.[168] The prognosis of NSIP in the connective tissue diseases is similar to that in idiopathic cases.[169]

ACUTE INTERSTITIAL PNEUMONIA (IDIOPATHIC DIFFUSE ALVEOLAR DAMAGE)

Acute interstitial pneumonia (AIP) differs from the other idiopathic interstitial pneumonias in that it presents as acute respiratory failure rather than chronic lung disease. The pathological basis is DAD, which has many well-recognised causes as well as the idiopathic variety now under discussion (see Box 4.2, p. 143).

Clinical features

As opposed to other interstitial lung diseases, AIP has an acute presentation and shows a rapid clinical progression.[170] The clinical features are very similar to those described by Hamman and Rich[171–173] but minor differences have been described.[174] AIP starts with a flulike episode, which is succeeded by rapidly progressive severe dyspnoea, often leading to death from respiratory failure. The age range is wide but the mean is approximately 50 years and there is no sex predilection. By definition, patients are previously healthy and have no underlying disease.[170,174] HRCT shows bilateral ground-glass opacification and dependent consolidation while in the organising phase there is reticular opacification with traction bronchiectasis and ultimately cystic change.

Histopathology

The histological features are those of DAD, as described in Chapter 4 (p. 136). DAD differs from UIP in its lack of established fibrosis and the presence of hyaline membranes in most cases, while long-term survivors lack the temporal heterogeneity of UIP. The organising phase of DAD may resemble organising pneumonia[175] and the late features may be indistinguishable from fibrotic NSIP.[148] It is important to exclude infection and special stains should be applied accordingly. Indeed, most biopsies come from the intensive care unit, with a view to confirming the presence of DAD and excluding infection, acute eosinophilic pneumonia and occult malignancy.

Prognosis

Mortality in AIP is reported as varying between 12 and 70%,[26,170,174] with survivors showing either complete recovery or residual fibrosis.

IDIOPATHIC BRONCHIOLOCENTRIC INTERSTITIAL PNEUMONIA

Centriacinar inflammation and fibrosis are features of many lung diseases, being seen for example in viral infections, bronchiectasis, aspiration, respiratory bronchiolitis-associated interstitial lung disease, extrinsic allergic alveolitis, Langerhans cell histiocytosis, rheumatoid disease and pneumoconiosis. Several of these conditions abate to leave only non-specific centriacinar scarring and reports of an idiopathic form of bronchiolocentric interstitial pneumonia may therefore engender initial scepticism. However, a few workers have reported small groups of patients with such pathological changes and distinctive demographic and clinical features.[176–178] The majority of these patients were middle-aged women with restrictive respiratory impairment and bilateral, predominantly lower-lobe interstitial infiltrates, airway thickening and traction bronchiectasis. No cause was apparent. Many of the patients died of their disease within a few years of presentation. At present it is uncertain whether these features represent a new pattern of idiopathic interstitial pneumonia or the end-result of a variety of previously described conditions, not least as several so-described patients had possible environmental exposures.[178]

EXTRINSIC ALLERGIC ALVEOLITIS (HYPERSENSITIVITY PNEUMONIA)

The synonymous terms 'extrinsic allergic alveolitis' and 'hypersensitivity pneumonia' are applied to a chronic granulomatous disease of the lungs that results from the inhalation of any of a wide variety of organic substances that are capable of acting as a foreign antigen and triggering a local hypersensitivity reaction.[179] Farmer's lung[180] is the archetypal example but there are numerous different circumstances and allergens, frequently designated by exotic names such as paprika pod splitter's lung, maple bark stripper's lung and the like (Table 6.1.4). Budgerigar-fancier's lung and summer-type hypersensitivity pneumonitis are respectively the commonest varieties of extrinsic allergic alveolitis in the UK and Japan.[181,182] In the USA farmer's lung is the commonest nationally[183] but at the Mayo Clinic avian proteins accounted for 34% of cases, 'hot tub' mycobacteria (see below) for 21%, farmer's lung for 11% and household moulds for 9%, with the causative agent unidentified in 25%.[184] No matter what the antigen, the pathology is identical in them all and a more meaningful division is into those of sudden onset (acute), those which come on gradually (subacute) and those with long-standing disease (chronic). Thus, the pigeon fancier with a large flock is likely to relate the onset of his symptoms to mucking out his loft a few hours previously, whereas the owner of a single budgerigar will probably not suspect that her gradually increasing breathlessness is attributable to the pet she has succoured without ill-effect for many years. In each case the allergen consists of avian protein in the bird droppings.

Clinical features

Atopy is not a prerequisite for extrinsic allergic alveolitis. Anyone may develop this disease but certain alleles of the major histocompatibility complex (MHC) appear to increase genetic susceptibility. Conversely, smoking appears to confer protection as the disease is unusual in smokers.[185] Patients with low constant exposure to the relevant allergen complain of slowly progressive breathlessness and are more likely to undergo lung biopsy than those with acute forms of the disease, which can generally be diagnosed from the occupational and clinical histories. Farmer's lung provides a typical example. This disease is liable to develop if hay has to be gathered when it is still damp, as often happens after a wet summer, in which circumstances thermophilic bacteria grow on it during storage. Subsequent handling in late winter may raise a fine dust which, if inhaled, can produce acute respiratory disease. This usually begins a few hours after exposure, with fever and a rigor, followed by cough, dyspnoea and, perhaps, expectoration of blood-stained sputum. About half such patients show transient pulmonary opacities on X-ray examination. Mild attacks clear up in 2–3 weeks but further attacks may be more severe and protracted, and recovery may never be complete. Occasional patients develop jejunal villous atrophy and suffer from intestinal malabsorption, as in coeliac disease.[186] The slowly progressive dyspnoea that results from constant low exposure is the result of a

Table 6.1.4 Some aetiological agents in extrinsic allergic alveolitis. Although this list is far from complete, byssinosis and humidifier fever are omitted intentionally, being dealt with on page 358

Antigen	Source	Disease
Thermophilic bacteria		
Micropolyspora faeni	Mouldy hay	Farmer's lung
Thermoactinomyces vulgaris	Mouldy grain	Grain handler's lung
M. faeni, T. vulgaris	Mushroom compost	Mushroom worker's lung
T. sacchari	Mouldy sugar cane (bagasse)	Bagassosis
T. vulgaris, T. thalpophilus	Contaminated water	Air conditioner lung
Other bacteria		
Bacillus subtilis	Biological washing powder	Detergent packer's lung
Cryptostroma corticale		
Bacillus subtilis		
Mycobacterium avium complex	Hot tubs	Hot tub lung
Fungi		
Cryptostroma corticale	Mouldy maple bark	Maple bark stripper's lung
Aspergillus clavatus	Mouldy malt or barley	Malt worker's lung
Aureobasidium pullulans	Mouldy redwood dust	Sequoiosis
Penicillium casei	Cheese mould	Cheese washer's lung
Penicillium frequentans	Mouldy cork dust	Suberosis
Trichosporon asahii	House dust, bird droppings	Summer-type pneumonitis
Animal proteins		
Avian serum and excreta	Pigeons, budgerigars	Bird fancier's lung
Feathers, serum	Chickens, turkeys	Chicken/turkey handler's lung
Rat urine and serum	Rats	Rodent handler's lung
Sitophilus granarius	Infested wheat flour	Wheat weevil lung
Porcine or ovine protein	Pituitary snuff	Pituitary snuff-taker's lung
Drugs, including methotrexate, procarbazine, trimethoprim, gold thiomalate		

Figure 6.1.17 Extrinsic allergic alveolitis. In the acute phase of the disease high-resolution computed tomography shows a generalised increase in the density of the lung parenchyma and faint nodularity. In this example, several thin-walled cystic air spaces are also evident, an occasional feature of the disease.

Figure 6.1.18 Extrinsic allergic alveolitis. A poorly formed non-necrotising giant cell granuloma (bottom right) is associated with widespread interstitial pneumonitis.

Figure 6.1.19 Extrinsic allergic alveolitis showing a collection of Schaumann bodies. *(Courtesy of Dr Nassif Ibrahim, Bristol, UK.)*

Figure 6.1.20 Extrinsic allergic alveolitis. To the right a giant cell contains two acicular crystal clefts while Masson bodies (*bourgeons conjonctifs*) representing organisation of luminal exudates are seen centre left.

restrictive respiratory defect with decreased lung compliance and reduced gas diffusion.

Radiologically, acute disease is characterised by generalised ground-glass opacification with small centrilobular nodules whereas in chronic cases the process often affects the upper lobes and HRCT shows a reticular pattern, reflecting the development of fibrosis (Fig. 6.1.17).[187] A mosaic pattern of attenuation may also be seen reflecting the bronchiolitic component of the disease. As with many diffuse diseases of the pulmonary parenchyma the advent of HRCT has resulted in many cases being diagnosed without recourse to biopsy. Bronchoalveolar lavage shows a lymphocytosis with a predominance of CD8 suppressor/cytotoxic T cells (see Table A2, p. 759). Skin tests and serology may provide further evidence in support of the diagnosis but there are many more antigens in nature than in the immunologist's armamentarium and often the responsible antigen is never identified.[65]

Histological appearances[65,66,153,188–191]

The lung is seldom biopsied in the acute forms of the disease and there are consequently few descriptions of the pathological features in these patients but the authors have encountered prominent necrotising granulomas in such a case. Others have reported capillaritis in an early acute fatal case[192] and following provocation tests.[193] DAD was reported in a further fatal case.[188]

Lung biopsies taken during the first few months of extrinsic allergic alveolitis show poorly formed non-necrotising granulomas. These are generally smaller and less frequent than those seen in sarcoidosis and are accompanied by widespread thickening of the alveolar walls by a diffuse lymphocytic infiltrate (Fig. 6.1.18). No fungal elements are found, but small fragments of foreign material may be present. Schaumann bodies may also be observed (Fig. 6.1.19). Isolated giant cells with cytoplasmic clefts are frequently observed: these are suggestive of the diagnosis but not specific (Fig. 6.1.20). In contrast to sarcoidosis, the hilar lymph nodes are unaffected. The diffuse background interstitial inflammation is another feature distinguishing the condition from sarcoidosis as it is only seen in the latter if biopsy is undertaken very early in the course of the disease. A further difference is the presence of knots of granulation tissue within alveoli and respiratory bronchioles (see Fig. 6.1.20), evidence of organisation of luminal exudates and responsible for the accumulation of lipid-laden

Figure 6.1.21 Extrinsic allergic alveolitis. The inflammatory infiltrate is maximal around bronchioles.

Figure 6.1.22 Lung biopsy in a chronic case of extrinsic allergic alveolitis shows cystic change and patchy bronchiolocentric inflammation (arrows).

Table 6.1.5 Biopsy findings in 60 patients with farmer's lung[189]

Interstitial pneumonitis	60	(100%)
Interstitial fibrosis	39	(66%)
Intra-alveolar fibrosis	39	(66%)
Foam cells	39	(66%)
Bronchiolitis obliterans	30	(50%)
Granulomas	42	(70%)
Solitary giant cells	32	(53%)
Vasculitis	0	

Table 6.1.6 A comparison of the histological features of pulmonary sarcoidosis, extrinsic allergic alveolitis (EAA) and lymphoid interstitial pneumonia (LIP)

	Sarcoid	EAA	LIP
Granulomas	Persistent, well formed	Evanescent, poorly formed	Persistent, poorly formed
Interstitial pneumonitis	Inconspicuous	Prominent, peribronchiolar	Very prominent, diffuse
Intraluminal fibrosis	Minimal	Moderate	Absent
Lymph node involvement	Prominent	Absent	Absent
Fibrosis	Dense in advanced cases	Dense in advanced cases	Slight

Progression and distribution of the lesions within the lungs

The granulomas resolve within about 6 months, unless there is further exposure, but the inflammation may progress to irreversible scarring, which in biopsy material is an adverse prognostic factor.[194] The fibrosis may show a histological pattern of either UIP or fibrotic NSIP.[65,66,191,195] In advanced cases, the lungs show end-stage features such as honeycombing. The upper lobes are affected more than the bases, although in acute cases chest radiographs show a basal preponderance. Whereas UIP is basal and affects a peripheral subpleural rim of lung, burnt-out extrinsic allergic alveolitis affects the upper lobes more than the lower and is patchy and irregular in its distribution, with central portions affected as much as the periphery (Fig. 6.1.23). Also, the fibrosis is often more bronchocentric in distribution, rather than being predominantly subpleural and paraseptal as in UIP.

Aetiology[196,197]

The role of an inhaled agent in provoking extrinsic allergic alveolitis has been demonstrated with inhalation tests. For example, extracts of mouldy hay produced characteristic reactions in 12 of 15 patients with farmer's lung compared with none of 20 control individuals,[198] but such testing would now be regarded as unethical due to the danger of permanent lung damage.

macrophages (endogenous lipid pneumonia) which may also be evident.

The granulomas tend to resolve with time but the diagnosis may still be suggested by the inflammatory process being peribronchiolar (Figs 6.1.21 and 6.1.22), these airways being the portal of entry of the aetiological agent. The peribronchiolar distribution of the inflammation also helps to distinguish extrinsic allergic alveolitis from NSIP and LIP. LIP is a condition that may also show poorly formed granulomas but it is characterised by a more diffuse, intense infiltrate that is seldom accompanied by any appreciable degree of fibrosis. The differential diagnosis also includes mycobacterial and fungal infection and adverse drug reactions to agents as diverse as methotrexate, interferon and tumour necrosis factor-α antagonists (see p. 389).

The histological features of extrinsic allergic alveolitis are summarised in Table 6.1.5 and contrasted with those of sarcoidosis and LIP in Table 6.1.6. Although they are characteristic of extrinsic allergic alveolitis and permit a confident histological diagnosis, exhaustive environmental and serological investigations quite commonly fail to identify the cause.[65,184]

Figure 6.1.23 Farmer's lung. Honeycombing is maximal in the upper lobe. *(Courtesy of Dr RME Seal, Cardiff, UK.)*

A feature of all forms of extrinsic allergic alveolitis is the presence of serum precipitins against extracts of the substances known to produce symptoms of the disease and because of this the disease is widely believed to represent an immune complex disorder, with the antigen–antibody complexes forming locally rather than being filtered from the circulation. The precipitins are well demonstrated by double diffusion (Ochterlony) testing or by immunoelectrophoresis, whereby, for example, avian antigens give a pattern of precipitin arcs with serum from cases of bird fancier's lung (Fig. 6.1.24). However, it should be noted that many exposed persons have circulating precipitins but few show evidence of disease. In support of an immune complex aetiology, biopsies from patients with farmer's lung subjected to provocation tests have shown immunoglobulin and complement around blood vessels.[193] The peribronchiolar/periarterial preponderance is explained by the antigen diffusing from the airways meeting antibodies diffusing from the blood at this site. Although granulomas are better known in cellular hypersensitivity states, they are quite compatible with immune complex disease, as it has been shown that they form when antigen and antibody are present in a particular ratio that renders them insoluble.[199]

On the other hand, there is considerable evidence to support cellular immune mechanisms playing an important role in extrinsic allergic alveolitis. In addition to the granulomas, most of the lymphocytes recovered by alveolar lavage are T-suppressor/cytotoxic cells (see Table A3, p. 760). Furthermore, in a study of symptomatic and

Figure 6.1.24 Extrinsic allergic alveolitis. Immunoelectrophoresis showing precipitation arcs where antibodies from the patient's serum have encountered the test antigen. *(Courtesy of Dr J Longbottom, Brompton, UK.)*

asymptomatic pigeon breeders, lymphocyte stimulation by pigeon serum extracts was only obtained in the first group, regardless of the presence or absence of precipitins, thus supporting a direct role of T-cell-mediated immunity in the aetiology of pigeon breeder's disease.[200] Further support for this comes from experiments producing hypersensitivity pneumonitis in athymic mice.[201]

Thus there is evidence that immune complexes and cellular hypersensitivity are both involved[179] and it is probably naive to conceive any immune process as being wholly humoral or wholly cellular. Furthermore, non-immunological mechanisms involving activation of complement by the alternate pattern have also been implicated in the pathogenesis of extrinsic allergic alveolitis.[196] Impaired lung immunity may explain the apparent protection against extrinsic allergic alveolitis observed in smokers.[185]

'Hot tub lung'

'Hot tub lung' is caused by the inhalation of *Mycobacterium avium-cellulare* from an infected spa pool and, although this bacterium can often be isolated from the patient's lungs, the condition is widely believed to represent extrinsic allergic alveolitis rather than infection. This is largely because it frequently resolves with corticosteroids, or even by avoiding exposure to the infected hot tub; antimycobacterial treatment does not appear to be required.[202] Patients complain of dyspnoea, cough, weight loss and fever while HRCT demonstrates centrilobular nodules and ground-glass opacification. The pathological changes consist of florid, non-necrotising granulomatous disease centred on the conducting airways. The granulomas are well formed and are frequently situated within the airway lumina. They are more prominent than is usually the case in extrinsic allergic alveolitis and the widespread interstitial inflammation characteristic of such alveolitis is not a feature – on the other hand, neither is the prominent necrosis that is commonly seen in mycobacterial infection. Culture and a history of exposure are necessary for the diagnosis as the bacteria are seldom identified on special stains of tissue sections. Sarcoidosis is the principal differential diagnosis, the distinction from which is often determined by the environmental history and culture.[202–208]

SARCOIDOSIS

Sarcoidosis is a multisystem granulomatous disease of unknown cause that is characterised by enhanced cellular hypersensitivity at sites of involvement. Elsewhere in the body cellular hypersensitivity is depressed so that reactions to common allergens such as tuberculin are consistently negative.

The lesions of sarcoidosis may be confined to one organ or disseminated widely. Autopsy studies show that asymptomatic sarcoidosis is much commoner than is realised clinically.[209] Lymph nodes, the lungs, liver, spleen, skin and eyes are the organs most commonly affected but virtually any part of the body may be involved. The distribution of the lesions is consistent with the lungs being the portal entry of the unknown causative agent, the lymph nodes being affected by lymphatic spread from the lungs, and other organs being involved by a combination of lymphatic and blood spread, a situation entirely analogous with that in tuberculosis.

The minimal criteria for an established diagnosis of sarcoidosis[210] are:

- consistent clinicoradiological features
- histological evidence of non-necrotising epithelioid cell granulomas
- exclusion of agents known to cause granulomatous disease

but the diagnosis may be made in biopsy-negative patients if there are appropriate clinical features and other supportive investigations.

The Kveim test has been largely abandoned because of fears of prion transmission: the inoculum consists of supposedly sterilised human splenic tissue affected by sarcoidosis.

Epidemiology

Sarcoidosis occurs worldwide but is more prevalent in the higher latitudes; northern Europe and North America have prevalence rates in the range of 10–40 per 100 000. The incidence and severity of the disease vary considerably between different racial groups living in the same geographical area. West Indian and Asian immigrants living in London have a 10-fold higher incidence than the native white population.[211] Similarly, black Americans have more sarcoidosis than whites, whilst the disease is quite rare in native Americans. It is also rare in Eskimos, Arabs and the Chinese. Negroes are affected more acutely and more severely than other races.

Aetiology

The aetiology of sarcoidosis is obscure; no single factor is known. The racial differences referred to above have generally been attributed to genetic factors,[212-215] Associations have been shown with the major histocompatibility complex (MHC), in particular the class II MHC alleles, several of which confer susceptibility (HLA-DR11,12,14,15,17) while others appear to be protective (HLA-DR1, DR4 and possibly HLA-DQ*0202).[216-218] Familial sarcoidosis has also been described, and variably ascribed to either genetic or shared environmental factors.[219-222] A comparison of monozygotic and dizygotic twin pairs suggests that genetic factors account for two-thirds of the susceptibility to sarcoidosis and environmental factors for one-third.[223]

Environmental factors are also suspected of playing a role in the aetiology of sarcoidosis, probably involving the uptake and processing of as yet unknown antigens, particularly by the respiratory system. Granulomas are of course found in a variety of conditions, notably tuberculosis, some fungal infections and chronic berylliosis. They may also be found in the vicinity of tumours. The granulomas of primary biliary cirrhosis resemble those of sarcoid and occasional patients have features of both these diseases.[224] Pulmonary granulomas have also been reported in HIV-infected patients receiving antiretroviral therapy[225] and in leukaemic patients being treated with interferon-α.[226]

Some authors regard sarcoidosis as an anomalous form of tuberculosis for occasional cases seem to swing from one of these conditions to the other and back again.[227,228] Acid-fast bacterial L forms have been cultured from the blood of patients with sarcoidosis,[229] and the application of molecular probes for mycobacterial nucleic acids to granulomatous tissue from patients with sarcoidosis has given positive results in a variable proportion of cases.[230-232] However, positive cultures are very rare, antituberculous treatment is ineffective and there are notable differences in the distribution of the two diseases: for example, there is a high incidence of uveitis in sarcoidosis that is not seen in tuberculosis. Another bacterium for which there is similar genomic but negative cultural evidence in sarcoid tissue is the epidermal agent *Propionibacterium acnes*.[233,234] Other agents suggested as having a role in the aetiology of sarcoidosis are listed in Table 6.1.7.

As noted above, sarcoidosis is characterised by anomalous immunological reactions. For example, the intracutaneous tuberculin reaction is generally negative, despite contact with tubercle bacilli, a phenomenon known as anergy. An explanation for this is provided by study of T-lymphocyte subsets.[235] In the blood, the suppressor cell (CD8):helper cell (CD4) ratio is increased in sarcoidosis whereas in bronchoalveolar lavage fluid the ratio alters in the opposite direction (see Table A3, p. 760). Analysis of lymphocyte subsets within the granuloma (see below) is in accordance with the lavage findings. The increase in CD4 helper T cells is seen especially in acute disease. When suitably stimulated these cells show a type I cytokine response, releasing cytokines such as IL-2, interferon-γ and IL-16 that attract other mononuclear cells into the granulomas. Cytokine profiles also cor-

Table 6.1.7 Sarcoidosis: proposed causative agents

Infective agents	Inorganic agents	Organic agents
Mycobacterium tuberculosis	Aluminium	Pine pollen
Other mycobacteria	Zirconium	
Propionibacterium acnes	Talc	
Borrelia burgdorferi		
Mycoplasma		
Herpes virus		
Epstein–Barr virus		
Coxsackie B virus		
Cytomegalo virus		

Figure 6.1.25 Sarcoidosis. High-resolution computed tomography shows numerous small nodules, some of which involve the interlobular septa (arrow). Note the enlarged lymph node immediately anterior to the trachea.

relate with disease progression. For example, increased IL-2 secretion is associated with a poor prognosis, whilst transforming growth factor-β is associated with spontaneous remission.[236]

Clinical features

Sarcoidosis usually appears early in adult life.[210] It affects the sexes equally.[12] Cigarette smokers appear to be less likely to develop sarcoidosis.[237] The presenting features are extremely varied, as may be expected of a disease so varied in its distribution. Most commonly, patients complain of fatigue, weight loss and a dry cough. Dyspnoea usually indicates more advanced disease. About one-third of patients develop erythema nodosum and this may be the presenting feature. Other extrapulmonary features include visual disturbances, neurological manifestations, arthralgia, parotid enlargement, hepatomegaly and cardiac dysrhythmia. Disfiguring indurated lesions on the cheeks and nose, known as lupus pernio, may develop. The onset of sarcoidosis is sometimes first evident in old tattoos or in scars containing foreign material such as road gravel that gained access years previously. Serum levels of calcium, angiotensin-converting enzyme and gamma-globulin levels are often elevated.

In the lungs, a multiplicity of small nodules comparable in size to miliary tubercles develops (Fig. 6.1.25). As with other granulomatous diseases of the lungs, the upper lobes are more severely affected than the lower lobes. The mediastinal lymph nodes often form large masses readily detectable by chest radiograph[238] and increasingly accessed by ultrasound-guided transbronchial needle aspiration.[239,240a] Sometimes the pulmonary lesions form large masses in what is known as a nodular or conglomerate form of the disease.[238,241] Occasionally the disease is centred on the airways and the patient has obstructive rather than restrictive respiratory impairment.[242,243]

Some degree of pulmonary hypertension is found in most patients whose sarcoidosis has progressed to irreversible pulmonary fibrosis.[244,245] However, fibrosis cannot be the only mechanism as pulmonary hypertension is sometimes found in the absence of such advanced disease.[246] The granulomatous impingement on pulmonary blood vessels described below offers an alternative explanation.[247,248] Compression of pulmonary arteries by enlarged mediastinal lymph nodes, sarcoid-related mediastinal fibrosis and left ventricular failure due to cardiac involvement are further mechanisms by which sarcoidosis may cause pulmonary hypertension.[248a]

Figure 6.1.26 Sarcoidosis. On the left granulomas have coalesced to form a mass lesion while the right side shows a more typical lymphatic distribution.

Pathological findings[249,250]

The histological hallmark of sarcoidosis is the granuloma, many of which are generally seen scattered throughout otherwise unremarkable lung tissue (Figs 6.1.26 and 6.1.27). They are generally confined to the interstitium and only rarely involve air spaces. The granulomas are preceded by a lymphocytic infiltrate[251] but this is transient and is seldom evident by the time lung biopsy is undertaken. Indeed, in contrast to extrinsic allergic alveolitis, the histopathology of pulmonary sarcoidosis is generally notable in that it lacks a diffuse lymphocytic infiltrate (Fig. 6.1.27).

Sarcoid granulomas closely resemble early tubercles microscopically; they differ from tubercles in that they do not undergo caseation, although a little central necrosis is occasionally seen microscopically (Fig. 6.1.28). Epithelioid cells and multinucleate giant cells of Langhans or foreign-body type are found in the centres of the granulomas. The giant cells often contain Schaumann and asteroid bodies (Figs 6.1.29 and 6.1.30) but these are not pathognomonic of sarcoidosis, for they may be found in other forms of granulomatous inflammation. Schaumann bodies represent lysosomal residual bodies,[252,253] whilst asteroid bodies are aggregates of vimentin microfilaments

Figure 6.1.27 Pulmonary sarcoidosis. The lung is studded with discrete non-necrotising epithelioid and giant cell granulomas. Intervening alveolar walls are unaffected. Two granulomas are closely applied to a bronchiole.

Figure 6.1.29 Pulmonary sarcoid showing an asteroid body within a giant cell.

Figure 6.1.30 Pulmonary sarcoidosis in an advanced stage. The granulomas have healed, leaving only the central calcified Schaumann bodies and extensive fibrosis that has destroyed the pulmonary parenchyma.

Figure 6.1.28 Sarcoid granulomas occasionally show a little central necrosis.

and microtubules derived from the cytosphere, the radial arrangement of which determines the bodies' stellate form.[254] Lymph nodes draining sarcoid tissue often contain small brown Hamazaki–Wesenberg bodies, which represent lysosomal ceroid pigment formed through the oxidation and polymerisation of unsaturated fatty acids. More often the follicular architecture of the hilar lymph nodes is completely effaced by numerous non-necrotising sarcoid granulomas (Fig. 6.1.31).

Figure 6.1.31 Nodal sarcoidosis. The lymph node contains numerous sarcoid granulomas.

Figure 6.1.32 Electron micrographs of epithelioid cells in a pulmonary sarcoid granuloma. (A) An immature epithelioid cell showing abundant rough endoplasmic reticulum. The lysosomal dense bodies that characterise a macrophage are not evident. The electron-dense structures are mitochondria. (B) A mature epithelioid cell showing an abundance of vesicles and Golgi apparatus. *(Courtesy of Dr C Danel and Miss A Dewar, Brompton, UK.)*

Epithelioid cells are derived from macrophages but such is the transformation they undergo during this development that there are few ultrastructural similarities: gone are the phagosomes and lysosomes of a macrophage, replaced by cytoplasmic organelles more in keeping with a secretory cell. The immature epithelioid cell is rich in rough endoplasmic reticulum, as seen in cells synthesising a proteinaceous secretion. Golgi apparatus and storage vesicles then appear, and in the mature epithelioid cell these organelles predominate (Fig. 6.1.32).[255] These cells secrete a variety of proinflammatory cytokines and fibrogenic cytokines, for example, transforming growth factor-β, tumour necrosis factor-α, RANTES and nitric oxide synthase.[256–261] The enzyme dipeptidyl carboxypeptidase (EC3.4.15.1), which acts as a kininase but is best known by its trivial name angiotensin-converting enzyme, has been localised to the cytoplasm of the epithelioid cells,[262] which would therefore appear to be the source of the high serum levels of this enzyme that characterise granulomatous disease in general and sarcoidosis in particular. The granulomas are also responsible for the final hydroxylation and hence activation of vitamin D,[263] thereby accounting for the hypercalcaemia that is so frequently found in sarcoidosis.[264]

Closely associated with the centrally situated epithelioid cells are T-helper lymphocytes. T-suppressor lymphocytes are fewer in number and more peripherally situated.[265,266] Cytokine studies suggest that the T-helper lymphocytes are mainly of the Th1 phenotype, producing IL-2 and interferon-γ.[267,268] Tissue gene expression analysis has shown a gene network engaged in Th1-type responses to be significantly overexpressed in pulmonary sarcoidosis, with proteins MMP-12 and ADAMDEC1 emerging as likely mediators of lung damage and remodelling.[269] A switch to predominantly Th2 lymphocytes may underlie a change from healing by resolution to healing by fibrosis. Antigen-presenting reticular cells are found at the periphery of the granulomas and B lymphocytes between the granulomas.[270]

At first sight the granulomas appear to be scattered haphazardly in the lung but in fact they are most numerous along the lymphatics and are therefore particularly well seen in relation to the centriacinar bronchioloarterial bundles (Fig. 6.1.33) and in the interlobular septa. The bronchi are richly supplied with lymphatics and the granulomas are accordingly well developed there, so this is a condition in which small fibreoptic bronchial biopsies frequently provide sufficient tissue for diagnostic purposes (Fig. 6.1.34).[271] Also, because of their distribution along lymphatics, the granulomas come very close to arteries and

veins and quite frequently involve all coats of these vessels in a granulomatous angiitis (see Fig. 6.1.33).[250,272,273] All sizes of vessel, from large elastic arteries to venules and lymphatics, may be affected, but veins are the vessels most commonly involved.[273] Indeed, sarcoidosis can sometimes cause veno-occlusive disease.[274] Right heart strain has been attributed to this vascular involvement.[247,248] Rarely, sarcoidosis is combined with disseminated visceral giant cell angiitis (see p. 445).

The granulomas may be so numerous that they become confluent, and rarely, large masses of sarcoid tissue are formed, the so-called nodular or conglomerate form of sarcoidosis (see Fig. 6.1.26).[238,241] Spontaneous resolution is common, suggesting that the granulomas often resolve but in other patients healing is by fibrosis, often with 'honeycombing' (Figs 6.1.35 and 6.1.36). The latter process involves progressive hyalinisation and Schaumann bodies may provide the only indication that extensive scarring is the result of granulomatous disease (see Fig. 6.1.30). However, active and healed granulomas are often seen together, suggesting that the unknown stimulus to the disease is a continuing one. Furthermore, early clinical disease may show fibrosis histologically, indicating that the disease may be quite advanced before it causes symptoms.

Figure 6.1.33 Pulmonary sarcoidosis. (A) The granulomas are clustered around small pulmonary blood vessels, where lymphatics are found. (B) Granulomas within and alongside a small vein, the lumen of which is occluded and the wall partly destroyed. Elastin-van Gieson stain.

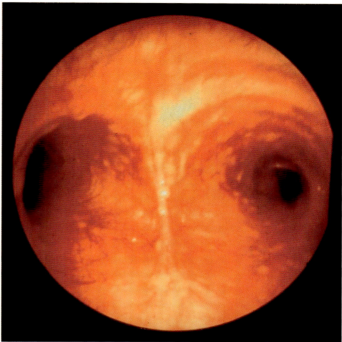

Figure 6.1.34 Sarcoidosis. Bronchoscopy shows yellow nodules studding the mucosa of the distal trachea and both main stem bronchi. (Reproduced from Häussinger et al. (2003)[433] with permission of Elsevier.)

Differential diagnosis

Infections such as tuberculosis always have to be considered in the differential diagnosis of sarcoidosis. The only conclusive histological distinction is the identification of *Mycobacterium tuberculosis* by Ziehl–Neelsen staining but features that favour sarcoidosis include granulomatous involvement of blood vessels and the presence of Schaumann bodies.[271] Necrotising sarcoid granulomatosis resembles tuberculosis in showing large tracts of necrosis but is widely considered to represent a form of conglomerate sarcoidosis (see p. 443).

Sarcoidosis also has to be distinguished from a giant cell reaction to foreign material, for which polarising filters are indispensable (not forgetting that fragmented Schaumann bodies are usually birefringent). However, as noted above, the onset of sarcoidosis is sometimes first evident in old scars containing foreign material, such as road gravel that gained access years previously. In general, sarcoid granulomas are more florid than the ordinary reaction to foreign material.

Sarcoid granulomas are also a well-known phenomenon in lymph nodes draining tumours. They may also be seen close to a tumour in organs such as the lung and may even mask the tumour.[275] Overlooking lymphoma in a lymph node showing florid secondary granulomas is a notorious trap for the unwary. Reports of sarcoidosis being associated with lymphoma should only be accepted if the two diseases affect anatomically distinct sites and the appropriate clinical, radiographic and serological features of each disease are present.[276]

Sarcoid-like granulomas characterise extrinsic allergic alveolitis but are generally more poorly formed, scanty, and seen on a background of diffuse chronic interstitial pneumonia, in contrast to sarcoidosis in which well-formed granulomas are usually studded throughout otherwise normal alveolar tissue. Even in very late sarcoidosis, lesions are generally recognisable as burnt-out granulomas, whereas in extrinsic allergic alveolitis the granulomas resolve without trace within a few months of last exposure to the responsible antigen. In both conditions, lymphocytes are increased in bronchoalveolar lavage fluid but in sarcoid the helper-cell:suppressor-cell ratio is high, whereas in extrinsic allergic alveolitis it is low (see Table A3, p. 60).

Course and prognosis

The course of the disease is unpredictable. In about 60% of cases the lesions regress over a period of 2–5 years and the patient recovers. After spontaneous improvement relapse is unusual. Sometimes, however, the lungs become progressively infiltrated and there is extensive fibrosis resulting in upper-lobe volume loss and traction bronchiectasis. Based on the radiographic changes, four stages of thoracic sarcoidosis have been described:

1. bilateral hilar lymphadenopathy (Löfgren's syndrome)
2. bilateral hilar lymphadenopathy and lung involvement
3. lung involvement without hilar lymphadenopathy
4. irreversible pulmonary fibrosis.

However, except that stage 4 is obviously preceded by stages 2 or 3, these are modes of presentation rather than successive

Figure 6.1.35 Late-stage pulmonary sarcoidosis. A whole lung slice showing fibrosis maximal in the upper lobe. *(Courtesy of Dr N Gubbay, Cheltenham, UK.)*

stages: lung involvement is not necessarily preceded by hilar lymphadenopathy.

An acute onset with erythema nodosum or asymptomatic bilateral hilar lymphadenopathy usually heralds a self-limiting course, whereas an insidious onset, especially with multiple extrapulmonary lesions, is more likely to be followed by relentless pulmonary fibrosis. Older patients and blacks do less well than the young and whites. Advanced pulmonary sarcoidosis is characterised by 'honeycombing', which may be complicated by life-threatening saprophytic aspergillosis (Fig. 6.1.37). An increased risk of pulmonary lymphoma and carcinoma has been identified in some studies[277,278] but not others.[279]

Because limited disease often resolves spontaneously the decision to treat must be weighed against the risks of drug side-effects. In those patients who require therapy, corticosteroids are the drugs of choice. Patients with progressive disease may require additional therapy with drugs such as chloroquine, azathioprine and cyclophosphamide. Drugs that suppress tumour necrosis factor-α may also be of benefit in steroid-refractory disease.[280]

The disease carries a mortality of about 5%, most of the deaths being attributable to either cardiac involvement or pulmonary fibrosis causing respiratory failure.[281–283] Rare causes of death include chronic renal failure due to nephrosclerosis and the cerebral effects of meningovascular sarcoidosis. If transplantation is undertaken the disease may develop in the new lungs and there is evidence that it derives from recipient immune cells.[284,285]

Figure 6.1.36 Late-stage pulmonary sarcoidosis. A paper-mounted whole-lung section showing fibrosis and 'honeycombing' maximal at the apex of the lung. Solid nodules at the upper end of the interlobar fissure are enlarged hilar lymph nodes, also involved by sarcoidosis.

PULMONARY LANGERHANS CELL HISTIOCYTOSIS (PULMONARY HISTIOCYTOSIS X, EOSINOPHILIC GRANULOMA OF THE LUNG)[286–290]

During the 1940s it became clear that three previously described clinical conditions, Hand–Schüller–Christian disease, Letterer–Siwe disease and eosinophilic granuloma, had much in common patho-

Figure 6.1.37 Pulmonary sarcoidosis complicated by saprophytic aspergillosis. An irregular fungus ball occupies a cavity just above the interlobar fissure. Elsewhere the lung shows irregular pale fibrosis, the result of long-standing sarcoidosis.

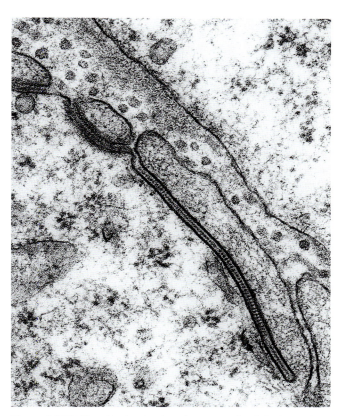

Figure 6.1.38 The ultrastructural marker organelle of the Langerhans cell (the Birbeck granule) is a pentalaminar structure with regularly spaced cross-striations. *(Reproduced from Corrin and Basset (1979)[287] with permission from Investigative Cell Pathology.)*

logically, and in 1953 the term 'histiocytosis X' was introduced to encompass all three.[291] This grouping subsequently derived support from the electron microscopic identification of a distinctive cytoplasmic marker organelle in all forms of the disease, the Birbeck granule (Fig. 6.1.38).[292] In normal tissues this marker organelle has been described only in Langerhans cells, the implication of this being that histiocytosis X represents a pathological proliferation of Langerhans cells. Accordingly, the term 'Langerhans cell histiocytosis' (or granulomatosis) is now preferred (Table 6.1.8). However, a distinction is drawn between pulmonary and extrapulmonary Langerhans cell histiocytosis. The latter mainly affects children and is thought to be neoplastic whereas pulmonary Langerhans cell histiocytosis is largely confined to young adult cigarette smokers and is thought to be reactive despite evidence of clonality in some of the pulmonary nodules.[293,294]

Langerhans cells are a constant feature of the normal epidermis and are occasionally found in the dermis. They are believed to be involved in delayed hypersensitivity reactions, particularly the transport of antigen from the skin to the draining lymph nodes (see p. 28). Langerhans cells are rarely identified in completely normal lung but they appear there in response to cigarette smoke.[295] They have also been observed in the lung in various pulmonary diseases, both reactive[296] and neoplastic.[297] Epithelial hyperplasia and metaplasia induced by tobacco smoke are particularly likely to be targeted by

Langerhans cells,[295,298] which appear to be attracted by the altered airway epithelium expressing granulocyte–macrophage colony-stimulating factor.[299] IL-2 has an inhibitory effect on Langerhans cells and it is notable that tobacco smoke constituents impair IL-2 production.[300,301] In pulmonary Langerhans cell histiocytosis electron micro-

Table 6.1.8 The different forms of Langerhans cell histiocytosis

Clinical form	Age	Organs commonly involved	Prognosis
Generalised diffuse (Letterer–Siwe disease)	Infancy	Bone, bone marrow, skin, lymph nodes, liver, spleen, thymus, lung	Usually lethal
Generalised multifocal (Hand–Schüller–Christian disease)	Childhood, young adults	Bone, skin, lung	Chronic disabling disease
Localised (eosinophilic granuloma of bone)	Childhood, young adults	Bone	Variable. May stabilise or remit
Localised (eosinophilic granuloma of lung)	Young adult smokers	Lung	Variable. May stabilise or remit

scopy shows that the Langerhans cells are in close contact with lymphocytes that have been previously characterised as T-helper cells: it is therefore suggested that the disease represents a hyperimmune response in which the Langerhans cells serve as accessory cells.[302]

Langerhans cells and their pathological counterpart have a moderate amount of light eosinophilic cytoplasm that is devoid of pigment, and a single nucleus with an indented cerebriform outline and a finely dispersed chromatin pattern. They carry surface receptors for Fc and C3 but are poorly phagocytic. Electron microscopy shows that they have few lysosomes but contain elongated pentalaminar structures of constant width (40–45 nm) with a longitudinal periodicity (10 nm) in their central laminae, the Birbeck granules (see Fig. 6.1.38).[292,303] Interdigitating dendritic cells are functionally related and morphologically similar to Langerhans cells but lack this marker organelle.[292] Both these cells express S-100 protein but CD1a, fascin and langerin are specific immunocytochemical markers of Langerhans cells.[304–308]

Clinical features

The lungs may be involved in the disseminated forms of Langerhans cell histiocytosis but they are most often affected in isolation. Young adults are affected most frequently but there is a wide age distribution. The great majority of patients are cigarette smokers.[237,309] Males outnumber females in most series but the more recent literature suggests a trend to a more equal sex distribution, reflecting the increasing number of women who smoke.

Non-specific chest complaints such as cough and dyspnoea are often accompanied by multiple pneumothoraces and sometimes by general symptoms such as weight loss and fever.[286] Some patients are asymptomatic despite radiographic evidence of lung disease. One previously asymptomatic patient presented with bilateral pneumothoraces and rapidly succumbed.[310] Chest radiographs typically show bilateral reticulonodular shadowing, most marked in the mid-zones[311] with sparing of the costophrenic angles, this last forming a useful point of distinction from IPF. HRCT shows features that reflect the stage of disease, ranging from nodules in the early stages to cysts at a later stage, again sparing the costophrenic angles. The cysts vary in shape, size and wall thickness (Fig. 6.1.39).[312] In a smoker, these features are highly specific and often obviate the need for biopsy.[313] Rarely, the disease may present as a solitary pulmonary nodule or with tracheal obstruction.[314,315] With advancing disease, the cysts enlarge and all zones of the lung become involved. Lung function tests usually show restrictive impairment. Pulmonary hypertension is a common feature and is often severe.[316] Blood eosinophilia is never found and, if present, should suggest alternative diagnoses such as eosinophilic pneumonia. Extrapulmonary involvement occurs in up to 15% of cases, when features such as lytic bone lesions or diabetes insipidus may give a clue to the diagnosis.

Course of the disease and response to therapy

The natural history of Langerhans cell histiocytosis of the lungs varies considerably (Table 6.1.9).[286,317–319] A few patients follow a rapidly downhill course and die early, while others improve spontaneously and become symptom-free with disappearance of the radiological changes. Others experience spontaneous remissions and relapses and slowly deteriorate, but the disease may arrest at any stage. Such patients are left with residual functional incapacity but suffer no further progression of the disease. Unfavourable prognostic features include generalised multisystem disease, prolonged fever and weight loss, widespread involvement of the lungs, multiple pneumothoraces, poor lung function, pulmonary hypertension and extremes of age.[286,316,317,319] In one study the overall median survival was 12.5 years, considerably shorter than expected.[319]

Figure 6.1.39 Langerhans cell histiocytosis. High-resolution computed tomography shows irregular cystic changes and scattered nodules.

Table 6.1.9 Evolution of the disease in 67 patients with pulmonary Langerhans cell histiocytosis[286]		
Evolution	**No. of patients**	**%**
Improved	9	14
Stabilised	27	40
Deteriorated	14	21
Died	17	25

Cytotoxic drugs have only been beneficial in Letterer–Siwe disease. Claims that steroids are beneficial are not substantiated in other series.[286] Generalised disease has been treated by bone marrow transplantation[320] and advanced pulmonary disease by lung transplantation, but some patients undergoing transplantation have developed the disease in their new lungs.[321] It seems sensible to advise patients with pulmonary Langerhans cell histiocytosis to stop smoking and there is anecdotal evidence that this is helpful. An infant with osseous Langerhans cell histiocytosis is reported to have responded well to IL-2 therapy; the relevance of IL-2 therapy to Langerhans cell proliferation is referred to above.[300]

Rare cases have been reported in which Langerhans cell histiocytosis has been associated with malignant lymphoma or leukaemia, the association following various patterns: the histiocytosis may follow, precede or develop at the same time as the lymphoma or leukaemia.[322,323] The basis of this association is unclear and may be multifactorial.[289] In one study of 102 adults with pulmonary Langerhans cell histiocytosis, six haematological cancers were identified.[319] A hypothetical relationship between Langerhans cell histiocytosis of the lung and pulmonary carcinoma may be explained by the sharing of an aetiological agent, such as cigarette smoking, rather than there being a direct cause-and-effect relationship.[324]

Pathological findings[286,287,325–327]

Microscopically, early lesions show a focal interstitial infiltrate of mitotically active Ki51- and Ki67-positive Langerhans cells intermingled with eosinophils (Fig. 6.1.40). The lesions are centred on the

Figure 6.1.40 Langerhans cell histiocytosis. (A) The Langerhans cells have vesicular nuclei and a moderate amount of pale cytoplasm that is devoid of phagocytosed material. Numerous eosinophils are also present. Immunostaining for S-100 (B) and CD1a (C) highlights the Langerhans cells.

Figure 6.1.41 Langerhans cell histiocytosis. The lesions are focal, peribronchiolar and interstitial.

Figure 6.1.42 Langerhans cell histiocytosis. A mixed mononuclear interstitial infiltrate has destroyed part of the bronchiolar wall. *(Reproduced from Corrin and Basset (1979)[287] with permission from* Investigative Cell Pathology.*)*

bronchioles (Figs 6.1.41 and 6.1.42), which are often weakened so that small cavities develop (Fig. 6.1.43). The cavitation may ultimately progress to gross cystic change (Fig. 6.1.44), which is responsible for the repeated pneumothoraces that are such a prominent clinical feature of the disease.

As the lesions heal, their appearances alter and they assume the form of stellate fibrous scars (Figs 6.1.45 and 6.1.46) in which Langerhans cells and eosinophils are no longer readily apparent, having been replaced by pigment-laden macrophages, lymphocytes, plasma cells and fibroblasts. The pigment in the macrophages is partly exogenous, and is largely derived from the cigarette smoke to which these patients have almost always been exposed, and partly endogenous – this component is generally Perls- and periodic acid–Schiff-positive and diastase-resistant. Old and active lesions are often found in the same specimen. At autopsy, interstitial fibrosis is widespread and there may be marked 'honeycombing': nevertheless, the predilection for the mid- and upper zones with sparing of the costophrenic angles, evident in life radiographically, is often still apparent after death (see Fig. 6.1.44). The fibrosis may be attributable

Figure 6.1.43 Langerhans cell histiocytosis showing microcystic change.

Figure 6.1.45 Pulmonary Langerhans cell histiocytosis. Older lesions often have a characteristically stellate outline.

Figure 6.1.44 Langerhans cell histiocytosis of the lung at autopsy. Severe fibrocystic change is seen at the apex of the upper lobe.

Figure 6.1.46 Pulmonary Langerhans cell histiocytosis. Small stellate scars on the cut surface represent healed lesions.

to fibroblast-stimulating cytokines such as platelet-derived growth factor, transforming growth factor-β, tumour necrosis factor-α and IL-1[97,328,329] and the cavitation to collagenolytic activity mediated by matrix metalloproteinases,[330,331] all of which have been demonstrated in Langerhans cells within active lesions.

The pulmonary hypertension is reflected in a proliferative vasculopathy involving both arteries and veins. It is suggested that this represents intrinsic pulmonary vascular disease, in which the pulmonary circulation is involved independently of the airway and parenchymal changes.[316]

Differential diagnosis

Differential pathological diagnoses include eosinophilic pneumonia (see p. 461), reactive eosinophilic pleuritis (see p. 711) and various patterns of interstitial pneumonia. The interstitial rather than intraluminal location of the eosinophils should indicate Langerhans cell histiocytosis (eosinophilic granuloma) rather than eosinophilic pneumonia, whereas an associated blood eosinophilia would favour the latter condition. HRCT patterns for these two disorders are also notably different. Reactive eosinophilic pleuritis is caused by pneumothorax and is limited to the pleura and subpleural lung tissue. IPF/UIP and fibrotic NSIP lack the focal centriacinar distribution of the lesions of eosinophilic granuloma. When Langerhans cell histiocytosis is completely inactive and the lung has reached an end stage of widespread 'honeycombing' common to many diseases, a definite histological diagnosis may no longer be possible but before this the focal distribution and stellate outline of the scars are very suggestive of burnt-out Langerhans cell histiocytosis.

The characteristic lesions are focal and may be obscured by other changes attributable to cigarette smoking, particularly smokers' macrophages filling the adjacent alveoli. DIP and respiratory bronchiolitis-associated interstitial lung disease (see pp. 311 and 313) often accompany Langerhans cell histiocytosis and hinder its recognition in this way.[332]

The immunocytochemical demonstration of CD1a, S-100 protein or fascin may be used to augment routine light microscopy[304-306] but positive results are only of significance in the right pathological setting. Langerhans cells and the related S-100-positive interdigitating dendritic cells are widely distributed and increased in a variety of reactive and neoplastic diseases[296,333]: CD1a, fascin and langerin are more specific than S-100 and can be detected in paraffin sections.[304-308] Negative results for these markers raise the possibility of histiocytic sarcoma which is exceptionally rare in the lung. However, it is recorded there, closely resembling Langerhans cell histiocytosis both clinically and histologically.[334] Langerhans cell sarcoma is quite different.[335] This sarcoma is also exceptionally rare in the lung but cases complicating pulmonary Langerhans cell histiocytosis are recorded.[336] It is distinguished from Langerhans cell histiocytosis histologically by the overt malignancy of its Langerhans cells, the nature of which may only be recognized by the characteristic staining reactions described above. Erdheim–Chester disease (see p. 492) is a further systemic histiocytic proliferation that may involve the lung. The cells are morphologically identical to those of Langerhans cell histiocytosis but, although they stain for S-100, they do not stain for CD1a and they lack Birbeck granules on electron microscopy. The distribution of disease is also different, following the path of the lymphatics rather than being primarily bronchiolocentric and partly cystic.[337,338]

The diagnosis has been made on transbronchial biopsy but surgical lung biopsy is generally required for a definite tissue diagnosis. Histological diagnosis is most difficult in the healing phase when Langerhans cells are poorly represented. At this stage immunocytochemistry is least helpful. The optimal applications of immunocytochemistry are probably in the examination of small fibreoptic specimens, in which the valuable architectural features evident in a surgical lung biopsy cannot be assessed, and in the evaluation of bronchoalveolar lavage cells.[339,340] Electron microscopy may also be used to identify Langerhans cells in lavage specimens but immunocytochemistry is more suited to the enumeration of lavage cells that is necessary for diagnosis. Patients with pulmonary Langerhans cell histiocytosis have an increased but variable number of Langerhans cells in their lavage fluid (1–25%) compared to normal non-smokers (fewer than 1%) and to normal smokers and patients with other interstitial lung diseases (up to 3%) (see Table A3, p. 760).[339,340] Thus, the sensitivity is low and lavage is therefore of limited diagnostic use.[313]

LYMPHANGIOLEIOMYOMATOSIS

Lymphangioleiomyomatosis is a rare but distinctive disease that in its fully developed state combines widespread proliferation of unusual smooth muscle in the lungs with lymphangioleiomyomas in thoraco-

abdominal lymph nodes.[341] However, either the lungs or the lymph nodes may be affected in isolation. A notable feature is that the disease is largely confined to women in the reproductive years. Onset is rare before the menarche[342] and after the menopause,[343-345] although it is being increasingly recognised in older women.[346] Very few men have been affected.[347-349] Of 243 patients enrolled in a national registry over a 3-year period, all were women. Their ages ranged from 18 to 76 years and the average age at onset of symptoms was 39 years.[350] Tuberous sclerosis was evident in 15%.

Aetiology

The fact that lymphangioleiomyomatosis is largely confined to women in the reproductive years suggests that it has a hormonal basis and this is supported by reports of exacerbations of the disease during pregnancy[351,352] and the menses,[353] and following oestrogen therapy.[354,355] Further support comes from the identification of oestrogen or progesterone receptors in the diseased lung tissue, and this presumably is responsible for the peculiar sex distribution.[356]

Lymphangioleiomyomatosis has long been recognised as having an intriguing relationship to tuberous sclerosis[341,357] and this has now been substantiated by molecular studies identifying mutation of a tuberous sclerosis gene in lung tissue showing lymphangioleiomyomatosis.[358-362] Stemming from these studies, two forms of tuberous sclerosis are now recognised (Table 6.1.10).[341,363-372] One is a dominant hereditary condition caused by mutation of the *TSC1* gene situated on chromosome 9. In these patients, the brain, skin and kidney are chiefly affected. Pulmonary lymphangioleiomyomatosis is clinically evident in only 2.3% of such patients[367] (but accounts for 10% of deaths).[364] In the second form of tuberous sclerosis, attributable to mutation of the *TSC2* gene located on chromosome 16, lymphangioleiomyomatosis is the dominant clinical manifestation and is responsible for most deaths.

The products of the *TSC1* and *TSC2* genes, respectively known as hamartin and tuberin, form a coiled complex that functions in multiple tumour suppressor roles in cell cycle control.[373] It is therefore not surprising that mutation of either gene results in increased cell growth. The *TSC2* form of tuberous sclerosis is often termed the sporadic form of pulmonary lymphangioleiomyomatosis. It would appear that the *TSC2* mutation is confined to certain somatic cells as this form of tuberous sclerosis is not hereditary: there is as yet no record of a woman suffering from sporadic pulmonary lymphangioleiomyomatosis giving birth to an affected child.

The demonstration of identical *TSC2* mutations in the pulmonary and renal lesions of a patient with sporadic lymphangioleiomyomatosis indicated that their constituent cells were derived from the same source and led to the suggestion that those comprising the pulmonary lesions had metastasised from the renal angiomyolipoma.[360] Metastatic spread (from lung to lung) also appears to be the explanation for recurrent lymphangioleiomyomatosis following transplantation, identical mutations being identified in the native and donor lungs, and angiomyolipoma being excluded at autopsy.[374,375] Clusters of the lesional cells enveloped by lymphatic endothelial cells have been identified within distant lymphatics and within chylous pleural and peritoneal fluid, suggesting that dissemination of the disease is by means of these smooth-muscle/lymphoendothelial cell packets.[376]

Tuberous sclerosis is referred to again on page 488 where further pulmonary manifestations are described.

Clinical features

Early studies indicated that patients with pulmonary lymphangioleiomyomatosis presented at an average age of 32–34 years[344,377-380] but with increasing recognition of the condition in older women the

Table 6.1.10 A comparison of the two forms of tuberous sclerosis[341,363–371]

	TSC1	TSC2 (sporadic lymphangioleiomyomatosis)
Family history	Common	Absent
Sex incidence	Equal	Almost exclusively female
Cerebral 'gliomas'	Present	Absent
Facial angiofibromas	Frequent	Absent
Cardiac rhabdomyomas	Occasionally present	Absent
Angiomyolipomas	Frequent	Frequent
Lymph node angioleiomyomatosis	Occasionally present	Occasionally present
Pulmonary lymphangioleiomyomatosis	Occasionally present	Present – the dominant feature
Multifocal type II pneumocyte hyperplasia	Occasionally present	Absent

If attention is concentrated on the occasional patients with classic (TSC1) tuberous sclerosis who have pulmonary involvement it is found that neurological disorders are rare and the sex incidence is overwhelmingly female. Clinically evident pulmonary lymphangioleiomyomatosis is initially found in only 2.3% of patients with classic (TSC1) tuberous sclerosis[367] but may be detected by computed tomography in 34–39% of women with this form of the disease[370,371] and accounts for 10% of deaths.

average age at presentation has shifted to 39–43 years.[346,350] Patients complain of breathlessness of insidious onset and are liable to develop any of three complications: repeated pneumothoraces, chylous effusions and pulmonary haemorrhage, all of which are satisfactorily explained by the pathological features of the disease, as outlined below.[341] The functional features are variable and may indicate obstructive, restrictive or mixed disease, generally with markedly reduced diffusing capacity, and a normal or mildly increased total lung capacity.[369,379,381–384] Bronchoalveolar lavage typically recovers haemosiderin-laden macrophages. Radiographically, the lungs show a reticular pattern but unlike fibrotic lungs they appear enlarged and ultimately show gross cystic change.[382] Septal lines (Kerley B) may be seen as a result of the lymphatic obstruction. The appearance on computed tomography is virtually diagnostic in the appropriate clinical context.[369,385] Thin-walled, well-defined cysts of fairly uniform size are evenly distributed throughout all lung zones: nodules are not a feature (Fig. 6.1.47).

The natural course of the disease is one of inexorable decline in respiratory function over a period of several years, inevitably culminating in death except in patients who reach the menopause, when the clinical state stabilises.[341,377,386] However, the rate of decline is very variable. Survival figures have progressively improved, probably due to a combination of improved patient management and early radiographic identification of the disease in asymptomatic women. Thus, 10-year survival figures of 20% were reported in 1975, 40% in 1995 and 79% in 1999.[341,352,387] Severe cystic change indicates advanced disease and a correspondingly worse prognosis.[387] Conversely, those patients in whom the lungs are spared and only extrapulmonary lymphatics are affected have a relatively good prognosis.[386,388] Treatment possibilities are discussed below.

Pathological findings

The essential pathological feature is a proliferation of unusual smooth-muscle cells that involves all parts of the lungs,[341,381,382] often in a focal manner. The smooth-muscle nature of the cells is not immediately apparent and they may be mistaken for fibroblasts. They are generally plump and spindle-shaped with pale eosinophilic cytoplasm (Fig. 6.1.48) but the cytoplasm may be clear and the cells polygonal in outline so that they appear epithelioid. Electron microscopy shows

Figure 6.1.47 Pulmonary lymphangioleiomyomatosis. Computed tomography shows thin-walled cystic spaces with no zonal distribution and no accompanying nodules.

them to have all the features of smooth muscle.[389] Immunostaining is in accord with this, both cell types being strongly positive for smooth-muscle actin.[390] However, an unusual feature is that 17–67% of the proliferating cells also react for the melanoma-related marker human melanin black-45 (HMB-45) (Fig. 6.1.49).[369,391–395] Electron microscopy shows the HMB-45 immunoreactivity to be localised to cytoplasmic inclusions similar to premelanosomes.[391] HMB-45 reactivity is a feature that lymphangioleiomyomatosis shares with the angiomyolipomas of tuberous sclerosis, benign clear cell tumour of the lung (see p. 625) and certain clear cell tumours at other sites, both benign and malignant.[396] The term 'perivascular epithelioid cell' has been applied as an encompassing term for the cell type from which these entities derive, although there is no normal counterpart; it is described as a mesenchymal cell that is either spindle-shaped or has a plump, glycogen-rich epithelioid phenotype, and variably

Figure 6.1.48 Pulmonary lymphangioleiomyomatosis. Spindle cells infiltrate the alveolar walls.

coexpresses actin, HMB-45, S-100, CD1a and cathepsin-k.[368,397-401] It is reported that HMB-45 and the receptors for oestrogen and progesterone are confined to the plump epithelioid cells whereas metalloproteases and proliferating-cell nuclear antigen are confined to the spindle cells.[368,391,402,403]

The alveolar walls are infiltrated by the unusual smooth-muscle cells and consequently thickened, often in nodular fashion. Narrow lymphatic channels are often evident within these cell collections.[404] At the periphery of the lesions the walls of bronchioles may be similarly infiltrated.[341] The interstitial connective tissue is increased[405] and structurally abnormal,[389,406] probably due to the protease activity exhibited by the spindle cells.[403,407] Consequent breakdown of the alveolar walls leads to focal cystic change, which ultimately culminates in gross 'honeycombing' throughout the lungs (Fig. 6.1.50). Airway collapse consequent upon this cystic change is the principal mechanism contributing to airflow limitation.[408] Rupture of the cysts explains the frequent pneumothoraces which are one of the distinctive complications of this disease. A histological score based on the severity of the cystic change and the degree of smooth-muscle infiltration has been shown to be of prognostic value.[409]

The proliferating cells also infiltrate blood vessels and the use of elastic stains demonstrates that small veins are often totally obliterated (Fig. 6.1.51).[341] This veno-occlusive process and perhaps direct capillary damage cause pulmonary haemorrhage, so explaining the haemoptyses that complicate the breathlessness. They also cause haemosiderosis (Fig. 6.1.52) and occasionally this is sufficiently severe to encrust the elastic laminae of pulmonary blood vessels with iron and calcium. Fragmentation of the encrusted elastin elicits a foreign-body giant cell reaction (so-called endogenous pneumoconiosis; see p. 449).

Involvement of lymphatics in the myoproliferative process and the development of lymphangioleiomyomas in mediastinal lymph nodes explain the frequent chylothoraces (Fig. 6.1.53).[341,410] Chyloptysis, chylous ascites and even chyluria may also develop.[353] The chylous effusions contain free-floating clumps of the lesional cells, so providing a useful source of these cells for special studies, but it is notable that mesothelial seedlings are not a feature of lymphangioleiomyomatosis.

The focal nature of the disease means that it may be difficult to identify the lesions in small biopsies, in which case the immunomarkers described above can be helpful, particularly smooth-muscle actin, HMB-45 and cathepsin-k.[400]

Figure 6.1.49 Pulmonary lymphangioleiomyomatosis. (A) Spindle cells evident in the walls of cystic spaces (arrows) stain for HMB-45(G). *(Case of Dr D. Schneider Coventry, UK.)*

Variant forms of the disease

In rare cases the lesional cells have a clear, glycogen-rich cytoplasm reminiscent of those comprising another form of 'PEComa', namely the clear cell tumour of the lung described on page 625.[411] Another unusual patient showed both a clear cell tumour and lymphangioleiomyomatosis limited to the right upper and middle lobes.[412] Occasionally pulmonary lymphangioleiomyomatosis is associated with micronodular type II pneumocyte hyperplasia (see p. 701) but this is to be regarded as an independent manifestation of tuberous sclerosis rather than a component of lymphangioleiomyomatosis.

Differential diagnosis

One of the conditions that histologically enters the differential diagnosis is IPF showing reactive hyperplasia of bronchiolar and vascular

Figure 6.1.51 Pulmonary lymphangioleiomyomatosis. Elastin staining reveals that small postcapillary blood vessels are infiltrated and their lumen markedly narrowed.

Figure 6.1.52 Pulmonary lymphangioleiomyomatosis. Occlusion of postcapillary blood vessels results in capillary rupture and haemosiderosis.

Figure 6.1.50 Pulmonary lymphangioleiomyomatosis. Infiltration of the alveolar walls weakens them, causing focal cystic change (A) and ultimately gross honeycombing (B). *(B courtesy of the late Dr AA Liebow, San Diego, USA.)*

Figure 6.1.53 Lymphangioleiomyoma of a mediastinal lymph node.

smooth muscle (so-called muscular cirrhosis of the lung, see Fig. 6.1.8C). However, the reactive smooth-muscle hyperplasia that accompanies fibrosis is quite mature and readily recognisable as such, whereas this is not the case in lymphangioleiomyomatosis. IPF also has an inflammatory component, which is not seen in lymphangioleiomyomatosis, and the reactive smooth muscle of IPF does not express HMB-45 or cathepsin-k. If doubt remains, HRCT will probably establish the diagnosis. Indeed, few cases now come to biopsy because of the high specificity of the imaging features, those that do often being smokers with a differential diagnosis of emphysema, which may coexist with lymphangioleiomyomatosis.

A further condition to be distinguished is that of so-called benign mestastasising leiomyomas (see p. 686).[413,414] This also affects women in the reproductive years and both conditions are to some extent hormonally dependent. However, the metastasising leiomyomas form distinct tumours – sharply outlined spherical masses that usually exceed 2 cm in diameter and may rarely be cystic. Histologically, they exactly reproduce the appearances of benign myometrial fibroids, containing smooth muscle that is readily recognisable as such, unlike the immature cells of lymphangioleiomyomatosis. Leiomyomas are also HMB-45-negative and the patients either have uterine fibroids or have had them removed. Although immature, lymphangioleiomyomatosis cells lack the atypia of a sarcoma, which was the diagnosis in what was probably the first report of the condition.[415] Lymphangiomatosis (see p. 632) is distinguished from lymphangioleiomyomatosis by being evidently vascular, confined to the major connective tissue planes of the lung and lacking the distinctive HMB-45-positive cells. Emphysema also lacks these cells, as do the metastases of endometrial stromal sarcoma,[416,417] two further conditions that have been mistaken for lymphangioleiomyomatosis.

Treatment

Because the disease is largely confined to women in the reproductive years attempts have been made to arrest the condition by oophorectomy, ovarian ablation with X-rays and hormonal manipulation.[418–423] Response has been varied and sometimes unrelated to sex steroid receptor analysis.[424] The oestrogen antagonist, tamoxifen, has often been employed but is probably best avoided as it may have agonist activity. Progesterone has also been widely employed but without significant benefit and few specialist centres now recommend hormonal therapy.[425,426]

For patients with progressive disease, lung transplantation offers an alternative treatment. It has been successfully performed in several patients[427] but recurrence in the allograft has been encountered, even with lungs obtained from male donors.[374,428,429] The source of the recurrent disease is discussed under aetiology.

The elucidation of the molecular mechanisms underlying tuberous sclerosis and lymphangioleiomyomatosis has led to the introduction of drugs targeting the growth factor that is normally inhibited by the hamartin/tuberin protein product of the tuberous sclerosis genes referred to above. One such agent is the mammalian target of rapamycin (mTOR) inhibitor sirolimus and trials of this drug are currently underway.[345,430,430a]

Metalloproteinases appear to play a role in the pathogenesis of lymphangioleiomyomatosis and because an ancillary action of the tetracycline antibiotic doxycyclin is the inhibition of these enzymes it has been proposed for the treatment of lymphangioleiomyomatosis.[431] Trials to assess the efficacy of doxycycline in lymphangioleiomyomatosis are currently underway.[430a]

Further in the future, the lymphangiogenic vascular endothelial growth factors C and D represent possible pharmacotherapeutic targets following the recent recognition that they are involved in the pathogenesis of lymphangioleiomyomatosis.[432]

Concern that children born to affected patients may suffer from tuberous sclerosis appears to be unwarranted and genetic counselling is not currently considered necessary, although pregnancy itself may be inadvisable because of reports of the lung disease being exacerbated during childbearing. An informative patient support group may be consulted at http://lam.uc.

REFERENCES

Usual interstitial pneumonia and idiopathic pulmonary fibrosis

1. Idiopathic pulmonary fibrosis: Diagnosis and treatment – International consensus statement. Am J Respir Crit Care Med 2000;161:646–64.
2. American Thoracic Society/European Respiratory. Society international multidisciplinary consensus classification of the idiopathic interstitial pneumonias. Am J Respir Crit Care Med 2002;165:277–304.
3. Raghu G, Collard HR, Egan J, et al. Idiopathic pulmonary fibrosis: evidence based guidelines for diagnosis and management. A joint ATS/ERS/JRS/ALAT statement. Am J Respir Crit Care Med, in press.
4. Flaherty KR, Travis WD, Colby TV, et al. Histopathologic variability in usual and nonspecific interstitial pneumonias. Am J Respir Crit Care Med 2001;164:1722–7.
5. Nicholson AG, Colby TV, Dubois RM, et al. The prognostic significance of the histologic pattern of interstitial pneumonia in patients presenting with the clinical entity of cryptogenic fibrosing alveolitis. Am J Respir Crit Care Med 2000;162:2213–17.
6. Katzenstein ALA, Zisman DA, Litzky LA, et al. Usual interstitial pneumonia – histologic study of biopsy and explant specimens. Am J Surg Pathol 2002;26:1567–77.
7. Monaghan H, Wells AU, Colby TV, et al. Prognostic implications of histologic patterns in multiple surgical lung. biopsies from patients with idiopathic interstitial pneumonias. Chest 2004;125:522–6.
8. Bjoraker JA, Ryu JH, Edwin MK, et al. Prognostic significance of histopathologic subsets in idiopathic pulmonary fibrosis. Am J Respir Crit Care Med 1998;157:199–203.
9. Travis WD, Matsui K, Moss J, et al. Idiopathic nonspecific interstitial pneumonia: Prognostic significance of cellular and fibrosing patterns – Survival comparison with usual interstitial pneumonia and desquamative interstitial pneumonia. Am J Surg Pathol 2000;24:19–33.
10. Hartman TE, Primack SL, Kang EY, et al. Disease progression in usual interstitial pneumonia compared with desquamative interstitial pneumonia: assessment with serial CT. Chest 1996;110:378–82.
11. Akira M, Yamamoto S, Hara H, et al. Serial computed tomographic evaluation in desquamative interstitial pneumonia. Thorax 1997;52:333–7.
12. Gribbin J, Hubbard RB, Le Jeune I, et al. Incidence and mortality of idiopathic pulmonary fibrosis and sarcoidosis in the UK. Thorax 2006;61:980–5.
13. Carrington CB, Gaensler EA, Coutu RE, et al. Natural history and treated course of usual and desquamative interstitial pneumonia. N Engl J Med 1978;298:801–9.
14. Turner-Warwick M, Burrows B, Johnson A. Cryptogenic fibrosing alveolitis: clinical

features and their influence on survival. Thorax 1980;35:171–80.

15. Baumgartner KB, Samet JM, Stidley CA, et al. Cigarette smoking: a risk factor for idiopathic pulmonary fibrosis. Am J Respir Crit Care Med 1997;155:242–8.

16. Johnston IDA, Prescott RJ, Chalmers JC, et al. British Thoracic Society study of cryptogenic fibrosing alveolitis: current presentation and initial management. Thorax 1997;52:38–44.

17. Hubbard R, Johnston I, Coultas DB, et al. Mortality rates from cryptogenic fibrosing alveolitis in seven countries. Thorax 1996;51:711–16.

18. Olson AL, Swigris JJ, Lezotte DC, et al. Mortality from pulmonary fibrosis increased in the United States from 1992 to 2003. Am J Respir Crit Care Med 2007;176:277–84.

19. Marshall RP, Puddicombe A, Cookson WOC, et al. Adult familial cryptogenic fibrosing alveolitis in the United Kingdom. Thorax 2000;55:143–6.

20. Lee HL, Ryu JH, Wittmer MH, et al. Familial idiopathic pulmonary fibrosis: clinical features and outcome. Chest 2005;127:2034–41.

21. Fishbein MC. Diagnosis: To biopsy or not to biopsy: assessing the role of surgical lung biopsy in the diagnosis of idiopathic pulmonary fibrosis. Chest 2005;128:520S-525.

22. Flaherty KR, Thwaite EL, Kazerooni EA, et al. Radiological versus histological diagnosis in UIP and NSIP: survival implications. Thorax 2003;58:143–8.

23. Rudd RM, Prescott RJ, Chalmers JC, et al. British Thoracic Society Study on cryptogenic fibrosing alveolitis: Response to treatment and survival. Thorax 2007;62:62–6.

24. Kondoh Y, Taniguchi H, Kawabata Y, et al. Acute exacerbation in idiopathic pulmonary fibrosis – analysis of clinical and pathologic findings in three cases. Chest 1993;103:1808–12.

25. Akira M. Computed tomography and pathologic findings in fulminant forms of idiopathic interstitial pneumonia. J Thorac Imaging 1999;14:76–84.

26. Vourlekis JS, Brown KK, Cool CD, et al. Acute interstitial pneumonitis. Case series and review of the literature. Medicine (Baltimore) 2000;79:369–78.

27. Ambrosini V, Cancellieri A, Chilosi M, et al. Acute exacerbation of idiopathic pulmonary fibrosis: report of a series. 22nd ed. 2003. p. 821–6.

28. Rice AJ, Wells AU, Bouros D, et al. Terminal diffuse alveolar damage in relation to interstitial pneumonias. An autopsy study. Am J Clin Pathol 2003;119:709–14.

29. Parambil JG, Myers JL, Ryu JH. Histopathologic features and outcome of patients with acute exacerbation of idiopathic pulmonary fibrosis undergoing surgical lung biopsy. Chest 2005;128:3310–15.

30. Parambil JG, Myers JL, Aubry MC, et al. Causes and prognosis of diffuse alveolar damage diagnosed on surgical lung biopsy. Chest 2007;132:50–7.

31. Collard HR, Moore BB, Flaherty KR, et al. Acute exacerbations of idiopathic pulmonary fibrosis. Am J Respir Crit Care Med 2007;176:636–43.

32. Daniels CE, Yi ES, Ryu JH. Autopsy findings in 42 consecutive patients with idiopathic pulmonary fibrosis. Eur Respir J 2008;32:170–4.

33. Douglas WW, Ryu JH, Schroeder DR. Idiopathic pulmonary fibrosis – impact of oxygen and colchicine, prednisone, or no therapy on survival. Am J Respir Crit Care Med 2000;161:1172–8.

34. Ziesche R, Hofbauer E, Wittmann K, et al. A preliminary study of long-term treatment with interferon gamma-1b and low-dose prednisolone in patients with idiopathic pulmonary fibrosis. N Engl J Med 1999;341:1264–9.

35. King TE Jr, Albera C, Bradford WZ, et al. Effect of interferon gamma-1b on survival in patients with idiopathic pulmonary fibrosis (INSPIRE): a multicentre, randomised, placebo-controlled trial. Lancet 2009;374:222–8.

36. Raghu G, Brown KK, Costabel U, et al. Treatment of idiopathic pulmonary fibrosis with etanercept: an exploratory, placebo-controlled trial. Am J Respir Crit Care Med 2008;178:948–55.

37. Daniels CE, Lasky JA, Limper AH, et al. Imatinib treatment for IPF: randomized placebo controlled trial results. Am J Respir Crit Care Med 2010;181:601–10.

38. Demedts M, Behr J, Buhl R, et al. High-dose acetylcysteine in idiopathic pulmonary fibrosis. N Engl J Med 2005;353:2229–42.

39. King TE Jr, Behr J, Brown KK, et al. BUILD-1: a randomized placebo-controlled trial of bosentan in idiopathic pulmonary fibrosis. Am J Respir Crit Care Med 2008;177:75–81.

40. Azuma A, Nukiwa T, Tsuboi E, et al. Double-blind, placebo-controlled trial of pirfenidone in patients with idiopathic pulmonary fibrosis. Am J Respir Crit Care Med 2005;171:1040–7.

41. Taniguchi H, Ebina M, Kondoh Y, et al. Pirfenidone in idiopathic pulmonary fibrosis. Eur Respir J 2010.

42. Kubo H, Nakayama K, Yanai M, et al. Anticoagulant therapy for idiopathic pulmonary fibrosis. Chest 2005;128:1475–82.

43. Honore I, Nunes H, Groussard O, et al. Acute respiratory failure after interferon-gamma therapy of end-stage pulmonary fibrosis. Am J Respir Crit Care Med 2003;167:953–7.

44. Selman M, Thannickal VJ, Pardo A, et al. Idiopathic pulmonary fibrosis: pathogenesis and therapeutic approaches. Drugs 2004;64:405–30.

45. Bajwa EK, Ayas NT, Schulzer M, et al. Interferon-gamma1b therapy in idiopathic pulmonary fibrosis: a metaanalysis. Chest 2005;128:203–6.

46. Williams TJ, Wilson JW. Challenges in pulmonary fibrosis: 7–Novel therapies and lung transplantation. Thorax 2008;63:277–84.

47. Maher TM, Wells AU, Laurent GJ. Idiopathic pulmonary fibrosis: multiple causes and multiple mechanisms? Eur Respir J 2007;30:835–9.

48. Yamashita M, Yamauchi K, Chiba R, et al. The definition of fibrogenic processes in fibroblastic foci of idiopathic pulmonary fibrosis based on morphometric quantification of extracellular matrices. Human Pathology 2009;40:1278–87.

49. Nicholson AG, Fulford LG, Colby TV, et al. The relationship between individual histologic features and disease progression in idiopathic pulmonary fibrosis. Am J Respir Crit Care Med 2002;166:173–7.

50. Tiitto L, Bloigu R, Heiskanen U, et al. Relationship between histopathological features and the course of idiopathic pulmonary fibrosis/usual interstitial pneumonia. Thorax 2006;61:1091–5.

51. Collard HR, Cool CD, Leslie KO, et al. Organizing pneumonia and lymphoplasmacytic inflammation predict treatment response in idiopathic pulmonary fibrosis. Histopathology 2007;50:258–65.

52. Hanak V, Ryu JH, de Carvalho E, et al. Profusion of fibroblast foci in patients with idiopathic pulmonary fibrosis does not predict outcome. Respiratory Medicine 2008;102:852–6.

53. Song JW, Do KH, Kim MY, et al. Pathologic and radiologic differences between idiopathic and collagen vascular disease-related usual interstitial pneumonia. Chest 2009;136:23–30.

54. Katzenstein ALA, Myers JL. Idiopathic pulmonary fibrosis: clinical relevance of pathologic classification. Am J Respir Crit Care Med 1998;157:1301–15.

55. Yousem SA. Eosinophilic pneumonia-like areas in idiopathic usual interstitial pneumonia. Modern Pathol 2000;13:1280–4.

56. Kawabata Y, Hoshi E, Murai K, et al. Smoking-related changes in the background lung of specimens resected for lung cancer: a semiquantitative study with correlation to postoperative course. Histopathology 2008;53:707–14.

57. Coalson JJ. The ultrastructure of human fibrosing alveolitis. Virchows Arch A Pathol Anat Histopathol 1982;395:181–99.

58. Corrin B, Dewar A, Rodriguez-Roisin R, et al. Fine structural changes in

cryptogenic fibrosing alveolitis and asbestosis. J Pathol 1985;147: 107–19.

59. Katzenstein ALA. Pathogenesis of 'fibrosis' in interstitial pneumonia: an electron microscopic study. Hum Pathol 1985;16:1015–24.

60. Scadding JG, Hinson KFW. Diffuse fibrosing alveolitis (diffuse interstitial fibrosis of the lungs): correlation of histology at biopsy with prognosis. Thorax 1967;22:291–304.

61. Stack BHR, Choo-Kang YFJ, Heard BE. The prognosis of cryptogenic fibrosing alveolitis. Thorax 1972;27:535–42.

62. Nicholson AG, Addis BJ, Bharucha H, et al. Inter-observer variation between pathologists in diffuse parenchymal lung disease. Thorax 2004;59:500–5.

62a. Cavazza A, Rossi G, Carbonelli C, Spaggiari L, Paci M, Roggeri A. The role of histology in idiopathic pulmonary fibrosis: An update. Respiratory Medicine 2010;104:S11–22.

63. Katzenstein ALA, Mukhopadhyay S, Myers JL. Diagnosis of usual interstitial pneumonia and distinction from other fibrosing interstitial lung diseases. Hum Pathol 2008;39:1275–94.

64. Katzenstein ALA, Mukhopadhyay S, Myers JL. Erratum to 'Diagnosis of usual interstitial pneumonia and distinction from other fibrosing interstitial lung diseases' [Hum Pathol 39 (2008) 1275–1294]. Human Pathology 2008;39:1562–81.

65. Coleman A, Colby TV. Histologic diagnosis of extrinsic allergic alveolitis. Am J Surg Pathol 1988;12:514–18.

66. Churg A, Muller NL, Flint J, et al. Chronic hypersensitivity pneumonitis. Am J Surg Pathol 2006;30:201–8.

67. Silva CI, Muller NL, Lynch DA, et al. Chronic hypersensitivity pneumonitis: differentiation from idiopathic pulmonary fibrosis and nonspecific interstitial pneumonia by using thin-section CT. Radiology 2008;246:288–97.

68. Corte TJ, Wort SJ, Gatzoulis MA, et al. Pulmonary vascular resistance predicts early mortality in patients with diffuse fibrotic lung disease and suspected pulmonary hypertension. Thorax 2009;64:883–8.

69. Hardie WD, Glasser SW, Hagood JS. Emerging concepts in the pathogenesis of lung fibrosis. Am J Pathol 2009;175: 3–16.

70. Strieter RM, Mehrad B. New mechanisms of pulmonary fibrosis. Chest 2009;136:1364–70.

71. Scadding JG. Fibrosing alveolitis. BMJ 1964;2:686.

72. Turner-Warwick M, Doniach D. Auto-antibody studies in interstitial pulmonary fibrosis. BMJ 1965;1:886–91.

73. Wallace WAH, Roberts SN, Caldwell H, et al. Circulating antibodies to lung

protein(s) in patients with cryptogenic fibrosing alveolitis. Thorax 1994;49:218–24.

74. Wallace WAH, Schofield JA, Lamb D, et al. Localisation of a pulmonary autoantigen in cryptogenic fibrosing alveolitis. Thorax 1994;49:1139–45.

75. Haslam PL, Thompson B, Mohammed I, et al. Circulating immune complexes in patients with cryptogenic fibrosing alveolitis. Clin Exp Immunol 1979;37:381–90.

76. Schwarz MI, Dreisin RB, Pratt DS, et al. Immunofluorescent patterns in the idiopathic interstitial pneumonias. J Lab Clin Med 1978;91:929–38.

77. Fox B, Shousha S, James KR, et al. Immunohistological study of human lungs by immunoperoxidase technique. J Clin Pathol 1982;35:144–50.

78. Hubbard R, Lewis S, Richards K, et al. Occupational exposure to metal or wood dust and aetiology of cryptogenic fibrosing alveolitis. Lancet 1996;347:284–9.

79. Hubbard R. Occupational dust exposure and the aetiology of cryptogenic fibrosing alveolitis. Eur Resp J 2001;18: 119S–21S.

80. Tobin RW, Pope CE, Pellegrini CA, et al. Increased prevalence of gastroesophageal reflux in patients with idiopathic pulmonary fibrosis. Am J Respir Crit Care Med 1998;158:1804–8.

81. Meliconi R, Andreone P, Fasano L, et al. Incidence of hepatitis C virus infection in Italian patients with idiopathic pulmonary fibrosis. Thorax 1996;51:315–17.

82. Kuwano K, Nomoto Y, Kunitake R, et al. Detection of adenovirus E1A DNA in pulmonary fibrosis using nested polymerase chain reaction. Eur Resp J 1997;10:1445–9.

83. Yonemaru M, Kasuga I, Kusumoto H, et al. Elevation of antibodies to cytomegalovirus and other herpes viruses in pulmonary fibrosis. Eur Resp J 1997;10:2040–5.

84. Tsukamoto K, Hayakawa H, Sato A, et al. Involvement of Epstein–Barr virus latent membrane protein 1 in disease progression in patients with idiopathic pulmonary fibrosis. Thorax 2000;55:958–61.

85. Bando M, Ohno S, Oshikawa K, et al. Infection of TT virus in patients with idiopathic pulmonary fibrosis. Resp Med 2001;95:935–42.

86. Kelly BG, Lok SS, Hasleton PS, et al. A rearranged form of Epstein–Barr virus DNA is associated with idiopathic pulmonary fibrosis. Am J Respir Crit Care Med 2002;166:510–3.

87. Hubbard R, Venn A, Smith C, et al. Exposure to commonly prescribed drugs and the etiology of cryptogenic fibrosing alveolitis: A case-control study. Am J Respir Crit Care Med 1998;157:743–7.

88. Britton J, Hubbard R. Recent advances in the aetiology of cryptogenic fibrosing

alveolitis. Histopathology 2000;37:387–92.

89. Elicker BM, Golden JA, Ordovas KG, et al. Progression of native lung fibrosis in lung transplant recipients with idiopathic pulmonary fibrosis. Respiratory Medicine 2010;104:426–33.

90. Steele MP, Speer MC, Loyd JE, et al. Clinical and pathologic features of familial interstitial pneumonia. Am J Respir Crit Care Med 2005;172:1146–52.

91. Musk AW, Zilko PJ, Manners P, et al. Genetic studies in familial fibrosing alveolitis. Possible linkage with immunoglobulin allotypes (Gm). Chest 1986;89:206–10.

92. Geddes DM, Webley M, Brewerton DA, et al. alpha 1-antitrypsin phenotypes in fibrosing alveolitis and rheumatoid arthritis. Lancet 1977;2:1049–51.

93. Lane KB, Marney A, Phillips JA, et al. Familial interstitial pulmonary fibrosis and linkage to chromosome 14. Chest 2001;120:75S–6S.

94. Thomas AQ, Lane K, Phillips J III, et al. Heterozygosity for a surfactant protein C gene mutation associated with usual interstitial pneumonitis and cellular nonspecific interstitial pneumonitis in one kindred. Am J Respir Crit Care Med 2002;165:1322–8.

95. Armanios MY, Chen JJ, Cogan JD, et al. Telomerase mutations in families with idiopathic pulmonary fibrosis. N Engl J Med 2007;356:1317–26.

96. Rosas IO, Ren P, Avila NA, et al. Early interstitial lung disease in familial pulmonary fibrosis. Am J Respir Crit Care Med 2007;176:698–705.

97. Corrin B, Butcher D, McAnulty BJ, et al. Immunohistochemical localization of transforming growth factor- beta(1) in the lungs of patients with systemic sclerosis, cryptogenic fibrosing alveolitis and other lung disorders. Histopathology 1994;24:145–50.

98. Wallace WAH, Howie SEM. Upregulation of tenascin and TGF beta production in a type II alveolar epithelial cell line by antibody against a pulmonary auto-antigen. J Pathol 2001;195:251–6.

99. Bergeron A, Soler P, Kambouchner M, et al. Cytokine profiles in idiopathic pulmonary fibrosis suggest an important role for TGF-beta and IL-10. Eur Resp J 2003;22:69–76.

100. Giaid A, Michel RP, Stewart DJ, et al. Expression of endothelin-1 in lungs of patients with cryptogenic fibrosing alveolitis. Lancet 1993;341: 1550–4.

101. Nash JRG, McLaughlin PJ, Butcher D, et al. Expression of tumour necrosis factor-alpha in cryptogenic fibrosing alveolitis. Histopathology 1993;22:343–7.

102. Uh ST, Inoue Y, King TE, et al. Morphometric analysis of insulin-like growth factor-I localization in lung tissues

of patients with idiopathic pulmonary fibrosis. Am J Respir Crit Care Med 1998;158:1626–35.

103. Kimura T, Ishii Y, Yoh K, et al. Overexpression of the transcription factor GATA-3 enhances the development of pulmonary fibrosis. Am J Pathol 2006;169:96–104.

104. Koli K, Myllarniemi M, Vuorinen K, et al. Bone morphogenetic protein-4 inhibitor gremlin is overexpressed in idiopathic pulmonary fibrosis. Am J Pathol 2006;169:61–71.

105. Pan LH, Yamauchi K, Uzuki M, et al. Type II alveolar epithelial cells and interstitial fibroblasts express connective tissue growth factor in IPF. Eur Resp J 2001;17:1220–7.

106. Choi ES, Pierce EM, Jakubzick C, et al. Focal interstitial CC chemokine receptor 7 (CCR7) expression in idiopathic interstitial pneumonia. J Clin Pathol 2006;59:28–39.

107. Fukuda Y, Ishizaki M, Kudoh S, et al. Localization of matrix metalloproteinases-1, -2, and -9 and tissue inhibitor of metalloproteinase-2 in interstitial lung diseases. Lab Invest 1998;78:687–98.

108. Thannickal VJ, Toews GB, White ES, et al. Mechanisms of pulmonary fibrosis. Annu Rev Med 2004;55:395–417.

109. Burkhardt A. Alveolitis and collapse in the pathogenesis of pulmonary fibrosis. Am Rev Respir Dis 1989;140:513–24.

110. Basset F, Ferrans VJ, Soler P, et al. Intraluminal fibrosis in interstitial lung disorders. Am J Pathol 1986;122:443–61.

111. Kondo A, Saiki S. Acute exacerbation in idiopathic interstitial pneumonia. In: Harasawa M, Fukuchi Y, Morinari H, editors. Interstitial Pneumonia of Unknown Etiology. Tokyo: University of Tokyo Press; 1989. p. 33–42.

113. Fukuda Y, Basset F, Ferrans VJ, et al. Significance of early intra-alveolar fibrotic lesions and integrin expression in lung biopsy specimens from patients with idiopathic pulmonary fibrosis. Hum Pathol 1995;26:53–61.

114. King TE, Schwarz MI, Brown K, et al. Idiopathic pulmonary fibrosis – relationship between histopathologic features and mortality. Am J Respir Crit Care Med 2001;164:1025–32.

115. Enomoto N, Suda T, Kato M, et al. Quantitative analysis of fibroblastic foci in usual interstitial pneumonia. Chest 2006;130:22–9.

116. Brody AR, Craighead JE. Interstitial associations of cells lining air spaces in human pulmonary fibrosis. Virchows Arch A Pathol Anat Histopathol 1976;372:39–49.

117. Adamson IYR, Hedgecock C, Bowden DH. Epithelial cell–fibroblast interactions in lung injury and repair. Am J Pathol 1990;137:385–92.

118. Guarino M, Tosoni A, Nebuloni M. Direct contribution of epithelium to organ fibrosis: epithelial-mesenchymal transition. Human Pathology 2009;40:1365–76.

119. Harada T, Nabeshima K, Hamasaki M, et al. Epithelial–mesenchymal transition in human lungs with usual interstitial pneumonia: quantitative immunohistochemistry. Pathol Int 2010;60:14–21.

120. Maher TM, Wells AU. Optimal treatment for idiopathic pulmonary fibrosis. Thorax 2008;63:1120–1.

121. Selman M, Pardo A, Barrera L, et al. Gene expression profiles distinguish idiopathic pulmonary fibrosis from hypersensitivity pneumonitis. Am J Respir Crit Care Med 2006;173:188–98.

122. Kradin RL, Divertie MB, Colvin RB, et al. Usual interstitial pneumonitis is a T cell alveolitis. Clin Immunol Immunopathol 1986;40:224–35.

123. Wells AU, Lorimer S, Majumdar S, et al. Fibrosing alveolitis in systemic sclerosis: increase in memory T-cells in lung interstitium. Eur Respir J 1995;8:266–71.

124. Kallenberg CGM, Schilizzi BM, Beaumont F, et al. Expression of class II major histocompatibility complex antigens on alveolar epithelium in interstitial lung disease: relevance to pathogenesis of idiopathic pulmonary fibrosis. J Clin Pathol 1987;40:725–33.

125. Komatsu T, Yamamoto M, Shimokata K, et al. Phenotypic characterization of alveolar capillary endothelial cells, alveolar epithelial cells and alveolar macrophages in patients with pulmonary fibrosis with special reference to MHC class II antigens. Virchows Arch A Pathol Anat Histopathol 1989;415:79–90.

126. Jakubzick C, Choi ES, Kunkel SL, et al. Augmented pulmonary IL-4 and IL-13 receptor subunit expression in idiopathic interstitial pneumonia. J Clin Pathol 2004;57:477–86.

127. Obayashi Y, Yamadori I, Fujita J, et al. The role of neutrophils in the pathogenesis of idiopathic pulmonary fibrosis. Chest 1997;112:1338–43.

128. Martin WJ. Neutrophils kill pulmonary endothelial cells by a hydrogen-peroxide-dependent pathway. An in vitro model of neutrophil-mediated lung injury. Am Rev Respir Dis 1984;130:209–13.

129. Ayars GH, Altman LC, Rosen H, et al. The injurious effect of neutrophils on pneumocytes in vitro. Am Rev Respir Dis 1984;130:964–73.

130. Donaldson K, Slight J, Brown GM, et al. The ability of inflammatory bronchoalveolar leucocyte populations elicited with microbes or mineral dust to injure alveolar epithelial cells and degrade extracellular matrix in vitro. Br J Exp Pathol 1988;69:327–38.

131. Chanez P, Lacoste JY, Guillot B, et al. Mast cells' contribution to the fibrosing

alveolitis of the scleroderma lung. Am Rev Respir Dis 1993;147:1497–502.

132. Hunt LW, Colby TV, Weiler DA, et al. Immunofluorescent staining for mast cells in idiopathic pulmonary fibrosis – quantification and evidence for extracellular release of mast cell tryptase. Mayo Clin Proc 1992;67:941–8.

133. Heard BE, Dewar A, Corrin B. Apposition of fibroblasts to mast cells and lymphocytes in normal human lung and in cryptogenic fibrosing alveolitis – ultrastructure and cell perimeter measurements. J Pathol 1992;166:303–10.

134. Inoue Y, King TE, Tinkle SS, et al. Human mast cell basic fibroblast growth factor in pulmonary fibrotic disorders. Am J Pathol 1996;149:2037–54.

135. Inoue Y, King TE, Barker E, et al. Basic fibroblast growth factor and its receptors in idiopathic pulmonary fibrosis and lymphangioleiomyomatosis. Am J Respir Crit Care Med 2002;166:765–73.

136. Edwards ST, Cruz AC, Donnelly S, et al. c-Kit immunophenotyping and metalloproteinase expression profiles of mast cells in interstitial lung diseases. J Pathol 2005;206:279–90.

137. Spencer H. Interstitial pneumonia. Ann Rev Med 1967;18:423–42.

138. Magro CM, Allen J, PopeHarman A, et al. The role of microvascular injury in the evolution of idiopathic pulmonary fibrosis. Am J Clin Pathol 2003;119:556–67.

139. Renzoni EA. Neovascularization in idiopathic pulmonary fibrosis: too much or too little? Am J Respir Crit Care Med 2004;169:1179–80.

140. Hubbard R, Venn A, Lewis S, et al. Lung cancer and cryptogenic fibrosing alveolitis – A population- based cohort study. Am J Respir Crit Care Med 2000;161:5–8.

141. Park J, Kim DS, Shim TS, et al. Lung cancer in patients with idiopathic pulmonary fibrosis. Eur Resp J 2001;17:1216–9.

142. Turner-Warwick M, Lebowitz M, Burrows B, et al. Cryptogenic fibrosing alveolitis and lung cancer. Thorax 1980;35:496–9.

143. Harris JM, Johnston IDA, Rudd R, et al. Cryptogenic fibrosing alveolitis and lung cancer: the BTS study. Thorax 2010;65:70–6.

144. Hojo S, Fujita J, Yamadori I, et al. Heterogeneous point mutations of the p53 gene in pulmonary fibrosis. Eur Resp J 1998;12:1404–8.

145. Kumar P, Goldstraw P, Yamada K, et al. Pulmonary fibrosis and lung cancer: risk and benefit analysis of pulmonary resection. J Thorac Cardiovasc Surg 2003;125:1321–7.

146. Nicholson AG, Wotherspoon AC, Jones AL, et al. Pulmonary B-cell non-Hodgkin's lymphoma associated with autoimmune

disorders: a clinicopathological review of six cases. Eur Respir J 1996;9:2022–5.

Non-specific interstitial pneumonia

147. Ognibene FP, Masur H, Rogers P, et al. Nonspecific interstitial pneumonitis without evidence of *Pneumocystis carinii* in asymptomatic patients infected with human immunodeficiency virus (HIV). Ann Intern Med 1988;109:874–9.

148. Katzenstein ALA, Fiorelli RF. Nonspecific interstitial pneumonia/fibrosis – histologic features and clinical significance. Am J Surg Pathol 1994;18:136–47.

149. Daniil ZD, Gilchrist FC, Nicholson AG, et al. A histologic pattern of nonspecific interstitial pneumonia is associated with a better prognosis than usual interstitial pneumonia in patients with cryptogenic fibrosing alveolitis. Am J Respir Crit Care Med 1999;160:899–905.

150. Nagai S, Kitaichi M, Itoh H, et al. Idiopathic nonspecific interstitial pneumonia/fibrosis: comparison with idiopathic pulmonary fibrosis and BOOP. Eur Resp J 1998;12:1010–9.

151. Travis WD, Hunninghake G, King TE Jr, et al. Idiopathic nonspecific interstitial pneumonia: report of an American Thoracic Society Project. Am J Respir Crit Care Med 2008;177:1338–47.

152. Park IN, Jegal Y, Kim DS, et al. Clinical course and lung function change of idiopathic nonspecific interstitial pneumonia. Eur Respir J 2009;33: 68–76.

153. Lima MS, Coletta EN, Ferreira RG, et al. Subacute and chronic hypersensitivity pneumonitis: histopathological patterns and survival. Respir Med 2009;103:508–15.

154. Flaherty KR, Martinez FJ. Nonspecific interstitial pneumonia. Semin Respir Crit Care Med 2006;27:652–8.

155. Tansey D, Wells AU, Colby TV, et al. Variations in histological patterns of interstitial pneumonia between connective tissue disorders and their relationship to prognosis. Histopathology 2004;44:585–96.

156. Nicholson AG, Wells AU. Nonspecific interstitial pneumonia – Nobody said it's perfect. Am J Respir Crit Care Med 2001;164:1553–4.

157. Hartman TE, Swensen SJ, Hansell DM, et al. Nonspecific interstitial pneumonia: variable appearance at high-resolution chest CT. Radiology 2000;217:701–5.

158. Bouros D, Wells AU, Nicholson AG, et al. Histopathologic subsets of fibrosing alveolitis in patients with systemic sclerosis and their relationship to outcome. Am J Respir Crit Care Med 2002;165:1581–6.

159. Douglas WW, Tazelaar HD, Hartman TE, et al. Polymyositis-dermatomyositis-associated interstitial lung disease. Am J Respir Crit Care Med 2001;164:1182–5.

160. Ito I, Nagai S, Kitaichi M, et al. Pulmonary manifestations of primary sjögren's syndrome: a clinical, radiologic, and pathologic study. Am J Respir Crit Care Med 2005;171:632–8.

161. Lee HK, Kim DS, Yoo B, et al. Histopathologic pattern and clinical features of rheumatoid arthritis-associated interstitial lung disease. Chest 2005;127:2019–27.

162. Kinder BW, Collard HR, Koth L, et al. Idiopathic nonspecific interstitial pneumonia: lung manifestation of undifferentiated connective tissue disease? Am J Respir Crit Care Med 2007;176:691–7.

163. Craig PJ, Wells AU, Doffman S, et al. Desquamative interstitial pneumonia, respiratory bronchiolitis and their relationship to smoking. Histopathology 2004;45:275–82.

164. Cottin V, Donsbeck AV, Revel D, et al. Nonspecific interstitial pneumonia: Individualization of a clinicopathologic entity in a series of 12 patients. Am J Respir Crit Care Med 1998;158: 1286–93.

165. Veeraraghavan S, Latsi PI, Wells AU, et al. BAL findings in idiopathic nonspecific interstitial pneumonia and usual interstitial pneumonia. Euro Resp J 2003;22:239–44.

166. MacDonald SL, Rubens MB, Hansell DM, et al. Nonspecific interstitial pneumonia and usual interstitial pneumonia: comparative appearances at and diagnostic accuracy of thin-section CT. Radiology 2001;221:600–5.

167. Akira M, Inoue G, Yamamoto S, et al. Non-specific interstitial pneumonia: findings on sequential CT scans of nine patients. Thorax 2000;55:854–9.

168. Park IN, Kim DS, Shim TS, et al. Acute exacerbation of interstitial pneumonia other than idiopathic pulmonary fibrosis. Chest 2007;132:214–20.

169. Park JH, Kim DS, Park IN, et al. Prognosis of fibrotic interstitial pneumonia: idiopathic versus collagen vascular disease-related subtypes. Am J Respir Crit Care Med 2007;175:705–11.

Acute interstitial pneumonia (idiopathic diffuse alveolar damage)

170. Katzenstein A-LA, Myers JL, Mazur MT. Acute interstitial pneumonia. A clinicopathologic, ultrastructural, and cell kinetic study. Am J Surg Pathol 1986;10:256–67.

171. Hamman L, Rich AR. A clinico-pathological conference. Internat Clin 1933;1:197.

172. Hamman L, Rich AR. Fulminating diffuse interstitial fibrosis of the lungs. Trans Am Clin &Climatol Assn 1935;51:154.

173. Hamman L, Rich AR. Acute diffuse interstitial fibrosis of the lungs. Bull Johns Hopkins Hospital 1944;74:177–212.

174. Olson J, Colby TV, Elliott CG. Hamman–Rich syndrome revisited. Mayo Clin Proc 1990;65:1538–48.

175. Colby TV. Pathologic aspects of bronchiolitis obliterans organizing pneumonia. Chest 1992;102:S38-43.

Idiopathic bronchiolocentric interstitial pneumonia

176. Yousem SA, Dacic S. Idiopathic bronchiolocentric interstitial pneumonia. Modern Pathol 2002;15:1148–53.

177. deCarvalho MEP, Kairalla RA, Capelozzi VL, et al. Centrilobular fibrosis: A novel histological pattern of idiopathic interstitial pneumonia. Pathol Res Pract 2002;198:577–83.

178. Churg A, Myers J, Suarez T, et al. Airway-centered interstitial fibrosis – A distinct form of aggressive diffuse lung disease. Amer J Surg Pathol 2004;28: 62–8.

Extrinsic allergic alveolitis (hypersensitivity pneumonia)

179. Bourke SJ, Dalphin JC, Boyd G, et al. Hypersensitivity pneumonitis: current concepts. Eur Resp J 2001;18:81S–92S.

180. Hapke EJ, Seal RME, Thomas GO, et al. Farmer's lung. Thorax 1968;23:451–68.

181. Hendrick DJ, Faux JA, Marshall R. Budgerigar-fancier's lung: the commonest variety of allergic alveolitis in Britain. BMJ 1978;2:81–4.

182. Ando M, Arima K, Yoneda R, et al. Japanese summer-type hypersensitivity pneumonitis – geographic distribution, home environment, and clinical characteristics of 621 cases. Am Rev Respir Dis 1991;144:765–9.

183. Bang KM, Weissman DN, Pinheiro GA, et al. Twenty-three years of hypersensitivity pneumonitis mortality surveillance in the United States. Am J Ind Med 2006;49:997–1004.

184. Hanak V, Golbin JM, Ryu JH. Causes and presenting features in 85 consecutive patients with hypersensitivity pneumonitis. Mayo Clin Proc 2007;82:812–6.

185. Warren CPW. Extrinsic allergic alveolitis: a disease commoner in non-smokers. Thorax 1977;32:567–9.

186. Godfrey RC, Evans CC. A national survey of bird fanciers' lung: including its possible association with jejunal villous atrophy. Br J Dis Chest 1984;78:75–88.

187. Franquet T, Hansell DM, Senbanjo T, et al. Lung cysts in subacute hypersensitivity pneumonitis. J Comput Assist Tomogr 2003;27:475–8.

188. Seal RME, Hapke EJ, Thomas GO, et al. The pathology of the acute and chronic stages of farmer's lung. Thorax 1968;23:469–89.

189. Reyes CN, Wenzel FJ, Lawton BR, et al. The pulmonary pathology of farmer's lung disease. Chest 1982;81:142–6.

190. Kawanami O, Basset F, Barrios R, et al. Hypersensitivity pneumonitis in man. Light- and electron-microscopic studies of 18 lung biopsies. Am J Pathol 1983;110:275–89.

191. Takemura T, Akashi T, Ohtani Y, et al. Pathology of hypersensitivity pneumonitis. Curr Opin Pulm Med 2008;14:440–54.

192. Barrowcliff DF, Arblaster PG. Farmer's lung: a study of an early acute fatal case. Thorax 1968;23:490–3.

193. Ghose T, Landrigan P, Killeen R, et al. Immunopathological studies in patients with farmer's lung. Clin Allergy 1974;4:119–29.

194. Vourlekis JS, Schwarz MI, Cherniack RM, et al. The effect of pulmonary fibrosis on survival in patients with hypersensitivity pneumonitis. Am J Med 2004;116:662–8.

195. Lima MS, Coletta ENAM, Ferreira RG, et al. Subacute and chronic hypersensitivity pneumonitis: Histopathological patterns and survival. Respiratory Medicine 2009;103:508–15.

196. Pepys J. Clinical and therapeutic significance of patterns of allergic reactions of the lungs to extrinsic agents. Am Rev Respir Dis 1977;116:573–88.

197. Roberts RC, Moore VL. Immunopathogenesis of hypersensitivity pneumonitis. Am Rev Respir Dis 1977;116:1075–90.

198. Williams JV. Inhalation and skin tests with extracts of hay and fungi in patients with farmer's lung. Thorax 1963;18:182–96.

199. Spector WG, Heesom N. The production of granulomata by antigen-antibody complexes. J Pathol 1969;98:31–9.

200. Hansen PJ, Penny R. Pigeon-breeder's disease. Study of the cell-mediated immune response to pigeon antigens by the lymphocyte culture technique. Int Arch Allergy Appl Immunol 1974;47:498–507.

201. Takizawa H, Ohta K, Horiuchi T, et al. Hypersensitivity pneumonitis in athymic nude mice – additional evidence of T-cell dependency. Am Rev Respir Dis 1992;146:479–84.

202. Hanak V, Kalra S, Aksamit TR, et al. Hot tub lung: presenting features and clinical course of 21 patients. Respir Med 2006;100:610–5.

203. Kahana LM, Kay JM, Yakrus MA, et al. Mycobacterium avium complex infection in an immunocompetent young adult related to hot tub exposure. Chest 1997;111:242–5.

204. Khoor A, Leslie KO, Tazelaar HD, et al. Diffuse pulmonary disease caused by nontuberculous mycobacteria in immunocompetent people (Hot tub lung). Am J Pathol 2001;115:755–62.

205. Kahana LM, Kay JM. Pneumonitis due to Mycobacterium avium complex in hot tub water: infection or hypersensitivity? Chest 1997;112:1713–4.

206. Marras TK, Wallace RJ Jr, Koth LL, et al. Hypersensitivity pneumonitis reaction to Mycobacterium avium in household water. Chest 2005;127:664–71.

207. Cappelluti E, Fraire AE, Schaefer OP. A case of 'hot tub lung' due to Mycobacterium avium complex in an immunocompetent host. Arch Intern Med 2003;163:845–8.

208. Zota V, Angelis SM, Fraire AE, et al. Lessons from Mycobacterium avium complex-associated pneumonitis: a case report. J Med Case Reports 2008;2:152.

Sarcoidosis

209. Hagerstrand I, Linell F. The prevalence of sarcoidosis in the autopsy material from a Swedish town. Acta Med Scand 1964;425:171.

210. Joint statement. The American Thoracic Society (ATS), the European Respiratory Society (ERS) and the World Association of Sarcoidosis and Other Granulomatous Disorders (WASOG) on sarcoidosis. Am J Respir Crit Care Med 1999;160:736–55.

211. Edmondstone WM, Wilson AR. Sarcoidosis in caucasians, blacks and Asians in London. Br J Dis Chest 1985;79:27–36.

212. Luisetti M, Beretta A, Casali L. Genetic aspects in sarcoidosis. Eur Resp J 2000;16:768–80.

213. Schurmann M, Reichel P, MullerMyhsok B, et al. Results from a genome-wide search for predisposing genes in sarcoidosis. Am J Respir Crit Care Med 2001;164:840–6.

214. Verleden GM, Dubois RM, Bouros D, et al. Genetic predisposition and pathogenetic mechanisms of interstitial lung diseases of unknown origin. Eur Resp J 2001;18:17S–29S, 17S–29S.

215. Moller DR, Chen ES. Genetic basis of remitting sarcoidosis – Triumph of the trimolecular complex? Am J Respir Cell Molec Biol 2002;27:391–5.

216. Grutters JC, Sato H, Welsh KI, et al. The importance of sarcoidosis genotype to lung phenotype. Amer J Resp Cell Molec Biol 2003;29:S59–62.

217. Grunewald J, Eklund A, Olerup O. Human leukocyte antigen class I alleles and the disease course in sarcoidosis patients. Amer J Resp Crit Care Med 2004;169:696–702.

218. Baughman RP, Lower EE, du Bois RM. Sarcoidosis. Lancet 2003;361:1111–8.

219. Parkes SA, Baker SBD, Bourdillon RE, et al. Epidemiology of sarcoidosis in the Isle of Man – 1: A case controlled study. Thorax 1987;42:420–6.

220. Hills SE, Parkes SA, Baker SBD. Epidemiology of sarcoidosis in the Isle of Man – 2: Evidence for space-time clustering. Thorax 1987;42:427–30.

221. McGrath DS, Daniil Z, Foley P, et al. Epidemiology of familial sarcoidosis in the UK. Thorax 2000;55:751–4.

222. Rybicki BA, Iannuzzi MC, Frederick MM, et al. Familial aggregation of sarcoidosis – A Case-Control Etiologic Study of Sarcoidosis (ACCESS). Am J Respir Crit Care Med 2001;164:2085–91.

223. Sverrild A, Backer V, Kyvik KO, et al. Heredity in sarcoidosis: a registry-based twin study. Thorax 2008;63:894–6.

224. Fagan EA, Moore-Gillon JC, Turner-Warwick M. Multiorgan granulomas and mitochondrial antibodies. N Engl J Med 1983;308:572–5.

225. Naccache JM, Antoine M, Wislez M, et al. Sarcoid-like pulmonary disorder in human immunodeficiency virus- infected patients receiving antiretroviral therapy. Am J Respir Crit Care Med 1999;159:2009–13.

226. Pietropaoli A, Modrak J, Utell M. Interferon-alpha therapy associated with the development of sarcoidosis. Chest 1999;116:569–72.

227. Scadding JG. Mycobacterium tuberculosis in the aetiology of sarcoidosis. BMJ 1960;2:1617–23.

228. Wong CF, Yew WW, Wong PC, et al. A case of concomitant tuberculosis and sarcoidosis with mycobacterial DNA present in the sarcoid lesion. Chest 1998;114:626–9.

229. Almenoff PL, Johnson A, Lesser M, et al. Growth of acid fast L forms from the blood of patients with sarcoidosis. Thorax 1996;51:530–3.

230. Wilsher ML, Menzies RE, Croxson MC. Mycobacterium tuberculosis DNA in tissues affected by sarcoidosis. Thorax 1998;53:871–4.

231. Ikonomopoulos JA, Gorgoulis VG, Zacharatos PV, et al. Multiplex polymerase chain reaction for the detection of mycobacterial DNA in cases of tuberculosis and sarcoidosis. Modern Pathol 1999;12:854–62.

232. Gupta D, Agarwal R, Aggarwal AN, et al. Molecular evidence for the role of mycobacteria in sarcoidosis: a meta-analysis. Eur Respir J 2007;30:508–16.

233. Eishi Y. Sarcoidosis and Propionibacterium acnes. Nippon Naika Gakkai Zasshi 2003;92:1182–9.

234. Eishi Y, Suga M, Ishige I, et al. Quantitative analysis of mycobacterial and propionibacterial DNA in lymph nodes of Japanese and European patients with sarcoidosis. J Clin Microbiol 2002;40:198–204.

235. Hunninghake GW, Crystal RG. Pulmonary sarcoidosis. A disorder mediated by excess helper T-lymphocyte activity at sites of disease activity. N Engl J Med 1981;305:429–34.

236. Ziegenhagen MW, Muller-Quernheim J. The cytokine network in sarcoidosis and its clinical relevance. J Intern Med 2003;253:18–30.

237. Hance AJ, Basset F, Saumon G, et al. Smoking and interstitial lung disease. The effect of cigarette smoking on the incidence of pulmonary histiocytosis X and sarcoidosis. Ann N Y Acad Sci 1986;465:643–56.

238. Abramowicz MJ, Ninane V, Depierreux M, et al. Tumour-like presentation of pulmonary sarcoidosis. Eur Respir J 1992;5:1286–7.

239. Garwood S, Judson MA, Silvestri G, et al. Endobronchial ultrasound for the diagnosis of pulmonary sarcoidosis. Chest 2007;132:1298–304.

240. Tremblay A, Stather DR, Maceachern P, et al. A randomized controlled trial of standard vs endobronchial ultrasonography-guided transbronchial needle aspiration in patients with suspected sarcoidosis. Chest 2009;136:340–6.

240a. Nakajima T, Yasufuku K, Kurosu K, et al. The role of EBUS-TBNA for the diagnosis of sarcoidosis – comparisons with other bronchoscopic diagnostic modalities. Respiratory Medicine 2009;103: 1796–800.

241. Malaisamy S, Dalal B, Bimenyuy C, et al. The clinical and radiologic features of nodular pulmonary sarcoidosis. Lung 2009;187:9–15.

242. McCann BG, Harrison BDW. Bronchiolar narrowing and occlusion in sarcoidosis – correlation of pathology with physiology. Respir Med 1991;85:65–7.

243. Polychronopoulos VS, Prakash UBS. Airway involvement in sarcoidosis. Chest 2009;136:1371–80.

244. Shorr AF, Helman DL, Davies DB, et al. Pulmonary hypertension in advanced sarcoidosis: epidemiology and clinical characteristics. Eur Respir J 2005;25:783–8.

245. Handa T, Nagai S, Miki S, et al. Incidence of pulmonary hypertension and its clinical relevance in patients with sarcoidosis. Chest 2006;129:1246–52.

246. Nunes H, Humbert M, Capron F, et al. Pulmonary hypertension associated with sarcoidosis: mechanisms, haemodynamics and prognosis. Thorax 2006;61:68–74.

247. Battesi JP, Georges R, Basset F, et al. Chronic cor pulmonale in pulmonary sarcoidosis. Thorax 1978;33:76–84.

248. Rodman DM, Lindenfeld JA. Successful treatment of sarcoidosis-associated pulmonary hypertension with corticosteroids. Chest 1990;97:500–2.

248a. Toonkel RL, Borczuk AC, Pearson GD, Horn EM, Thomashow BM. Sarcoidosis-associated fibrosing mediastinitis with resultant pulmonary hypertension: a case report and review of the literature. Respiration 2010;79:341–5.

249. Mitchell DN, Scadding JG, Heard BE, et al. Sarcoidosis: histopathological definition and clinical diagnosis. J Clin Pathol 1977;30:395–408.

250. Rosen Y, Vuletin JC, Pertschuk LP, et al. Sarcoidosis: from the pathologist's vantage point. Pathol Annu 1979;14:405–39.

251. Rosen Y, Athanassiades TJ, Moon S, et al. Nongranulomatous interstitial pneumonitis in sarcoidosis. Relationship to development of epithelioid granulomas. Chest 1978;74:122–5.

252. Reid JD, Andersen ME. Calcium oxalate in sarcoid granulomas. With particular reference to the small ovoid body and a note on the finding of dolomite. Am J Clin Pathol 1988;90:545–58.

253. Visscher D, Churg A, Katzenstein ALA. Significance of crystalline inclusions in lung granulomas. Mod Pathol 1988;1:415–9.

254. Cain H, Kraus B. Immunofluorescence microscopic demonstration of vimentin filaments in asteroid bodies of sarcoidosis. Comparison with electron microscopic findings. Virchows Arch B Cell Pathol 1983;42:213–26.

255. De Vos R, de Wolf-Peeters C, Facchetti F, et al. Plasmacytoid monocytes in epithelioid cell granulomas: ultrastructural and immunoelectron microscopic study. Ultrastruct Pathol 1990;14:291–302.

256. Mornex JF, Leroux C, Greenland T, et al. From granuloma to fibrosis in interstitial lung diseases – molecular and cellular interactions. Eur Respir J 1994;7:779–85.

257. Myatt N, Coghill G, Morrison K, et al. Detection of tumour necrosis factor alpha in sarcoidosis and tuberculosis granulomas using in situ hybridisation. J Clin Pathol 1994;47:423–6.

258. Petrek M, Pantelidis P, Southcott AM, et al. The source and role of RANTES in interstitial lung disease. Eur Resp J 1997;10:1207–16.

259. Tolnay E, Kuhnen C, Voss B, et al. Expression and localization of vascular endothelial growth factor and its receptor flt in pulmonary sarcoidosis. Virchows Archiv 1998;432:61–5.

260. Shigehara K, Shijubo N, Hirasawa M, et al. Immunolocalization of extracellular matrix proteins and integrins in sarcoid lymph nodes. Virchows Archiv 1998;433:55–61.

261. Facchetti F, Vermi W, Fiorentini S, et al. Expression of inducible nitric oxide synthase in human granulomas and histiocytic reactions. Am J Pathol 1999;154:145–52.

262. Pertschuk LP, Silverstein E, Friedland J. Immunohistologic diagnosis of sarcoidosis. Detection of angiotensin-converting enzyme in sarcoid granulomas. Am J Clin Pathol 1981;75:350–4.

263. Adams JS, Sharma OP, Glacad MA, et al. Metabolism of 25-hydroxyvitamin D3 by cultured pulmonary alveolar macrophages in sarcoidosis. J Clin Invest 1983;72:1856–60.

264. Papapoulos SE, Frahjer LJ, Sandler LM, et al. 1,25-dihydroxycholecalciferol in the pathogenesis of the hypercalcemia of sarcoidosis. Lancet 1979;ii:627–30.

265. van den Oord JJ, de Wolf-Peeters C, Facchetti F, et al. Cellular composition of hypersensitivity-type granulomas: immunohistochemical analysis of tuberculous and sarcoidal lymphadenitis. Hum Pathol 1984;15:559–65.

266. van Maarsseven ACMT, Mullink H, Alons CL, et al. Distribution of T-lymphocyte subsets in different portions of sarcoid granulomas: Immunohistologic analysis with monoclonal antibodies. Hum Pathol 1986;17:493–500.

267. Baumer I, Zissel G, Schlaak M, et al. Th1/Th2 cell distribution in pulmonary sarcoidosis. Am J Respir Cell Molec Biol 1997;16:171–7.

268. Minshall EM, Tsicopoulos A, Yasruel Z, et al. Cytokine mRNA gene expression in active and nonactive pulmonary sarcoidosis. Eur Resp J 1997;10:2034–9.

269. Crouser ED, Culver DA, Knox KS, et al. Gene expression profiling identifies MMP-12 and ADAMDEC1 as potential pathogenic mediators of pulmonary sarcoidosis. Am J Respir Crit Care Med 2009;179:929–38.

270. Fazel SB, Howie SEM, Krajewski AS, et al. Lymphocyte-B accumulations in human pulmonary sarcoidosis. Thorax 1992;47:964–7.

271. Hsu RM, Connors AF, Tomashefski JF. Histologic, microbiologic, and clinical correlates of the diagnosis of sarcoidosis by transbronchial biopsy. Arch Pathol Lab Med 1996;120:364–8.

272. Michaels L, Brown NJ, Cory-Wright M. Arterial changes in pulmonary sarcoidosis. Arch Pathol 1960;69:741–9.

273. Takemura T, Matsui Y, Saiki S, et al. Pulmonary vascular involvement in sarcoidosis – a report of 40 autopsy cases. Hum Pathol 1992;23:1216–23.

274. Jones RM, Dawson A, Jenkins GH, et al. Sarcoidosis-related pulmonary veno-occlusive disease presenting with recurrent haemoptysis. Eur Respir J 2009;34: 517–20.

275. Risbano MG, Groshong SD, Schwarz MI. Lung nodules in a woman with a history of breast cancer. Chest 2007;132:1697–701.

276. Karakantza M, Matutes E, Maclennan K, et al. Association between sarcoidosis and lymphoma revisited. J Clin Pathol 1996;49:208–12.

277. Askling J, Grunewald J, Eklund A, et al. Increased risk for cancer following sarcoidosis. Am J Respir Crit Care Med 1999;160:1668–72.

278. Bouros D, Hatzakis K, Labrakis H, et al. Association of malignancy with diseases causing interstitial pulmonary changes. Chest 2002;121:1278–89.

279. Seersholm N, Vestbo J, Viskum K. Risk of malignant neoplasms in patients with pulmonary sarcoidosis. Thorax 1997;52:892–4.

280. Baughman RP, Drent M, Kavuru M, et al. Infliximab therapy in patients with chronic sarcoidosis and pulmonary involvement. Am J Respir Crit Care Med 2006;174:795–802.

281. Huang CT, Heurich AE, Sutton AL, et al. Mortality in sarcoidosis. A changing pattern of the causes of death. Eur J Respir Dis 1981;62:231–8.

282. Perry A, Vuitch F. Causes of death in patients with sarcoidosis: a morphologic study of 38 autopsies with clinicopathologic correlations. Arch Pathol Lab Med 1995;119:167–72.

283. Iwai K, Tachibana T, Takemura T, et al. Pathological studies on sarcoidosis autopsy. I. Epidemiological features of 320 cases in Japan. Acta Pathol Jpn 1993;43:372–6.

284. Johnson BA, Duncan SR, Ohori NP, et al. Recurrence of sarcoidosis in pulmonary allograft recipients. Am Rev Respir Dis 1993;148:1373–7.

285. Milman N, Andersen CB, Burton CM, et al. Recurrent sarcoid granulomas in a transplanted lung derive from recipient immune cells. Eur Respir J 2005;26:549–52.

Langerhans cell histiocytosis

286. Basset F, Corrin B, Spencer H. Pulmonary histiocytosis X. Am Rev Respir Dis 1978;118:811–20.

287. Corrin B, Basset F. A review of histiocytosis X with particular reference to eosinophilic granuloma of the lung. Invest Cell Pathol 1979;2:137–46.

288. Tazi A, Soler P, Hance AJ. Adult pulmonary Langerhans' cell histiocytosis. Thorax 2000;55:405–16.

289. Vassallo R, Ryu JH, Colby TV, et al. Medical progress: Pulmonary Langerhans'-cell histiocytosis. N Engl J Med 2000;342:1969–78.

290. Sundar KM, Gosselin MV, Chung HL, et al. Pulmonary Langerhans cell histiocytosis: Emerging concepts in pathobiology, radiology, and clinical evolution of disease. Chest 2003;123:1673–83.

291. Lichtenstein L. Histiocytosis X. Integration of eosinophilic granuloma of bone, 'Letterer–Siwe disease' and 'Schuller–Christian disease' as related manifestations of a single nosologic entity. Arch Pathol 1953;56:84–102.

292. Birbeck MS, Breathnach AS, Everall JD. An electron microscopic study of basal melanocytes and high level clear cells (Langerhans' cell) in vitiligo. J Invest Dermatol 1961;37:51.

293. Yousem SA, Colby TV, Chen YY, et al. Pulmonary Langerhans' cell histiocytosis – Molecular analysis of clonality. Amer J Surg Pathol 2001;25:630–6.

294. Weiss LM, Grogan TM, Muller-Hermelink HK, et al. Langerhans cell histiocytosis. In: World Health Organization Classification of Tumours: Tumours of haematopoietic and lymphoid tissue. Lyons: IARC Press; 2001. p. 280–2.

295. Casolaro MA, Bernaudin J-F, Saltini C, et al. Accumulation of Langerhans' cells on the epithelial surface of the lower respiratory tract in normal subjects in association with cigarette smoking. Am Rev Respir Dis 1988;137:406–11.

296. Kawanami O, Basset F, Ferrans VJ, et al. Pulmonary Langerhans' cells in patients with fibrotic lung disorders. Lab Invest 1981;44:227.

297. Furukawa T, Watanabe S, Kodama T, et al. T-zone histiocytes in adenocarcinoma of the lung in relation to postoperative prognosis. Cancer 1985;56:2651–6.

298. Soler P, Moreau A, Basset F, et al. Cigarette smoking-induced changes in the number and differentiated state of pulmonary dendritic cells/Langerhans cells. Am Rev Respir Dis 1989;139:1112–7.

299. Tazi A, Bonay M, Bergeron A, et al. Role of granulocyte-macrophage colony stimulating factor (GM-CSF) in the pathogenesis of adult pulmonary histiocytosis X. Thorax 1996;51:611–4.

300. Hirose M, Saito S, Yoshimoto T, et al. Interleukin-2 therapy of Langerhans cell histiocytosis. Acta Paediatr 1995;84:1204–6.

301. Rajagopol J, Shepard JAO, Mark EJ, et al. A 58-year-old man with interstitial pulmonary disease. Eosinophilic granuloma, late (Burned-out) stage. N Engl J Med 2002;347:1262–8.

302. Tazi A, Bonay M, Gransaigne M, et al. Surface phenotype of Langerhans cells and lymphocytes in granulomatous lesions from patients with pulmonary histiocytosis-X. Am Rev Respir Dis 1993;147:1531–6.

303. Robb IA, Jimenez CL, Carpenter BF. Birbeck granules or Birbeck junctions – intercellular zipper-like lattice junctions in eosinophilic granuloma of bone. Ultrastruct Pathol 1992;16:423–8.

304. Krenacs L, Tiszalvicz L, Krenacs T, et al. Immunohistochemical detection of CD1A antigen in formalin-fixed and paraffin-embedded tissue sections with monoclonal antibody 010. J Pathol 1993;171:99–104.

305. Emile JF, Wechsler J, Brousse N, et al. Langerhans' cell histiocytosis: definitive diagnosis with the use of monoclonal antibody 010 on routinely paraffin-embedded samples. Am J Surg Pathol 1995;19:636–41.

306. Pinkus GS, Lones MA, Matsumura F, et al. Langerhans cell histiocytosis – Immunohistochemical expression of fascin, a dendritic cell marker. Am J Clin Pathol 2002;118:335–43.

307. Sholl LM, Hornick JL, Pinkus JL, et al. Immunohistochemical analysis of langerin in Langerhans cell histiocytosis and pulmonary inflammatory and infectious diseases. Am J Surg Pathol 2007;31:947–52.

308. Lau SK, Chu PG, Weiss LM. Immunohistochemical expression of langerin in Langerhans cell histiocytosis and non-Langerhans cell histiocytic disorders. Am J Surg Pathol 2008;32:615–9.

309. Lieberman PH, Jones CR, Steinman RM, et al. Langerhans cell (eosinophilic) granulomatosis: a clinicopathologic study encompassing 50 years. Am J Surg Pathol 1996;20:519–52.

310. Nakhla H, Jumbelic MI. Sudden death of a patient with pulmonary Langerhans cell histiocytosis. Arch Pathol Lab Med 2005;129:798–9.

311. Lacronique J, Roth C, Battesti J-P, et al. Chest radiological features of pulmonary histiocytosis X: a report based on 50 adult cases. Thorax 1982;37:104–9.

312. Abbott GF, Rosado-de-Christenson ML, Franks TJ, et al. From the archives of the AFIP: pulmonary Langerhans cell histiocytosis. Radiographics 2004;24:821–41.

313. Tazi A. Adult pulmonary Langerhans' cell histiocytosis. Eur Respir J 2006;27:1272–85.

314. Fichtenbaum CJ, Kleinman GM, Haddad RG. Eosinophilic granuloma of the lung presenting as a solitary pulmonary nodule. Thorax 1990;45:905–6.

315. Fridlender ZG, Glazer M, Amir G et al. Obstructing tracheal pulmonary Langerhans cell histiocytosis. Chest 2005;128:1057–8.

316. Fartoukh M, Humbert M, Capron F, et al. Severe pulmonary hypertension in histiocytosis X. Am J Respir Crit Care Med 2000;161:216–23.

317. Delobbe K, Durieu J, Duhamel A, et al. Determinants of survival in pulmonary Langerhans' cell granulomatosis (histiocytosis X). Eur Respir J 1996;9:2002–6.

318. Tazi A, Montcelly L, Bergeron A, et al. Relapsing nodular lesions in the course of adult pulmonary Langerhans cell histiocytosis. Am J Respir Crit Care Med 1998;157:2007–10.

319. Vassallo R, Ryu JH, Schroeder DR, et al. Clinical outcomes of pulmonary Langerhans'-cell histiocytosis in adults. N Engl J Med 2002;346:484–90.

320. Stoll M, Freund M, Schmid H, et al. Allogeneic bone marrow transplantation for Langerhans' cell histiocytosis X. Cancer 1990;66:284–8.

321. Habib SB, Congleton J, Carr D, et al. Recipient Langerhans cell histiocytosis recurring following bilateral lung transplantation. Thorax 1998;53:323–5.

322. Li SY, Borowitz MJ. CD79a(+) T-cell lymphoblastic lymphoma with coexisting Langerhans cell histiocytosis – A short case report and review of the literature. Arch Pathol Lab Med 2001;125:958–60.

323. Christie LJ, Evans AT, Bray SE, et al. Lesions resembling Langerhans cell histiocytosis in association with other lymphoproliferative disorders: a reactive or neoplastic phenomenon? Human Pathology 2006;37:32–9.

324. Sadoun D, Vaylet F, Valeyre D, et al. Bronchogenic carcinoma in patients with

pulmonary histiocytosis-X. Chest 1992;101:1610–3.

325. Sakuma N, Kamei T, Ohta M, et al. Immunohistochemical and ultrastructural examination of histiocytosis-X cells in pulmonary eosinophilic granuloma. Acta Pathol Jpn 1992;42:719–26.

326. Travis WD, Borok Z, Roum JH, et al. Pulmonary Langerhans cell granulomatosis (histiocytosis-X) – a clinicopathologic study of 48 cases. Am J Surg Pathol 1993;17:971–86.

327. Kambouchner M, Basset FO, Marchal L, et al. Three-dimensional characterization of pathologic lesions in pulmonary Langerhans cell histiocytosis. Am J Respir Crit Care Med 2002;166:1483–90.

328. Asakura S, Colby TV, Limper AH. Tissue localization of transforming growth factor-beta 1 in pulmonary eosinophilic granuloma. Am J Respir Crit Care Med 1996;154:1525–30.

329. de Graaf JH, Tamminga RYJ, Dam-Meiring A, et al. The presence of cytokines in Langerhans' cell histiocytosis. J Pathol 1996;180:400–6.

330. Rousseau-Merck MF, Barbey S, Mouly H, et al. Collagenolytic activity of eosinophilic granuloma in vitro. Experientia 1979;35:1226–7.

331. Hayashi T, Rush WL, Travis WD, et al. Immunohistochemical study of matrix metalloproteinases and their tissue inhibitors in pulmonary Langerhans' cell granulomatosis. Arch Pathol Lab Med 1997;121:930–7.

332. Vassallo R, Jensen EA, Colby TV, et al. The overlap between respiratory bronchiolitis and desquamative interstitial pneumonia in pulmonary Langerhans cell histiocytosis – High-resolution CT, histologic, and functional correlations. Chest 2003;124:1199–205.

333. Shimizu S, Yoshinouchi T, Ohtsuki Y, et al. The appearance of S-100 protein-positive dendritic cells and the distribution of lymphocyte subsets in idiopathic nonspecific interstitial pneumonia. Resp Med 2002;96:770–6.

334. Stacher E, Beham-Schmid C, Terpe HJ, et al. Pulmonary histiocytic sarcoma mimicking pulmonary Langerhans cell histiocytosis in a young adult presenting with spontaneous pneumothorax: a potential diagnostic pitfall. Virchows Archiv 2009;455:187–90.

335. Pileri SA, Grogan TM, Harris NL, et al. Tumours of histiocytes and accessory dendritic cells: an immunohistochemical approach to classification from the International Lymphoma Study Group based on 61 cases. Histopathology 2002;41:1–29.

336. Lee JS, Ko GH, Kim HC, et al. Langerhans cell sarcoma arising from Langerhans cell histiocytosis: a case report. J Korean Med Sci 2006;21:577–80.

337. Egan AJM, Boardman LA, Tazelaar HD, et al. Erdheim–Chester disease – Clinical, radiologic, and histopathologic findings in five patients with interstitial lung disease. Am J Surg Pathol 1999;23:17–26.

338. Rush WL, Andriko JAW, GalateauSalle F, et al. Pulmonary pathology of Erdheim–Chester disease. Modern Pathol 2000;13:747–54.

339. Danel C, Israelbiet D, Costabel U, et al. The clinical role of BAL in pulmonary histiocytosis-X. Eur Respir J 1990;3:949–50.

340. Auerswald U, Barth J, Magnussen H. Value of CD-1-positive cells in bronchoalveolar lavage fluid for the diagnosis of pulmonary histiocytosis-X. Lung 1991;169:305–9.

Lymphangioleiomyomatosis

341. Corrin B, Liebow AA, Friedman PJ. Pulmonary lymphangiomyomatosis. Am J Pathol 1975;79:347–82.

342. Ciftci AO, Sanlialp I, Tanyel FC, et al. The association of pulmonary lymphangioleiomyomatosis with renal and hepatic angiomyolipomas in a prepubertal girl: a previously unreported entity. Respiration 2007;74:335–7.

343. Baldi S, Papotti M, Valente ML, et al. Pulmonary lymphangioleiomyomatosis in postmenopausal women: report of two cases and review of the literature. Eur Respir J 1994;7:1013–6.

344. Johnson SR, Tattersfield AE. Clinical experience of lymphangioleiomyomatosis in the UK. Thorax 2000;55:1052–7.

345. Johnson SR. Lymphangioleiomyomatosis. Eur Respir J 2006;27:1056–65.

346. Cohen MM, Pollock-BarZiv S, Johnson SR. Emerging clinical picture of lymphangioleiomyomatosis. Thorax 2005;60:875–9.

347. Aubry MC, Myers JL, Ryu JH, et al. Pulmonary lymphangioleiomyomatosis in a man. Am J Respir Crit Care Med 2000;162:749–52.

348. Kim NR, Chung MP, Park CK, et al. Pulmonary lymphangioleiomyomatosis and multiple hepatic angiomyolipomas in a man. Pathol Int 2003;53:231–5.

349. Schiavina M, Di Scioscio V, Contini P, et al. Pulmonary lymphangioleiomyomatosis in a karyotypically normal man without tuberous sclerosis complex. Am J Respir Crit Care Med 2007;176:96–8.

350. Ryu JH, Moss J, Beck GJ, et al. The NHLBI lymphangioleiomyomatosis registry: characteristics of 230 patients at enrollment. Am J Respir Crit Care Med 2006;173:105–11.

351. Hughes E, Hodder RV. Pulmonary lymphangiomyomatosis complicating pregnancy. A case report. J Reprod Med 1987;32:553.

352. Urban T, Lazor R, Lacronique J, et al. Pulmonary lymphangioleiomyomatosis. A

study of 69 patients. Groupe d'Etudes et de Recherche sur les Maladies 'Orphelines' Pulmonaires (GERM'O'P). Medicine (Baltimore) 1999;78:321–37.

353. Gray SR, Carrington CB, Cornog JL. Lymphangiomyomatosis. Report of a case with ureteral involvement and chyluria. Cancer 1975;35:490–8.

354. Shen A, Iseman ID, Waldron JA, et al. Exacerbation of pulmonary lymphangioleiomyomatosis by exogenous estrogens. Chest 1987;91:782–5.

355. Yano S. Exacerbation of pulmonary lymphangioleiomyomatosis by exogenous oestrogen used for infertility treatment. Thorax 2002;57:1085–6.

356. Berger U, Khaghani A, Pomerance A, et al. Pulmonary lymphangioleiomyomatosis and steroid receptors. An immunocytochemical study. Am J Clin Pathol 1990;93:609–14.

357. Valensi QJ. Pulmonary lymphangiomyoma, a probable forme fruste of tuberous sclerosis: a case report and survey of the literature. Am Rev Respir Dis 1973;108:1411–5.

358. European Chromosome 16 Consortium. Identification and characterization of the tuberous sclerosis gene on chromosome 16. Cell 1993;75:1305–15.

359. Menchine M, Emelin JK, Mischel PS, et al. Tissue and cell-type specific expression of the tuberous sclerosis gene, TSC2, in human tissues. Mod Pathol 1996;9:1071–80.

360. Carsillo T, Astrinidis A, Henske EP. Mutations in the tuberous sclerosis complex gene TSC2 are a cause of sporadic pulmonary lymphangioleiomyomatosis. Proc Natl Acad Sci U S A 2000;97:6085–90.

361. Maruyama H, Seyama K, Sobajima J, et al. Multifocal micronodular pneumocyte hyperplasia and lymphangioleiomyomatosis in tuberous sclerosis with a TSC2 gene. Modern Pathol 2001;14:609–14.

362. Yu J, Astrinidis A, Henske EP. Chromosome 16 loss of heterozygosity in tuberous sclerosis and sporadic lymphangiomyomatosis. Am J Respir Crit Care Med 2001;164:1537–40.

363. Lie JT, Miller RD, Williams DE. Cystic disease of the lungs in tuberous sclerosis. Clinicopathologic correlation, including body plethysmographic lung function tests. Mayo Clin Proc 1980;55:547–53.

364. Shepherd CW, Gomez MR, Lie JT, et al. Causes of death in patients with tuberous sclerosis. Mayo Clin Proc 1991;66:792–6.

365. Bernstein SM, Newell JD, Adamczyk D, et al. How common are renal angiomyolipomas in patients with pulmonary lymphangiomyomatosis? Am J Respir Crit Care Med 1995;152:2138–43.

366. Maziak DE, Kesten S, Rappaport DC, et al. Extrathoracic angiomyolipomas in

lymphangioleiomyomatosis. Eur Respir J 1996;9:402–5.

367. Castro M, Shepherd CW, Gomez MR, et al. Pulmonary tuberous sclerosis. Chest 1995;107:189–95.

368. Bonetti F, Chiodera P. The lung in tuberous sclerosis. In: Corrin B, editor. Pathology of Lung Tumors. London: Churchill Livingstone; 1997. p. 225–40.

369. Chu SC, Horiba K, Usuki J, et al. Comprehensive evaluation of 35 patients with lymphangioleiomyomatosis. Chest 1999;115:1041–52.

370. Franz DN, Brody A, Meyer C, et al. Mutational and radiographic analysis of pulmonary disease consistent with lymphangioleiomyomatosis and micronodular pneumocyte hyperplasia in women with tuberous sclerosis. Am J Respir Crit Care Med 2001;164:661–8.

371. Moss J, Avila NA, Barnes PM, et al. Prevalence and clinical characteristics of lymphangioleiomyomatosis (LAM) in patients with tuberous sclerosis complex. Am J Respir Crit Care Med 2001;164:669–71.

372. Chorianopoulos D, Stratakos G. Lymphangioleiomyomatosis and tuberous sclerosis complex. Lung 2008;186: 197–207.

373. PachecoRodriguez G, Kristof AS, Stevens LA, et al. Genetics and gene expression in Lymphangioleiomyomatosis. Chest 2002;121:56S–60S.

374. Bittmann I, Rolf B, Amann G, et al. Recurrence of lymphangioleiomyomatosis after single lung transplantation: New insights into pathogenesis. Hum Pathol 2003;34:95–8.

375. Karbowniczek M, Astrinidis A, Balsara BR, et al. Recurrent lymphangiomyomatosis after transplantation – Genetic analyses reveal a metastatic mechanism. Am J Respir Crit Care Med 2003;167:976–82.

376. Kumasaka T, Seyama K, Mitani K, et al. Lymphangiogenesis-mediated shedding of LAM cell clusters as a mechanism for dissemination in lymphangioleiomyomatosis. Am J Surg Pathol 2005;29:1356–66.

377. Taylor JR, Ryu J, Colby TV, et al. Lymphangioleiomyomatosis. Clinical course in 32 patients. N Engl J Med 1990;323:1254–60.

378. Johnson S. Rare diseases – 1 – Lymphangioleiomyomatosis: clinical features, management and basic mechanisms. Thorax 1999;54:254–64.

379. Sullivan EJ. Lymphangioleiomyomatosis – a review. Chest 1998;114:1689–703.

380. Oh YM, Mo EK, Jang SH, et al. Pulmonary lymphangioleiomyomatosis in Korea. Thorax 1999;54:618–21.

381. Vadas G, Pare JAP, Thurlbeck WM. Pulmonary and lymph node myomatosis: review of the literature and report of a case. Can Med Assoc J 1967;96: 420–4.

382. Carrington CB, Cugell DW, Gaensler EA, et al. Lymphangioleiomyomatosis. Physiologic–pathologic–radiologic correlations. Am Rev Respir Dis 1977;116:977–95.

383. Burger CD, Hyatt RE, Staats BA. Pulmonary mechanics in lymphangioleiomyomatosis. Am Rev Respir Dis 1991;143:1030–3.

384. Crausman RS, Jennings CA, Irvin CG, et al. Lymphangioleiomyomatosis: the pathophysiology of diminished exercise capacity. Am J Respir Crit Care Med 1996;153:1368–76.

385. Aberle DR, Hansell DM, Brown K, et al. Lymphangiomyomatosis: CT, chest radiographic, and functional correlations. Radiology 1990;176:381–7.

386. Silverstein EF, Ellis K, Wolff M, et al. Pulmonary lymphangiomyomatosis. AJR Am J Roentgenol 1974;120:832–50.

387. Kitaichi M, Nishimura K, Itoh H, et al. Pulmonary lymphangioleiomyomatosis: a report of 46 patients including a clinicopathologic study of prognostic factors. Am J Respir Crit Care Med 1995;151:527–33.

388. Bhattacharyya AK, Balogh K. Retroperitoneal lymphangioleiomyomatosis. Cancer 1985;56:1144–6.

389. Basset F, Soler P, Marsac J, et al. Pulmonary lymphangiomyomatosis. Three new cases studied with electron microscopy. Cancer 1976;38: 2357–66.

390. Matthews TJ, Hornall D, Sheppard MN. Comparison of the use of antibodies to alpha-smooth muscle actin and desmin in pulmonary lymphangioleiomyomatosis. J Clin Pathol 1993;46:479–80.

391. Bonetti F, Chiodera PL, Pea M, et al. Transbronchial biopsy in lymphangiomyomatosis of the lung – HMB45 for diagnosis. Am J Surg Pathol 1993;17:1092–102.

392. Hoon V, Thung SN, Kaneko M, et al. HMB-45 reactivity in renal angiomyolipoma and lymphangiomyomatosis. Arch Pathol Lab Med 1994;118:732–4.

393. Chan JKC, Tsang WYW, Pau MY, et al. Lymphangiomyomatosis and angiomyolipoma: closely related entities characterized by hamartomatous proliferation of HMB-45-positive smooth muscle. Histopathology 1993;22: 445–55.

394. Tanaka H, Imada A, Morikawa T, et al. Diagnosis of pulmonary lymphangioleiomyomatosis by HMB45 in surgically treated spontaneous pneumothorax. Eur Respir J 1995;8:1879–82.

395. Kalassian KG, Doyle R, Kao P, et al. Lymphangioleiomyomatosis: new insights. Am J Respir Crit Care Med 1997;155:1183–6.

396. Hornick JL, Fletcher CD. PEComa: what do we know so far? Histopathology 2006;48:75–82.

397. Bonetti F, Pea M, Martignoni G, et al. Clear cell ('sugar') tumor of the lung is a lesion strictly related to angiomyolipoma – the concept of a family of lesions characterized by the presence of the perivascular epithelioid cells (PEC). Pathology 1995;26:230–6.

398. Pea M, Martignoni G, Zamboni G, et al. Perivascular epithelioid cell. Am J Surg Pathol 1996;20:1149–53.

399. Adachi Y, Horie Y, Kitamura Y, et al. CD1a expression in PEComas. Pathology International 2008;58:169–73.

400. Chilosi M, Pea M, Martignoni G, et al. Cathepsin-k expression in pulmonary lymphangioleiomyomatosis. Mod Pathol 2009;22:161–6.

401. Folpe AL, Kwiatkowski DJ. Perivascular epithelioid cell neoplasms: pathology and pathogenesis. Human Pathology 2010;41:1–15.

402. Matsumoto Y, Horiba K, Usuki J, et al. Markers of cell proliferation and expression of melanosomal antigen in lymphangioleiomyomatosis. Am J Respir Cell Molec Biol 1999;21:327–36.

403. Matsui K, Takeda K, Yu ZX, et al. Downregulation of estrogen and progesterone receptors in the abnormal smooth muscle cells in pulmonary lymphangioleiomyomatosis following therapy – An immunohistochemical study. Am J Respir Crit Care Med 2000;161:1002–9.

404. Kumasaka T, Seyama K, Mitani K, et al. Lymphangiogenesis in lymphangioleiomyomatosis: its implication in the progression of lymphangioleiomyomatosis. Am J Surg Pathol 2004;28:1007–16.

405. Merrilees MJ, Hankin EJ, Black JL, et al. Matrix proteoglycans and remodelling of interstitial lung tissue in lymphangioleiomyomatosis. J Pathol 2004;203:653–60.

406. Fukuda Y, Kawamoto M, Yamamoto A, et al. Role of elastic fiber degradation in emphysema-like lesions of pulmonary lymphangiomyomatosis. Hum Pathol 1990;21:1252–61.

407. Hayashi T, Fleming MV, Stetler-Stevenson WG, et al. Immunohistochemical study of matrix metalloproteinases (MMPs) and their tissue inhibitors (TIMPs) in pulmonary lymphangioleiomyomatosis (LAM). Hum Pathol 1997;28:1071–8.

408. Sobonya RE, Quan SF, Fleishman JS. Pulmonary lymphangioleiomyomatosis: quantitative analysis of lesions producing airflow limitation. Hum Pathol 1985;16:1122–8.

409. Matsui K, Beasley MB, Nelson WK, et al. Prognostic significance of pulmonary lymphangioleiomyomatosis histologic score. Amer J Surg Pathol 2001;25:479–84.

410. Matsui K, Tatsuguchi A, Valencia J, et al. Extrapulmonary lymphangioleiomyomatosis (LAM): Clinicopathologic features in 22 cases. Hum Pathol 2000;31:1242–8.

411. Pileri SA, Cavazza A, Schiavina M, et al. Clear-cell proliferation of the lung with lymphangioleiomyomatosis-like change. Histopathology 2004;44:156–63.

412. Hironaka M, Fukayama M. Regional proliferation of HMB-45-positive clear cells of the lung with lymphangioleiomyomatosislike distribution, replacing the lobes with multiple cysts and a nodule. Am J Surg Pathol 1999;23:1288–93.

413. Steiner PE. Metastasizing fibroleiomyoma of the uterus – report of a case and review of the literature. Am J Pathol 1939;15:89–109.

414. Spiro RH, McPeak CJ. On the so-called metastasizing leiomyoma. Cancer 1966;19:544–8.

415. Burrel LST, Ross JM. A case of chylous effusion due to leiomyosarcoma. Br J Tuberc Dis Chest 1937;31:38–9.

416. Itoh T, Mochizuki M, Kumazaki S, et al. Cystic pulmonary metastases of endometrial stromal sarcoma of the uterus, mimicking lymphangiomyomatosis: A case report with immunohistochemistry of HMB45. Pathol Int 1997;47:725–9.

417. Mahadeva R, Stewart S, Wallwork J. Metastatic endometrial stromal sarcoma masquerading as pulmonary lymphangioleiomyomatosis. J Clin Pathol 1999;52:147–8.

418. Svendsen TL, Viskum K, Hansborg N, et al. Pulmonary lymphangioleiomyomatosis: a case of progesterone receptor positive lymphangioleiomyomatosis treated with medroxyprogesterone, oophorectomy and tamoxifen. Br J Dis Chest 1984;78: 264–71.

419. Westermann CJJ, Oostveen ACM, Wagenaar SSC, et al. Pulmonary tuberous sclerosis treated with tamoxifen and progesterone. Thorax 1986;41: 892–3.

420. Kitzsteiner KA, Mallen RG. Pulmonary lymphangiomyomatosis: treatment with castration. Cancer 1980;46:2248–9.

421. Banner A, Carrington CB, Emory WB, et al. Efficacy of oophorectomy in lymphangioleiomyomatosis and benign metastasizing leiomyoma. N Engl J Med 1981;305:204–9.

422. Adamson D, Heinrichs WL, Raybin DM, et al. Successful treatment of pulmonary lymphangiomyomatosis with oophorectomy and progesterone. Am Rev Respir Dis 1985;132:916–21.

423. Urban T, Kuttenn F, Gompel A, et al. Pulmonary lymphangiomyomatosis – follow-up and long-term outcome with antiestrogen therapy – a report of 8 cases. Chest 1992;102:472–6.

424. Dishner W, Cordasco EM, Blackburn J, et al. Pulmonary lymphangiomyomatosis. Chest 1984;85:796–9.

425. Taveira-DaSilva AM, Stylianou MP, Hedin CJ, et al. Decline in lung function in patients with lymphangioleiomyomatosis treated with or without progesterone. Chest 2004;126:1867–74.

426. Johnson SR, Cordier JF, Lazor R, et al. European Respiratory Society guidelines for the diagnosis and management of lymphangioleiomyomatosis. Eur Respir J 2010;35:14–26.

427. Boehler A, Speich R, Russi EW, et al. Lung transplantation for lymphangioleiomyomatosis. N Engl J Med 1996;335:1275–80.

428. Nine JS, Yousem SA, Paradis IL, et al. Lymphangioleiomyomatosis recurrence after lung transplantation. J Heart Lung Transplant 1994;13:714–9.

429. O'Brien JD, Lium JH, Parosa JF, et al. Lymphangiomyomatosis recurrence in the allograft after single-lung transplantation. Am J Respir Crit Care Med 1995;151:2033–6.

430. Bissler JJ, McCormack FX, Young LR, et al. Sirolimus for angiomyolipoma in tuberous sclerosis complex or lymphangioleiomyomatosis. N Engl J Med 2008;358:140–51.

430a. Glasgow CG, Steagall WK, Taveira-DaSilva A, et al. Lymphangioleiomyomatosis (LAM): Molecular insights lead to targeted therapies. Respiratory Medicine 2010; 104:S45–58.

431. Moses MA, Harper J, Folkman J. Doxycycline treatment for lymphangioleiomyomatosis with urinary monitoring for MMPs. N Engl J Med 2006;354:2621–2.

432. Issaka RB, Oommen S, Gupta SK, et al. Vascular endothelial growth factors C and D induces proliferation of lymphangioleiomyomatosis cells through autocrine crosstalk with endothelium. Am J Pathol 2009;175:1410–20.

433. Häussinger K, Kohlhäuffl M, Bolliger CT. Diagnostic bronchoscopy. In: Gibson GJ, Geddes DM, Costabel U, et al, editors. Respiratory Medicine. 3rd ed. London: Saunders; 2003. p. 415–30.

6.2 Alveolar filling defects

CRYPTOGENIC ORGANISING PNEUMONIA (IDIOPATHIC BRONCHIOLITIS OBLITERANS ORGANISING PNEUMONIA)

The first description of this alveolar filling defect should probably be attributed to Liebow and Carrington,[1] who used the title interstitial pneumonia with bronchiolitis obliterans (BIP) despite the predominant involvement of air spaces rather than the interstitium. Subsequent workers drew attention to the corticosteroid-sensitivity of the condition[2,3] and the terms cryptogenic organising pneumonia (COP)[4] and bronchiolitis obliterans organising pneumonia (BOOP)[5] followed, the latter covering both the idiopathic variety and those of known causation. The emphasis on bronchiolar involvement in the term

BOOP inevitably led to confusion with bronchiolitis obliterans affecting proximal bronchioles and therefore characterised by airflow obstruction. Whilst it is true that the luminal fibrosis of organising pneumonia extends proximally into alveolar ducts, respiratory bronchioles and even membranous bronchioles, it remains limited to relatively peripheral air spaces and the functional deficit is restrictive rather than obstructive. An appreciation of the geometry of the airways (see Table 1.2, p. 3) helps in understanding the different functional and clinical effects of proximal and distal airway obliteration.

The corticosteroid-sensitivity of COP is probably attributable to its collagen being of type III (newly formed, flexible and susceptible to enzymatic digestion) rather than the more mature type I, and the abundance of proteolytic enzymes within the Masson bodies.[6] This corticosteroid-sensitivity probably applies to organising pneumonia irrespective of the cause of the initial exudate.

Clinical features

COP presents a distinct clinicopathological syndrome, recognition of which is important because it is responsive to corticosteroid-responsiveness.[2-4] Men and women are affected equally and most are in the 40–60-year age group. Persistent cough, shortness of breath and malaise are common complaints. The onset is insidious. Chest radiographs show widespread blotchy opacities, which regress in some places whilst progressing in others and developing anew elsewhere.[7] High-resolution computed tomography (HRCT) scans typically show bilateral consolidation, which has a predominantly subpleural and peribronchial distribution (Fig. 6.2.1). Reticular changes, localised nodules and ground-glass opacification are less common. The changes wax and wane, unlike those of bronchioloalveolar carcinoma, which COP may otherwise resemble radilgraphically. Pulmonary function tests generally show a predominantly restrictive ventilatory defect but some patients have a mixed obstructive and restrictive pattern. The erythrocyte sedimentation rate is elevated but no evidence of infection can be detected, either by culture or serologically. Bronchoalveolar lavage shows a lymphocytosis with a low T-helper/suppressor cell ratio (see Table A3, p. 760).[8,9]

Some patients are affected each spring and in these there is an intriguing association with cholestasis.[10] Circulating immune complexes have been identified in some patients.[11] Another intriguing

Figure 6.2.1 Cryptogenic organising pneumonia. High-resolution computed tomography shows patchy bilateral air space consolidation with a predominantly subpleural distribution. Focal ground-glass shadows are also seen.

observation is that postirradiation organising pneumonia appears to 'prime' the non-irradiated areas of the lungs as these may subsequently develop the same changes,[12–14] a point of difference from the usual form of radiation pneumonitis which is generally confined to the irradiated area of lung. One woman suffered self-limited attacks a few days before each menstrual period.[15]

The prognosis is usually excellent, particularly with corticosteroid therapy, but patients may relapse when these are withdrawn. Rare patients have unusually severe disease and deteriorate rapidly despite treatment. Autopsy in such cases has shown interstitial fibrosis rather than the intra-alveolar fibrosis seen on biopsy.[16]

Histopathology[4,5,17,17a]

Various conditions cause organising pneumonia (Box 6.2.1) but, whatever its aetiology, biopsy shows micropolypoid buds of granulation tissue (*bourgeons conjonctifs* or Masson bodies) in the air spaces (Fig. 6.2.2). The buds may extend from one alveolus to the next through the pores of Kohn (which were first identified by this process). Alveoli are mainly affected but the process also involves respiratory bronchioles and the more peripheral membranous bronchioles. Occasionally, residual fibrin is seen in or near the connective tissue buds, which also contain small numbers of lymphocytes, plasma cells, neutrophils, macrophages and fibroblasts. The inflammatory cells tend to cluster in the centres of the buds. Chronic inflammation and interstitial fibrosis of the alveolar walls may also be seen but the predominant change is that within the air spaces. The alveoli are often lined by reactive type II cells. Electron microscopy shows evidence of acute alveolar epithelial injury.[18]

Differential diagnosis

A striking histological feature of organising pneumonia is its temporal homogeneity, which gives the impression of damage occurring at a single moment. This contrasts with usual interstitial pneumonia (UIP), where fibroblastic foci lie adjacent to areas of well-established interstitial fibrosis. However, in time, the intra-alveolar granulation tissue of organising pneumonia may be incorporated into the alveolar wall by an accretive process, resulting in interstitial fibrosis and a similarity to UIP, with a correspondingly worse prognosis.[16,19] In such cases, HRCT may reveal more typical features elsewhere in the lungs.

Box 6.2.1 Conditions resulting in organising pneumonia

	Suggestive histological features
Bacterial pneumonia	Neutrophilia, organisms on special stains
Bronchial obstruction, chronic bronchiolitis	Lipid-laden macrophages
Diffuse alveolar damage (organising phase)	More diffuse low-power distribution, exudative foci
Radiation	
Aspiration pneumonia	Foreign material
Fume and toxin exposure	
Connective tissue disease	Other manifestations of such disease (e.g. rheumatoid nodules)
Extrinsic allergic alveolitis	Bronchocentricity, granulomas
Pulmonary eosinophilia	Eosinophils
Drug reactions	Eosinophils
Transplantation (bone marrow, lung, kidney)	
Inflammatory bowel disease	
Adjacent disease, e.g. Abscess	
Wegener's granulomatosis	Vasculitis, granulomas
Neoplasms	Tumour
Langerhans cell histiocytosis	Langerhans cells
Cryptogenic	

Organising pneumonia is easily distinguished from the exudative phase of diffuse alveolar disease (DAD) by an absence of hyaline membranes but the organising phase of DAD may show organising pneumonia and only be separable by review of the clinical data. Features that favour COP over organising DAD include a patchy peribronchiolar distribution and relatively little expansion of the interstitium by oedematous fibroinflammatory tissue. IgG$_4$-related systemic sclerosing disease, which is dealt with on page 485, may also be confused with organising pneumonia as intra-alveolar organisation may be part of its spectrum of presentation in the lung. It is characterised by a heavy infiltrate of IgG$_4$-bearing plasma cells, the recognition of which is key to the diagnosis, along with obliterative phlebitis and involvement of other organs such as the pancreas. In similar fashion, organising pneumonia may mask underlying Langerhans cell histiocytosis, lymphoma and vasculitis,[20] so the background lung should be carefully scrutinised in any case showing organising pneumonia.

Pathologists conducting necropsies on patients dying of bronchopneumonia will be familiar with the histological pattern of organising pneumonia but, before dismissing it in a biopsy as yet another example of healing bacterial pneumonia, they should ask themselves why a condition that is usually diagnosed without such recourse should be so investigated. Consultation with the clinician may lead to a diagnosis of COP and successful treatment with corticosteroids. Many causes of organising pneumonia are only identifiable clinically. Without clinical input, a reasonable pathological conclusion is 'organising pneumonia, aetiology not apparent'.

Figure 6.2.2 Cryptogenic organising pneumonia. (A) Air space consolidation is evident on low-power microscopy. (B) Higher power shows buds of granulation tissue within alveoli adjacent to a bronchovascular bundle. (C) Partial epithelialisation of the periphery of the granulation tissue buds may occur. (D) An elastin stain highlights the intra-alveolar rather than interstitial location.

Acute fibrinous and organising pneumonia

On occasion organising pneumonia may be associated with prominent knots of fibrin, resulting in a histological pattern that has been termed acute fibrinous and organising pneumonia (Fig. 6.2.3).[21,22] The clinical features and course of the disease are more those of acute alveolar injury but the hyaline membranes of diffuse alveolar damage are not evident and there is no eosinophilia. Cases have been described in association with drug toxicity and following stem cell transplanta-tion, associations that are also seen with the more typical pattern of organising pneumonia described above. Other associations have included collagen vascular disease, bacterial infection, lymphoma and a variety of environmental and occupational exposures.[22] Acute fibri-nous and organising pneumonia probably represents a florid variant of organising pneumonia rather than a different disease. Imaging shows bilateral basal opacities that are either diffuse or reticulo-nodular. The prognosis is poor, similar to that seen in acute lung injury of any cause.

Figure 6.2.3 Acute fibrinous and organising pneumonia. The alveoli contain both fibrin and buds of granulation tissue.

Figure 6.2.4 'Desquamative' interstitial pneumonia represents an alveolar filling defect rather than an interstitial disease.

DESQUAMATIVE INTERSTITIAL PNEUMONIA

Desquamative interstitial pneumonia (DIP) is characterised by an excess of alveolar macrophages so marked that the alveoli are practically filled by these cells. This is accompanied by only a mild degree of chronic interstitial inflammation so that the alveolar walls are only slightly thickened, if at all. The adjective 'interstitial' therefore puts the wrong emphasis on what is essentially an alveolar filling defect (Fig. 6.2.4). Furthermore, the term 'desquamative' is quite inappropriate. It was introduced[23] in the belief that the free cells were exfoliated (desquamated) alveolar epithelial cells, a misconception that is easy to understand when only routinely stained sections are examined (Fig. 6.2.5): the true nature of the free cells was shown first by electron microscopy[24,25] and then by immunocytochemistry (Fig. 6.2.6), which demonstrate that they are macrophages. Nevertheless, although the term 'alveolar macrophage pneumonia' has been suggested, the consensus view is to continue with the more familiar, if histogenetically incorrect, term of DIP.[26]

Aetiology

The nature of DIP is not well understood but its recognised associations suggest that it is a pathological response to a variety of pulmonary insults rather than a specific disease. In adults it mainly affects cigarette smokers and in these individuals it may be regarded merely as an excessive macrophage response to inhaled smoke.[27] DIP is also seen in workers exposed to exceptionally dusty environments.[25,28,29] Others apparently develop DIP in response to relatively low levels of atmospheric pollution, presumably being hypersensitive to dust.[30] Long-term therapy with drugs such as nitrofurantoin may also result in DIP.[31] A minority of patients have connective tissue disorders, although it remains uncertain whether this association is coincidental, represents a direct effect or is related to smoking.[32–34] A role has also been proposed for osteopontin, raised levels of which have been identified in bronchoalveolar lavage from patients with both DIP and Langerhans cell histiocytosis.[35] DIP is also encountered in children, sometimes as a manifestation of surfactant apoprotein B deficiency. Other children with DIP have had lipid storage diseases and it is possible that unrecognised metabolic defects may be responsible for

Figure 6.2.5 'Desquamative' interstitial pneumonia. The alveoli are filled by mononuclear cells that morphologically resemble the adjacent hyperplastic alveolar type II epithelial cells and it is easy to imagine a desquamative process.

other cases (see p. 46). There remains a small group of patients, who despite all clinical investigations have no evidence of any potential causative association and may therefore be regarded as having idiopathic DIP.[36]

Clinical features

Most patients with DIP are middle-aged cigarette smokers who complain of breathlessness and cough of insidious onset. Chest radiographs show hazy 'ground-glass' opacification of the lower lung fields, sometimes accompanied by reticular markings and cystic change (Fig. 6.2.7).[37–39] Pulmonary function tests show a restrictive pattern with a reduction in diffusing capacity. Hypoxaemia is often evident on blood gas analysis. Bronchoalveolar lavage shows increased numbers of macrophages, eosinophils (mean 18%) and neutrophilis

Figure 6.2.6 'Desquamative' interstitial pneumonia. Immunostaining for (A) the macrophage marker CD68 and (B) the epithelial (cytokeratin) marker MNF116 shows that the cells filling the alveoli are macrophages rather than desquamated epithelial cells.

Figure 6.2.7 'Desquamative' interstitial pneumonia. High-resolution computed tomography shows patchy peripheral ground-glass shadowing.

Figure 6.2.8 'Desquamative' interstitial pneumonia. The macrophages that fill the alveoli include multinucleate forms.

Figure 6.2.9 'Desquamative' interstitial pneumonia. Lymphoid foci representing follicular bronchiolitis stand out against the general consolidation.

(mean 11%).[39] Most patients respond well to corticosteroids,[26,38,40–42] especially if they quit smoking. They may recover completely, or stabilise, but relapse many years later is recorded,[43,44] even after lung transplantation.[45] In a minority of patients the disease progresses slowly to interstitial fibrosis,[37,46] ultimately proving fatal after, on average, 12 years.[40] The outcome is worse in children, especially in infants and those with familial disease.

Pathological features

The principal histopathological feature is consolidation of the lung by large numbers of alveolar macrophages, which may be multinucleate (see Figs 6.2.4, 6.2.5 and 6.2.8). This is accompanied by an interstitial lymphocytic infiltrate and fibrosis, both of which are usually mild. There is often also follicular bronchiolitis, the scattered lymphoid follicles contrasting with the diffuse macrophage accumulation (Fig. 6.2.9). The macrophages have abundant eosinophilic cytoplasm, which often contains brown granules that stain variably with both Perls and periodic acid–Schiff reagents (Fig. 6.2.10). Eosinophils are occasionally evident, but not so many in lung tissue as on lavage. Centriacinar emphysema may be seen as an independent smoking-related condition.[36]

Figure 6.2.10 'Desquamative' interstitial pneumonia. Endogenous cytoplasmic pigment granules are strongly stained by the periodic acid–Schiff reaction.

Differential diagnosis

As well as being a response to extrinsic stimuli such as smoke, dust and drugs, DIP, or an appearance very like it, often accompanies other lung diseases, which it may mask.[47] For example, the small focal lesions of Langerhans cell histiocytosis are often accompanied by an excess of alveolar macrophages and may consequently be overlooked.[48] Similarly, alveolar macrophages are often considerably increased near a tumour and may be the only abnormality evident in a small biopsy: if a neoplasm is suspected clinically but only an excess of macrophages is found, a further biopsy should be advised rather than proffering a diagnosis of DIP. In resolving eosinophilic pneumonia eosinophils may be scanty and macrophages numerous so that the appearances simulate DIP.

The frequent association of DIP with cigarette smoking is also seen in respiratory bronchiolitis-associated interstitial lung disease (RBILD: see below), which it closely resembles histologically, the principal differences being the centriacinar concentration of the macrophages and the mild peribronchiolar fibrosis of the latter condition. The term 'smoking-related interstitial lung disease' has been proposed to encompass DIP, RBILD and Langerhans cell histiocytosis,[34,49,50] but there are differences in the spectrum of associated clinical disorders.[26]

UIP may be associated with considerable numbers of alveolar macrophages and therefore resemble DIP but the latter is more uniform in its distribution and appearance: the patchy subpleural preponderance of UIP is not seen in DIP. Any fibrosis that develops in DIP is diffuse and temporally uniform, resembling non-specific interstitial pneumonia more than UIP, and possibly representing a further effect of smoking.[36]

If multinucleate macrophages are prominent, the giant cell interstitial pneumonia of cobalt workers may be considered but the multinucleate epithelial cells that characterise this condition are not evident in DIP.

A lipidosis may result in a pattern resembling DIP. Cytoplasmic vacuolation of the alveolar macrophages favours such a diagnosis, especially if there is no evidence of airway obstruction, which commonly causes the accumulation of foamy macrophages.

Lastly, DIP may be mimicked by an unusual pattern of carcinoma, one in which the neoplastic cells are poorly cohesive and fill rather than destroy the alveoli. Immunostaining for epithelial and macrophage markers (cytokeratin and CD67 respectively) readily distinguishes the two.[51]

RESPIRATORY BRONCHIOLITIS AND RESPIRATORY BRONCHIOLITIS-ASSOCIATED INTERSTITIAL LUNG DISEASE

The term 'respiratory bronchiolitis' (RB) was coined in 1974 to describe the presence of pigmented macrophages within the respiratory bronchioles of healthy young cigarette smokers.[52] RB was subsequently recognised in patients with evidence of mild respiratory dysfunction and the term 'respiratory bronchiolitis-associated interstitial lung disease' or RBILD was introduced for this clinical syndrome.[53] RBILD has been regarded as the clinical correlate of RB, and RB as the histopathological basis of RBILD, but attention is increasingly being drawn to centriacinar interstitial fibrosis in cigarette smokers, thus extending the histopathological basis of RB-ILD.[54–56] Patients with RB or RBILD are almost universally heavy cigarette smokers.[27,50] Conversely, RB is present in almost all heavy smokers but not all smokers develop RBILD.

RBILD is considered in this chapter rather than that preceding because of its link to RB and hence DIP, both of which affect the air spaces more than the interstitium. These diseases all largely affect smokers and are characterised by an accumulation of smokers' macrophages. They also show considerable clinical and radiological overlap.[27,36,54] It may be that DIP is a particularly florid form of RB.[57,58] Many cases formerly identified as DIP would now be regarded as showing RB or RBILD and the three may merely be regarded as different aspects of 'smoking-related interstitial lung disease'.[34,50,59]

Clinical features

Patients with RB are often asymptomatic and unaware that there is anything amiss with their lungs whereas those with RBILD generally complain of cough and mild breathlessness.[53,57] Other symptoms include chest pain, weight loss and, rarely, fever and haemoptysis. Crepitations are heard on auscultation but clubbing is unusual. Chest radiographs usually show airway thickening but may be normal. There may also be linear opacities suggestive of interstitial lung disease. HRCT scans show varying degrees of patchy ground-glass opacity and centrilobular nodules (Fig. 6.2.11).[60] Lung function tests may be normal or show a mild restrictive defect. If the patient gives up smoking or receives corticosteroids the changes largely clear: the prognosis is good.[27,57]

Pathology

In both RB and DIP the predominant change is an excess of alveolar macrophages but in RB the changes are centriacinar, the excess macrophages filling the lumina of the respiratory bronchioles and alveoli surrounding the terminal and respiratory bronchioles rather than being diffusely distributed throughout the acinus (Fig. 6.2.11). In both diseases the macrophages contain an abundance of brown smoke particles. The interstitial component of RBILD consists of a variable degree of fibrosis around the bronchioles and involving the walls of adjacent alveoli. The fibrosis is described as hyaline, hypocellular and resembling amyloid.[55] The peripheral pulmonary parenchyma is usually normal but rare cases may show patchy subpleural fibrosis. 'Honeycombing' is not a feature and if present suggests that the RB is an incidental finding.[55,60]

Differential diagnosis

RB and RBILD are distinguished from DIP by the distribution of the pigmented macrophages, as outlined above, while RBILD also has its

Figure 6.2.11 Respiratory bronchiolitis-associated interstitial lung disease. (A) High-resolution computed tomography shows patchy ground-glass attenuation with evidence of air-trapping. (B) Microscopy shows alveolar filling by macrophages and mild focal thickening of the interstitium by chronic inflammation and fibrosis. Unlike desquamative interstitial pneumonia, the distribution is centriacinar rather than diffuse (compare with Fig. 6.2.4). (C) Peribronchiolar fibrosis may also be seen. (D) Brown (smoker's) pigment is evident in the cytoplasm of the macrophages.

interstitial component. The distinction of RB and RBILD from other patterns of interstitial pneumonia is the same as for DIP but some workers stress the hypocellular nature of the fibrosis.[55] RB often accompanies other smoking-related changes and if seen alone in a biopsy from a patient who has been confidently diagnosed as having another smoking-related disease there has probably been a sampling error. Thus, RB may accompany and obscure the focal lesions of Langerhans cell histiocytosis, which is also strongly related to cigarette smoking. Other independent smoking-related changes such as emphysema may also accompany RB. Inflammation and fibrosis of the bronchiolar wall are also described in cigarette smokers[61] and may therefore be associated with RB.

EXOGENOUS LIPID PNEUMONIA

Exogenous lipid pneumonia results from the aspiration or inhalation of oils, which may be animal, vegetable or mineral. A common example is liquid paraffin, which gains access to the lungs via the trachea when it is taken orally as a lubricant for constipation and inadvertently aspirated,[62–67] or when it is used as a vehicle for drugs administered by a nasal spray. It is not very irritative and the patient is often unaware that aspiration is occurring. Aspiration of the ingested oil occurs during sleep and is especially likely if there is achalasia of the cardia or hiatus hernia with reflux.[65] Aspiration of petroleum jelly applied to the nose has also led to exogenous lipid pneumonia.[68] Examples of animal or vegetable fat being aspirated include milk[69] or fatty dietary supplements such as ghee[70] entering the lungs of debilitated children with feeding difficulties. The aspiration of vegetable oil also occurred in the past from the use of menthol in olive oil for the treatment of tuberculous laryngitis, and occasionally from the use of iodinated vegetable oils for bronchography.[71,72] Unusual causes of exogenous lipid pneumonia include occupational exposure to oil mists[73] and the smoking of blackfat tobacco,[74] while an acute form may occur after massive aspiration by fire-eaters.[75] Clinically, patients typically present with non-resolving consolidation (Fig. 6.2.12) but occasionally a localised mass mimicking malignancy may occur.

In the lungs, the oil gives rise to a chronic granulomatous lesion that radiologically may simulate a carcinoma, and in some such cases lobectomy has been undertaken unnecessarily.[62] The term 'paraffinoma' is often applied to localised tumour-like lesions caused by the aspiration of liquid paraffin. In other cases, a widespread 'pneumonia' has proved fatal, its true nature only being recognised postmortem (see Fig. 6.2.12).[64]

Histologically, droplets of oil are surrounded by macrophages and foreign-body giant cells. The droplets may form a fine sieve-like pattern, but adjoining droplets tend to coalesce, with the result that many alveoli are filled by a single large globule (Fig. 6.2.13A). Since the oil is dissolved out in histological processing, the alveoli appear empty and may be mistakenly thought to have contained air rather than lipid. Attention may then be concentrated on the relatively minor interstitial changes and the alveolar filling may be overlooked. On closer examination, however, multinucleated giant cells are evident stretched around the globules, and this should suggest the true diagnosis. If reserve tissue is available, frozen sections may be stained for fat (Fig. 6.2.13B).

In contrast to the relatively inactive long-chain saturated hydrocarbons of mineral derivation, animal oils may cause intense inflammation and even necrosis. This is caused by injurious free fatty acids, which may be present in the oil itself, or released by enzymatic action within the lungs. Most animal and vegetable oils contain unsaturated lipids, which are osmiophilic, whereas mineral oils such as liquid paraffin that are fully saturated do not stain with osmic acid. Halogenated hydrocarbons such as the bronchography medium lipiodol (iodized poppy seed oil) can be differentially stained with brilliant cresyl blue.[76] In a few cases, infrared spectrophotometry has been used to identify the nature of the oils.[63,65,66]

In infants the presence of foamy macrophages in the sputum or bronchoalveolar lavage is often taken to indicate gastric reflux and poorly defined respiratory problems are then ascribed to the aspiration of gastric material,[77,78] but this cannot go unchallenged as macrophage clearance is one of the ways the lung normally rids itself of spent surfactant, resulting in lipid-laden foamy macrophages.

ENDOGENOUS LIPID PNEUMONIA (OBSTRUCTIVE PNEUMONITIS)

The lung generates considerable amounts of lipid to reduce alveolar surface tension. Much of this lipid is recycled by the alveolar epithelium but some is cleared through the airways and, if these are obstructed, for example by a tumour, the spent surfactant accumulates in alveolar macrophages. These cells then increase in number and size and take on the usual appearance of lipophages, developing a voluminous foamy cytoplasm (Fig. 6.2.14). The alveoli become filled with these cells and macroscopically the affected area shows yellow consolidation, sometimes referred to as golden or obstructive pneumonia.[79,80] Similar changes develop when the alveolar architecture is

Figure 6.2.12 Exogenous lipid pneumonia that was only recognised postmortem. Subsequent enquiries established that, unknown to her medical attendants, the patient had been ingesting massive amounts of liquid paraffin to counter constipation.

disrupted, impairing the clearance of lung lipids, as in diffuse fibrosis. In long-standing cases foamy macrophages may distend the interstitium rather than the air spaces and the appearances simulate those of diffuse panbronchiolitis (see p. 124). Endogenous and exogenous lipid are compared in Table 6.2.1.

Chronic interstitial pneumonia generally develops, and if the obstruction is not relieved, infection is almost inevitable, causing acute pneumonia, which may progress to abscess formation or bronchiectasis. Occasionally granulomatous inflammation destroys the walls of airways beyond the obstruction, closely simulating the appearances of bronchocentric granulomatosis. Sometimes the foamy

Figure 6.2.13 Exogenous lipid pneumonia. (A) What might appear at first sight to be air spaces represent dissolved globules of liquid paraffin; multinucleate foreign-body giant cells stretched around the globules provide a clue to the diagnosis. (B) Oil red O fat stain performed on frozen section showing that the spaces contain lipid rather than air.

Figure 6.2.14 Endogenous lipid pneumonia due to bronchial obstruction. The clearance of lung lipids, chiefly spent surfactant, is impaired and foamy macrophages fill the alveoli (A). (B) In contrast to exogenous lipoid pneumonia the cytoplasm shows fine vacuolation.

macrophages disintegrate to release their charge of ingested lipid and the accumulation of this material may closely simulate the appearances of alveolar lipoproteinosis, which is described next, even to the extent of including cholesterol crystals. Endogenous lipid pneumonia may also develop without airway obstruction in lipidoses such Niemann–Pick disease[81] and in response to amphiphilic drugs such as amiodarone (Table 6.2.2).

ALVEOLAR LIPOPROTEINOSIS

Alveolar lipoproteinosis is a rare condition characterised by finely granular eosinophilic material filling the air spaces. It was first named, and is still generally known as, pulmonary alveolar proteinosis,[82,83] but lipoproteinosis reflects better the chemical composition of the alveolar material. The nature of the lipoprotein varies and several causes are now recognised. Since its initial description in 1958 over 400 cases have been reported.[83]

Table 6.2.1 Comparison of exogenous and endogenous lipid pneumonia

	Exogenous	**Endogenous**
Foamy macrophages	Intra-alveolar and interstitial	Intra-alveolar
Giant cells	Around droplets	Absent (except around cholesterol crystals)
Extracellular fat droplets	Many and varied in size	Absent
Obstructing lesion	Absent	Present
Lipid	Usually mineral (saturated and therefore non-osmiophilic)	Animal (unsaturated and therefore osmiophilic)

Table 6.2.2	Causes of endogenous lipoid pneumonia
Localised	Airway obstruction (usually tumour) Successful tumour ablation
Bronchocentric	Diffuse panbronchiolitis
Diffuse	Drug reaction (e.g. amiodarone) Inborn error of metabolism (e.g. Niemann–Pick)

Aetiology and pathogenesis

Alveolar lipoproteinosis has long been regarded as representing a failure of the alveolar macrophages to rid the lungs of spent surfactant[84–86] and it is now recognised that this defect generally has an autoimmune basis. In most cases the condition is attributable to the development of autoantibodies that neutralise granulocyte–macrophage colony-stimulating factor (GM-CSF) and so impair macrophage function.[87–91] An alveolar CD4 lymphocytosis is evident once the alveoli have been cleared of the lipoproteinaceous material.[92]

In other patients the condition is secondary to heavy dust exposure.[93–97] Here it appears to be due to hypersecretion of surfactant exceeding the capability of the normal clearance mechanism. Evidence for this derives from animal dusting experiments leading to alveolar lipoproteinosis in which it was found that surfactant synthesis trebled whereas macrophage clearance only doubled.[98,99] Such experiments also show that the condition evolves through a stage of endogenous lipid pneumonia characterised by the accumulation of large lipid-laden macrophages that eventually break down to release their burden of spent surfactant.[100,101] At first the released material is loosely floccular and weakly staining but it gradually condenses to assume the characteristic staining properties of alveolar lipoproteinosis described below.[102] Some patients exhibit both alveolar lipoproteinosis and endogenous lipid pneumonia.[103]

In a further animal model, rats given high doses of amphiphilic drugs such as chlorphentermine, iprindole and amiodarone over long periods developed endogenous lipid pneumonia[104–106] and occasionally this progressed to alveolar lipoproteinosis.[107] These drugs block lysosomal sphingomyelinase and phospholipase and the material that accumulates in the alveoli of these animals represents the accumulated substrate of these lipases. The process here is analogous to the lipid storage disorders, except that the lysosomal deficiency is acquired rather than inborn.

Alveolar lipoproteinosis has also been reported in children with various enzyme defects, notably those that result in deficiency of surfactant proteins (see p. 46).[108–113] It seems likely that in these children the alveolar lipoproteinosis represents a compensatory hypersecretion of surfactant. Again there is an initial stage of endogenous lipid pneumonia, representing macrophage ingestion of the excess surfactant. Alveolar lipoproteinosis has also been reported in patients with lysinuric protein intolerance, appearing first in either childhood[114–116] or adult life.[117] It is uncertain whether the lipoproteinosis in these patients results from a defect in surfactant synthesis or faulty macrophage function. Other children with alveolar lipoproteinosis show mutation of the gene responsible for the β-chain of the GM-CSF receptor.[118] Genetic defects presumably account for rare familial cases reported in the older literature.[119,120]

Other patients with alveolar lipoproteinosis have leukaemia, lymphoma or other diseases characterised by immunosuppression,[121–124] In these patients surfactant is only weakly represented in the alveolar material[125,126] and there is also interstitial pneumonia or fibrosis.[127]

Figure 6.2.15 Alveolar lipoproteinosis. High-resolution computed tomography shows a 'crazy paving' pattern of opacification.

The pathogenesis in these patients is poorly understood but the lipoprotein may represent autophagosomal residual bodies extruded from degenerate alveolar cells.[128] A similar mechanism may operate in the rare cases that complicate pulmonary infection[129] or lung transplantation.[116,130]

Appearances very similar to those of alveolar lipoproteinosis may result from bronchial obstruction, as described above under endogenous lipid pneumonia. They have also been described in association with a surfactant-secreting bronchioloalveolar cell carcinoma.[131]

One conclusion to be drawn from these varied observations is that alveolar lipoproteinosis represents a clinicopathological syndrome of multiple causation rather than a single disease.

Clinical features

Alveolar lipoproteinosis may affect patients of any age, but in one large cohort the median age at diagnosis was 51 years and men outnumbered women by 2 to 1.[91] However, the genetic defects referred to above generally manifest themselves in childhood. Most studies report an increased incidence of smoking.[132,133]

The main symptom is slowly increasing dyspnoea.[91] Radiographically, alveolar lipoproteinosis is often characterised by patches of consolidation alternating with normal lung, although in the first case to be described there were perihilar feathery opacities that suggested oedema.[82] However, no cause for oedema was apparent and no evidence of oedema is ever found on auscultation. HRCT scan is characteristic, showing a 'crazy paving' pattern of alveolar 'ground-glass' consolidation with interlobular septal thickening (Fig. 6.2.15).[133–135] The diagnosis may be established by alveolar lavage (Fig. 6.2.16),[132,136–138] while the identification of autoantibodies against GM-CSF is diagnostic in those cases in which these antibodies play a causative role.[139]

Spontaneous remission occurs in about a third of patients with the autoimmune form of the disease, a further third stabilise, and the remainder progress.[140] These last patients formerly died of the disease but therapeutic lung lavage[136,141–143] has transformed the prognosis. More recently the administration of GM-CSF by either subcutaneous injection or aerosol has been introduced as a further treatment

Figure 6.2.16 Alveolar lipoproteinosis. Lung lavage shows clumps of acellular proteinaceous debris with very few inflammatory cells.

Figure 6.2.17 Alveolar lipoproteinosis. Therapeutic bronchoalveolar lavage recovers an opalescent, white fluid.

option.[92,144–146] The regulatory relationship between interleukin-10 and GM-CSF suggest that levels of interleukin-10 and anti-GM-CSF titres are indicative of response to GM-CSF therapy.[143,147,148]

Therapeutic lavage is performed under general anaesthesia, one lung being washed out at a time with up to 30 litres of saline introduced through a cuffed double-lumen tube that permits respiration to continue in the other lung.[136,141] The recovered lavage fluid is milky white and with time white flocculent material precipitates out (Fig. 6.2.17). Residual saline is rapidly absorbed.[149] Lavage may be repeated if the disease recurs and ultimately this treatment generally proves effective. Some patients have undergone lung transplantation but recurrent alveolar lipoproteinosis is recorded, even following double-lung transplantation.[150]

Pathological features

Chemical analysis of material washed from patients' lungs shows considerable amounts of lipids, including those that normally lower the alveolar surface tension. However, the lavage material is deficient in such physical properties, perhaps due to lysosomal activity within alveolar macrophages, but its surface activity can be restored by ethanol.[151]

Histologically, the alveoli are filled with a finely granular acellular deposit that is eosinophilic, and generally periodic acid–Schiff-positive and diastase-resistant (Fig. 6.2.18A, B).[82,121] The staining with periodic acid–Schiff reagents is explained by the presence of large amounts of surfactant apoprotein, which is heavily glycosylated. The surfactant apoprotein can also be demonstrated immunohistochemically (Fig. 6.2.18C).[125,126] Electron microscopy shows that the alveolar deposit consists of innumerable osmiophilic lamellar bodies consistent with denatured surfactant.(Fig. 6.2.19).[136] Foamy macrophages and cholesterol crystal clefts are often found within the granular material together with eosinophilic globules, the latter representing surfactant apoprotein-D, in contrast to the granular material which stains

for surfactant apoprotein-A.[152] The alveolar walls are generally unremarkable and the condition is essentially an alveolar filling defect. However, those cases in which the disease complicates immunosuppression differ in that surfactant apoprotein is only weakly represented[126] and there is also interstitial pneumonia or fibrosis.[126–128] At autopsy the lungs are heavy, firm and yellow on the cut surface (Fig. 6.2.20).

Differential diagnosis

The differential diagnosis of alveolar lipoproteinosis is from *Pneumocystis jirovecii* pneumonia and pulmonary oedema, but the alveolar material is granular rather than foamy or amorphous, and is associated with cholesterol crystal clefts and foamy macrophages that are not found in either of these conditions. In children the possibility of a surfactant protein gene mutation needs to be considered.

Complications

Opportunistic infections represent the major complication of alveolar lipoproteinosis. *Nocardia* and fungi are mainly involved but mycobacterial infection may also develop.[153–155] It is notable that the growth of these microbes is enhanced in vitro if their culture medium is enriched with the lipoproteinaceous material obtained at lavage.[156] Infection is also promoted by abnormalities in surfactant apoprotein and poor macrophage function impairing host defence.[84–86]

Figure 6.2.18 Alveolar lipoproteinosis. The alveoli are filled by eosinophilic amorphous or finely granular material in which there are the acicular clefts of dissolved cholesterol. The alveolar walls are unremarkable. (A) Haematoxylin and eosin stain. (B) Periodic acid–Schiff stain. (C) Immunoperoxidase stain for surfactant apoprotein.

Figure 6.2.19 Alveolar lipoproteinosis. Electron microscopy of the alveolar material recovered in lung washings. The granular material is lamellar and osmiophilic. The appearances are those of a complex lipid and are consistent with the material representing denatured surfactant.

CHOLESTEROL PNEUMONITIS

Cholesterol accumulation in the lung is manifest in paraffin sections as sheaves of acicular crystal clefts in both the alveolar spaces and interstitium (Fig. 6.2.21). The cholesterol crystals are frequently attended by foreign-body giant cells and a non-specific chronic inflammatory infiltrate. Large numbers of cholesterol crystals may be seen in obstructive pneumonitis, and also without recognised cause.[157] Disruption of the alveolar architecture, as in diffuse fibrosis, impairs the clearance of lung lipids and leads to the accumulation of surfactant, which may be manifest as focal alveolar lipoproteinosis and cholesterol pneumonitis. Diffuse pulmonary fibrosis is often accompanied by type II cell hyperplasia and the metabolic activity of these surfactant synthesising cells may also contribute to the accumulation of cholesterol and other lipids.[158]

Scanty cholesterol crystal clefts are often a feature of extrinsic allergic alveolitis and are occasionally seen in other granulomatous conditions, for example, sarcoid. They are also recorded in pulmonary hypertension,[159,160] and localised collections are found in necrotic foci such as chronic tuberculous lesions and progressive massive fibrosis of coal-workers.

A review[161] of idiopathic cholesterol pneumonitis identified it as a disease of the elderly, particularly men who were heavy smokers, but the disease is also encountered in children, sometimes in siblings. In children it may sometimes coexist with or progress to alveolar lipoproteinosis (see Figs 6.2.20 and 6.2.21).[162] The relationship of cholesterol pneumonitis to alveolar lipoproteinosis is also demon-

Figure 6.2.20 Alveolar lipoproteinosis. At autopsy the lungs are heavy, firm and yellow on the cut surface.

Figure 6.2.21 Cholesterol pneumonitis. Numerous elongated clefts of dissolved cholesterol crystals are evident in this lung biopsy of a young girl who within 4 years had died of alveolar lipoproteinosis (shown in Fig. 6.2.20).

Figure 6.2.22 Corpus amylaceum. Corpora amylacea are sometimes found incidentally in the lungs, free in the alveoli. This one has a central black particle, which has possibly acted as the starting point on which the body has formed.

strated by the development of either condition in patients with errors in surfactant synthesis and lysinuric protein intolerance.[114,115,117]

Changes resembling those of cholesterol pneumonitis are found in alkane lipogranulomatosis but this is a generalised storage disorder that affects many other organs as well as the lungs (see p. 492).

CORPORA AMYLACEA

Corpora amylacea identical to those more commonly seen in the prostate were first described in the lungs by Friedrich in 1856.[163] They are an incidental finding, more common in the elderly, and on occasion they may be observed in the sputum.[164] They are round, intra-alveolar structures, 50–150 µm in diameter (Fig. 6.2.22), which stain uniformly with both eosin and Congo red. With the latter stain, polarisers show both the birefringence and dichroism of amyloid,[164] which immunocytochemically is shown to be derived from β_2 macroglobulin.[165] Polarising filters also show both radial striations and circumferential lamellae,[164] the latter representing periodic precipitation zones (Liesegang rings) that occur spontaneously in colloidal solutions.[166] Electron microscopy[164] shows that the bodies consist largely of sheaves of microfibrils, possibly representing cytokeratin derived from alveolar epithelial cells. Elongated macrophages occasionally adhere to the surface of the bodies. Occasionally a central

black spherule is evident, suggesting that a dust particle has provided a nidus on which alveolar secretions of cellular components may have precipitated (see Fig. 6.2.22).[164,167] Corpora amylacea are merely microscopic curiosities that have no clinical importance, unless they are mistaken for fungal spores or parasitic ova.

ALVEOLAR MICROLITHIASIS

Alveolar microlithiasis is a rare condition characterised by extensive alveolar accumulation of calcified microliths. It was first described in 1918[168] and received its current designation in 1933.[169] Virtually any age group may be affected but the third and fourth decades are most frequently involved.[170-173] Both sporadic and familial cases are reported, the latter reflecting autosomal-recessive inheritance.[170,171,174,175] Males outnumber females in the sporadic cases whereas the reverse is true when the disease is familial. There is a wide geographical distribution but exceptionally high numbers are reported from Turkey, Italy and the USA.[175-177] The cause appears to be mutation of the type IIb sodium phosphate co-transporter gene *SLC34A2*.[178,179] This is involved in phosphate homeostasis in several organs, including the lung where its gene product, which is expressed by type II alveolar epithelial cells, controls uptake of the phosphate required for surfactant synthesis. Loss of function of the gene product results in calcium chelation and hence microlith formation.

The disease is characterised by a distinctive fine micronodular calcification in the lungs that is heaviest basally or around the hila but may be so extensive as to produce almost complete radiographic opacification. Lymph nodes are not enlarged. The condition may be symptomless and discovered by chance on routine chest radiography. HRCT shows dense alveolar calcification with a perilobular and bronchovascular distribution.[180] The disease may stabilise at any time but more often over a period of many years it progressively restricts lung movement and impairs gas diffusion until it eventually leads to severe dyspnoea and death from respiratory and cardiac failure.[171,181,182] Serum levels of surfactant proteins A and D correlate with progression of the disease, and may provide a useful monitoring tool. No effective medical treatment has yet been reported except for regression of the opacification in one patient treated with disodium editronate, an agent that inhibits the microcrystalline growth of hydroxyapatite.[183] Lung transplantation has proved successful in some cases.[184,185]

Most cases have been diagnosed at necropsy, when the lungs are rock-hard and extremely heavy, and a band saw is generally needed to cut them into slices. However, with greater recognition of the disorder, diagnosis is now usually made on either transbronchial biopsy or bronchoalveolar lavage, or, when other family members are affected, by HRCT alone.[177] In decalcified sections, enormous numbers of wavy concentrically laminate microliths, up to 300 μm in diameter, can be seen filling the alveoli (Fig. 6.2.23). The alveolar walls surrounding them may undergo fibrosis. In less advanced areas, only occasional microliths are scattered among otherwise normal air spaces. Rarely, the microliths are also present in the alveolar interstitium and bronchial mucosa.[186] Sometimes they are identified in the sputum,[171,187] where they are to be distinguished from the larger 'liths' that derive from a focus of dystrophic calcification eroding a bronchus.[188,189] Analysis shows them to consist of calcium and phosphorus salts in the form of carboxyapatite.[173,190,191]

Figure 6.2.23 Alveolar microlithiasis. (A) High-resolution computed tomography shows patchy alveolar shadowing with dense subpleural and septal opacification. (B) The alveoli are filled by innumerable heavily calcified lamellar bodies of wavy configuration.

CALCOSPHERITES (CONCHOIDAL BODIES)

The term 'calcospherite' or 'conchoidal body' is applied to certain laminated calcified structures found in either the air spaces or the tissues of the lung, where they are respectively known as blue bodies and Schaumann bodies.

'Blue bodies'

Blue bodies are laminated intra-alveolar structures that are usually found in focal collections (Fig. 6.2.24).[192-194] Individually, they measure 15–40 μm in diameter and are hence smaller than microliths or corpora amylacea. The name blue body derives from their weak haematoxyphilia. Calcium carbonate in a mucopolysaccharide matrix is the major component but there is also an outer rim of iron. Blue bodies are most frequently found when there is an excessive number of alveolar macrophages, as in DIP; they probably represent the extruded residual bodies of lysosomes. They are a histopathological curio of no clinical importance, unless mistaken for life-threatening conditions such as alveolar microlithiasis (see above).[195]

Schaumann bodies

Schaumann bodies are found within connective tissue rather than the air spaces but will be dealt with here as they are similar to blue bodies. They are commonly found in granulomas and, like blue bodies, they probably represent the residuum of lysosomal activity. They may be found in large numbers in the scars of healed sarcoidosis or berylliosis (see Fig. 6.1.31). They are larger than blue bodies, measuring up to 80 μm in diameter, and are more distinctly laminate and calcific. Similar calcospherites are sometimes found within the stroma of papillary tumours, in both the lung and other organs.

Figure 6.2.24 Alveolar calcospherites. These structures probably derive from alveolar macrophage lysosomal activity, being found in conditions marked by increased numbers of these cells. Their haematoxyphilia is responsible for their colloquial name of 'blue bodies'.

Figure 6.2.25 Alveolar ossification. An incidental finding in the lungs of a man dying of unrelated causes.

ALVEOLAR OSSIFICATION

Dystrophic ossification is common in the lung but is interstitial and is therefore dealt with elsewhere (see p. 149). This section deals with isolated foci of laminated bone that are found on occasion within alveoli of otherwise normal appearance (Fig. 6.2.25).[196,197] This form of ossification is commonest in the elderly and particularly in association with prolonged pulmonary congestion or thromboembolism. It is therefore likely to represent a form of acquired metaplasia rather than a congenital heterotopia. It is generally an incidental finding of no clinical consequence.

REFERENCES

Cryptogenic organising pneumonia (idiopathic bronchiolitis obliterans organising pneumonia)

1. Liebow AA, Carrington CB. The interstitial pneumonias. In: Simon M, editor. Frontiers of Pulmonary Radiology. New York: Grune & Stratton; 1969. p. 102–41.
2. Otto H, Mieth I. Morphology and therapeutic chances of interstitial lung disease. Respiration 1979;38:171–6.
3. Grinblat J, Mechlis S, Lewitus Z. Organizing pneumonia-like process. An unusual observation in steroid responsive cases with features of chronic interstitial pneumonia. Chest 1981;80: 259–63.
4. Davison AG, Heard BE, McAllister WAC, et al. Cryptogenic organizing pneumonitis. Q J Med 1983;52:382–94.
5. Epler GR, Colby TV, McLoud TC, et al. Bronchiolitis obliterans organizing pneumonia. N Engl J Med 1985;312:152–8.
6. Fukuda Y, Ishizaki M, Kudoh S, et al. Localization of matrix metalloproteinases-1, -2, and -9 and tissue inhibitor of metalloproteinase-2 in interstitial lung diseases. Lab Invest 1998;78:687–98.

7. King TE. BOOP: an important cause of migratory pulmonary infiltrates? Eur Respir J 1995;8:193–5.
8. Costabel U, Teschler H, Guzman J. Bronchiolitis obliterans organizing pneumonia (BOOP) – the cytological and immunocytological profile of bronchoalveolar lavage. Eur Respir J 1992;5:791–7.
9. Cordier JF. Organising pneumonia. Thorax 2000;55:318–28.
10. Spiteri MA, Klenerman P, Sheppard MN, et al. Seasonal cryptogenic organising pneumonia with biochemical cholestasis – a new clinical entity. Lancet 1992;340:281–4.
11. Miyagawa Y, Nagata N, Shigematsu N. Clinicopathological study of migratory lung infiltrates. Thorax 1991;46:233–8.
12. Crestani B, Kambouchner M, Soler P, et al. Migratory bronchiolitis obliterans organizing pneumonia after unilateral radiation therapy for breast carcinoma. Eur Respir J 1995;8:318–21.
13. Bayle JY, Nesme P, Bejui-Thivolet F, et al. Migratory organizing pneumonitis 'primed' by radiation therapy. Eur Respir J 1995;8:322–6.
14. Stover DE, Milite F, Zakowski M. A newly recognized syndrome – Radiation related bronchiolitis obliterans and organizing

pneumonia. Respiration 2001;68: 540–4.
15. Yigla M, BenItzhak O, Solomonov A, et al. Recurrent, self-limited, menstrual-associated bronchiolitis obliterans organizing pneumonia. Chest 2000;118:253–6.
16. Cohen AJ, King TE Jr, Downey GP. Rapidly progressive bronchiolitis obliterans with organizing pneumonia. Am J Respir Crit Care Med 1994;149:1670–5.
17. Colby TV. Pathologic aspects of bronchiolitis obliterans organizing pneumonia. Chest 1992;102:S38–43.
17a. Yi E, Aubry MC. Pulmonary pseudoneoplasms. Arch Pathol Lab Med 2010;134:417–26.
18. Myers JL, Katzenstein ALA. Ultrastructural evidence of alveolar epithelial injury in idiopathic bronchiolitis obliterans-organizing pneumonia. Am J Pathol 1988;132:102–9.
19. Yousem SA, Lohr RH, Colby TV. Idiopathic bronchiolitis obliterans organizing pneumonia/ cryptogenic organizing pneumonia with unfavorable outcome: Pathologic predictors. Modern Pathol 1997;10:864–71.
20. Uner AH, Rozumslota B, Katzenstein ALA. Bronchiolitis obliterans-organizing pneumonia (BOOP)-like variant of

Wegener's granulomatosis: a clinicopathologic study of 16 cases. Am J Surg Pathol 1996;20:794–801.

Acute fibrinous and organising pneumonia

21. Yoshinouchi T, Ohtsuki Y, Kubo K, et al. Clinicopathological study on two types of cryptogenic organizing pneumonitis. Respir Med 1995;89:271–8.

22. Beasley MB, Franks TJ, Galvin JR, et al. Acute fibrinous and organizing pneumonia – A histologic pattern of lung injury and possible variant of diffuse alveolar damage. Arch Pathol Lab Med 2002;126:1064–70.

Desquamative interstitial pneumonia

23. Liebow AA. Definition and classification of interstitial pneumonias in human pathology. Prog Resp Res 1975;8:1–33.

24. Leroy EP. Desquamative interstitial pneumonia. Virchows Arch A Pathol Anat Histopathol 1969;348:117–30.

25. Corrin B, Price AB. Electron microscopic studies in desquamative interstitial pneumonia associated with asbestos. Thorax 1972;27:324–31.

26. American Thoracic Society/European Respiratory. Society international multidisciplinary consensus classification of the idiopathic interstitial pneumonias. Am J Respir Crit Care Med 2002;165:277–304.

27. Ryu JH, Myers JL, Capizzi SA, et al. Desquamative interstitial pneumonia and respiratory bronchiolitis-associated interstitial lung disease. Chest 2005;127:178–84.

28. Herbert A, Sterling G, Abraham J, et al. Desquamative interstitial pneumonia in an aluminum welder. Hum Pathol 1982;13:694–9.

29. Freed JA, Miller A, Gordon RE, et al. Desquamative interstitial pneumonia associated with chrysotile asbestos fibres. Br J Ind Med 1991;48:332–7.

30. Abraham JL, Hertzberg MA. Inorganic particulates associated with desquamative interstitial pneumonia. Chest 1981;80S:67S–70S.

31. Bone RC, Wolfe J, Sobonya RE, et al. Desquamative interstitial pneumonia following long-term nitrofurantoin therapy. Am J Med 1976;60:697–701.

32. Tubbs RR, Benjamin SP, Reich NE, et al. Desquamative interstitial pneumonitis: cellular phase of fibrosing alveolitis. Chest 1977;72:159–65.

33. Ishii H, Iwata A, Sakamoto N, et al. Desquamative interstitial pneumonia (DIP) in a patient with rheumatoid arthritis: is DIP associated with autoimmune disorders? Intern Med 2009;48:827–30.

34. Vassallo R, Ryu JH. Tobacco smoke-related diffuse lung diseases. Semin Respir Crit Care Med 2008;29:643–50.

35. Prasse A, Stahl M, Schulz G, et al. Essential role of osteopontin in smoking-related interstitial lung diseases. Am J Pathol 2009;174:1683–91.

36. Craig PJ, Wells AU, Doffman S, et al. Desquamative interstitial pneumonia, respiratory bronchiolitis and their relationship to smoking. Histopathology 2004;45:275–82.

37. Hartman TE, Primack SL, Kang EY, et al. Disease progression in usual interstitial pneumonia compared with desquamative interstitial pneumonia: assessment with serial CT. Chest 1996;110:378–82.

38. Akira M, Yamamoto S, Hara H, et al. Serial computed tomographic evaluation in desquamative interstitial pneumonia. Thorax 1997;52:333–7.

39. Kawabata Y, Takemura T, Hebisawa A, et al. Eosinophilia in bronchoalveolar lavage fluid and architectural destruction are features of desquamative interstitial pneumonia. Histopathology 2008;52:194–202.

40. Carrington CB, Gaensler EA, Coutu RE, et al. Natural history and treated course of usual and desquamative interstitial pneumonia. N Engl J Med 1978;298:801–9.

41. Turner-Warwick M, Burrows B, Johnson A. Cryptogenic fibrosing alveolitis: clinical features and their influence on survival. Thorax 1980;35:171–80.

42. Nicholson AG, Colby TV, du Bois RM, et al. The prognostic significance of the histologic pattern of interstitial pneumonia in patients presenting with the clinical entity of cryptogenic fibrosing alveolitis. Am J Respir Crit Care Med 2000;162:2213–7.

43. Hunter AM, Lamb D. Relapse of fibrosing alveolitis (desquamative interstitial pneumonia) after twelve years. Thorax 1979;34:677–9.

44. Lipworth BJ, Woodcock A, Addis B, et al. Late relapse of desquamative interstitial pneumonia. Am Rev Respir Dis 1987;136:1253–5.

45. Verleden GM, Sels F, VanRaemdonck D, et al. Possible recurrence of desquamative interstitial pneumonitis in a single lung transplant recipient. Eur Resp J 1998;11:971–4.

46. McCann BG, Brewer DB. A case of desquamative interstitial pneumonia progressing to 'honeycomb lung'. J Pathol 1974;112:199–202.

47. Bedrossian CWM, Kuhn C, Luna MA, et al. Desquamative interstitial pneumonia-like reaction accompanying pulmonary lesions. Chest 1977;72:166–9.

48. Vassallo R, Jensen EA, Colby TV, et al. The overlap between respiratory bronchiolitis and desquamative interstitial pneumonia in pulmonary Langerhans cell histiocytosis – High-resolution CT, histologic, and functional correlations. Chest 2003;124:1199–205.

49. Ryu JH, Colby TV, Hartman TE, et al. Smoking-related interstitial lung diseases: a concise review. EurRespJ 2001;17:122–32.

50. Wells AU, Nicholson AG, Hansell DM. Challenges in pulmonary fibrosis 4: Smoking-induced diffuse interstitial lung diseases. Thorax 2007;62:904–10.

51. Mutton AE, Hasleton PS, Curry A, et al. Differentiation of desquamative interstitial pneumonia (DIP) from pulmonary adenocarcinoma by immunocytochemistry. Histopathology 1998;33:129–35.

Respiratory bronchiolitis and respiratory bronchiolitis-associated interstitial lung disease

52. Niewoehner DE, Kleinerman J, Rice DB. Pathologic changes in the peripheral airways of young cigarette smokers. N Engl J Med 1974;291:755.

53. Myers JL, Veal CF, Shin MS, et al. Respiratory bronchiolitis causing interstitial lung disease. A clinicopathological study of six cases. Am Rev Respir Dis 1987;135:880–4.

54. Fraig M, Shreesha U, Savici D, et al. Respiratory bronchiolitis – A clinicopathologic study in current smokers, ex-smokers, and never-smokers. Am J Surg Pathol 2002;26:647–53.

55. Yousem SA. Respiratory bronchiolitis-associated interstitial lung disease with fibrosis is a lesion distinct from fibrotic nonspecific interstitial pneumonia: a proposal. Mod Pathol 2006;19:1474–9.

56. Kawabata Y, Hoshi E, Murai K, et al. Smoking-related changes in the background lung of specimens resected for lung cancer: a semiquantitative study with correlation to postoperative course. Histopathology 2008;53:707–14.

57. Yousem SA, Colby TV, Gaensler EA. Respiratory bronchiolitis-associated interstitial lung disease and its relationship to desquamative interstitial pneumonia. Mayo Clin Proc 1989;64:1373–80.

58. Katzenstein ALA. Idiopathic interstitial pneumonia: classification and diagnosis. In: Churg A, Katzenstein ALA, editors. The Lung: Current Concepts. Baltimore: Williams & Wilkins; 1993. p. 1–31.

59. Heyneman LE, Ward S, Lynch DA, et al. Respiratory bronchiolitis, respiratory bronchiolitis-associated interstitial lung disease, and desquamative interstitial pneumonia: different entities or part of the spectrum of the same disease process? Am J Roentgenol 1999;173:1617–22.

60. Moon J, Dubois RM, Colby TV, et al. Clinical significance of respiratory bronchiolitis on open lung biopsy and its relationship to smoking related interstitial lung disease. Thorax 1999;54:1009–14.

61. Adesina AM, Vallyathan V, McQuillen EN, et al. Bronchiolar inflammation and

fibrosis associated with smoking – a morphologic cross-sectional population analysis. Am Rev Respir Dis 1991;143:144–9.

Exogenous lipid pneumonia

62. Wagner JC, Adler DI, Fuller DN. Foreign body granulomata of the lungs due to liquid paraffin. Thorax 1955;10: 157–70.

63. Elston CW. Pneumonia due to liquid paraffin: with chemical analysis. Arch Dis Child 1966;41:428–34.

64. Salm R, Hughes EW. A case of chronic paraffin pneumonitis. Thorax 1970;25:762–8.

65. Fox B. Liquid paraffin pneumonia – with chemical analysis and electron microscopy. Virchows Arch A Pathol Anat Histopathol 1979;382:339–46.

66. Corrin B, Crocker PR, Hood BJ, et al. Paraffinoma confirmed by infrared spectrophotometry. Thorax 1987;42:389–90.

67. Midulla F, Strappini PM, Ascoli V, et al. Bronchoalveolar lavage cell analysis in a child with chronic lipid pneumonia. Eur Resp J 1998;11:239–42.

68. Brown AC, Slocum PC, Putthoff SL, et al. Exogenous lipoid pneumonia due to nasal application of petroleum jelly. Chest 1994;105:968–9.

69. Gibson JB. Infection of the lungs by 'saprophytic' mycobacteria in achalasia of the cardia, with report of a fatal case showing lipoid pneumonia due to milk. J Pathol Bacteriol 1953;65:239–51.

70. Annobil SH, Morad NA, Khurana P, et al. Reaction of human lungs to aspirated animal fat (ghee): a clinicopathological study. Virchows Arch 1995;426:301–5.

71. Felton WL. The reaction of pulmonary tissue to lipiodol. J Thorac Surg 1953;25:530–42.

72. Greenberg SD, Spjut HJ, Hallman GL. Experimental study of bronchographic media on lung. Arch Otolaryngol Head Neck Surg 1966;83:276–82.

73. Skorodin MS, Chandrasekhar AJ. An occupational cause of exogenous lipoid pneumonia. Arch Pathol Lab Med 1983;107:610–1.

74. Miller GJ, Ashcroft MT, Beadnell HMSG, et al. The lipoid pneumonia of blackfat tobacco smokers in Guyana. Q J Med 1971;40:457–70.

75. Trullas Vila JC, Pizarro SS, Nogue XS, et al. Acute exogenous lipoid pneumonia in 'fire-eaters'. Description of two cases. Rev Clin Esp 2007;207:240–2.

76. Felton WL. A method for the identification of lipiodol in tissue sections. Lab Invest 1952;1:364–7.

77. Nussbaum E, Maggi JC, Mathis R, et al. Association of lipid-laden alveolar macrophages and gastroesophageal reflux in children. J Pediatr 1987;110: 190–4.

78. Moran JR, Block SM, Lyerly AD, et al. Lipid-laden alveolar macrophages and lactose assay as markers of aspiration in neonates with lung disease. J Pediatr 1988;112:643–5.

Endogenous lipid pneumonia

79. De Navasquez SJ, Trounce JR, Wayte AB. Lipoid pneumonia (non-inhalation) in carcinoma of the lung treated by radiotherapy. Lancet 1951;1:1206–8.

80. De Navasquez SJ, Haslewood GAD. Endogenous lipoid pneumonia with special reference to carcinoma of the lung. Thorax 1954;9:35–7.

81. Nicholson AG, Wells AU, Hooper J, et al. Successful treatment of endogenous lipoid pneumonia due to Niemann–Pick type B disease with whole-lung lavage. Am J Respir Crit Care Med 2002;165: 128–31.

Alveolar lipoproteinosis

82. Rosen SH, Castleman B, Liebow AA. Pulmonary alveolar proteinosis. N Engl J Med 1958;258:1123–42.

83. Seymour JF, Presneill JJ. Pulmonary alveolar proteinosis – progress in the first 44 years. Am J Respir Crit Care Med 2002;166:215–35.

84. Golde DW, Territo M, Finley TN, et al. Defective lung macrophages in pulmonary alveolar proteinosis. Ann Intern Med 1976;85:304–9.

85. Nugent KM, Pesanti EL. Macrophage function in pulmonary alveolar proteinosis. Am Rev Respir Dis 1983;127:780–1.

86. Gonzalez-Rothi RJ, Harris JO. Pulmonary alveolar proteinosis. Further evaluation of abnormal alveolar macrophages. Chest 1986;90:656–661.

87. Dranoff G, Crawford AD, Sadelain M, et al. Involvement of granulocyte-macrophage colony-stimulating factor in pulmonary homeostasis. Science 1994;264:713–6.

88. Seymour JF, Begley CG, Dirksen U, et al. Attenuated hematopoietic response to granulocyte-macrophage colony-stimulating factor in patients with acquired pulmonary alveolar proteinosis. Blood 1998;92:2657–67.

89. Kitamura T, Tanaka N, Watanabe J, et al. Idiopathic pulmonary alveolar proteinosis as an autoimmune disease with neutralizing antibody against granulocyte/macrophage colony-stimulating factor. J Exp Med 1999;190:875–80.

90. Trapnell BC, Whitsett JA, Nakata K. Pulmonary alveolar proteinosis. N Eng J Med 2003;349:2527–39.

91. Inoue Y, Trapnell BC, Tazawa R, et al. Characteristics of a large cohort of patients with autoimmune pulmonary alveolar proteinosis in Japan. Am J Respir Crit Care Med 2008;177:752–62.

92. Schoch OD, Schanz U, Koller M, et al. BAL findings in a patient with pulmonary alveolar proteinosis successfully treated with GM-CSF. Thorax 2002;57:277–80.

93. Buechner HA, Ansari A. Acute silico-proteinosis. Dis Chest 1969;55:274–84.

94. Xipell JM, Ham KN, Price CG, et al. Acute silicolipoproteinosis. Thorax 1977;32:104–11.

95. Suratt PM, Winn WC, Brody AR, et al. Acute silicosis in tombstone sandblasters. Am Rev Respir Dis 1977;115:521–9.

96. Miller RR, Churg AM, Hutcheon M, et al. Case report: pulmonary alveolar proteinosis and aluminum dust exposure. Am Rev Respir Dis 1984;130:312–5.

97. McDonald JW, Alvarez F, Keller CA. Pulmonary alveolar proteinosis in association with household exposure to fibrous insulation material. Chest 2000;117:1813–7.

98. Heppleston AG, Fletcher K, Wyatt I. Changes in the composition of lung lipids and the 'turnover' of dipalmitoyl lecithin in experimental alveolar lipo-proteinosis induced by inhaled quartz. Br J Exp Pathol 1974;55:384–95.

99. Miller BE, Bakewell WE, Katyal SL, et al. Induction of surfactant protein (SP-A) biosynthesis and SP-A mRNA in activated type II cells during acute silicosis in rats. Am J Respir Cell Mol Biol 1990;3: 217–26.

100. Gross P, De Treville RTP. Alveolar proteinosis. Its experimental production in rodents. Arch Pathol 1968;86:255–61.

101. Corrin B, King E. Experimental endogenous lipid pneumonia and silicosis. J Pathol 1969;97:325–30.

102. Corrin B, King E. Pathogenesis of experimental pulmonary alveolar proteinosis. Thorax 1970;25:230–6.

103. McDonald JW, Roggli VL, Bradford WD. Coexisting endogenous and exogenous lipoid pneumonia and alveolar proteinosis in a patient with neurodevelopmental disease. Pediatr Pathol 1993;14:505–11.

104. Heath D, Smith P, Hasleton PS. Effects of chlorphentermine on the rat lung. Thorax 1973;28:551–8.

105. Vijeyaratnam GS, Corrin B. Fine structural alterations in the lungs of iprindole-treated rats. J Pathol 1974;114:233–9.

106. Costa-Jussa FR, Corrin B, Jacobs JM. Amiodarone lung toxicity: a human and experimental study. J Pathol 1984;144:73–9.

107. Vijeyaratnam GS, Corrin B. Pulmonary alveolar proteinosis developing from desquamative interstitial pneumonia in long term toxicity studies of iprindole in the rat. Virchows Arch A Pathol Anat Histopathol 1973;358:1–10.

108. Nogee LM, Demello DE, Dehner LP, et al. Brief report – deficiency of pulmonary surfactant protein-B in congenital alveolar proteinosis. N Engl J Med 1993;328:406–10.

109. Demello DE, Nogee LM, Heyman S, et al. Molecular and phenotypic variability in the congenital alveolar proteinosis syndrome associated with inherited surfactant protein B deficiency. J Pediatr 1994;125:43–50.

110. Nogee L, Garnier G, Dietz H, et al. A mutation in the surfactant protein B gene responsible for fatal neonatal respiratory disease in multiple kindreds. J Clin Invest 1994;93:1860–3.

111. Demello DE, Heyman S, Phelps DS, et al. Ultrastructure of lung in surfactant protein B deficiency. Am J Respir Cell Mol Biol 1994;11:230–9.

112. Ball R, Chetcuti PAJ, Beverley D. Fatal familial surfactant protein B deficiency. Arch Dis Child 1995;73:F53.

113. Mildenberger E, Demello DE, Lin ZW, et al. Focal congenital alveolar proteinosis associated with abnormal surfactant protein B messenger RNA. Chest 2001;119:645–7.

114. Parto K, Kallajoki M, Aho H, et al. Pulmonary alveolar proteinosis and glomerulonephritis in lysinuric protein intolerance: case reports and autopsy findings of four pediatric patients. Hum Pathol 1994;25:400–7.

115. McManus DT, Moore R, Hill CM, et al. Necropsy findings in lysinuric protein intolerance. J Clin Pathol 1996;49: 345–7.

116. Santamaria F, Brancaccio G, Parenti G, et al. Recurrent fatal pulmonary alveolar proteinosis after heart–lung transplantation in a child with lysinuric protein intolerance. J Pediatr 2004;145:268–72.

117. Parto K, Maki L, Pelliniemi LJ, et al. Abnormal pulmonary macrophages in lysinuric protein intolerance: ultrastructural, morphometric, and X-ray microanalytic study. Arch Pathol Lab Med 1994;118:536–41.

118. Dirksen U, Nishinakamura R, Groneck P, et al. Human pulmonary alveolar proteinosis associated with a defect in GM-CSF/IL-3/IL-5 receptor common beta chain expression. J Clin Invest 1997;100:2211–7.

119. Webster JR, Battifora H, Furey C, et al. Pulmonary alveolar proteinosis in two siblings with decreased immunoglobulin A. Am J Med 1980;69:786–9.

120. Teja K, Cooper PH, Squires JE, et al. Pulmonary alveolar proteinosis in four siblings. N Engl J Med 1981;305:1390–2.

121. Williams GE, Medley DRK, Brown R. Pulmonary alveolar proteinosis. Lancet 1960;i:1385–8.

122. Carnovale R, Zornoza J, Goldman AM, et al. Pulmonary alveolar proteinosis: its association with hematologic malignancy and lymphoma. Radiology 1977;122:303–6.

123. Bedrossian CWM, Luna MA, Conklin RH, et al. Alveolar proteinosis as a consequence of immunosuppression. A hypothesis based on clinical and pathologic observations. Hum Pathol 1980;11:527–35.

124. Ruben FL, Talamo TS. Secondary pulmonary alveolar proteinosis occurring in two patients with acquired immune deficiency syndrome. Am J Med 1986;80:1187–90.

125. Singh G, Katyal SL. Surfactant apoprotein in nonmalignant pulmonary disorders. Am J Pathol 1980;101:51–62.

126. Singh G, Katyal SL, Bedrossian CWM, et al. Pulmonary alveolar proteinosis. Chest 1983;83:82–6.

127. Hudson AR, Halprin GM, Miller JA, et al. Pulmonary interstitial fibrosis following alveolar proteinosis. Chest 1974;65: 700–2.

128. Jacobovitz-Derks D, Corrin B. Degenerative processes in the pathogenesis of pulmonary alveolar lipoproteinosis. Virchows Arch A Pathol Anat Histopathol 1977;376:165–74.

129. Butnor KJ, Sporn TA. Human parainfluenza virus giant cell pneumonia following cord blood transplant associated with pulmonary alveolar proteinosis. Arch Pathol Lab Med 2003;127:235–8.

130. Yousem SA. Alveolar lipoproteinosis in lung allograft recipients. Hum Pathol 1997;28:1383–6.

131. Vazquez M, Sidhu GS. Surfactant production by neoplastic type II pneumocytes. Ultrastruct Pathol 1988;12:605–12.

132. du Bois RM, McAllister WAC, Branthwaite MA. Alveolar proteinosis: diagnosis and treatment over a 10-year period. Thorax 1983;38:360–3.

133. Shah PL, Hansell D, Lawson PR, et al. Pulmonary alveolar proteinosis: clinical aspects and current concepts on pathogenesis. Thorax 2000;55:67–77.

134. Rossi SE, Erasmus JJ, Volpacchio M, et al. 'Crazy-paving' pattern at thin-section CT of the lungs: radiologic-pathologic overview. Radiographics 2003;23:1509–19.

135. Holbert JM, Costello P, Li W, et al. CT features of pulmonary alveolar proteinosis. AJR Am J Roentgenol 2001;176:1287–94.

136. Costello JF, Moriarty DC, Branthwaite MA, et al. Diagnosis and management of alveolar proteinosis: the role of electron microscopy. Thorax 1975;30:121–32.

137. Milleron BJ, Costabel U, Teschler H, et al. Bronchoalveolar lavage cell data in alveolar proteinosis. Am Rev Respir Dis 1991;144:1330–2.

138. Mikami T, Yamamoto Y, Yokoyama M, et al. Pulmonary alveolar proteinosis: diagnosis using routinely processed smears of bronchoalveolar lavage fluid. J Clin Pathol 1997;50:981–4.

139. Bonfield TL, Russell D, Burgess S, et al. Autoantibodies against granulocyte macrophage colony-stimulating factor are diagnostic for pulmonary alveolar proteinosis. Am J Respir Cell Molec Biol 2002;27:481–6.

140. Larson RK, Gordinier R. Pulmonary alveolar proteinosis: report of six cases, review of the literature, and formulation of a new theory. Ann Intern Med 1965;62:292–312.

141. Danel C, Israel-Biet D, Costabel U, et al. Therapeutic applications of bronchoalveolar lavage. Eur Respir J 1992;5:1173–5.

142. Beccaria M, Luisetti M, Rodi G, et al. Long-term durable benefit after whole lung lavage in pulmonary alveolar proteinosis. Eur Resp J 2004;23:526–31.

143. Morgan C. The benefits of whole lung lavage in pulmonary alveolar proteinosis. Eur Respir J 2004;23:503–5.

144. Barraclough RM, Gillies AJ. Pulmonary alveolar proteinosis: a complete response to GM-CSF therapy. Thorax 2001;56:664–5.

145. Venkateshiah SB, Yan TD, Bonfield TL, et al. An open-label trial of granulocyte macrophage colony stimulating factor therapy for moderate symptomatic pulmonary alveolar proteinosis. Chest 2006;130:227–37.

146. Wylam ME, Ten R, Prakash UBS, et al. Aerosol granulocyte-macrophage colony-stimulating factor for pulmonary alveolar proteinosis. Eur Respir J 2006;27:585–93.

147. Bonfield TL, Kavuru MS, Thomassen MJ. Anti-GM-CSF titer predicts response to GM-CSF therapy in pulmonary alveolar proteinosis. Clin Immunol 2002;105:342–50.

148. Thomassen MJ, Raychaudhuri B, Bonfield TL, et al. Elevated IL-10 inhibits GM-CSF synthesis in pulmonary alveolar proteinosis. Autoimmunity 2003;36:285–90.

149. Chesnutt MS, Nuckton TJ, Golden J, et al. Rapid alveolar epithelial fluid clearance following lung lavage in pulmonary alveolar proteinosis. Chest 2001;120:271–4.

150. Parker LA, Novotny DB. Recurrent alveolar proteinosis following double lung transplantation. Chest 1997;111: 1457–8.

151. McClenahan JB, Mussenden R. Pulmonary alveolar proteinosis. Arch Intern Med 1974;133:284–7.

152. Kobayashi M, Takeuchi T, Ohtsuki Y. Differences in the immunolocalization of surfactant protein (SP)-A, SP-D, and KL-6 in pulmonary alveolar proteinosis. Pathology International 2008;58: 203–7.

153. Burbank B, Morrione TG, Cutler SS. Pulmonary alveolar proteinosis and nocardiosis. Am J Med 1960;28: 1002–7.

154. Summers JE. Pulmonary alveolar proteinosis. Review of the literature with follow-up studies and report of two new cases. Calif Med 1966;104:428–36.

155. Reyes JM, Putong PB. Association of pulmonary alveolar lipoproteinosis with mycobacterial infection. Am J Clin Pathol 1980;74:478–85.

156. Ramirez RJ, Savard EV, Hawkins JE. Biological effects of pulmonary washings from cases of alveolar proteinosis. Am Rev Respir Dis 1966;94:244–6.

Cholesterol pneumonitis

157. Waddell WR, Sniffen RC, Sweet RH. Chronic pneumonitis: its clinical and pathologic importance. Report of ten cases showing interstitial pneumonitis and unusual cholesterol deposits. J Thorac Surg 1949;18:707–37.

158. Kay JM, Heath D, Hasleton PS, et al. Aetiology of pulmonary cholesterol-ester granulomas. Br J Dis Chest 1970;64:55–7.

159. Fischer EG, Marek JM, Morris A, et al. Cholesterol granulomas of the lungs associated with microangiopathic hemolytic anemia and thrombocytopenia in pulmonary hypertension – A case report and review of the literature. Arch Pathol Lab Med 2000;124:1813–5.

160. Nolan RL, McAdams HP, Sporn TA, et al. Pulmonary cholesterol granulomas in patients with pulmonary artery hypertension: chest radiographic and CT findings. AJR Am J Roentgenol 1999;172:1317–9.

161. Lawler W. Idiopathic cholesterol pneumonitis. Histopathology 1977;1:385–95.

162. Sato K, Takahashi H, Amano H, et al. Diffuse progressive pulmonary interstitial and intra-alveolar cholesterol granulomas in childhood. Eur Respir J 1996;9:2419–22.

Corpora amylacea

163. Friedreich N. Corpora amylacea in den Lungen. Arch Path Anat 1856;9:613–8.

164. Michaels L, Levene C. Pulmonary corpora amylacea. J Path Bact 1957;74:49–56.

165. Rocken C, Linke RP, Saeger W. Corpora amylacea in the lung, prostate and uterus – a comparative and immunohistochemical study. Pathol Res Pract 1996;192:998–1006.

166. Tuur SM, Nelson AM, Gibson DW, et al. Liesegang rings in tissue. How to distinguish Liesegang rings from the giant kidney worm, Dioctophyma renale. Am J Surg Pathol 1987;11:598–605.

167. Hollander DH, Hutchins GM. Central spherules in pulmonary corpora amylacea. Arch Pathol Lab Med 1978;102:629–30.

Alveolar microlithiasis

168. Harbitz F. Extensive calcification of the lungs as a distinct disease. Arch Intern Med 1918;21:139–46.

169. Puhr L. Mikrolithiasis alveolaris pulmonum. Virchows Arch A Pathol Anat Histopathol 1933;290:156–60.

170. Sosman MC, Dodd GD, Jones WD. The familial occurrence of pulmonary alveolar microlithiasis. AJR 1957;77:947–1012.

171. Prakash UBS, Barham SS, Rosenow EC, et al. Pulmonary alveolar microlithiasis: a review including ultrastructural and pulmonary function studies. Mayo Clin Proc 1983;58:290–300.

172. Volle E, Kaufmann HJ. Pulmonary alveolar microlithiasis in pediatric patients. Review of the world literature and two new observations. Pediatr Radiol 1987;17:439–42.

173. Moran CA, Hochholzer L, Hasleton PS, et al. Pulmonary alveolar microlithiasis: A clinicopathologic and chemical analysis of seven cases. Arch Pathol Lab Med 1997;121:607–11.

174. Mariotta S, Guidi L, Mattia P, et al. Pulmonary microlithiasis – report of two cases. Respiration 1997;64:165–9.

175. Senyigit A, Yaramis A, Gurkan F, et al. Pulmonary alveolar microlithiasis: A rare familial inheritance with report of six gases in a family – Contribution of six new cases to the number of case reports in Turkey. Respiration 2001;68:204–9.

176. Lauta VM. Pulmonary alveolar microlithiasis: an overview of clinical and pathological features together with possible therapies. Resp Med 2003;97:1081–5.

177. Castellana G, Lamorgese V. Pulmonary alveolar microlithiasis. World cases and review of the literature. Respiration 2003;70:549–55.

178. Corut A, Senyigit A, Ugur SA, et al. Mutations in SLC34A2 cause pulmonary alveolar microlithiasis and are possibly associated with testicular microlithiasis. Am J Hum Genet 2006;79:650–6.

179. Huqun, Izumi S, Miyazawa H, et al. Mutations in the SLC34A2 gene are associated with pulmonary alveolar microlithiasis. Am J Respir Crit Care Med 2007;175:263–8.

180. Cluzel P, Grenier P, Bernadac P, et al. Pulmonary alveolar microlithiasis: CT findings. J Comput Assist Tomogr 1991;15:938–42.

181. Balikian JP, Fuleihan FJD, Nucho CN. Pulmonary alveolar microlithiasis. Report of five cases with special reference to roentgen manifestations. Amer J Roentgenol 1968;103:509–18.

182. O'Neil RP, Cohn JE, Pellegrino ED. Pulmonary alveolar microlithiasis. A family study. Ann Intern Med 1967;67:957–67.

183. Ozcelik U, Gulsun M, Gocmen A, et al. Treatment and follow-up of pulmonary alveolar microlithiasis with disodium editronate: radiological demonstration. Pediatr Radiol 2002;32:380–3.

184. Edelman JD, Bavaria J, Kaiser LR, et al. Bilateral sequential lung transplantation for pulmonary alveolar microlithiasis. Chest 1997;112:1140–4.

185. Tachibana T, Hagiwara K, Johkoh T. Pulmonary alveolar microlithiasis: review and management. Curr Opin Pulm Med 2009;15:486–90.

186. Sears MR, Chang AR, Taylor AJ. Pulmonary alveolar microlithiasis. Thorax 1971;26:704–11.

187. Tao LC. Microliths in sputum specimens and their relationship to pulmonary alveolar microlithiasis. Am J Clin Pathol 1978;69:482–5.

188. Pritzker KPH, Desai SD, Patterson MC, et al. Calcite sputum lith. Characterization by analytic scanning electron microscopy and X-ray diffraction. Am J Clin Pathol 1981;75:253–7.

189. Samson IM, Rossoff LJ. Chronic lithoptysis with multiple bilateral broncholiths. Chest 1997;112:563–5.

190. Barnard NJ, Crocker PR, Blainey AD, et al. Pulmonary alveolar microlithiasis. A new analytical approach. Histopathology 1987;11:639–45.

191. Pracyk JB, Simonson SG, Young SL, et al. Composition of lung lavage in pulmonary alveolar microlithiasis. Respiration 1996;63:254–60.

Calcospherites

192. Dail D, Liebow AA. Intraalveolar conchoidal bodies. Am J Pathol 1976;82:43–4a.

193. Gardiner IT, Uff JS. 'Blue bodies' in a case of cryptogenic fibrosing alveolitis (desquamative type) – an ultra-structural study. Thorax 1978;33:806–13.

194. Koss MN, Johnson FB, Hochholzer L. Pulmonary blue bodies. Hum Pathol 1981;12:258–66.

195. Ratjen FA, Schoenfeld B, Wiesemann HG. Pulmonary alveolar microlithiasis and lymphocytic interstitial pneumonitis in a 10 year old girl. Eur Respir J 1992;5:1283–5.

Alveolar ossification

196. Green JD, Harle TS, Greenberg SD, et al. Disseminated pulmonary ossification. A case report with demonstration of electron-microscopic features. Am Rev Respir Dis 1970;101:293–8.

197. Gortenuti G, Portuese A. Disseminated pulmonary ossification. Eur J Radiol 1985;5:14.

Chapter | 7 |

Occupational, environmental and iatrogenic lung disease

7.1 Occupational disease

This chapter deals with the pneumoconioses, occupational asthma, occupational fevers and the effects of toxic fume and gases. Occupational diseases of the lung considered elsewhere include the effects of atmospheric pressure changes (see p. 368), extrinsic allergic alveolitis (see p. 279), carcinoma of the lung (see p. 534) and asbestos-induced pleural disease (see pp. 714–729). Dusty occupations in general are also associated with an increased risk of chronic obstructive pulmonary disease.[1,2]

PNEUMOCONIOSIS: GENERAL FEATURES

Definition of pneumoconiosis

The term 'pneumoconiosis' is an abbreviation (and etymological corruption) of Zenker's pneumonokoniosis,[3] which derives from *pneumon* (lung) and *konis* (dust) and therefore translates as dusty lung;

©2010 Elsevier Ltd
DOI: 10.1016/B978-0-7020-3369-8.00007-0

in practice the term is confined to the effects of mineral dust on the lungs. Diseases caused by organic dusts are not included among the pneumoconioses and, in medicolegal practice at least, the presence of dust alone is insufficient to indicate pneumoconiosis: for compensation to be considered, the mineral dust must alter the structure of the lung and cause disability. The British Industrial Injuries Advisory Council defined pneumoconiosis as 'permanent alteration of lung structure due to the inhalation of mineral dust and the tissue reactions of the lung to its presence, excluding bronchitis and emphysema'.[4] Parkes recommends that cancer and asthma caused by mineral dust should also be excluded from the definition, an opinion with which we concur.[5]

Dust deposition in the lung

To reach the lung, dust particles have to be very small. Particle density and shape also affect the aerodynamic properties of dust. Host factors such as airflow characteristics, airway branching patterns and airway disease also affect dust deposition. Three deposition mechanisms are recognised (Fig. 7.1.1):

1. Inertial impaction: When air streams change direction or velocity, the inertia of the entrained particles causes them to maintain their original direction for a distance that depends upon their density and the square of their diameter. The same rules govern a car approaching a bend too fast: the car crashes into the outside of the bend.
2. Sedimentation (gravitational settlement): Under the influence of gravity, particles settle with a speed that is proportional to their density and the square of their diameter.
3. Diffusion: Very small airborne particles acquire a random motion as a result of bombardment by the surrounding gas molecules.

Inhaled dust particles are liable to sediment out in the alveoli if they have a diameter in the range of 1–5 μm, are roughly spherical in shape, and in density approximate to that of water. Larger or denser particles impact or precipitate on the walls of the conductive airways and are rapidly removed by ciliary action. Smaller particles may reach the alveoli but do not sediment so readily and many are therefore exhaled. Very small particles are deposited on the walls of alveoli by diffusion but because they are so small the total amount of dust deposited in this way is insignificant compared with that deposited by sedimentation (Fig. 7.1.2). Direct measurement shows that most lung dust (96%) has a particle diameter less than 2.5 μm.[6]

Fibrous dust particles behave differently. Fibres over 100 μm in length may reach the alveoli if they are very thin and remain aligned with the air stream. Fibre penetration is inversely related to path length and the number of bifurcations.[7] Tall people have longer conductive airways and experience more deposition in these sites than short people who have greater alveolar deposition for the same level of exposure.[8]

Slightly more dust is deposited in the right lung than the left, probably because the right main bronchus is more in line with the trachea, and is broader and shorter than the left, and carries 55% of the inhaled air.[9,10]

Dust clearance from the lung

Inhaled dust that settles in the conductive airways is removed within a day or two by ciliary action. Only dust that reaches the alveoli is liable to cause pneumoconiosis and much of this is also removed, but the clearance rate here is much slower: many coalminers continue to expectorate mine dust years after retirement. Alveolar clearance is

Impaction

Sedimentation

Gravity

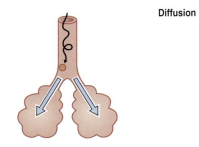

Diffusion

Figure 7.1.1 Mechanisms of particle deposition in the respiratory tract.

largely effected by macrophages, principally via the airways to the pharynx but also via lymphatics to the regional lymph nodes. The airway and interstitial routes interconnect at the bronchiolar level[11] where some dust-laden macrophages leave the interstitium for the air space.[12] This interconnection is probably the route utilised by circulating macrophages clearing other parts of the body of endogenous or exogenous particulate matter via the lung.[13] Long asbestos fibres present a particular problem to macrophage clearance. Some minerals, notably chrysotile asbestos, undergo slow physicochemical dissolution in the lungs.

Only a small fraction of the inhaled dust gains access to the interstitium, a necessary step if it is to cause pneumoconiosis. Some free dust enters through the bronchus-associated lymphoid tissue[11,12] and some is taken up by, or pierces, the alveolar epithelium (Fig. 1.34, p. 21).[14–16] Some of this is transported within hours to the hilar lymph nodes.[17] So rapid is this translocation that it is thought not to involve

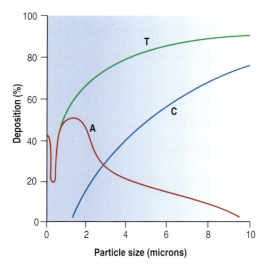

Figure 7.1.2 Percentage dust deposition in the respiratory tract according to particle diameter. The major alveolar impact is that of particles 1–3 μm diameter. Submicron particles are of negligible mass. T, total dust deposition; C, deposition on the ciliated epithelium; A, alveolar deposition.

phagocytes, although interstitial macrophages are undoubtedly important in continuing the transportation of dust to the nodes. Ultrafine dust particles are particularly liable to be transported across the alveolar epithelium.[11] The integrity of the alveolar epithelium is very important to dust translocation from the air spaces to the interstitium. Much more dust reaches the interstitium if the epithelium is damaged.[18,19]

It is widely thought that macrophages that have left the interstitium for the alveolar space never return,[17,20] but this is probably untrue.[21] Heavily laden macrophages accumulate in alveoli bordering the terminal and respiratory bronchioles, eventually filling them completely. Erosion of the alveolar epithelium permits re-entry of these macrophages into the interstitium,[22] very close to foci of bronchial mucosa-associated lymphoid tissue (MALT), which are found near the terminal bronchioles.[23] These aggregates guard the mouths of lymphatics, which commence at this point; alveoli are devoid of lymphatics. Dust-laden interstitial macrophages accumulate in and around the bronchial MALT, which Macklin therefore referred to as dust sumps.[24] Most pneumoconiotic lesions are found in the region of the dust sumps and are therefore focal. Asbestosis is diffuse rather than focal because the long asbestos fibres are not readily mobilised and cannot be concentrated in the centriacinar dust sumps. This is also seen on occasion with platy non-fibrous dusts such as talc, mica, kaolinite and feldspar.[25–33] Within the dust sumps the dust particles are not static. They are constantly being freed and reingested by interstitial macrophages and, because these cells are mobile, successively inhaled dusts soon become intimately mixed.[34] Macrophages play an important role in pneumoconiosis and if the dust is fibrogenic the repeated phagocytosis of indestructible mineral particles results in constant fibroblast stimulation.

The zonal distribution of pneumoconiosis

Pneumoconiosis affects both lungs but seldom evenly and some pneumoconioses show characteristic patterns of lung involvement. In most, the lesions are more numerous and better developed in the upper lobes than the bases but the reverse is true of asbestosis. The reasons for this are complex but undoubtedly involve the dust deposition:clearance ratio for the effect of the dust will depend upon both its amount and the duration of its stay in the lungs. There are well-recognised regional differences in the distribution and clearance of inhaled material, which in turn are dependent upon man's upright posture, the consequent gravitational forces being maximal at the apices.[35] When standing at rest, the apices of the lungs are hardly perfused, so that lymph formation and clearance are much better at the bases.[36–38] Similarly, the apices are relatively less well aerated; alveoli in the lower lobes receive more air than those in the upper lobes.[37,39] The greater respiratory excursions at the bases are thought to promote macrophage mobility there. It is to be expected therefore that the bases would both receive and clear more dust than the apices, rendering it difficult to predict on theoretical grounds which parts of the lungs carry the heaviest dust burden. In fact, more dust of all types is found in the upper lobes, the part most severely affected by every type of pneumoconiosis except asbestosis.[40,41] The predilection of asbestos to affect the periphery of the lower lobes is attributed to the dangerous long asbestos fibres preponderating there.[41,42]

Pulmonary reactions to mineral dust

The main tissue reaction to mineral dust is fibrosis. Silica is highly fibrogenic and is therefore very likely to cause pneumoconiosis. Carbon is non-fibrogenic and therefore, unless there are complications, coal pneumoconiosis causes little disability. Tin too is harmless, and stannosis therefore unimportant, although the chest radiograph is highly abnormal because tin is very radiopaque. Stannosis is one of several terms that specify pneumoconiosis due to a particular mineral, the best known being silicosis, asbestosis and anthracosis. Table 7.1.1 summarises the various pulmonary reactions to mineral dust.

Identification of the dust

The blackness of carbon and red-brown colour of iron give ample evidence, both naked-eye and microscopically, of the type and amount of these dusts when they are present in the lung (Fig. 7.1.3), but other inorganic dusts may be more difficult to identify. However, a flick-out substage condenser and Polaroid filters to test for refractility and birefringence respectively are useful adjuncts that are too often neglected by the histopathologist. Crystalline silica is traditionally regarded as being only weakly birefringent, in contrast to silicates which generally show up brightly with simple crossed Polaroid filters.[43] However, with modern microscope lamps, if the light source is set at high intensity when using Polaroid filters, both silica and silicates are birefringent.[44] Mineralogists use polarising microscopy for analysis, but only by studying large polished crystals with controlled orientation of the light. The small dust particles found in tissue sections are too small to permit analysis by this technique but it is nevertheless very useful for detecting their presence (Fig. 7.1.4).

Particle shape gives a useful indication of mineral type but appearances are sometimes deceptive: the plate-like crystals of talc are seldom observed as such, usually being viewed edge-on, when they appear to be needle-shaped. Occasionally, stains can be used to identify minerals, e.g. a modified Perls' reaction for inhaled iron, and Irwin's aluminon stain for aluminium, but these too have largely been replaced by modern analytical techniques.

Table 7.1.1 Pulmonary reactions to mineral dust

Pulmonary reaction	Examples
Macrophage accumulation with a little reticulin deposition	Anthracosis Siderosis Stannosis Baritosis Coal pneumoconiosis (macules) Aluminium pneumoconiosis (granular aluminium)
Nodular or massive fibrosis	Silicosis Mixed-dust pneumoconiosis Coal pneumoconiosis (nodules)
Diffuse fibrosis	Asbestosis Hard-metal pneumoconiosis Aluminium pneumoconiosis (aluminium fume and stamped aluminium)
Epithelioid and giant cell granulomas	Chronic berylliosis
Alveolar lipoproteinosis	'Acute' silicosis, but also seen with heavy exposure to other dusts (see p. 317)
Small-airway disease	Various dusts (see p. 123)

Microincineration combined with dark-field microscopy can also be used to demonstrate small particles. Incombustible mineral particles that cannot be seen with bright-field or polarising microscopy are rendered visible by this technique and their position on the slide can be compared with tissue reactions evident in a serial section that has not been incinerated. Microincineration has, however, also been largely replaced by modern analytical techniques that will now be considered.

Analytical electron microscopy is very helpful in identifying minerals, whether applied to lung digests or tissue sections.[45-48] Scanning electron microscopy permits the examination of thicker sections than transmission electron microscopy but does not detect very small particles. However, scanning electron microscopy allows more tissue to be examined and avoids the difficulty of cutting mineral particles with an ultramicrotome.

Mineral particles in a 5-µm thick deparaffinised section can be recognised in a scanning electron microscope set to collect the back-scattered electrons.[46] The instrument can then be focused on points of potential interest and switched to X-ray diffraction, which provides information on crystal structure (Fig. 7.1.5). Alternatively, elemental analysis may be undertaken with either energy-dispersive or wavelength-dispersive X-ray spectroscopy. With energy-dispersive X-ray spectroscopy, all elements of atomic number above 11 are identified, whilst with wavelength-dispersive X-ray spectroscopy the section can be scanned for one particular element. With the former technique different elements are shown graphically as individual

Figure 7.1.3 (A) Coal and (B) haematite miner's lungs. The respective black and red colours of these lungs give a good indication of their mineral content. Paper-mounted whole-lung sections. *(Courtesy of WGJ Edwards, London, UK.)*

Figure 7.1.4 Talc pneumoconiosis. Only carbon is evident when the lesions are viewed with (A) non-polarised light, whereas the abundant talc particles are readily seen when (B) polarised light is employed.

Figure 7.1.5 Electron diffraction patterns of gold, used for calibration purposes. The ring pattern (A) indicates that the material is polycrystalline and the spot pattern (B) indicates that it is a single crystal: amorphous materials give no regular pattern. The spacing of the rings gives information on crystalline structure and can be usefully applied to distinguish the various crystalline forms of silica (quartz, tridymite, cristobalite) for example. *(Courtesy of Dr M Wineberg, London, UK.)*

peaks, the heights of which are proportional to the amounts of the different elements within the particle studied, thereby giving information on probable molecular formula (Fig. 7.1.6). Thus, different silicates can be distinguished from each other and also from silica, which registers as pure silicon, oxygen (atomic number 8) not being detected. The fact that the elements of low atomic number that constitute organic chemicals are not detected means that any minerals present (except beryllium, atomic number 4) can be recognised easily in tissue sections. Only particles can be analysed however: elements present in only molecular amounts cannot be detected by X-ray analysis.

The detection of trace amounts of substances such as beryllium requires bulk chemical analysis or techniques that are not widely available such as atomic absorption spectrometry, neutron activation analysis and microprobe mass spectrometry.[49,50] The last of these techniques can also provide molecular (as opposed to elemental) analysis of organic as well as inorganic particles.[51] Another analytical technique of interest is microscopic infrared spectroscopy which provides data on the compound nature of microscopic particles in tissue sections (Fig. 7.1.7). Micro-Raman spectroscopy is also useful in this respect. Some metals cause hypersensitivity, which can be identified by exposing the patient's lymphocytes to metals and measuring their reaction in vitro.[52]

Radiological grading of pneumoconiosis

A scheme for grading pneumoconiosis radiologically by comparison with standard radiographs has been adopted by the International Labour Organisation (ILO) and is widely used.[53] Small opacities (up to 1 cm diameter) are graded by their profusion, 1, 2 and 3 indicating

Figure 7.1.6 Dust particles in the lung: electron microprobe analysis. (A) The secondary (scanning) electron microscopic image of a deparaffinised 5-µm-thick section of lung showing clumps of macrophages in an alveolar lumen. (B) Back-scattered scanning electron microscopic image showing three of the macrophages at higher power: several bright particles worthy of further attention are evident. (C) X-ray energy spectrum of one of the particles showing it to be a silicate. The section had been transferred from a glass to a Perspex slide to avoid background signals, glass being siliceous. Each element emits a unique energy pattern when bombarded by electrons while the number of counts is in proportion to the amount of the particular element that is present in the particle. *(Courtesy of Professor DA Levison, Dundee, UK.)*

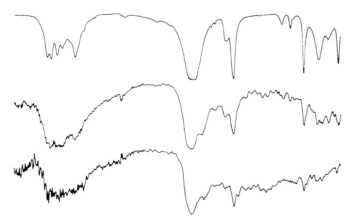

Figure 7.1.7 Infrared spectra of calcium oxalate. Top, reference standard; centre and bottom, crystals in human tissue sections. *(Courtesy of Professor DA Levison, Dundee, UK.)*

increasing numbers, and by their size, increasing through p, q and r if rounded and s, t and u if irregular. Type p opacities are described as punctiform and measure up to 1.5 mm in diameter; larger lesions up to 3 mm in diameter (type q) are described as micronodular or miliary; and those over 3 mm and up to 1 cm in diameter (type r) are described as nodular. Irregular opacities cannot be sized so accurately, s, t and u indicating fine, medium and coarse respectively. Large opacities (over 1 cm diameter) are graded by their combined size, increasing through A, an opacity measuring between 1 and 5 cm in diameter; B, one or more opacities whose combined area does not exceed the equivalent of one-third of the area of the right lung field (when they are regrouped in the mind's eye or measured with a transparent ruler); and C, one or more opacities whose combined area exceeds one-third of the area of the right lung field (when similarly regrouped). In coalworkers, small opacities (up to 1 cm diameter) correspond to simple coalworker's pneumoconiosis and large opacities (over 1 cm diameter) to complicated coalworker's pneumoconiosis, which is also known as progressive massive fibrosis.

SILICOSIS[43]

Mineralogy

Silicosis is caused by the inhalation of silica (silicon dioxide, SiO_2), which is to be distinguished from the silicates, these being more complex compounds in which silicon and oxygen form an anion combined with cations such as aluminium and magnesium: talc, for example, is a hydrated magnesium silicate with the formula $Mg_3Si_4O_{10}(OH)_2$. The element silicon is also to be distinguished from the synthetic organic polymer silicone, used in implants.

Crystalline silica is highly fibrogenic whereas amorphous silica and silicates other than asbestos are relatively inert. Silica exists in several crystalline forms, of which quartz, cristobalite and tridymite are the most important: tridymite is the most fibrogenic and cristobalite more so than quartz.[43,54]

Occupations at risk

Silicotic lesions have been identified in the lungs of Egyptian mummies, and the injurious effects on the lungs of inhaling mine dust have been recognised for more than 400 years. As long ago as the sixteenth century in Joachimsthal, Bohemia (now Jachymov, Czech Republic), diseases of miners' lungs were attributed to the dust the miners breathed. Silicosis, tuberculosis and lung cancer are all now known to have been prevalent among the miners in this region, the cancer being largely attributable to the high level of radioactivity in the mines.

Silicosis was recognised in the UK soon after the discovery in 1720 that the addition of calcined flint to the clay from which china is made produced a finer, whiter and tougher ware. The preparation and use of this flint powder were highly dangerous, causing the condition known as potter's rot, one of the first of the many trade names by which silicosis has since been known. Aluminium oxide (alumina) now provides a safe, effective substitute for flint in this industry.

In 1830 it was noted that Sheffield fork grinders who used a dry grindstone died early, and amongst other preventive measures it was recommended that the occupation should be confined to criminals: fortunately for them, the substitution of carborundum (silicon carbide) for sandstone was effective enough. However, silicosis still occurs in some miners, tunnellers, quarrymen, stone dressers and metal workers.

Silica in one form or another is used in many trades – in the manufacture of glass and pottery, in the moulds used in iron foundries, as an abrasive in grinding and sandblasting, and as a furnace lining that is refractory to high temperatures. Rocks such as granite and sandstone are siliceous and their dusts are encountered in many mining and quarrying operations. In coal mining in the UK the highest incidence of the disease was in pits where the thinness of the coal seams required the removal of a large amount of siliceous rock, a process known as 'hard heading'. In South Africa, silicosis causes a high mortality among the gold miners on the Witwatersrand, where the metallic ore is embedded in quartz. Slate is a metamorphic rock that contains both silica and silicates, and slateworkers develop both silicosis and mixed-dust pneumoconiosis.[55,56] Nor are rural industries immune from the disease, particularly if ventilation is inadequate, as it is in certain African huts where stone implements are used to pound meal and the occupants develop mixed-dust pneumoconiosis.[57] Silicosis and mixed-dust pneumoconiosis have also been reported in dental technicians.[58]

Desert sand is practically pure silica but the particles are generally too large to reach the lungs. However, silicosis has been reported in inhabitants of the Sahara, Libyan and Negev deserts and those living in windy valleys high in the Himalayan mountains,[59–65] whilst in California the inhalation of dust raised from earth has led to silicate pneumoconiosis in farm workers,[66] horses[67] and a variety of zoo animals.[68]

The silica in rocks such as granite, slate and sandstone is largely in the form of quartz and this is therefore the type of silica encountered in most of the industries considered above. Cristobalite and tridymite, which are possibly even more fibrogenic than quartz, are more likely to be encountered in the ceramic, refractory and diatomaceous earth industries where processing involves high temperatures.

Clinical features

Many workers with silicosis are asymptomatic. As a general rule, exposure to silica dust extends over many years, often 20 or more, before the symptoms of silicosis first appear: by the time the disease becomes overt clinically, much irreparable damage has been inflicted on the lungs. The initial symptoms are cough and breathlessness. From then onwards, respiratory disability progresses, even if the patient is no longer exposed to silica dust. Ultimately, there may be distressing dyspnoea with even the slightest exercise.

Silicosis sometimes develops more rapidly, perhaps within a year or so of first exposure. Such 'acute silicosis' was observed in the scouring powder industry in the 1930s when these cleansing agents consisted of ground sandstone mixed with a little soap and washing soda.[69,70] The additives were considered to have rendered the silica in the sandstone more dangerous but it is possible that the rapidity of onset of the disease merely reflected the intensity of the dust cloud to which the packers were exposed. Confusingly, the term 'acute silicosis' has since been applied to a further effect of heavy dust exposure in tunnellers, sand blasters and silica flour workers, namely pulmonary alveolar lipoproteinosis (see below),[71,72] whilst the terms 'accelerated silicosis' or 'cellular phase silicosis' have been substituted for 'acute silicosis' in referring to the rapid development of early cellular lesions.[43,73]

The time from first exposure to the development of symptoms (the latency period) is inversely proportional to the exposure level. However, it is evident that a certain amount of silica can be tolerated in the lungs without fibrosis developing, indicating either a time factor in the pathogenetic process or a threshold dust load that has to be reached before fibrosis develops.

Pathological findings

Silica particles that are roughly spherical in shape and of a diameter in the range of 1–5 μm sediment out in the alveoli and are concentrated within macrophages at Macklin's dust sumps, as explained previously (see p. 27). Early lesions, as seen in so-called accelerated or cellular phase silicosis, consist of collections of macrophages separated by only an occasional wisp of collagen. The early lesions have been likened to granulomas and on occasion have been mistaken for Langerhans cell histiocytosis or a storage disorder, but Langerhans cells are scanty and the histiocytes contain dust particles rather than accumulated lipid or polysaccharide. The macrophages of the early lesion are gradually replaced by fibroblasts and collagen is laid down in a characteristic pattern. The mature silicotic nodule is largely acellular and consists of hyaline collagen arranged in a whorled pattern, the whole lesion being well demarcated (Fig. 7.1.8) and sometimes calcified. Small numbers of birefringent crystals are generally evident within the nodules when polarising filters are used, but these mainly represent silicates such as mica and talc, inhaled with the silica. Silica particles are generally considered to be only weakly birefringent,[43] but fairly strong birefringence is evident in strong light (see above).[44]

Figure 7.1.8 A silicotic nodule consisting of hyaline collagen arranged in a whorled pattern.

The silicotic nodules are situated in the centres of the pulmonary acini and are more numerous in the upper zones than the bases (Fig. 7.1.9A). They measure up to 5 mm across and are hard and easily palpable. They are grey if caused by relatively pure silica but black in coalminers and red in haematite miners.

Silicotic nodules develop first in the hilar lymph nodes and are generally better developed there than in the lungs.[74–76] Indeed, silicotic nodules are occasionally found in the hilar lymph nodes of persons who have no occupational history of exposure to silica and whose lungs are free of such lesions, the silica in the nodes being presumed to represent inhaled particles derived from quartz-rich soil.[77] Severely affected lymph nodes often calcify peripherally, giving a characteristic eggshell-like radiographic pattern. This is sometimes the only radiological abnormality.[76] Such enlarged lymph nodes may occasionally press upon and obstruct adjacent large bronchi[78] or result in a left recurrent laryngeal nerve palsy,[79] so simulating malignancy.[80] Sometimes the nodules develop within the walls of major bronchi, occasionally causing a middle-lobe syndrome (see p. 92).[81] Silicotic nodules are also found along the lines of the pleural lymphatics[75,82] where they have been likened to drops of candle wax on the visceral pleura. Very rarely, silica-induced fibrosis is more pronounced in the pleura than in the lungs.[83]

Lung tissue between the nodules is often quite normal and not until the process is very advanced is there any disability (Fig. 7.1.9B). In severe cases large masses of fibrous tissue are formed, which may undergo central necrosis and cavitation (Fig. 7.1.10).[84] On close inspection it is evident that these consist of conglomerations of many silicotic nodules closely packed together. In such severe cases cor pulmonale develops. Occasionally, silicotic nodules develop in the abdominal as well as the thoracic lymph nodes, and in the liver, spleen, peritoneum and bone marrow.[85–89]

In about 10% of cases, the typical pulmonary nodules that predominantly affect the upper lobes are accompanied by diffuse fibrosis that is maximal in the lower lobes.[27,33,90–92] The latter may show 'honeycombing' and closely resemble idiopathic pulmonary fibrosis. The association is too common to be explained by chance and the diffuse fibrosis is therefore regarded as a further manifestation of the pneumoconiosis, possibly due to an interaction between the dust and the immunological factors discussed below.

Pathogenesis

The pathogenesis of silicosis has excited much interest and many different theories have been advanced over the years. An early theory held

Figure 7.1.9 Silicosis. (A) The nodules are most numerous in the upper part of the lung where there is a conglomerate silicotic mass at one point. Paper-mounted whole-lung section. (B) Microscopy shows silicotic nodules scattered throughout otherwise normal lung tissue.

that the hardness of the silica was responsible, but this was discounted by the observation that silicon carbide (carborundum) is harder than silica but is non-fibrogenic. Theories based on the piezoelectric property and on the solubility of silica were successively abandoned although the latter had a long period of popularity. It gained

Figure 7.1.10 Silicosis. (A) The nodules are larger than in Figure 7.1.9a and have fused together. Cavitating conglomerate silicosis destroys most of the upper lobe. Paper-mounted whole-lung section. (B) Microscopy of conglomerate silicosis.

support from Kettle's experiments which showed that fibrosis developed about chambers placed in an animal's peritoneal cavity if the chambers contained silica powder sealed in by a collodion membrane through which solutes such as silicic acid could pass. However, it was later shown that the pores in a collodion membrane are quite irregular in size and when the experiments were repeated using chambers guarded by millipore membranes, no fibrosis developed, despite solutes being able to diffuse out.[93] The solubility theory also fails to take account of the differing fibrogenicity of the various forms of silica despite them being of similar solubility.[54] Furthermore, if the outer, more soluble layer of the particles is removed by etching, fibrogenicity is increased although solubility is decreased. In line with this, freshly fractured crystalline silica is more pathogenic in every respect than its aged equivalent,[94] which may partly explain the severity of silicosis in trades such as sandblasting. These observations suggest that the fibrogenicity of silica is connected with its surface configuration.

It is now known that uptake of the silica by macrophages is necessary for silicosis to develop. If silica and macrophages are enclosed together in peritoneal millipore chambers, a soluble product of the macrophages diffuses out and causes fibrosis. This observation led to the realisation that the fibrogenicity of the various crystalline forms of silica correlated well with their toxicity to macrophages and for a time macrophage death was thought to be necessary.[95] It is now considered that before the macrophages are killed by the ingested silica, they are stimulated to secrete factors that both damage other constituents of the lung and promote fibrosis.[96–102] Transforming growth factor-β is one fibrogenic factor that has been implicated in the pathogenesis of silicosis.[103–105]

Toxic damage to macrophages is due to silica particles injuring the phagolysosomal membranes, so releasing acid hydrolases into the cytoplasm.[95] It is important in the pathogenesis of the disease indirectly because when the macrophage crumbles, the silica particles are taken up by fresh macrophages and the fibrogenic process continues. It has been suggested that early involvement of the hilar lymph nodes in the fibrogenic process promotes the development of the disease in the lung by delaying dust clearance.[74]

Immunological aspects of silicosis

Immunological factors have been implicated in the pathogenesis of silicosis because many patients with silicosis have polyclonal hyper-gammaglobulinaemia, rheumatoid factor or antinuclear antibodies, and because there is a well-recognised association between auto-immune diseases such as systemic sclerosis and rheumatoid disease and exposure to silica.[43,106–109] The relation of immunity to dust exposure appears to be a reciprocal one: on the one hand, the presence of dust results in rheumatoid lesions in the lungs being more florid (see Caplan's syndrome, p. 341), whilst on the other, non-specific immunisation of rabbits with horse serum results in experimental silicotic lesions being larger and more collagenous.[110] It is doubtful whether pneumoconiosis and autoimmune disease play a causative role in each other but one seems to aggravate the other and may lead to its earlier development.

Tuberculosis complicating silicosis (silicotuberculosis)

One of the commonest and most feared complications of silicosis is chronic respiratory tuberculosis.[109] Once this infection has been added to the silicosis, the prognosis rapidly worsens. It is thought that in the presence of silica, the tubercle bacilli proliferate more rapidly because the ingested silica particles damage phagolysosomal membranes and thereby interfere with the defensive activity of the macrophages. The synergistic action of silica dust has long been held responsible for the inordinately high incidence of respiratory tuberculosis in mining communities. Many former South African gold miners now have acquired immunodeficiency syndrome (AIDS) as well as silicosis and tuberculosis has consequently reached almost epidemic proportions amongst these men. Phagocyte damage by ingested dust particles may also cause some cases of chronic necrotising aspergillosis complicating pneumoconiosis.[111]

Silica-induced lung cancer

A series of studies suggesting that there might be a link between silica inhalation and lung cancer was reviewed by the International Agency for Research on Cancer in 1987, leading to the conclusion that the evidence for carcinogenicity of crystalline silica in experimental animals was sufficient, while in humans it was limited.[112] Subsequent epidemiological publications were reviewed in 1996, when it was concluded that the epidemiological evidence linking exposure to silica to the risk of lung cancer had become somewhat stronger[113] but that in the absence of lung fibrosis remained scanty.[113] The pathological evidence in humans is also weak in that premalignant changes around silicotic nodules are seldom evident.[114] Nevertheless, on this rather insubstantial evidence, lung cancer in the presence of silicosis (but not coal or mixed-dust pneumoconiosis) has been accepted as a prescribed industrial disease in the UK since 1992.[115] Some subsequent studies have provided support for this decision.[116] In contrast to the sparse data on classic silicosis, the evidence linking carcinoma of the lung to the rare diffuse pattern of fibrosis attributed to silica and mixed dusts is much stronger and appears incontrovertible.[33,92]

Alveolar lipoproteinosis in response to heavy dust exposure

A further complication of exposure to silica is the development of alveolar lipoproteinosis (see p. 317).[71,72,117,118] Very heavy experimental exposure to silica, and indeed other dusts, stimulates hypersecretion of alveolar surfactant to such an extent that the normal clearance mechanism is overwhelmed.[119-125] Alveolar macrophages are enlarged by numerous phagolysosomes distended by lamellar bodies that represent ingested surfactant. The alveoli are filled by such cells and, having a foamy cytoplasm, they produce the appearances of endogenous lipid pneumonia, similar to that more usually encountered as part of an obstructive pneumonitis distal to a bronchial tumour. The macrophages gradually disintegrate and the free denatured surfactant slowly becomes compacted, during which time its staining with both eosin and the periodic acid–Schiff reagents intensifies until the appearances are finally those of alveolar lipoproteinosis. This process prevents the aggregation and concentration of the dust in the usual foci and thereby hinders the development of silicosis. Lipoproteinosis and silicosis may be seen in conjunction but, more often, different areas of the lung show one or the other. The lipoproteinosis has its own severe impact on lung function, but, unlike silicosis, is potentially reversible (by massive alveolar lavage).

Silica-induced renal disease

Occasional patients exposed to silica develop renal disease.[126-129] Two mechanisms appear to operate. First, translocation of silica particles from the lungs leads to their deposition in the renal interstitium with resultant nephrotoxicity. Second, silica stimulates an autoimmune response characterised by the formation of various antibodies, notably rheumatoid factor and antinuclear antibodies, which leads to the development of immune complex-mediated glomerulonephritis.[128,129]

Figure 7.1.11 Diatomaceous earth. (A) Scanning electron micrograph showing the calcified diatoms, ×15 000. (B) Electron microprobe analysis shows only silicon (Si); the oxygen with which silicon is combined in silica (silicon dioxide, SiO_2) is of too low an atomic number to register. The titanium (Ti) peak derives from the sample holder. *(Courtesy of Dr D Dinsdale, Leicester, UK and Professor B Nemery, Leuven, Belgium.)*

Amorphous silica

Manmade submicron forms of silica, variously known as amorphous, vitreous, colloidal, synthetic or precipitated silica, are widely used in industry. They consist of pure non-crystalline silicon dioxide. Particle size ranges from 5 to 200 nm but aggregates of the particles measure from 1 to 10 μm. Industrial surveys suggest that inhalation of such dust is harmless, observations that are in accord with the results of animal experiments.[54]

Diatomaceous earth (keiselguhr)

An amorphous silica is the principal component of the fossilised remains of diatoms that constitute the sedimentary rock, diatomite (Fig. 7.1.11). This is generally obtained by open-cast mining, following which the rock is crushed and calcined. The calcined product is used in filters, insulation material and as a filler. Being amorphous, the silica in diatomite is harmless, but calcining (>1000°C) results in its conversion to crystalline forms of silica. Diatomaceous earth pneumoconiosis is unusual and its risk appears to be related to the amount of cristobalite and tridymite (two forms of crystalline silica) produced in the calcining process.[130]

SILICATES[43]

The silicates are complex compounds in which silicon and oxygen form an anion combined with cations such as aluminium and magnesium: talc, for example, is a hydrated magnesium silicate with the formula $Mg_3Si_4O_{10}(OH)_2$. Silicates include fibrous forms (asbestos and the zeolites), plate-like forms (talc and mica) and clays (kaolinite and fuller's earth). In histological sections, the platy talc and mica particles are generally cut tangentially and therefore appear needle-shaped (see Fig. 7.1.4). They are strongly birefringent whereas the clays are only weakly so. Talc particles in the lung exceeding 5 µm in length should arouse suspicion of intravenous drug abuse.[131]

Of the fibrous silicates, zeolite is used as a building material in certain communities, notably in central Turkey. Pneumoconiosis is not a problem but zeolites are of medical interest because, like asbestos, they present a mesothelioma risk. Asbestos is dealt with separately (see below).

Pneumoconiosis has been described with various non-fibrous silicates, notably in the rubber industry, which uses talc and, less commonly, mica as lubricants. Other occupations posing a risk include the extraction of kaolinite from china clay (kaolin),[27,132,133] and in the open-cast and underground mining of fuller's earth (montmorillonite, bentonite and attapulgite clays, which were originally used in 'fulling' (degreasing) wool).[134,135] However, all these substances are commonly contaminated with silica, asbestos or both, and it has been questioned whether in pure state they are at all fibrogenic. The modifying effect of inert substances such as iron on that of silica is well known (see mixed-dust pneumoconiosis, below) and it has been suggested that talc, mica and fuller's earth act in a similar way in regard to their more fibrogenic contaminants, the pneumoconioses attributed to them in reality representing mixed-dust pneumoconiosis or asbestosis. Contrary evidence comes from reports of pulmonary fibrosis in persons heavily exposed to pure talc, mica or kaolin.[32]

All these silicates are evident in the tissues as plate-like birefringent crystals which often provoke a foreign-body giant cell reaction (see Fig. 7.1.3) and may result in fibrotic nodules. Large focal lesions resembling the progressive massive fibrosis of coalworkers may be produced, and also a diffuse 'asbestosis-like' form of pneumoconiosis, the latter attributed to poor macrophage mobilisation of the plate-like particles.[27–32,132–138] It would appear therefore that silicates are indeed fibrogenic if enough is inhaled; they appear to vary in fibrogenicity but in all cases they are less fibrogenic than silica.

INERT DUSTS

Inert dusts are non-fibrogenic and therefore of little clinical consequence, although elements of high atomic number can give rise to a striking chest radiograph.[139] It should be noted however that inert or lowly fibrogenic materials may be associated with substances of medical importance, for example, kaolin, bentonite and barytes (barite) may all be contaminated with silica[27,134,140] and talc may be contaminated with asbestos.

The best known of the inhaled inert mineral dusts is carbon while, of the remainder, iron is the most widespread. Others include tin and barium. With all these dusts, particles retained in the lung are gathered at Macklin's dust sumps by heavily laden macrophages which are lightly bound together there by a few reticulin fibres. Collagen is not formed and the worker suffers no ill-effects. The lungs take on the colour of the dust and in siderosis assume a deep brick-red hue.

Carbon deposition is commonly found in the lungs, particularly those of city dwellers and tobacco smokers. It is also the principal constituent of coal, which is dealt with separately below, and large amounts of pure carbon may be inhaled by workers involved in the manufacture of carbon black, carbon electrodes and charcoal.[141–144] Although carbon is regarded as being non-fibrogenic, the very heavy lung burdens encountered in industries such as these may lead to the complicated form of pneumonconiosis known as progressive massive fibrosis that is more commonly encountered in coal workers (see p. 340). Heavy pure carbon deposition may also be acquired domestically when wood is burnt in buildings devoid of a chimney, so-called 'hut lung',[145] a term that is also applied to the domestic acquisition of carbon mixed with silica or silicates, resulting in forms of mixed-dust pneumoconiosis.[57,64,65]

Anthracofibrosis is a term introduced by Chinese bronchoscopists for bronchial stenosis or obliteration associated with carbon pigmentation of the mucosa.[146] Although the original description incriminated tuberculosis, mixtures of various mineral dusts acquired at work or domestically are a more likely cause.[147–150]

Iron dust in the lungs was first described by Zenker in 1867, when he also introduced the terms siderosis and pneumonokoniosis.[3] Zenker was describing a woman who coloured paper with iron oxide powder ('rouge'), a substance which is still encountered by some workers engaged in polishing silver, glass, stone and cutlery. Siderosis is also found in welders, iron foundry fettlers, steel workers, boiler scalers and haematite miners and crushers. Iron dust particles are reddish-brown but in the lung may be masked by carbon[151]: when evident, or revealed by microincineration, they resemble haemosiderin and generally give a positive Perls' reaction, but particularly with haematite, heat (60–80°C) and concentrated (12N) hydrochloric acid may be necessary.[152]

Haematite miners in both the UK (Cumbria) and France (Lorraine) have an increased risk of bronchial carcinoma, but radon gas rather than haematite is the suspected carcinogen. Radon is a decay product of uranium. Minute amounts are present in all rocks but local concentrations occur and these are liable to build up in mines if ventilation is limited.

Silver, as well as iron, is found in the lungs of silver polishers, where it stains elastin in alveolar walls and pulmonary vessels grey. Such argyrosiderosis is as harmless as siderosis.

Tin miners are subject to silicosis but not stannosis because the ore, which is found in association with siliceous rocks, contains only low concentrations of the metal. Tin smelters, on the other hand, and factory workers exposed to high concentrations of tin dust or fume, are liable to inhale large amounts of this inert metal and develop the striking chest radiograph of stannosis. They remain in good health however for tin is completely non-fibrogenic. Tin particles in the lung resemble carbon but are strongly birefringent and remain after microincineration: microprobe analysis provides positive identification.

Other inert dusts include barium, which also has a high atomic number and is therefore radiopaque,[139] and minerals of low radiodensity such as limestone, marble and cement (all chiefly composed of calcium carbonate) and gypsum (hydrated calcium sulphate). However, the extraction of barium ore (almost entirely in the form of barium sulphate, which is known as barytes in Europe and barite in the USA) may entail exposure to silica and silicates. Pure baritosis resembles stannosis and siderosis.

MIXED-DUST PNEUMOCONIOSIS

The term 'mixed-dust pneumoconiosis' refers to the changes brought about by inhaling a mixture of silica and some other less fibrogenic substance such as iron, carbon, kaolin or mica.[33,151,153–155] The proportion of silica is usually less than 10%. Typical occupations include foundry work and welding and the mining of coal, haematite, slate, shale and china clay.

The action of the silica is modified and, although fibrotic nodules are formed, they lack the well-demarcated outline and concentric pattern of classic silicosis. The lesions are found in a centriacinar position and are stellate in outline with adjacent scar emphysema. They are firm and generally measure no more than 5 mm in diameter. They closely resemble the fibrotic nodules of simple coal pneumoconiosis (see below). Confluent lesions also occur on occasions. These resemble the progressive massive fibrosis of coalworkers and appear to represent a single large lesion rather than a conglomeration of individual nodules, as in advanced silicosis. Abundant dust is generally evident in lesions of all sizes; this consists of black carbon or brown iron mixed with crystals of varying degrees of birefringence, silicates generally being strongly birefringent and silica weakly so. Calcification is unusual. Mixed-dust pneumoconiosis carries an increased risk of pulmonary tuberculosis, but not to the same degree as silicosis. In some cases the stellate nodules are accompanied by diffuse fibrosis, as in silicosis and again possibly involving interactions between the dust and immunological factors. Involvement of the bronchi with consequent stenosis (so-called anthracofibrosis) is described above.

COAL PNEUMOCONIOSIS[156]

The term 'anthracosis' was initially applied to changes observed in a coalminer's lung[157] but is now often extended to include the common carbon pigmentation of city dwellers' lungs, and the term 'coal pneumoconiosis' is more appropriate to a special form of pneumoconiosis to which coalworkers are subject, particularly those who work underground. The principal constituent of coal, carbon, is non-fibrogenic, so suspicion has naturally fallen on the ash content of mine dust, some of which derives from the coal, some from adjacent rock strata and some from stone dust laid in the roadways to minimise the risk of coal dust explosions. Coal itself appears to be the responsible agent because coal-trimmers, working in the docks and not exposed to rock dust, also develop the disease.[158] Coalminers encountering siliceous rock are, of course, also liable to develop silicosis like other underground workers.

Mineralogy

Coal consists largely of elemental carbon, oxygen and hydrogen with traces of iron ore and clays such kaolinite, muscovite and illite, but no silica. The mineral content varies with the type and rank (calorific value) of the coal. All coal derives from peat, the youngest type being lignite and the oldest anthracite, with bituminous (house) coal in between. As it ages, the oxygen and mineral constituents diminish and the coal hardens. Lignite is soft and said to be of low rank, anthracite hard and of high rank, with bituminous coal intermediate.

Although high-rank coal is of low mineral content, its dust is more toxic to macrophages in vitro and is cleared more slowly in vivo. This observation may explain why, in the UK, high-rank coal is associated with a higher prevalence of coal pneumoconiosis.

The low mineral content of high-rank coal is reflected in the mineral content of the lungs of those who hew such coal in the UK, but in the Ruhr, in Germany, and in Pennsylvania, in the USA, anthracite miners' lungs contain more silica than those who hew bituminous coal, the silica presumably deriving from other sources. Not surprisingly, the presence of silica is reflected in the tissue reaction to the inhaled dust, resulting in a more fibrotic reaction very analogous to mixed-dust pneumoconiosis. A spectrum of changes is therefore encountered in

coalminers' lungs, ranging from coal pneumoconiosis through mixed-dust pneumoconiosis to silicosis; the findings in any individual depend upon the nature of the coal being mined and the type of work undertaken.

In high-rank British collieries the development of coal pneumoconiosis appears to depend on the total mass of dust inhaled, whereas in low-rank British collieries the mineral content of the lung dust appears to be more important.[159] This may explain apparently contrary data drawn from different coalfields – data based on coals of different composition that are not strictly comparable. Some workers have stressed the importance of silica in the dust whereas others, particularly in the high-rank coalfields of south Wales, have been unable to detect any association between silica and the level of pneumoconiosis. Both findings may be correct, but only for the particular group of miners examined in each case.[160]

Pathology

The lesions of coal pneumoconiosis are generally focal and fall into one or other of two major types, simple and complicated, depending upon whether the lesions measure up to or over 1 cm; simple corresponds to categories 1–3 of the ILO grading system (see p. 331) and complicated, which is also known as progressive massive fibrosis, to ILO categories A–C. More diffuse interstitial fibrosis has been reported in about 16% of Welsh and West Virginian coalminers, usually involving those carrying a particularly heavy dust burden; it runs a more benign course than non-occupational interstitial fibrosis (idiopathic pulmonary fibrosis).[161] Similar findings have been reported from France.[162]

Simple coal pneumoconiosis consists of focal dust pigmentation of the lungs, which may be associated with a little fibrosis and varying degrees of emphysema. Its clinical effects are relatively minor. Some degree of black pigmentation (anthracosis) of the lungs is common in the general urban population, especially in industrial areas, but much denser pigmentation is seen in coalminers, whose lungs at necropsy are black or slate-grey. Black pigment is evident in the visceral pleura along the lines of the lymphatics and on the cut surface where it outlines the interlobular septa and is concentrated in Macklin's centriacinar dust sumps (Fig. 7.1.12). The dust is generally more plentiful in the upper parts of the lungs and in the hilar lymph nodes, possibly due to poorer perfusion and consequently poorer lymphatic drainage there (see p. 21).[162]

Two forms of coal dust foci are recognised, macules and nodules, the former being soft and impalpable and the latter hard due to substantial amounts of collagen. Both lesions are typically stellate but the more fibrotic the nodules, the more rounded they become, until it is difficult to distinguish them macroscopically from those of silicosis. In these circumstances reliance has to be placed on the whorled pattern of the collagen that is evident microscopically in silicosis. The stellate nodules are analogous to those seen in mixed-dust pneumoconiosis caused by mixtures of silica and inert dusts other than carbon (see above). With polarising filters, small numbers of birefringent crystals may be seen in both macules and nodules, usually representing mica or kaolinite derived from rock that bordered the coal.

Macules consist of closely packed dust particles, free or within heavily laden macrophages, so that the lesion appears black throughout (Fig. 7.1.13). Appropriate stains show that the dust-laden macrophages and free dust are lightly bound by reticulin. Very little collagen is evident. Although striking in their appearance, dust macules are thought to have little effect on lung function.

Nodules contain substantial amounts of collagen and are thought to have an adverse, but limited, effect on respiration. They vary from a heavily pigmented, stellate lesion, which apart from its collagen content resembles the dust macule (Fig. 7.1.14), to one that is less

Figure 7.1.12 A coalminer's lung showing heavy dust deposition in the centres of the acini (Macklin's dust sumps). On palpation the dust deposits felt soft and were consequently described as macules rather than nodules. Despite the heavy dust deposition, there is minimal pneumoconiosis. Part of a paper-mounted whole-lung section.

Figure 7.1.13 Coal macule. A centriacinar dust deposit of stellate outline consisting of macrophages heavily laden with coal dust and bound together by only a little reticulin. Collagen is not a feature.

pigmented and more circumscribed. The stellate, heavily pigmented type of nodule is seen in lungs that have a relatively low ash content whilst the more rounded and less pigmented nodule is seen in lungs with relatively high ash loads.[163]

Radiologically (see p. 321), p-type opacities correspond to macules, q-type opacities to the stellate nodules that resemble those of mixed-dust pneumoconiosis and r-type opacities to the rounded nodules that resemble those of silicosis.[53,164] Thus, the radiological changes of simple coalworker's pneumoconiosis are due to the dust and the small amount of collagen present and do not reflect any emphysema that may also be present. However, pulmonary dust foci are often associated with emphysema (Fig. 7.1.15) and the severity of the emphysema appears to correlate with the dust load. The prevalence of chronic bronchitis and emphysema is high in the coal industry and it has long been debated whether occupation or cigarette smoking is the major factor contributing to emphysema in coalminers.[165–168] As well as mineral dust, nitrous fumes from shot-firing form another occupational hazard of coal mining.

Heppleston made a special study of the emphysema found in coalminers, claiming that it differs from centriacinar emphysema, as seen in smokers in the general population, and attributing it to the dust.[169] He introduced the term 'focal emphysema of coalworkers' to describe this special process. Others find it very difficult to identify any convincing difference between the emphysema of coalworkers and that encountered outside the industry but Heppleston based his claims on the study of serial sections. By this means he showed that, although both forms affect respiratory bronchioles, the focal emphysema of coalworkers affects more proximal orders of these airways and is not associated with the bronchiolitis seen with centriacinar emphysema. Furthermore, focal emphysema is a dilatation lesion whereas

Figure 7.1.14 Coal nodule. A centriacinar dust nodule of stellate outline in which coal dust-laden macrophages are mixed with moderate amounts of collagen.

Figure 7.1.15 Coalworker's pneumoconiosis – simple type, consisting of coal macules and nodules associated with focal emphysema. Paper-mounted whole-lung section.

Figure 7.1.16 Coal pneumoconiosis – complicated type. In addition to the focal dust deposits there is a large area of progressive massive fibrosis in the upper lobe. Paper-mounted whole-lung section.

centriacinar emphysema involves destruction of adjacent alveolar walls. By definition, therefore, focal emphysema is not a true emphysema at all (see p. 102). However, it has been shown that mineral dusts cause elastin and collagen breakdown in the rat lung.[170] Focal emphysema may progress to the destructive centriacinar form and this has strengthened claims that mine dust plays a causal role in centriacinar emphysema.[1,171–176] In the UK, these claims have been accepted and chronic bronchitis and emphysema in coalminers and metal production workers have been accepted as prescribed industrial diseases since 1992.[177] In Germany too, chronic obstructive pulmonary disease is now compensatable as an occupational disease. The conditions for compensation in the UK were initially:

- underground coal mining for a minimum of 20 years in aggregate
- forced expiratory volume in 1 second at least 1 litre below that expected or less than 1 litre in total
- radiological category of at least 1/1.

However the last of these criteria has now been dropped. The inclusion of a time element and the omission of some estimate of dust load (such as radiological category) have been criticised, with some justification.[178] As with lung cancer caused by chromates benefit is paid irrespective of smoking habits.

Whereas simple coal pneumoconiosis, particularly the macular variety, has little effect on lung function, complicated coal pneumo-coniosis, also known as progressive massive fibrosis, can have very serious consequences. Particularly when the lesions are large, it is associated with productive cough, breathlessness, significant impairment of lung function and premature death. The major factor accounting for the development of progressive massive fibrosis appears to be the sheer bulk of coal dust in the lung, rather than coal rank or the silica content of the mine dust.[179] Progressive massive fibrosis has occasionally been recorded in dockers loading silica-free coal into the holds of ships[158] and in workers exposed to pure carbon in the manufacture of carbon black and carbon electrodes.[141–143]

Progressive massive fibrosis is characterised by large (over 1 cm) black masses, situated anywhere in the lungs but most common in the upper lobes. The lesions may be solitary or multiple and very large, occupying most of the lobe and even crossing an interlobar fissure to involve an adjacent lobe (Figs 7.1.3B, 7.1.16). They cut fairly easily, often with the release from a central cavity of black fluid flecked by cholesterol crystals. For many years it was believed that the condition was the result of synergism between mycobacterial infection and dust but the failure of the attack rate to decrease as tuberculosis declined negated this view.[180] Today, more emphasis is placed on total dust load for the lesions tend to affect lungs that carry an unduly heavy dust burden. If the remainder of the lung shows little evidence of dust accumulation, the possibility of the masses representing Caplan-type lesions (see below) should be considered.

Microscopically, the lesions consist of dust and connective tissue intermixed in a random fashion. Central necrosis and cavitation commonly occur. The necrosis is thought to be ischaemic.[181] It is amorphous or finely granular, and eosinophilic apart from abundant dust particles and cholesterol crystal clefts. The fibrotic component in a complicated pneumoconiotic lesion is rich in fibronectin, with collagen only more abundant at the periphery.[182] Two types of progressive massive fibrosis are recognisable, corresponding to the two types of nodule described in simple coal pneumoconiosis.[163] The first appears to have arisen by enlargement of a single nodule, whereas the second is a conglomeration of individual lesions, each of which corresponds to the more circumscribed type of nodule seen in simple coal pneumoconiosis. The ash content of the lungs bearing these two types of progressive massive fibrosis varies in the same way as with the two types of simple pneumoconiotic nodules, the enlarged single lesion being found in lungs with a relatively low ash content, and the conglomerate lesion in lungs with a relatively high ash content. The second type resembles the conglomerate nodules of large silicotic lesions but lacks the characteristic whorled pattern of the latter.

The diffuse interstitial fibrosis found in a minority of coalworkers is associated with heavy dust deposition. It may progress to honeycombing but, as with the focal forms and unlike idiopathic interstitial fibrosis, it is better developed in the upper zones, the reasons for which are discussed above (see the zonal distribution of pneumoconiosis, p. 329).

Pathogenesis

The pathogenesis of coal pneumoconiosis has much in common with that of silicosis, and indeed many other pneumoconioses. It involves the promotion of fibrogenic factor synthesis and release by cells phagocytosing the inhaled dust. Several such factors have now been identified, the degree of fibrosis produced varying with the amount of dust inhaled and the ability of its constituents to promote the production of the responsible cytokines. These include platelet-derived growth factor, insulin-like growth factors 1 and 6, transforming growth factor-β and tumour necrosis factor-α.[101,183,184] As with other minerals, the indestructability of the dust perpetuates the process.

As in silicosis, immunological factors appear to be involved, for there is an increased prevalence of rheumatoid arthritis[185] and of circulating autoantibodies[186-188] in miners with coal pneumoconiosis. Rheumatoid factor has also been demonstrated within the lung lesions.[189] These abnormalities are generally more pronounced in miners with complicated pneumoconiosis but are also found in those with the simple variety. It is also possibly pertinent to the immunological basis of coal pneumoconiosis that some of the pulmonary manifestations of rheumatoid disease are more pronounced in coalminers. This was first pointed out by Caplan and will be considered next.

Pneumoconiosis and rheumatoid disease (Caplan's syndrome)

Caplan described distinctive radiographic opacities in the lungs of coalminers with rheumatoid disease,[190] and it is now recognised that similar lesions may develop in rheumatoid patients exposed to siliceous dusts. The development of such rheumatoid pneumoconiosis does not correlate with the extrapulmonary or serological activity of the rheumatoid process. Nor is there a strong relation to dust burden: Caplan lesions are characteristically seen in chest radiographs that show little evidence of simple coal pneumoconiosis.

Figure 7.1.17 Caplan lesions in a coalminer's lung, which characteristically shows only light dust deposition. *(Courtesy of Dr R Seal, formerly of Penarth, UK.)*

Figure 7.1.18 A Caplan lesion, characterised by successive bands of dust within the centre of a large necrobiotic nodule.

Pathologists recognise the lesions as particularly large necrobiotic nodules similar to those seen in rheumatoid patients who are not exposed to dust (Fig. 7.1.17). However, because of their large size (up to 5 cm diameter) they may be confused with progressive massive fibrosis undergoing central ischaemic necrosis (see above) or silicosis complicated by caseating tuberculosis. Such errors will be less likely if the radiological evolution of the lesions is considered for they tend to cavitate and undergo rapid remission, only to be succeeded by others. They are also well demarcated radiologically. Pathologically, they resemble rheumatoid nodules in showing peripheral palisading but differ in their large size and the presence of dust.[191] The dust accumulates in circumferential bands or arcs within the necrotic centres of the lesion (Fig. 7.1.18), an arrangement that suggests periodic episodes of inflammatory activity. Caplan lesions differ from tuberculosis in lacking satellite lesions and tubercle bacilli, and from progressive massive fibrosis in showing characteristic bands of dust pigmentation (Table 7.1.2) and only light dust deposition in the surrounding lung.

Table 7.1.2 Histological features of Caplan lesions, silicotuberculosis and progressive massive fibrosis

	Caplan lesions	Silicotuberculosis	Progressive massive fibrosis
Palisading	+	–	–
Dust banding	+	–	–
Satellite tubercles	–	+	–
Necrosis	+	+	+
Cholesterol crystals	+	±	+
Calcification	+	+	±

+ present; ± poorly represented; – absent.

Table 7.1.3 Asbestos production by country, 2000[194]

Country	Tons
Russia	752 000
China	350 000
Canada	320 000
Brazil	209 000
Kazakhstan	179 000
Zimbabwe	152 000
Others	88 000

ASBESTOSIS

Asbestosis is defined as diffuse interstitial fibrosis of the lung caused by exposure to asbestos dust.[192,193] It does not cover asbestos-induced carcinoma of the lung or asbestos-induced pleural disease. The development of asbestosis depends on the presence of fairly large dust burdens: this is in contrast to mesothelioma and other forms of asbestos-induced pleural disease, which, although also dose-related, occur following the inhalation of far smaller amounts of asbestos dust.

Asbestos types and production

Asbestos is a generic term for more than 30 naturally occurring fibrous silicates, fibre being defined as an elongated particle with a length-to-breadth (aspect) ratio of at least 3. Asbestos fibres have a high aspect ratio, generally over 8. Based on their physical configuration they can be divided into two major groups, serpentine and amphibole. The physical dimensions and configuration of asbestos fibres are strongly linked to their pathogenicity.

Chrysotile (white asbestos) is the only important serpentine form. It accounts for most of the world production of asbestos of all types (Table 7.1.3).[194] Being a serpentine mineral, chrysotile consists of long, curly fibres that can be carded, spun and woven like cotton (Fig. 7.1.19). The curly chrysotile fibres are carried into the lungs less readily than the straight amphibole asbestos fibres, and once there undergo physicochemical dissolution and are cleared more readily.

Figure 7.1.19 A sample of Quebec chrysotile showing the fibrous nature of the ore.

They readily fragment into short particles that are easily ingested by macrophages and in the acidic environment of the macrophage phagolysosome they are particularly unstable. The half-life of chrysotile in the lungs is estimated to be in the order of only a few months.[195,196] Not surprisingly therefore chrysotile is the least harmful type of asbestos in respect of all forms of asbestos-induced pleuropulmonary disease.[197–199] It may nevertheless cause pulmonary fibrosis if sufficient is inhaled.[200,201]

In contrast to chrysotile, amphibole forms of asbestos consist of straight rigid fibres that are stable within the lung. They do not fragment, they are insensitive to chemical attack and their clearance half-lives are in the order of decades rather than months.[196] The main amphibole forms of asbestos of commercial importance are crocidolite (blue asbestos) and amosite (brown asbestos). Crocidolite, reputedly the most dangerous in regard to all forms of asbestos-related disease, was formerly mined in Western Australia (Wittenoom) and South Africa (Cape Province and the Transvaal); it was the principal amphibole used in the UK. Amosite, the name of which derives from the acronym for the former Asbestos Mines of South Africa company in the Transvaal, was the principal amphibole used in North America. Amphiboles are no longer imported by the developed countries but much remains in old lagging and presents a considerable dust hazard when this is removed. Tremolite, a further amphibole asbestos, contaminates Quebec chrysotile deposits, Montana vermiculite and many forms of commercial (non-cosmetic) talc and is responsible for much of the asbestos-related disease in chrysotile miners and millers.[202] Another amphibole asbestos, anthophyllite, was formerly mined in Finland. It causes pleural plaques (see p. 716) but not lung disease, possibly because its fibres are relatively thick (Fig. 7.1.20).[203]

Erionite is a zeolite rather than a type of asbestos but is comparable in form to amphibole asbestos and is also biopersistent. It is found

Figure 7.1.20 Electron micrographs of dispersed samples of asbestos. (A) Chrysotile; (B) crocidolite; (C) amosite; (D) anthophyllite, all ×2800, the bar representing 10 μm. *(Reproduced from Wagner et al. (1980)[203] by permission of Professor FD Pooley and the British Medical Bulletin.)*

Table 7.1.4 Asbestos consumption by country, 2000[194]

Country	Tons	kg/capita/year
Russia	447 000	3.4
China	410 000	0.4
Brazil	182 000	1.3
India	125 000	0.2
Thailand	121 000	3.0
Japan	99 000	1.5
Indonesia	55 000	0.3
South Korea	29 000	1.9
Mexico	27 000	0.4
Others	178 000	

in parts of central Turkey where it causes both mesothelioma and a pattern of interstitial pulmonary fibrosis that is comparable to asbestosis.[204,205]

Asbestos use and exposure

Exposure to asbestos occurs in countries where it is extracted (Table 7.1.3), which is mostly by the open-cast method, and in those countries that continue to use this mineral (Table 7.1.4). The developed nations have largely ceased to use asbestos but countries keen to develop their industrial base and less concerned with health issues continue to use considerable amounts in a vast range of trades. Asbestos is used particularly for fireproofing, in heat and sound insulation and for strengthening plastics and cement. Thus, unless adequate precautions are taken, exposure is experienced by dockers unloading asbestos in the close confines of a ship's hold, by thermal insulation workers (laggers and strippers) in shipyards, power stations, train maintenance depots, factories and other large buildings, by construction workers such as carpenters cutting asbestos building panels, and by workers making asbestos products such as fireproof textiles, brake and clutch linings, and specialised cement.

As well as such direct exposure, exposure may also be:

- indirect, as experienced by the families of asbestos workers
- paraoccupational, as experienced by those working alongside an asbestos worker
- neighbourhood, as experienced by those living downwind of an asbestos works or mine
- ambient, as experienced by those living or working in a building containing asbestos.

Exposure to asbestos incorporated in the structure of a building carries a negligible health risk if the asbestos material is well maintained to prevent shedding of dust. Stripping asbestos out is more dangerous than maintaining it in situ, but maintenance is sometimes neglected. The near indestructibility of asbestos accentuates the health problems that its ubiquity poses.

Asbestos bodies

Because of their aerodynamic properties, fibres of 100 μm or more in length may reach the finer bronchioles and alveoli. Once impacted, the sharp asbestos fibres become coated with a film of protein that is rich in iron. The coating is thickest at the ends of the fibres, giving a dumb-bell appearance. In time, a distinctive segmentation of this outer layer develops (Fig. 7.1.21). These coated structures are termed 'asbestos bodies'. Because other fibres may gain a similar coat, the non-specific term 'ferruginous body' has been advocated. However, coated carbon fibres (so-called coal bodies) are easily recognised as such by their black core.[206] In practice, ferruginous bodies with the appearance of asbestos bodies almost always prove to have an asbestos core.[207,208] Long fibres are more likely to be coated than short ones, which are cleared more quickly: in one study few fibres less than 5 μm in length were coated and few fibres over 40 μm in length were uncoated.[209] Amphiboles form bodies more readily than chrysotile. A comparison of light and electron microscopic fibre counts found that 0.14% of chrysotile, 5% of crocidolite and 26.5% of amosite formed bodies.[210] Nevertheless, sufficient chrysotile fibres are coated to permit recognition of asbestosis by standard histological criteria (diffuse fibrosis and asbestos bodies), even if chrysotile is the only asbestos present.[211] Despite the biodegradability of chrysotile, asbestos body numbers do not materially diminish with time.[212] Very occasionally however a patient with diffuse pulmonary fibrosis and a history of asbestos exposure has no evident asbestos bodies but analysis shows a fibre burden within the range found in asbestosis, justifying fibre analysis in such cases.[212a]

There is evidence that alveolar macrophages are involved in the coating of asbestos fibres to form asbestos bodies and that the bodies are less harmful to the macrophages than uncoated fibres.[213] Asbestos bodies give a Prussian blue reaction for iron when stained by Perls' method and their yellow-brown colour makes them easily recognisable in unstained films of sputum or in unstained histological sections. Sections may be cut 30 μm thick to increase the yield and help identify bodies that lie at an angle to the microtome blade. There is a good correlation between the numbers of asbestos bodies seen in lung sections and those in tissue digests.[214,215] The bodies may be found singly or in irregular clumps or stellate clusters. They are unevenly distributed but in well-established asbestosis they are easily found. If they are not evident, asbestos burden may be assessed quantitatively in tissue digests (see below). Their presence in lung tissue, sputum or bronchoalveolar lavage fluid merely confirms exposure, not the presence of disease. However, the number of asbestos bodies in lavage fluid correlates well with lung asbestos burden[216,217] and the number in sputum correlates with the duration and intensity of exposure.[216–218]

Fibre counts[193,208,219–223]

Quantitation is desirable in certain circumstances (Box 7.1.1), in which case it is best effected on 2-cm³ blocks of fixed or fresh lung tissue obtained from three different sites, avoiding tumour and thickened pleura. The tissue blocks are digested with caustic soda or bleach, following which the fibres may be collected on a millipore membrane or viewed in suspension in a red blood cell-counting chamber. If phase contrast optics are used both coated and uncoated fibres can be assessed.[219] Alternatively, dark ground illumination can be used to demonstrate uncoated fibres.[221] However, electron microscopy is to be preferred as it detects far more fibres than are visible by light microscopy and can also provide information on fibre type. It is important that the laboratory is well practised in fibre analysis and has established its own control range for the general population as well as asbestosis as most lungs contain some asbestos.

Ambient fibres are generally shorter than 5 μm and some workers therefore confine their counts to fibres that are at least as long as this.[224] Justification for this comes from animal experiments demonstrating that long fibres cause more inflammation, chromosomal damage, fibrosis, lung tumours and mesotheliomas than short fibres,[225–228] and from studies in humans suggesting that long fibres

Figure 7.1.21 Asbestos bodies seen by light microscopy in (A) an unstained 30-µm-thick paraffin section; (B) by scanning electron microscopy in the digest of an asbestos worker's lung and (C) by transmission electron microscopy in lung tissue. The asbestos fibres have acquired the iron-protein coating that characterises an asbestos body. In most places the coating has become segmented, giving rise to bead-like formations, a change accompanying ageing of the bodies. *((B) Courtesy of Dr B Fox, London, UK and (C) courtesy of Miss A Dewar, Brompton, UK.)*

Box 7.1.1 Circumstances in which asbestos fibre counts are desirable

Quantitation desirable	Quantitation unnecessary
Mesothelioma if exposure is disputed and asbestos bodies are not evident	Mesothelioma if there is a history of exposure or asbestos bodies are evident
Pulmonary fibrosis (with or without carcinoma of the lung) in an asbestos worker but asbestos bodies are not evident	If there is obvious asbestosis
Carcinoma of the lung in an asbestos worker if there is no fibrosis	

---

are responsible for asbestosis.[229] Other human studies have shown that, although asbestos load is maximal in the upper lobes, more long fibres are found at the bases, where fibrosis is most marked.[41,230] A further reason for limiting attention to the longer fibres is that the shorter ones are cleared more easily and their number therefore varies with the time lapsed since last exposure. For these reasons asbestos regulations in many countries now limit attention to fibres that are over 5 µm in length and have a length-to-diameter (aspect) ratio greater than 3: such fibres have become known as regulatory or World Health Organization (WHO) fibres.

Values are best expressed as fibres/g dry lung. By light microscopy, normal values range up to 50 000: over 20 000 is seen with mesotheliomas, and over 1 000 000 in asbestosis (Table 7.1.5).[216,224,231,232] However, compared with electron microscopy, light microscopy is relatively insensitive, showing only 26.5% of the amosite, 5% of the crocidolite and 0.14% of the chrysotile.[210] Light microscopic counts correlate poorly with severity of asbestosis[219] and electron microscopy

Table 7.1.5 Lung asbestos fibre counts per gram of dried lung

	Light microscopy	Electron microscopy
Normal city dwellers	Up to 50 000	Up to 5 000 000
Mesothelioma	Over 20 000	Over 1 000 000
Asbestosis (minimal)	Over 100 000	Over 10 000 000
Asbestosis (established)	Over 1 000 000	Over 100 000 000

The light microscopic counts include total fibres (coated and uncoated). The electron microscopic counts include only amphibole asbestos. Results from different laboratories vary and these figures, derived from several sources,[216,231,232] provide only a general guide. Reliable results depend upon counts being made regularly and the normal range from that laboratory being ascertained. Ratios of counts obtained by electron and light microscopy vary greatly but approximate to 100.

Figure 7.1.22 At high magnification chysotile fibres are seen to be tubular. Transmission electron micrograph ×51 000. *(Courtesy of Miss A Dewar, Brompton, UK.)*

is better in this respect.[197–199] By transmission electron microscopy, values may range up to 5 000 000 in controls, with asbestosis generally above 100 000 000 and mesotheliomas found at any level down to 1 000 000, all these figures representing amphibole fibres/g dried lung (see Table 7.1.5).[216,231,232] It should be noted that counts from different parts of the same lung may vary widely;[42,231–235] caution should therefore be exercised in interpreting a count obtained on a single sample. There is also wide discrepancy between laboratories, even when analysing the same sample.[234] Results obtained in an individual case therefore have to be evaluated against a standard set of values unique to that laboratory.

Electron microscopy also provides valuable information on the type of fibre. Chrysotile differs physically from the amphiboles in two respects: its fibres are both curved and hollow (Figs 7.1.20 and 7.1.22). With an electron microscope equipped for microprobe analysis, the various forms of asbestos may also be distinguished from other fibres and from each other (Box 7.1.2),[230,236] an important point as the amphibole forms of asbestos are far more dangerous than chrysotile (Table 7.1.6).[197–199]

Chrysotile	$Mg_3(Si_2O_5)(OH)_4$
Crocidolite	$Na_2Fe_5(Si_8O_{22})(OH)_2$
Amosite	$(Fe,Mg)_7(Si_8O_{22})(OH)_2$
Tremolite	$Ca_2Mg_5(Si_8O_{22})(OH)_2$

Table 7.1.6 Mean percentage lung fibre type by diagnostic category in a group of British asbestos factory workers compared to local controls[199]

Fibre type	Controls	Asbestosis	Carcinoma of the lung	Pleural mesothelioma
Crocidolite	2.8	60.1	56.7	20.2
Amosite	2.6	17.7	30.4	39.3
Chrysotile	25.9	4.0	6.9	17.0
Other (mainly fly ash)	68.7	18.2	6.0	23.5

Non-asbestos fibres commonly found in the lung include mullite, which derives from fly ash. This may constitute up to 70% of the total fibre burden (see Table 7.1.6) and is thought to be harmless. There is no firm evidence that manmade fibres present a health hazard[237] but in certain localities natural non-asbestos mineral fibres, zeolites for example, are important causes of mesothelioma (see p. 718) and also cause interstitial pulmonary fibrosis.[204]

Clinical and radiological features

In contrast to the first half of the twentieth century, much of the asbestosis encountered today is asymptomatic, identified radiologically or histologically in lungs resected for carcinoma or removed at autopsy. Symptomatic cases are characterised by an insidious onset of breathlessness, a dry cough and crackles over the lower lung fields. Finger clubbing is a variable feature. Lung function tests show a restrictive respiratory defect. Radiology initially shows small irregular basal opacities that gradually coalesce to become linear, coarsen and eventually progress to a honeycomb pattern of small cysts.

The principal differential diagnosis, both clinically and pathologically, is from idiopathic pulmonary fibrosis. This is aided by the slow progression of asbestosis, which often extends over 20 years, as opposed to an average course of 2–3 years from presentation to death for the idiopathic condition.

Most cases of asbestosis are diagnosed solely on the occupational history and these clinicoradiological features. Recourse to histology is unusual but biopsy (preferably as a wedge of lung) may be undertaken if the clinical features are atypical. Histology also arises when the pathologist samples lung parenchyma remote from a resected carcinoma (the universal importance of which cannot be overemphasised).

Figure 7.1.23 Asbestosis. Fine interstitial fibrosis is evident beneath the pleura at the base of the lung. Barium sulphate-impregnated specimen.

Box 7.1.3 Criteria for grading asbestosis[193,245,246]

Extent

A	None
B	Less than 25% of the lung substance involved
C	25–50% of the lung affected
D	More than 50% of the lung diseased

Severity[a]

0	No appreciable peribronchiolar fibrosis, or fibrosis confined to the bronchiolar walls
1[b]	Fibrosis confined to the walls of respiratory bronchioles and the first tier of adjacent alveoli
2[b]	Extension of fibrosis to involve alveolar ducts and/or two or more tiers of alveoli adjacent to the respiratory bronchiole, with sparing of at least some alveoli between adjacent bronchioles
3	Fibrotic thickening of the walls of all alveoli between at least two adjacent respiratory bronchioles
4	Honeycomb change

[a]An average score is obtained for an individual case by adding the scores for each slide (0–4), then dividing by the number of slides examined

[b]Grade 1 and, to a lesser extent, grade 2 need to be distinguished from smoking-induced peribronchiolar fibrosis and mixed-dust pneumoconiosis.

Coroners require autopsy verification of the diagnosis in all suspected cases and this also necessitates hystology.

Morbid anatomy

When the lungs from a patient with asbestosis are seen at autopsy, pleural fibrosis is often found, and although this may also be attributable to asbestos exposure it is to be regarded as an independent process and not part of the asbestosis: it is dealt with separately on page 715.

Slicing the lung affected by asbestosis shows a fine subpleural fibrosis, especially of the lower lobes (Fig. 7.1.23). In severe cases the fibrosis often extends upwards to involve the middle lobe and lingula, and sometimes the upper lobes also. Microcystic change associated with the fibrosis develops in advanced cases and in severe disease there may be cysts over 1 cm in diameter. However, these classic changes are seldom seen in developed countries today. Following decades of dust suppression in asbestos factories, current patients have mild to moderate asbestosis and are dying of related cancer or of non-pulmonary disease.[238] In some of these cases the asbestosis is only detectable microscopically. Fixation of the lungs through the bronchi and the use of Heard's barium sulphate impregnation technique facilitate demonstration of the fibrosis (see p. 757 and Fig. 7.1.23). The mild degree of asbestosis currently encountered is of little functional significance but is often critical in determining whether an associated carcinoma of the lung should be attributed to asbestos exposure (see below).

Histological appearances

The histological diagnosis of asbestosis requires an appropriate pattern of interstitial fibrosis associated with the presence of asbestos bodies. Both components must be present. The fibrosis is paucicellular, lacking any significant degree of inflammation and being collagenous rather than fibroblastic.

It is generally considered that asbestosis begins about the respiratory bronchioles and alveolar ducts where most of the asbestos fibres impact.[15] Alveolar walls attached to these bronchioles show fine interstitial fibrosis. However, this early lesion has to be interpreted with caution because it is not specific to asbestos, being found with other inhaled mineral dusts[239,240] and even in many cigarette smokers who have not been so exposed.[241] It more likely represents a non-specific reaction to a variety of inhaled particles. It may cause mild airflow obstruction but is not associated with the radiographic, clinical or restrictive changes of classic asbestosis.

As the disease progresses, the focal changes join up so that the basal subpleural regions show widespread interstitial fibrosis and eventually complete destruction of the alveolar architecture. In severe cases there may be honeycombing and metaplastic changes in the alveolar and bronchiolar epithelium. Apart from the presence of asbestos bodies the changes resemble those of non-specific interstitial pneumonia, or more rarely usual interstitial pneumonia. Fibroblastic foci may be found but they are uncommon. There is often an increase in alveolar macrophages but the desquamative interstitial pneumonia that has been reported in association with asbestos[242,243] is not to be regarded as a variant of asbestosis[192]; concomitant smoking is a more likely cause.[241] A variety of other non-specific inflammatory processes such as organising pneumonia have been reported in asbestos workers and if localised some have been suspected of representing malignancy until biopsied.[244]

Several schemes have been proposed for grading the extent and severity of asbestosis. These are of value in epidemiological studies but should only be applied to cases meeting the histopathological criteria for a diagnosis of asbestosis. One such scheme is shown in Box 7.1.3.[193,245,246]

In well-established asbestosis asbestos bodies are numerous and easy to find, aggregates of them sometimes forming clumps (Fig. 7.1.24). In earlier lesions a detailed search may be necessary, in which

Figure 7.1.24 Asbestosis. Interstitial fibrosis is associated with many asbestos bodies (A), which are shown in detail in (B).

Figure 7.1.25 Cytoplasmic hyaline in asbestosis. (A) Eosinophilic inclusions are seen in the cytoplasm of several hyperplastic type II pneumocytes. Haematoxylin & eosin. *(Courtesy of Professor VL Roggli, Durham, USA.)* (B) Electron microscopy shows that the inclusions represent a tangle of microfilaments. *(Courtesy of Professor D Henderson, Adelaide, Australia.)* *(Both images reproduced by permission of the publishers of* Archives of Pathology and Laboratory Medicine.[193]*)*

case the examination of unstained or Perls-stained sections facilitates their identification. Minimum criteria for the diagnosis of asbestosis require the identification of diffuse interstitial fibrosis in well-inflated lung tissue remote from a lung cancer or other mass lesion and the presence of either two or more asbestos bodies in tissue with a section area of 1 cm^2 or a count of uncoated asbestos fibres that falls in the range recorded for asbestosis by the same laboratory.[192,193] There are marked variations in the concentration of asbestos fibres between samples from the same lung[216,235] and it is therefore recommended that at least three areas be sampled, the apices of the upper and lower lobes and the base of the lower lobe.[223]

The equivalent of Mallory's alcoholic hyalin of the liver has been described in the lungs in asbestosis,[193,247] and subsequently in other pulmonary conditions.[248-251] It is seen as small eosinophilic cytoplasmic inclusions within hyperplastic type II alveolar epithelial cells (Fig. 7.1.25A). Electron microscopy shows that the inclusions consist of a tangle of tonofilaments (Fig. 7.1.25B) and by immunocytochemistry a positive reaction is obtained with antibodies to cytokeratin, both these features being typical of Mallory's hyalin in the liver. The inclusions also react for ubiquitin, the accumulation of which is indicative of cellular damage, in particular faulty proteinolysis.[251]

Differential diagnosis

The differential diagnosis of asbestosis includes pulmonary fibrosis due to many other causes, any of which may of course affect an asbestos worker as much as members of the general population. The proportion of diffuse pulmonary fibrosis in asbestos workers that is not attributable to asbestos has been estimated to be as high as 5% and likely to rise as the risk of asbestosis diminishes with better industrial hygiene.[252]

The principal differential diagnosis of asbestosis is from idiopathic pulmonary fibrosis. Both diseases affect the bases and periphery of the lungs predominantly. In the late stages, cystic change is more evident in idiopathic pulmonary fibrosis but this criterion is not totally reliable. Nor is the presence of pleural fibrosis, although it is usually present in asbestosis and is seldom found in idiopathic pulmonary fibrosis. Asbestosis seldom progresses or does so very slowly after exposure ceases[253,254] whereas idiopathic pulmonary fibrosis typically proves fatal within 3–4 years from onset. The fibrosis of asbestosis is generally paucicellular: inflammation is not a feature and the fibroblastic foci that characterise the usual interstitial pneumonia pattern of fibrosing alveolitis are seldom observed in asbestosis.

Very often the distinction from idiopathic pulmonary fibrosis has to be based on the amount of asbestos in the lung and, if asbestos bodies are not readily identifiable, this has to depend on fibre counts. Errors are made both by overlooking substantial numbers of asbestos bodies completely and by ascribing undue importance to scanty bodies. If considering the possibility of minimal asbestosis (to justify attributing carcinoma of the lung to asbestos, for example) it should be remembered that a little peribronchiolar fibrosis is also characteristic of smokers' lungs, centriacinar emphysema and early mixed-dust pneumoconiosis.[239–241,255] As described above, at least two asbestos bodies/cm^2 in the presence of interstitial fibrosis distant from any lung cancer or other mass lesion is required for a diagnosis of asbestosis.[192]

Pathogenesis

Although the causes of asbestosis and idiopathic pulmonary fibrosis are very different, they resemble each other in several ways, suggesting that similar pathogenetic mechanisms may operate.[105,256–258] In both these diseases there is degeneration of the alveolar epithelium and capillary endothelium, with patchy loss of the former,[256] and bronchoalveolar lavage shows an increase in macrophages that might perpetuate the damage by releasing lysosomal enzymes, nitric oxide and hydroxyl radicals.[257,259–261] Both diseases are also characterised by an increased prevalence of circulating non-organ-specific autoantibodies.[262] Experimentally, asbestos exposure leads to the activation of a variety of fibrogenic cytokines at sites of lung injury.[105,263–268]

Inhaled asbestos activates a complement-dependent chemoattractant for macrophages[269] and macrophage stimulation involves the secretion of fibroblast stimulating factors,[270–272] asbestos being intermediate between haematite and silica in regard to macrophage-mediated fibrogenicity.[273] The epithelial damage could be mediated directly by the needle-like asbestos fibres or indirectly through enhanced phagocyte generation of free radicals (which is much greater with amphibole asbestos than with either chrysotile or silica).[268,274] Fibrogenic cytokines released by activated pulmonary phagocytes and regenerating alveolar epithelial cells in asbestosis include tumour necrosis factor-α and transforming growth factor-β,[268] as in idiopathic pulmonary fibrosis.

Asbestos-induced lung cancer

As a result of better industrial hygiene, asbestosis is less severe today than in earlier years when it followed much heavier exposure, with the consequence that death from respiratory failure and cor pulmonale is less common and sufferers are surviving longer. There is therefore now a greater risk of asbestos-related cancer eventually developing.

Table 7.1.7 Excess mortality from carcinoma of the lung attributable to asbestos exposure and cigarette smoking in insulation workers.[278] Together, these factors have a multiplicative rather than additive effect

Group	Mortality ratio
Non-smoking controls	1
Non-smoking asbestos workers	5
Cigarette-smoking controls	11
Cigarette-smoking asbestos workers	53

Asbestos exposure predisposes to two varieties of malignant neoplasm, carcinoma of the lung and mesothelioma of the pleura and peritoneum. The risk of malignancy increases with dose but the relative risk of carcinoma is much smaller than that of mesothelioma. For example, with heavy exposure, as in lagging, the risk of mesothelioma is increased 1000-fold whereas it is increased only fivefold for lung cancer. Hence, with light exposure there is a substantial risk of mesothelioma but only a small risk of lung cancer. Asbestosis requires heavy exposure and in one group of patients with asbestosis, 39% died of pulmonary carcinoma, 10% of mesothelioma and 19% of other respiratory diseases.[238] Although there were many earlier reports, the link with carcinoma of the lung may be considered to have been firmly established by 1955,[275] that between crocidolite asbestos and mesothelioma by 1960,[276] and that between amosite asbestos and mesothelioma by 1972.[277] Mesothelioma is considered on page 717.

In regard to carcinoma of the lung, asbestos is not such a potent pulmonary carcinogen as cigarette smoke but together their effects are multiplicative rather than additive (Table 7.1.7).[278,279] However, the risk attributable to asbestos is the same regardless of smoking history, being increased fivefold in both smokers and non-smokers. There is usually a latent period in excess of 20 years between first exposure to asbestos and the development of lung cancer and the risk increases the greater the cumulative exposure. The increased risk involves carcinomas of all the histological types encountered in the lung, although adenocarcinoma has been disproportionately overrepresented.[245,280–285]

It is uncertain[114] whether the increased risk of carcinoma is caused by the asbestos[192,286–291] or the asbestosis.[292–299] The latter view envisages the carcinoma arising in the foci of alveolar epithelial hyperplasia and dysplasia that commonly accompany any interstitial fibrosis (see carcinoma complicating idiopathic pulmonary fibrosis, p. 275). However, most carcinomas complicating asbestosis arise in the bronchi rather than the alveolar tissue. On the other hand, more arise in the sites worst affected by asbestosis, the lower lobes and the periphery of the lung, than in the general population (Fig. 7.1.26).[238,245,281–285]

The majority view has been that asbestosis is a necessary precursor of the carcinoma but evidence to the contrary is finding increasing support (Table 7.1.8).[192] In the UK, industrial compensation was formerly only awarded to an asbestos worker for carcinoma of the lung if there was also asbestosis or diffuse pleural fibrosis but new rules were introduced in 2006. Asbestosis remains a sufficient criterion but diffuse pleural thickening is not and asbestosis is no longer a necessary criterion: asbestos is deemed to have been responsible if the patient worked in asbestos textile manufacture, spraying, lagging or gas mask manufacture for at least 5 years before 1975 or 10 years after 1975. The basis for these changes is the premise that heavy asbestos exposure is sufficient in itself to account for carcinoma of the lung.

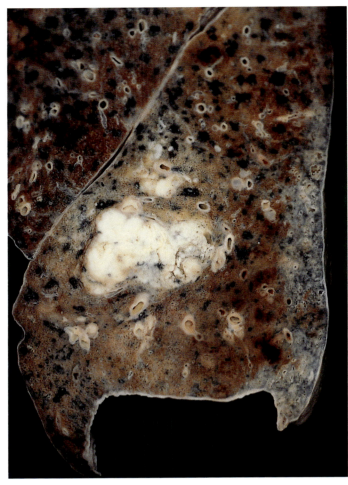

Figure 7.1.26 Asbestosis associated with carcinoma of the lung. The asbestosis has been highlighted by barium sulphate impregnation and is seen as a grey subpleural band to the right of the picture. Although the carcinoma has arisen in the same lobe as the asbestosis it has not obviously arisen in an area affected by asbestosis.

Table 7.1.8 Requirements for attributing carcinoma of the lung to asbestos

The traditional view that the carcinoma complicates asbestosis	The Helsinki criteria,[192] which are based upon substantial exposure
1. Asbestosis and 2. A minimum lag time of 20 years	1. Asbestosis diagnosed clinically, radiologically or histologically or A minimum count of 5000 asbestos bodies per gram dry lung tissue (/g dry), or an uncoated asbestos fibre burden of 2 million amphibole fibres more than 5 μm in length/g dry, or 5 million amphibole fibres more than 1 μm in length/g dry or Estimated cumulative exposure to asbestos of at least 25 fibres/ml-years or An occupational history of 1 year of heavy exposure to asbestos (e.g. manufacture of asbestos products, asbestos spraying) or 5–10 years of moderate exposure (e.g. construction or ship-building) and 2. A minimum lag time of 10 years

> **Box 7.1.4 Compensation standards for asbestos-associated lung cancer in different countries[289]**
>
> Government standards vary considerably and in the civil courts claims are often based on lesser evidence. Some examples of government standards are:
>
> **UK**
>
> Asbestosis or employment in a specified industry for a specified time (see text)
>
> **USA**
>
> The presence of asbestos-related bilateral pleural plaques or asbestos-related bilateral pleural thickening and occupational exposure and a lag time of at least 12 years
>
> **Germany**
>
> The presence of asbestosis or pleural plaques or diffuse pleural thickening or fibre-years of exposure
>
> **Denmark**
>
> Only fibre-years of exposure are taken into account
>
> **Finland**
>
> Exposure, at least 10 years' latency and asbestos-related pleural or parenchymal changes
>
> **Sweden**
>
> Asbestosis is not required but smoking is taken into consideration
>
> **Norway**
>
> Attempts are made to quantify separately the attributability to asbestos, smoking and other factors (e.g. radon)

Lung fibre counts in the asbestosis range (see Table 7.1.5) provide valuable evidence of such exposure. Compensation standards for asbestos-associated lung cancer in different countries are shown in Box 7.1.4.[192,289]

Asbestos-induced airway disease

Although asbestosis causes a restrictive respiratory defect, airflow limitation is also seen in this disease. Much of the airflow limitation is attributable to cigarette smoking but it is also seen in non-smoking asbestos workers and is worse in those with asbestosis.[300] The pathological basis of this appears to be small-airways disease (see p. 123).[301] It is possibly a non-specific reaction to inhaled dust or cigarette smoke.[302] Because it is not established that this lesion progresses to interstitial alveolar fibrosis (asbestosis) the term 'asbestos airways disease' is suggested.[302] Fibrosis limited to the bronchioles is specifically excluded from the definition of asbestosis in the latest guidelines (although these retain grade 0 for fibrosis limited to the bronchiolar walls).[193] It should also be noted that, although emphysema is considered to be a destructive rather than fibrotic condition, a little focal fibrosis is generally evident in this common condition[255] and does not necessarily indicate early asbestosis.

ALUMINIUM

Aluminium has been implicated in the development of respiratory disease during the refining of its principal ore, bauxite, to yield various aluminium oxides (aluminas), in the preparation of the metal by smelting alumina, in the production of corundum abrasive and in the production of special aluminium powders used in explosives.

Refining of bauxite

Bauxite is a mixture of various aluminium oxides, hydroxides and silicates, iron oxide and titanium dioxide. The oxides of aluminium are obtained by differential heating of the ore and the respiratory effects of this work appear to be no more than mild airway irritation. It is generally accepted that aluminium oxide is inert.

Aluminium smelting

Aluminium is prepared by the electrolytic reduction of its oxide dissolved in sodium aluminium fluoride (cryolite), a process releasing a considerable amount of fluoride-rich effluent. Exposed workers have complained of what is termed pot-room asthma. The pathology of this condition is not well described but the pathogenesis is thought to involve irritation rather than allergy.[303]

Abrasive manufacture

The abrasive corundum is formed from bauxite mixed with coke and iron heated in an electric arc furnace, a process in which workers may be exposed to the fumes of alumina and free silica. In the past some of these workers developed diffuse pulmonary fibrosis (Shaver's disease)[369] and, although this was initially attributed to the aluminium, it is now agreed that the free silica was the responsible agent. The exposure to free silica has been reduced and the disease is now regarded as historic.

Aluminium powder

Aluminium powder holds a paradoxical position in regard to lung disease. In certain industries it has caused very severe pulmonary fibrosis, yet in others it has proved harmless. Indeed, at one time Canadian miners breathed aluminium dust before work, in the belief that this would reduce the danger of silica in the mine dust[304] and more recently silicosis has been treated by such means in France.[305] It is questionable whether this practice is effective but it at least appears to cause no harm. The explanation for these contradictory observations probably lies in differing methods of manufacture of aluminium powder.

Aluminium metal appears to be an inert substance but this is only because it has a high affinity for oxygen and the surface layer of aluminium oxide so formed is firmly bound to the underlying metal, unlike ferric oxide which permits further rusting of iron. Granular aluminium powders, produced in a ball mill or from a jet of molten aluminium, therefore acquire a protective coat of surface oxide and are inert. With stamped aluminium powders, however, surface oxidation is prevented by lubricants added to aid the separation of these flake-like particles. The usual lubricant (stearin) contains stearic acid and this polar compound combines with the underlying metal, which is thereby protected from both atmospheric oxidation and the

action of body fluids when such dust is inhaled. In certain circumstances, however, non-polar lubricants in the form of mineral oils have been substituted for stearin. This happened in Germany during the Second World War when munition production was stepped up but stearin was difficult to obtain,[306,307] and in the UK in the 1950s to make the powder darker for purely commercial reasons.[308] In vitro, oil-coated stamped aluminium powder reacts with water to produce aluminium hydroxide, which affords the underlying metal no protection against further attack, so that aluminium hydroxide continues to be formed.[309] This substance is a protein denaturant, once used in the tanning industry, and it is believed that this property underlies the very exceptional cases of severe pulmonary fibrosis that have occurred in connection with stamped aluminium powder produced with mineral oil rather than stearin.[309,310] The fibrosis has a very characteristic pattern, affecting the upper lobes and progressing rapidly, the interval from onset of symptoms to death being as short as 2 years.[308] There is marked shrinkage of the lungs with gross elevation of the diaphragm and buckling of the trachea (Fig. 7.1.27). The lungs are grey (Fig. 7.1.28) and microscopically, numerous small black jagged particles are seen. These can be shown to contain aluminium with Irwin's aluminon stain or by microprobe analysis.[311]

What appears to be a different pathological effect of aluminium dust on the lungs is the rare development of granulomatous disease resembling sarcoidosis and berylliosis.[312,313] This represents hypersensitivity to the metal, amenable to confirmation with a lymphocyte transformation test similar to that used to diagnosis berylliosis (see below).

Aluminium welding

Rare cases of desquamative interstitial pneumonia and pulmonary fibrosis have been reported in aluminium welders.[311,314]

RARE EARTH (CERIUM) PNEUMOCONIOSIS

Elements with atomic numbers from 57 (lanthanum) to 71 (lutetium) are known as the lanthanides or rare earth metals. They are used in many manufacturing processes, including the production of high-temperature ceramics and the grinding of optical lenses. Carbon arc lamps used in reproduction photography emit appreciable quantities of oxidised lanthanides, particularly cerium oxide, and there are reports of pneumoconiosis in exposed individuals.[315] The pathological changes reported have varied from granulomatous nodules to diffuse interstitial fibrosis indistinguishable from the idiopathic variety except for the presence of rare earth elements (usually cerium) detected by polarising light microscopy and electron microprobe analysis.[315]

HARD-METAL DISEASE (COBALT LUNG)

Hard metal is a tungsten alloy containing small amounts of cobalt, titanium, molybdenum and nickel. It is exceptionally tough and once formed can only be worked with diamond. It is used in the tips of drill bits, on abrasive wheels and discs, and in armaments. Interstitial lung disease is liable to arise in its manufacture or in those using hard metal as an abrasive.[316] Experimental work suggests that cobalt is the dangerous constituent[317] but this element is soluble and, unless industrial contact has been recent, analysis of lung tissue usually shows tungsten and titanium but no cobalt. The role of cobalt is also

Figure 7.1.27 Aluminium pneumoconiosis. (A) A chest radiograph showing opacification of the lung apices. (B) A barium swallow showing severe buckling of the oesophagus due to fibrous contracture of the lung apices and adjacent mediastinal tissues, as seen in Figure 7.1.B. *(Courtesy of the late Professor RE Lane, Manchester, UK.)*

Figure 7.1.28 Aluminium pneumoconiosis. The lungs postmortem show severe fibrosis of the apex and overlying pleura. *(Courtesy of the late Dr G Manning, Bolton, UK.)*

indicated by the development of similar interstitial lung disease in diamond polishers using high-speed polishing discs made with a diamond-cobalt surface that lacked tungsten carbide and the other constituents of hard metal.[318,319]

Hard-metal lung disease and cobalt lung take two forms, an industrial asthma and interstitial fibrosis. The latter has a diffuse lower zonal distribution and the appearances mimic idiopathic pulmonary fibrosis. However, an unusual feature is the presence of moderate, or perhaps only small numbers, of giant cells (Fig. 7.1.29A, B).[316,320] Not only are there multinucleate alveolar macrophages but syncytial cell forms develop in the alveolar epithelium. Electron microscopy confirms that these are multinucleate type II pneumocytes (Fig. 7.1.29C).[316] Such epithelial changes are well known in measles pneumonia but the viral inclusion bodies that characterise this infection are not found in hard-metal pneumoconiosis. The changes are those initially described as a particular pattern of idiopathic interstitial pneumonia termed giant cell interstitial pneumonia or GIP (see p. 264). Elemental analysis shows that many, but not all, cases of GIP represent hard-metal disease. The exceptions seldom give a history of cobalt exposure and must be presumed to represent true idiopathic cases. Conversely, epithelial giant cells are not always found in hard-metal pneumoconiosis and so their presence, although highly characteristic, is neither totally specific nor totally sensitive.

BERYLLIOSIS

Beryllium is the lightest of metals. It has an atomic weight of 4 and special properties that make it especially useful in many applications. It is more rigid than steel, has a high melting point and is an excellent conductor of heat and electricity. Unfortunately, the inhalation of beryllium dust or fume is exceedingly dangerous.[321,322] Those who worked with beryllium compounds before precautionary measures were taken suffered a high morbidity and mortality. Sometimes, the escape of dangerous fumes from the factories was on such a scale that people living in nearby houses, downwind from the places in which these materials were being worked, contracted and occasionally died from berylliosis ('neighbourhood cases').[323] Alternatively, contamination of a beryllium worker's clothes might lead to berylliosis in a

Figure 7.1.29 Giant cell interstitial pneumonia in hard-metal workers. (A) There is interstitial pneumonia and fibrosis and several alveolar epithelial cells are multinucleate (arrows). (B) Higher magnification shows a light lymphocytic infiltrate, numerous alveolar macrophages and several multinucleate giant cells.

relative.[324] Beryllium compounds may also cause contact dermatitis and conjunctivitis.[325] Beryllium is also classified as a probable pulmonary carcinogen,[326] but this is controversial.

Two forms of berylliosis are recognised, acute and chronic. Acute berylliosis was first reported in Germany in 1933[327] and is now largely of historical interest, being only encountered as a result of rare accidental or unexpected exposure. It follows the inhalation of a soluble beryllium salt and represents chemical injury, the pathology being that of diffuse alveolar damage (see p. 136). Further consideration will be confined to chronic berylliosis, which is allergic in nature.

Uses of beryllium and occupations at risk

Chronic berylliosis was first reported in 1946 in the fluorescent lamp industry.[328] Beryllium has now been replaced in this application but it has since proved to be of great value in the nuclear, electronic, computer and aerospace industries and the production of refractory materials and crucibles that are to be subjected to particularly high temperatures. The alloys of beryllium are also now widely used, especially those with copper, on which it confers elasticity and resistance to fatigue. Alloy manufacture and the machining of beryllium alloys are therefore further activities that entail a risk of berylliosis, as is the recovery of the metal in the recycling of scrapped electronic and computer parts. Seemingly innocuous occupations such as dental laboratory technician are not without risk of chronic berylliosis.[329]

Pathogenesis

There are good grounds for regarding chronic berylliosis as being an allergic condition. Many of those affected react strongly to skin tests with dilute solutions of beryllium salts, although these must be undertaken with care: occasionally in a highly sensitised person even so small an exposure may evoke a systemic reaction. The skin reaction is of the delayed type, occurs in only 5% of exposed individuals, is not associated with a clear-cut dose–response curve and represents a granulomatous response. Further evidence for the disease having an allergic basis derives from bronchoalveolar lavage, which demonstrates an excess of T-helper lymphocytes that proliferate in vitro on exposure to beryllium salts.[330] A positive transformation test given by these lymphocytes is a more reliable indicator of disease than in vitro blood lymphocyte transformation testing,[52] which is safe but not wholly reliable and indicates only sensitization, rather than berylliosis.

Susceptibility to berylliosis varies widely from person to person and it is notable that chronic pulmonary disease is strongly associated with the HLA antigen DPβ1 and the *Glu69* gene.[331,332] The importance of genetic factors is supported by a report of the disease in identical twins.[333]

Chronic berylliosis is thought to be initiated by the metal binding to tissue proteins and acting as a hapten to initiate a delayed hypersensitivity response characterised by a proliferation of T-helper lymphocytes. These sensitised cells in turn secrete a variety of cytokines (e.g. interleukin-2, tumour necrosis factor-α and interferon-γ) that recruit and activate macrophages, which mature into epithelioid cells. The resultant epithelioid cell granulomas destroy the lung tissue and lead to pulmonary fibrosis.

Pathological changes

If beryllium enters the subcutaneous tissues through a cut or abrasion, as often happened in the earlier days of fluorescent lamp manufacture, a sarcoid-like granuloma soon appears at the site; in time, the overlying epidermis may break down to form an ulcer.

Even more serious are the lesions produced by the inhalation of beryllium. Chronic pulmonary berylliosis takes the form of a widespread granulomatous pneumonia with a histological picture identical to that of sarcoidosis (Fig. 7.1.30A). Both berylliosis and sarcoidosis affect the upper lobes more than the lower (Fig. 7.1.30B) and in both diseases the granulomas are preferentially distributed along lymphatics and may involve adjacent blood vessels. In neither condition is there widespread necrosis but in both diseases the granulomas occasionally display a little central necrosis or hyalinisation. As in sarcoidosis, the hilar lymph nodes may be involved but, unlike sarcoidosis, not in isolation.

Over a period of many years, the sarcoid-like granulomas gradually undergo progressive fibrosis, with consequent impairment of pulmonary function. In the later stages, when the disease has become chronic, dispersal of beryllium from its site of initial absorption may lead to generalisation of the disease and to the appearance of similar granulomas elsewhere, particularly in the liver, kidneys, spleen and skin, but this is unusual.

Figure 7.1.30 Chronic berylliosis. (A) Numerous non-necrotising epithelioid and giant cell granulomas are seen in the lungs. (B) The upper and middle lobes and the apex of the lower lobe are contracted by extensive fibrosis. Paper mounted whole lung section.

Clinical features

Chronic berylliosis is characterised by the gradual onset of cough, shortness of breath, chest pain, night sweats and fatigue. These symptoms may develop within a few weeks of exposure or many years later. Once the worker is exposed, the beryllium is retained in the tissues

and there is a lifelong risk of disease. Progression often entails alternating exacerbations and remissions, long after exposure has ceased.

Analysis

In keeping with the view that berylliosis is a hypersensitivity reaction, very little beryllium is necessary to cause the disease. Particulate beryllium is so scanty in the affected tissues and the atomic number of beryllium so low that electron microprobe analysis is generally unsuitable for its detection. Furthermore conventional detectors are protected by a beryllium window. However, the substitution of a polymeric window has enabled beryllium to be detected by electron microprobe analysis, presumably in a patient with fairly heavy exposure.[334] Ion or laser microprobe mass spectroscopy can also detect very small amounts of beryllium in tissue sections but these techniques are not widely available.

Differential diagnosis

The differential diagnosis of chronic berylliosis is from sarcoidosis, to which it is identical morphologically.[335–337] However, as noted above, it is unusual for berylliosis to cause significant hilar lymphadenopathy in the absence of pulmonary disease, which is a common feature of sarcoidosis. Extrathoracic granulomas, erythema nodosum and uveitis, which are all common in sarcoidosis, are unusual in berylliosis. However, one group found that 6% of patients initially diagnosed as having sarcoidosis actually had chronic berylliosis.[338] Similar findings have been reported by others.[324,339] Any patient thought to have sarcoidosis who has worked with or near metals should be offered a beryllium lymphocyte transformation test. A list of laboratories performing this test can be found at www.dimensional.com/~mhj/medical_testing.html.

POLYVINYL CHLORIDE PNEUMOCONIOSIS

Although polyvinyl is not a mineral and the reaction of the lungs to its presence is therefore not a true pneumoconiosis, it is generally so termed and is dealt with here for convenience. Workers are exposed to polyvinyl chloride dust in the milling and bagging of this plastic and micronodular opacities may be detected in their lungs radiologically. However, the material is non-fibrogenic and histology merely shows a foreign-body reaction to the dust particles.[340] The radiological opacities may abate when exposure ceases.[341] Nevertheless, one polyvinyl chloride worker developed systemic sclerosis,[342] which is a recognised complication of silicosis (see p. 335). Polyvinyl chloride is produced from vinyl chloride monomer, which has a causal association with angiosarcoma of the liver and probably other forms of cancer, including carcinoma of the lung (see p. 534).

FLOCK WORKER'S LUNG

In the late 1990s a characteristic lung disease was identified in workers at several factories producing plush material by spraying nylon flock on to an adhesive backing material.[343–346] The flock fibres are too large to be inspired but may be mixed with smaller nylon shards of respirable size. The workers complained of cough and breathlessness and were found to have a restrictive ventilatory defect with interstitial markings on radiography. Their symptoms improved on removal from the workplace but relapsed on return to work. Pathologically, there was lymphocytic bronchiolitis and peribronchiolitis with widespread lymphoid hyperplasia represented by lymphoid aggregates.

Granulomas were not identified. The histological appearances suggest a severe immunological reaction and raise possibilities such as rheumatoid disease and Sjögren's syndrome but consideration of the clinical and serological setting and the occupation should permit recognition of the cause.

POPCORN WORKER'S LUNG

The industrial production of popcorn and other foodstuffs appears to carry a risk of obstructive airway disease.[347-350] Biopsy of affected workers has shown peribronchiolar fibrosis and granulomas and air sampling has identified many volatile organic compounds, of which the flavouring agent diacetyl (2,3-butanedione) is suspected of being responsible for the bronchiolitis.

PAINT SPRAYING

It is difficult to continue paint spraying (air brushing, aerographics) without adequate respiratory protection but in the early 1990s several small aerographic factories operated in the neighbourhood of Alicante, southeastern Spain without any concern for the workers' health. The workers were required to paint patterns on textiles using a hand-held spray gun. The atmospheric pollution was intense but complaints of respiratory difficulties were met with reassurances and the workers urged to continue. This they did because of the otherwise poor economy, often returning to work when disabling breathlessness had settled down. A change of paint (to Acramin F) may have contributed because the worst-affected workers were employed at two plants that had made this switch. Their illness has been described as the 'Ardystil syndrome' after the name of one of these factories. Some workers were left with permanent respiratory disability. One required a lung transplant and 6 others died.[351-354] Transbronchial biopsy showed organising pneumonia, which in the fatal cases had progressed to irreversible interstitial fibrosis. A similar outbreak of respiratory disease was subsequently reported in Algerian textile factories where Acromin F was applied by the same technique.[355,356] Acromin F is marketed as a paste and used as such without ill-effect. Its use in heavy spray form appears to be responsible for the 'Ardystil syndrome'.

MINERAL OILS AND PETROLEUM

Workers in engineering workshops may be exposed to the prolonged inhalation of fine sprays or mists of the longer-chain hydrocarbons that constitute many mineral oils. This may result in exogenous lipid pneumonia,[357] which is described on page 314, or extrinsic allergic alveolitis.[358-360] The vapour of shorter-chain hydrocarbons such as paraffin oil (kerosene: C_{10-16}) and petrol (gasoline: C_{4-12}) and gaseous hydrocarbons such as propane may act as acute asphyxiants or central nervous system depressants but have negligible pulmonary toxicity. However, if they are ingested or aspirated in their liquid form they are acutely toxic to the lungs, producing a chemical pneumonitis with the features of diffuse alveolar damage. Ingestion may be accidental or deliberate (see Fig. 4.19, p. 142) whereas aspiration is generally inadvertent, occurring in siphoning accidents, such as those experienced by fairground operatives who 'breath or eat fire' ('fire-eater's lung').[361,362] Animal experiments involving the intratracheal injection of kerosene resulted in acute pulmonary exudates, which cleared except for residual bronchiolitis.[363]

Table 7.1.9 Principal respiratory risks of welding

Source	Derivative	Effect
Metals being welded	Iron	Siderosis
	Zinc	Metal fume fever
	Beryllium	Berylliosis (acute or chronic)
	Chrome, nickel	Asthma
	Cadmium, manganese	Diffuse alveolar damage
	Chrome, nickel, arsenic	Lung cancer
Burning of adjacent surfaces	Isocyanates	Asthma
	Phosgene	Bronchitis, bronchiolitis
	Tetrafluoroethylene	Polymer fume fever
	Oxides of nitrogen	Bronchitis
Electrode insulation Protective clothes	Asbestos	Mesothelioma
Gas used to prevent oxidation	Carbon dioxide	Asphyxia
Combustive gas	Carbon monoxide	Carbon monoxide poisoning
Ultraviolet light	Ozone	Bronchitis
Various	Silica, silicates	Silicosis, mixed-dust pneumoconiosis

WELDING

Welder's pneumoconiosis, first recognised in 1936,[364] essentially represents the fairly harmless deposition of iron in the lungs (siderosis – see p. 337). However, welders may suffer various ill-effects from the inhalation of substances other than iron (Table 7.1.9). Some of these are para-occupational risks, that is, encountered by welders because they work near another process and are inadvertently exposed: thus, shipyard welders may be exposed to asbestos,[365] and those in foundries to silica. Welders may therefore develop a mixed-dust pneumoconiosis (see p. 337), rather than just siderosis. However, one analytical investigation identified excess amounts of iron alone in association with pulmonary fibrosis; the silicon content did not differ from that in controls.[366]

More directly, welders may be exposed to asbestos insulation that they themselves use, while welders of special steel alloys run the risk of metal-induced asthma, metal fume fever, polymer fume fever and the consequences of toxic metal fume inhalation,[367] all of which are described separately in this chapter, as is lung disease in aluminium welders. Chronic bronchitis has been attributed to the inhalation of low concentrations of irritants such as ozone and nitrogen dioxide by welders but this risk is unproven and the subject of much controversy. Welders may also inhale carcinogenic hexavalent chromium compounds in the course of their work and therefore develop lung cancer. The term 'welder's lung' is often applied indiscriminately to any of these diseases and, as it has no specific meaning, is best avoided.

TOXIC FUMES AND GASES

Dust, fume and gas are some of the terms used to describe different physical forms of respirable agents. They are defined in Table 7.2.1 on page 372. The parts of the respiratory tract at which they exert their maximal effect are influenced by particle size and solubility (see Table 7.2.2 and Fig. 7.2.2, p. 372).

Toxic metal fume[368]

The finely divided fume of several metals is highly toxic to the lungs and capable of producing severe acute and chronic damage to both the conductive airways and the alveoli, resulting in acute tracheo-bronchitis and bronchiolitis, diffuse alveolar damage, obliterative bronchiolitis and pulmonary fibrosis. Important metal fumes in this respect include aluminium, which is released together with silica fume in bauxite smelting (see Shaver's disease,[369] above), cadmium from welding or cutting special steels, chromium from cutting its alloys or in the manufacture of chromates, cobalt released in the production and use of its alloys (see hard-metal disease, above), mercury released in various industries and in the home,[370] nickel carbonyl released during the purification of metallic nickel or the manufacture of nickel alloys[371] and beryllium (see above).

Toxic gases

Many irritant gases cause severe acute and chronic damage to both the conductive airways and alveoli. The changes are non-specific and similar to those wrought by toxic metal fumes (see above) and viruses amongst other agents. They consist of acute tracheobronchitis and bronchiolitis, obliterative bronchiolitis, diffuse alveolar damage and pulmonary fibrosis.

The gases liable to produce such damage include oxides of nitrogen, sulphur dioxide, ozone, phosgene, chlorine, ammonia and various constituents of smoke, notably acrolein. Some of these are also touched upon in Chapter 7.2 because they are of general as well as occupational importance, although there is no rigid difference between general and occupational pollution.

Ozone, sulphur dioxide and nitrogen dioxide are oxidising gases that may be found together as industrial atmospheric pollutants. Each is capable of producing diffuse alveolar damage by means of its oxidising properties and the release of free active radicals. In addition, they cause damage to distal airways, particularly terminal and respiratory bronchioles, with resulting bronchiolitis.

Oxides of nitrogen may be encountered with fatal consequences by farmhands seeking to free a blockage in a silo when they encounter pockets of this gas that have accumulated on top of the fermenting silage: the term 'silo-filler's disease' is generally applied to the initial haemorrhagic oedema or the obliterative bronchiolitis that develops in those who survive the initial chemical injury.[372-375] Asphyxia due to the farmhand encountering pockets of carbon dioxide is a further hazard within agricultural silos. Other farmhands have suffered from the inhalation of toxic gases or bacteria when handling liquid manure.[376-379] Welding, which is considered below, may also involve exposure to toxic gases such as oxides of nitrogen.

Ozone, the principal oxidant gas of photochemical smog, produces pulmonary changes at relatively low levels and may be encountered at higher concentrations in various industries. Potentially dangerous levels of ozone are produced from atmospheric oxygen by ultraviolet radiation given off in welding while ozone is used in industry to sterilise water, bleach paper, flour and oils, and mask the odour of organic effluents. The damage wrought by ozone is predominantly centriacinar in distribution, affecting terminal and respiratory bronchiolar epithelium and proximal alveolar epithelium.[380-382] There is loss of cilia and necrosis of centriacinar alveolar type I epithelial cells. The changes are dose-dependent and, in one study, the youngest animals

were most sensitive.[383] In long-term experiments, hyperplastic bronchiolar Clara and ciliated cells extended peripherally to line alveolar ducts.[384] The role of granulocytes is stressed in some experimental studies[385] and it is notable that neutrophil migration is prominent when the human lungs are damaged by ozone.[386]

Aldehydes such as acetaldehyde, formaldehyde and acrylic aldehyde (acrolein) are widely used in the plastics and chemical industries. The first is a liquid and the others are water-soluble gases. Pathologists are of course familiar with formaldehyde solution from its use as a disinfectant and histological fixative. All these aldehydes are intensely irritant and their acute effects generally prevent prolonged exposure to high concentrations. Chronic effects include skin sensitivity and asthma, and in rats nasal carcinoma. However, the doses to which these experimental animals were exposed far exceed any that are likely to be encountered by humans, in whom there is no convincing evidence of aldehyde-induced cancer.[387]

Ammonia gas is extensively used in industry as a raw material, notably in the manufacture of nitrogenous products such as fertilisers and plastics. It is highly soluble and its acute irritative effects are mainly felt in the eyes, nose and throat, but high levels affect the major airways, possibly leading to them being blocked by exudates. Survival usually brings full recovery but bronchiectasis and obliterative bronchiolitis have been described.

Chlorine gas is widely used in the chemical industry. It is transported and stored under pressure in liquid form. Heavy exposure through its accidental release or use as a war gas has proved fatal through its acute toxicity causing exudative airway occlusion and pulmonary oedema. Survivors usually recover completely but, as with nitrogen dioxide and ammonia, there is a risk of obliterative bronchiolitis.

Phosgene (carbonyl chloride, $COCl_2$) is a poisonous, colourless gas that was responsible for thousands of deaths during World War I, when it was used in chemical warfare. It is used industrially in the preparation of some organic chemical compounds and is formed, perhaps inadvertently,[388] by the combustion of methylene chloride in products such as paint strippers. Phosgene causes injury to terminal bronchioles and alveoli, with resulting oedema and hyaline membrane formation. The mechanism of cell damage is uncertain but it may depend on inactivation of intracellular enzymes by the gas. Long-term problems are rare but chronic bronchitis and emphysema have been described in survivors.

Mustard gas (bichloroethyl sulphide, $C_4H_8Cl_2S$) is a further agent that has been used in chemical warfare. It is primarily a skin vesicant but when inhaled it results in widespread epithelial destruction and pulmonary oedema. Survivors may be left with irritant-induced asthma (reactive airways dysfunction), chronic bronchitis, tracheo-bronchomalacia, bronchiectasis and bronchiolitis obliterans.[389-391]

Thionyl chloride is used in the manufacture of lithium batteries where it is liable to result in the release of sulphur dioxide and hydrochloric acid fumes. Workers in such factories have developed lung injury varying from mild, reversible interstitial disease to severe obliterative bronchiolitis.[392]

Hydrogen sulphide is the principal chemical hazard of natural gas production. High levels of the gas also buid up in sheds housing large numbers of pigs, the source here being the pig manure. Once inhaled the gas is rapidly absorbed into the blood stream. The effects are therefore widespread but include the usual respiratory effects of irritant gases, varying from sneezing to pulmonary oedema and acute respiratory distress, depending upon the exposure. In Alberta 221 cases were identified over a 5-year period. The overall mortality was 6%; 5% of victims were dead on arrival at hospital. Most required admission to hospital but the survivors experienced no long-term adverse effects.[392a]

Table 7.1.10 Work-related respiratory disease in the UK[394]	
Disease	**Estimated annual number of cases**
Occupational asthma	941
Non-malignant pleural disease	730
Mesothelioma	644
Pneumoconiosis	341
Inhalation accidents	280
Lung cancer	70
Infectious disease	59
Extrinsic allergic alveolitis	46
Bronchitis	38
Byssinosis	1
Other diagnoses	117
Total	3207

Table 7.1.11 Agents that cause occupational asthma and examples of the occupations involved[397]	
Causative agent	**Occupations involved**
High-molecular-weight agents (patients are usually atopic)	
Laboratory animals	Laboratory animal handling
Flour and grain	Baking, milling, farming
Enzymes	Detergent and drug manufacture, baking
Seafoods	Food processing
Gums	Carpet and drug manufacture
Low-molecular-weight agents (patients are not necessarily atopic)	
Isocyanates	Foam and plastic manufacture, spray painting, insulation
Anhydrides	Plastic and epoxy resin handling
Wood dusts	Forestry, carpentry
Soldering fluxes	Electronics
Formaldehyde, glutaraldehyde	Histopathology, nursing, radiography
Amines	Shellac and lacquer handling, soldering
Chloramine	Cleaning
Dyes	Textiles
Acrylates	Adhesive application
Metals	Solderers, refiners
Drugs	Pharmaceutical work

ANOXIC ASPHYXIA

The danger of asphyxia from the inhalation of gases devoid of oxygen is fairly widespread in industry.[393] It generally arises from the use of inert gases, which, being non-toxic, give a false sense of security. Pockets of these gases tend to form in confined spaces. Anoxic death from the accumulation of methane is well known in mines and has also occurred in slurry pits and sewers. Anoxic asphyxia in diving (and anaesthesia) has resulted from the incorrect connection of gas cylinders or failure to notice that a mixed gas contains insufficient oxygen. Deaths have occurred in welding when argon or carbon dioxide has been used to shield the weld and prevent oxidation of the metals at the high temperatures employed. Deaths have also resulted from inadvertent entry to discharged oil tanks filled with nitrogen to reduce the risk of explosions, or from the formation of pockets of nitrogen gas applied in liquid form to freeze the contents of damaged pipes so that they can be repaired without the necessity to drain down.

The respiration of a gas devoid of oxygen causes loss of consciousness within seconds because it not only fails to provide oxygen but removes that present in the pulmonary arterial blood. The changes at autopsy are those common to cellular hypoxia. They include cerebral and serosal petechiae and pulmonary congestion and haemorrhage but these features are not specific and are not always present. The cause of death can generally only be surmised from the circumstances surrounding the death.

OCCUPATIONAL ASTHMA

Occupational asthma is the commonest cause of work-related respiratory disease in many western countries (Table 7.1.10).[394-396] The reported incidence ranges from 13 per million workers in South Africa to 174 per million workers in Finland.[395,396] It occurs in many industries (Table 7.1.11)[397] and occupational factors can be identified as contributing to asthma in about 15% of adult cases.[398] Over 250 aetio-logical agents have been identified.[399] In the UK a third are organic, a third chemical, 6% metallic and the rest miscellaneous. The commonest, in descending order, are isocyanates, flour and grain, laboratory animals, glutaraldehyde, solder or colophony and hardening agents.[400]

Atopy appears to predispose to occupational asthma when the allergen is of high molecular weight but not when it is of low molecular weight. For example, atopic individuals are particularly prone to develop asthma if employed in the manufacture of biological detergents, whereas atopy does not increase the risk of asthma from sensitisation to toluene di-isocyanate, which is a serious health problem in the manufacture of polyurethane. Similarly, platinum salts are such potent sensitising agents that nearly all those exposed to them develop asthma. Asthma-provoking metals other than platinum include chromium, cobalt, nickel and vanadium, all of which are used in steel alloys, and possibly aluminium (see pot-room asthma, p. 357). Other asthma-inducing factors encountered in industry include grain and flour dust, certain wood dusts, soldering fluxes containing colophony (pine resin), epoxy resin hardeners such as phthallic anhydride, isocyanate-containing foams and paints, formaldehyde and the excreta of laboratory animals. Contaminated humidifiers may cause occupational asthma as well as humidifier fever and extrinsic allergic alveolitis.[401] Pathologically, occupational asthma is identical to non-occupational asthma (see p. 109).

Byssinosis

Byssinosis is a further form of occupational asthma,[402] one encountered in the cotton industry. The sensitising agent is a component of the cotton bract, which is the part of the cotton harvest other than the cotton fibre. Bract consists of dried leaf, other plant debris and soil particles and contains a variety of fungal and bacterial residues, including lipopolysaccharide endotoxin, but the exact nature of the sensitising agent remains unknown.[403] The endotoxin is unlikely to be responsible for byssinosis but may be the cause of so-called mill fever, a self-limiting illness characterised by malaise, fever and leukocytosis that is experienced by many people on first visiting a cotton mill.

Dust levels and the risk of byssinosis are particularly high in the carding rooms where the raw cotton is teased out before it is spun. Affected workers are worse when they return to work after the weekend break, a feature attributed to antibody levels having built up during this brief respite from the cotton dust. There is no link with atopy and the fluctuating antibodies are precipitins of the immunoglobulin G class. Complement activation by both arms of the complement cascade has been reported.[404,405]

When the Lancashire economy was largely cotton-based, necropsies on workers suffering from byssinosis generally showed gross emphysema, and this came to be accepted as evidence of byssinosis. However, it is now realised that in this heavily industrialised part of the UK, emphysema is as common in the general population as in cotton workers and it can no longer be considered a component of byssinosis. Other findings in byssinosis are more commensurate with asthma, namely an increase in bronchial muscle and mucous cells.[406] No granulomas or other evidence of extrinsic allergic alveolitis are found.

OCCUPATIONAL FEVERS

Fever may be the predominant feature in a variety of occupational illnesses and the unifying term 'inhalation fever' has been proposed.[407] However, the individual occupations are of interest and these conditions will therefore be considered separately. Mill fever has been mentioned above under byssinosis.

Humidifier fever[408]

Humidifier fever is an acute illness characterised by malaise, fever, myalgia, cough, tightness in the chest and breathlessness, all of which are worse on Monday mornings if the humidifier responsible is at work rather than home. The chest complaints, and their aggravation on return to work after the weekend, are features shared with byssinosis (see above) but the general complaints fit better with extrinsic allergic alveolitis (see p. 279). Humidifier fever develops in circumstances that also lead to the development of a form of extrinsic allergic alveolitis, and not surprisingly the same name has been extended to this latter condition, with inevitable confusion. Both diseases are caused by microbiological contamination of humidifiers or air conditioners so that a fine spray of microorganisms is emitted into the office, factory or home. Investigations have generally shown the baffle plates of the air conditioner to be covered with a slime of bacteria, fungi or protozoa (mainly amoeba and ciliates), and extracts of this have been used to identify precipitins in the patient's sera, as in extrinsic allergic alveolitis. However, unlike extrinsic allergic alveolitis, humidifier fever resolves within a day and leaves no permanent injury. For this reason there is seldom the opportunity to study the tissue changes, and partly for this reason it remains unclear whether the disease is mediated by immune complexes, as in extrinsic allergic alveolitis, or by endotoxins derived from the contaminants.

Pulmonary mycotoxicosis

A febrile illness occurring in precipitin-negative farm-workers after heavy exposure to fungi in their silos was attributed to inhaled fungal toxins and named pulmonary mycotoxicosis.[409] It is also known as precipitin test-negative farmer's lung and organic dust toxic syndrome.[410] The condition is generally self-limiting and is seldom biopsied but desquamative interstitial pneumonia and diffuse alveolar damage have been reported.[411,412]

Metal fume fever

This is a self-limiting acute illness characterised by fever, sweating, myalgia, chest pain, headache and nausea, that comes on Monday mornings when occupational exposure is experienced after a weekend's respite, as with bysinnosis and humidifier fever; during the week tolerance develops.[368,413] The disease involves the release of cytokines such as tumour necrosis factor and is presumed to have an allergic basis.[414] The metals involved are chiefly zinc, copper and magnesium, and, to a lesser extent, aluminium, antimony, iron, manganese and nickel. Occupations at risk include any that generate such metal fumes, but particularly welding. It is most commonly associated with welding zinc-coated surfaces. If the symptoms persist, alternative diagnoses, such as acute cadmium poisoning and other specific toxic metal fume diseases, should be suspected: these are not self-limiting and may cause severe bronchiolitis or diffuse alveolar damage (see above).

Polymer fume fever

This illness resembles metal fume fever except that it occurs without regard to previous exposure: no tolerance develops and there is therefore no particular susceptibility on Mondays. The polymers concerned are quite inert, except when heated to produce fume: polytetrafluorethylene (PTFE, Teflon, Fluon, Halon) is a notable example. As with other self-limiting diseases, little is known of the tissue changes.

REFERENCES

Pneumoconiosis: general features

1. Oxman AD, Muir DCF, Shannon HS, et al. Occupational dust exposure and chronic obstructive pulmonary disease – a systematic overview of the evidence. Am Rev Respir Dis 1993;148:38–48.
2. Blanc PD, Iribarren C, Trupin L, et al. Occupational exposures and the risk of COPD: dusty trades revisited. Thorax 2009;64:6–12.
3. Meiklejohn A. The origin of the term 'pneumonokoniosis'. Br J Ind Med 1960;17:155–60.
4. Industrial Injuries Advisory Council. Pneumoconiosis and byssinosis. London: HMSO; 1973. p. 1.
5. Parkes WR. Aerosols: their deposition and clearance. In: Parkes WR, editor. Occupational Lung Disorders. 3rd ed. Oxford: Butterworth Heinemann; 1994. p. 35.
6. Churg A, Brauer M. Human lung parenchyma retains PM2.5. Amer J Respir Crit Care Med 1997;155:2109–11.
7. Pinkerton KE, Plopper CG, Mercer RR, et al. Airway branching patterns influence asbestos fiber location and the extent of tissue injury in the pulmonary parenchyma. Lab Invest 1986;55:688–95.

8. Becklake MR, Toyota B, Stewart M, et al. Lung structure as a risk factor in adverse pulmonary responses to asbestos exposure. A case-referent study in Quebec chrysotile miners and millers. Am Rev Respir Dis 1983;128:385–8.

9. Schlesinger MR, Lippman M. Particle deposition in casts of the human upper tracheobronchial tree. Am Ind Hyg Assoc J 1972;33:237–50.

10. Pityn P, Chamberlain MJ, King ME, et al. Differences in particle deposition between the two lungs. Respir Med 1995;89: 15–9.

11. Ferin J, Oberdorster G, Penney DP. Pulmonary retention of ultrafine and fine particles in rats. Am J Respir Cell Mol Biol 1992;6:535–42.

12. Brundelet PJ. Experimental study of the dust-clearance mechanism of the lung. Acta Path Microbiol Scand 1965;7–141.

13. Cordingley JL, Nicol T. The lung: an excretory route for macromolecules and particles. J Physiol (London) 1967; 190:7.

14. Corrin B. Phagocytic potential of pulmonary alveolar epithelium with particular reference to surfactant metabolism. Thorax 1970;25:110–5.

15. Brody AR, Hill LH, Adkins B, et al. Chrysotile asbestos inhalation in rats: deposition pattern and reaction of alveolar epithelium and pulmonary macrophages. Am Rev Respir Dis 1981;123:670–8.

16. Churg A. The uptake of mineral particles by pulmonary epithelial cells. Amer J Respir Crit Care Med 1996;154:1124–40.

17. Lehnert BE, Valdez YE, Stewart CC. Translocation of particles to the tracheobronchial lymph nodes after lung deposition: kinetics and particle-cell relationships. Exp Lung Res 1986;10:245–66.

18. Adamson IYR, Hedgecock C. Patterns of particle deposition and retention after instillation to mouse lung during acute injury and fibrotic repair. Exp Lung Res 1995;21:695–709.

19. Adamson IYR, Prieditis H. Silica deposition in the lung during epithelial injury potentiates fibrosis and increases particle translocation to lymph nodes. Exp Lung Res 1998;24:293–306.

20. Gross P, Westrick M. The permeability of lung parenchyma to particulate matter. Am J Pathol 1954;30:195–207.

21. Corry D, Kulkarni P, Lipscomb MF. The migration of bronchoalveolar macrophages into hilar lymph nodes. Am J Pathol 1984;115:321–8.

22. Policard A, Collet A, Pregermain S, et al. Etude au microscope electronique du granulome pulmonaire silicotique experimental. Presse Med 1957;65: 121–4.

23. Emery JL, Dinsdale F. The postnatal development of lymphoreticular aggregates and lymph nodes in infants' lungs. J Clin Pathol 1973;26:539–45.

24. Macklin CS. Pulmonary sumps, dust accumulations, alveolar fluid and lymph vessels. Acta Anat 1955;23:1–33.

25. O'Driscoll BRC, Cooke RDP, Mamtora H, et al. Candida lung abscesses complicating parenteral nutrition. Thorax 1988;43:418–9.

26. Pintar K, Funahashi A, Siegesmund KA. A diffuse form of pulmonary silicosis in foundry workers. Arch Pathol Lab Med 1976;100:535–8.

27. Wagner JC, Pooley FD, Gibbs A, et al. Inhalation of china stone and china clay dusts: relationship between mineralogy of dust retained in the lungs and pathological changes. Thorax 1986;41:190–6.

28. Kleinfeld M, Giel CP, Majeranowski JF, et al. Talc pneumoconiosis. A report of six patients with postmortem findings. Arch Env Health 1963;7:101–15.

29. Ruttner JR, Spycher MA, Sticher H. Diffuse 'asbestosis-like' interstitial fibrosis of the lung. Pathol Microbiol 1972;38: 250–7.

30. Vallyathan NV, Craighead JE. Pulmonary pathology in workers exposed to nonasbestiform talc. Hum Pathol 1981;12:28–35.

31. Davies D, Cotton R. Mica pneumoconiosis. Br J Ind Med 1983;40:22–7.

32. Gibbs AE, Pooley FD, Griffiths DM, et al. Talc pneumoconiosis – a pathologic and mineralogic study. Hum Pathol 1992;23:1344–54.

33. Honma K, Chiyotani K. Diffuse interstitial fibrosis in nonasbestos pneumoconiosis – a pathological study. Respiration 1993;60:120–6.

34. Heppleston AG. The disposal of coal and haematite dusts inhaled successively. J Pathol Bacteriol 1958;75:113–26.

35. Glazier JB, Hughes JMB, Maloney JE, et al. Vertical gradient of alveolar size in lungs of dogs frozen intact. J Appl Physiol 1967;23:694–705.

36. Dock W. Apical localization of phthisis. Am Rev Tuberc 1946;53:297–305.

37. West JB, Dollery CT. Distribution of blood flow and ventilation perfusion ratio in the lung, measured with radioactive CO_2. J Appl Physiol 1960;15:405–10.

38. Goodwin RA, Des Prez RM. Apical localization of pulmonary tuberculosis, chronic pulmonary histoplasmosis, and progressive massive fibrosis of the lung. Chest 1983;83:801–5.

39. Bake B, Wood L, Murphy B, et al. Effect of inspiratory flow rate on the regional distribution of inspired gas. J Appl Physiol 1974;37:8–17.

40. Davson J, Susman W. Apical scars and their relationship to siliceous dust accumulation in non-silicotic lungs. J Path Bact 1937;45:597–612.

41. Sebastien P, Fondimare A, Bignon J, et al. Topographic distribution of asbestos fibres in human lung in relation to occupational and non-occupational exposure. In: Walton WH, editor. Inhaled Particles IV. Oxford: Pergamon; 1977. p. 435–46.

42. Churg A. The distribution of amosite asbestos in the periphery of the normal human lung. Br J Ind Med 1990;47:677–81.

43. Silicosis and Silicate Disease Committee. Diseases associated with exposure to silica and nonfibrous silicate minerals. Arch Pathol Lab Med 1988;112:673–720.

44. McDonald JW, Roggli VL. Detection of silica particles in lung tissue by polarizing light microscopy. Arch Pathol Lab Med 1995;119:242–6.

45. Crocker PR, Doyle DV, Levison DA. A practical method for the identification of particulate and crystalline material in paraffin-embedded tissue specimens. J Pathol 1980;131:165–73.

46. Crocker PR, Toulson E, Levison DA. Particles in paraffin sections demonstrated in the backscattered electron image [BEI]. Micron 1982;13:437–46.

47. Abraham JL, Burnett BR. Quantitative analysis of inorganic particulate burden in situ in tissue sections. Scanning Electron Microsc 1983;II:681–96.

48. Levison DA. Microanalysis in histopathology. J Pathol 1989;157:95–7.

49. Abraham JL, Rossi R, Marquez N, et al. Ion microprobe mass analysis of beryllium in situ in human lung: preliminary results. Scanning Electron Microsc 1976;III: 501–6.

50. Jones-Williams W, Wallach ER. Laser probe mass spectrometry (LAMMS) analysis of beryllium, sarcoidosis and other granulomatous diseases. Sarcoidosis 1991;6:111–7.

51. DeNollin S, Poels K, VanVaeck L, et al. Molecular identification of foreign inclusions in inflammatory tissue surrounding metal implants by Fourier transform laser microprobe mass spectrometry. Pathol Res Pract 1997;193:313–8.

52. Jones Williams W, Williams WR. Value of beryllium lymphocyte transformation test in chronic beryllium disease and in potentially exposed workers. Thorax 1983;38:41–4.

53. Vallyathan V, Brower PS, Green FHY, et al. Radiographic and pathologic correlation of coal workers' pneumoconiosis. Amer J Respir Crit Care Med 1996;154:741–8.

Silicosis

54. King EJ, Mohanty GP, Harrison CV, et al. The action of different forms of pure silica on the lungs of rats. Br J Ind Med 1953;10:9–17.

55. Gibbs AR, Craighead JE, Pooley FD, et al. The pathology of slate workers' pneumoconiosis in North Wales and Vermont. Ann Occup Hyg 1988;32: 273–8.

56. Craighead JE, Emerson RJ, Stanley DE. Slateworker's pneumoconiosis. Hum Pathol 1992;23:1098–105.

57. Palmer PES, Daynes G. Transkei silicosis. S Afr Med J 1967;41:1182–8.

58. Selden A, Sahle W, Johansson L, et al. Three cases of dental technician's pneumoconiosis related to cobalt-chromium-molybdenum dust exposure: diagnosis and follow-up. Chest 1996;109:837–42.

59. Policard A, Collet A. Deposition of silicosis dust in the lungs of the inhabitants of the Sahara regions. Arch Ind Hyg Occup Med 1952;5:527–34.

60. Fossati C. Sulla possibilita e sulla frequenza della silicosi pulmonare tra gli abitanti del deserto libico. Med Lav 1969;60:144–9.

61. Hirsch M, Bar-Ziv J, Lehmann E, et al. Simple siliceous pneumoconiosis of Bedouin females in the Negev desert. Clin Radiol 1974;25:507–10.

62. Bar-Ziv J, Goldberg G. Simple siliceous pneumoconiosis in Negev Bedouins. Arch Environ Health 1974;29:121–6.

63. Fennerty A, Hunter AM, Smith AP, et al. Silicosis in a Pakistani farmer. BMJ 1983;ii:648.

64. Norboo T, Angchuk PT, Yahya M, et al. Silicosis in a Himalayan village population – role of environmental dust. Thorax 1991;46:341–3.

65. Saiyed HN, Sharma YK, Sadhu HG, et al. Non-occupational pneumoconiosis at high altitude villages in central Ladakh. Br J Ind Med 1991;48:825–9.

66. Sherwin RP, Barman ML, Abraham JL. Silicate pneumoconiosis of farm workers. Lab Invest 1979;40:576–82.

67. Schwartz LW, Knight HD, Malloy RL, et al. Silicate pneumoconiosis and pulmonary fibrosis in horses from the Monterey-Carmel peninsula. Chest 1981;80:82S–5S.

68. Brambilla C, Abraham J, Brambilla E, et al. Comparative pathology of silicate pneumoconiosis. Am J Pathol 1979;96:149–70.

69. MacDonald G, Piggot AP, Gilder FW. Two cases of acute silicosis – with a suggested theory of causation. Lancet 1930;2:846–8.

70. Chapman EM. Acute silicosis. JAMA 1932;98:1439–41.

71. Vincent M, Arthaud Y, Crettet G, et al. Silicose aigue fatale par inhalation volontaire de poudre à recurer. Rev Mal Resp 1995;12:499–502.

72. Suratt PM, Winn WC, Brody AR, et al. Acute silicosis in tombstone sandblasters. Am Rev Respir Dis 1977;115:521–9.

73. Seaton A, Legge JS, Henderson J, et al. Accelerated silicosis in Scottish stonemasons. Lancet 1991;337:341–4.

74. Murray J, Webster I, Reid G, et al. The relation between fibrosis of hilar lymph glands and the development of parenchymal silicosis. Br J Ind Med 1991;48:267–9.

75. Hessel PA, Sluis-Cremer GK, Lee SL. Distribution of silicotic collagenization in relation to smoking habits. Am Rev Respir Dis 1991;144:297–301.

76. Baldwin DR, Lambert L, Pantin CFA, et al. Silicosis presenting as bilateral hilar lymphadenopathy. Thorax 1996;51:1165–7.

77. Tosi P, Franzinelli A, Miracco C, et al. Silicotic lymph node lesions in non-occupationally exposed lung carcinoma patients. Eur J Respir Dis 1986;68:362–9.

78. Kampalath BN, McMahon JT, Cohen A, et al. Obliterative central bronchitis due to mineral dust in patients with pneumoconiosis. Arch Pathol Lab Med 1998;122:56–62.

79. Lardinois D, Gugger M, Balmer MC, et al. Left recurrent laryngeal nerve palsy associated with silicosis. Eur Resp J 1999;14:720–2.

80. Argani P, Ghossein R, Rosai J. Anthracotic and anthracosilicotic spindle cell pseudotumors of mediastinal lymph nodes: Report of five cases of a reactive lesion that simulates malignancy. Hum Pathol 1998;29:851–5.

81. Chien HP, Lin TP, Chen HL, et al. Right middle lobe atelectasis associated with endobronchial silicotic lesions. Arch Pathol Lab Med 2000;124:1619–22.

82. Rashid AMH, Green FHY. Pleural pearls following silicosis: a histological and electronmicroscopic study. Histopathology 1995;26:84–7.

83. Zeren EH, Colby TV, Roggli VL. Silica-induced pleural disease: An unusual case mimicking malignant mesothelioma. Chest 1997;112:1436–8.

84. Ng TP, Chan SL. Factors associated with massive fibrosis in silicosis. Thorax 1991;46:229–32.

85. Lynch KM. Silicosis of systemic distribution. Am J Pathol 1942;18:313–31.

86. Langlois SLEP, Sterrett GF, Henderson DW. Hepatosplenic silicosis. Australas Radiol 1977;21:143–9.

87. Carmichael GP, Targoff C, Pintar K et al. Hepatic silicosis. Am J Clin Pathol 1980;73:720–2.

88. Eide J, Gylseth B, Skaug V. Silicotic lesions of the bone marrow: histopathology and microanalysis. Histopathology 1984;8:693–703.

89. Miranda RN, McMillan PN, Pricolo VE, et al. Peritoneal silicosis. Arch Pathol Lab Med 1996;120:300–2.

90. Harding HE, McLaughlin AIG. Pulmonary fibrosis in non-ferrous foundry workers. Br J Ind Med 1955;12:92–9.

91. Cockcroft AE, Wagner JC, Seal EM, et al. Irregular opacities in coalworkers' pneumoconiosis – correlation with pulmonary function and pathology. Ann Occup Hyg 1982;26:767–87.

92. Katabami M, Dosakaakita H, Honma K, et al. Pneumoconiosis-related lung cancers – Preferential occurrence from diffuse interstitial fibrosis-type pneumoconiosis. Amer J Respir Crit Care Med 2000;162:295–300.

93. Rowsell EV, Nagelschmidt G, Curran RC. The effects of dusts on peritoneal cells within diffusion chambers. J Pathol Bacteriol 1960;80:337–44.

94. Vallyathan V, Castranova V, Pack D, et al. Freshly fractured quartz inhalation leads to enhanced lung injury and inflammation: potential role of free radicals. Am J Respir Crit Care Med 1995;152:1003–9.

95. Allison AC, Harington JS, Birbeck M. An examination of the cytotoxic effects of silica on macrophages. J Exp Med 1966;124:141–54.

96. Heppleston AG, Styles JA. Activity of macrophage factor in collagen formation by silica. Nature 1967;214:521–2.

97. Aalto M, Kulonen E. Fractionation of connective-tissue-activating factors from the culture medium of silica-treated macrophages. Acta Path Microbiol Scand Sect C 1979;87:241–50.

98. Aalto M, Turakainen H, Kulonen E. Effect of SiO_2-liberated macrophage factor on protein synthesis in connective tissue in vitro. Scand J Clin Lab Invest 1979;39:205–13.

99. Lugano EM, Dauber JH, Elias JA, et al. The regulation of lung fibroblast proliferation by alveolar macrophages in experimental silicosis. Am Rev Respir Dis 1984;129:767–71.

100. Donaldson K, Slight J, Brown GM, et al. The ability of inflammatory bronchoalveolar leucocyte populations elicited with microbes or mineral dust to injure alveolar epithelial cells and degrade extracellular matrix in vitro. Br J Exp Pathol 1988;69:327–38.

101. Vanhee D, Gosset P, Boitelle A, et al. Cytokines and cytokine network in silicosis and coal workers' pneumoconiosis. Eur Respir J 1995;8:834–42.

102. Claudio E, Segade F, Wrobel K, et al. Activation of murine macrophages by silica particles in vitro is a process independent of silica-induced cell death. Am J Respir Cell Mol Biol 1995;13:547–54.

103. Mariani TJ, Roby JD, Mecham RP, et al. Localization of type I procollagen gene expression in silica-induced granulomatous lung disease and implication of transforming growth factor-beta as a mediator of fibrosis. Am J Pathol 1996;148:151–64.

104. Jagirdar J, Begin R, Dufresne A, et al. Transforming growth factor-beta (TGF-beta) in silicosis. Amer J Respir Crit Care Med 1996;154:1076–81.

105. Mossman BT, Churg A. Mechanisms in the pathogenesis of asbestosis and silicosis. Amer J Respir Crit Care Med 1998;157:1666–80.

106. Erasmus LD. Scleroderma in gold-miners on the Witwatersrand with particular reference to pulmonary manifestations. S Afr J Lab Clin Med 1957;3:209–31.

107. Vigliani EC, Pernis B. Immunological factors in the pathogenesis of the hyaline tissue of silicosis. Br J Ind Med 1958;15:8–14.

108. Scheule RK, Holian A. Mini-review – immunologic aspects of pneumoconiosis. Exp Lung Res 1991;17:661–85.

109. Beckett W, Abraham J, Becklake M, et al. Adverse effects of crystalline silica exposure. Amer J Respir Crit Care Med 1997;155:761–8.

110. Powell DEB, Gough J. Br J Exp Pathol 1959;40:40–3.

111. Kato T, Usami I, Morita H, et al. Chronic necrotizing pulmonary aspergillosis in pneumoconiosis – clinical and radiologic findings in 10 patients. Chest 2002;121:118–27.

112. International Agency for Research on Cancer (Lyons). Silica and some silicates. Monographs on the evaluation of the carcinogenic risk of chemicals to humans 1987;42.

113. Weill H, McDonald JC. Occupational lung disease: 1. exposure to crystalline silica and risk of lung cancer: the epidemiological evidence. Thorax 1996;51:97–102.

114. Craighead JE. Do silica and asbestos cause lung cancer? Arch Pathol Lab Med 1992;116:16–20.

115. Department of Social Security. Lung cancer in relation to occupational exposure to silica. Report by the Industrial Injuries Advisory Council in accordance with Section 171 of the Social Security Administration Act 1992 on the question whether lung cancer in relation to occupational exposure to silica should be prescribed. London: HMSO; 1992. p. 1–5.

116. Checkoway H, Hughes JM, Weill H, et al. Crystalline silica exposure, radiological silicosis, and lung cancer mortality in diatomaceous earth industry workers. Thorax 1999;54:56–9.

117. Buechner HA, Ansari A. Acute silico-proteinosis. Dis Chest 1969;55:274–84.

118. Xipell JM, Ham KN, Price CG, et al. Acute silicolipoproteinosis. Thorax 1977;32:104–11.

119. Heppleston AG. Atypical reaction to inhaled silica. Nature 1967;213:199.

120. Gross P, De Treville RTP. Alveolar proteinosis. Its experimental production in rodents. Arch Pathol 1968;86:255–61.

121. Corrin B, King E. Experimental endogenous lipid pneumonia and silicosis. J Pathol 1969;97:325–30.

122. Corrin B, King E. Pathogenesis of experimental pulmonary alveolar proteinosis. J Pathol 1970;25:230–6.

123. Heppleston AG, Fletcher K, Wyatt I. Changes in the composition of lung lipids and the 'turnover' of dipalmitoyl lecithin in experimental alveolar lipo-proteinosis induced by inhaled quartz. Br J Exp Pathol 1974;55:384–95.

124. Miller RR, Churg AM, Hutcheon M, et al. Case report: pulmonary alveolar proteinosis and aluminum dust exposure. Am Rev Respir Dis 1984;130:312–5.

125. Miller BE, Bakewell WE, Katyal SL, et al. Induction of surfactant protein (SP-A) biosynthesis and SP-A mRNA in activated type II cells during acute silicosis in rats. Am J Respir Cell Mol Biol 1990;3:217–26.

126. Hauglustaine D, Van Damme B, Daenens P, et al. Silicon nephropathy: a possible occupational hazard. Nephron 1980;26:219–24.

127. Bolton WK, Suratt PM, Strugill BC. Rapidly progressive silicon nephropathy. Am J Med 1981;71:823–8.

128. Osorio AM, Thun MJ, Novak RF, et al. Silica and glomerulonephritis: case report and review of the literature. Am J Kidney Dis 1987;9:224–30.

129. Sherson D, Jorgensen F. Rapidly progressive crescenteric glomerulonephritis in a sandblaster with silicosis. Br J Ind Med 1989;46:675–6.

130. Dutra FR. Diatomaceous earth pneumoconiosis. Arch Env Health 1965;11:613–9.

Silicates

131. Abraham JL, Brambilla C. Particle size for differentiation between inhalation and injection pulmonary talcosis. Environ Res 1980;21:94–6.

132. Lapenas DJ, Gale PN. Kaolin pneumoconiosis. A case report. Arch Pathol Lab Med 1983;107:650–3.

133. Lapenas D, Gale P, Kennedy T, et al. Kaolin pneumoconiosis. Radiologic, pathologic and mineralogic findings. Am Rev Respir Dis 1984;130:282–8.

134. Phibbs BP, Sundin RE, Mitchell RS. Silicosis in Wyoming bentonite workers. Am Rev Respir Dis 1971;103:1–17.

135. Sakula A. Pneumoconiosis due to Fuller's earth. Thorax 1961;16:176–9.

136. Wells IP, Dubbins PA, Whimster WF. Pulmonary disease caused by the inhalation of cosmetic talcum powder. Br J Radiol 1979;52:586–8.

137. Berner A, Gylseth B, Levy F. Talc dust pneumoconiosis. Acta Path Microbiol Scand 1981;89:17–21.

138. Landas SK, Schwartz DA. Mica-associated pulmonary interstitial fibrosis. Am Rev Respir Dis 1991;144:718–21.

Inert dusts

139. Doig AT. Baritosis: a benign pneumoconiosis. Thorax 1976;31:30–9.

140. Seaton A, Ruckley VA, Addison J, et al. Silicosis in barium miners. Thorax 1986;41:591–5.

141. Watson AJ, Black J, Doig AT, et al. Pneumoconiosis in carbon electrode makers. Br J Ind Med 1959;16:274.

142. Miller AA, Ramsden F. Carbon pneumoconiosis. Br J Ind Med 1961;18:103–13.

143. Gaensler EA, Cadigan JB, Sasahara AA, et al. Graphite pneumoconiosis of electrotypers. Am J Med 1966;41:864–82.

144. Diaz JV, Koff J, Gotway MB, et al. Case report: a case of wood-smoke-related pulmonary disease. Environ Health Perspect 2006;114:759–62.

145. Gold JA, Jagirdar J, Hay JG, et al. Hut lung. A domestically acquired particulate lung disease. Medicine (Baltimore) 2000;79:310–7.

146. Chung MP, Kim H, Rhee CH, et al. Bronchial stenosis due to anthracofibrosis. Chest 1998;113:344–50.

147. Naccache JM, Monnet I, Nunes H, et al. Anthracofibrosis attributed to mixed mineral dust exposure: report of three cases. Thorax 2008;63:655–7.

148. Wynn GJ, Turkington PM, O'Driscoll BR. Anthracofibrosis, bronchial stenosis with overlying anthracotic mucosa: possibly a new occupational lung disorder. Chest 2008;134:1069–73.

149. Naccache JM, Monnet I, Guillon F, et al. Occupational anthracofibrosis. Chest 2009;135:1694.

150. Wynn GJ, Turkington PM, O'Driscoll BR. Response. Chest 2009;135:1694–5.

151. McLaughlin AIG, Harding HE. Pneumoconiosis and other causes of death in iron and steel foundry workers. Arch Ind Health 1956;14:350–78.

152. Highman B. Histochemical study of certain iron ore dusts. Bull Internat Assoc Med museums 1951;32:97–9.

Mixed-dust pneumoconiosis

153. Honma K, Abraham JL, Chiyotani K, et al. Proposed criteria for mixed-dust pneumoconiosis: definition, descriptions, and guidelines for pathologic diagnosis and clinical correlation. Hum Pathol 2004;35:1515–23.

154. Arakawa H, Johkoh T, Honma K, et al. Chronic interstitial pneumonia in silicosis and mix-dust pneumoconiosis: its prevalence and comparison of CT findings with idiopathic pulmonary fibrosis. Chest 2007;131:1870–6.

155. Honma K, Abraham JL, Chiyotani K, et al. Proposed criteria for mixed-dust pneumoconiosis: Definition, descriptions, and guidelines for pathologic diagnosis and clinical correlation. Human Pathology 2004;35:1515–23.

Coal pneumoconiosis

156. Green FHY, Laqueur WA. Coal workers' pneumoconiosis. Pathol Annu 1980;15:333–410.

157. Stratton TML. Edin Med Surg J 1838;49:490.

158. Gough J. Pneumoconiosis in coal trimmers. J Pathol Bacteriol 1940;51:277–85.

159. Douglas AN, Robertson A, Chapman JS, et al. Dust exposure, dust recovered from the lung, and associated pathology in a group of British coalminers. Br J Ind Med 1986;43:795–801.

160. Davis JMG. The relationship between the mass and composition of coal mine dust and the development of pneumoconiosis. In: Rom WN, Archer VE, editors. Health Implication of New Energy Technologies. Ann Arbor: Butterworth; 1980. p. 283–92.

161. McConnochie K, Green FHY, Vallyathan V, et al. Interstitial fibrosis in coal miners – experience in Wales and West Virginia. Ann Occup Hyg 1988;32:553–60.

162. Remy-Jardin M, Degreef JM, Beuscart R, et al. Coal worker's pneumoconiosis: CT assessment in exposed workers and correlation with radiographic findings. Radiology 1990;177:363–71.

163. Davis JMG, Chapman J, Collings P, et al. Variations in the histological patterns of the lesions of coal workers' pneumoconiosis in Britain and their relationship to lung dust content. Am Rev Respir Dis 1983;128:118–24.

164. Ruckley VA, Fernie JM, Chapman JS, et al. Comparison of radiographic appearances with associated pathology and lung dust content in a group of coalworkers. Br J Ind Med 1984;41:459–67.

165. Churg A, Wright JL, Wiggs B, et al. Small airways disease and mineral dust exposure. Prevalence, structure and function. Am Rev Respir Dis 1985;131:139–43.

166. Morgan WKC. Coal mining, emphysema, and compensation revisited. Br J Ind Med 1993;50:1051–2.

167. Seaton A. Coal mining, emphysema, and compensation revisited – reply. Br J Ind Med 1993;50:1052–3.

168. Coggon D, Taylor AN. Coal mining and chronic obstructive pulmonary disease: a review of the evidence. Thorax 1998;53:398–407.

169. Heppleston AG. The pathogenesis of simple pneumokoniosis in coal workers. J Path Bact 1954;67:51–63.

170. Li K, Keeling B, Churg A. Mineral dusts cause elastin and collagen breakdown in the rat lung: a potential mechanism of dust-induced emphysema. Am J Respir Crit Care Med 1996;153:644–9.

171. Ryder R, Lyons JP, Campbell H, et al. Emphysema in coal workers' pneumoconiosis. BMJ 1970;3:481–7.

172. Lyons JP, Ryder R, Campbell H, et al. Pulmonary disability in coal workers' pneumoconiosis. BMJ 1972;i:713–6.

173. Leigh J, Outhred KG, McKenzie HI, et al. Quantified pathology of emphysema, pneumoconiosis, and chronic bronchitis in coal workers. Br J Ind Med 1983;40:258–63.

174. Ruckley VA, Gauld SJ, Chapman JS, et al. Emphysema and dust exposure in a group of coal workers. Am Rev Respir Dis 1984;129:528–32.

175. Nemery B. Coal worker's lung: not only black, but also full of holes. Am J Respir Crit Care Med 2009;180:199–200.

176. Kuempel ED, Wheeler MW, Smith RJ, et al. Contributions of dust exposure and cigarette smoking to emphysema severity in coal miners in the United States. Am J Respir Crit Care Med 2009;180:257–64.

177. Department of Social Security. Chronic bronchitis and emphysema. Report by the Industrial Injuries Advisory Council in accordance with Section 171 of the Social Security Administration Act 1992 on the question whether bronchitis and emphysema in coal miners and metal production workers should be prescribed. London: HMSO; 1992. p. 1.

178. Seaton A. The new prescription: industrial injuries benefits for smokers? Thorax 1998;53:335–6.

179. Hurley JF, Alexander WP, Hazledine DJ, et al. Exposure to respirable coalmine dust and incidence of progressive massive fibrosis. Br J Ind Med 1987;44:661–72.

180. Cochrane AL. The attack rate of progressive massive fibrosis. Br J Ind Med 1962;19:52–64.

181. Theodos PA, Cathcart RT, Fraimow W. Ischemic necrosis in anthracosilicosis. Arch Env Health 1961;2:609–19.

182. Wagner JC, Wusterman FS, Edwards JH, et al. The composition of massive lesions in coal miners. Thorax 1975;30:382–8.

183. Vanhee D, Gosset P, Wallaert B, et al. Mechanisms of fibrosis in coal workers' pneumoconiosis: increased production of platelet-derived growth factor, insulin-like growth factor type I, and transforming growth factor beta and relationship to disease severity. Am J Respir Crit Care Med 1994;150:1049–55.

184. Vanhee D, Gosset P, Marquette CH, et al. Secretion and mRNA expression of TNF alpha and IL-6 in the lungs of pneumoconiosis patients. Am J Respir Crit Care Med 1995;152:298–306.

185. Caplan A, Payne RB, Withey JL. A broader concept of Caplan's syndrome related to rheumatoid factors. Thorax 1962;17:205–12.

186. Ball J. Differential agglutination test in rheumatoid arthritis complicated by pneumoconiosis. Ann Rheum Dis 1955;14:159–61.

187. Soutar CA, Turner-Warwick M, Parkes WR. Circulating antinuclear antibody and rheumatoid factor in coal pneumoconiosis. BMJ 1974;3:145–52.

188. Pearson DJ, Mentnech MS, Elliott JA, et al. Serologic changes in pneumoconiosis and progressive massive fibrosis of coal workers. Am Rev Respir Dis 1981;124:696–9.

189. Wagner JC, McCormick JN. Immunological investigations of coalworkers' disease. J R Coll Physicians Lond 1967;2:49–56.

190. Caplan A. Certain unusual radiological appearances in the chest of coal-miners suffering from rheumatoid arthritis. Thorax 1953;8:29–37.

191. Gough J, Rivers D, Seal RME. Pathological studies of modified pneumoconiosis in coal-miners with rheumatoid arthritis (Caplan's syndrome). Thorax 1955;10:9–18.

Asbestosis

192. Asbestos, asbestosis, and cancer: the Helsinki criteria for diagnosis and attribution. Scand J Work Environ Health 1997;23:311–6.

193. Roggli VL, Gibbs AR, Attanoos R, et al. Pathology of asbestosis: an update of the diagnostic criteria. Report of the Asbestosis Committee of the College of American Pathologists and Pulmonary Pathology Society. Arch Pathol Lab Med 2010;134:462–80.

194. LaDou J. The asbestos cancer epidemic. Environ Health Perspect 2004;112:285–90.

195. Churg A, Wright JL, Gilks B, et al. Rapid short-term clearance of chrysotile compared with amosite asbestos in the guinea pig. Am Rev Respir Dis 1989;139:885–90.

196. Churg A, Wright JL. Persistence of natural mineral fibers in human lungs: an overview. Environ Health Perspect 1994;102:229–33.

197. Wagner JC, Pooley FD, Berry G, et al. A pathological and mineralogical study of asbestos-related deaths in the United Kingdom in 1977. Ann Occup Hyg 1982;26:423–31.

198. Wagner JC, Moncrieff CB, Coles R, et al. Correlation between fibre content of the lungs and disease in naval dockyard workers. Br J Ind Med 1986;43:391–5.

199. Wagner JC, Newhouse ML, Corrin B, et al. Correlation between fibre content of the lung and disease in east London asbestos factory workers. Br J Ind Med 1988;45:305–8.

200. Wagner JC, Berry G, Skidmore JW, et al. The effects of the inhalation of asbestos in rats. Br J Cancer 1974;29:252–69.

201. Davis JMG, Beckett ST, Bolton RE, et al. Mass and number of fibres in the pathogenesis of asbestos related lung disease in rats. Br J Cancer 1978;37:673–88.

202. Churg A, Wright JL, Vedal S. Fiber burden and patterns of asbestos-related disease in chrysotile miners and millers. Am Rev Respir Dis 1993;148:25–31.

203. Wagner JC, Berry G, Pooley FD. Carcinogenesis and mineral fibres. Br Med Bull 1980;36:53–6.

204. Emri S, Demir A, Dogan M, et al. Lung diseases due to environmental exposures to erionite and asbestos in Turkey. Toxicol Lett 2002;127:251–7.

205. Baris YI, Grandjean P. Prospective study of mesothelioma mortality in Turkish villages with exposure to fibrous zeolite. J Natl Cancer Inst 2006;98:414–7.

206. Dodson RF, O'Sullivan M, Corn CJ, et al. Analysis of ferruginous bodies in bronchoalveolar lavage from foundry workers. Br J Ind Med 1993;50:1032–8.

207. Warnock ML. Analysis of the cores of ferruginous (asbestos) bodies from the general population. Lab Invest 1979;40:622–6.

208. Churg A. Fiber counting and analysis in the diagnosis of asbestos-related disease. Hum Pathol 1982;13:381–92.

209. Morgan A, Holmes A. Concentrations and dimensions of coated and uncoated asbestos fibres in the human lung. Br J Ind Med 1980;37:25–32.

210. Pooley FD, Ranson DL. Comparison of the results of asbestos fibre dust counts in lung tissue obtained by analytical electron microscopy and light microscopy. J Clin Pathol 1986;39:313–7.

211. Holden J, Churg A. Asbestos bodies and the diagnosis of asbestosis in chrysotile workers. Environ Res 1986;39:232–6.

212. Johansson LG, Albin MP, Jakobsson KM, et al. Ferruginous bodies and pulmonary fibrosis in dead low to moderately exposed asbestos cement workers: histological examination. Br J Ind Med 1987;44:550–8.

212a. Schneider F, Sporn TA, Roggli VL. Asbestos fiber content of lungs with diffuse interstitial fibrosis: an analytical scanning electron microscopic analysis of 249 cases. Archives of Pathology & Laboratory Medicine 2010;134:457–61.

213. McLemore TL, Roggli V, Marshall MV, et al. Comparison of phagocytosis of uncoated versus coated asbestos fibers by cultured human pulmonary alveolar macrophages. Chest 1981;80:39S-42S.

214. Roggli VL, Pratt PC. Numbers of asbestos bodies on iron-stained tissue sections in relation to asbestos body counts in lung tissue digests. Hum Pathol 1983;14:355–61.

215. Roggli VL, Pratt PC, Brody AR. Asbestos content of lung tissue in asbestos associated diseases: a study of 110 cases. Br J Ind Med 1986;43:18–28.

216. Gibbs AR, Pooley FD. Analysis and interpretation of inorganic mineral particles in 'lung' tissues. Thorax 1996;51:327–34.

217. Karjalainen A, Piipari R, Mantyla T, et al. Asbestos bodies in bronchoalveolar lavage in relation to asbestos bodies and asbestos fibres in lung parenchyma. Eur Respir J 1996;9:1000–5.

218. Paris C, GalateauSalle F, Creveuil C, et al. Asbestos bodies in the sputum of asbestos workers: correlation with occupational exposure. Eur Resp J 2002;20:1167–73.

219. Ashcroft T, Heppleston AG. The optical and electron microscopic determination of pulmonary asbestos fibre concentration and its relation to human pathology reaction. J Clin Pathol 1973;26:224–34.

220. Davis JMG, Glyseth B, Morgan A. Assessment of mineral fibres from human lung tissue. Thorax 1986;41:167–75.

221. James KR, Bull TB, Fox B. Detection of asbestos fibres by dark ground microscopy. J Clin Pathol 1987;40:1259–60.

222. Churg A. Analysis of lung asbestos content. Br J Ind Med 1991;48:649–52.

223. De Vuyst P, Karjalainen A, Dumortier P, et al. Guidelines for mineral fibre analyses in biological samples: report of the ERS Working Group. Eur Resp J 1998;11:1416–26.

224. Whitwell F, Scott J, Grimshaw M. Relationship between occupations and asbestos-fibre content of the lungs in patients with pleural mesothelioma, lung cancer, and other diseases. Thorax 1977;32:377–86.

225. Donaldson K, Brown GM, Brown DM, et al. Inflammation-generating potential of long and short-fibre amosite asbestos samples. Br J Ind Med 1989;46:271–6.

226. Donaldson K, Li XY, Dogra S, et al. Asbestos-stimulated tumour necrosis factor release from alveolar macrophages depends on fibre length and opsonization. J Pathol 1992;168:243–8.

227. Davis JMG, Addison J, Bolton RE, et al. The pathogenicity of long versus short fibre amosite asbestos administered to rats by inhalation and intra-peritoneal injection. Br J Exp Pathol 1986;67:415–30.

228. Donaldson K, Golyasnya N. Cytogenetic and pathogenic effects of long and short amosite asbestos. J Pathol 1995;177:303–7.

229. Green FHY, Harley R, Vallyathan V, et al. Exposure and mineralogical correlates of pulmonary fibrosis in chrysotile asbestos workers. Occup Environ Medicine 1997;54:549–59.

230. Pooley FD, Clark NJ. Quantitative assessment of inorganic fibrous particulates in dust samples with an analytical transmission electron microscope. Ann Occup Hyg 1979;22:253–71.

231. Gibbs AR, Stephens M, Griffiths DM, et al. Fibre distribution in the lungs and pleura of subjects with asbestos related diffuse pleural fibrosis. Br J Ind Med 1991;48:762–70.

232. Dawson A, Gibbs AR, Pooley FD, et al. Malignant mesothelioma in women. Thorax 1993;48:269–74.

233. Churg A, Wood P. Observations on the distribution of asbestos fibres in human lungs. Environ Res 1983;31:374–80.

234. Gylseth B, Churg A, Davis JMG, et al. Analysis of asbestos fibres and asbestos bodies in tissue samples from human lung: an international interlaboratory trial. Scand J Work Environ Health 1985;11:107–10.

235. Morgan A, Holmes A. Distribution and characteristics of amphibole asbestos fibres in the left lung of an insulation worker measured with the light microscope. Br J Ind Med 1983;40:45–50.

236. Pooley FD. The identification of asbestos dust with an electron microprobe analyser. Ann Occup Hyg 1975;13:181–6.

237. Doll R. Symposium on man-made mineral fibres, Copenhagen, October 1986: overview and conclusions. Ann Occup Hyg 1987;31:805–20.

238. Coutts II, Gilson JC, Kerr IH, et al. Mortality in cases of asbestosis diagnosed by a pneumoconiosis medical panel. Thorax 1987;42:111–6.

239. Churg A, Wright JL. Small-airway lesions in patients exposed to nonasbestos mineral dusts. Hum Pathol 1983;14:688–93.

240. Churg A, Wright JL. Small airways disease and mineral dust exposure. Pathol Annu 1983;18:233–51.

241. Auerbach O, Garfinkel L, Hammond EC. Relation of smoking and age to findings in lung parenchyma: a microscopic study. Chest 1974;65:29–35.

242. Corrin B, Price AB. Electron microscopic studies in desquamative interstitial pneumonia associated with asbestos. Thorax 1972;27:324–31.

243. Freed JA, Miller A, Gordon RE, et al. Desquamative interstitial pneumonia associated with chrysotile asbestos fibres. Br J Ind Med 1991;48:332–7.

244. Hammar SP, Hallman KO. Localized inflammatory pulmonary disease in subjects occupationally exposed to asbestos. Chest 1993;103:1792–9.

245. Hinson KFW, Otto H, Webster I, et al. Criteria for the diagnosis and grading of asbestosis. In: Bogovski P, Gilson JC, Timbrell V, et al, editors. Biological Effects of Asbestos IARC Lyon Scientific publications no8. Oxford: Pergamon; 1973. p. 54–7.

246. Craighead JE, Abraham JL, Churg A, et al. The pathology of asbestos-associated diseases of the lung and pleural cavities: diagnostic criteria and proposed grading schema. Report of the Pneumoconiosis Committee of the College of American Pathologists and the National Institute for Occupational Safety and Health. Arch Pathol Lab Med 1982;106:544–96.

247. Kuhn C, Kuo TT. Cytoplasmic hyalin in asbestosis. Arch Pathol 1973;95:190–4.

248. Warnock ML, Press M, Churg A. Further observations on cytoplasmic hyaline in the lung. Hum Pathol 1980;11:59–65.

249. Franks TJ, Chong PY, Chui P, et al. Lung pathology of severe acute respiratory

syndrome (SARS): A study of 8 autopsy cases from Singapore. Hum Pathol 2003;34:743–8.

250. Nicholls JM, Poon LL, Lee KC, et al. Lung pathology of fatal severe acute respiratory syndrome. Lancet 2003;361:1773–8.

251. Yamada T, Uehara K, Kawanishi R, et al. Immunohistochemical detection of ubiquitin-positive intracytoplasmic eosinophilic inclusion bodies in diffuse alveolar damage. Histopathology 2006;48:846–54.

252. Gaensler EA, Jederlinic PJ, Churg A. Idiopathic pulmonary fibrosis in asbestos-exposed workers. Am Rev Respir Dis 1991;144:689–96.

253. Berry G. Mortality of workers certified by pneumoconiosis medical panels as having asbestosis. Br J Ind Med 1981;38:130–7.

254. Jones RN, Diem JE, Ziskand MM, et al. Radiographic evidence of asbestos effects in American marine engineers. J Occup Med 1984;26:281–4.

255. Thurlbeck WM. Morphology of emphysema and emphysema-like conditions. In: Thurlbeck WM, editor. Chronic airflow obstruction in lung disease. Philadelphia: Saunders; 1976. p. 98–9.

256. Corrin B, Dewar A, Rodriguez-Roisin R, et al. Fine structural changes in cryptogenic fibrosing alveolitis and asbestosis. J Pathol 1985;147:107–19.

257. Gadek J, Hunninghake G, Schoenberger C, et al. Pulmonary asbestosis and idiopathic pulmonary fibrosis: pathogenetic parallels. Chest 1981;80:63S–4S.

258. Adamson IYR, Bowden DH. Crocidolite-induced pulmonary fibrosis in mice. Cytokinetic and biochemical studies. Am J Pathol 1986;122:261–7.

259. Schapira RM, Ghio AJ, Effros RM, et al. Hydroxyl radicals are formed in the rat lung after asbestos instillation invivo. Am J Respir Cell Mol Biol 1994;10:573–9.

260. Thomas G, Ando T, Verma K, et al. Asbestos fibers and interferon-gamma up-regulate nitric oxide production in rat alveolar macrophages. Am J Respir Cell Mol Biol 1994;11:707–15.

261. Kinnula VL. Oxidant sand antioxidant mechanisms of lung disease caused by asbestos fibres. Eur Resp J 1999;14:706–16.

262. Turner-Warwick M, Haslam P. Antibodies in some chronic fibrosing lung diseases. Clin Allergy 1971;1:83–95.

263. Janssen YMW, Driscoll KE, Howard B, et al. Asbestos causes translocation of p65 protein and increases NF-kappa B DNA binding activity in rat lung epithelial and pleural mesothelial cells. Am J Pathol 1997;151:389–401.

264. Liu JY, Morris GF, Lei WH, et al. Rapid activation of PDGF-A and -B expression at sites of lung injury in asbestos-exposed rats. Am J Respir Cell Molec Biol 1997;17:129–40.

265. Lasky JA, Tonthat BH, Liu JY, et al. Upregulation of the PDGF-alpha receptor precedes asbestos-induced lung fibrosis in rats. Amer J Respir Crit Care Med 1998;157:1652–7.

266. Liu JY, Brass DM, Hoyle GW, et al. TNF-alpha receptor knockout mice are protected from the fibroproliferative effects of inhaled asbestos fibers. Am J Pathol 1998;153:1839–47.

267. Tsuda A, Stringer BK, Miljailovich SM, et al. Alveolar cell stretching in the presence of fibrous particles induces interleukin-8 responses. Am J Respir Cell Molec Biol 1999;21:455–62.

268. Kamp DW, Weitzman SA. The molecular basis of asbestos induced lung injury. Thorax 1999;54:638–52.

269. Warheit DB, George G, Hill LH, et al. Inhaled asbestos activates a complement-dependent chemoattractant for macrophages. Lab Invest 1985;52:505–14.

270. Lemaire I, Beaudoin H, Masse S, et al. Alveolar macrophage stimulation of lung fibroblast growth in asbestos-induced pulmonary fibrosis. Am J Pathol 1986;122:205–11.

271. Rom WN, Travis WD, Brody AR. Cellular and molecular basis of the asbestos-related diseases. Am Rev Respir Dis 1991;143:408–22.

272. Liu JY, Morris GF, Lei WH, et al. Up-regulated expression of transforming growth factor-α in the bronchiolar-alveolar duct regions of asbestos-exposed rats. Am J Pathol 1996;149:205–17.

273. Bateman ED, Emerson RJ, Cole PJ. A study of macrophage-mediated initiation of fibrosis by asbestos and silica using a diffusion chamber technique. Br J Exp Pathol 1982;63:414–25.

274. Vallyathan V, Mega JF, Shi XL, et al. Enhanced generation of free radicals from phagocytes induced by mineral dusts. Am J Respir Cell Mol Biol 1992;6:404–13.

275. Doll R. Mortality from lung cancer in asbestos workers. Br J Ind Med 1955;12:81–6.

276. Wagner JC, Sleggs CA, Marchand P. Diffuse pleural mesotheliomas and asbestos exposure in Northwestern Cape Province. Br J Ind Med 1960;17:260–71.

277. Selikoff IJ, Hammond EC, Churg J. Carcinogenicity of amosite asbestos. Arch Env Health 1972;25:183–6.

278. Hammond EC, Selikoff IJ, Seidman H. Asbestos exposure, cigarette smoking and death rates. Ann N Y Acad Sci 1979;330:473–90.

279. de Klerk NH, Musk AW, Armstrong BK, et al. Smoking, exposure to crocidolite, and the incidence of lung cancer and asbestosis. Br J Ind Med 1991;48:412–7.

280. Kannerstein M, Churg J. Pathology of carcinoma of the lung associated with asbestos exposure. Cancer 1972;30:14–21.

281. Whitwell F, Newhouse ML, Bennett DR. A study of the histological cell types of lung cancer in workers suffering from asbestosis in the United Kingdom. Br J Ind Med 1974;31:298–303.

282. Churg A. Lung cancer cell type and asbestos exposure. JAMA 1985;253:2984–5.

283. Johansson L, Albin M, Jakobsson K, et al. Histological type of lung carcinoma in asbestos cement workers and matched controls. Br J Ind Med 1992;49:626.

284. Raffn E, Lynge E, Korsgaard B. Incidence of lung cancer by histological type among asbestos cement workers in Denmark. Br J Ind Med 1993;50:85–9.

285. Raffn E, Villadsen E, Engholm G, et al. Lung cancer in asbestos cement workers in Denmark. Occup Environ Med 1996;53:399–402.

286. De Vos Irvine H, Lamont DW, Hole DJ, et al. Asbestos and lung cancer in Glasgow and the west of Scotland. BMJ 1993;306:1503–6.

287. de Klerk NH, Musk AW, Eccles JL, et al. Exposure to crocidolite and the incidence of different histological types of lung cancer. Occup Environ Med 1996;53:157–9.

288. Rudd R. Asbestos and lung cancer. Thorax 1997;52:306.

289. Henderson DW, de Klerk NH, Hammar SP, et al. Asbestos and lung cancer: is it attributable to asbestosis or to asbestos fibre burden? In: Corrin B, editor. Pathology of Lung Tumours. London: Churchill Livingstone; 1997. p. 83–118.

290. Pohlabeln H, Wild P, Schill W, et al. Asbestos fibreyears and lung cancer: a two phase case-control study with expert exposure assessment. Occup Environ Med 2002;59:410–4.

291. Hodgson JT, Darnton A. The quantitative risks of mesothelioma and lung cancer in relation to asbestos exposure. Ann Occup Hyg 2000;44:565–601.

292. Browne K. Is asbestos or asbestosis the cause of the increased risk of lung cancer in asbestos workers? Br J Ind Med 1986;43:145–9.

293. Sluis-Cremer GK, Bezuidenhout BN. Relation between asbestosis and bronchial cancer in amphibole asbestos miners. Br J Ind Med 1989;46:537–40.

294. Hughes JM, Weill H. Asbestosis as a precursor of asbestos related lung cancer – results of a prospective mortality study. Br J Ind Med 1991;48:229–33.

295. Jones RN, Hughes JM, Weill H. Asbestos exposure, asbestosis, and asbestos-attributable lung cancer. Thorax 1996;51:S9–S15.

296. Jones RN. Asbestos and lung cancer – Reply. Thorax 1997;52:306.

297. Cagle PT. Criteria for attributing lung cancer to asbestos exposure. Am J Clin Pathol 2002;117:9–15.

298. Weiss W. Asbestosis: A marker for the increased risk of lung cancer among workers exposed to asbestos. Chest 1999;115:536–49.

299. Hessel PA, Gamble JF, McDonald JC. Asbestos, asbestosis, and lung cancer: a critical assessment of the epidemiological evidence. Thorax 2005;60:433–6.

300. Begin R, Cantin A, Berthiaume Y, et al. Airway function in lifetime-nonsmoking older asbestos workers. Am J Med 1983;75:631–8.

301. Wright JL, Churg A. Severe diffuse small airways abnormalities in long term chrysotile asbestos miners. Br J Ind Med 1985;42:556.

302. Wright JL, Churg A. Morphology of small-airway lesions in patients with asbestos exposure. Hum Pathol 1984;15:68–74.

Aluminium

303. Abramson MJ, Wlodarczyk JH, Saunders NA, et al. Does aluminum smelting cause lung disease? Am Rev Respir Dis 1989;139:1042–57.

304. Crombie DW, Blaischell JL, MacPherson G. The treatment of silicosis by aluminum powder. Can Med Assoc J 1944;50:318–28.

305. Duchange L, Brichet A, Lamblin C, et al. Silicose aigue. Caractéristiques cliniques, radiologiques, fonctionnelles et cytologiques du liquide broncho-alveolaire. A propos de 6 observations. Rev Mal Resp 1998;15:527–34.

306. Goralewski G, Jaeger R. Zur Klinik, Pathologie and Pathogenesis der Aluminiumlunge. Arch Gewerbepath Hyg 1941;11:102–5.

307. Goralewski G. Die Aluminiumlunge – eine neue Gewerbeerkrankung. Z f d ges Inn Med 1947;2:665–73.

308. Mitchell J, Manning GB, Molyneux M, et al. Pulmonary fibrosis in workers exposed to finely powdered aluminium. Br J Ind Med 1961;18:10–20.

309. Corrin B. Aluminium pneumoconiosis I. in vitro comparison of stamped aluminium powders containing different lubricating agents and a granular aluminium powder. Br J Ind Med 1963;20:264–7.

310. Corrin B. Aluminium pneumoconiosis II. Effect on the rat lung of intratracheal injections of stamped aluminium powders containing different lubricating agents and of a granular aluminium powder. Br J Ind Med 1963;20:268–76.

311. Herbert A, Sterling G, Abraham J, et al. Desquamative interstitial pneumonia in an aluminum welder. Hum Pathol 1982;13:694–9.

312. Vuyst P, Dumortier P, Schandene L, et al. Sarcoidlike lung granulomatosis induced by aluminum dusts. Am Rev Respir Dis 1987;135:493–7.

313. Chen W-J, Monnat RJ, Chen M, et al. Aluminum induced pulmonary granulomatosis. Hum Pathol 1978;9:705–11.

314. Hull MJ, Abraham JL. Aluminum welding fume-induced pneumoconiosis. Hum Pathol 2002;33:819–25.

Rare earth (cerium) pneumoconiosis

315. McDonald JW, Ghio AJ, Sheehan CE, et al. Rare earth (cerium oxide) pneumoconiosis: analytical scanning electron microscopy and literature review. Mod Pathol 1995;8:859–65.

Hard metal disease (cobalt lung)

316. Davison AG, Haslam PL, Corrin B, et al. Interstitial lung disease and asthma in hard-metal workers: bronchoalveolar lavage, ultrastructural, and analytical findings and results of bronchial provocation tests. Thorax 1983;38:119–28.

317. Schepers GWH. The biological action of tungsten carbide and cobalt: studies on experimental pulmonary histopathology. Arch Ind Health 1955;12:140–6.

318. Demedts M, Gheysens B, Nagels J, et al. Cobalt lung in diamond polishers. Am Rev Respir Dis 1984;130:130–5.

319. Nemery B, Nagels J, Verbeken E, et al. Rapidly fatal progression of cobalt lung in a diamond polisher. Am Rev Respir Dis 1990;141:1373–8.

320. Rolfe MW, Paine R, Davenport RB, et al. Hard metal pneumoconiosis and the association of tumor necrosis factor-alpha. Am Rev Respir Dis 1992;146:1600–2.

Berylliosis

321. Kriebel D, Brain JD, Sprince NL, et al. The pulmonary toxicity of beryllium. Am Rev Respir Dis 1988;137:464–73.

322. Meyer KC. Beryllium and lung disease. Chest 1994;106:942–6.

323. Maier LA, Martyny JW, Liang J, et al. Recent chronic beryllium disease in residents surrounding a beryllium facility. Am J Respir Crit Care Med 2008;177:1012–7.

324. Newman LS, Kreiss K. Nonoccupational beryllium disease masquerading as sarcoidosis – identification by blood lymphocyte proliferative response to beryllium. Am Rev Respir Dis 1992;145:1212–4.

325. Williams WJ. Beryllium disease. Postgrad Med J 1988;64:511–6.

326. International Agency for Research on Cancer. An evaluation of carcinogenic risk to humans. Overall evaluation of carcinogenicity: an updating of IARC monographs vols 1–42. Supplement 7. Lyons: IARC; 1987.

327. Weber HH, Englehardt WE. Uber eine Apparatur zur Erzeugung niedriger Staubkonzentrationen von grosser Konstanz und eine Methode zur mikrogravinctrischen Staubbestemmung. Anwendung bei der Untersuchung von Stauben aus der Beryllliumsgewinnung. Zentbl GewHyg Unfallerhut 1933;10:41–7.

328. Hardy HL, Tabershaw IR. Delayed chenical pneumonitis occurring in workers exposed to beryllium compounds. J Ind Hyg Toxicol 1946;28:197–211.

329. Kotloff RM, Richman PS, Greenacre JK, et al. Chronic beryllium disease in a dental laboratory technician. Am Rev Respir Dis 1993;147:205–7.

330. Saltini C, Winestock K, Kirby M, et al. Maintenance of alveolitis in patients with chronic beryllium disease by beryllium-specific helper T cells. N Engl J Med 1989;320:1103–9.

331. Richeldi L, Sorrentino R, Saltini C. HLA-DPB1 glutamate 69: a genetic marker of beryllium disease. Science 1993;262:242–8.

332. Saltini C, Amicosante M, Franchi A, et al. Immunogenetic basis of environmental lung disease: lessons from the beryllliosis model. Eur Resp J 1998;12:1463–75.

333. McConnochie K, Williams WR, Kilpatrick GS, et al. Beryllium disease in identical twins. Br J Dis Chest 1988;82:431–5.

334. Butnor KJ, Sporn TA, Ingram P, et al. Beryllium detection in human lung tissue using electron probe X-ray microanalysis. Mod Pathol 2003;16:1171–7.

335. Jones Williams W. Diagnostic criteria for chronic beryllium disease (CBD) based on the UK Registry 1945–1991. Sarcoidosis 1993;10:41–3.

336. Jones Williams W. United Kingdom beryllium registry: mortality and autopsy study. Environ Health Perspect 1996;104:949–51.

337. Alberts WM. Lung disease and the lightest of metals. Chest 2004;126:1730–2.

338. Fireman E, Haimsky E, Noiderfer M, et al. Misdiagnosis of sarcoidosis in patients with chronic beryllium disease. Sarcoidosis Vasc Diffuse Lung Dis 2003;20:144–8.

339. Muller-Quernheim J, Gaede KI, Fireman E, et al. Diagnoses of chronic beryllium disease within cohorts of sarcoidosis patients. Eur Respir J 2006;27:1190–5.

Polyvinyl chloride pneumoconiosis

340. Arnaud A, Pommier de Santi P, Garbe L, et al. Polyvinyl chloride pneumoconiosis. Thorax 1978;33:19–25.

341. White NW, Ehrlich RI. Regression of polyvinylchloride polymer pneumoconiosis. Thorax 1997;52:748–9.

342. Studnicka MJ, Menzinger G, Drlicek M, et al. Pneumoconiosis and systemic sclerosis following 10 years of exposure to polyvinyl chloride dust. Thorax 1995;50:583–5.

Flock workers' lung

343. Eschenbacher WL, Kreiss K, Lougheed MD, et al. Nylon flock-associated interstitial

lung disease. Am J Respir Crit Care Med 1999;159:2003–8.

344. Boag AH, Colby TV, Fraire AE, et al. The pathology of interstitial lung disease in nylon flock workers. Am J Surg Pathol 1999;23:1539–45.

345. Kern DG, Kuhn C, Ely EW, et al. Flock worker's lung: broadening the spectrum of clinicopathology, narrowing the spectrum of suspected etiologies [see comments]. Chest 2000;117:251–9.

346. Barroso E, Ibanez MD, Aranda FI, et al. Polyethylene flock-associated interstitial lung disease in a Spanish female. Eur Resp J 2002;20:1610–2.

Popcorn workers' lung

347. Kreiss K, Gomaa A, Kullman G, et al. Clinical bronchiolitis obliterans in workers at a microwave-popcorn plant. N Engl J Med 2002;347:330–8.

348. Kreiss K, Gomaa A, Kullman G, et al. Clinical bronchiolitis obliterans in workers at a microwave-popcorn plant. N Engl J Med 2002;347:330–8.

349. Akpinar-Elci M, Travis WD, Lynch DA, et al. Bronchiolitis obliterans syndrome in popcorn production plant workers. Eur Respir J 2004;24:298–302.

350. Hendrick DJ. 'Popcorn worker's lung' in Britain in a man making potato crisp flavouring. Thorax 2008;63:267–8.

Paint spraying

351. Sanz P, Prat A. Toxicity in textile air-brushing in Spain. Lancet 1993;342:240.

352. Moya C, Anto JM, Taylor AJN, et al. Outbreak of organising pneumonia in textile printing sprayers. Lancet 1994;344:498–502.

353. Sole A, Cordero PJ, Morales P, et al. Epidemic outbreak of interstitial lung disease in aerographics textile workers – the 'Ardystil syndrome': a first year follow up. Thorax 1996;51:94–5.

354. Romero S, Hernandez L, Gil J, et al. Organizing pneumonia in textile printing workers: a clinical description. Eur Resp J 1998;11:265–71.

355. Kadi OF, Mohammed-Brahim B, Fyad A, et al. Outbreak of pulmonary disease in textile dye sprayers in Algeria. Lancet 1994;344:962–3.

356. Kadi FO, Abdesslam T, Nemery B. Five-year follow-up of Algerian victims of the "Ardystil syndrome". Eur Respir J 1999;13:940–1.

Mineral oils and petroleum

357. Skorodin MS, Chandrasekhar AJ. An occupational cause of exogenous lipoid pneumonia. Arch Pathol Lab Med 1983;107:610–1.

358. Bernstein DI, Lummus ZL, Santilli G, et al. Machine operator's lung. A hypersensitivity pneumonitis disorder associated with exposure to metalworking fluid aerosols. Chest 1995;108:636–41.

359. Kreiss K, Cox-Ganser J. Metalworking fluid-associated hypersensitivity pneumonitis: a workshop summary. Am J Ind Med 1997;32:423–32.

360. Bracker A, Storey E, Yang C, et al. An outbreak of hypersensitivity pneumonitis at a metalworking plant: a longitudinal assessment of intervention effectiveness. Appl Occup Environ Hyg 2003;18: 96–108.

361. Brander PE, Taskinen E, Stenius-Aarniala B. Fire-eater's lung. Eur Respir J 1992;5:112–4.

362. Gentina T, Tillie-Leblond I, Birolleau S, et al. Fire-eater's lung: seventeen cases and a review of the literature. Medicine (Baltimore) 2001;80:291–7.

363. Scharf SM, Prinsloo I. Pulmonary mechanics in dogs given different doses of kerosene intratracheally. Am Rev Resp Dis 1982;126:695–700.

Welding

364. Doig MB, McLaughlin ALG. X-ray appearance of the lungs of electric arc welders. Lancet 1936;i:771–5.

365. McMillan GH. The health of welders in naval dockyards: the risk of asbestos-related diseases occurring in welders. J Soc Occup Med 1983;25:727–30.

366. Funahashi A, Schlueter DP, Pintar K, et al. Welders' pneumoconiosis: tissue elemental microanalysis by energy dispersive X ray analysis. Br J Ind Med 1988;45:14–8.

367. Sferlazza SJ, Beckett WS. The respiratory health of welders. Am Rev Respir Dis 1991;143:1134–48.

Toxic fumes and gases

368. Nemery B. Metal toxicity and the respiratory tract. Eur Respir J 1990;3:202–19.

369. Shaver CG, Riddell AR. Lung changes associated with the manufacture of alumina abrasives. Am J Med Sci 1947;29:145–57.

370. Asano S, Eto K, Kurisaki E, et al. Acute inorganic mercury vapor inhalation poisoning. Pathol Int 2000;50:169–74.

371. Sunderman FW, Kincaid JF. Nickel poisoning II. Studies on patients suffering from acute exposure to vapors of nickel carbonyl. JAMA 1954;155:889–94.

372. Lowry T, Schuman LM. Silo-filler's disease – a syndrome caused by nitrogen dioxide. JAMA 1956;162:153.

373. Ramirez RJ, Dowell AR. Silo-filler's disease: nitrogen dioxide-induced lung injury. Ann Intern Med 1971;74:569–76.

374. Douglas WW, Hepper NGG, Colby TV. Silo filler's disease. Mayo Clin Proc 1989;64:291–304.

375. Zwemer FL, Pratt DS, May JJ. Silo-filler's disease in New York state. Am Rev Respir Dis 1992;146:650–3.

376. Osbern L, Crapo R. Dung lung: a report of toxic exposure to liquid manure. Ann Intern Med 1981;95:312–4.

377. Morse DL, Woodbury MA, Rentmeester K, et al. Death caused by fermenting manure. JAMA 1981;245:63–4.

378. Donham KJ, Knapp LW, Monson R, et al. Acute toxic exposure to gases from liquid manure. J Occup Med 1982;24:142–5.

379. Fahy JV, Walley T, Gibney RTN, et al. 'Slurry lung': a report of three cases. Thorax 1991;46:394–5.

380. Plopper CG, Dungworth DL, Tyler WS. Pulmonary lesions in rats exposed to ozone. Am J Pathol 1973;71:375–94.

381. Pratt PC. Pathology of adult respiratory distress syndrome. In: Thurlbeck WM, Abell MR, editors. The Lung. Baltimore: Williams and Wilkins; 1978. p. 43–57.

382. Harkema JR, Plopper CG, Hyde DM, et al. Response of macaque bronchiolar epithelium to ambient concentrations of ozone. Am J Pathol 1993;143: 857–66.

383. Bils RF. Ultrastructural alterations of alveolar tissue of mice. Arch Env Health 1970;20:468–80.

384. Pinkerton KE, Dodge DE, Cederdahl-Demmler J, et al. Differentiated bronchiolar epithelium in alveolar ducts of rats exposed to ozone for 20 months. Am J Pathol 1993;142:947–56.

385. Hyde DM, Hubbard WC, Wong V, et al. Ozone-induced acute tracheobronchial epithelial injury – relationship to granulocyte emigration in the lung. Am J Respir Cell Mol Biol 1992;6:481–97.

386. Aris RM, Christian D, Hearne PQ, et al. Ozone-induced airway inflammation in human subjects as determined by airway lavage and biopsy. Am Rev Respir Dis 1993;148:1363–72.

387. Gardner MJ, Pannett B, Winter PD, et al. A cohort study of workers exposed to formaldehyde in the British chemical industry – an update. Br J Ind Med 1993;50:827–34.

388. Snyder RW, Mishel HS, Christensen GC. Pulmonary toxicity following exposure to methylene chloride and its combustion product, phosgene. Chest 1992;102: 1921.

389. Emad A, Rezaian GR. The diversity of the effects of sulfur mustard gas inhalation on respiratory system 10 years after a single, heavy exposure: analysis of 197 cases. Chest 1997;112:734–8.

390. Ghanei M, Moqadam FA, Mohammad MM, et al. Tracheobronchomalacia and air trapping after mustard gas exposure. Am J Respir Crit Care Med 2006;173:304–9.

391. Ghanei M, Tazelaar HD, Chilosi M, et al. An International collaborative pathologic study of surgical lung biopsies from mustard gas-exposed patients. Respiratory Medicine 2008;102:825–30.

392. Konichezky S, Schattner A, Ezri T, et al. Thionyl-chloride-induced lung injury and bronchiolitis obliterans. Chest 1993;104:971–3.

392a. Burnett WW, King EG, Grace M, Hall WF. Hydrogen sulfide poisoning: review of 5 years' experience. Can Med Assoc J 1977;117:1277–80.

Anoxic asphyxia

393. James PB, Calder IM. Anoxic asphyxia – a cause of industrial fatalities: a review. J R Soc Med 1991;84:493.

Occupational asthma

394. Ross DJ, Sallie BA, McDonald JC. SWORD '94: surveillance of work-related and occupational respiratory disease in the UK. Occup Med 1995;45:175–8.

395. Hnizdo E, Esterhuizen TM, Rees D, et al. Occupational asthma as identified by the Surveillance of Work-related and Occupational Respiratory Diseases programme in South Africa. Clin Exp Allergy 2001;31:32–9.

396. Karjalainen A, Kurppa K, Virtanen S, et al. Incidence of occupational asthma by occupation and industry in Finland. Am J Ind Med 2000;37:451–8.

397. Sallie BA, Ross DJ, Meredith SK, et al. SWORD '93: surveillance of work-related and occupational respiratory disease in the UK. Occup Med 1994;44:177–82.

398. Balmes J, Becklake M, Blanc P, et al. American Thoracic Society Statement: Occupational contribution to the burden of airway disease. Am J Respir Crit Care Med 2003;167:787–97.

399. Chanyeung M, Malo JL. Aetiological agents in occupational asthma. Eur Respir J 1994;7:346–71.

400. McDonald JC, Keynes HL, Meredith SK. Reported incidence of occupational asthma in the United Kingdom, 1989–97. Occup Environ Med 2000;57:823–9.

401. Burge PS, Finnegan M, Horsefield N, et al. Occupational asthma in a factory with a contaminated humidifier. Thorax 1985;40:248–54.

402. Rooke GB. The pathology of byssinosis. Chest 1981;79:67S-71S.

403. Niven RM, Pickering CAC. Byssinosis: a review. Thorax 1996;51:632–7.

404. Mundie TG, Boackle RJ, Ainsworth SK. In vitro alternative and classical activation of complement by extracts of cotton mill dust: a possible mechanism in the pathogenesis of byssinosis. Environ Res 1983;32:47–56.

405. Kutz SA, Olenchok SA, Elliot JA, et al. Antibody independent complement activation by card-room cotton dust. Environ Res 1979;19:405–14.

406. Edwards C, Macartney J, Rooke G, et al. The pathology of the lung in byssinotics. Thorax 1975;30:612–23.

Occupational fevers

407. Raskandersen A, Pratt DS. Inhalation fever – a proposed unifying term for febrile reactions to inhalation of noxious substances. Br J Ind Med 1992;49:40.

408. MRC Symposium. Humidifier fever. Thorax 1977;32:653–63.

409. Emanuel DA, Wenzel FJ, Lawton BR. Pulmonary mycotoxicosis. Chest 1975;67:293–7.

410. May JJ, Stallones L, Darrow D, et al. Organic dust toxicity (pulmonary mycotoxicosis) associated with silo unloading. Thorax 1986;41:919–23.

411. Lougheed MD, Roos JO, Waddell WR, et al. Desquamative interstitial pneumonitis and diffuse alveolar damage in textile workers: potential role of mycotoxins. Chest 1995;108:1196–200.

412. Perry LP, Iwata M, Tazelaar HD, et al. Pulmonary mycotoxicosis: A clinicopathologic study of three cases. Modern Pathol 1998;11:432–6.

413. Vogelmeier C, Konig G, Bencze K, et al. Pulmonary involvement in zinc fume fever. Chest 1987;92:946–8.

414. Blanc PD, Boushey HA, Wong H, et al. Cytokines in metal fume fever. Am Rev Respir Dis 1993;147:134–8.

Chapter | 7 |

7.2 Environmental lung disease

ENVIRONMENTAL IRRADIATION

Environmental irradiation chiefly affects the skin but in some parts of the world rocks near the surface release significant amounts of radon gas. This carcinogen is liable to accumulate in buildings and be inhaled, so subjecting the occupants to an increased risk of lung cancer. The installation of underfloor ventilation is therefore advocated in such areas. This subject is explored more fully on page 533.

ATMOSPHERIC PRESSURE CHANGES

The body is vulnerable to both increases and decreases in pressure and it is the lungs that often bear the brunt of the damage. Increased pressure may result in blast injury or crushing of the chest while decreased pressure may result in the lungs literally bursting or dissolved gases being released within the blood (caisson disease), or the vascular alterations that underlie mountain sickness developing. Some of these pressure changes entail a risk of pneumothorax and it is essential that this is properly investigated postmortem by the chest being opened under a water seal. Loud music has been incriminated as a specific form of air pressure change causing pneumothorax and metereologists have shown that 'spontaneous' pneumothoraces tend to occur in clusters associated with natural drops in atmospheric pressure.[1,2]

Blast injury

Explosions may cause injury by the body being violently thrown against a less moveable object, by objects being thrown against the body or by the blast wave hitting the body. These mechanisms often act together but sometimes there is only blast injury, to which the lungs are particularly vulnerable. For a time it was considered that the damage was direct, the blast wave travelling down the airways to injure the lungs. However, at the start of the Second World War, experiments conducted in the UK showed that the lungs were injured indirectly, the blast wave being transmitted to them through the chest wall: pulmonary blast injury is worst on the side of the body towards the explosion, and can be reduced by protective clothing.[3] Underwater explosions are particularly dangerous because water is incompressible. There may be severe internal injury but no external evidence of damage other than a trickle of blood from the mouth or nose. This is because the injury is rate-dependent. Quite small thoracic deformation may produce severe pulmonary damage if peak compression is attained very quickly, typically in less than 5 ms. Conversely, severe chest wall distortion may produce only minor pulmonary contusion if this time is extended beyond 20 ms.[4]

At necropsy, the lungs are contused, with blood evident in the airways and parenchyma. Depending on the force of the blast, the haemorrhage may be pinpoint, patchy or confluent. It tends to follow the lines of the ribs and may be accompanied by pleuropulmonary lacerations having the same distribution. In this case there will also be haemothorax, pneumothorax and possibly air embolism. Patchy pulmonary haemorrhages cuff the blood vessels.[5,6] In patients who survive for a few days, the lungs resemble the liver macroscopically and histologically show chronic interstitial inflammation and fibrosis as well as haemorrhage.[7] Other injuries are often present and fat embolism, aspiration pneumonia, fluid overload and infection may all be added to the effects of the blast wave.

Chest squeeze

'Chest squeeze' is another form of barotrauma caused by high pressure but here the body is compressed rather than subject to a sudden wave of pressure as in blast injury. It is experienced by divers who descend very deeply, thereby subjecting their bodies to such high pressure that their chest walls are literally crushed, so that their ribs break and their lungs are severely compressed. More common mishaps experienced by divers include drowning and decompression sickness, both of which are dealt with below, and neurological syndromes such as nitrogen narcosis, which will not be considered further.[8]

Burst lung

'Burst lung' is the most acute form of decompression sickness.[9] It is experienced by divers and submariners making rapid ascents from depth and by aviators who ascend too rapidly in unpressurised aeroplanes, experience failure of a plane's pressure system or have to eject at high altitudes. Injury to the lung is caused by trapped alveolar gas expanding so rapidly that it exceeds total lung capacity before it can escape through the trachea. The lungs literally burst: the alveolar walls rupture and blood mixes directly with alveolar air. The victim experiences chest pain and there may be blood-stained froth at the mouth or frank haemoptysis. Air may enter the alveolar walls to cause interstitial emphysema or air embolism. Asthmatics may be at particular risk because of regional air-trapping.[10]. Diving mammals such as porpoises and whales are protected from such dangers of peripheral air-trapping by cartilage extending far out into the finest conductive airways so that these passages never close, even at the end of full expiration (Fig. 7.2.1).[11,12]

Patients requiring positive-pressure artificial respiration are also at risk of burst lung, but the complications of the resultant interstitial emphysema differ from those experienced by divers. In divers, the chest wall is buttressed by the surrounding water and air in the interstitium is liable to track towards the hilum of the lungs and enter pulmonary veins, with resultant cerebral and coronary air embolism, either of which may prove fatal.[13] Iatrogenic burst lung, on the other hand, takes place in patients whose chest wall is not so buttressed, and then outward rupture of the interstitial air is more likely, resulting in pneumothorax. Extension of the interstitial emphysema to the mediastinum, neck and chest wall is also more likely in such patients, resulting in surgical emphysema at these sites. However, there are exceptional cases marked by both cerebral embolism and extensive air tracking.[14]

Figure 7.2.1 Sea lion lung. The smallest airways of deep-diving mammals such as the sea lion are buttressed by cartilage to ensure that all air is evacuated from the lungs when the animal is at depth to prevent the lungs bursting on rapid ascent. In humans there are several generations of airways that lack cartilage (the bronchioles) and consequently close before exhalation is complete. The trapped gas (the residual volume) is normally of no consequence but it poses a danger that the lungs may burst or of decompression sickness if ascent is rapid, whether in the sea or by air. *(Courtesy of Professor D Denison, Brompton, UK.)*

Decompression sickness (caisson disease)

The same circumstances that lead to burst lung may also cause decompression sickness, which is also known as caisson disease.[9] In this condition there is a sudden release of nitrogen gas that has gone into solution in the lipids of adipose tissue and of myelinated nervous tissue at the higher pressure: the released nitrogen gains access to the blood stream in which it forms bubbles.[15] Doppler ultrasound techniques show that this is quite customary when divers ascend from depth,[16] but the lungs generally provide an effective filter so that there are no untoward systemic effects, although there may be sudden chest pain on deep inspiration ('the chokes'). Gradual decompression permits the nitrogen to diffuse across the alveolar membranes and be exhaled. If, however, substantial amounts of nitrogen are released from solution, sufficient pulmonary arteries may be blocked to cause pulmonary hypertension, with resultant opening of arteriovenous communications or a patent foramen ovale, so permitting the gas to enter the systemic circulation. This is often followed by limb pains ('the bends') and perhaps cerebral symptoms ('the staggers'). Fatal cases are characterised by gas bubbles within blood vessels throughout the body and froth in the heart chambers. Delayed effects include ischaemic necrosis of bones and other tissues.[17]

Deep-diving mammals are protected by the same mechanism that prevents them suffering from burst lung. They exhale before diving and during the dive the chest is compressed to the extent that virtually all the gas in the lungs passes into the cartilage-buttressed non-respiratory airways (see Fig. 7.2.1), resulting in very little to be absorbed by the blood. The pulmonary collapse also serves to reduce buoyancy. The distribution of the little gas that is absorbed is minimised by bradycardia.[18] Many viscera experience anaerobic respiration but hypoxia is minimised in the heart and musculature by high levels of haemoglobin and myoglobin. The brain is further protected by the supplying arteries drawing on oxygen stored in an unusual sponge-like cervical organ known as the rete mirabilis.

Mountain sickness

Mountain sickness is due to reduced atmospheric pressure brought about more slowly than that responsible for decompression sickness[19,20] It may be acute or chronic.

Acute mountain sickness

Acute mountain sickness is likely to be experienced by anyone who ascends above 3000–4000 m without a period of acclimatisation at intermediate levels. Symptoms are as liable to occur in people born at high altitude who return after a few weeks spent at sea level as in those who go to the mountains for the first time: acclimatisation is obviously short-lived and is therefore necessary whenever an ascent is to be made. The ill-effects are commonly precipitated by exercise. In the susceptible, acute mountain sickness commonly appears within 3 days of ascent.

The basis of acute mountain sickness is tissue hypoxia. It results in deteriorating intellectual and psychological function, headache, nausea, vomiting, and more rarely pulmonary and cerebral oedema. High-altitude pulmonary oedema is characterised by increasing dyspnoea, cyanosis and a dry cough, and later the production of copious, frothy sputum, which sometimes becomes blood-stained.[21] The pulmonary artery pressure is markedly raised but wedge pressures are normal, indicating that the left side of the heart is unaffected and that pulmonary venous constriction is unlikely to be an important contributory factor.

The pulmonary oedema fluid has a high protein content[22] and the condition has been characterised as a non-cardiogenic high-permeability oedema associated with excessive pulmonary hypertension.[23,24] Hypoxia is a well-known cause of pulmonary arteriolar constriction but in acute mountain sickness the vascular response appears to be exaggerated for the pulmonary artery pressure is considerably higher than is usual for the altitude. An association with certain HLA complexes (HLA-DR6 and HLA-DQ4) suggests that this has a genetic basis.[25] Although arteriolar constriction only tends to protect the pulmonary capillaries, it could explain the oedema if the process was patchy – as is the resultant oedema – for patchy arteriolar constriction would subject the rest of the lung to abnormally high pressures and lead to capillary stress failure in these areas (see pp. 402 and 448).[26,27] Measurements of capillary pressure suggest that this is indeed the case.[28] Furthermore, vasodilators such as calcium channel blocking agents and inhaled nitric oxide gas[23,29,30] have been used with success to counter acute mountain sickness, supporting the idea that hypoxic vasoconstriction plays a central role.

Autopsy shows the lungs to be heavy and firm. The cut surface weeps oedema fluid, which is often blood-stained, but a striking feature is the patchy distribution of the changes. Areas of haemorrhagic oedema alternate with others that contain clear oedema fluid and others that are normal apart from overinflation. Pulmonary arterial thrombi are commonly found. Microscopy confirms the presence of haemorrhagic oedema and may show neutrophils and hyaline membranes in the alveoli. The alveolar capillaries are congested and may contain thrombi. There may also be an increase in mast cells and rarely pulmonary infarction. The right ventricle is commonly dilated whereas the left ventricle is normal. Highlanders generally show right ventricular hypertrophy and increased muscle in their pulmonary arteriesm, changes that are not apparent in lowlanders.[31,32]

Chronic mountain sickness

Prolonged residence at high altitude leads to hypoxic pulmonary hypertension (see p. 424), an increase in red cell mass and cor pulmonale. Livestock taken from lowland plains to high-altitude pastures suffer similarly but the natural stock of the Himalayas and Ethiopian highlands are apparently immune. So too are other species long established at high altitude such as the llama and yak. These species are said to have adapted to their climate, that is, the forces of natural selection have bred out the pulmonary vasoconstrictive response to hypoxia. Cattle of European origin and humans acclimatise to high altitude by processes such as increasing their red cell mass but generally they are not adapted like native species and suffer hypoxic pulmonary hypertension at altitudes in excess of 3000 m. Certain Himalayan highlanders may be an exception to this in that their small pulmonary arteries are reported not to show the muscularisation that characterises hypoxic pulmonary hypertension.[33]

In cattle of European origin, the dependent oedema of right-sided cardiac failure caused by hypoxic pulmonary hypertension affects the breast (brisket) particularly and in the Rocky Mountains of North America such cattle are said to have 'brisket disease'.[34] A human counterpart of this has been described in children of Chinese ancestry who have been taken to reside in Tibet and who have developed a fatal form of subacute infantile mountain sickness.[35]

A small minority of permanent residents in the Andes develop the changes of chronic mountain sickness to a marked degree and are said to suffer from Monge's disease.[36] The basis of this is alveolar hypoventilation, which leads to a progressive fall in systemic arterial oxygen saturation and elevation of haemoglobin concentration to an unusually severe degree. The latter averages about 25 g/dl, which exceeds even the 20 g/dl found in healthy high-altitude residents. Patients with Monge's disease are so deeply cyanosed that their lips are virtually black. Their pulmonary artery resistance is also markedly raised. The cause of the alveolar hypoventilation is uncertain but the only cases of Monge's disease that have come to necropsy had conditions such as kyphoscoliosis that predispose to alveolar hypoxia.

DROWNING

Drowning is defined as suffocation by submersion, and usually occurs in water. It is the commonest cause of accidental death among divers but 96% of drowning accidents do not involve deep descents. Falling into quite shallow water is a particularly common cause of drowning in young children. In adults, men outnumber women by 4 to 1. More die in fresh water than the sea, not because it is more hazardous to the lungs than sea water, but because unguarded inland waters and swimming pools are visited more frequently. Alcohol consumption contributes to many deaths by drowning.

Drowning is not simply a matter of being unable to keep one's head above water. This may be merely a secondary event. For example, the entry dive may result in underwater head injury, or the exertion of swimming may precipitate a heart attack. Furthermore, the struggling swimmer going down for the third time ('drowning not waving') is the exception: most drowning is characterised by the swimmer failing to surface or quietly dropping beneath the surface without anyone noticing.

Swimming underwater can be extremely hazardous if it is preceded by hyperventilation, a danger that needs to be more widely appreciated. Hyperventilation results in undue loss of carbon dioxide so that instead of hypercapnia forcing the swimmer to surface to breathe, progress under water may be continued until hypoxia causes sudden loss of consciousness.

Panic contributes to many swimming accidents and is often precipitated by the inadvertent aspiration of just a little water. Most people are naturally buoyant, but only slightly so. With the lungs fully expanded the average adult has a positive buoyancy of about 2.5 kg, which is sufficient to keep the head out of the water if the rest of the body is submerged. If an arm (weight about 3 kg) is raised to wave for help, the head will go down. If the swimmer shouts, exhalation reduces buoyancy to neutral at normal end-expiration and to negative at residual volume. Buoyancy cannot be regained when the head is submerged and unless able to swim to the surface, the person will continue to sink.

Autopsy generally shows that the lungs are full of water, but some victims die of 'dry drowning' due to laryngospasm. Events may also be modified by the temperature of the water. Sudden immersion in cold water may result in tachycardia, hypertension and hyperventilation, making it difficult for the victim to keep the airways free of water. It may also result in sudden death due to ventricular fibrillation. Even a good swimmer loses consciousness within an hour of immersion in very cold water. Drowning is then inevitable unless a correctly fitted life jacket is worn, in which case there is a danger of death from hypothermia. However, as in open heart surgery, cold prolongs the interval before there is irreversible brain damage.

If the person is rescued, water in the lungs is quickly absorbed, even if it is saline, and therefore hyperosmolar:aspirated sea water is quickly equilibrated by pure water joining it from the blood but the alveolar epithelial barrier remains impermeable to protein and once osmotic equilibrium is reached, all is quickly reabsorbed.[37-39] Fresh water is absorbed even more quickly. It is unnecessary to tip the patient to hasten this process. Any water recovered in this way comes from the stomach and time that should be devoted to mouth-to-mouth breathing and cardiac massage is lost. These resuscitative efforts may need to be prolonged as fresh water in particular inactivates alveolar surfactant, leading to alveolar collapse which persists until the surfactant is replenished. Very few victims who are resuscitated on site fail to survive, and very few who cannot be resuscitated on site recover later.

Interchange of fluid between the blood and air spaces may cause major fluctuations in plasma volume with consequent changes in ionic concentrations and haemolysis. Hypervolaemia may cause circulatory problems but hyperkalaemia consequent upon the haemolysis is not thought to be as important as was formerly believed: ventricular fibrillation following submersion is more likely to be a complication of hypothermia than of electrolyte imbalance.

Circulatory collapse may ensue shortly after rescue. This is due to loss of the circulatory support provided by the pressure the water exerts on the body, which results in a considerable increase in cardiac output while the body is immersed. On leaving the water the loss of this support results in a tendency to venous pooling. Although this is countered by baroreceptor responses, these are reduced by prolonged immersion in cold water. Circulatory collapse is believed to be the cause of death in many persons who perish within minutes of rescue. To counter this effect, patients should be lifted out of the water in the prone position.

It can be seen that, in fatal cases, the pathologist is faced with several possibilities. Thus, death may have been due to:

- natural causes before the body entered the water
- unnatural causes before entry, the body merely being disposed of in the water
- natural causes in the water
- injuries received in the water from impact with rocks, a boat or a ship's propeller, or in tropical waters from predators such as a crocodile or a shark (any of which may also be incurred after death, as may disfigurement by fish and rats)

- 'dry drowning'
- true drowning
- hypothermia
- circulatory failure after rescue.

True drowning is indicated by froth in the airways and heavy water-filled lungs. Both fresh and salt water contain numerous microscopic algae known as diatoms and those representative of the water in which the drowning occurred are found in the lungs. Unless death occurred before submersion, diatoms are also found in other viscera because these tiny life forms easily enter the circulation. Thus, the presence of diatoms in digests of organs such as the kidneys, liver, brain and bone marrow suggests that death was due to drowning. Because they have a siliceous capsule, diatoms are resistant to putrefaction as well as digestion and can be identified in the body long after death. However, a positive test is not always accepted as proof of drowning and a negative test does not exclude drowning.

INHALED TOXIC AGENTS

The various physical forms in which respirable environmental agents may be encountered are defined in Table 7.2.1. Some effects of inhalant lung injury are recognised as distinct disease entities and are dealt with elsewhere: for example, the pneumoconioses on page 327, extrinsic allergic alveolitis on page 279, chronic bronchitis on page 98 and lung cancer on page 532. Other respirable agents, such as lead fume and carbon monoxide gas, exert their harmful effects elsewhere in the body and will not be considered further. This section is concerned with toxic substances that may be inhaled by the general public. Those that are more likely to be encountered in the workplace or in war zones are considered on page 355.

The lungs have a rather stereotyped pattern of response to inhaled toxins, displaying degenerative changes and inflammation of varying degree, the former sometimes amounting to necrosis. In general, the site of maximal absorption or injury is related to solubility (for gases and vapours) and particle size (for aerosols such as dusts, fog, fumes, mists, smog and smoke): the less water-soluble and the smaller the particle size, the further down the respiratory tract the agent will penetrate (Fig. 7.2.2 and Table 7.2.2).[40-42] Thus, ammonia produces intense congestion of the upper respiratory passages and laryngeal oedema whereas phosgene has little effect on these sites but causes pulmonary oedema.[40]

Air pollution[43-47]

The toxic (as opposed to allergenic) air pollutants thought to pose the greatest threat to the lungs comprise smoke particles, sulphur dioxide, oxides of nitrogen, various aldehydes and ozone. Smoke and sulphur dioxide derive particularly from the combustion of fossil fuels in domestic fires and power stations, nitrogen dioxide is an important car exhaust and domestic gas appliance pollutant and ozone is the principal photochemical product of smog. Aldehydes such as formaldehyde and acrylic aldehyde (acrolein) also contribute to general air pollution because they are released in the combustion of diesel oil and petrol. Collectively, these pollutants have been incriminated in the exacerbation (rather than causation) of asthma. They also predispose to respiratory infection and result in airway inflammation and hypersecretion.[48,49] Their effect on children is of particular concern because development of the lungs is known to continue well into childhood and damage to the lungs before their growth is complete

Table 7.2.1	Definitions of respirable agents by physical form
Gas	A formless compressible fluid in which all molecules of the agent move freely at room temperature (25°C) and standard pressure (760 mmHg) to fill the space available
Vapour	Gaseous state of an agent which is normally liquid or solid at room temperature and standard pressure
Aerosol	Dispersion of solid or liquid particles of microscopic size in a gaseous medium. The following are all examples:
Dust	Dispersion of solid particles. Those of respirable size are not readily seen with the naked eye unless they are bathed in bright light
Fog	Dispersion of liquid particles generated by condensation from the vapour state
Fume	Dispersion of solid particles generated by condensation from the vapour state
Mist	Dispersion of liquid particles generated by condensation or mechanical means (e.g. nebulisation). The droplets are generally larger than those of a fog and may be visible individually to the naked eye
Smog	Mixture of smoke and fog, the former being the result of industrial pollution, the latter of natural climatic factors
Smoke	Dispersion of small particles (usually less than 0.1 μm diameter) resulting from incomplete combustion of organic substances

Gas	Henry's constant at 37°C	Major site of absorption or toxicity
Ammonia	0.0011	Upper respiratory tract
Sulphur dioxide	0.05	Upper respiratory tract and trachea
Formaldehyde	0.56	Upper respiratory tract and trachea
Ozone	6.4	Tracheobronchial
Nitrogen dioxide	8.8	Tracheobronchial and pulmonary
Oxygen	42	Pulmonary
Nitrogen	77	Pulmonary

Table 7.2.2 Relation of solubility of an inhaled gas to its major site of absorption or toxicity[41]

Henry's constant: moles/l(air)/moles/l(water).

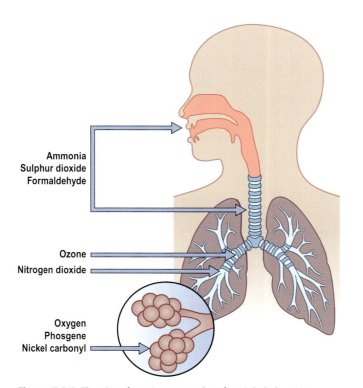

Ammonia
Sulphur dioxide
Formaldehyde

Ozone
Nitrogen dioxide

Oxygen
Phosgene
Nickel carbonyl

Figure 7.2.2 The site of maximum uptake of an inhaled gas is dependent upon its solubility. Thus, ammonia, sulphur dioxide and formaldehyde, which are highly soluble, have their major impact on the upper respiratory tract and trachea whereas oxygen, phosgene ($COCl_2$) and nickel carbonyl ($Ni(CO)_4$), which are less soluble, are taken up in the alveoli, where their toxicity is mainly experienced.

is likely to be irreparable. At the other extreme of life episodes of severe air pollution are known to hasten the deaths of many patients with chronic airway disease. Particularly high concentrations of the agents responsible for air pollution may be encountered in industry and their effects are therefore also considered in Chapter 7.1, on occupational diseases of the lung. Many of the polycyclic hydrocarbons found in polluted air are carcinogenic (see p. 532) and it is therefore not surprising that urban air pollution has been found to be associated with excess mortality from lung cancer.[50]

Domestic air pollution is rife in many of the poorer parts of the world due to the burning of biomass (wood, dried cow dung, bagasse, straw) in unventilated living rooms for heating and cooking. The women are particularly at risk of developing chronic bronchitis while their children have an increased incidence of acute respiratory infections.[51,52,52a]

Volcanic ash (tephra) irritates the eyes, skin and respiratory tract and in some eruptions may contain much free silica (e.g. Montserrat in 1995 and Mount St Helens, Washington state, USA in 1980) or be associated with the release of radon gas (e.g. the Azores in 1957).[53] The destruction of the World Trade Center in 2001 caused massive air pollution of New York city that had lasting respiratory effects on survivors, rescue workers and local residents.[54-56] At the time of the disaster there was much smoke from combustion of aeroplane fuel and flammable materials in the building while the collapse of the twin towers released dust from cement and dry-wall partitions that was highly alkaline.[57-59] This caused considerable irritation of the eyes and the conductive airways. A year later many victims were still suffering from bronchial hyperreactivity and poor ventilatory function, in a so-called reactive airways dysfunction syndrome[54,55] and there was continuing spirometric decline 5 years later.[60] The respirable portion of the dust formed only a small fraction of the whole but given the level of exposure its future effects cannot be discounted, particularly as it contained substances such as asbestos. Unusual effects attributed to the disaster include acute eosinophilic pneumonia and granulomatous pneumonitis.[61,62]

Allergenic air pollutants are dealt with in detail in the sections on asthma (see p. 109) and extrinsic allergic alveolitis (see p. 279). Allergenic air pollution is generally occupational or domestic but periodic widespread air pollution was responsible for the epidemics

Respiratory diseases caused by smoking

Carcinoma

Chronic obstructive lung disease

Chronic bronchitis

'Small-airways disease'

Emphysema

Respiratory bronchiolitis

Desquamative interstitial pneumonia

Respiratory diseases that are commoner or worse in smokers

Adult respiratory distress syndrome

Respiratory infections

Common cold

Influenza

Varicella pneumonia

Bacterial pneumonia

Tuberculosis

Pneumothorax

Cryptogenic fibrosing alveolitis

Langerhans cell histiocytosis

Asbestosis

Goodpasture's disease

Respiratory diseases that are less common or less severe in smokers

Extrinsic allergic alveolitis

Sarcoidosis

Quite advanced interstitial fibrosis has been reported in smokers with no clinical evidence of interstitial lung disease.[69b] Early changes detectable in smokers include chronic bronchiolitis, fibrosis of the bronchiolar wall and mild peribronchiolar interstitial fibrosis.[70,71] Even earlier changes are detectable at the molecular level: as many as 152 smoking-responsive genes that are significantly up-regulated or down-regulated have been identified in normal cigarette smokers.[72] There is marked individual variation, which may explain why many lifelong heavy smokers experience no respiratory problems.

Histological evidence that a patient smokes is provided by an increase in the number of alveolar macrophages and a characteristic brown discoloration of cytoplasm due to the phagocytosis of tar and other particulate matter derived from tobacco smoke (Fig. 7.2.3).

Cigarette smokers are at greater risk of lung disease than cigar and pipe smokers, probably because they inhale more deeply. They do this because cigarette smoke is more acid than cigar and pipe smoke and its nicotine content is therefore absorbed more easily through the lungs than the buccal mucosa. Smokers obviously put their own health at greatest risk but the lesser hazards of passive smoking are now well recognized (see p. 532). Passive smoking involves both the smoke exhaled by others and that coming from smouldering tobacco between puffs, the latter being known as sidestream smoke. The harmful effects of maternal smoking on the unborn child also come in this category. They include increased airway responsiveness and reduced lung function during the neonatal period and an increased risk of sudden infant death syndrome. Reduced numbers of alveolar attachments to the bronchioles have been demonstrated in such infants.[73] Smoking is also associated with disease of other organs (e.g. carcinoma of the oesophagus and bladder) but these are outwith the remit of this text.

Tobacco smoking by waterpipe (shisha, hubble-bubble) is enjoying a rise in popularity, both in its heartland, the Middle East, and western countries, and wherever it is practised it is widely perceived as being less dangerous than smoking cigarettes.[74] This is probably a misconception. What evidence there is suggests that water-pipe tobacco smoking is just as harmful as cigarette smoking, if not more so.[75]

of asthma seen in Barcelona in the 1980s, which were eventually traced to ships discharging cargoes of soya flour (see p. 114).

Tobacco smoke

Smoking-related diseases figure large throughout this book and in this section they are merely summarised collectively. Of the greatest importance, both in the number of patients they affect and in their clinical effects on the individual, are the various forms of chronic obstructive lung disease and lung cancer, but there are many other respiratory diseases associated with smoking, and a few that are less common in smokers (Box 7.2.1).[63] Not surprisingly, these diseases are often encountered in combination and sometimes one may obscure another. For example, a cigarette smoker may have emphysema in the upper lobes and idiopathic pulmonary fibrosis in the lower lobes.[64,65] Alternatively, Langerhans cell histiocytosis and desquamative interstitial pneumonia may affect the same parts of the lungs, in which case the focal lesions of the former may be masked by the latter condition.[63]

The term 'smoking-related interstitial lung disease' has been introduced to cover a spectrum of interstitial diseases related to smoking[63,66,67] as well as being used in a more restricted sense to describe a combination of air space enlargement and interstitial fibrosis predominantly affecting the lower lobes.[68,69,69a]

Burns and smoke inhalation

The lungs may be injured in burned patients in many ways (Box 7.2.2)[76,77] but an important consideration when a body is recovered from a fire is whether death was due to the fire or took place beforehand, the latter raising the possibility of foul play. A vital reaction to the skin burns and the presence of soot in the lower airways provide evidence that death occurred in the fire but an absence of soot from the airways may be due to death occurring rapidly, from asphyxia or poisoning by gases released in the conflagration. Soot is cleared rapidly and if the patient survives a few days an absence of soot from the airways is to be expected.[76]

Lung injury may result directly from heat and smoke inhalation or indirectly from the release of mediators associated with blast injury or shock. Although air temperature in a fire may reach very high temperatures thermal injury seldom extends beyond the carina but more extensive injury from heat alone was seen in men exposed to steam escaping from a fractured boiler pipe.[78] Those dying immediately showed coagulative necrosis of the respiratory mucosa down to the level of the alveolar ducts and alveolar congestion and oedema, while those surviving a little longer exhibited diffuse alveolar damage. The diffuse alveolar damage probably represented a manifestation of shock from their extensive cutaneous scalding whereas the mucosal necrosis is directly attributable to heat. Diffuse alveolar damage is

Figure 7.2.3 Macrophages of a heavy cigarette smoker. (A) Numerous brown macrophages fill the alveoli. Electron microscopy shows that the lysosomal dense bodies are increased in number and contain lipidic 'tar bodies' (B) or the needle-shaped crystals of kaolinite (C). *(Transmission electron micrographs, courtesy of Miss A Dewar, Brompton, UK.)*

usually part of systemic multiorgan failure in these patients, and is the leading cause of death in burns.[79]

The ubiquity of plastics today means that smoke contains numerous irritants, including isocyanates, aldehydes and fluorinated organic chemicals. Irritant smoke products have two principal effects. Firstly, they cause an immediate painful stimulation of the eyes and respiratory tract which at low concentrations may prevent escape and at high concentrations may cause laryngeal spasm and death. Secondly, they cause bronchopulmonary injury some hours after exposure. Burned patients dying within 4–12 days often show tracheobronchial necrosis and diffuse alveolar damage with prominent hyaline membranes.[76,77,80] Secondary herpesvirus infection is often present.[81,82]

The respiratory changes caused by heat and smoke are non-specific and careful consideration of the many causes of lung injury in burned patients listed in Box 7.2.2 and of the clinical circumstances and management is generally required. Often it will be concluded that the cause of the lung injury is multifactorial. Long-term consequences of smoke inhalation include bronchiectasis and obliterative bronchiolitis.[83]

Methyl isocyanate, the chemical released at Bhopal

The Bhopal catastrophe of 1984 was caused by the accidental release of 30 tons of methyl isocyanate gas ($CH_3–N=C=O$) from a pesticide plant.[84] Over 200 000 people were exposed, of whom 2500 died, mostly within hours of exposure, and 60 000 were seriously injured. The victims complained of intense ocular and respiratory irritation. Some survivors were left with persistent respiratory impairment, which was thought to be due to obliterative bronchiolitis.[85,86]

Methyl isocyanate is an extremely potent respiratory irritant, destroying the epithelium throughout the conducting airways, with comparatively less parenchymal injury. In survivors, epithelial regeneration, often involving squamous metaplasia, quickly commences, but not before endobronchial granulation tissue projections have developed, resulting in obliterative bronchiolitis.

Tear gas

Tear gases are chemical irritants delivered as an aerosol for the purpose of riot control. They react with mucocutaneous sensory nerve receptors causing intense irritation of the eyes, mucous membranes and skin. The respiratory effects are mainly concentrated on the upper tract so that there is violent sneezing, severe rhinorrhoea and cough but there may also be tracheobronchitis and rarely pulmonary oedema.[87] Patients with pre-existent asthma or chronic obstructive pulmonary disease are most severely affected while others may be left with reactive airways dysfunction.

INGESTED TOXIC AGENTS

Toxins reaching the lungs via the blood stream may be drugs, food contaminants, metabolites produced elsewhere in the body, or chemicals ingested intentionally or accidentally, either in the home or the workplace.

The lungs are selectively damaged by certain blood-borne toxins for a variety of reasons. For example, the herbicide paraquat is preferentially taken up by the lungs because of its molecular homology with certain endogenous substances. As detailed below, the type I alveolar epithelial cells are the cells that bear the brunt of the damage in paraquat poisoning. On the other hand, the alveolar capillary endothelium has its own selective uptake mechanisms (see Metabolic functions of the pulmonary endothelium, p. 23) which may be responsible for it being selectively damaged by other chemicals.

The bronchiolar Clara cells are selectively injured by some ingested chemicals because they are equipped to deal with inhaled xenobiotics, but occasionally this activity results in metabolites that are extremely toxic. An example of this from veterinary medicine is provided by the furan-derivative 4-ipomeanol, which is found in mouldy sweet potatoes and results in acute pulmonary oedema in cattle fed such a diet. When this chemical is injected into mice, the bronchioles are denuded of Clara cells whereas the intervening ciliated cells are completely unaffected. The selective damage to the bronchiolar Clara cells appears to stem from the oxidative efficiency of their P-450 cytochromes,[88] which is much higher than those of the liver. Chemicals having a similarly selective effect on bronchiolar Clara cells include 3-methylfuran, carbon tetrachloride, naphthalene and 1,1-dichloroethylene, the last of which is a volatile compound that is widely used in the plastics industry. Procarcinogens may be activated in the airways by similar mechanisms.

Paraquat

Paraquat is a dipyridylium compound that is widely used in agriculture as a herbicide. It kills all green plants but is inactivated on contact with the soil. It is applied as a spray and if the manufacturer's instructions are followed there is no danger to health. Most fatal cases of paraquat poisoning, both accidental and suicidal, have been due to ingestion of the 20% aqueous solution Gramoxone. The less concentrated granular form Weedol is unlikely to be ingested accidentally but may be taken suicidally.[89] Paraquat is not absorbed by the intact skin but repeated or prolonged application damages the epidermis so that absorption into the blood stream with consequent systemic effects is possible, but rare.[90]

Although paraquat has toxic effects on the liver, kidneys and myocardium, these are transient and attention has centred on the pulmonary changes, which are usually fatal. Following suicidal ingestion of large amounts of paraquat, death from multiorgan failure and pulmonary haemorrhage occurs within a few days, whereas most

Figure 7.2.4 Formulae of paraquat and the endogenous oligoamines putrescine, spermine and spermidine showing the molecular similarities. The name paraquat derives from the chemical's *para*-methyl groups and its *quat*ernary nitrogen atoms.

victims of accidental paraquat poisoning die from progressive pulmonary fibrosis between 10 and 14 days after ingestion. In those who survive longer, a honeycomb pattern of pulmonary fibrosis may be apparent.[91]

Paraquat is a powerful oxidant and owes its toxicity to the production of active oxygen radicals. The lungs are particularly susceptible because paraquat is concentrated there by an active uptake mechanism in the alveolar epithelium. The inadvertent uptake of paraquat probably stems from a similarity between the molecular arrangement of its quaternary nitrogen atoms and the amine groups of endogenous oligoamines such as putrescine, spermidine and spermine, which are concerned in alveolar epithelial cell division and differentiation (Fig. 7.2.4).[92] This results in paraquat levels being 6–10 times higher in the lung than in the plasma. Once taken up by the lung, paraquat is not metabolised but participates in redox cycling so that superoxide radicals are constantly produced. Epithelial injury is proportional to the concentration of paraquat, while it is lessened by hypoxia and antioxidants such as superoxide dismutase, and potentiated by increased concentrations of oxygen.[93-96] The high concentration of oxygen in the alveoli is a further reason why the lungs are particularly vulnerable to paraquat.

Knowledge of the toxic effects of paraquat comes from observations on autopsy series[89,97,98] and from experimental studies that have enabled the sequence of pulmonary changes to be observed.[99-102] In accordance with paraquat being taken up by the alveolar epithelium, electron microscopy shows that these cells suffer more profound damage than the endothelium.[99] Type I epithelial cells swell and undergo necrosis (Fig. 7.2.5),[103] whilst type II cells, although remaining capable of proliferation, show ultrastructural evidence of damage with derangement of cell organelles.[99,100] Histological changes in the lungs follow the pattern of diffuse alveolar damage, with a characteristic feature of the early exudative phase being intense vascular congestion and alveolar haemorrhage.[89,97,104] Hyaline membranes are most clearly seen by about 5 days (Fig. 7.2.6) and epithelial proliferation and fibrosis are conspicuous by about 14 days.

The pattern of pulmonary fibrosis in paraquat poisoning has been disputed. Some authors have stressed its interstitial position, whereas others have clearly demonstrated that it is intra-alveolar.[98,102,104-107] However, as described on page 148, it generally assumes an obliterative pattern of intra-alveolar fibrosis in which the lumina of several adjacent alveoli are totally effaced, rendering them completely airless (see Fig. 4.24, p. 148).

Toxic oil syndrome

A new multisystem disease appeared abruptly in the environs of Madrid in 1981.[108-110] Over 20 000 people were affected and about 1

Figure 7.2.5 Paraquat poisoning. After initial swelling of the cytoplasm (A) the type I alveolar epithelial cells proceed to complete necrosis (B), exposing the basement membrane (arrow) they share with the alveolar capillary endothelium to alveolar air. Flecks of fibrin are seen in the alveolus. Intact endothelium and part of an erythrocyte are seen beneath the denuded basement membrane. *(Reproduced by permission of the editors of the* Journal of Pathology[99] *and* Progress in Respiratory Research.[103]*)*

Figure 7.2.6 Suicidal paraquat poisoning. The ingestion of large amounts of the chemical has led to death from pulmonary haemorrhage and diffuse alveolar damage within 3 days. Note the hyaline membrane formation and early interstitial fibrosis. *(Courtesy of Dr D Melcher, Brighton, UK.)*

in 60 died. The disease was initially thought to be *Mycoplasma* pneumonia but was soon found to be associated with the use of adulterated oil sold illicitly by door-to-door salesmen. Although it was sold for culinary purposes the oil had been produced for industrial use in steel manufacture. It consisted of rapeseed and olive oil mixed with liquified animal fat, aniline and other organic chemicals. It has not been possible to identify the exact chemical responsible for the disease or to reproduce the changes in other species but the later induction of similar pathological changes by another substance contaminated with an aniline derivative is possibly relevant (see L-tryptophan-induced eosinophilia–myalgia syndrome, p. 389).[111] Some clinical and pathological features of the disease suggest that immune mechanisms may also be involved.

The initial clinical features included fever, respiratory distress, cough, haemoptysis, skin eruptions and marked eosinophilia. Radiographs suggested pulmonary oedema and sometimes showed pleural effusion. About 5% of patients died at this stage but most recovered quickly. However, within a few weeks many were readmitted to hospital with nausea, vomiting, diarrhoea and abdominal pain. About a quarter then proceeded to develop weakness, myalgia, weight loss, scleroderma-like skin signs and pulmonary hypertension.[112,113] Many of these patients died after a long, wasting illness or are permanently disabled with neurological and hepatic disorders.

In the early phase the lungs showed the most severe changes, which consisted of a combination of diffuse alveolar damage, eosinophilic infiltrates and arterial luminal narrowing by endothelial swelling and vacuolation, intimal foam cell infiltration and a non-necrotising vasculitis.[109,112,114] There was also capillary thrombosis, which later extended into arteries and veins, culminating in fibrosing obliteration of these blood vessels. In some patients dying of haemoptysis, dilated thin-walled blood vessels were identified in the mucosa of major blood-filled airways. Late features in the lungs included plexogenic arteriopathy (see p. 420), possibly secondary to changes in the liver. Similar inflammatory and vascular changes were seen in many other tissues. Notable extrapulmonary features included fasciitis, vasculitis, neuronal degeneration, perineuritis, hepatic injury and tissue eosinophilia.

Sauropus androgynus

Sauropus androgynus is a vegetable that is widely cultivated for the table in many south-eastern Asian countries. It is apparently harmless when cooked but recently there has been a vogue in Taiwan for consuming large amounts of its unprocessed juice, blended with that of guavas or pineapple, because of its supposed efficacy as a slimming aid and in blood pressure control. Coincident with this fad there has been an upsurge in patients with symptoms of obstructive lung disease. Within a 4-month period more than 60 such patients were seen at one hospital.[115–117] They had four features in common: recent consumption of uncooked *S. androgynus* juice, fixed ventilatory obstruction, radiological evidence of bilateral bronchiectasis and an absence of any previous chronic respiratory disease. Four patients agreed to undergo open-lung biopsy. This showed chronic bronchiolitis or obliterative bronchiolitis of constrictive pattern. The lymphocytes were mainly T cells but immunofluorescent and electron microscopy showed no evidence of an immune process. Four patients underwent single-lung transplantation. The excised lungs showed sclerotic obliteration of bronchial arteries in the walls of bronchi 4–5 mm in diameter with segmental necrosis of bronchi 2–4 mm in diameter. The changes were considered to fit best with segmental ischaemic necrosis of bronchi at the watershed zone of the bronchial and pulmonary vasculature.[118] Further patients have required lung transplantation but public education of the dangers of this herbal medicine now appears to have been successful.[119]

RECREATIONAL DRUGS

Alcohol and nicotine outstrip all other recreational drugs in popularity and their effects are of course well known. Those of tobacco smoking are summarised above and dealt with in detail in the chapters on obstructive lung disease (Chapter 3) and carcinoma of the lung (Chapter 12.1). Less well known is the lung disease that results from smoking Blackfat tobacco, a practice popular with Guyanese Indians. Blackfat is the trade name of a type of tobacco that is flavoured with mineral oil, some of which vaporises and is inhaled when the tobacco is smoked, to cause exogenous lipid pneumonia (see p. 314 [Ch8]).[120] In recent years the smoking of two other substances, marijuana and cocaine, has gained in popularity. It would not be surprising if the long-term effects of smoking these substances were similar to those of cigarette smoking but as yet it is too early to judge. However, the short-term effects are similar to those of tobacco smoking and this bodes badly for their ultimate effects.

Marijuana

Marijuana consists of the dried leaves of the cannabis plant, also known as hemp, as opposed to hashish, which is the plant's resin, and a further extract known as 'weed oil'. All these substances are smoked because they contain cannabis alkaloids which have psychoactive effects. However, this habit also exposes the lungs to many of the same respiratory irritants that are found in tobacco smoke. Initial exposure to marijuana smoke often results in coughing while habitual smokers produce black sputum. Bronchial biopsy shows inflammation and squamous metaplasia and bronchoalveolar lavage demonstrates increased numbers of cells, which are predominantly macrophages but also include neutrophils.[121-125] These changes are virtually identical to the short-term effects of tobacco smoke and are therefore likely to be similarly followed by the development of chronic obstructive lung disease and lung cancer. Indeed, the dangers of smoking marijuana are probably greater than those of smoking tobacco as compared with tobacco smoking it is associated with a fivefold greater increase in blood carboxyhaemoglobin and a threefold increase in the amount of tar inhaled.[126] It is estimated that three cannabis cigarettes result in the same degree of bronchial damage as 20 tobacco cigarettes.[127] There is also evidence that the effects of smoking marijuana and tobacco are additive.[128]

Not surprisingly therefore, epidemiological studies report a dose-related impairment of large-airway function in marijuana smokers.[129] There are also several reports attributing pneumothorax to marijuana smoking (Fig. 7.2.7).[130,131] The pneumothorax may be spontaneous or develop during the deep, sustained inspiratory effort involved in smoking marijuana (or cocaine), which may be enhanced by a partner applying positive ventilatory pressure by mouth-to-mouth contact. Thoracoscopy in such cases has shown predominantly apical, irregular bullous emphysema, while lung biopsy has demonstrated widespread alveolar filling by heavily pigmented macrophages.[131,132] Evidence is also beginning to accumulate that long-term cannabis use increases the risk of lung cancer.[133] Smoking cannabis in the form of weed oil is also reported to result in exogenous lipid pneumonia.[134]

Cocaine

Cocaine hydrochloride is a fine white powder derived from the leaves of the plant *Erythroxolon coca* by a complex chemical process. It is heat-labile and therefore cannot be smoked. Users inject it intravenously or inhale it unheated through the nose, the latter practice

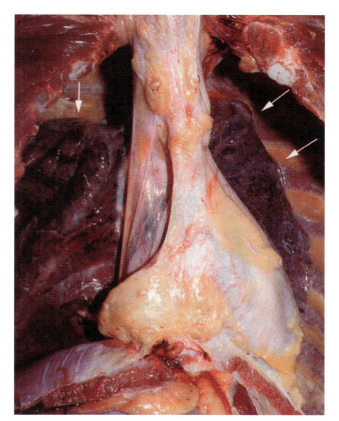

Figure 7.2.7 Bilateral pneumothoraces in a 23-year-old man who died suddenly while smoking marijuana. The collapsed lungs (arrows) have retracted towards the mediastinum. *(Courtesy of Dr JF Tomashefski Junior, Cleveland, USA.[131])*

being known as 'snorting'. However, a heat-stable free-base form that can be smoked is easily prepared from the hydrochloride with baking powder and a solvent such as ether. This process results in a crystalline deposit that is known as 'rock' because of its appearance or 'crack' because of the crackling sound it emits when heated. When smoked, the cocaine is readily absorbed and an intense surge of euphoria is experienced within 8 seconds. The intravenous route takes twice as long and 'snorting' several minutes. The hard addict therefore prefers to smoke 'crack'.

A variety of pulmonary complications of smoking free-base cocaine has been reported.[128,135-144] Acute effects include cough, shortness of breath, chest pain and haemoptysis. Asthma may be aggravated, black sputum is produced, and pneumothorax and interstitial emphysema have resulted from Valsalva manoeuvres undertaken in the belief that they promote even more rapid absorption. Biopsy has shown pulmonary congestion and oedema, organising pneumonia, haemorrhage, haemosiderosis, diffuse alveolar damage and interstitial pneumonia or fibrosis. Less common effects include eosinophilic pneumonia, extrapulmonary eosinophilic angiitis, medial thickening of pulmonary arteries and the barotrauma described above (see Fig. 7.2.7). Severe burning of the airways has also been seen due to 'crack' being smoked before all the ether used in its preparation has evaporated.

'Snorting' unheated cocaine has its own complications: substances such as cellulose or talc with which the drug is 'cut' (mixed as a diluent) are liable to provoke a foreign-body giant cell reaction in the lungs (Fig. 7.2.8).[145] However, particles of foreign material larger than those in the usual respirable range (allowing for the fibrous shape of substances such as cellulose) should suggest intravenous use (see 'Filler embolism', below).

Heroin

Heroin is usually injected, but it may be smoked, when, as with marijuana, it is liable to lead to a very pronounced macrophage response. Intravenous heroin abuse sometimes causes the sudden onset of a potentially fatal high-permeability pulmonary oedema (Fig. 7.2.9). Intravenous abuse of heroin and other drugs is also liable to cause 'filler embolism', which will now be considered.

'Filler embolism'

'Filler embolism' is the result of illicit drug usage in which compounds designed for oral use are injected intravenously to heighten their effects. Oral preparations consist largely of fillers such as talc or starch and this insoluble particulate matter accumulates in the pulmonary capillaries. It provokes a foreign-body giant cell reaction, thrombosis and fibrosis and may cause pulmonary hypertension (Fig. 7.2.10 and see Fig. 8.1.13, p. 412).[146–153] The various materials may be distinguished by their morphology, staining characteristics (see Fig. 7.2.10

and Table 7.2.3) and elemental composition, as studied by X-ray spectroscopy (see p. 330).

4-methyl-aminorex

This 'designer' drug, taken for its central stimulant activity (street names 'ice' or 'U-4-E-uh', pronounced euphoria), is related to the appetite suppressor aminorex, discussed on page 424, and has similarly been associated with pulmonary hypertension.[154]

Figure 7.2.9 Frothy oedema fluid protrudes from the nostrils of a person who died while injecting heroin intravenously. Similar froth filled the whole respiratory tract. (*Courtesy of Dr JF Tomashefski Junior, Cleveland, USA.*[131])

Figure 7.2.8 A foreign-body granulomatous response in the lungs to cellulose filler inhaled by a cocaine sniffer. Section viewed by partially polarised light microscopy.

Table 7.2.3 Tablet filler materials

Filler	Shape	Size	Polarisation	Histochemistry
Starch	Round	8–12 µm	Maltese cross	d-PAS
Talc	Platy but seen edge-on as needles	5–15 µm	Strong	None
Cellulose	Fibrous	25–200 µm	Strong	PAS, Congo red
Crosprovidone	Globular or coral-like	100 µm	Negative	Mucicarmine, Congo red
Magnesium stearate	Irregular	5–10 µm	Positive	None
Silica	Irregular	10–20 µm	Positive	None
d-PAS, diastase-controlled periodic acid–Schiff.				

Figure 7.2.10 Tablet filler materials in the lungs. (a) Intravascular and perivascular deposits of the tablet dispersant crospovidone eliciting a foreign-body giant cell reaction. (b) A crosprovidone granuloma stained with mucicarmine. (c) A starch granuloma stained with periodic acid–Schiff reagents. (d) The Maltese cross birefringence of starch viewed by polarized light. *(Courtesy of Dr JF Tomashefski Junior, Cleveland, USA.[131])*

REFERENCES

Atmospheric pressure changes

1. Noppen M, Verbanck S, Harvey J, et al. Music: a new cause of primary spontaneous pneumothorax. Thorax 2004;59:722–4.

2. Alifano M, Forti Parri SN, Bonfanti B, et al. Atmospheric pressure influences the risk of pneumothorax: beware of the storm! Chest 2007;131:1877–82.

3. Zuckerman S. Experimental study of blast injuries to the lungs. Lancet 1940;2:219–24.

4. Cooper GJ, Taylor DEM. Biophysics of impact injury to the chest and abdomen. J R Army Med Corps 1989;135:58–67.

5. Tsokos M, Paulsen F, Petri S, et al. Histologic, immunohistochemical, and ultrastructural findings in human blast lung injury. Amer J Respir Crit Care Med 2003;168:549–55.

6. Tsokos M, Paulsen F, Petri S, et al. Histologic, immunohistochemical, and ultrastructural findings in human blast lung injury. Am J Respir Crit Care Med 2003;168:549–55.

7. Brown RFR, Cooper GJ, Maynard RL. The ultrastructure of rat lung following acute primary blast injury. Int J Exp Pathol 1993;74:151–62.

8. Nadel JA, Denison D. Disorders associated with diving. In: Murray JF, Nadel JA, editors. Textbook of Respiratory Medicine. 2nd ed. Philadelphia: Saunders; 1994. p. 2099–116.

9. Kidd DJ, Elliott DH. Decompression disorders in divers. In: Bennett PB, Elliott DH, editors. The Physiology and Medicine of Diving and Compressed Air Work. 2nd ed. London: Bailliere Tindall; 1975. p. 471–95.

10. Liebow AA, Stark JE, Vogel J, et al. Intrapulmonary air trapping in submarine escape training casualties. U S Armed Forces Med J 1959;10:265–89.

11. Denison DM, Warrell DA, West JB. Airway structure and alveolar emptying in the

lungs of sea lions and dogs. Respir Physiol 1971;13:253–60.

12. Denison DM, Kooyman GL. The structure and function of the small airways in pinniped and sea otter lungs. Respir Physiol 1973;17:1–10.

13. Cooperman EM, Hogg J, Thurlbeck WM. Mechanisms of death in shallow-water scuba diving. Can Med Assoc J 1968;99:1128–31.

14. Broome CR, Jarvis LJ, Clark RJ. Pulmonary barotrauma in submarine escape training. Thorax 1994;49:186–7.

15. Elliott DH, Hallenbeck JM. The pathophysiology of decompression sickness. In: Bennett PB, Elliott DH, editors. The Physiology and Medicine of Diving and Compressed Air Work. 2nd ed. London: Bailliere Tindall; 1975. p. 435–55.

16. Boussuges A, Blanc F, Carturan D. Hemodynamic changes induced by recreational scuba diving. Chest 2006;129:1337–43.

17. McCallum RI. Dysbaric osteonecrosis: aseptic necrosis of bone. In: Bennett PB, Elliott DH, editors. The Physiology and Medicine of Diving and Compressed Air Work. 2nd ed. London: Bailliere Tindall; 1975. p. 504–21.

18. Fahlman A, Olszowka A, Bostrom B, et al. Deep diving mammals: Dive behavior and circulatory adjustments contribute to bends avoidance. Respir Physiol Neurobiol 2006;153:66–77.

19. Hackett PH, Roach RC. Current concepts: High-altitude illness. N Engl J Med 2001;345:107–14.

20. Schoene RB. Illnesses at high altitude. Chest 2008;134:402–16.

21. Bartsch P. High altitude pulmonary edema. Respiration 1997;64:435–43.

22. Schoene RB, Hackett PH, Henderson WR, et al. High altitude pulmonary oedema; characteristics of lung lavage fluid. JAMA 1986;256:63–9.

23. Bartsch P, Maggiorini M, Ritter M, et al. Prevention of high-altitude pulmonary edema by nifedipine. N Engl J Med 1991;325:1284–9.

24. Naeije R. Pulmonary circulation at high altitude. Respiration 1997;64:429–34.

25. Hanaoka M, Kubo K, Yamazaki Y, et al. Association of high-altitude pulmonary edema with the major histocompatibility complex. Circulation 1998;97:1124–8.

26. West JB, Colice GL, Lee YJ, et al. Pathogenesis of high-altitude pulmonary oedema: direct evidence of stress failure of pulmonary capillaries. Eur Respir J 1995;8:523–9.

27. Hultgren HN. High-altitude pulmonary edema: current concepts. Annu Rev Med 1996;47:267–84.

28. Maggiorini M, Melot C, Pierre S, et al. High-altitude pulmonary edema is initially caused by an increase in capillary pressure. Circulation 2001;103:2078–83.

29. Reeves JT, Schoene RB. When lungs on mountains leak – studying pulmonary edema at high altitudes. N Engl J Med 1991;325:1306–7.

30. Scherrer U, Vollenweider L, Delabays A, et al. Inhaled nitric oxide for high-altitude pulmonary edema. N Engl J Med 1996;334:624–9.

31. Hultgren HN, Wilson R, Kosek JC. Lung pathology in high-altitude pulmonary edema. Wilderness Environ Med 1997;8:218–20.

32. Droma Y, Hanaoka M, Hotta J, et al. Pathological features of the lung in fatal high altitude pulmonary edema occurring at moderate altitude in Japan. High Alt Med Biol 2001;2:515–23.

33. Gupta ML, Rao KS, Anand IS, et al. Lack of smooth muscle in the small pulmonary arteries of the native Ladakhi – is the Himalayan highlander adapted? Am Rev Respir Dis 1992;145:1201–4.

34. Harris P. Evolution, hypoxia and high altitude. In: Heath D, editor. Aspects of Hypoxia. Liverpool: Liverpool University Press; 1986. p. 207–16.

35. Heath D, Harris P, Sui GJ, et al. Pulmonary blood vessels and endocrine cells in subacute infantile mountain sickness. Respir Med 1989;83:77–81.

36. Harris P, Heath D. The Human Pulmonary Circulation: Its Form and Function in Health and Disease. 3rd ed. Edinburgh: Churchill Livingstone; 1986.

Drowning

37. Cohen DS, Matthay MA, Cogan MG, et al. Pulmonary edema associated with salt water near-drowning – new insights. Am Rev Respir Dis 1992;146:794–6.

38. Folkesson HG, Kheradmand F, Matthay MA. The effect of salt water on alveolar epithelial barrier function. Am J Respir Crit Care Med 1994;150:1555–63.

39. Gregorakos L, Markou N, Psalida V, et al. Near-drowning: clinical course of lung injury in adults. Lung 2009;187:93–7.

Inhaled toxic agents

40. Haggard HW. Action of irritant gases upon the respiratory tract. J Indust Hyg 1924;5:390.

41. Miller FJ, Overton JH, Kimbell JS, et al. Regional respiratory tract absorption of inhaled reactive gases. In: Gardner DE, Crapo JD, McClellan RO, editors. Toxicology of the Lung. 2nd ed. New York: Raven Press; 1993.

42. Newman Taylor AJ. Respiratory irritants encountered at work. Thorax 1996;51:541–5.

43. Bascom R, Bromberg PA, Hill C, et al. Health effects of outdoor air pollution. Am J Respir Crit Care Med 1996;153:3–50; 477–98.

44. Committee of the Environmental and Occupational Health Assembly of the American Thoracic Society. Health effects of outdoor air pollution. Am J Respir Crit Care Med 1996;153:3–50.

45. Committee of the Environmental and Occupational Health Assembly of the American Thoracic Society. Health effects of outdoor air pollution. Part 2. Am J Respir Crit Care Med 1996;153:477–98.

46. Samet JM, Dominici F, Curriero FC, et al. Fine particulate air pollution and mortality in 20 US Cities, 1987–1994. N Engl J Med 2000;343:1742–9.

47. Sydbom A, Blomberg A, Parnia S, et al. Health effects of diesel exhaust emissions. Eur Resp J 2001;17:733–46.

48. Souza MB, Saldiva PHN, Pope CA, et al. Respiratory changes due to long-term exposure to urban levels of air pollution: A histopathologic study in humans. Chest 1998;113:1312–8.

49. Sherwin RP, Richters V, Everson RB, et al. Chronic glandular bronchitis in young

individuals residing in a metropolitan area. Virchows Archiv 1998;433:341–8.

50. Dockery DW, Pope CA, Xu XP, et al. An association between air pollution and mortality in 6 United States cities. N Engl J Med 1993;329:1753–9.

51. Akhtar T, Ullah Z, Khan MH, et al. Chronic bronchitis in women using solid biomass fuel in rural peshawar, Pakistan. Chest 2007;132:1472–5.

52. Emmelin A, Wall S. Indoor air pollution: a poverty-related cause of mortality among the children of the world. Chest 2007;132:1615–23.

52a. Hu G, Zhou Y, Tian J, et al. Risk of COPD from exposure to biomass smoke. Chest 2010;138:20–31.

53. Weinstein P, Cook A. Human health impacts of volcanic activity. Histopathology 2002;41:329–33.

54. Banauch GI, Alleyne D, Sanchez R, et al. Persistent hyperreactivity and reactive airway dysfunction in firefighters at the World Trade Center. Am J Respir Crit Care Med 2003;168:54–62.

55. Reibman J, Lin S, Hwang SA, et al. The World Trade Center residents' respiratory health study: new-onset respiratory symptoms and pulmonary function. Environ Health Perspect 2005;113:406–11.

56. Banauch GI, Hall C, Weiden M, et al. Pulmonary function after exposure to the World Trade Center collapse in the New York City Fire Department. Am J Respir Crit Care Med 2006;174:312–9.

57. Lioy PJ, Weisel CP, Millette JR, et al. Characterization of the dust/smoke aerosol that settled east of the World Trade Center (WTC) in lower Manhattan after the collapse of the WTC 11 September 2001. Environ Health Perspect 2002;110:703–14.

58. McGee JK, Chen LC, Cohen MD, et al. Chemical analysis of World Trade Center fine particulate matter for use in toxicologic assessment. Environ Health Perspect 2003;111:972–80.

59. Landrigan PJ, Lioy PJ, Thurston G, et al. Health and environmental consequences of the World Trade Center disaster. Environ Health Perspect 2004;112:731–9.

60. Skloot GS, Schechter CB, Herbert R, et al. Longitudinal assessment of spirometry in the World Trade Center medical monitoring program. Chest 2009;135:492–8.

61. Rom WN, Weiden M, Garcia R, et al. Acute eosinophilic pneumonia in a New York City firefighter exposed to World Trade Center dust. Am J Respir Crit Care Med 2002;166:797–800.

62. Safirstein BH, Klukowicz A, Miller R, et al. Granulomatous pneumonitis following exposure to the World Trade Center collapse. Chest 2003;123:301–4.

63. Ryu JH, Colby TV, Hartman TE, et al. Smoking-related interstitial lung diseases: a concise review. Eur Resp J 2001;17:122–32.
64. Grubstein A, Bendayan D, Schactman I, et al. Concomitant upper-lobe bullous emphysema, lower-lobe interstitial fibrosis and pulmonary hypertension in heavy smokers: report of eight cases and review of the literature. Respir Med 2005;99:948–54.
65. Jankowich MD, Polsky M, Klein M, et al. Heterogeneity in combined pulmonary fibrosis and emphysema. Respiration 2008;75:411–7.
66. Nagai S, Hoshino Y, Hayashi M, et al. Smoking-related interstitial lung diseases. Curr Opin Pulm Med 2000;6:415–9.
67. Wells AU, Nicholson AG, Hansell DM. Challenges in pulmonary fibrosis 4: Smoking-induced diffuse interstitial lung diseases. Thorax 2007;62:904–10.
68. Cottin V, Nunes H, Brillet PY, et al. Combined pulmonary fibrosis and emphysema: a distinct underrecognised entity. Eur Respir J 2005;26:586–93.
69. Kawabata Y, Hoshi E, Murai K, et al. Smoking-related changes in the background lung of specimens resected for lung cancer: a semiquantitative study with correlation to postoperative course. Histopathology 2008;53:707–14.
69a. Balbi B, Cottin V, Singh S, et al. Clinical Assembly contribution to the celebration of 20 years of the ERS. Smoking-related lung diseases: a clinical perspective. Eur Respir J 2010;35:231–3.
69b. Katzenstein ALA, Mukhopadhyay S, Zanardi C, et al. Clinically occult interstitial fibrosis in smokers: classification and significance of a surprisingly common finding in lobectomy specimens. Hum Path 2010;41:316–25.
70. Adesina AM, Vallyathan V, McQuillen EN, et al. Bronchiolar inflammation and fibrosis associated with smoking – a morphologic cross-sectional population analysis. Am Rev Respir Dis 1991;143:144–9.
71. Auerbach O, Garfinkel L, Hammond EC. Relation of smoking and age to findings in lung parenchyma: a microscopic study. Chest 1974;65:29–35.
72. Ammous Z, Hackett NR, Butler MW, et al. Variability in small airway epithelial gene expression among normal smokers. Chest 2008;133:1344–53.
73. Elliot JG, Carroll NG, James AL, et al. Airway alveolar attachment points and exposure to cigarette smoke in utero. Am J Respir Crit Care Med 2003;167:45–9.
74. Warren CW, Jones NR, Eriksen MP, et al. Patterns of global tobacco use in young people and implications for future chronic disease burden in adults. The Lancet 367:749–53.
75. Maziak W, Ward KD, Afifi Soweid RA, et al. Tobacco smoking using a waterpipe: a

re-emerging strain in a global epidemic. Tob Control 2004;13:327–33.
76. Foley FD, Moncrief JA, Mason AD. Pathology of the lung in fatally burned patients. Ann Surg 1968;167:251–64.
77. Toor AH, Tomashefski JF, Kleinerman J. Respiratory tract pathology in patients with severe burns. Hum Pathol 1990;21:1212–20.
78. Brinkmann B, Puschel K. Heat injuries to the respiratory system. Virchows Arch A Pathol Anat Histopathol 1978;379:299–311.
79. Sheridan RL, Ryan CM, Yin LM, et al. Death in the burn unit: sterile multiple organ failure. Burns 1998;24:307–11.
80. Nash G, Foley FD, Langlinais PC. Pulmonary interstitial edema and hyaline membranes in adult burn patients. Hum Pathol 1975;5:149–60.
81. Hayden FG, Himel HN, Heggers JP. Herpesvirus infections in burn patients. Chest 1994;106:S15-21.
82. Byers RJ, Hasleton PS, Quigley A, et al. Pulmonary herpes simplex in burns patients. Eur Respir J 1996;9:2313–7.
83. Tasaka S, Kanazawa M, Mori M, et al. Long-term course of bronchiectasis and bronchiolitis obliterans as late complication of smoke inhalation. Respiration 1995;62:40–2.
84. Weill H. Disaster at Bhopal: the accident, early findings and respiratory health outlook in those injured. Bull Eur Physiopath Resp 1987;23:587–90.
85. Vijayan VK, Sankaran K, Sharma SK, et al. Chronic lung inflammation in victims of toxic gas leak at Bhopal. Respir Med 1995;89:105–11.
86. Cullinan P, Acquilla S, Ramana Dhara V. Respiratory morbidity 10 years after the Union Carbide gas leak at Bhopal: a cross sectional survey. BMJ 1997;314:338–42.
87. Carron PN, Yersin B. Management of the effects of exposure to tear gas. BMJ 2009;338:b2283.

Ingested toxic agents

88. Boyd MR. Evidence for the Clara cell as a site of cytochrome P450-dependent mixed-function oxidase activity in lung. Nature 1977;269:713–5.
89. Rebello G, Mason JK. Pulmonary histological appearances in fatal paraquat poisoning. Histopathology 1977;2:53–66.
90. Papiris SA, Maniati MA. Kyriakidis V, et al. Pulmonary damage due to paraquat poisoning through skin absorption. Respiration 1995;62:101–3.
91. Hudson M, Patel SB, Ewen SWB, et al. Paraquat induced pulmonary fibrosis in three survivors. Thorax 1991;46:201–4.
92. Hoet PHM, Dinsdale D, Lewis CPL, et al. Kinetics and cellular localisation of putrescine uptake in human lung tissue. Thorax 1993;48:1235–41.

93. Fisher HK, Clements JA, Wright RR. Enhancement of oxygen toxicity by the herbicide paraquat. Am Rev Respir Dis 1973;107:246–52.
94. Rhodes ML, Zavala DC, Brown D. Hypoxic protection in paraquat poisoning. Lab Invest 1976;35:496–500.
95. Raffin TA, Simon LM, Douglas WHJ, et al. The effects of variable O_2 tension and of exogenous superoxide dismutase on type II pneumocytes exposed to paraquat. Lab Invest 1980;42:205.
96. Skillrud DM, Martin WJ. Paraquat-induced injury of type II alveolar cells. Am Rev Respir Dis 1984;129:995–9.
97. Parkinson C. The changing pattern of paraquat poisoning in man. Histopathology 1980;4:171–83.
98. Takahashi T, Takahashi Y, Nio M. Remodeling of the alveolar structure in the paraquat lung of humans: a morphometric study. Hum Pathol 1994;25:702–8.
99. Vijeyaratnam GS, Corrin B. Experimental paraquat poisoning. J Pathol 1971;103:123–9.
100. Smith P, Heath D, Kay JM. The pathogenesis and structure of paraquat-induced pulmonary fibrosis in rats. J Pathol 1974;114:57–67.
101. Sykes BI, Purchase IFH, Smith LL. Pulmonary ultrastructure after oral and intravenous dosage of paraquat to rats. J Pathol 1977;121:233–41.
102. Fukuda Y, Ferrans VJ, Schoenberger CI, et al. Patterns of pulmonary structural remodeling after experimental paraquat toxicity. Am J Pathol 1985;118:452–75.
103. Corrin B, Vijeyaratnam GS. Experimental models of interstitial pneumonia: paraquat, iprindole. Prog Resp Res 1975;8:107–20.
104. Toner PG, Vetters JM, Spilg WGS, et al. Fine structure of the lung lesion in a case of paraquat poisoning. J Pathol 1970;102:182–3.
105. Copland GM, Kolin A, Shulman HS. Fatal pulmonary intra-alveolar fibrosis after paraquat ingestion. N Engl J Med 1974;291:290–2.
106. Smith P, Heath D. Paraquat lung: a reappraisal. Thorax 1974;29:643–53.
107. Hara H, Manabe T, Hayashi T. An immunohistochemical study of the fibrosing process in paraquat lung injury. Virchows Arch A Pathol Anat Histopathol 1989;415:357–66.
108. Tabuenca JM. Toxic-allergic syndrome caused by ingestion of rapeseed oil denatured with aniline. Lancet 1981;2:567–8.
109. Martinez-Tello FJ, Navas-Palacios JJ, Ricoy JR, et al. Pathology of a new toxic syndrome caused by ingestion of adulterated oil in Spain. Virchows Arch A Pathol Anat Histopathol 1982;397:261–85.
110. Kilbourne EM, Rigaue-Perez JG, Heath CW, et al. Clinical epidemiology of toxic oil

syndrome. N Engl J Med 1983;309:1408–14.

111. Mayeno AN, Belongia EA, Lin F, et al. 3-(phenylamino)alanine, a novel aniline-derived amino acid associated with the eosinophilia-myalgia syndrome – a link to the toxic oil syndrome. Mayo Clin Proc 1992;67:1134–9.

112. Gomez-Sanchez MA, de Juan MJM, Gomez-Pajuelo C, et al. Pulmonary hypertension due to toxic oil syndrome. A clinicopathologic study. Chest 1989;95:325–31.

113. Cheng TO. Pulmonary hypertension in patients with eosinophilia–myalgia syndrome or toxic oil syndrome. Mayo Clin Proc 1993;68:823.

114. Fernandez-Segoviano P, Esteban A, Martinez-Cabruja R. Pulmonary vascular lesions in the toxic oil syndrome in Spain. Thorax 1983;38:724–9.

115. Lai R-S, Chiang AA, Wu M-T, et al. Outbreak of bronchiolitis obliterans associated with consumption of *Sauropus androgynus* in Taiwan. Lancet 1996;348:83–5.

116. Chang H, Wang JS, Tseng HH, et al. Histopathological study of *Sauropus androgynus*-associated constrictive bronchiolitis obliterans: a new cause of constrictive bronchiolitis obliterans. Am J Surg Pathol 1997;21:35–42.

117. Wang JS, Tseng HH, Lai RS, et al. *Sauropus androgynus*-constrictive obliterative bronchitis/bronchiolitis – histopathological study of pneumonectomy and biopsy specimens with emphasis on the inflammatory process and disease progression. Histopathology 2000;37:402–10.

118. Chang YL, Yao YT, Wang NS, et al. Segmental necrosis of small bronchi after prolonged intakes of *Sauropus androgynus* in Taiwan. Am J Respir Crit Care Med 1998;157:594–8.

119. Wang JS, Tseng HH, Lai RS. *Sauropus* bronchiolitis – Reply. Am J Surg Pathol 1998;22:380–1.

Recreational drugs

120. Miller GJ, Ashcroft MT, Beadnell HMSG, et al. The lipoid pneumonia of blackfat tobacco smokers in Guyana. Q J Med 1971;40:457–70.

121. Hyashi M, Sornberger GC, Huber GL. A morphometric analysis of the male and female tracheal epithelium after experimental exposure to marijuana smoke. Lab Invest 1980;42:65–9.

122. Barbers RG, Gong H, Tashkin DP, et al. Differential examination of bronchoalveolar lavage cells in tobacco cigarette and marijuana smokers. Am Rev Respir Dis 1987;135:1271–5.

123. Gong H, Fligiel S, Tashkin DP, et al. Tracheobronchial changes in habitual, heavy smokers of marijuana with and without tobacco. Am Rev Respir Dis 1987;136:142–9.

124. Roth MD, Arora A, Barsky SH, et al. Airway inflammation in young marijuana and tobacco smokers. Am J Respir Crit Care Med 1998;157:928–37.

125. Just N, Delourme J, Delattre C, et al. An unusual cause of patchy ground-glass opacity. Thorax 2009;64:12 & 74.

126. Wu TC, Tashkin DP, Djahed B, et al. Pulmonary hazards of smoking marijuana as compared with tobacco. N Engl J Med 1988;318:347–51.

127. British Lung Foundation. A smoking gun? 2003. Available online at: www.lunguk.org/news/index.html.

128. Fligiel SEG, Roth MD, Kleerup EC, et al. Tracheobronchial histopathology in habitual smokers of cocaine, marijuana, and/or tobacco. Chest 1997;112:319–26.

129. Aldington S, Williams M, Nowitz M, et al. Effects of cannabis on pulmonary structure, function and symptoms. Thorax 2007;62:1058–63.

130. Johnson MK, Smith RP, Morrison D, et al. Large lung bullae in marijuana smokers. Thorax 2000;55:340–2.

131. Tomashefski JF Jr, Felo JA. The pulmonary pathology of illicit drug and substance abuse. Current Diagnostic Pathology 2004;10:413–26.

132. Gill AF. Bong lung: regular smokers of cannabis show relatively distinctive histologic changes that predispose to pneumothorax. American Journal of Surgical Pathology 2005;29:980–2.

133. Aldington S, Harwood M, Cox B, et al. Cannabis use and risk of lung cancer: a case-control study. Eur Respir J 2008;31:280–6.

134. Vethanayagam D, Pugsley S, Dunn EJ, et al. Exogenous lipid pneumonia related to smoking weed oil following cadaveric renal transplantation. Can Respir J 2000;7:338–42.

135. Ettinger NA, Albin RJ. A review of the respiratory effects of smoking cocaine. Am J Med 1989;87:664–8.

136. Jentzen J. Medical complications of cocaine abuse. Am J Clin Pathol 1993;100:475–6.

137. Greenebaum E, Copeland A, Grewal R. Blackened bronchoalveolar lavage fluid in crack smokers – a preliminary study. Am J Clin Pathol 1993;100:481–7.

138. Bailey ME, Fraire AE, Greenberg SD, et al. Pulmonary histopathology in cocaine abusers. Hum Pathol 1994;25:203–7.

139. Haim DY, Lippmann ML, Goldberg SK, et al. Pulmonary complications of crack cocaine: a comprehensive review. Chest 1995;107:233–40.

140. Orriols R, Munoz X, Ferrer J, et al. Cocaine-induced Churg–Strauss vasculitis. Eur Respir J 1996;9:175–7.

141. Murray RJ, Smialek JE, Golle M, et al. Pulmonary artery medial hypertrophy in cocaine users without foreign particle microembolization. Chest 1989;96:1050–3.

142. Forrester JM, Steele AW, Waldron JA, et al. Crack lung: an acute pulmonary syndrome with a spectrum of clinical and histopathologic findings. Am Rev Respir Dis 1990;142:462–7.

143. Tashkin DP, Kleerup EC, Hoh CK, et al. Effects of 'crack' cocaine on pulmonary alveolar permeability. Chest 1997;112:327–35.

144. Perez GMGR, Bragado FG, Gil AMP. Pulmonary hemorrhage and antiglomerular basement membrane antibody-mediated glomerulonephritis after exposure to smoked cocaine (crack): A case report and review of the literature. Pathol Int 1997;47:692–7.

145. Cooper CB, Bai TR, Heyderman E, et al. Cellulose granulomas in the lungs of a cocaine sniffer. BMJ 1983;286:2021–2.

146. Arnett EN, Battle WE, Russo JV, et al. Intravenous injection of talc-containing drugs intended for oral use. A cause of pulmonary granulomatosis and pulmonary hypertension. Am J Med 1976;60:711–8.

147. Gross EM. Autopsy findings in drug addicts. Pathol Annu 1978;13:35–67.

148. Pare JAP, Fraser RG, Hogg JC, et al. Pulmonary 'mainline' granulomatosis: talcosis of intravenous methadone abuse. Medicine (Baltimore) 1979;58:229–39.

149. Waller BF, Brownlee WJ, Roberts WC. Self induced pulmonary granulomatosis. A consequence of intravenous injection of drugs intended for oral use. Chest 1980;78:90–4.

150. Tomashefski JF Jr, Hirsch CS. The pulmonary vascular lesions of intravenous drug abuse. Hum Pathol 1980;11:133–45.

151. Tomashefski JF, Hirsch CS, Jolly PN. Microcrystalline cellulose pulmonary embolism and granulomatosis. Arch Pathol Lab Med 1981;105:89–93.

152. Farber HW, Fairman RP, Glauser FL. Talc granulomatosis: laboratory findings similar to sarcoidosis. Am Rev Respir Dis 1982;125:258–61.

153. Rajs J, Harm T, Ormstad K. Postmortem findings of pulmonary lesions of older datum in intravenous drug addicts. A forensic-pathologic study. Virchows Arch A Pathol Anat Histopathol 1984;402:405–14.

154. Gaine SP, Rubin LJ, Kmetzo JJ, et al. Recreational use of Aminorex and pulmonary hypertension. Chest 2000;118:1496–500.

Chapter | 7 |

7.3 Iatrogenic lung disease

ADVERSE DRUG REACTIONS

It is estimated that 5% of all hospital admissions are due to effects of therapeutic drugs, that 10–18% of inpatients experience a drug reaction and that 3% of deaths in hospital may be related to drug therapy.[1-4] The lungs are often involved in these adverse reactions.

Mechanisms of adverse drug reactions[5]

The mechanism of an adverse drug reaction may be based on:

- overdosage: toxicity linked to excess dose, or impaired excretion, or both
- side-effect: undesirable pharmacological effect at recommended dose
- interaction with other drugs

and in susceptible individuals only:

- intolerance (representing a low threshold to the normal action of the drug)
- idiosyncrasy (an abnormal reaction based on a genetically determined metabolic or enzymic deficiency)
- allergy in the form of any of the four main hypersensitivity reactions:
  1. immediate IgE-mediated hypersensitivity
  2. IgG- or IgM-mediated cytotoxicity
  3. IgG- or IgM-mediated immune complex disease
  4. T-cell-mediated cellular hypersensitivity
- pseudoallergic reaction: A reaction with the same clinical manifestations as an allergic reaction (e.g. as a result of histamine release) but lacking immunological specificity.

Classification of adverse drug reactions

One classification of adverse drug reactions is that based upon the type of drug (Box 7.3.1).[6] This is not adopted here but in passing it is worth noting that pharmacists are generally very helpful in supplying details of adverse reactions to specific drugs. Alternatively, information on the long list of potentially pneumotoxic drugs may be obtained at http://www.pneumotox.com. A useful scheme for

Box 7.3.1 Principal therapeutic agents known to cause pulmonary disease[6]

Chemotherapeutic drugs

Azathioprine
Bleomycin
Busulphan
Chlorambucil
Cyclophosphamide
Etoposide
Ifosfamide
Melphalan
Mitomycin
Nitrosoureas
Procarbazine
Vinblastine
Cytosine arabinoside
Methotrexate

Antibiotics

Amphotericin B
Nitrofurantoin
Sulphasalazine
Sulphonamides
Pentamidine

Anti-inflammatory drugs

Acetylsalicylic acid
  (aspirin)
Gold
Methotrexate
*Non-steroidal anti-
  inflammatory agents*
Penicillamine

Immunosuppressive drugs

Ciclosporin
Interleukin-2

Analgesics

Diamorphine (heroin)
Ethchlorvynol
Methadone
Naloxone
Propoxyphene
Salicylates

Cardiovascular drugs

Amiodarone
*Angiotensin-converting enzyme
  inhibitors*
Anticoagulants
β-antagonists

Fibrinolytic agents

Protamine
Tocainide

Inhalants

Aspirated mineral oil
Oxygen

Intravenous agents

Ethanolamine oleate (sodium morrhuate)
Iodised oil (lymphangiography)
Fat emulsion

Miscellaneous

Bromocriptine
Dantrolene
Hydrochlorothiazide
Methysergide
Oral contraceptives
Tocolytic agents
Tricyclics
L-Tryptophan
X-irradiation

Particularly common agents are italicized.

Table 7.3.1 Pathological patterns of drug-induced lung disease

Pathological pattern	Prototypic drug(s)
Cytotoxicity 　Diffuse alveolar damage 　Interstitial fibrosis (NSIP, UIP, mixed) 　Organising pneumonia	Chemotherapy
Phospholipidosis	Amiodarone
Alveolar proteinosis	Chemotherapy
Eosinophilic pneumonia	Nitrofurantoin
Eosinophilia–myalgia syndrome	L-tryptophan
Granulomatous alveolitis	Methotrexate
Aspiration lesions	Liquid paraffin
Pulmonary vascular disease 　Hypertension 　Thromboembolism 　Haemorrhage	 Aminorex Oestrogen Anticoagulants
Opportunistic infection	Immunosuppressive agents
Metastatic calcification	Vitamin D
Carcinoma of the lung	Arsenicals
Pleural disease	Practolol

NSIP, non-specific interstitial pneumonia; UIP, usual interstitial pneumonia.

Reduced respiratory drive

Central depression of respiration occurs as a side-effect of barbiturates, morphine and its derivatives, and even mild sedatives, and may be particularly troublesome in patients suffering from chronic obstructive lung disease. Ventilation in such patients may be largely dependent on hypoxic respiratory drive and treatment with oxygen may therefore also have an adverse effect on respiration by lowering the degree of hypoxia and so diminishing the stimulation of the respiratory centre. Peripheral impairment of the respiratory drive may be brought about by aminosides and other antibiotics, while corticosteroids may result in a myopathy affecting the respiratory muscles. Other iatrogenic hazards affecting the peripheral nerves controlling respiration include nerve root disease complicating immunisation and surgical damage to the spinal and phrenic nerves.

Drug-induced bronchospasm

Asthmatic patients are particularly susceptible to exacerbations of their disease by drugs (Box 7.3.2). This effect may occur either as a predictable pharmacological side-effect of the drug or as an idiosyncratic response. Examples of the former include β-adrenergicic antagonists and cholinergic agents while examples of the latter include sensitivity to the colouring agent tartrazine, for which reason many manufacturers have eliminated tartrazine from their red, orange and yellow tablets. Allergic bronchoconstriction also forms part of generalised anaphylactic reactions induced by vaccines and antisera and occurs as a localised response to penicillin, iodine-containing contrast media, iron dextran and other medicaments. Bronchospasm may also be initiated by the non-specific irritant effect of inhaling nebulised drugs if they are prepared as a hypotonic solution, a side-effect that is prevented by using isotonic solutions.

assessing whether a particular clinical manifestation represents an adverse drug reaction considers previous experience with the drug, alternative aetiological agents, the timing of events, drug levels, and the effect of withdrawing the drug and rechallenge with the drug.[7] It is worth bearing in mind that:

- One drug may cause several patterns of disease.
- One pattern of disease may be produced by a variety of drugs.
- A drug reaction may develop long after the drug has been withdrawn.
- A drug reaction may develop suddenly even though the dose of the drug has not been altered.
- Drug effects may be augmented by factors such as age, previous radiotherapy and elevated oxygen levels.
- Drug reactions may be localised.
- Many drugs cross the placenta to affect the fetus.

An alternative classification of adverse drug reactions, which is more appropriate to pathology practice and which will be followed here, is one based on the pattern of disease. Some pathological patterns of drug-induced lung disease are shown in Table 7.3.1.

Aspirin-induced asthma has been recognised for many years and more recently several of the newer anti-inflammatory drugs have been found to exacerbate asthma in certain sensitive individuals. The basis for this is uncertain but the likelihood of an individual anti-inflammatory drug provoking an asthmatic response is related to its potency as an inhibitor of prostaglandin cyclooxygenase pathway, resulting in the production of leukotrienes.[8–10]

As well as asthma being exacerbated by drugs, the disease has been caused by occupational exposure in the pharmaceutical industry to certain drugs which can be inhaled during manufacture, notably penicillin, cephalosporin, methyldopa, cimetidine and piperazine.

Obliterative bronchiolitis

Obliterative bronchiolitis of the constrictive type has been reported with penicillamine[11,12] and gold[13,14] but in many cases it is possibly the underlying condition rather than the drug that is responsible (see p. 123). This is often rheumatoid disease, which is sometimes complicated by bronchiolitis obliterans whether the patient is under treatment or not.[15]

Organising pneumonia extending into peripheral bronchioles (see p. 120) may be seen with a variety of drugs but results in a restrictive rather than obstructive lung defect and is to be regarded as a cytotoxic effect of the drug acting primarily at the alveolar level (see below).

Raw *Sancropus androgyns* taken as a slimming aid causes severe obliterative bronchiolitis (see p. 376).

Cytotoxic effects of drugs

The cytotoxic effects of drugs may be acute or chronic, leading to changes as varied as pulmonary oedema, diffuse alveolar damage, pulmonary haemorrhage and haemosiderosis, organising pneumonia, interstitial pneumonitis and interstitial fibrosis.[16,17] Some of the most severe acute effects are seen with the chemotherapeutic agents used in malignant disease[18] but they are also recorded with drugs that are not traditionally thought to be cytotoxic, e.g. desferri-oxamine administered as a prolonged intravenous infusion in acute iron poisoning.[19]

Pulmonary toxicity due to busulphan was first described in 1961,[20] and has been the subject of several subsequent studies.[21–24] It remains the mainstay of treatment for chronic myeloid leukaemia. Like other alkylating agents, it acts by cross-linking DNA strands. Clinical estimates of the incidence of pulmonary toxicity vary around 4% but subclinical damage is thought to be much more common. Although not strictly dose-dependent, toxicity is rarely seen with a total cumulative dose of less than 500 mg. Synergy with radiation and other cytotoxic drugs occurs.[25] Similar effects have been reported for most cytotoxic agents, particularly bleomycin.[26] Pulmonary toxic-ity is seen less commonly with other alkylating agents, such as cyclo-phosphamide and melphalan.[27–30]

Bleomycin is a cytotoxic antibiotic derived from *Streptomyces* species. It is widely used in the treatment of neoplasms such as lymphomas and germ cell tumours, and is thought to produce its therapeutic and toxic effects by altering the normal balance between oxidants (active oxygen radicals) and antioxidant systems.[26] Bleomycin produces superoxide radicals when incubated with oxygen and iron in vitro. Oxygen enhances its effects,[31] a fact well known to anaesthetists who accordingly take care to limit concentrations of inspired oxygen to 30% in patients on bleomycin who are undergoing surgery.[32–34] Radiotherapy and cytotoxic agents such as bleomycin are also synergistic. Bleomycin is preferentially concentrated in the lungs and pulmonary fibrosis can be produced in animals when it is adminis-tered intravenously, intraperitoneally or by intratracheal instillation. Electron microscopy shows that the early changes consist of swelling and vesiculation of endothelial cells, interstitial oedema and type I epithelial cell necrosis.[35,36] The reported incidence of bleomycin toxicity varies from 2 to 40% depending on the type of patient being treated and on dosage. In general, toxic effects increase with age and cumulative dose: above a total dose of about 500 units they rise significantly.

The acute morphological changes attributable to drugs include pulmonary oedema and diffuse alveolar damage. Acute pulmonary oedema is seen in heroin addicts who die while injecting themselves intravenously but it is also seen in patients administered a variety of drugs therapeutically, for example hydrochlorothiazide, salicylate, opiates, vinorelbine,and desferrioxamine. The oedema is of the high permeability type (see p. 402), rich in protein, and is occasionally haemorrhagic or accompanied by the hyaline membranes of diffuse alveolar damage.

Diffuse alveolar damage has alveolar epithelial necrosis as its basis (Figs 7.3.1 and 7.3.2). However, the continuing action of many cyto-toxic drugs affects the regeneration process so that atypical type II epithelial cells develop, a characteristic feature that was first described with busulphan and subsequently with bleomycin.[21,37] These two drugs differ chemically but both act (by different mechanisms) on DNA. The atypical cells have abundant deeply eosinophilic or amphophilic cytoplasm and large nuclei, which may be multiple but are usually single. The nuclei measure up to 12 μm and are densely stained throughout or contain either large homogeneous deeply eosi-nophilic inclusions or clear vacuoles (Fig. 7.3.3). Electron microscopy distinguishes the inclusions from nucleoli and shows them to consist of tubular aggregates derived from the internal nuclear membrane.[37] Airway epithelium shows similar nuclear changes and often undergoes squamous metaplasia. The presence of such cells in sputum specimens submitted for cytology can lead to a misdiagnosis of malignancy.

Fibrosis may follow diffuse alveolar damage or develop insidiously, perhaps many years after drug therapy ceased (Fig. 7.3.4).[38] It may be both interstitial and intra-alveolar. The interstitial component is often accompanied by a non-specific chronic inflammatory infiltrate. The proportions of inflammation, which is potentially reversible, and fibrosis, which when collagenous is irreversible, obviously bear on the prognosis. However, most case reports antedate the recent

Figure 7.3.1 Drug toxicity. A cancer patient administered a cocktail of cytotoxic drugs developed acute respiratory distress and biopsy showed loss of the type I alveolar epithelial cells when examined by electron microscopy. The alveolar basement membrane is bare on its alveolar aspect (above). Capillary endothelial cells show cytoplasmic swelling. *(Courtesy of Miss A Dewar, Brompton, UK.)*

Figure 7.3.2 Amiodarone toxicity resulting in diffuse alveolar damage characterised by hyaline membrane formation.

Figure 7.3.3 Busulphan toxicity. The alveoli are lined by regenerating epithelial cells and the central cell has a very prominent nucleus.

Figure 7.3.4 Fatal pulmonary fibrosis resulting from busulphan therapy, which had been administered for 2 years several years previously.

classification of interstitial pneumonia described in Chapter 6 and it is uncertain how their pathological appearances would now be classified. The majority lack the classic features of usual interstitial pneumonia and fibrotic non-specific interstitial pneumonia. Many show overlapping patterns of intersitital pneumonia and this alone should arouse suspicion that a drug may have been responsible. However,

Some cytotoxic drugs result in pulmonary changes by more than one mechanism: for example, methotrexate may produce hypersensitivity reactions with granuloma formation[41–44] or pulmonary eosinophilia[45] as well as diffuse alveolar damage. Pulmonary toxicity is also occasionally seen in patients undergoing treatment with gold salts for rheumatoid disease: in addition to diffuse alveolar damage, there may be eosinophilia and dermatitis in these cases, again indicating possible hypersensitivity.[46] Nitrofurantoin is another example of a drug resulting in a variety of patterns of alveolar injury: diffuse alveolar damage, desquamative interstitial pneumonia, giant cell interstitial pneumonia, organising pneumonia and eosinophilic pneumonia have all been recorded in association with this drug.[47–49]

It should also be noted that in patients with neoplastic disease, clinical features suggestive of a pulmonary drug reaction may be due to factors other than drugs. In leukaemic patients, for example, these include direct infiltration of the lungs by leukaemic cells, opportunist infection and, if bone marrow transplantation has been undertaken, the effects of irradiation and possibly graft-versus-host disease.

Phospholipidosis

Phospholipidosis is encountered with drugs such as the antidysrhythmic agent amiodarone,[50] which block lysosomal enzymes involved in the breakdown of complex lipids. This leads to their accumulation throughout the body but the effect is most marked in tissues that take up the drug and contain cells rich in lysosomes. The lung fulfils both these requirements through its rich complement of alveolar macrophages. These cells accumulate the enzyme substrate (phospholipid) in their cytoplasm with the result that large foam cells fill the alveoli (Fig. 7.3.6). The appearances are those of endogenous lipid pneumonia, similar to that seen in obstructive pneumonitis. However, with amiodarone cytoplasmic vacuolation is also seen in epithelial and interstitial cells. The phospholipid inclusions contained within the vacuoles are particularly well seen in unstained frozen sections viewed by polarised light.[51] Identical changes to those induced by amiodarone were seen in the lungs of rats exposed to very high levels of the antidepressant drug iprindole[52] and the anorectic drug chlorphentermine.[53] These three compounds, iprindole, chlorphentermine and amiodarone, all belong to the amphiphilic group of drugs which block lysosomal phospholipase and sphingomyelinase. Although their pharmacological actions are very different, a molecular homology is apparent (Fig. 7.3.7).

It is likely that all patients receiving substantial amounts of amiodarone develop phospholipidosis throughout the body, but this is generally well tolerated. Only a minority experience respiratory impairment and in these there is also evidence of pulmonary inflammation and fibrosis, which is possibly mediated immunologically.[54] These patients generally have a restrictive lung deficit, the onset of which may be acute or chronic. Bronchoalveolar lavage shows foamy macrophages but these cells indicate exposure to the drug rather than drug toxicity; nor are they specific to amiodarone, being observed on occasion with other drugs. Lymphocytes of suppressor type may also be detected on lavage.[54] Histologically, amiodarone toxicity is diagnosed on a combination of phospholipidosis and interstitial pneumonia and fibrosis. Occasionally the hyaline membranes of diffuse alveolar damage are superimposed on the interstitial changes (see Fig. 7.3.2).[55–57] In some patients the fibrosis is intraalveolar rather than interstitial and the appearances are those of organising pneumonia.[58] The process may be localised and mimic a neoplasm radiologically.[59,60]

Amiodarone toxicity is probably dose-dependent but there is considerable individual variation in the amount required,[61,62] which appears to be under genetic control.[63] Amiodarone toxicity is uncommon in patients taking daily doses of 200 mg or less whereas the

Figure 7.3.5 Nitrofurantoin toxicity. The lung shows patchy subpleural fibrosis (A) with fibroblastic foci (B). These are the classic features of usual interstitial pneumonia but lung function improved after withdrawal of the drug.

there are drugs that undoubtedly cause a usual interstitial pneumonia pattern, for example the chemotherapeutic agents and nitrofurantoin (Fig. 7.3.5), while others, for example the statins, are recorded as having induced a non-specific interstitial pneumonia pattern.[39] A drug history is therefore imperative when assessing any patient with diffuse parenchymal lung disease.

Organising pneumonia similar to the cryptogenic condition described on page 308, and probably similarly reversible with steroids, has been encountered with a variety of drugs, including amiodarone, sulphasalazine and pencillamine.[40] Penicillamine has also been incriminated in the development of both diffuse alveolitis and bronchiolitis obliterans, but both these changes could well be due to the underlying rheumatoid disease for which the pencillamine is administered.[15] In busulphan lung there may be an organising intraalveolar fibrinous exudate,[21] which at its most extreme results in irreversible effacement of the alveolar architecture by sheets of loose connective tissue (see p. 148).

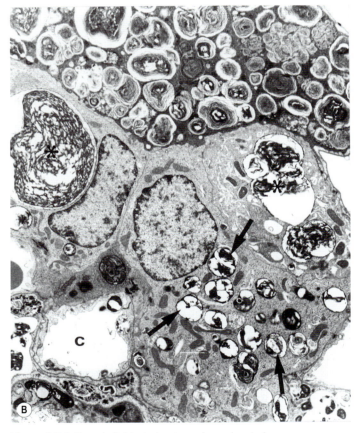

Figure 7.3.6 Phospholipidosis due to prolonged amiodarone administration. Amiodarone blocks lysosomal phospholipases, leading to the accumulation of phospholipids in many organs. In the lung this is manifest as endogenous lipid pneumonia. (A) By light microscopy the alveoli are filled with foamy macrophages. (B) Electron micrograph showing an alveolar macrophage (top) packed with osmiophilic lamellar bodies. The macrophage covers several type II pneumocytes that, in addition to their normal surfactant inclusions (arrows), contain large lamellated drug-induced inclusions (asterisks), which are also seen in capillary endothelial cells. C, capillary. *(Reproduced with permission from Costa-Jussa et al. (1984).[50])*

Amiodarone

Iprindole

Chlorphentermine

Figure 7.3.7 Formulae of several amphiphilic drugs, all of which block lysosomal phospholipases and cause endogenous lipid pneumonia. The pharmacological actions of these drugs differ but a molecular homology is evident.

prevalence of the disease exceeds 50% in patients treated with doses of 1200 mg/day. Duration is also important: it may require 2–3 years for a patient on 200 mg/day to develop symptoms but only 10 months for one on 400 mg/day. The drug has a long half-life and may take weeks to clear the body completely. Previous pulmonary injury renders the lung unduly sensitive to amiodarone. Acute toxicity has been encountered in patients on moderate doses who have experienced recent or even concomitant pulmonary procedures such as intubation, lobectomy or ventilation with high concentrations of oxygen.[64]

Alveolar proteinosis

With continued experimental administration of the drug iprindole mentioned above, the phospholipidosis it produced gradually evolved into alveolar proteinosis (more properly called lipoproteinosis; see p. 316),[65] but this has not been reported as a drug effect in humans. Alveolar proteinosis has however been recognised in a number of patients receiving chemotherapy for conditions such as leukaemia. The mechanism here is probably based on the cytotoxic action of the drug and the material filling the alveoli may represent the detritus of degenerate alveolar cells rather than excess pulmonary surfactant, as in the primary auto-immune form of alveolar proteinosis.

Eosinophilic pneumonia

Eosinophilic pneumonia, the pathology of which is described on page 461, may be caused by several drugs, including nitrofurantoin, *para*-aminosalicylic acid, sulphasalazine, phenylbutazone, gold compounds, aspirin and penicillin (see Box 9.3, p. 460).[66,67] It may also follow radiation to the chest.[68] The tissue eosinophilia is generally accompanied by a rise in the number of eosinophils in the blood. The clinical picture varies from transient asymptomatic opacities on a chest radiograph to a life-threatening illness with severe respiratory distress and hypoxaemia, so-called acute eosinophilic pneumonia (see p. 462). The reaction is often associated with a florid rash. Withdrawal of the drug may be all that is required to effect resolution but corticosteroids are usually given as they produce a marked improvement.

Churg–Strauss syndrome

This syndrome of necrotising granulomatosis, vasculitis and eosinophilia in asthmatic patients, which is described more fully on page 465, has been reported when leukotriene receptor antagonists have been used to treat asthma. However, it is likely that the syndrome has been merely unmasked by the antileukotriene permitting a reduction in corticosteroid dose rather than representing a direct effect of the antileukotriene.[69,70] Mesalazine has also been implicated in inducing a vasculitis during treatment for inflammatory bowel disease.[71]

Eosinophilia–myalgia syndrome

The eosinophilia–myalgia syndrome was identified in the USA in 1989 and quickly identified as being due to the ingestion of L-tryptophan from one particular Japanese supplier. Withdrawal of this substance led to the virtual elimination of the disease, but not before 2000 patients had been affected, 1 in 60 fatally.[72–76] Cases were subsequently described in Europe where there were further fatalities.

L-tryptophan is an essential amino acid that is freely available to the public: its purchase does not require a medical prescription. It has been promoted as a dietary supplement and as an agent against insomnia and premenstrual tension. Women in the reproductive years preponderated in the patients affected by the resultant eosinophilia–myalgia. The clinicopathological features of the syndrome are similar to those of the Spanish toxic oil syndrome (see p. 375) and differ more in degree than type. The discovery of an aniline-derived contaminant in the tryptophan-induced condition is a further link connecting these two syndromes.[77] An immune basis is suggested by the identification of T lymphocytes activated against fibroblasts in the eosinophilia–myalgia syndrome.[78]

The illness is a multisystem disorder and besides blood eosinophilia and myalgia there may be arthralgia, fever, rash and involvement of the lungs, liver and central nervous system. As in the toxic oil syndrome, there is fasciitis, wasting and muscle pain associated with blood and tissue eosinophilia. The lungs are affected in 60% of cases. Pulmonary symptoms have included cough, dyspnoea and chest pain. Radiographs have shown diffuse bilateral infiltrates and pulmonary hypertension has been documented in a few cases.[79]

Histology of the lungs shows an oedematous myxoid intimal thickening affecting small pulmonary blood vessels and a diffuse interstitial lymphocytic and eosinophilic infiltrate.[72,73,75,76,80] These cells may also be seen within the walls of the thickened blood vessels (Fig. 7.3.8).[72,76] Massive ingestion of L-tryptophan has resulted in the appearances of an organising pneumonia.[81]

Granulomatous alveolitis

As an adverse drug reaction, granulomatous alveolitis is best exemplified by the extrinsic allergic alveolitis of pituitary snuff-takers, but it is also encountered on rare occasions with cytotoxic and other drugs, including methotrexate, bacille Calmette–Guérin (BCG) immunisation, interferons, ciprofloxacin, antiviral therapy and tumour necrosis factor antagonists.[42–44,48,82–90] The histological appearances may suggest extrinsic allergic alveolitis or sarcoidosis but the centri-

Figure 7.3.8 L-tryptophan toxicity. (A) There is a diffuse interstitial infiltrate of lymphocytes with smaller numbers of eosinophils. (B) The same infiltrate involves pulmonary blood vessels. *(Courtesy of Dr TV Colby, Scottsdale, USA.)*

acinar or lymphangitic concentration of these conditions is usually lacking. However, unless an infective agent can be demonstrated the diagnosis generally requires consideration of the clinical and environmental details, including any drug regimen.

Aspiration lesions

Exogenous lipid pneumonia may result from the unintentional aspiration of various fat-based medicaments such as liquid paraffin, oily nose drops and petroleum jelly or of fat-rich dietary supplements in the form of ghee.[91–97] The consumption of liquid paraffin as an aperient is common in some countries and may be taking place without the knowledge of the patient's medical practitioner. Regurgitation and aspiration of ingested oil are especially likely to happen during sleep in the presence of a hiatus hernia or when the oesophagus fails to empty completely into the stomach because of achalasia of the cardia. The aspiration of vegetable oil occurred in the past from the use of menthol in olive oil for the treatment of tuberculous laryngitis, and occasionally from the use of iodinated vegetable oils for bronchography.[98–101] More recently exogenous lipid pneumonia has developed from the constant sucking of lollipops formulated for the administration of the analgesic fentanyl but also containing a stearate component.[102] The treatment of epistaxis by nasal packing with paraffin gauze has also led to exogenous lipid pneumonia. The pathology of exogenous lipid pneumonia is described on page 314. Other medicines may also be aspirated unwittingly, for example a ferrous sulphate tablet may cause brown iron staining and necrosis of the bronchus at the point of impact, progressing to bronchial stenosis.[103–105] Distal infection is then likely, as with any foreign body. Barium sulphate aspiration may complicate gastrointestinal radiography.[106] Large amounts may impair ventilation but being inert there is no permanent injury to the lungs, although the striking changes are evident on the chest radiograph.

Pulmonary hypertension

An outbreak of pulmonary hypertension affecting many Swiss, Austrian and German patients in the period 1966–68 was probably due to the anorectic drug aminorex,[107] which was accordingly withdrawn with regression in the number of new cases. The pathology in these patients was identical to that of primary pulmonary hypertension (see p. 420) and it proved impossible to reproduce the condition in laboratory animals but the epidemiological evidence that aminorex was to blame is very strong. Fenfluramine and phentermine, further anorectic drugs that are chemically similar to aminorex, have also been associated with such plexogenic pulmonary hypertension,[108–112] and with fibroproliferative plaque on the tricuspid valve and pulmonary arteries.[113]

Pulmonary hypertension due to pulmonary veno-occlusive disease has sometimes complicated the use of cytotoxic chemotherapeutic agents[114] or followed bone marrow transplantation.[115]

Non-steroidal anti-inflammatory agents such as indomethacin and diclofenac cross the placenta and, if given in late pregnancy, may cause premature closure of the ductus arteriosus, resulting in severe neonatal pulmonary hypertension.[116,117]

Pulmonary hypertension is a well-recognised association of human immunodeficiency virus (HIV) infection but until recently has been unexplained. Now, however, evidence is emerging that the highly active antiretroviral therapy administered to HIV-positive patients might be responsible for the pulmonary hypertension.[118]

Pulmonary embolism

The older high-oestrogen contraceptive drugs carried a slight risk of thromboembolism but this is not seen with the newer preparations. Pulmonary thromboembolism has also occurred with a drug-induced lupus syndrome associated with anticardiolipin antibodies. Chemotherapeutic drugs such as mitomycin may cause widespread small-vessel thrombosis resulting in the haemolytic–uraemic (thrombotic microangiopathic) syndrome. There is prominent involvement of pulmonary vessels and patients often suffer from respiratory as well as renal insufficiency, and pulmonary hypertension. The syndrome can develop during treatment or up to several months after the drug has been withdrawn. Pulmonary thromboembolism is also recorded as a complication of immunoglobulin infusion.[119]

Non-traumatic fat embolism has resulted from the agglutination or 'creaming' of fat emulsions administered intravenously as a source of calories to debilitated patients.[120–125] The agglutinated liposomes occlude fine blood vessels throughout the body, causing effects such as priapism, osteonecrosis and pancreatitis. They may be demonstrated in the pulmonary capillaries but the lungs have considerable vascular reserve and it is uncertain what effect the vascular occlusion has on pulmonary function. Agglutination of these fat emulsions is particularly common in severely ill patients and this has been attributed to the elevated blood levels of acute-phase proteins, especially C-reactive protein, that are found in the very ill. The agglutination is also induced by calcium and may be brought about by

Figure 7.3.9 Agglutination of emulsified fat administered intravenously. (A) With haematoxylin and eosin staining, seemingly empty vacuoles appear to occupy the alveolar capillaries. (B) The agglutinated fat has not been dissolved in processing and can be demonstrated by Sudan black. *(Courtesy of Dr G Hulman, Nottinghamshire, UK.)*

administering calcium and other mineral supplements through the same venous line as the fat. Once agglutinated, the fat is less soluble and may be demonstrated in paraffin sections. Sudan black is especially useful for this purpose (Fig. 7.3.9). Microvascular crystal embolism is a further risk of parenteral nutrition, the crystals representing various calcium salts that may precipitate in the circulation.[126]

Transient diffusion abnormalities attributed to oil embolism are very common in patients undergoing lymphangiography but serious respiratory impairment is limited to those patients with pre-existing lung disease or in whom substantial amounts of contrast medium are injected rapidly.[127–130]

Other emboli of an iatrogenic nature described in pulmonary arteries include the broken-off ends of intravenous catheters and cannulas, particles from dialysis tubing,[131] prosthetic implants of substances such as Teflon and silicone[88,132–135] and various materials injected to occlude abnormal blood vessels.[136,137]

Diffuse pulmonary haemorrhage

Diffuse pulmonary haemorrhage may result from interference with the clotting mechanism by anticoagulants[138] or from widespread pulmonary capillaritis, the latter reported in leukaemic patients treated with retinoic acid.[139] Pulmonary haemorrhage has also been reported as an idiosyncratic reaction to lymphangiography media[140] and as a complication of immunoglobulin infusion,[141] while the development of anti-basement membrane antibodies resulting in Goodpasture's syndrome has been attributed to penicillamine.[141a]

Opportunistic infection

Infection is a common pulmonary hazard in any patient receiving corticosteroids, chemotherapy or any other immunosuppressant drug. Viral, bacterial, fungal and protozoal infections, often in combination, may all develop in the lungs of such patients and tissue reactions may be atypical. *Pneumocystis jiroveci*, for example, may elicit a granulomatous reaction or cause diffuse alveolar damage rather than the usual foamy alveolar exudate (see p. 226).

Metastatic calcification

Metastatic calcification, described on page 489, may result from any drug causing hypercalcaemia, e.g. high doses of vitamin D, calcium and inorganic phosphate or excessive alkali intake in the treatment of peptic ulceration.

Carcinoma of the lung

Carcinoma of the lung may be promoted by drugs. Arsenicals cause squamous metaplasia of the bronchi and occasionally squamous carcinoma, while peripheral scar cancers, usually adenocarcinomas, have developed in lungs showing fibrosis due to drugs such as busulphan.

Pleural disease

Drugs may result in a variety of pleural diseases.[142] Common examples include effusions, chronic inflammation and fibrosis. These are usually encountered in isolation but may be associated with chronic interstitial pneumonia or fibrosis. Sometimes there is also serological evidence of systemic lupus erythematosus: many drugs, including hydantoin, practolol, procainamide, hydralazine and sulphonamides, are associated with the development of a syndrome resembling systemic lupus erythematosus that includes pleural disease. Whether the drugs are directly responsible for the syndrome or merely promote the development of latent natural disease is uncertain.

Ergotamine derivatives such as methysergide and bromocriptine are notable for the production of pleural fibrosis, which is sometimes associated with mediastinal and retroperitoneal fibrosis large amounts or prolonged treatment are generally required to produce this effect.[143-145] In patients given practolol, pleural thickening has become evident several years after the drug was discontinued. This shows the need for a careful drug history in any patient with unexplained pleural fibrosis.

RADIATION INJURY

Reports of radiation-induced lung damage began to appear soon after ionising radiation became widely used in the treatment of malignant disease.[146-148] Despite refinements in radiotherapy techniques it is often impossible to avoid irradiating small areas of lung when treating cancer of the lung, breast, spine, thymus and oesophagus. Parts of the lungs are also included in 'mantle' irradiation of mediastinal lymph nodes affected by lymphoma. Occasionally, the whole of both lungs is irradiated, as in the treatment of widespread pulmonary metastases or as part of whole-body irradiation prior to marrow transplantation for the treatment of leukaemia. Radiation pneumonitis, usually localised, is estimated to affect about 8% of patients.[149]

Therapeutic irradiation is given as divided doses over several weeks in order to minimise damage to adjacent tissue. The effects of such fractionated treatment are cumulative. In the lungs an early exudative phase soon passes and progressive damage becomes apparent only after months or even years.[150,151] The changes are generally confined to the area of lung that is irradiated but are widespread when the whole body is irradiated prior to bone marrow transplantation or there is accidental whole-body irradiation. However, localised irradiation of the lung has been followed by abnormalities in non-irradiated areas. These include bilateral alveolar exudates,[152] migratory organising pneumonia affecting both lungs[153,154] and fulminant bilateral interstitial pneumonia.[155] The likelihood of lung injury is increased by the simultaneous use of cytotoxic drugs and oxygen therapy.[156] Furthermore, chemotherapy following irradiation may result in exacerbation of the injury in areas previously irradiated, a phenomenon termed 'recall pneumonitis'.[157,158] In the long term, irradiation also results in an increased incidence of lung carcinoma. This was seen in patients given therapeutic irradiation to the spine for ankylosing spondylitis[159] and is still encountered on occasion following irradiation for breast cancer.[160] The pathogenesis of radiation injury is described on page 146.

Radiation damage to the lung is traditionally separated into fulminant acute injury coming on within days, subacute pneumonitis developing within several weeks (typically 2–3 months) and interstitial fibrosis slowly evolving from the subacute stage or making itself apparent years later. The migratory organising pneumonia referred to above is an unusual further effect, as is chronic eosinophilic pneumonia.[68] In the pleura, radiation causes fibrinous effusions and adhesions. Pleural effusion and pulmonary oedema may be augmented by the long-term effects of radiation on the heart.

Fulminant acute injury is an unusual and unexpected effect of therapeutic radiation but one that is likely to come to the attention of the pathologist as an autopsy is often requested. The clinical features are those of acute lung injury and the pathological changes are those of diffuse alveolar damage. The cause is likely to be accidental overdosage, augmentation of the radiation damage by accompanying oxygen therapy or treatment with cytotoxic drugs. Occasionally however these factors can be excluded, in which case the damage has to be ascribed to 'hypersensitivity'.

Subacute radiation pneumonitis is encountered more commonly. After an interval of about 2–3 months the patient complains of shortness of breath and a non-productive cough. The chest radiograph shows hazy opacification proceeding to more dense consolidation. Lung biopsy shows alveolar and interstitial oedema, possibly with residual hyaline membranes, proliferation of atypical alveolar epithelial cells and interstitial fibroblasts and organising thrombosis. Later, as the process advances, there is widespread fibrosis comparable to that illustrated in Figure 4.24 on page 148 and ultimately dense scarring (Fig. 7.3.10).

Tracheal and aortic injury may complicate radiation treatment of tracheal lesions, sometimes resulting in an aortotracheal fistula.[161]

RESPIRATOR LUNG AND OXYGEN TOXICITY

Patients requiring mechanical ventilation are liable to suffer lung injury in a number of ways. In addition to effects of barotrauma such as pneumothorax and surgical emphysema, they often develop diffuse alveolar damage. The high oxygen tension that is often combined with

Figure 7.3.10 Radiation damage. A dense scar is seen in an area of the lung that had been irradiated previously.

mechanical ventilation is a major factor[162-164] but mechanical forces other than the high pressures responsible for barotrauma can also contribute to this form of lung injury, notably by resulting in excessive end-expiratory stretch and repeated collapse/recruitment of the alveolar walls.[165,166] Low tidal volume ventilation is therefore a fundamental part of the management of diffuse alveolar damage.

Although oxygen is necessary to life, it is cytotoxic in high concentrations. Severe hyperoxia damages DNA, inhibits cellular proliferation and ultimately kills cells. Its toxicity is thought to be due to the intracellular production of active oxygen radicals, some of which derive from activated neutrophils attracted to the site of injury.[167-170] Under normal conditions most of the oxygen is reduced to water by cytochrome oxidase, and any active radicals produced are eliminated by superoxide dismutase, catalase and other antioxidants. However, these defence mechanisms may prove inadequate when active radicals are produced in excess.[171]

Problems are likely to arise in clinical practice when lung disease necessitates the concentration of oxygen in the inspired air being raised in order to maintain normal blood levels of oxygen and prevent cerebral hypoxia.[172-174] A 'safe' level for oxygen administration is not firmly established and, because of species differences in susceptibility to oxygen, caution is needed in extrapolating from animal studies. However, animal experiments have shown that previous damage to the lungs renders them unduly sensitive to oxygen[175,176] and conversely that prior exposure to high levels of oxygen confers some resistance to subsequent oxygen exposure.[177] Clinical studies suggest that less than 50% oxygen (at atmospheric pressure) can be tolerated for long periods without ill effect. Little, if any, serious lung damage results from administration of 100% oxygen for up to 48 hours but concentrations between 50% and 100% carry a risk of damage if this period is exceeded.[171,178] Extracorporeal oxygenation of the blood circumvents the problem but if it is to be prolonged it becomes a

major undertaking that poses its own hazards; it is therefore generally reserved for patients who remain hypoxaemic despite other measures.[179] Intravenous blood oxygenators are employed to minimise the supplementation of inspired oxygen and partial liquid ventilation utilising perfluorocarbon has also been used.[180] Experimentally, disruption of CD40 binding to reduce the release of proinflammatory cytokines has shown promising results in blunting oxygen-induced lung injury.[181]

None of the morphological changes attributable to oxygen toxicity is specific.[174] The earliest ultrastructural change in experimental oxygen poisoning is swelling of endothelial cells, the cytoplasm of which becomes grossly oedematous and vacuolated. Swelling and fragmentation of type I epithelial cells follow and these cells become separated from their basement membrane, which is then coated by thin strands of protein.[178] This coating is replaced by proliferating type II cells by the 12th day. With recovery in room air the lungs practically return to normal.[182] The full clinical picture of oxygen poisoning is the acute respiratory distress syndrome and the corresponding pathological changes are those of diffuse alveolar damage,[174] as described on page 136.

BLOOD TRANSFUSION

Patients with hypovolaemic shock or undergoing major surgery often require massive blood transfusions and this provides another possible cause of pulmonary damage. Although hypervolaemia is the commonest cause of pulmonary oedema after blood transfusion, transfusion-related acute lung injury is more often fatal. Platelet and white cell aggregates are known to develop in stored blood, but a relationship between the number of microaggregates transfused and the degree of respiratory impairment has not been convincingly demonstrated. Leukocyte antibodies are a more likely cause of lung injury in these patients. Such antibodies are often found in multiparous female donors as a result of sensitisation by fetal white cells during pregnancy. Alternatively, the recipient may have developed them during pregnancy or as a result of previous blood transfusions. The implicated antibodies are thought to initiate alveolar capillary damage within hours of transfusion by stimulating granulocyte aggregation.[183,184] Electron microscopy has shown capillary endothelial damage with activated granulocytes in contact with alveolar basement membranes.[185]

CARDIOPULMONARY BYPASS

Cardiopulmonary bypass entails oxygenation and circulation of the blood by extracorporeal devices, so permitting major heart surgery. In the early days of such surgery it was not unusual for patients to develop fatal respiratory insufficiency in the postoperative period. This led to the term 'postperfusion lung'. Electron microscopic studies showed alveolar damage with degranulation of neutrophils in pulmonary capillaries.[186,187] The syndrome is now less common but infants remain susceptible.[188]

The most likely explanation is that the synthetic materials with which blood comes into contact during the bypass procedure are able to activate complement. This is mediated by Hageman factor (factor XII) and the alternative pathway. Aggregation of neutrophils leads to their sequestration in the lungs and damage results from their release of lysosomal enzymes and active radicals.[188-190] The process is delayed by hypothermia.[189]

COMPLICATIONS OF CARDIAC INJURY

A postcardiac injury syndrome develops after a variety of myocardial or pericardial injuries: it has been described after cardiac surgery (post-pericardiotomy syndrome), myocardial infarction (Dressler's syndrome), blunt trauma to the chest, percutaneous puncture of the heart and implantation of a pacemaker.[191] There is a delay of anything between a few days and a few months between the cardiac injury and the onset of symptoms, which comprise chest pain, breathlessness, dyspnoea and fever. Examination usually reveals haemorrhagic pleural or pericardial effusions and pulmonary infiltrates. The syndrome usually resolves spontaneously and few pathological studies have therefore been conducted. However, the changes of diffuse alveolar damage have been reported, principally hyaline membrane formation and type II pneumocyte hyperplasia.[192] The pathogenesis is obscure. Antibodies reacting with myocardial antigens often develop after cardiac surgery but there is no relationship between these and the development of the syndrome.[192–194]

COMPLICATIONS OF RADIOFREQUENCY ABLATION

This minimally invasive technique is used to destroy lesions as varied as pulmonary metastases and the connection between the left atrium and ectopic foci in the muscular sleeves that surround the terminations of the pulmonary veins (see p. 76). The former may be complicated by pneumothorax and the latter by pulmonary vein stenosis.[195,196]

COMPLICATIONS OF CENTRAL VASCULAR CANNULATION

Central venous cannulation (synonym: catheterisation) is widely used in treating seriously ill patients and may give rise to serious complications. The commonest early complications related to the respiratory tract are caused by local trauma: they include pneumothorax, subcutaneous emphysema, haemothorax and air embolism. Infection occurs later, causing endocarditis, septic emboli and lung abscesses.[197] Thrombosis is another common late complication: one autopsy study of patients with central venous lines showed that 15% had major pulmonary emboli and 65% had microscopic emboli in their pulmonary arteries.[198] Pulmonary artery cannulation, for example with a Swan–Ganz catheter, may result in pulmonary infarction or any of the traumatic complications of central venous catheterisation mentioned above.

COMPLICATIONS OF TRACHEAL MANIPULATIONS[199,200]

Tracheotomy entails a small immediate risk of haemorrhage from damaged subthyroidal arteries, while an endotracheal tube predisposes to infection, as with all foreign bodies. Infection is also promoted by the filtering action of the upper respiratory air passages being bypassed. The latter factor also necessitates humidification of the inspired air and on occasion the humidifier or ventilator has become contaminated so that an aerosol of bacteria is introduced directly into the lower respiratory tract.[201] High-pressure ventilation

Figure 7.3.11 Tracheal stenosis following prolonged intubation. The tracheal wall shows fibrosis while the tracheal cartilage is dysplastic and shows osseous metaplasia, appearances similar to those seen in relapsing polychondritis (compare with Fig. 3.4, p. 95).

may also lead to interstitial emphysema, pneumothorax and surgical emphysema.

Asphyxia may follow an endotracheal tube becoming blocked by secretions or through it being badly positioned. Secretions need to be constantly removed yet repeated suctioning to achieve this has led to cardiac dysrrythmia and even cardiac arrest.[202]

If the balloon on the endotracheal tube is too near the tracheostomy it may act as a fulcrum, causing the tip of the tube to press into the tracheal wall. Pressure necrosis and perforation may follow, leading to mediastinitis, tracheo-oesophageal fistula or erosion of a large blood vessel. These are also complications of tracheobronchial laser therapy.

Pressure from the balloon may lead to a tracheal diverticulum and after the tube is withdrawn the trachea may become narrowed at either the site of the incision or further down where the balloon on the tracheal tube causes pressure. Small, shallow ulcers generally heal quickly but deeper ulcers cause necrosis of the tracheal cartilage, and healing is then often accompanied by fibrous stenosis (Fig. 7.3.11) or web formation. This results in wheezing and dyspnoea but not before the trachea has narrowed to 30% of its original size, which may take months. Earlier narrowing may be caused by oedema or a fibrinous pseudomembrane.[203,204] Sometimes the stenosis takes the form of a large mass of granulation tissue at the tracheostomy site, a so-called granuloma ball. In children especially, intubation may lead to tracheomalacia so that after the tube is removed the airway collapses.[205] Necrotising sialometaplasia is a further complication of prolonged intubation.[206] The incidence of such posttracheostomy complications can be minimised by careful placement of the stoma and tube, avoidance of large apertures and high cuff pressures, elimination of heavy connecting equipment and meticulous care of the tracheostomy.

Nasogastric feeding tubes may of course lead to aspiration lesions in the lungs and even fatal asphyxia if they are inadvertently allowed to enter the trachea rather than the oesophagus.

COMPLICATIONS OF BRONCHOSCOPY

Bronchoscopy is generally a safe, almost routine procedure. A review of 23 862 patients who underwent bronchoscopy identified severe complications in 152 (0.637%), of whom three died.[207] The fatal cases comprised a 78-year-old with coronary heart disease who developed cardiac arrest and two patients who had had tracheal transplantation for oesophageal cancer and required bronchoscopic laser treatment but died of airway obstruction.

COMPLICATIONS OF THORACIC DRAINAGE TUBES

The pleural cavity is intubated in the treatment of pneumothorax and pleural effusions the tube being placed anteriorly to drain air and posteriorly to drain fluid. Complications include laceration of an intercostal artery or vein, the lung, the diaphragm and the heart.

PNEUMONECTOMY[208]

Pneumonectomy has been practised since the 1930s, since when the mortality associated with this operation has dropped from over 50% to near zero in the best hospitals. Risk factors include underlying lung disease, other medical conditions and more extensive procedures such as pleuropneumonectomy and pneumonectomy combined with chest wall resection.

The anatomical changes that take place soon after pneumonectomy have been extensively studied by radiologists who describe the air-filled postpneumonectomy space gradually filling with fluid and contracting as the mediastinum shifts and the ipsilateral dome of the diaphragm rises.[209] Much of the space is filled by fluid within 2 weeks but complete opacification may take up to 6 months. Rapid filling in the immediate postoperative period suggests haemorrhage or chylothorax. However, fluid accumulation is normally rapid after pleuro-

pneumonectomy and may compromise the function of the other lung.

Pathologists conducting autopsies long after the operation may find complete fibrous obliteration of the postpneumonectomy space, coupled with mediastinal shift and elevation of the hemidiaphragm, but often there is persistent brown fluid, which may be clear, cloudy or occasionally purulent.[210] The remaining lung is generally enlarged, with its volume greater than predicted. Animal studies have shown that if one lung is excised early in life the enlargement is partly due to enhanced growth but later it represents only dilatation of existing air spaces. Hepatocyte growth factor is thought to be involved in the proliferation of residual lung cells following pneumonectomy.[211]

Pulmonary complications include those typically seen after other thoracic procedures, such as haemorrhage and infection, and those unique to the postpneumonectomy state, namely anastomotic dehiscence and postpneumonectomy pulmonary oedema. The latter presents as the acute respiratory distress syndrome and represents the early stages of diffuse alveolar damage. It follows severe shift of the heart and mediastinum, which is commoner in children and young adults, in whom the tissues are more compliant.[212–215] The condition complicates up to 4% of lung resections[216,217] and is commoner following excision of the right lung when severe herniation of the left lung into the postpneumonectomy space stretches the trachea and left main bronchus and the latter is compressed between the left pulmonary artery in front and the arch of the aorta behind. In the long term the compression can result in bronchomalacia and postobstructive bronchiectasis. If postpneumonectomy oedema develops the immediate postoperative mortality is high – 50% following pneumonectomy, 42% following lobectomy and 22% following sublobar resections.[217,218] The pathogenesis is probably multifactorial but apart from factors such as fluid overload and high inspired oxygen concentrations there is probably an element of alveolar wall injury, induced by oxidant generation secondary to lung stretching and general surgical trauma.[219,220]

REFERENCES

Adverse drug reactions

1. Shapiro S, Slone D, Lewis GP, et al. Fatal drug reactions among medical inpatients. JAMA 1971;216:467–72.
2. Roughead EE, Gilbert AL, Primrose JG, et al. Drug-related hospital admissions: a review of Australian studies published 1988–1996. Med J Aust 1998;168:405–8.
3. Lazarou J, Pomeranz BH, Corey PN. Incidence of adverse drug reactions in hospitalized patients: a meta-analysis of prospective studies (see comments). JAMA 1998;279:1200–5.
4. Wilson RM, Runciman WB, Gibberd RW, et al. The Quality in Australian Health Care Study. Med J Aust 1995;163: 458–71.
5. Vervloet D, Durham S. Adverse reactions to drugs. BMJ 1998;316:1511–4.
6. Rosenow EC, Myers JL, Swensen SJ, et al. Drug-induced pulmonary disease – an update. Chest 1992;102:239–50.
7. Hutchinson TA, Leventhal JM, Kramer MS, et al. An algorithm for the operational assessment of adverse drug reactions. II. Demonstration of reproducibility and validity. JAMA 1979;242:633–8.

8. Van Arsdel PP. Aspirin idiosyncrasy and tolerance. J Allergy Clin Immunol 1984;73:431–4.
9. Ameisen JC, Capron A, Joseph M, et al. Aspirin-sensitive asthma: abnormal platelet response to drugs inducing asthmatic attacks; diagnostic and physiopathological implications. Int Arch Allergy Appl Immunol 1985;78:438–48.
10. Lee TH. Mechanism of aspirin sensitivity. Am Rev Respir Dis 1992;145:S34–6.
11. Epler GR, Snider GL, Gaensler EA, et al. Bronchiolitis and bronchitis in connective tissue disease. A possible relationship to the use of penicillamine. JAMA 1979;242:528–32.
12. Boehler A, Vogt P, Speich R, et al. Bronchiolitis obliterans in a patient with localized scleroderma treated with D-penicillamine. Eur Respir J 1996;9:1317–9.
13. Schwartzman KJ, Bowie DM, Yeadon C, et al. Constrictive bronchiolitis obliterans following gold therapy for psoriatic arthritis. Eur Respir J 1995;8:2191–3.
14. Tomioka H, King TE. Gold-induced pulmonary disease: clinical features,

outcome, and differentiation from rheumatoid lung disease. Amer J Respir Crit Care Med 1997;155:1011–20.
15. Geddes DM, Corrin B, Brewerton DA, et al. Progressive airway obliteration in adults and its association with rheumatoid disease. Q J Med 1977;46:427–44.
16. Camus P, Foucher P, Bonniaud P, et al. Drug-induced infiltrative lung disease. Eur Resp J 2001;18:93S–100S.
17. Camus P, Bonniaud P, Fanton A, et al. Drug-induced and iatrogenic infiltrative lung disease. Clin Chest Med 2004;25:479–519, vi.
18. Camus P, Kudoh S, Ebina M. Interstitial lung disease associated with drug therapy. Br J Cancer 2004;91:S18–23.
19. Tenenbein M, Kowalski S, Sienko A, et al. Pulmonary toxic effects of continuous desferrioxamine administration in acute iron poisoning. Lancet 1992;339:699–701.
20. Oliner H, Schwartz R, Rubio R, et al. Interstitial pulmonary fibrosis following busulfan therapy. Am J Med 1961;31:134–9.
21. Heard BE, Cooke RA. Busulphan lung. Thorax 1968;23:187–93.

22. Burns WA, McFarland W, Matthews MJ. Busulphan-induced pulmonary disease. Report of a case and review of the literature. Am Rev Respir Dis 1970;101:408–13.

23. Podoll LN, Winkler SS. Busulfan lung: report of two cases and review of the literature. AJR Am J Roentgenol 1974;120:151–6.

24. Elias AD, Mark EJ, Trotman-Dickenson B. A 60-year-old man with pulmonary infiltrates after a bone marrow transplantation – Busulfan pneumonitis. N Engl J Med 1997;337:480–9.

25. Cooper JAD, White DA, Matthay RA. Drug-induced pulmonary disease. Am Rev Respir Dis 1986;133:321–40.

26. Moseley PL, Shasby DM, Brady M, et al. Lung parenchymal injury induced by bleomycin. Am Rev Respir Dis 1984;130:1082–6.

27. Slavin RE, Millan JC, Mullins CM. Pathology of high dose intermittent cyclophosphamide therapy. Hum Pathol 1975;6:693–709.

28. Mark GJ, Lehimgar-Zaden A, Ragsdale BD. Cyclophosphamide pneumonitis. Thorax 1978;33:89–93.

29. Taetle R, Dickman PS, Feldman PS. Pulmonary histopathologic changes associated with melphalan therapy. Cancer 1978;42:1239–45.

30. Goucher G, Rowland V, Hawkins J. Melphalan-induced pulmonary interstitial fibrosis. Chest 1980;77:805–6.

31. Tryka AF, Skornik WA, Godlaski JJ, et al. Potentiation of bleomycin-induced lung injury by exposure to 70% oxygen. Am Rev Respir Dis 1982;126:1074–9.

32. Goldiner PL, Carlon GC, Cvitkovik E, et al. Factors influencing postoperative morbidity and mortality in patients treated with bleomycin. BMJ 1978;i:1664–7.

33. Alan SC, Riddell GS, Butchart EG. Bleomycin therapy and anaesthesia. Anaesthesia 1981;36:60–3.

34. Hulbert JC, Grossman JE, Cummings KB. Risk factors of anesthesia and surgery in bleomycin-treated patients. J Urol 1983;130:163–4.

35. Adamson IYR, Bowden DH. The pathogenesis of bleomycin-induced pulmonary damage in mice. Am J Pathol 1974;77:185–97.

36. Bedrossian CWM, Greenberg SD, Yawn DH, et al. Experimentally induced bleomycin sulfate toxicity. Arch Pathol Lab Med 1977;101:248–54.

37. Gyorkey F, Gyorkey P, Sinkovics JG. Origin and significance of intranuclear tubular inclusions in type II pulmonary alveolar epithelial cells of patients with bleomycin and busulfan toxicity. Ultrastruct Pathol 1980;1:211–21.

38. Hasleton PS, O'Driscoll BR, Lynch P, et al. Late BCNU lung – a light and ultrastructural study on the delayed effect of BCNU on the lung parenchyma. J Pathol 1991;164:31–6.

39. Lantuejoul S, Brambilla E, Brambilla C, et al. Statin-induced fibrotic nonspecific interstitial pneumonia. Eur Resp J 2002;19:577–80.

40. Camus P, Lombard JN, Perrichon M, et al. Bronchiolitis obliterans organizing pneumonia during treatment with acebutolol and amiodarone. Thorax 1989;44:711–5.

41. Sastman HD, Matthay RA, Putman CE. Methotrexate-induced pneumonitis (Baltimore). Medicine (Baltimore) 1976;55:371–88.

42. White DA, Rankin JA, Stover DE, et al. Methotrexate pneumonitis. Bronchoalveolar lavage findings suggest an immunologic disorder. Am Rev Respir Dis 1989;139:18–21.

43. Leduc D, Devuyst P, Lheureux P, et al. Pneumonitis complicating low-dose methotrexate therapy for rheumatoid arthritis – discrepancies between lung biopsy and bronchoalveolar lavage findings. Chest 1993;104:1620–3.

44. Imokawa S, Colby TV, Leslie KO, et al. Methotrexate pneumonitis: review of the literature and histopathological findings in nine patients. Eur Resp J 2000;15:373–81.

45. Ginsberg SJ, Comis RL. The pulmonary toxicity of antineoplastic agents. Semin Oncol 1982;9:34–5.

46. Scott DL, Bradby GVH, Aitman TJ, et al. Relationship of gold and penicillamine therapy to diffuse interstitial lung disease. Proc Soc Exp Biol Med 1981;40:136–41.

47. Bone RC, Wolfe J, Sobonya RE, et al. Desquamative interstitial pneumonia following long-term nitrofurantoin therapy. Am J Med 1976;60:697–701.

48. Magee F, Wright JL, Chan N, et al. Two unusual pathological reactions to nitrofurantoin: case reports. Histopathology 1986;10:701–6.

49. Cameron RJ, Kolbe J, Wilsher ML, et al. Bronchiolitis obliterans organising pneumonia associated with the use of nitrofurantoin. Thorax 2000;55:249–51.

50. Costa-Jussa FR, Corrin B, Jacobs JM. Amiodarone lung toxicity: a human and experimental study. J Pathol 1984;144:73–9.

51. Jacobson W, Stewart S, Gresham GA, et al. Effect of amiodarone on the lung shown by polarized light microscopy. Arch Pathol Lab Med 1997;121:1269–71.

52. Vijeyaratnam GS, Corrin B. Fine structural alterations in the lungs of iprindole-treated rats. J Pathol 1974;114:233–9.

53. Heath D, Smith P, Hasleton PS. Effects of chlorphentermine on the rat lung. Thorax 1973;28:551–8.

54. Akoun GM, Gauthier-Rahman S, Milleron BJ, et al. Amiodarone-induced hypersensitivity pneumonitis. Evidence of an immunological cell-mediated mechanism. Chest 1984;85:133–5.

55. Darmanata JI, van Zandwijk N, Duren DR, et al. Amiodarone pneumonitis: three further cases with a review of published reports. Thorax 1984;39:57–64.

56. Dean PJ, Groshart KD, Porterfield JG, et al. Amiodarone-associated pulmonary toxicity. A clinical and pathologic study of eleven cases. Am J Clin Pathol 1987;87:7–13.

57. Myers JL, Kennedy JI, Plumb VJ. Amiodarone lung: pathologic findings in clinically toxic patients. Hum Pathol 1987;18:349–54.

58. Oren S, Turkot S, Golzman B, et al. Amiodarone-induced bronchiolitis obliterans organizing pneumonia (BOOP). Respir Med 1996;90:167–9.

59. Kimura T, Kuramochi S, Katayama T, et al. Amiodarone-related pulmonary mass and unique membranous glomerulonephritis in a patient with valvular heart disease: Diagnostic pitfall and new findings. Pathol Int 2008;58:657–63.

60. Ruangchira-Urai R, Colby TV, Klein J, et al. Nodular amiodarone lung disease. Am J Surg Pathol 2008;32:1654–60.

61. Polkey MI, Wilson POG, Rees PJ. Amiodarone pneumonitis: no safe dose. Respir Med 1995;89:233–5.

62. Hargreaves MR, Benson MK. Amiodarone pneumonitis: no safe dose. Respir Med 1996;90:119.

63. Wilson BD, Lippmann ML. Susceptibility to amiodarone-induced pulmonary toxicity: relationship to the uptake of amiodarone by isolated lung cells. Lung 1996;174:31–41.

64. Handschin AE, Lardinois D, Schneiter D, et al. Acute amiodarone-induced pulmonary toxicity following lung resection. Respiration 2003;70:310–12.

65. Vijeyaratnam GS, Corrin B. Pulmonary alveolar proteinosis developing from desquamative interstitial pneumonia in long term toxicity studies of iprindole in the rat. Virchows Arch A Pathol Anat Histopathol 1973;358:1–10.

66. Allen JN, Davis WB. Eosinophilic lung diseases. Am J Respir Crit Care Med 1994;150:1423–38.

67. Tanigawa K, Sugiyama K, Matsuyama H, et al. Mesalazine-induced eosinophilic pneumonia. Respiration 1999;66:69–72.

68. Cottin V, Frognier R, Monnot H, et al. Chronic eosinophilic pneumonia after radiation therapy for breast cancer. Eur Resp J 2004;23:9–13.

69. Wechsler ME, Finn D, Gunawardena D, et al. Churg–Strauss syndrome in patients receiving montelukast as treatment for asthma. Chest 2000;117:708–13.

70. LeGall C, Pham S, Vignes S, et al. Inhaled corticosteroids and Churg–Strauss syndrome: a report of five cases. Eur Resp J 2000;15:978–81.

71. Faller M, Gasser B, Massard G, et al. Pulmonary migratory infiltrates and pachypleuritis in a patient with Crohn's disease. Respiration 2000;67:459–63.

72. Tazelaar HD, Myers JL, Drage CW, et al. Pulmonary disease associated with L-tryptophan-induced eosinophilic myalgia syndrome. Clinical and pathologic features. Chest 1990;97:1032–6.

73. Flannery MT, Wallach PM, Espinoza LR, et al. A case of the eosinophilia-myalgia syndrome associated with use of an L-tryptophan product. Ann Intern Med 1990;112:300–1.

74. Belongia EA, Hedberg CW, Gleich GJ, et al. An investigation of the cause of the eosinophilia–myalgia syndrome associated with tryptophan use. N Engl J Med 1990;323:357–65.

75. Herrick MK, Chang Y, Horoupian DS, et al. L-tryptophan and the eosinophilia–myalgia syndrome: pathologic findings in eight patients. Hum Pathol 1991;22:12–21.

76. Winkelmann RK, Connolly SM, Quimby SR, et al. Histopathologic features of the L-tryptophan-related eosinophilia–myalgia (fasciitis) syndrome. Mayo Clin Proc 1991;66:457–63.

77. Mayeno AN, Belongia EA, Lin F, et al. 3-(phenylamino)alanine, a novel aniline-derived amino acid associated with the eosinophilia–myalgia syndrome – a link to the toxic oil syndrome. Mayo Clin Proc 1992;67:1134–9.

78. Illa I, Dinsmore S, Dalakas MC. Immune-mediated mechanisms and immune activation of fibroblasts in the pathogenesis of eosinophilia-myalgia syndrome induced by L-tryptophan. Hum Pathol 1993;24:702–9.

79. Cheng TO. Pulmonary hypertension in patients with eosinophilia–myalgia syndrome or toxic oil syndrome. Mayo Clin Proc 1993;68:823.

80. Tazelaar HD, Myers JL, Strickler JG, et al. Tryptophan-induced lung disease – an immunophenotypic, immunofluorescent, and electron microscopic study. Mod Pathol 1993;6:56–60.

81. Mar KE, Sen P, Tan K, et al. Bronchiolitis obliterans organizing pneumonia associated with massive L-tryptophan ingestion. Chest 1993;104:1924–6.

82. Clarysse AM, Cathey WJ, Cartwright GE, et al. Pulmonary disease complicating intermittent therapy with methotrexate. JAMA 1969;209:1861–4.

83. Hasan FM, Mark EJ. Case records of the Massachusetts General Hospital. A 28-year-old man with increasing dyspnea, dry cough, and fever after chemotherapy for lymphoma. N Engl J Med 1990;323:737–47.

84. Pietropaoli A, Modrak J, Utell M. Interferon-alpha therapy associated with the development of sarcoidosis. Chest 1999;116:569–72.

85. Ayers MM, Jeffery PK. Proliferation and differentiation in mammalian airway epithelium. Eur Respir J 1988;1:58–80.

86. Naccache JM, Antoine M, Wislez M, et al. Sarcoid-like pulmonary disorder in human immunodeficiency virus-infected patients receiving antiretroviral therapy. Amer J Respir Crit Care Med 1999;159:2009–13.

87. Steiger D, Bubendorf L, Oberholzer M, et al. Ciprofloxacin-induced acute interstitial pneumonitis. Eur Resp J 2004;23:172–4.

88. Vavricka SR, Wettstein T, Speich R, et al. Pulmonary granulomas after tumour necrosis factor alpha antagonist therapy. Thorax 2003;58:278–9.

89. O'Shea FD, Marras TK, Inman RD. Pulmonary sarcoidosis developing during infliximab therapy. Arthritis Rheum 2006;55:978–81.

90. Kudrin A, Chilvers ER, Ginawi A, et al. Sarcoid-like granulomatous disease following etanercept treatment for RA. J Rheumatol 2007;34:648–9.

91. Elston CW. Pneumonia due to liquid paraffin: with chemical analysis. Arch Dis Child 1966;41:428–34.

92. Salm R, Hughes EW. A case of chronic paraffin pneumonitis. Thorax 1970;25:762–8.

93. Fox B. Liquid paraffin pneumonia – with chemical analysis and electron microscopy. Virchows Arch A Pathol Anat Histopathol 1979;382:339–46.

94. Corrin B, Crocker PR, Hood BJ, et al. Paraffinoma confirmed by infrared spectrophotometry. Thorax 1987;42:389–90.

95. Wagner JC, Adler DI, Fuller DN. Foreign body granulomata of the lungs due to liquid paraffin. Thorax 1955;10:157–70.

96. Brown AC, Slocum PC, Putthoff SL, et al. Exogenous lipoid pneumonia due to nasal application of petroleum jelly. Chest 1994;105:968–9.

97. Annobil SH, Morad NA, Khurana P, et al. Reaction of human lungs to aspirated animal fat (ghee): a clinicopathological study. Virchows Arch 1995;426:301–5.

98. Rayl JE. Clinical reactions following bronchography. Ann Otol Rhinol Laryngol 1965;74:1120–32.

99. Felton WL. The reaction of pulmonary tissue to lipiodol. J Thorac Surg 1953;25:530–42.

100. Greenberg SD, Spjut HJ, Hallman GL. Experimental study of bronchographic media on lung. Arch Otolaryngol Head Neck Surg 1966;83:276–82.

101. Felton WL. A method for the identification of lipiodol in tissue sections. Lab Invest 1952;1:364–7.

102. Mathai SK, Rubinowitz AN, Homer RJ, et al. Of Lungs, Lipids, and Lollipops. Chest 2009;136:1420–3.

103. Lamaze R, Trechot P, Martinet Y. Bronchial necrosis and granuloma induced by the aspiration of a tablet of ferrous sulphate. Eur Respir J 1994;7:1710–1.

104. Lee P, Culver DA, Farver C, et al. Syndrome of iron pill aspiration. Chest 2002;121:1355–7.

105. Sundar KM, Elliott CG, Thomsen GE. Tetracycline aspiration – Case report and review of the literature. Respiration 2001;68:416–9.

106. Tamm I, Kortsik C. Severe barium sulfate aspiration into the lung: Clinical presentation, prognosis and therapy. Respiration 1999;66:81–4.

107. Kay JM, Smith P, Heath D. Aminorex and the pulmonary circulation. Thorax 1971;26:262–70.

108. Douglas JG, Munro JF, Kitchin AH, et al. Pulmonary hypertension and fenfluramine. BMJ 1981;283:881–3.

109. McMurray J, Bloomfield P, Miller HC. Irreversible pulmonary hypertension after treatment with fenfluramine. BMJ 1986;292:239–40.

110. Kay JM. Dietary pulmonary hypertension. Thorax 1994;49:S33–8.

111. Abenhaim L, Moride Y, Brenot F, et al. Appetite-suppressant drugs and the risk of primary pulmonary hypertension. N Engl J Med 1996;335:609–16.

112. Mark EJ, Patalas ED, Chang HT, et al. Fatal pulmonary hypertension associated with short-term use of fenfluramine and phentermine. N Engl J Med 1997;337:602–6.

113. Tomita T, Zhao Q. Autopsy findings of heart and lungs in a patient with primary pulmonary hypertension associated with use of fenfluramine and phentermine. Chest 2002;121:649–52.

114. Lombard CM, Churg A, Winokur S. Pulmonary veno-occlusive disease following therapy for malignant neoplasms. Chest 1987;92:871–6.

115. Williams LM, Fussell S, Veith RW, et al. Pulmonary veno-occlusive disease in an adult following bone marrow transplantation: case report and review of the literature. Chest 1996;109:1388–91.

116. Moise KJ Jr, Huhta JC, Sharif DS, et al. Indomethacin in the treatment of premature labor. Effects on the fetal ductus arteriosus. N Engl J Med 1988;319:327–31.

117. Auer M, Brezinka C, Eller P, et al. Prenatal diagnosis of intrauterine premature closure of the ductus arteriosus following maternal diclofenac application. Ultrasound Obstet Gynecol 2004;23:513–6.

118. Wang X, Chai H, Lin PH, et al. Roles and mechanisms of human immunodeficiency virus protease inhibitor ritonavir and other anti-human immunodeficiency virus drugs in endothelial dysfunction of porcine pulmonary arteries and human pulmonary artery endothelial cells. Am J Pathol 2009;174:771–81.

119. Alliot C, Rapin JP, Besson M, et al. Pulmonary embolism after intravenous immunoglobulin. J R Soc Med 2001;94:187–8.

120. Barson AJ, Chiswick ML, Doig CM. Fat embolism in infancy after intravenous fat infusions. Arch Dis Child 1978;53:218–23.

121. Levene MI, Wigglesworth JS, Desai R. Pulmonary fat accumulation after Intralipid infusion in the preterm infant. Lancet 1980;II:815–8.

122. Hulman G, Levene M. Intralipid microemboli. Arch Dis Child 1986;61:702–3.

123. Hulman G. The pathogenesis of fat embolism. J Pathol 1995;176:3–9.

124. Kitchell CC, Balogh K. Pulmonary lipid emboli in association with long-term hyperalimentation. Hum Pathol 1986;17:83–5.

125. Lekka ME, Liokatis S, Nathanail C, et al. The impact of intravenous fat emulsion administration in acute lung injury. Am J Resp Crit Care Med 2004;169:638–44.

126. Reedy JS, Kuhlman JE, Voytovich M. Microvascular pulmonary emboli secondary to precipitated crystals in a patient receiving total parenteral nutrition – A case report and description of the high-resolution CT findings. Chest 1999;115:892–5.

127. Gough JH, Gough MH, Thomas ML. Pulmonary complications following lymphangiography with a note on technique. Br J Radiol 1964;37: 416–21.

128. Fraimow W, Wallace S, Lewis P, et al. Changes in pulmonary function due to lymphangiography. Radiology 1965;85:231–41.

129. Davidson JW. Pulmonary complications of lymphangiography. N Engl J Med 1971;285:237.

130. Silvestri RC, Hyseby JS, Rughani I, et al. Respiratory distress syndrome from lymphangiography contrast medium. Am Rev Respir Dis 1980;122:543–9.

131. Leong AS-Y, Disney APS, Gove DW. Spallation and migration of silicone from blood-pump tubing in patients on hemodialysis. N Engl J Med 1982;306:135–40.

132. Chastre J, Basset F, Viau F, et al. Acute pneumonitis after subcutaneous injections of silicone in transsexual men. N Engl J Med 1983;308:764–7.

133. Robinson MJ, Nestor M, Rywlin AM. Pulmonary granulomas secondary to embolic prosthetic valve material. Hum Pathol 1981;12:759–62.

134. Mittleman RE, Marraccini JV. Pulmonary Teflon granulomas following periurethral Teflon injection for urinary incontinence. Arch Pathol Lab Med 1983;107:611–2.

135. Lai YF, Chao TY, Wong SL. Acute pneumonitis after subcutaneous injections of silicone for augmentation mammaplasty. Chest 1994;106:1152–5.

136. Fairfax AJ, Ball J, Batten JC, et al. A pathological study following bronchial artery embolization for haemoptysis in cystic fibrosis. Br J Dis Chest 1980;74:345–52.

137. Coard K, Silver MD, Perkins G, et al. Isobutyl-2-cyanoacrylate pulmonary emboli associated with occlusive embolotherapy of cerebral arteriovenous malformations. Histopathology 1984;8:917–26.

138. Lena H, Desrues B, Quinquenel ML, et al. Hemorragie alveolaire diffuse secondaire a l'utilisation d'anticoagulants oraux. Rev Mal Resp 1995;12:496–8.

139. Nicolls MR, Terada LS, Tuder RM, et al. Diffuse alveolar hemorrhage with underlying pulmonary capillaritis in the retinoic acid syndrome. Amer J Respir Crit Care Med 1998;158:1302–5.

140. Wiertz LM, Gagnon JH, Anthonisen NR. Intrapulmonary hemorrhage with anemia after lymphangiography. N Engl J Med 1971;285:1364–5.

141. Kalra S, Bell MR, Rihal CS. Alveolar hemorrhage as a complication of treatment with abciximab. Chest 2001;120:126–31.

141a. Sternlick I, Bennett B, Scheinberg JH. D-penicillamine induced Goodpasture's syndrome in Wilson's disease. Ann Intern Med 82:673–6.

142. Morelock SY, Sahn SA. Drugs and the pleura. Chest 1999;116:212–21.

143. Pfitzenmeyer P, Foucher P, Dennewald G, et al. Pleuropulmonary changes induced by ergoline drugs. Eur Respir J 1996;9:1013–9.

144. Comet R, Domingo C, Such JJ, et al. Pleuropulmonary disease as a side-effect of treatment with bromcriptine. Resp Med 1998;92:1172–4.

145. Danoff SK, Grasso ME, Terry PB, et al. Pleuropulmonary disease due to pergolide use for restless legs syndrome. Chest 2001;120:313–6.

Radiation injury

146. Hines LE. Fibrosis of the lung following roentgen-ray treatments for tumor. JAMA 1922;79:720–2.

147. Warren S, Spencer J. Radiation reaction in the lung. AJR Am J Roentgenol 1940;43:682–701.

148. Warren S, Gates O. Radiation pneumonitis: experimental and pathologic observations. Arch Pathol Lab Med 1940;30:440–60.

149. Roach M III, Gandara DR, Yuo HS, et al. Radiation pneumonitis following combined modality therapy for lung cancer: analysis of prognostic factors. J Clin Oncol 1995;13:2606–12.

150. Gross NJ. The pathogenesis of radiation-induced lung damage. Lung 1981;159:115–25.

151. Chandler Smith J. Radiation pneumonitis: a review. Am Rev Respir Dis 1963;87:647–55.

152. Fulkerson WJ, McLendon RE, Proznitz LR. Adult respiratory distress syndrome after limited thoracic radiotherapy. Cancer 1986;57:1941–6.

153. Crestani B, Kambouchner M, Soler P, et al. Migratory bronchiolitis obliterans organizing pneumonia after unilateral radiation therapy for breast carcinoma. Eur Respir J 1995;8:318–21.

154. Bayle JY, Nesme P, Bejui-Thivolet F, et al. Migratory organizing pneumonitis 'primed' by radiation therapy. Eur Respir J 1995;8:322–6.

155. Wharton SP, Rogers TK. Hamman–Rich syndrome 'primed' by radiation? Resp Med 1999;93:136–7.

156. Ma LD, Taylor GA, Wharam MD, et al. 'Recall' pneumonitis: adriamycin potentiation of radiation pneumonitis in two children. Radiology 1993;187: 465–7.

157. Thomas PS, Agrawal S, Gore M, et al. Recall lung pneumonitis due to carmustine after radiotherapy. Thorax 1995;50: 1116–8.

158. Movsas B, Raffin TA, Epstein AH, et al. Pulmonary radiation injury. Chest 1997;111:1061–76.

159. Court-Brown WM, Doll R. Mortality from cancer and other causes after radiotherapy for ankylosing spondylitis. BMJ 1965;2:1327–32.

160. Neugut AI, Murray T, Santos J, et al. Increased risk of lung cancer after breast cancer radiation therapy in cigarette smokers. Cancer 1994;73:1615–20.

161. Allende DS, Rodriguez ER, Tan CD. Aortotracheal fistula secondary to bacterial aortitis. Arch Pathol Lab Med 2009;133:983–6.

Respirator lung and oxygen toxicity

162. Nash G, Bowen JA, Langlinais PC. Respirator lung – a misnomer. Arch Pathol Lab Med 1972;21:234–8.

163. Pratt PC. Pathology of adult respiratory distress syndrome. In: Thurlbeck WM, Abell MR, editors. The Lung. Baltimore: Williams and Wilkins; 1978. p. 43–57.

164. Pratt PC, Vollmer RT, Shelburne JD, et al. Pulmonary morphology in a multihospital collaborative extracorporeal membrane oxygenation project. Am J Pathol 1979;95:191–214.

165. Slutsky AS. Lung injury caused by mechanical ventilation. Chest 1999;116:9S-15S.

166. Ricard JD, Dreyfuss D, Saumon G. Ventilator-induced lung injury. Eur Resp J 2003;22:2S–9S.

167. Sacks T, Moldow CF, Craddock PR, et al. Oxygen radicals mediate endothelial cell damage by complement-stimulated granulocytes. J Clin Invest 1978;61:1161–7.

168. Johnson KJ, Fantone JC, Daplan J, et al. In vitro damage of rat lungs by oxygen metabolites. J Clin Invest 1981;67:983–93.

169. Wegner CD, Wolyniec WW, Laplante AM, et al. Intercellular adhesion molecule-1 contributes to pulmonary oxygen toxicity in mice – role of leukocytes revised. Lung 1992;170:267–79.

170. Kang BH, Crapo JD, Wegner CD, et al. Intercellular adhesion molecule-1 expression on the alveolar epithelium and

its modification by hyperoxia. Am J Respir Cell Mol Biol 1993;9:350–5.

171. Deneke SM, Fanburg BL. Normobaric oxygen toxicity of the lung. N Engl J Med 1980;303:76–86.

172. Kapanci Y, Tosco R, Eggermann J, et al. Oxygen pneumonitis in man. Chest 1972;62:162–9.

173. Pratt PC. Pathology of pulmonary oxygen toxicity. Am Rev Respir Dis 1974;110:51–7.

174. Katzenstein ALA, Bloor CM, Liebow AA. Diffuse alveolar damage – the role of oxygen, shock and related factors. Am J Pathol 1976;85:210–22.

175. Haschek WM, Brody AR, Klein-Szanto AJP, et al. Diffuse interstitial pulmonary fibrosis. Pulmonary fibrosis in mice induced by treatment with butylated hydroxytoluene and oxygen. Am J Pathol 1981;105:334–5.

176. Witschi HR, Haschek WM, Klein-Szanto AJP, et al. Potentiation of diffuse lung damage by oxygen: determining values. Am Rev Respir Dis 1981;123:98–103.

177. Yamamoto E, Wittner M, Rosenbaum RM. Resistance and susceptibility to oxygen toxicity by cell types of the gas–blood barrier of the rat lung. Am J Pathol 1970;59:409–36.

178. Gould VE, Tosco R, Wheelis RF, et al. Oxygen pneumonitis in man. Ultrastructural observations on the development of the alveolar lesions. Lab Invest 1972;26:499–508.

179. Peek GJ, Moore HM, Moore N, et al. Extracorporeal membrane oxygenation for adult respiratory failure. Chest 1997;112:759–64.

180. Bruch LA, Flint A, Hirschl RB. Pulmonary pathology of patients treated with partial liquid ventilation. Mod Pathol 1997;10:463–8.

181. Adawi A, Zhang Y, Baggs R, et al. Disruption of the CD40-CD40 ligand system prevents an oxygen-induced respiratory distress syndrome. Am J Pathol 1998;152:651–7.

182. Kapanci Y, Weibel ER, Kaplan HP, et al. Pathogenesis and reversibility of the pulmonary lesions of oxygen toxicity in monkeys. II Ultrastructural and morphometric studies. Lab Invest 1969;20:101–18.

Blood transfusion

183. Popovsky MA, Abel MD, Moore SB. Transfusion-related acute lung injury associated with passive transfer of antileukocyte antibodies. Am Rev Respir Dis 1983;128:185–9.

184. Divertie MB. Diffuse alveolar damage, respiratory failure and blood transfusion. Mayo Clin Proc 1984;59:643–4.

185. Dry SM, Bechard KM, Milford EL, et al. The pathology of transfusion-related acute lung injury. Amer J Clin Pathol 1999;112:216–21.

Cardiopulmonary bypass

186. Ratliff NB, Youg WG, Hackol DB, et al. Pulmonary injury – secondary to extracorporeal circulation. J Thorac Cardiovasc Surg 1973;65:425–32.

187. Asada S, Yamaguchi M. Fine structural changes in the lungs following cardiopulmonary bypass. Chest 1971;59:478–83.

188. Westaby S. Complement and the damaging effects of cardiopulmonary bypass. Thorax 1983;38:321–5.

189. Tonz M, Mihaljevic T, Vonsegesser LK, et al. Acute lung injury during cardiopulmonary bypass: are the neutrophils responsible? Chest 1995;108:1551–6.

190. Wan S, LeClerc JL, Vincent JL. Inflammatory response to cardiopulmonary bypass: Mechanisms involved and possible therapeutic strategies. Chest 1997;112:676–92.

Complications of cardiac injury

191. Stelzner TJ, King TE, Antony VB, et al. The pleuropulmonary manifestations of the postcardiac injury syndrome. Chest 1983;84:383.

192. Weiser NJ, Kantor M, Russell HK, et al. The postmyocardial infarction syndrome. The nonspecificity of the pulmonary manifestations. Circulation 1962;25:643–50.

193. Khan AH. The postcardiac injury syndromes. Clin Cardiol 1992;15:67–72.

194. Akl ES, Latif N, Dunn MJ, et al. Antiheart antibodies following open heart surgery: incidence and correlation with postpericardiotomy syndrome. Eur J Cardiothorac Surg 1992;6:503–7.

Complications of radiofrequency ablation

195. Gillams AR, Lees WR. Analysis of the factors associated with radiofrequency ablation-induced pneumothorax. Clin Radiol 2007;62:639–44.

195a. Yang HM, Lai CK, Patel J, et al. Irreversible intrapulmonary vascular changes after pulmonary vein stenosis complicating catheter ablation for atrial fibrillation. Cardiovasc Pathol 2007;16:51–5.

196. Kojodjojo P, Wong T, Wright AR, et al. Pulmonary venous stenosis after treatment for atrial fibrillation. BMJ 2008;336:830–2.

Complications of central vascular cannulation

197. Rowley KM, Clubb BSS, Smith GJW, et al. Right sided infective endocarditis as a consequence of flow directed pulmonary artery catheterisation. N Engl J Med 1984;311:1152–6.

198. Connors AF Jr, Castele RJ, Farhat NZ, et al. Complication of right heart catherisation. Chest 1985;88:567–72.

Complications of tracheal manipulations

199. Stauffer JL, Olson DE, Petty TL. Complications and consequences of endotracheal intubation and tracheotomy. A prospective study of 150 critically ill adult patients. Am J Med 1981;70:65–75.

200. Vanheurn LWE, Theunissen PHMH, Ramsay G, et al. Pathologic changes of the trachea after percutaneous dilatational tracheotomy. Chest 1996;109:1466–9.

201. Phillips I. Pseudomonas aeruginosa respiratory tract infections in patients receiving mechanical ventilation. J Hyg 1967;65:229–35.

202. Skim C. Cardiac arrhythmias resulting from tracheal suctioning. Ann Intern Med 1969;71:1149–53.

203. Deslee G, Brichet A, Lebuffe G, et al. Obstructive fibrinous tracheal pseudomembrane – A potentially fatal complication of tracheal intubation. Amer J Respir Crit Care Med 2000;162:1169–71.

204. Francois B, Bellissant E, Gissot V, et al. 12-h pretreatment with methylprednisolone versus placebo for prevention of postextubation laryngeal oedema: a randomised double-blind trial. Lancet 2007;369:1083–9.

205. Jacobs IN, Wetmore RF, Tom LW, et al. Tracheobronchomalacia in children. Arch Otolaryngol Head Neck Surg 1994;120:154–8.

206. Romagosa V, Bella MR, Truchero C, et al. Necrotizing sialometaplasia (adenometaplasia) of the trachea. Histopathology 1992;21:280–2.

Complications of bronchoscopy

207. Jin F, Mu D, Chu D, et al. Severe complications of bronchoscopy. Respiration 2008;76:429–33.

Pneumonectomy

208. Kopec SE, Irwin RS, UmaliTorres CB, et al. The postpneumonectomy state. Chest 1998;114:1158–84.

209. Biondetti PR, Fiore D, Sartori F, et al. Evaluation of post-pneumonectomy space by computed tomography. J Comput Assist Tomogr 1982;6:238–42.

210. Suarez J, Clagett T, Brown AL Jr. The postpneumonectomy space: factors influencing its obliteration. J Thorac Cardiovasc Surg 1969;57:539–42.

211. Sakamaki Y, Matsumoto K, Mizuno S, et al. Hepatocyte growth factor stimulates proliferation of respiratory epithelial cells during postpneumonectomy compensatory lung growth in mice. Amer J Respir Cell Molec Biol 2002;26:525–33.

212. Adams HD, Junod F, Aberdeen E, et al. Severe airway obstruction caused by mediastinal displacement after right pneumonectomy in a child. A case report. J Thorac Cardiovasc Surg 1972;63:534–9.

213. Grillo HC, Shepard JA, Mathisen DJ, et al. Postpneumonectomy syndrome: diagnosis,

management, and results. Ann Thorac Surg 1992;54:638–50.

214. Cordova FC, Travaline JM, O'Brien GM, et al. Treatment of left pneumonectomy syndrome with an expandable endobronchial prosthesis. Chest 1996;109:567–70.

215. Boiselle PM, Shepard JA, McLoud TC, et al. Postpneumonectomy syndrome: another twist. J Thorac Imaging 1997;12:209–11.

216. Kutlu CA, Williams EA, Evans TW, et al. Acute lung injury and acute respiratory distress syndrome after pulmonary resection. Ann Thorac Surg 2000;69:376–80.

217. Tang SS, Redmond K, Griffiths M, et al. The mortality from acute respiratory distress syndrome after pulmonary resection is reducing: a 10-year single institutional experience. Eur J Cardiothorac Surg 2008;34:898–902.

218. Dulu A, Pastores SM, Park B, et al. Prevalence and mortality of acute lung injury and ARDS after lung resection. Chest 2006;130:73–8.

219. Williams EA, Quinlan GJ, Anning PB, et al. Lung injury following pulmonary resection in the isolated, blood-perfused rat lung. Eur Resp J 1999;14:745–50.

220. Jordan S, Mitchell JA, Quinlan GJ, et al. The pathogenesis of lung injury following pulmonary resection. Eur Resp J 2000;15:790–9.

Chapter | 8 |

Vascular disease

8.1 Congestion and oedema; thrombosis, embolism and infarction; aneurysms

This section deals with several important pulmonary vascular diseases but some others are dealt with elsewhere – congenital anomalies of pulmonary vessels in Chapter 2, shock in Chapter 4 and vascular tumours of the lung in Chapter 12.3.

PULMONARY CONGESTION AND OEDEMA

Congestion of the lungs may be active or passive, the former accompanying inflammation and the latter the result of an increase in pressure in the pulmonary veins, typically due to failure of the left ventricle or mitral stenosis. The active variety includes the congestive atelectasis that results from circulatory shock (see p. 143).

At necropsy the pulmonary vessels are engorged, the lungs are heavy and blood can be expressed from the cut surface. Histologically the capillaries are distended. Pulmonary congestion is often associated with pulmonary oedema and haemosiderosis.

Pulmonary oedema

Pathogenesis

In accordance with Starling's law, water moves between the vascular and interstitial compartments of the lung in response to net hydrostatic and osmotic forces acting across the vessel wall, modulated by the permeability of this membrane. The capillaries constitute the main site of microvascular fluid exchange, but small arteries and veins are also involved. Water movement chiefly takes place through the endothelial cell junctions; beyond these the endothelial basement membrane offers no barrier to fluid transport.[1] Within the interstitium, water again flows along a hydrostatic gradient, in this case to the corners of the alveoli, and thence to the connective tissue surrounding the arteries and bronchioles at the centres of the acini and the veins in the interlobular septa.[2,3] These are the sites where lymphatics commence.[3,4] There is considerable reserve in the clearance capacity of the pulmonary lymphatics, which may increase their load 10-fold when pulmonary oedema threatens,[5] but above this, spillover

©2010 Elsevier Ltd
DOI: 10.1016/B978-0-7020-3369-8.00008-2

into the alveoli is inevitable. Before this the lungs sound dry on auscultation but the patient may nevertheless be breathless because the increased interstitial pressure triggers juxtacapillary nociceptors, which are represented by fine nerve terminals in the alveolar interstitium.[6,7]

In circumstances that involve only pressure changes, the oedema fluid is generally similar to normal interstitial fluid but in other circumstances the permeability of the vessels is increased and blood cells and high-molecular-weight plasma proteins, such as fibrinogen, escape into the tissues. Two main types of pulmonary oedema are therefore described, haemodynamic and cytotoxic (or irritant), characterised by the escape of low- and high-molecular-weight blood substances respectively. Electron microscopy shows that in haemodynamic oedema there is widening of the interstitial spaces in the alveolar walls by fluid, with separation of the collagen and elastin fibres, but that this is confined to the thick side of the air–blood barrier. In contrast, in cytotoxic oedema fluid also accumulates in the thin part of the air–blood barrier so that the endothelial cells are detached from their basement membranes and are often stretched over large subendothelial blebs of fluid (Fig. 8.1.1),[8] changes that do not occur in uncomplicated haemodynamic pulmonary oedema.[9]

The separation of haemodynamic and cytotoxic oedema is not absolute: large haemodynamic forces alone can result in the escape of high-molecular-weight blood proteins.[10,11] Electron microscopy shows that when the alveolar capillary pressure is raised above 40 mmHg in anaesthetised rabbits, breaks develop in both the endothelium of the alveolar capillaries and the alveolar epithelium.[12-16] Such stress failure results in high-permeability pulmonary oedema, and even frank alveolar haemorrhage. This explains why the oedema fluid of mitral stenosis is often tinged with blood, and why haemosiderosis is seen in other diseases characterised by raised pulmonary venous pressure, such as veno-occlusive disease (see p. 427) and lymphangioleiomyomatosis (see p. 293).

Stress failure of the alveoli also explains the occasional sudden demise of a thoroughbred racehorse from a 'burst blood vessel'.[17] These animals have been bred to such an extent that their cardiovascular systems develop very high pulmonary vascular pressures on exercise. Alveolar haemorrhage is common in these horses, although it is seldom apparent to their attendants. Similar exercise-induced pulmonary haemorrhage has also been described in racing greyhounds and it is possible that the lungs of top athletes may also develop stress failure on occasion.[15,18,19] Stress failure is also seen when there is overinflation of the lung, such as that which occurs when there is a sudden drop in atmospheric pressure (see 'burst lung', p. 369) or when alveolar gas pressures are raised unduly by mechanical respiratory assistance devices in intensive care units.

Specific causes of pulmonary oedema include:

- *Pulmonary venous hypertension.* This is the common factor by which conditions such as left ventricular failure, mitral stenosis and pulmonary veno-occlusive disease contribute to haemodynamic pulmonary oedema. A rise in pressure at the venous end of the pulmonary capillaries causes increased amounts of fluid to leave these vessels, with fluid that cannot be reabsorbed by the capillaries or drained by lymphatics accumulating as oedema. In left ventricular failure the accumulation of fluid is compounded by sodium retention, which is an important consequence of 'forward heart failure' through its effects on adrenocortical perfusion and aldosterone secretion.
- *Hypoproteinaemia.* This is a potential cause of haemodynamic pulmonary oedema, and underlies that occasionally observed in cirrhosis.

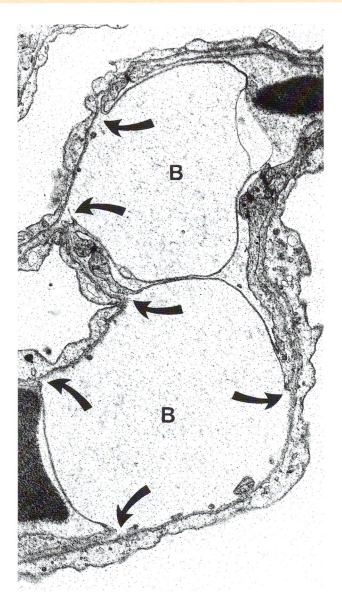

Figure 8.1.1 Cytotoxic oedema. Fluid has accumulated on the thin side of the air–blood barrier, raising the alveolar capillary endothelium off its basement membrane and producing two subendothelial blebs (B) which stretch right across the capillary. Arrows mark the points at which the endothelium is lifted off its basement membrane. Transmission electron micrograph of the lung of a rat that had been subjected to very high doses of the antidepressant drug iprindole. *(Courtesy of Dr GS Balasubramaniam, Melbourne, Australia.)*

- *Intravenous fluid overload.* Intravenous fluid overload may lead to pulmonary oedema by causing both left ventricular overload and dilution of the plasma proteins.
- *Re-expansion of the lungs.* Rapid drainage of a pleural effusion or the removal of a large pleural tumour occasionally alters pulmonary haemodynamics to such an extent that pulmonary oedema results.[20] The oedema fluid is rich in protein, suggesting that vascular permeability is increased and that there is stress failure of the alveolar walls.
- *Airway obstruction.* Suggested mechanisms involved in the pulmonary oedema that occasionally accompanies airway

obstruction include negative intrathoracic pressure causing transiently low interstitial pressure in the lungs, impaired left ventricular function and hypoxic postcapillary vasoconstriction.[21] Low protein levels in the oedema fluid favour a hydrostatic mechanism.[22]

- *Inhalation of irritant gases.* The accidental inhalation of gases such as ammonia, sulphur dioxide, chlorine, ozone and the oxides of nitrogen may cause widespread cytotoxic injury to the pulmonary capillaries as well as the alveolar epithelium, resulting in high-permeability pulmonary oedema.[23]
- *Oxygen.* Oxygen in high concentration, necessarily administered in some cases of severe lung injury, may further damage the lung and lead to cytotoxic pulmonary oedema.[24-26]
- *Acute pulmonary infection.* Oedema is a common feature of most pulmonary infections. It is attributable to the direct or indirect effects on the capillary endothelium and alveolar epithelium of toxins produced by the infective agent.
- *Chemotherapy.* Treatment with drugs such as busulphan is occasionally complicated by pulmonary oedema because of their cytotoxicity to alveolar endothelial and epithelial cells.
- *Shock lung.* This condition is characterised by severe cytotoxic pulmonary oedema. The endothelial damage is attributable to several factors, notably nitric oxide, which is released in large amounts by activated macrophages, and oxygen and hydroxyl neutrophils sequestered in the pulmonary capillaries. The detailed pathology of shock lung is described on page 142.
- *Renal failure.* Several mechanisms contribute to the development of pulmonary oedema in renal failure. They include fluid retention, hypertensive cardiac failure and hypoproteinaemia. The fluid is rich in protein, suggesting that cytotoxic factors or stress failure may also operate.[27,28]
- *High altitude.* The pulmonary oedema of acute mountain sickness (see p. 370) has a complex pathogenesis but the possibility that haemodynamic factors are involved is suggested by the undue susceptibility to the condition of persons with aplasia or hypoplasia of one pulmonary artery.[29,30] The lung lavage fluid is rich in protein[31] and electron microscopy shows subendothelial blebs characteristic of cytotoxic injury (see Fig. 8.1.1) or even disruption of the alveolar walls,[32] indicating that there is haemodynamic stress failure.[12,33] The oedema can be prevented or treated successfully with vasodilators such as calcium channel blocking agents taken orally[34,35] or inhaled nitric oxide,[36] suggesting that hypoxic vasoconstriction plays an important pathogenetic role. Hypoxia is a powerful stimulus to pulmonary vasoconstriction but it mainly affects precapillary vessels and would therefore seem to protect the capillary bed. This apparent anomaly may be explained by the patchy nature of the oedema. If the hypoxic vasoconstriction affected some pulmonary arteries more than others some capillaries would be protected and the remainder subjected to abnormally high pressures: patchy vasoconstriction would lead to patchy stress failure. Hypoxic venous constriction may also be involved[37] (relevant to which is evidence that flow through the valve-less pulmonary veins is controlled by sphincters[38]).
- *Cerebral injury.* Neurogenic pulmonary oedema is a well-recognised feature of cerebral damage, especially that caused by trauma or subarachnoid haemorrhage. Its pathogenesis appears to involve massive adrenergic release mediated by the hypothalamus.[39-41] This results in widespread vasoconstriction with marked systemic hypertension. Fluid then shifts from the systemic circulation to the relatively more compliant pulmonary circulation, with a resultant outpouring of fluid into the lung. Stress failure is invoked to explain the high-permeability nature of the oedema fluid.[12]

- *Heroin overdosage.* This is a well-recognised cause of pulmonary oedema. Its pathogenesis is not well understood but high protein levels in the oedema fluid suggest increased pulmonary capillary permeability.[42] Adrenergic hyperactivity similar to that envisaged in neurogenic injury may be involved.
- *Prostacyclin therapy.* Prostacyclin has been used to dilate the pulmonary arteries in patients with pulmonary hypertension but its continuous intravenous administration has been complicated by pulmonary oedema when the hypertension has been due to postcapillary obstruction, as in pulmonary veno-occlusive disease and pulmonary capillary haemangiomatosis.[43]

Pathological findings

At necropsy, an oedematous lung may weigh as much as 1 kg, nearly three times its normal weight. It feels firm and fails to collapse when the thorax is opened, so that the pleural surface remains smooth. Pleural effusion is often also present. Frothy fluid fills the airways and watery fluid escapes from the exposed cut surface. The fibrin-containing fluid of 'toxic' oedema does not run from the cut surface as freely as the watery fluid of haemodynamic oedema due to its high fibrin content. The appearances may simulate haemorrhage if red cells have escaped in large numbers into the fluid. Interstitial oedema is seen to distend the loose connective tissue of the interlobular septa and that around the airways and arteries. The subpleural lymphatics may be visibly distended and often the hilar lymph nodes are considerably enlarged, soft and moist.

Microscopically, the interlobular septa and the periarterial connective tissue sheaths are swollen and lymphatics within them are dilated (see Fig. 2.8). Alveolar oedema is seen as a homogeneous, eosinophilic proteinaceous material filling the air spaces (Fig. 8.1.2). Entrapped air bubbles are represented by rounded spaces within the proteinaceous contents of the alveoli. Only scanty threads of fibrin are generally found, but in severe cases, especially of the toxic variety, much fibrin is present in the fluid. The lungs are then particularly firm and have been described as showing 'congestive consolidation'. There may also be many red blood cells in the air spaces. Iron-containing macrophages may be found in chronic cases.[43a]

Organisation of the fibrinous material may occur, leading to fibrosis in the alveoli.[44] This takes the form of intra-alveolar plugs of oedematous granulation tissue known as *bourgeons conjonctifs* or Masson bodies.[45] Similar bodies develop in the bronchioles and the appearances closely mimic those found in healing bacterial pneumonia and in cryptogenic organising pneumonia. The connective tissue plugs may be incorporated into the alveolar walls, causing interstitial fibrosis by an accretive process.[46,47] Interstitial fibrosis may also arise as a direct consequence of interstitial oedema, so-called *gefässlose* (vessel-less) organisation.[48] The combination of haemosiderosis and fibrosis spawned the term 'brown induration of the lungs' for the changes that develop in long-standing mitral stenosis (Fig. 8.1.3).[49]

The vascular changes resulting from pulmonary venous hypertension are described in Chapter 8.2.

Radiological findings[44,50,51]

Interstitial oedema is recognisable in radiographs of the chest by a combination of hilar enlargement, caused by peribronchial and periarterial cuffing, and peripheral linear opacities resulting from oedema of the interlobular septa. There is a greater concentration of perivascular and peribronchial connective tissue at the hila and consequently the hilar opacities are enlarged, more dense and less well defined. Septal thickening is visualised radiologically as a series of non-branching, horizontal lines, 1–3 cm long, extending to the

Figure 8.1.2 Pulmonary oedema. Eosinophilic proteinaceous fluid fills many alveoli.

pleura at the lung bases. They are popularly known as Kerley B lines.

Alveolar oedema exaggerates the hilar prominence of the interstitial oedema that precedes it to produce a 'bat's wing' or 'butterfly' shadow. This picture was first described in cases of uraemia but is now known to occur with other causes of pulmonary oedema. The opacification is particularly marked in severe oedema, such as occurs in shock, when there may be a total 'white-out' of the lung fields except for patent bronchi which are seen as if forming a 'negative bronchogram'.

In addition to the features of oedema, the chest radiograph often shows enlargement of the heart and widening of vessels to upper zones of the lungs. The latter may be a direct effect of raised venous pressure on vessels that are normally at lower than alveolar pressure and therefore collapsed, or it may be a consequence of the vascular remodelling seen at the lung bases in pulmonary venous hypertension, which is described on page 427.

Clinical features

Breathlessness is an early feature of pulmonary oedema, encountered when the process is still interstitial because of stimulation of the juxtacapillary nociceptors.[6,7] With the onset of alveolar oedema crepitations are heard on auscultation and in severe cases watery sputum is produced, sometimes tinged by blood, and the patient is cyanosed and hypoxaemic. It is often essential to maintain cerebral oxygenation by augmenting the concentration of inspired oxygen despite the deleterious effect this may have on an already injured lung. Patients in left ventricular failure are prone to attacks of severe breathlessness when recumbent, typically at night. This is aptly termed paroxysmal nocturnal dyspnoea but is often still referred to by the older term 'cardiac asthma'. The distinction from bronchial asthma (see p. 109) may be blurred by oedematous swelling of the bronchial wall causing the patient to wheeze.

PULMONARY THROMBOSIS AND THROMBOEMBOLISM

Pulmonary thrombosis, as distinct from thromboembolism, is seldom symptomatic in the absence of other pulmonary vascular disease. It is most commonly encountered as a complication of pulmonary hypertension of any cause, and then confounds the histological distinction of thromboembolic pulmonary hypertension from that due to other causes, in particular the primary variety. It is necessary therefore to search for the specific histological features of the other varieties of pulmonary hypertension (which are dealt with in the next chapter) whenever pulmonary thrombosis is recognised. Although atheroma is a feature of pulmonary hypertension (see Fig. 8.2.17),[52] it is generally confined to the large elastic pulmonary arteries and seldom attains the advanced, ulcerated degree that predisposes to aortic thrombosis. Thrombosis complicating pulmonary hypertension probably commences in the smaller muscular pulmonary arteries, which narrow in this condition.

As well as complicating pulmonary hypertension, pulmonary thrombosis and infarction also develop in systemic lupus erythematosus,[53] sickle cell disease,[54–58] spherocytosis,[59] thalassaemia,[60,61] paroxysmal nocturnal haemoglobinuria,[62] the antiphospholipid antibody syndrome,[53,63] the hypereosinophilic syndrome,[64,65] rare varieties of pulmonary vasculitis that affect the large elastic arteries,[66,67] diffuse alveolar damage and unusual varieties of vascular infection.[68] Pulmonary thrombosis is also predisposed to by low blood flow, as in congenital anomalies such as pulmonary stenosis and in pulmonary aneurysms.

Thromboembolism

Aetiology

Pulmonary thromboembolism is rare in the third world but common in developed countries.[69] Economic development in Hong Kong has been accompanied by an increasing incidence of the disease[70,71] and in the USA the incidence of pulmonary thromboembolism among non-whites is much the same as in whites.[72]

In western countries, thrombotic pulmonary emboli, often unsuspected in life, are commonly encountered at necropsy, especially in elderly and obese people who have been confined to bed with congestive cardiac failure, and in adults of any age who have undergone major surgery, suffer from cancer or have been the victims of major trauma.[73–79] They develop in people who sleep in chairs that hinder venous return from the legs (e.g. deck chairs) and especially in air-travellers who are immobile for a long time. Nearly half prove fatal.[80] Pulmonary embolism is also prone to occur after childbirth. Contributing factors are listed in Box 8.1.1.[81–83] They operate in three ways, as described by Virchow in his well-known triad:

- by promoting blood stasis
- by damaging vascular endothelium
- by activatiing coagulation factors.

Thrombosis after operations and childbirth is promoted by the increased numbers of platelets that accompany any form of trauma. It often occurs in tributaries of the main veins of the legs and thighs, where the vascular stasis that follows immobilisation is known to be most pronounced. Puerperal thromboembolism is more frequent in women whose lactation has been suppressed by the administration of oestrogens than among those who breast-feed and in line with this it is known that the older high-oestrogen contraceptive pill carried a small risk of promoting thromboembolism by affecting the clotting factors VII and X and platelet aggregation. This risk is believed to be

Figure 8.1.3 'Brown induration' representing a combination of haemosiderosis and interstitial fibrosis due to chronic pulmonary congestion and oedema in patients with long-standing left-sided cardiac failure. (A) Paper-mounted whole-lung section showing brown discoloration. *(Courtesy of WG Edwards, London, UK.)* (B) Haematoxylin and eosin section showing septal fibrosis and increased numbers of brown alveolar macrophages. (C) An elastin van Geison stain shows intimal sclerosis of the pulmonary veins within the fibrosed interlobular septa. (D) A Perls stain shows marked haemosiderosis.

Box 8.1.1 Risk factors for venous thromboembolism[83]

Major risk factors
Surgery
- Major abdominal/pelvic surgery
- Hip/knee replacement
- Postoperative intensive care

Obstetrics
- Late pregnancy
- Caesarean section
- Puerperium

Lower-limb problems
- Fracture
- Varicose veins

Malignancy
- Abdominal/pelvic
- Advanced/metastatic

Reduced mobility
- Hospitalisation
- Institutional care

Miscellaneous
- Previous venous thromboembolism

Minor risk factors
Cardiovascular
- Congenital heart disease
- Congestive cardiac failure
- Hypertension
- Superficial venous thrombosis
- Indwelling central vein catheter

Oestrogens
- Oral contraceptive
- Hormone replacement therapy

Miscellaneous
- Chronic obstructive pulmonary disease
- Neurological disability
- Occult malignancy
- Thrombotic disorders
- Long-distance sedentary travel
- Obesity
- Other[a]

[a]Inflammatory bowel disease, nephrotic syndrome, chronic dialysis, myeloproliferative disorders, paroxysmal nocturnal haemoglobinuria, Behçet's disease.

Table 8.1.1 Deaths from pulmonary embolism per million population by age and sex in England and Wales

		Age (years)					
	All ages	<45	45–54	55–64	65–74	75–84	>84
Men	20	0	54	16	67	210	461
Women	33	1	4	12	61	218	497

Table 8.1.2 Deaths from pulmonary embolism by season[a]

Season	Deaths (n)
January to March	2898
April to June	2651
July to September	2646
October to December	2893

[a]11088 cases assembled from 23 reports from the northern hemisphere.[90]

Table 8.1.3 Incidence of pulmonary embolism according to the site of leg vein thrombosis[93]

Pulmonary embolism	Incidence
Calf vein thrombosis	0/21 patients
Calf and thigh vein thrombosis	8/15 patients

Pulmonary embolism detected by lung perfusion and ventilation scans.

Leg vein thrombosis detected by venography, impedance plethysmography and radiofibrinogen scanning.

of antithrombin III, factor V (Leiden), protein C and protein S. Usually these need to interact with acquired risk factors before thrombosis occurs, being otherwise uncommonly associated with idiopathic thromboembolism. For example, factor V (Leiden) defect in isolation increases the risk of thromboembolism 3–5-fold but in conjunction with oestrogen therapy 35-fold.[83] Further conditions characterised by hypercoaguability include the antiphospholipid syndrome and microalbuminuria.[63,86]

Despite the dangers of childbirth and oral contraception, the standardised mortality rate from thromboembolism is roughly the same for men and women; the increased risk of major trauma in young male adults balances the risks special to women. However, the crude death rate from thromboembolism is much greater in women than in men[87] because of the marked effect of advancing age on the incidence of thromboembolism and the greater number of elderly women in the population (Table 8.1.1). There is also a minor seasonal variation in the incidence of pulmonary thromboembolism, the risk being greater in the colder months (Table 8.1.2).[88–92]

It is when calf vein thrombi propagate proximally to reach the main veins of the thigh that they are most likely to break off and reach the lungs as emboli (Table 8.1.3).[93] Proximal propagation is encountered in approximately 20% of patients with calf vein thrombosis and

almost non-existent with the present low-oestrogen contraceptive pills.[84]

Hypercoaguability is fairly prevalent in the general population and presumably augments the other factors contributing to thrombosis listed in Box 8.1.1. It can be recognised in 25% of patients with venous thromboembolism and in an even higher number of patients whose thrombosis is otherwise unexplained. High levels of factors VIII and XI are fairly common in the general population (each has a prevalence of about 10%) but abnormalities in the levels of many other clotting factors are also recognised.[85] They include deficiencies

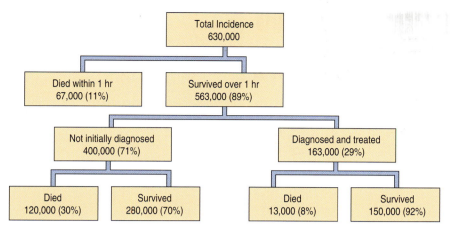

Figure 8.1.4 Annual incidence and survival in pulmonary thromboembolism in the USA. *(Reproduced from Dalen & Alpert (1975)[74] with permission.)*

approximately 50% of those with proximal leg vein thrombosis develop pulmonary embolism.[94] Residual deep-vein thrombosis can be demonstrated in most patients who have recently suffered pulmonary embolism.[95] The danger of leg vein thrombosis and embolism is lessened by the use of prophylactic massage and exercise. Treatment is mainly based on anticoagulation but may involve venous ligation proximal to the thrombus and thromboembolectomy. Leg vein thrombosis is nearly always bilateral and this should be kept in mind when ligation is being considered. Approximately 11% of patients with pulmonary thromboembolism die within 1 hour and only 29% of the remainder are correctly diagnosed and treated appropriately, which is unfortunate as there are 10 times as many deaths in the undiagnosed and untreated majority (Fig. 8.1.4).[74]

The periprostatic venous plexus is another source of pulmonary emboli, particularly multiple small emboli. Thrombosis here is promoted by local inflammation as well as by sluggish venous flow as in heart failure. Less often, thrombotic emboli originate in the veins of the arms or in the chambers on the right side of the heart. Other sources include intravenous cannulae and endocarditis affecting the valves on the right side of the heart. In one study 86% of thrombotic emboli reached the lungs via the inferior vena cava, 3% came via the superior vena cava, 3% originated in the heart and in 8% of cases the thrombosis was widespread.[96]

Clinical features

Sometimes the embolus is a massive one, and its lodgement in the pulmonary trunk or main pulmonary artery is immediately fatal because it obstructs the pulmonary circulation. In only 28% of such cases is a diagnosis of pulmonary thromboembolism made before death.[96] More frequently the embolus is small and without significant effect. Alternatively, the embolus may result in pulmonary infarction, which is indicated clinically by an attack of localised pleural pain, dyspnoea and haemoptysis. Often there is more than one embolic episode. Multiple microemboli as a cause of pulmonary hypertension is considered on page 426.

The high prevalence of unsuspected pulmonary thromboembolism evident at autopsy has been demonstrated in life with perfusion scans, emphasising that once a diagnosis of peripheral venous thrombosis has been established, anticoagulant therapy should be instituted without delay.[97] Thromboendartectomy is being increasingly undertaken.[98,99]

Distribution of the emboli

When clots are introduced into a rabbit's systemic vein, both the size of the clots and the anatomy of the pulmonary arterial tree affect their subsequent distribution in the lungs.[100] Whilst large emboli lodge in any of the main arteries, those of medium size are carried disproportionately often into the vessels of the posterior basal segments. In humans, pulmonary infarcts are commoner in the posterior basal segments of the lower lobes[96] and solitary metastatic tumours are more frequently basal than apical. The explanation lies in the anatomy of the pulmonary arteries: they have a large axial trunk that gives off its branches at an angle and terminates in the posterior basal segment.

Pathological findings

The sudden impaction of a large embolus in the pulmonary trunk brings the circulation virtually to a halt. The small volume of blood that can percolate past the thrombotic mass is quite insufficient to fill the left side of the heart and maintain normal systemic arterial pressure and an adequate circulation through the cerebral and coronary arteries. In such cases, the embolus is found at necropsy to be coiled on itself, straddling the bifurcation of the pulmonary trunk (Fig. 8.1.5). The chambers of the right side of the heart and the venae cavae are distended, the left atrium and ventricle contracted, and the lungs pale. The coiling distinguishes embolic thrombi from thrombi that have formed in the pulmonary arteries. When the embolus is removed from its site of impaction and is uncoiled it is seen to be of a diameter that corresponds to the calibre of the vessels in which it formed. Its surface is marked in correspondence with the venous valves: the broken ends of the thrombotic cast of the tributary veins can also be recognised and it may be possible to match these with the thrombus remaining in the veins.

Both thrombi formed in situ and thrombotic emboli are firm but friable, and show striae of Zahn, which are evident to the naked eye and indicative of their development during life (Fig. 8.1.6): these features distinguish them from clots, which are formed postmortem. Clots are shiny, soft and elastic: when pulled carefully from the vessels they show a characteristic 'horse's tail' appearance, their end being a cast of blood from the smaller branches of the pulmonary artery. Clots may show a transition from red to yellow, due to postmortem sedimentation of the cellular constituents of the stagnant blood, leaving a paler zone of serum in the eventual coagulum: this demarcation lacks the alternate white and red layers formed respectively of platelets

Figure 8.1.5 Massive pulmonary thromboembolism. Coiled thrombus occludes the pulmonary trunk and the main pulmonary arteries. *(Courtesy of Dr GA Russell, Tunbridge Wells, UK.)*

Figure 8.1.6 Thrombotic emboli showing the striae of Zahn. The striae represent successive layers of platelets and fibrin-enmeshed blood cells, indicating that the material was formed in life and therefore represents thrombus rather than clot. (A) Thrombus showing the striae is seen in pulmonary arteries on the cut surface of the lung (arrow). Note that the postmortem clot to the right lacks the striae. (B) Thrombus removed from the lung again shows the striae (centre).

and fibrin-enmeshed blood cells that characterise the striae of Zahn in a thrombus.

Fresh thrombus may fragment and disperse into smaller pulmonary arteries, of which there is a great reserve, but within a few days thrombotic emboli undergo organisation and become firmly adherent to the vessel wall.[98,99] In 4–6 weeks they are converted into fibrous tissue, often with recanalisation. Some emboli seem to disappear and it is presumed that they are destroyed by fibrinolysin. Thin fibrous bands stretching across the lumen of major pulmonary arteries are sometimes the only evidence of previous thromboembolism (Fig. 8.1.7A).[101] More often, the lumen of smaller arteries is divided up into multiple channels by the usual process of recanalisation (Fig. 8.1.7B).[102]

PULMONARY INFARCTION

Like other infarcts, those in the lungs are generally wedge-shaped. An occluded pulmonary artery is found at the apex of the infarct; the base of the infarct is on the pleura. Often the edge of a lobe is involved, in which case the lesion is diamond-shaped rather than wedge-shaped (Fig. 8.1.8). Any part of the lung may be affected but infarction is commonest at the bases, for the reasons explained above. Pulmonary infarcts are commonly multiple.

Partial and complete infarction

Completely infarcted tissue is beyond recovery and healing is only possible by repair (rather than by resolution), culminating in a fibrous scar. This is the situation in only a minority of pulmonary infarcts: most resolve completely, indicating that the lung tissue is not damaged irretrievably. The infarction is only partial. Frequently the lung escapes even this state of partial devitalisation, despite complete obstruction

of a pulmonary artery. The explanation for this is the dual blood supply to the lung and the lung's independence of the blood stream for oxygen. True infarction is therefore rare and to produce even a partial infarct some factor other than failure of the pulmonary arterial supply is required. This factor is frequently a cardiac condition compromising the bronchial arterial supply. Although bronchial arteries normally supply little blood to peripheral lung tissue, they are capable of supplying more should the pulmonary artery supply fail. A common clinical setting for pulmonary infarction is the patient confined to bed with heart failure. This promotes thromboembolism and at the same time compromises the bronchial arterial supply. Pulmonary infarction is very rare in the absence of passive pulmonary venous congestion.

Partial infarcts are initially characterised by oedema but within 48 hours capillaries rupture and the resultant lesions are intensely haemorrhagic, swollen, firm and dark red (see Fig. 8.1.8). The edge is sharply demarcated. Acute inflammation develops where infarcts border healthy lung and fibrin is found on the pleural surface of the involved area. Microscopically, the alveoli are filled with blood. Their walls are intact however and the basic architecture of the tissue is unaltered. Complete and rapid resolution is frequently observed radiologically and if the patient then dies, perhaps of a further massive embolism, no abnormality other than haemosiderin-laden macrophages can be detected in the recently infarcted area. Less often, necrosis is found, signifying true infarction. Healing is then by organi-

Figure 8.1.7 (A) Thin fibrous bands stretching across the lumen of pulmonary arteries may be the only remains of organised thrombotic emboli. (B) The bands are seen as intraluminal fibrous strands on microscopy.

Figure 8.1.8 Recent infarct of lung. The dark area is infarcted lung in which the air spaces have become filled with blood. Just above the lesion can be seen the supplying pulmonary artery occluded by thrombus. *(Reproduced by permission of the Curator of the Gordon Museum, Guy's Hospital, London, UK; courtesy of Miss P Turnbull, Charing Cross Hospital and Medical School, London.)*

sation, which is marked by slow paling and shrinkage, until eventually only a barely detectable scar remains. As with most scars in organs that are subject to constant movement, such as the lung and the heart, they are rich in elastin.[103] If the lesion is excised before it has been fully organised, the central necrosis is seen to be bordered by granulation tissue rich in foam cells and haemosiderin-laden macrophages. However, if these features are not well developed conditions such as Wegener's granulomatosis, rheumatoid nodule and chronic infection enter the differential diagnosis, especially if the classic wedge shape of an infarction is not well represented.[104] Basophilic karyorrhexis and chronic inflammation involving both the granulation tissue and the wall of the artery in which the embolus impacted may further the

impression of Wegener's while palisading of the reparative cells may suggest a rheumatoid nodule. In these circumstances the diagnosis of infarction is often no more than tentative, based partly upon negative features, such as an absence of extrapulmonary and serological evidence of Wegener's granulomatosis and rheumatoid disease and no evidence of infection being found.

If the embolus is infected, as may happen with abdominal sepsis, infected venous cannulae or bacterial endocarditis affecting the valves on the right side of the heart, septic infarction is likely. Suppuration soon causes this to resemble any other lung abscess. A few initially sterile lung infarcts become abscesses by colonisation of the devitalised tissue by airborne bacteria.

Pulmonary venous infarction

In contrast to the infarcts caused by pulmonary artery occlusion, pulmonary venous infarction is very rare. This is attributable to the rich network of venous collateral vessels that drain the lung. Most of the few reported cases have been due to sclerosing mediastinitis. Other recorded causes include left atrial myxoma, left atrial thrombosis complicating mitral stenosis, venous thrombosis following pulmonary resection and carcinoma of the lung.[105,106] The infarcts are similar to those caused by arterial occlusion. Chronic venous obstruction, as seen in pulmonary veno-occlusive disease (see p. 427) may result in interstitial fibrosis. These areas of scarring are rich in haemosiderin and possibly represent healed venous infarcts.

NON-THROMBOTIC PULMONARY EMBOLI

Pulmonary embolism may result from various kinds of material forming in, or gaining access to, the systemic veins. Apart from thrombi, these include fat droplets, various types of tissue, clumps of tumour cells, gas bubbles and a variety of foreign substances. In some parts of the world parasitic emboli are important: these include the eggs of schistosomes (p. 254) and the adult form of the canine heart worm *Dirofilaria immitis* (p. 258).[107] In contrast to thrombotic emboli, the effects of non-thrombotic emboli are not purely mechanical but are also linked to the nature of the embolus.

Fat embolism

Fat embolism is usually the result of bone or soft-tissue trauma, but other causes such as liposuction or bone marrow infarction complicating haemoglobinopathy are occasionally responsible (Box 8.1.2).[107-111] Under any of these circumstances, fat or oil globules enter the systemic veins and reach the lungs. Small fat globules can almost always be demonstrated in pulmonary capillaries after any fracture if frozen sections are stained appropriately and only a small proportion of patients develop symptoms referable to the embolism.

The classic fat embolism syndrome consists of hypoxaemia, cerebral disturbance, tachycardia and a petechial rash that is typically maximal over the front of the chest. The hypoxaemia is attributed to the emboli blocking pulmonary capillaries and causing pulmonary arteriovenous anastomoses to open so that venous blood bypasses the lungs. The extrapulmonary symptoms are attributed to emboli that have similarly bypassed the pulmonary capillaries to occlude small systemic arteries. The presence or absence of lesions is determined by the extent of vascular anastomoses in the organ concerned and the relative susceptibility of the tissue to oxygen lack. For these reasons the brain is particularly affected, showing petechial haemorrhages in the white

matter. However, the kidney is the best organ in which to identify systemic fat embolism microscopically because it filters the blood and the fat accumulates in the glomeruli.

Some patients with fat embolism develop severe respiratory failure. This is seldom due to extensive occlusion of the pulmonary circulation. More often it is caused by traumatic shock, which has its own profound effects on the lungs (see p. 142). Alternatively, it is suggested that the lungs are damaged by irritant fatty acids released by lysis of the fat.[112-114]

Microembolism of agglutinated fat emulsions[110,115,116] or of crystals derived from infusions during the course of total parenteral nutrition[117] is described on page 390.

Amniotic fluid embolism

Occasionally, during childbirth, amniotic fluid with its content of particulate debris, mostly epidermal squames and meconium, is forced by strong uterine contractions into the maternal circulation through small incomplete lower uterine tears, resulting in fatal microembolism of the mother's small pulmonary arteries.[118] The emboli may be quite sparse, suggesting that death is due to anaphylactic shock rather than pulmonary vascular occlusion, a possibility that is supported in some cases by the amniotic fluid embolism being accompanied by disseminated intravascular coagulation (see p. 144), mast cell degranulation and complement activation.[119] Recognition of the meconium mucus and epidermal squames is facilitated by the application of a mucous stain such as alcian blue and immunohistochemistry using antibodies against cytokeratin (coupled with an endothelial marker such as CD34 to distinguish the squames from degenerate exfoliated endothelial cells).

Trophoblastic embolism

Trophoblastic tissue may be found in the lungs in a large proportion of women who die during pregnancy or the puerperium.[120] It is particularly common in women suffering from eclampsia and in those undergoing uterine surgery for hydatidiform moles and as a side-effect of chemotherapy for choriocarcinoma.[121] Trophoblastic embolism is recognisable as isolated multinucleated syncytiotrophoblastic cells within pulmonary blood vessels (Fig. 8.1.9) and can be confirmed as such by the immunocytochemical demonstration of human chorionic gonadotrophin. Chorionic villi are not observed in the pulmonary vessels in normal pregnancies but are common in molar pregnancies.[122] It is believed that uterine contractions dislodge the trophoblastic tissue and enable it to enter the blood stream. The trophoblastic emboli cause no structural changes in the lung and appear to be immunologically inert, in spite of their fetal origin. They do not predispose to thrombosis and usually undergo early lysis[120] but rare fatal cases of massive trophoblastic embolism are recorded in which over 80% of the pulmonary vessels are occluded.[123] In exceptional cases of benign hydatidiform mole, it has been noted radiologically that masses within the lungs may persist for up to a year, but regress and totally disappear thereafter[124]; they presumably represent trophoblastic emboli that have gained a temporary foothold in the lungs.

Decidual embolism

Small foci of decidua are occasionally observed in the lungs in pregnancy. Such foci located immediately beneath the pleura[125] may represent focal metaplasia of the overlying serosa but deep in the lung an embolic aetiology is generally assumed, although the decidual tissue is usually extravascular. The nature of this tissue is discussed further under the subject of pleuropulmonary endometriosis (see p. 495).

Box 8.1.2 Causes of fat embolism[107]

Bone fracture
Soft-tissue trauma
Liposuction
Bone marrow infarction complicating haemoglobinopathy
Bone marrow harvest
Viral hepatitis affecting a fatty liver
Pancreatitis
Intravenous injection of various oils by accident or intent
Periurethral injection to treat stress incontinence
Breast augmentation

Figure 8.1.9 Trophoblast embolism. The trophoblast is recognisable as a clump of multinucleated syncytiotrophoblastic cells within a pulmonary artery.

Figure 8.1.10 Bone marrow embolism incurred as a terminal event during unsuccessful attempts at cardiac massage in which ribs were fractured.

Tumour embolism

Tumour emboli are common in the lungs. A few survive to form metastatic deposits but most die very soon after arriving in the lungs: the embolus then becomes enclosed by platelets and finally undergoes organisation.[126] Vascular occlusion by tumour emboli is sometimes so widespread that it leads to right-sided heart failure[127–133] whilst massive tumour emboli have sometimes proved fatal[134–136] or necessitated emergency embolectomy.[137] In other patients they have caused flitting radiographic opacities, which presumably represent infarcts.[138] Occlusion of the pulmonary arteries may be due to tumour alone or the tumour may promote thrombosis, organisation of which results in fibrocellular intimal thickening, so-called carcinomatous thrombotic microangiopathy or vascular intimal carcinomatosis (see p. 682).[139–142] Embolic sarcoma is distinguished from the primary sarcoma of the pulmonary arteries described on page 638 by the presence of an extrapulmonary source.

Other tissue embolism

Bone marrow is frequently seen plugging small pulmonary arteries postmortem when ribs have been broken during unsuccessful attempts at cardiac resuscitation or following trauma to other bones (Fig. 8.1.10). Other traumatic emboli may consist of brain tissue,[143,144] liver tissue,[145,145a] bile (Fig. 8.1.11),[146] bone fragments (Fig. 8.1.12) or very rarely atheromatous cholesterol crystals.[147] Haemorrhage has been ascribed to the last of these but none of the others is of clinical consequence; they merely represent incidental necropsy findings.

Foreign-body embolism

Some drug addicts break up preparations of drugs intended for oral use and inject an aqueous suspension intravenously. Substances used as fillers in the manufacture of tablets include starch, cellulose, talc and crosprovidone (poly[N-vinyl-2-pyrrolidone]). When injected intravenously, these lodge in pulmonary vessels and induce thrombosis and a local foreign-body granulomatous reaction (Fig. 8.1.13 and see Fig. 7.2.10, p. 379).[148–155] Pulmonary hypertension may result if

Figure 8.1.11 Bile embolism in a patient who died suddenly from rupture of a hepatic hydatid cyst. Partial organisation of the bile indicates that bile leakage had been occurring for some time before death. Haematoxylin and eosin. *(Courtesy of Dr T Jelihovsky, Sydney, Australia.)*

the injury to the vessels is extensive.[148] Widespread pulmonary fibrosis may also develop, occasionally mimicking pneumoconiotic progressive massive fibrosis.[156] Starch particles can be identified by their characteristic Maltese cross appearance on polarising microscopy, and talc by its platy form on polarising microscopy and by elemental electron microprobe analysis.[156] Cellulose fibres can be distinguish from platy crystals such as talc by their reaction with periodic acid–Schiff, silver methenamine and Congo red stains.[153,157] Crosprovidone is seen as basophilic, coral-like particles, the nature of which can be confirmed by infrared spectroscopy.[158] Any of these particles may leave the blood vessels and be found in the interstitial tissues and even air spaces. Talc particles in the lung exceeding 5 μm in length should arouse suspicion of intravenous drug abuse,[159] but cellulose fibres up to 120 μm in length may reach the lungs and cause granulomatosis in addicts who inhale their illicit drugs.[157,160]

Other embolic foreign bodies described in pulmonary arteries include airgun pellets,[161] shrapnel, whole bullets,[162] masonry and

Figure 8.1.12 Bone embolism. A fragment of bone is lodged in a pulmonary artery after failed resuscitation.

Figure 8.1.14 Embolised vegetable matter is present within a pulmonary artery in a patient who died of a ruptured oesophagus. *(Courtesy of Dr CA Seldenrijk, Nieuwegein, The Netherlands.)*

Figure 8.1.13 Drug addict's lung viewed with partially polarised light showing a granulomatous response to numerous birefringent plate-like talc crystals. Although reaching the lungs by the pulmonary arteries, the crystals work their way through the vessel walls and eventually become widely distributed in the lungs.

Figure 8.1.15 Therapeutic embolisation with foam introduced by percutaneous cannulation of the bronchial arteries in an unsuccessful attempt to stem haemorrhage into an aspergilloma cavity.

stone fragments, food particles (Fig. 8.1.14), the broken-off ends of intravenous catheters and cannulas, plastic particles from dialysis tubing and other intravascular devices,[163,163a] therapeutic injections or prosthetic implants of substances such as Teflon, hyaluronic acid and silicone,[164a,168a] lymphangiography contrast medium,[169–172] various materials injected to occlude abnormal blood vessels or deprive a tumour of its blood supply,[173,174] and mercury, this last generally introduced into the circulation with suicidal intent.[175] Patients with psychiatric problems have also injected themselves with various other substances, such as olive oil, resulting in pulmonary lipogranulomatosis.[176]

Bronchial, as opposed to pulmonary, artery embolisation is sometimes carried out therapeutically in an attempt to stem intractable haemorrhage from lesions that are difficult to resect, such as an aspergilloma.[177] The same technique is used on occasion to induce infarction of neoplasms. It involves the cannulation of bronchial arteries via a femoral artery and the aorta. Bronchial arteries are chosen because aspergillomas and tumours derive their blood supply from these systemic vessels, as is the case with most pulmonary disease. If the procedure fails to stem the haemorrhage and surgery is resorted to, or the patient dies, the pathologist may be asked to confirm that the bronchial arteries do contain the injected material. This is usually a synthetic foam and is easily recognised as such (Fig. 8.1.15), but Verhoeff–van Gieson staining is recommended as a means of facilitating its recognition.[178]

Air embolism

Venous air embolism may occur whenever a vein above the level of the heart is opened and exposed to the atmosphere, for example during operations on the head and neck or pelvic operations in which the patient is put in the Trendelenburg position. Air may also enter veins during peritoneal insufflation at laparoscopy or be inadvertently injected under pressure during urgent transfusions. A central venous pressure line carries a high risk of air embolism. Air embolism also occurs during high pressure mechanical ventilation or due to dramatic

Figure 8.1.16 Idiopathic aneurysm of the pulmonary artery. The patient died of respiratory failure secondary to scoliosis, which was also idiopathic.

Box 8.1.3 **Causes of pulmonary artery aneurysms**[182]

Congenital

with arteriovenous communication
Isolated
As part of hereditary haemorrhagic telangiectasia

without arteriovenous communication

Vasculitic

Infective
Syphilitic
Tuberculous
'Mycotic' (from septic emboli)

Non-infective
Behçet's syndrome
Hughes–Stovin syndrome
Tuberous sclerosis[185]

Hypertensive
Traumatic
Idiopathic[183,184]

changes in atmospheric pressure (see p. 368) or there is severe chest trauma.

Following venous air embolism, the fine bubbles into which the air is churned during its passage through the heart are carried into the pulmonary arteries. The cause of death is generally acute heart failure and the embolism is recognised by a frothy mixture of air and blood filling the chambers of the right side of the heart and pulmonary trunk. The volume of air needed to produce fatal air embolism in this way may be 100–200 ml or more. More rarely, air embolism results in pulmonary oedema.[181]

Systemic air embolism occurs most frequently during open-heart surgery but may also develop after chest trauma or as a sequel to venous air embolism in patients with an arteriovenous shunt (paradoxical air embolism). It is also recorded in aeroplane passengers with cystic lung disease.[179,180] A few millilitres of air introduced into the systemic arteries may prove fatal through obstruction of small vessels in the brain stem.

PULMONARY ANEURYSMS

An aneurysm is defined as a localised vascular dilatation but the term is usually confined to arterial dilatations. Localised venous dilatations are generally termed varices. Both are rare in the pulmonary circulation. Either may be saccular or fusiform.

Historically, most pulmonary aneurysms have been syphilitic or tuberculous but these causes are now very rare. Today, various other causes are recognised but sometimes no cause can be identified (Fig. 8.1.16 and Box 8.1.3).[182–185] The basic fault in all aneurysms is a localised defect in the arterial media. Most are dealt with elsewhere: arteriovenous on p. 76, infective on p. 437, Behçet's syndrome and Hughes–Stovin syndromes on pp. 447 and 479 and hypertensive on p. 431. Traumatic aneurysms may be true or false, the latter representing a haematoma alongside and communicating with the parent artery through a complete defect in the vessel wall but walled off externally by a fibrous capsule.

Dissecting aneurysms have also been reported in pulmonary arteries, usually complicating pulmonary hypertension.[186,187] They may also be encountered in a systemic vessel supplying an extralobar sequestration (Fig. 8.1.17).

Figure 8.1.17 Dissection of a systemic artery supplying a pulmonary sequestration. (A) Haematoxylin and eosin stain; (B) elastin van Gieson stain.

Figure 8.1.18 Pulmonary varix. (A) A circumscribed blood-filled cyst is present within the lower lobe. (B) Microscopy shows a thin fibrous wall, which contains variable amounts of disordered elastin fibres (c).

Pulmonary varix

A pulmonary varix is a localised dilatation of a pulmonary vein (Fig. 8.1.18).[188] Apart from rare examples that bleed, sometimes with fatal results, the condition is discovered incidentally at autopsy or by radiography.[189] In many cases the varix is assumed to represent a congenital anomaly or to develop postnatally because of a congenital defect in the vein wall. A substantial number of pulmonary varices, perhaps half, are secondary to mitral valve regurgitation.[190] Rarely, they are found in association with end-stage liver disease.[189]

REFERENCES

Pulmonary congestion and oedema

1. Schneeberger-Keeley EE, Karnovsky MJ. The ultrastructural basis of alveolar-capillary membrane permeability to peroxidase used as a tracer. J Cell Biol 1968;37:781–93.
2. Weibel ER, Bachofen H. Structural design of the alveolar septum and fluid exchange. In: Fishman ARE, editor. Pulmonary Edema. Baltimore: Williams and Wilkins; 1979. p. 1–20.
3. Michel RP, Meterissian S, Poulsen RS. Morphometry of the distribution of hydrostatic pulmonary oedema in dogs. Br J Exp Pathol 1986;67:865–77.
4. Staub NC, Nagano H, Pearce ML. Pulmonary edema in dogs, especially the sequence of fluid accumulation in lungs. J Appl Physiol 1967;22:227–40.
5. Staub NC. The pathophysiology of pulmonary edema. Hum Pathol 1970;1:419–32.
6. Spencer H, Leof D. The innervation of the human lung. J Anat 1964;98:599–609.
7. Fox B, Bull TB, Guz A. Innervation of alveolar walls in the human lung: an electron microscopical study. J Anat 1980;131:683–92.
8. Vijeyaratnam GS, Corrin B. Fine structural alterations in the lungs of iprindole-treated rats. J Pathol 1974;114:233–9.
9. Kay JM, Edwards FR. Ultrastructure of the alveolar-capillary wall in mitral stenosis. J Pathol 1973;111:239–45.
10. Pietra GG, Szidon JP, Leventhal MM, et al. Hemoglobin as a tracer in hemodynamic pulmonary edema. Science 1969;166:1643–6.
11. Schneeberger EE, Karnovsky MJ. The influence of intravascular fluid volume on the permeability of newborn and adult mouse lungs to ultrastructural protein tracers. J Cell Biol 1971;49:319–34.
12. West JB, Mathieu-Costello O. Stress failure of pulmonary capillaries – role in lung and heart disease. Lancet 1992;340: 762–7.
13. Bachofen H, Schurch S, Michel RP, et al. Experimental hydrostatic pulmonary edema in rabbit lungs – morphology. Am Rev Respir Dis 1993;147:989–96.

14. Bachofen H, Schurch S, Weibel ER. Experimental hydrostatic pulmonary edema in rabbit lungs – barrier lesions. Am Rev Respir Dis 1993;147:997–1004.

15. Mathieu-Costello OA, West JB. Are pulmonary capillaries susceptible to mechanical stress? Chest 1994;105:S102–S107.

16. Wu DXY, Weibel ER, Bachofen H, et al. Lung lesions in experimental hydrostatic pulmonary edema: an electron microscopic and morphometric study. Exp Lung Res 1995;21:711–30.

17. O'Callaghan MW, Pascoe JR, Tyler WS, et al. Exercise-induced pulmonary haemorrhage in the horse: results of a detailed clinical, post mortem and imaging study. VIII. Conclusions and implications. Equine Vet J 1987;19:428–34.

18. Weiler-Ravell D, Shupak A, Goldenberg I, et al. Pulmonary oedema and haemoptysis induced by strenuous swimming. BMJ 1995;311:361–2.

19. Ghio AJ, Ghio C, Bassett M. Exercise-induced pulmonary hemorrhage after running a marathon. Lung 2006;184:331–3.

20. Waller DA, Saunders NR. Unilateral pulmonary oedema following the removal of a giant pleural tumour. Thorax 1989;44:682–3.

21. Boykett M. Pulmonary oedema after acute asphyxia in a child. BMJ 1989;298:928.

22. Fremont RD, Kallet RH, Matthay MA, et al. Postobstructive pulmonary edema: a case for hydrostatic mechanisms. Chest 2007;131:1742–6.

23. Plopper CG, Dungworth DL, Tyler WS. Pulmonary lesions in rats exposed to ozone. Am J Pathol 1973;71:375–94.

24. Kapanci Y, Weibel ER, Kaplan HP, et al. Pathogenesis and reversibility of the pulmonary lesions of oxygen toxicity in monkeys. II Ultrastructural and morphometric studies. Lab Invest 1969;20:101–18.

25. Gould VE, Tosco R, Wheelis RF, et al. Oxygen pneumonitis in man. Ultrastructural observations on the development of the alveolar lesions. Lab Invest 1972;26:499–508.

26. Pratt PC. Pathology of pulmonary oxygen toxicity. Am Rev Respir Dis 1974;110:51–7.

27. Rocker GM, Morgan AG, Pearson D, et al. Pulmonary vascular permeability to transferrin in the pulmonary oedema of renal failure. Thorax 1987;42:620–3.

28. Crosbie WA, Snowden S, Parsons V. Changes in lung capillary permeability in renal failure. BMJ 1972;4:388–90.

29. Hackett PH, Creagh CE, Grover RF, et al. High altitude pulmonary edema in persons without the right pulmonary artery. N Engl J Med 1980;302:1070–3.

30. Fiorenzano G, Rastelli V, Greco V, et al. Unilateral high-altitude pulmonary edema in a subject with right pulmonary artery hypoplasia. Respiration 1994;61:51–4.

31. Schoene RB, Hackett PH, Henderson WR, et al. High altitude pulmonary oedema; characteristics of lung lavage fluid. JAMA 1986;256:63–9.

32. Heath D, Moosavi H, Smith P. Ultrastructure of high altitude pulmonary oedema. Thorax 1973;28:694–700.

33. West JB, Colice GL, Lee YJ, et al. Pathogenesis of high-altitude pulmonary oedema: direct evidence of stress failure of pulmonary capillaries. Eur Respir J 1995;8:523–9.

34. Bartsch P, Maggiorini M, Ritter M, et al. Prevention of high-altitude pulmonary edema by nifedipine. N Engl J Med 1991;325:1284–9.

35. Reeves JT, Schoene RB. When lungs on mountains leak – studying pulmonary edema at high altitudes. N Engl J Med 1991;325:1306–7.

36. Scherrer U, Vollenweider L, Delabays A, et al. Inhaled nitric oxide for high-altitude pulmonary edema. N Engl J Med 1996;334:624–9.

37. Wagenvoort CA, Wagenvoort N. Pulmonary veins in high-altitude residents: a morphometric study. Thorax 1982;37:931–5.

38. Schraufnagel DE, Patel KR. Sphincters in pulmonary veins. An anatomic study in rats. Am Rev Respir Dis 1990;141:721–6.

39. Editorial. Neurogenic pulmonary oedema. Lancet 1985;1:1430–1.

40. Wray NP, Nicotra MB. Pathogenesis of neurogenic pulmonary oedema. Am Rev Respir Dis 1978;118:783–6.

41. Carlson RW, Schaeffer RC, Michaels SG, et al. Pulmonary oedema following intracranial haemorrhage. Chest 1979;75:731–4.

42. Katz S, Aberman A, Frand UI, et al. Heroin pulmonary edema. Evidence for increased pulmonary capillary permeability. Am Rev Respir Dis 1972;106:472–4.

43. Humbert M, Maitre S, Capron F, et al. Pulmonary edema complicating continuous intravenous prostacyclin in pulmonary capillary hemangiomatosis. Am J Respir Crit Care Med 1998;157:1681–5.

43a. Zampieri FMDEC, Parra ER, Canzian M, et al. Biopsy-proven pulmonary determinants of heart disease. Lung 2010;188:63–70

44. Heard BE, Steiner RE, Herdan A, et al. Oedema and fibrosis of the lungs in left ventricular failure. Br J Radiol 1968;41:161–71.

45. Masson P, Riopelle JL, Martin P. Poumon rheumatismal. Ann Anat Path 1937;14:359–82.

46. Spencer H. Interstitial pneumonia. Ann Rev Med 1967;18:423–42.

47. Spencer H. Chronic interstitial pneumonia. In: Liebow AA, editor. The Lung. International Academy of Pathology monograph No.8. Baltimore: Williams & Wilkins; 1967. p. 134–50.

48. Eppinger H. Die Permeabilitatspathologie als die Lehre vom Krankheitsbeginn. Vienna: Springer; 1949.

49. Goyette EM, Farinacci CJ, Forsee JH, et al. The clinicopathologic correlation of lung biopsies in mitral stenosis. Am Heart J 1954;47:645–52.

50. Herrnheiser G, Hinson KFW. An anatomical explanation of the formation of butterfly shadows. Thorax 1954;9:198–210.

51. Grainger RG. Interstitial pulmonary oedema and its radiological diagnosis. A sign of pulmonary venous and capillary hypertension. Br J Radiol 1958;31:201–17.

Pulmonary thrombosis and thromboembolism

52. Moore GW, Smith RRL, Hutchins GM. Pulmonary artery atherosclerosis. Correlation with systemic atherosclerosis and hypertensive pulmonary vascular disease. Arch Pathol Lab Med 1982;106:378–80.

53. Boey ML, Colaco CB, Gharavi AE, et al. Thrombosis in systemic lupus erythematosus: striking association with the presence of circulating lupus anticoagulant. BMJ 1983;287:1021–3.

54. Oppenehimer EH, Esterly JR. Pulmonary changes in sickle cell disease. Am Rev Respir Dis 1971;103:858–9.

55. Collins FS, Orringer EP. Pulmonary hypertension and cor pulmonale in the sickle hemoglobinopathies. Am J Med 1982;73:814–21.

56. Athanasou NA, Hatton C, McGee JO, et al. Vascular occlusion and infarction in sickle cell crisis and the sickle chest syndrome. J Clin Pathol 1985;38:659–64.

57. Gray A, Anionwu EN, Davies SC, et al. Patterns of mortality in sickle cell disease in the United Kingdom. J Clin Pathol 1991;44:459–63.

58. Weil JV, Castro O, Malik AB, et al. Pathogenesis of lung disease in sickle hemoglobinopathies. Am Rev Respir Dis 1993;148:249–56.

59. Verresen D, Debacker W, Vanmeerbeeck J, et al. Spherocytosis and pulmonary hypertension: coincidental occurrence or causal relationship? Eur Respir J 1991;4:629–31.

61. Landing BH, Nadorra R, Hyman CB, et al. Pulmonary lesions of thalassemia major. In: Rosenberg HS, Bernstein J, editors. Respiratory and Alimentary Tract Diseases Volume 11 Perspectives in Pediatric Pathology. Basel: Karger; 1987. p. 82–96.

62. Heller PG, Grinberg AR, Lencioni M, et al. Pulmonary hypertension in paroxysmal nocturnal hemoglobinuria. Chest 1992;102:642–3.

63. Pilling J, Cutaia M. The antiphospholipid antibody syndrome – A vascular disease with pulmonary manifestations. Chest 1997;112:1451–3.

64. Chusid MJ, Dale DC, West BC, et al. The hypereosinophilic syndrome: analysis of fourteen cases with review of the literature. Medicine 1975;54:1–27.

65. Weller PF, Bubley GJ. The idiopathic hypereosinophilic syndrome. Blood 1994;83:2759–79.

66. Wagenaar SS, Westermann CJJ, Corrin B. Giant cell arteritis limited to large elastic pulmonary arteries. Thorax 1981;36:876–7.

67. Wagenaar SS, van den Bosch JMM, Westermann CJJ, et al. Isolated granulomatous giant cell vasculitis of the pulmonary elastic arteries. Arch Pathol Lab Med 1986;110:962–4.

68. Stermer E, Bassan H, Oliven A, et al. Massive thrombosis as a result of triple infestation of the pulmonary arterial circulation by Ascaris, Candida, and Mucor. Hum Pathol 1984;15:996–1001.

69. Thomas WA, Davies JNP, O'Neal RM, et al. Incidence of myocardial infarction correlated with venous and pulmonary thrombosis and embolism. A geographic study based on autopsies in Uganda, East Africa and St Louis, U.S.A. Am J Cardiol 1960;5:41–7.

70. Chau KY, Yuen ST, Ng THK, et al. An autopsy study of pulmonary thromboembolism in Hong-Kong Chinese. Pathology 1991;23:181–4.

71. Chan CW. Pulmonary thromboembolism in Hong-Kong Chinese. Pathology 1993;25:99–100.

72. Lilienfeld DE, Chan E, Ehland J, et al. Mortality from pulmonary embolism in the United States: 1962 to 1984. Chest 1990;98:1067–72.

73. Fleming HA, Bailey SM. Massive pulmonary embolism in healthy people. BMJ 1966;1:1322–6.

74. Dalen JE, Alpert JS. Natural history of pulmonary embolism. Prog Cardiovasc Dis 1975;17:259–70.

75. Saeger W, Genzkow M. Venous thromboses and pulmonary embolisms in post-mortem series – probable causes by correlations of clinical data and basic diseases. Pathol Res Pract 1994;190:394–9.

76. Geerts WH, Code KI, Jay RM, et al. A prospective study of venous thromboembolism after major trauma. N Engl J Med 1994;331:1601–6.

77. Baglin TP, White K, Charles A. Fatal pulmonary embolism in hospitalised medical patients. J Clin Pathol 1997;50:609–10.

78. Alikhan R, Peters F, Wilmott R, et al. Fatal pulmonary embolism in hospitalised patients: a necropsy review. J Clin Pathol 2004;57:1254–7.

79. Sweetland S, Green J, Liu B, et al. Duration and magnitude of the postoperative risk of venous thromboembolism in middle aged women: prospective cohort study. BMJ 2009;339:b4583.

80. Diebold J, Lohrs U. Venous thrombosis and pulmonary embolism – a study of 5039 autopsies. Pathol Res Pract 1991;187:260–6.

81. Connors AF Jr, Castele RJ, Farhat NZ, et al. Complication of right heart catherisation. Chest 1985;88:567–72.

82. Katsumura Y, Ohtsubo KI. Incidence of pulmonary thromboembolism, infarction and haemorrhage in disseminated intravascular coagulation: a necroscopic analysis. Thorax 1995;50:160–4.

83. British Thoracic Society Standards of Care Committee. BTS Guidelines for the Management of Suspected Acute Pulmonary Embolism. Thorax 2003;58:470–84.

84. Lidegaard O, Lokkegaard E, Svendsen AL, et al. Hormonal contraception and risk of venous thromboembolism: national follow-up study. BMJ 2009;339:557–60.

85. Dalen JE. Pulmonary embolism: What have we learned since Virchow? – Natural history, pathophysiology, and diagnosis. Chest 2002;122:1440–56.

86. Mahmoodi BK, Gansevoort RT, Veeger NJ, et al. Microalbuminuria and risk of venous thromboembolism. JAMA 2009;301:1790–7.

87. Office of Population Censuses and Surveys. Mortality statistics: cause 1988. London: HMSO; 1990.

88. Chau KY, Yuen ST, Wong MP. Seasonal variation in the necropsy incidence of pulmonary thromboembolism in Hong Kong. J Clin Pathol 1995;48:578–9.

89. Chau KY, Yuen ST, Wong MP. Seasonal variation in the necropsy incidence of pulmonary thromboembolism – comment. J Clin Pathol 1995;48:883.

90. Allan TM, Douglas AS. Seasonal variation in deep vein thrombosis. Fatal pulmonary embolism is increased in both autumn and winter. BMJ 1996;312:1227.

92. Stein PD, Kayali F, Beemath A, et al. Mortality from acute pulmonary embolism according to season. Chest 2005;128:3156–8.

93. Moser KM, LeMoine JR. Is embolic risk conditioned by location of deep venous thrombosis? Ann Intern Med 1981;94:439–44.

94. Hull RD, Raskob GE, Hirsh J. Prophylaxis of venous thromboembolism: an overview. Chest 1986;89:374S–83S.

95. Girard P, Musset D, Parent F, et al. High prevalence of detectable deep venous thrombosis in patients with acute pulmonary embolism. Chest 1999;116:903–8.

96. Morpurgo M, Schmid C. The spectrum of pulmonary embolism. Chest 1995;107:18S–20S.

97. Huisman MV, Buller HR, ten Cate JW, et al. Unexpected high prevalence of silent pulmonary embolism in patients with deep venous thrombosis. Chest 1989;95:498–502.

98. Blauwet LA, Edwards WD, Tazelaar HD, et al. Surgical pathology of pulmonary thromboendarterectomy: A study of 54 cases from 1990 to 2001. Hum Pathol 2003;34:1290–8.

99. Bernard J, Yi ES. Pulmonary thromboendarterectomy: a clinicopathologic study of 200 consecutive pulmonary thromboendarterectomy cases in one institution. Hum Pathol 2007;38:871–7.

100. Pryce DM, Heard BE. The distribution of experimental pulmonary emboli in the rabbit. J Pathol Bacteriol 1956;71:15–25.

101. Morrell MT, Dunnill MS. Fibrous bands in conducting pulmonary arteries. J Clin Pathol 1967;20:139–44.

102. Wagenvoort CA. Pathology of pulmonary thromboembolism. Chest 1995;107:S10–S17.

Pulmonary infarction

103. Castleman B. Healed pulmonary infarcts. Arch Pathol 1940;30:130–42.

104. Yousem SA. The surgical pathology of pulmonary infarcts: diagnostic confusion with granulomatous disease, vasculitis, and neoplasia. Mod Pathol 2009;22:679–85.

105. Williamson WA, Tronic BS, Levitan N, et al. Pulmonary venous infarction. Chest 1992;102:937–40.

106. Williamson WA, Tronic BS, Levitan N, et al. Pulmonary venous infarction secondary to squamous cell carcinoma. Chest 1992;102:950–2.

Non-thrombotic pulmonary emboli

107. Jorens PG, van Marck E, Snoeckx A, et al. Nonthrombotic pulmonary embolism. Eur Respir J 2009;34:452–74.

108. Sevitt S. The role of fat embolism in causation and of oxygen toxicity in the lung pathology. In: Williams WG, Smith RE, editors. Trauma of the Chest. Bristol: John Wright; 1977. p. 164–75.

109. Laub DR Jr, Laub DR. Fat embolism syndrome after liposuction: a case report and review of the literature. Ann Plast Surg 1990;25:48–52.

110. Hulman G. The pathogenesis of fat embolism. J Pathol 1995;176:3–9.

111. Zaidi Y, Sivakumaran M, Graham C, et al. Fatal bone marrow embolism in a patient with sickle cell beta(+) thalassaemia. J Clin Pathol 1996;49:774–5.

112. Baker PL. Free fatty acids, catecholamines, and arterial hypoxia in patients with fat embolism. The J Trauma 1971;11:1026–30.

113. Moylan JA, Birnbaum M, Katz A, et al. Fat emboli syndrome. J Trauma 1976;16:341–7.

114. Asnis DS, Saltzman HP, Melchert A. Shark oil pneumonia – an overlooked entity. Chest 1993;103:976–7.

115. Hulman G, Levene M. Intralipid microemboli. Arch Dis Child 1986;61:702–3.

116. Kitchell CC, Balogh K. Pulmonary lipid emboli in association with long-term hyperalimentation. Hum Pathol 1986;17:83–5.

117. Reedy JS, Kuhlman JE, Voytovich M. Microvascular pulmonary emboli secondary to precipitated crystals in a patient receiving total parenteral nutrition – A case report and description of the high-resolution CT findings. Chest 1999;115:892–5.

118. Attwood HD. Amniotic fluid embolism. Pathol Annu 1972;7:145–72.

119. Fineschi V, Riezzo I, Cantatore S, et al. Complement C3a expression and tryptase degranulation as promising histopathological tests for diagnosing fatal amniotic fluid embolism. Virchows Archiv 2009;454:283–90.

120. Attwood HD, Park WW. Embolism to the lung by trophoblast. J Obstet Gynaec Brit Commonw 1961;68:611–7.

121. Garner EI. Trophoblastic pulmonary embolization after hysterectomy for invasive complete mole. A case report. Journal of Reproductive Medicine 1999;44:908–12.

122. Attwood HD. Personal communication 1991.

123. Delmis J, Pfeifer D, Ivanisevic M, et al. Sudden death from trophoblastic embolism in pregnancy. Eur J Obstet Gynecol Reprod Biol 2000;92:225–7.

124. Savage MB. Trophoblastic lesions of the lungs following benign hydatidiform mole. Am J Obst Gyn 1951;62:346–52.

125. Park WW. The occurrence of decidual tissue within the lung: report of a case. J Pathol Bacteriol 1954;67:563–70.

126. Willis RA. The Spread of Tumours in the Human Body. 3 ed. London: Butterworths; 1973. p. 47–8.

127. Morgan AD. The pathology of subacute cor pulmonale in diffuse carcinomatosis of the lungs. J Pathol Bacteriol 1949;61:75–84.

128. Bagshawe KD, Brooks WDW. Subacute pulmonary hypertension due to chorionepithelioma. Lancet 1959;1:653–8.

129. He XW, Tang YH, Luo ZQ, et al. Subacute cor pulmonale due to tumor embolization to the lungs. Angiology 1989;40:11–7.

130. Seckl MJ, Rustin GJS, Newlands ES, et al. Pulmonary embolism, pulmonary hypertension, and choriocarcinoma. Lancet 1991;338:1313–5.

131. Veinot JP, Ford SE, Price RG. Subacute cor pulmonale due to tumor embolization. Arch Pathol Lab Med 1992;116:131–4.

132. Soares FA, Landell GAM, Deoliveira JAM. Pulmonary tumor embolism to alveolar septal capillaries – an unusual cause of sudden cor pulmonale. Arch Pathol Lab Med 1992;116:187–8.

133. Hibbert M, Braude S. Tumour microembolism presenting as 'primary pulmonary hypertension'. Thorax 1997;52:1016–7.

134. Storey PD, Goldstein W. Pulmonary embolization from primary hepatic carcinoma. Arch Intern Med 1962;110:262–9.

135. Wakasa K, Sakurai M, Uchida A, et al. Massive pulmonary tumor emboli in osteosarcoma: occult and fatal complication. Cancer 1990;66:583–6.

136. Ahmed AA, Heller DS. Fatal pulmonary tumor embolism caused by chondroblastic osteosarcoma – Report of a case and review of the literature. Arch Pathol Lab Med 1999;123:437–40.

137. Watanabe S, Shimokawa S, Sakasegawa K, et al. Choriocarcinoma in the pulmonary artery treated with emergency pulmonary embolectomy. Chest 2002;121:654–6.

138. Edmondstone WM. Flitting radiographic shadows: an unusual presentation of cancer in the lungs. Thorax 1998;53:906–8.

139. von Herbay A, Illes A, Waldherr R, et al. Pulmonary tumor thrombotic microangiopathy with pulmonary hypertension. Cancer 1990;66:587–92.

140. Systrom DM, Mark EJ, Bhalla M, et al. A 55-year-old woman with acute respiratory failure and radiographically clear lungs – pulmonary embolic and lymphangitic carcinomatosis of breast origin. N Engl J Med 1995;332:1700–7.

141. Sato Y, Marutsuka K, Asada Y, et al. Pulmonary tumor thrombotic microangiopathy. Pathol Int 1995;45:436–40.

142. Kobayashi H, Tamashima S, Shigeyama J, et al. Vascular intimal carcinomatosis: An autopsy case of unusual form of pulmonary metastasis of transitional cell carcinoma. Pathol Int 1997;47:655–7.

143. Levine SB. Embolism of cerebral tissue to lungs. Arch Pathol 1973;96:183–5.

144. Bohm N, Keller KM, Kloke WD. Pulmonary and systemic cerebellar tissue embolism due to birth injury. Virchows Arch A Pathol Anat Histopathol 1982;398:229–35.

145. Dunnill MS. The pathology of pulmonary embolism. Br J Surg 1968;55:790794.

145a. Mehta RI, Lai CK, Kee S, Fishbein MC. Intrapulmonary ectopic liver after orthotopic heart transplantation. Archives of Pathology & Laboratory Medicine 2010;134:1060–2.

146. Balogh K. Pulmonary bile emboli. Sequelae of iatrogenic trauma. Arch Pathol Lab Med 1984;108:814–6.

147. Sabatine MS, Oelberg DA, Mark EJ, et al. Pulmonary cholesterol crystal embolization. Chest 1997;112:1687–92.

148. Arnett EN, Battle WE, Russo JV, et al. Intravenous injection of talc-containing drugs intended for oral use. A cause of pulmonary granulomatosis and pulmonary hypertension. Am J Med 1976;60:711–8.

149. Gross EM. Autopsy findings in drug addicts. Pathol Annu 1978;13:35–67.

150. Pare JAP, Fraser RG, Hogg JC, et al. Pulmonary 'mainline' granulomatosis: talcosis of intravenous methadone abuse. Medicine (Baltimore) 1979;58:229–39.

151. Waller BF, Brownlee WJ, Roberts WC. Self induced pulmonary granulomatosis. A consequence of intravenous injection of drugs intended for oral use. Chest 1980;78:90–4.

152. Tomashefski JF Jr, Hirsch CS. The pulmonary vascular lesions of intravenous drug abuse. Hum Pathol 1980;11:133–45.

153. Tomashefski JF, Hirsch CS, Jolly PN. Microcrystalline cellulose pulmonary embolism and granulomatosis. Arch Pathol Lab Med 1981;105:89–93.

154. Farber HW, Fairman RP, Glauser FL. Talc granulomatosis: laboratory findings similar to sarcoidosis. Am Rev Respir Dis 1982;125:258–61.

155. Rajs J, Harm T, Ormstad K. Postmortem findings of pulmonary lesions of older datum in intravenous drug addicts. A forensic-pathologic study. Virchows Arch A Pathol Anat Histopathol 1984;402:405–14.

156. Crouch E, Churg A. Progressive massive fibrosis of the lung secondary to intravenous injection of talc. A pathologic and mineralogic analysis. Am J Clin Pathol 1983;80:520–6.

157. Cooper CB, Bai TR, Heyderman E, et al. Cellulose granulomas in the lungs of a cocaine sniffer. BMJ 1983;286:2021–2.

158. Ganesan S, Felo J, Saldana M, et al. Embolized crospovidone (poly[N-vinyl-2-pyrrolidone]) in the lungs of intravenous drug users. Mod Pathol 2003;16:286–92.

159. Abraham JL, Brambilla C. Particle size for differentiation between inhalation and injection pulmonary talcosis. Environ Res 1980;21:94–6.

160. Buchanan DR, Lamb D, Seaton A. Punk rocker's lung: pulmonary fibrosis in a drug snorting fire-eater. BMJ 1981;283:1661.

161. Lamb RK, Pawade A, Prior AL. Intravascular missile: apparent retrograde course from the left ventricle. Thorax 1988;43:499–500.

162. Nehme AE. Intracranial bullet migrating to pulmonary artery. J Trauma 1980;20:344–6.

163. Leong ASY, Disney APS, Gove DW. Spallation and migration of silicone from blood-pump tubing in patients on hemodialysis. N Engl J Med 1982;306:135–40.

163a. Mehta RI, Mehta RI, Solis OE, et al. Hydrophilic polymer emboli: an under-recognised iatrogenic cause of ischemia and infarct. Mod Pathol 2010;23:921–30.

164. Chastre J, Basset F, Viau F, et al. Acute pneumonitis after subcutaneous injections of silicone in transsexual men. N Engl J Med 1983;308:764–7.

165. Robinson MJ, Nestor M, Rywlin AM. Pulmonary granulomas secondary to embolic prosthetic valve material. Hum Pathol 1981;12:759–62.

166. Mittleman RE, Marraccini JV. Pulmonary Teflon granulomas following periurethral Teflon injection for urinary incontinence. Arch Pathol Lab Med 1983;107:611–2.

167. Lai YF, Chao TY, Wong SL. Acute pneumonitis after subcutaneous injections of silicone for augmentation mammaplasty. Chest 1994;106:1152–5.

168. Schmid A, Tzur A, Leshko L, et al. Silicone embolism syndrome: a case report, review of the literature, and comparison with fat embolism syndrome. Chest 2005;127:2276–81.

168a. Park HJ, Jung KH, Kim SY, Lee JH, Jeong JY, Kim JH. Hyaluronic acid pulmonary embolism: a critical consequence of an illegal cosmetic vaginal procedure. Thorax 2010;65:360–1.

169. Gough JH, Gough MH, Thomas ML. Pulmonary complications following lymphangiography with a note on technique. Br J Radiol 1964;37:416–21.

170. Fraimow W, Wallace S, Lewis P, et al. Changes in pulmonary function due to lymphangiography. Radiology 1965;85:231–41.

171. Davidson JW. Pulmonary complications of lymphangiography. N Engl J Med 1971;285:237.

172. Silvestri RC, Hyseby JS, Rughani I, et al. Respiratory distress syndrome from lymphangiography contrast medium. Am Rev Respir Dis 1980;122:543–9.

173. Coard K, Silver MD, Perkins G, et al. Isobutyl-2-cyanoacrylate pulmonary emboli associated with occlusive embolotherapy of cerebral arteriovenous malformations. Histopathology 1984;8:917–26.

174. Murakata LA, Lewin-Smith MR, Specht CS, et al. Characterization of acrylic polyamide plastic embolization particles in vitro and in human tissue sections by light microscopy, infrared microspectroscopy and scanning electron microscopy with energy dispersive X-ray analysis. Mod Pathol 2006;19:922–30.

175. Oliver RM, Thomas MR, Cornaby AJ, et al. Mercury pulmonary emboli following intravenous self-injection. Br J Dis Chest 1987;81:76–9.

176. Bhagat R, Holmes IH, Kulaga A, et al. Self-injection with olive oil: a cause of lipoid pneumonia. Chest 1995;107:875–6.

177. Fairfax AJ, Ball J, Batten JC, et al. A pathological study following bronchial artery embolization for haemoptysis in cystic fibrosis. Br J Dis Chest 1980;74:345–52.

178. Kepes JJ, Yarde WL. Visualization of injected embolic material (polyvinyl alcohol) in paraffin sections with Verhoeff–van Gieson elastica stain. Am J Surg Pathol 1995;19:709–11.

179. Zaugg M, Kaplan V, Widmer U, et al. Fatal air embolism in an airplane passenger with a giant intrapulmonary bronchogenic cyst. Am J Respir Crit Care Med 1998;157:1686–9.

180. Belcher E, Lawson MH, Nicholson AG, et al. Congenital cystic adenomatoid malformation presenting as in-flight systemic air embolisation. Eur Respir J 2007;30:801–4.

181. Fitchet A, Fitzpatrick AP. Central venous air embolism causing pulmonary oedema mimicking left ventricular failure. BMJ 1998;316:604–6.

Pulmonary aneurysms

182. Bartter T, Irwin RS, Nash G. Aneurysms of the pulmonary arteries. Chest 1988;94:1065–75.

183. Chiu B, Magil A. Idiopathic pulmonary arterial trunk aneurysm presenting as cor pulmonale: report of a case. Hum Pathol 1985;16:947–9.

184. Onorato E, Festa P, Bourlon F, et al. Idiopathic right pulmonary artery aneurysm with pulmonary valve insufficiency. Cathet Cardiovasc Diagn 1996;37:162–5.

185. Burrows NJ, Johnson SR. Pulmonary artery aneurysm and tuberous sclerosis. Thorax 2004;59:86.

186. Shanks JH, Coup A, Howat AJ. Dissecting aneurysm of the pulmonary artery associated with a large facial cavernous haemangioma. Histopathology 1997;30:390–2.

187. Inayama Y, Nakatani Y, Kitamura H. Pulmonary artery dissection in patients without underlying pulmonary hypertension. Histopathology 2001;38:435–42.

188. Bartram C, Strickland B. Pulmonary varices. Br J Radiol 1971;44:927–35.

189. Man KM, Keeffe EB, Brown CR, et al. Pulmonary varices presenting as a solitary lung mass in a patient with end-stage liver disease. Chest 1994;106:294–6.

190. Shida T, Ohashi H, Nakamura K, et al. Pulmonary varices associated with mitral valve disease: a case report and survey of the literature. Ann Thorac Surg 1982;34:452–6.

Chapter | 8 |

8.2 Pulmonary hypertension

Normally the pressure in the pulmonary artery seldom exceeds 30/15 mmHg but in a variety of cardiopulmonary diseases this figure can increase up to fourfold. Pulmonary hypertension is defined as a mean pulmonary artery pressure greater than or equal to 25 mmHg at rest.[1] The causes operate at the precapillary, capillary or postcapillary level, as listed in Table 8.2.1. Pre- and postcapillary forms of pulmonary hypertension are distinguished haemodynamically by capillary wedge pressures of ≤15 or >15 mmHg respectively.[2,3]

In diffuse fibrosis the pulmonary pathology is dominated by the parenchymal disease, but with the other causes the vascular changes preponderate. These fall into distinct categories that largely correspond to the cause of the hypertension, the principal ones being plexogenic, hypoxic, thromboembolic and venous, as indicated in Table 8.2.1 and Figure 8.2.1. Thus, to a large extent, the pathological changes indicate the cause of the hypertension, as well as its presence and severity.[4,5] This classification serves pathologists well but is apparently of less benefit to clinicians and a multispecialty international group has therefore devised an alternative classification, which is shown in Box 8.2.1.[6,7] This concentrates on clinical parameters rather than histological features and thus facilitates categorisation of the many patients who are not studied histologically. However, it may be noted that in this classification diseases that show the same histological pattern of vasculopathy (e.g. left-sided heart disease and compression of large veins) appear in different categories, whilst others that are profoundly different histologically are grouped together (e.g. plexogenic arteriopathy and pulmonary veno-occlusive disease).[8] We therefore adhere to the scheme depicted in Table 8.2.1 and Figure 8.2.1. Whichever classification is preferred, certain histological features are shared by all categories and these will be described first. An elastin stain is invaluable in appreciating the vascular changes.

The earliest vascular changes are not specific and are present irrespective of the cause. In mild pulmonary hypertension histological diagnosis will be entirely dependent on the recognition of these early changes. They consist of medial hypertrophy, which is followed by subendothelial intimal fibrosis (Fig. 8.2.2). Isolated intimal fibrosis is not indicative of pulmonary hypertension as it is merely a common age change encountered irrespective of the pressure in the lesser circulation. Medial thickening is not an age change but is due to prolonged contraction of its smooth muscle and represents a form of work hypertrophy, probably stimulated by mediators released by the endothelium, notably endothelin, which counters the action of the endothelium-derived vasodilatory agent nitric oxide.[9]

Medial thickening is conveniently quantitated by tracing the internal and external elastic laminae on a digitising tablet and using a computer to express the media as a proportion of the whole vessel in terms of either its diameter or area. The vessel is often collapsed and

Table 8.2.1 Causes of pulmonary hypertension and their principal pathological features

Cause	Pathology
Precapillary: constrictive	Plexogenic arteriopathy
Unknown (primary pulmonary hypertension)	
Hyperkinetic congenital heart disease	
Chronic liver disease with portosystemic venous shunting	
Human immunodeficiency virus infection	
Appetite-suppressing drugs (aminorex, fenfluramine)	
Hereditary haemorrhagic telangiectasia	
Connective tissue disease	
Precapillary: hypoxic	Peripheral extension of medial muscle and the development of longitudinal muscle within the intima
Prolonged residence at high altitude	
Chronic obstructive lung disease	
Sleep apnoea obesity syndrome	
Precapillary: embolic	Recanalisation
Thromboembolic	
Parasitic (schistosomal)	
Tumour emboli	
Capillary	
Widespread pulmonary fibrosis	
Capillary haemangiomatosis	
Diffuse smooth-muscle proliferation	
Postcapillary	Venous muscular hypertrophy and luminal obliteration
Left-sided heart disease	
Veno-occlusive disease	

Figure 8.2.1 Patterns of vasculopathy in pulmonary hypertension. (1) Plexogenic arteriopathy characterised by medial hypertrophy, concentric intimal fibrosis, necrotising arteritis and a variety of dilatation lesions. (2) Thromboembolic vasculopathy, characterised by eccentric intimal thickening and duplication of the lumen by intimal bands. (3) Venous hypertension characterised by medial hypertrophy and either eccentric or concentric thickening of the arterial media coupled with intimal sclerosis of the postcapillary vessels. (4) Hypoxic vasculopathy, characterised by mild medial hypertrophy and the development of longitudinal bundles of smooth muscle in the intima. *(Reproduced from Wagenvoort (1973)[4] by permission of the editor of* Chest.*)*

the elastic laminae consequently wrinkled but the computer can be programmed to express the diameter of the vessel as if it had been fixed in the filled state and the elastic laminae were smooth.[10] Normal values are best obtained by the same operator but the medial thickness of a normal muscular pulmonary artery has been given as 3–5% of its external diameter (compared with 15–20% in systemic arteries).[11]

PLEXOGENIC PULMONARY ARTERIOPATHY

The word 'plexogenic' indicates a potential to develop plexiform lesions rather than their presence and was chosen to identify the disease as a whole, including the early stages described above because the plexiform lesions occur only in the final stages of the disease.[12] It is notable that plexiform lesions are not encountered in chronic pulmonary venous hypertension, chronic hypoxic pulmonary hypertension or pulmonary hypertension due to chronic thromboembolic disease. They are limited to forms of pulmonary hypertension characterised by intense vasoconstriction, which are those listed under Precapillary: constrictive in Table 8.2.1.

In plexogenic arteriopathy the medial hypertrophy described above is followed in sequence by concentric intimal fibrosis, necrotising

fibrinoid arteriopathy (Fig. 8.2.3) and the development of characteristic dilatation lesions, some of which are plexiform.[12–15]

The cellular component of the concentric intimal fibrosis is made up of fibroblasts, myofibroblasts and smooth-muscle cells, largely derived from the media but with contributions from the endothelium and circulating stem cells.[16–19] Concentric intimal fibrosis is also encountered in some connective tissue disease, particularly systemic sclerosis (see p. 430).

The necrotising arteriopathy is very similar morphologically to the autoimmune arteritides dealt with in the next chapter but is to be regarded as a consequence of severe medial contraction rather than an immune process. It is seldom seen in isolation, nearly always being accompanied by the dilatation lesions that develop from it.

Dilatation lesions are thin-walled vascular structures that come off a greatly thickened muscular artery. Beyond their point of origin the parent artery is usually obliterated by intimal fibrosis (Fig. 8.2.4).[20] They are thought to represent 'blow-out lesions' at points of necrotising arteritis in the wall of the parent vessel.[14,20] It is therefore justifiable to condense into one the last three grades of the traditional Heath and Edwards grading system (Table 8.2.2),[14,21,22] which was devised specifically for patients with hyperkinetic pulmonary hypertension secondary to congenital heart disease but can be equally applied to plexogenic arteriopathy of whatever cause.

Dilatation lesions involve the supernumerary arteries where these vessels leave the axial arteries (see Fig. 8.2.4).[20,23] Supernumerary arteries differ from axial arteries in that they do not accompany bronchioles or branch at a narrow angle: they leave the axial vessel at

1. Pulmonary arterial hypertension (PAH)
    1.1. Idiopathic (IPAH)
    1.2. Familial (FPAH)
    1.3. Associated with (APAH):
        1.3.1. Collagen vascular disease
        1.3.2. Congenital systemic-to-pulmonary shunts
        1.3.3. Portal hypertension
        1.3.4. Human immunodeficiency virus (HIV) infection
        1.3.5. Drugs and toxins
        1.3.6. Other (thyroid disorders, glycogen storage disease, Gaucher disease, hereditary telangiectasia, haemoglobinopathies, myeloproliferative disorders, splenectomy)
    1.4. Associated with significant venous or capillary involvement
        1.4.1. Pulmonary veno-occlusive disease (PVOD)
        1.4.2. Pulmonary capillary haemangiomatosis (PCH)
    1.5. Persistent pulmonary hypertension of the newborn
2. Pulmonary hypertension with left heart disease
    2.1. Left-sided atrial or ventricular heart disease
    2.2. Left-sided valvular heart disease
3. Pulmonary hypertension associated with lung diseases and/or hypoxaemia
    3.1. Chronic obstructive pulmonary disease
    3.2. Interstitial lung disease
    3.3. Sleep-disordered breathing
    3.4. Alveolar hypoventilation disorders
    3.5. Chronic exposure to high altitude
    3.6. Developmental abnormalities
4. Pulmonary hypertension due to chronic thrombotic and/or embolic disease
    4.1. Thromboembolic obstruction of proximal pulmonary arteries
    4.2. Thromboembolic obstruction of distal pulmonary arteries
    4.3. Non-thrombotic pulmonary embolism (tumour, parasites, foreign material)
5. Miscellaneous
    Sarcoidosis, histiocytosis X, lymphangiomatosis, compression of pulmonary vessels (adenopathy, tumour, fibrosing mediastinitis)

Figure 8.2.3 (A) Necrotising arteritis in a patient with severe pulmonary hypertension secondary to a ventricular septal defect. (B) In another patient with pulmonary hypertension an early dilatation lesion has developed consequent upon the arterial wall being weakened by focal necrosis.

Figure 8.2.2 Pulmonary hypertension. There is marked medial hypertrophy and cellular intimal thickening. Pulmonary arteries normally have an extremely thin media and the thickening here represents marked hypertrophy. Its proximity to an airway indicates that this blood vessel is an artery rather than a vein.

an obtuse angle and feed alveolar capillaries soon after their origin.[24] Thus they rapidly narrow and there is considerable reduction in pressure over a short distance. When the arterial pressure is raised there is significant physical stress on these arteries and it is likely that this is involved in the development of the necrotising arteritis and the subsequent dilatation lesions.

Dilatation lesions are described as being simple, plexiform or angiomatoid. Simple dilatation lesions are saccular aneurysms, whereas plexiform lesions represent such aneurysms filled by connective tissue that is rich in myofibroblasts and is intersected by a complex of fine endothelium-lined spaces (Fig. 8.2.5).[16,25] It is reported that the endothelial cell proliferation is monoclonal in primary but not in secondary pulmonary hypertension.[26,27] Plexiform lesions often lead to wide thin-walled vessels which in turn feed into capillaries (Fig. 8.2.6).[20] They occasionally reach a diameter of 1 mm. The multiple fine channels probably represent organised and recanalised thrombi within an otherwise simple dilatation lesion. The narrow channels of

Figure 8.2.4 A computer-aided reconstruction of the distal pulmonary arteries in plexogenic pulmonary hypertension. Plexiform lesions (white) occur in supernumerary arteries just proximal to a point where the larger axial arteries are obliterated by intimal proliferation (green). Only a few patent vessels remain (arrows). *(Reproduced from Yaginuma et al. (1990)[20] by permission of the editor of* Thorax.*)*

Figure 8.2.5 A plexiform lesion. The media of this pulmonary artery is deficient on one side and here the lumen communicates with a plexus of fine channels. On the other side of the artery the media is greatly hypertrophied.

Table 8.2.2 Heath & Edwards[21] grading system of hypertensive pulmonary vascular disease. This system was designed for use in connection with congenital heart disease. It is applicable to other causes of plexogenic pulmonary arteriopathy but not to other causes of pulmonary hypertension. Because dilatation lesions are now thought to be due to fibrinoid necrosis,[14] grades 4–6 could well be condensed into one. The critical area regarding reversibility lies in the region of grades 2 and 3 and there is a case for dividing these according to the degree of luminal narrowing[22]

Grade	Histological criteria
1	Medial hypertrophy
2	Grade 1 plus cellular intimal thickening
3	Grade 1 plus fibrous intimal thickening
4	Grades 2 or 3 plus dilatation lesions
5	Grade 4 plus haemosiderosis
6	Grade 5 plus necrotising arteritis

Figure 8.2.6 A plexiform lesion. The point of origin from the adjacent artery is not evident but surrounding the plexiform lesion is a collection of wide thin-walled vessels.

Siderophages, cholesterol granulomas and focal fibrosis represent secondary changes consequent upon pulmonary haemorrhage, which may complicate severe or longstanding cases of plexogenic pulmonary hypertension.[15] Pulmonary arterial thrombosis, identical in appearance to thrombotic embolism, is generally a further secondary change[15] but in primary pulmonary hypertension it may be an inherent component of the pathogenetic process, as discussed below.[30]

Congenital heart disease

Congenital cardiovascular anomalies characterised by left-to-right shunting, such as patent ductus arteriosus and septal defects, result in a hyperkinetic form of pulmonary hypertension in which the blood enters the pulmonary arteries in greater volume or at a higher pressure than usual. In cases of atrial septal defect, blood passes from the left to the right atrium, and so adds to the quantity of blood entering the pulmonary artery. This can usually be accommodated because of the marked distensibility of the pulmonary vasculature and hypertension seldom develops before middle age. However, when there is a ven-

a plexiform lesion are probably responsible for the microangiopathic haemolytic anaemia that occasionally complicates plexogenic pulmonary arteriopathy.[28] The angiomatoid lesion consists of several thin-walled cavernous spaces linking a muscular pulmonary artery to its capillary bed and resembling a haemangioma (Fig. 8.2.7). They were once thought to represent congenital malformations but are now recognised to be acquired.

Plexiform lesions need to be distinguished from organised recanalised thrombus with florid endothelial cell proliferation. The essential difference is that plexiform lesions lie alongside the parent artery whereas organised thrombus is within. Elastin stains are helpful in that pulmonary arteries containing recanalised thrombus usually have intact internal and external elastic laminae whereas these structures are destroyed at the site of plexiform lesions.[29]

Figure 8.2.7 An angiomatoid lesion. A convoluted, wide, thin-walled vessel simulating a haemangioma leads directly off a hypertrophied pulmonary artery; the narrow sinusoids of a plexiform lesion are not apparent in this type of dilatation lesion.

Figure 8.2.8 Aorta (left) and pulmonary trunk (right) in congenital pulmonary hypertension secondary to a ventricular septal defect (A), and in acquired pulmonary hypertension secondary to bronchopulmonary disease that developed in adult life (B). The fragmented elastin pattern of the normal adult pulmonary trunk is maintained in acquired pulmonary hypertension but in patients in whom the pulmonary hypertension has been present from birth the fetal pattern (which is identical to that in the aorta) is maintained. Elastin van Gieson stain.

tricular septal defect or patent ductus arteriosus, the increase in the volume of the blood in the pulmonary circulation is accompanied by a substantial increase in pressure. The changes in the walls of the pulmonary arteries are consequently more severe and develop early in life. There is severe constriction of small muscular arteries, which undergo medial hypertrophy and raise the pulmonary resistance through their hypertonicity. At this stage they are still capable of relaxation and there is enough circulatory reserve to meet the needs of exercise, but when severe hypertension persists the lumen of the small muscular arteries becomes further narrowed by thickening of the intima. Initially this is due to concentric laminar cellular proliferation but later intimal fibrosis supervenes. The vessels are then less capable of adaptive dilatation, the hypertension becomes irreversible and the patient enters a perpetual state of high pulmonary resistance and low circulatory reserve. Further vascular changes are those described above under plexogenic arteriopathy. There may also be secondary pulmonary artery thrombosis, organisation of which leads to eccentric plaques of intimal fibrosis. The practical point is that the underlying congenital anomalies should be corrected before the pulmonary arteries are permanently narrowed by intimal fibrosis.

Lung biopsy can be useful in assessing the reversibility of hyperkinetic pulmonary hypertension,[31–33] but carries a risk of severe haemorrhage and most cases are now assessed by cardiac catheterisation. Histological features that are compatible with a successful corrective operation include medial hypertrophy, cellular concentric intimal thickening of moderate degree and eccentric intimal fibrosis consequent upon thrombosis. Conversely, severe intimal fibrosis, fibrinoid necrosis and dilatation lesions suggest that the pulmonary hypertension will progress despite corrective surgery. However, potential reversibility probably differs from safe operability. Medial hypertrophy is potentially reversible but may be associated with fatal pulmonary hypertensive crises at operation.[34]

The major pulmonary arteries are elastic vessels and at birth the pattern of their elastic laminae closely resembles that of the aorta. However, within the first few months of life there is fragmentation of the elastic fibres and an irreversible 'adult pattern' is reached by about the age of 6 months. This 'adult pattern' is maintained even if pulmonary hypertension develops in later life, whereas in congenital pulmonary hypertension the 'aortic pattern' found at birth persists (Fig. 8.2.8).

In conditions leading to low pulmonary flow rates or diminished pulmonary artery pulse pressure, such as congenital pulmonary stenosis, perhaps as part of Fallot's tetrad, the pulmonary arteries show changes the reverse of those described above, namely medial atrophy, so that they are extremely thin-walled. A media is sometimes not apparent. The low blood flow and the almost invariably raised haematocrit promote thrombosis and evidence of this in the form of eccentric intimal plaques or subdivision of the lumen is often apparent. However, this is seldom so extensive that it causes pulmonary hypertension, but corrective procedures entailing shunts may lead to plexogenic arteriopathy.

Primary pulmonary hypertension

The microscopic features of primary pulmonary hypertension are those of plexogenic pulmonary arteriopathy, as described above. They are indistinguishable from those seen in plexogenic pulmonary hypertension due to any of the other causes listed in Table 8.2.1. A diagnosis of primary pulmonary hypertension can therefore only be made when all other possible causes of plexogenic pulmonary arteriopathy have been excluded by full clinical and radiological examination, cardiac catheterisation and, if necessary, open-lung biopsy. Despite this, the term 'primary pulmonary hypertension' has been used by clinicians when the condition remains unexplained after investigations that fall short of histological assessment. Pathological examination in 156 such cases showed that 70% were plexogenic, 20% were thrombotic and 6% showed venous obliteration.[13] Similar heterogeneity has been reported in other series.[35] Although plexogenic, thromboembolic and veno-occlusive pulmonary hypertension cannot be distinguished without histological assessment, their histological distinction is often blurred by plexogenic arteriopathy being complicated by thrombosis,[30] by the changes of veno-occlusive disease extending proximally to involve arteries and by venous abnormalities being identified in plexogenic arteriopathy.[15] Some workers therefore regard primary plexogenic arteriopathy, thrombotic pulmonary vascular disease and veno-occlusion as facets of one condition and term this primary pulmonary hypertension, on the basis that the cause is unknown whatever the predominant histological pattern.[35–37] Thus, the term 'primary pulmonary hypertension' is currently used in three different ways, of which we prefer the first:

1. for primary plexogenic pulmonary hypertension
2. for pulmonary hypertension that cannot be explained despite full clinical investigation (but falling short of histological assessment)
3. for pulmonary hypertension due to intrinsic pulmonary vascular disease regardless of whether histology shows this to be thrombotic, plexogenic or veno-occlusive.

Primary plexogenic pulmonary hypertension can occur at any age but most commonly affects young adults, with women outnumbering men by about 2 to 1.[13,38] A family history is evident in approximately 6% of patients[38] but the identification first of the responsible gene on chromosome 2 (2q32-34),[39,40] and then its expression in seemingly sporadic cases of primary pulmonary hypertension,[41,42] suggests that the true prevalence of familial cases is considerably higher. The gene concerned encodes for bone morphogenetic receptor protein-II (BMPR2), which controls the action of transforming growth factor-β on the vessel wall.[43–46] It is therefore relevant that the genes for hereditary haemorrhagic teleangiectasia (Osler–Weber–Rendu disease – see pp. 76 and 481), of which plexogenic pulmonary hypertension is a rare feature, also control the vascular transforming growth factor-β pathway.[47,48] Mutation of the BMPR2 gene is found in 70% of patients with familial pulmonary hypertension and up to 10% of patients with sporadic primary pulmonary hypertension.[49]

Endothelial factors such as angiotensin-converting enzyme, endothelin and (deficiency of) nitric oxide are further likely mediators.[50–52] Female sex hormones may also play a role.[53] A reported increase in airway neuroendocrine cells[54–56] and the detection of Chlamydia pneumoniae in the hypertrophied pulmonary arteries of a patient dying of pulmonary hypertension[57] are of uncertain significance. Raynaud's phenomenon is found in 10% and a positive anti-nuclear antibody test in about 30% of patients with primary pulmonary hypertension.[38] There is also a high prevalence of autoimmune thyroid disease.[58] Pulmonary hypertension associated with more pronounced connective tissue disease is considered below.

Hepatic disease

The prevalence of plexogenic pulmonary hypertension in cirrhosis is in the order of 0.7%[59] and the fact that it takes this form of arteriopathy[60,61] suggests that it is vasoconstrictive, perhaps the result of metabolites that are normally inactivated in the liver. Paradoxically, some patients with cirrhosis of the liver develop pulmonary arterial dilatation and arteriovenous communications in the lungs[62–64] while

in one series pulmonary venous intimal thickening was identified in 65% of cirrhotic patients.[65]

Ingested agents

A notable increase in the incidence of 'primary' pulmonary hypertension occurred in Switzerland, Austria and Germany during the period 1966–68 when the anorectic drug aminorex was marketed.[66] It was not possible to reproduce the disease experimentally but the epidemiological evidence that aminorex fumarate was responsible for the pulmonary hypertension is strong. The drug had been on sale only in these three countries and the increase in the frequency of pulmonary hypertension closely followed the rise in its sale, while following its withdrawal there was a corresponding fall in the number of cases of pulmonary hypertension. Another anorectic drug, fenfluramine, has also been linked to the development of pulmonary hypertension.[67–70] Plexiform lesions have been described with both these drugs.[71]

Pulmonary hypertension formed part of the Spanish toxic oil episode and the L-tryptophan-induced eosinophilia–myalgia syndrome. The changes wrought by these 'dietary' supplements include a pulmonary vasculitis and differ from those of plexogenic arteriopathy. They are described on pages 375 and 389.

Pyrollizidine alkaloids derived from various species of Senecio (ragworts and groundsels) cause intense vasoconstrictive pulmonary hypertension in laboratory animals but there is no evidence that ingestion of these plants causes pulmonary hypertension in humans. Nevertheless, observations such as these support the histopathological evidence that primary plexogenic pulmonary hypertension is vaso-contrictive in nature due to an as yet unidentified neural or humoral agent.

Human immunodeficiency virus (HIV) infection

An association of pulmonary hypertension with HIV infection is well established but until recently has been unexplained.[72–75] The virus cannot be identified in the pulmonary vessels but tubuloreticular structures suggestive of cytokine accumulation have been identified there by electron microscopy in HIV-positive individuals.[76] Evidence now emerging suggests that it is the highly active antiretroviral drugs administered to HIV-infected patients that are responsible for the vascular injury rather than the virus itself.[77]

The incidence of pulmonary hypertension in HIV-positive patients is 1 in 200, the male-to-female ratio is 1.6:1 and the age range is 3–56 years, with a mean of 32 years.[78] The arteriopathy is generally plexogenic but thrombotic or veno-occlusive changes are described in 15% of cases.[78] Suggestions that Kaposi sarcoma herpesvirus is similarly associated with pulmonary hypertension have not been substantiated.[79]

HYPOXIC PULMONARY HYPERTENSION

The pulmonary circulation differs from the systemic circulation in that it reacts to hypoxia by vasoconstriction rather than vasodilatation. Hypoxia, whether due to high altitude or a ventilatory lung defect, causes the muscular pulmonary arteries to constrict and, although the consequent pulmonary hypertension may be life-threatening, the intense spasm that leads to necrotising arteriopathy and dilatation lesions of plexogenic arteriopathy is not a feature. The mechanism by which hypoxia leads to pulmonary artery constriction is unclear but

Figure 8.2.9 Normal precapillary blood vessels of the lungs. As pulmonary arteries narrow, the muscle of the media thins progressively and in vessels between 100 and 30 μm in diameter it is represented only by a spiral so that in cross-section arteries of this size are only muscularised for part of their circumference. Below 30 μm diameter, precapillary vessels have no muscle at all in their walls, which consist only of fibroelastic tissue.

Figure 8.2.10 Hypoxic pulmonary hypertension. Intralobular arteries smaller than 30 μm diameter with a well-developed medial coat indicative of pulmonary hypertension are especially found with hypoxia. Elastin van Gieson stain.

Figure 8.2.11 Hypoxic pulmonary hypertension. The arterial media is hypertrophied and longitudinal bundles of smooth muscle have developed in the intima.

it operates at the local level, affecting only those vessels in the immediate vicinity of airways with low oxygen tensions.[80,81] It is likely that it involves changes in the levels of vasoactive factors synthesised and released by the arterial endothelium, in particular nitric oxide, which has vasodilatory properties, and endothelin, which is a vasoconstrictor (see p. 24).[50,51,82–84] The arteries involved are principally small precapillary vessels[80,81] but small pulmonary veins are also affected.[85] However, the earliest morphological response to hypoxia is found in the carotid bodies, which undergo hyperplasia before any structural changes are detectable in the lungs.[86]

Ventilatory disorders causing pulmonary hypertension include chronic obstructive pulmonary disease (see p. 102), bronchiectasis (see p. 119) and extrapulmonary causes of poor ventilation such as kyphoscoliosis and obesity. In emphysema, there is no correlation between the extent of capillary loss and right ventricular weight[87,88]: vasoconstriction is held to be responsible, as in other forms of hypoxic pulmonary hypertension. It is also possible that cigarette smoke components may augment the hypoxia by acting directly on the artery wall.[89] In bronchiectasis, both hypoxia and left-to-right shunts consequent upon bronchopulmonary arterial anastomoses contribute to the pulmonary hypertension.

Morphological changes characteristic of hypoxic pulmonary hypertension include mild medial hypertrophy affecting the smallest precapillary vessels. Below 100 μm diameter, the medial muscle normally spirals out and none at all is normally seen in vessels below about 30 μm in diameter: between 100 and 30 μm diameter, muscle is normally limited to one side of the vessel (Fig. 8.2.9). Fully muscularised vessels below 100 μm diameter and partially muscularised vessels below 30 μm diameter therefore indicate medial hypertrophy (Fig. 8.2.10).

A further feature is the occasional development of longitudinal bundles of smooth muscle in the intima of small pulmonary arteries (Fig. 8.2.11).[90–93] It is suggested that the development of longitudinal smooth muscle in the intima is caused by repeated stretching of the small pulmonary vessels as a consequence of wide respiratory excursions: in some experimental models, stretching of vessels results in such laying-down of longitudinal muscle,[94] but this is not confirmed by others, who regard the process as a component of normal repair.[95] Longitudinal smooth muscle is found in pulmonary arteries in other forms of pulmonary hypertension,[15,96] but not so noticeably as in the

hypoxic forms. The arterial changes found in hypoxic pulmonary hypertension are reversible, but irreversible airway disease or prolonged residence at high altitude may result in death in right-sided heart failure that is directly attributable to the hypoxic pulmonary hypertension.

PULMONARY HYPERTENSION IN DIFFUSE PARENCHYMAL LUNG DISEASE

Pulmonary hypertension develops when there is widespread pulmonary destruction, whatever the cause, but particularly pulmonary fibrosis. Thus, it is seen in advanced idiopathic pulmonary fibrosis, sarcoidosis, pneumoconiosis and Langerhans cell histiocytosis. In the fibrotic parts of the lung, occlusive intimal fibroelastosis akin to endarteritis obliterans is evident at a relatively early stage. With advancing disease there is widespread loss of capillaries and in less

Figure 8.2.12 Pulmonary hypertension associated with diffuse smooth-muscle proliferation of the lungs. *(Courtesy of Dr M Goddard, Papworth, UK.)*

Figure 8.2.13 Thromboembolic pulmonary hypertension. The artery has a double lumen separated by a collagenous band that represents organised thrombus. Elastin van Gieson stain.

severely affected parts small precapillary vessels are fully muscularised. In sarcoidosis the granulomas may involve the media and even the intima of pulmonary blood vessels (see Fig. 6.1.33, p. 287).

Rare examples have been reported of middle-aged men with severe pulmonary hypertension and diffuse smooth-muscle cell proliferation of the lungs (Fig. 8.2.12).[97,98] The smooth-muscle cell proliferation involves bronchioles, alveoli and small pulmonary arteries and veins; the vascular involvement accounts for the severe pulmonary hypertension, which results in cor pulmonale. The changes differ from those of pulmonary lymphangioleiomyomatosis (see p. 293) but are nevertheless also considered to be hamartomatous.[98]

EMBOLIC PULMONARY HYPERTENSION

Pulmonary hypertension may result from progressive diminution of the pulmonary vascular bed by multiple emboli. Thrombotic emboli may be very numerous but small and clinically silent. In these circumstances lung biopsy may show occlusion of small pulmonary arteries by thrombi in various stages of organisation. Totally organised emboli appear as eccentric fibrotic intimal plaques or show the multiple new lumina that indicate recanalisation (Fig. 8.2.13).[99] Occasionally the organisation of the thrombus takes the form of multiple fine channels and the appearances mimic those of a plexiform lesion. However, the latter develops in a thrombosed dilatation lesion and is situated alongside the parent artery whereas organisation of thrombotic emboli is confined to the obliterated arterial lumen. The elastic laminae are intact in recanalised arteries but destroyed at the site of a plexiform lesion.[29] We do not support the view that thromboembolic pulmonary hypertension is characterised by plexiform lesions, as proposed by some workers.[100] As well as recanalisation by conventional thin-walled vessels, channels having a thick muscle coat and believed to be bronchial arteries are described within the fibrosed intima of affected pulmonary arteries (so-called vessel-within-vessel or double-media lesion).[101,102] However, although many pulmonary arteries may be occluded, the lesions are focal and beyond them distal branches appear quite normal, yet are non-functioning.

Changes such as these are generally taken to indicate thromboembolism[103] but could equally represent primary pulmonary thrombosis. Indeed, there are those who believe that thromboembolism is seldom the cause of pulmonary hypertension; evidence adduced in favour of this includes the observation that it is very difficult to induce pulmonary hypertension experimentally by repeated embolisation of thrombi.[104] This is in line with the third use of the term 'primary pulmonary hypertension' described above, namely it being applied irrespective of whether the changes are predominantly plexogenic, thrombotic or veno-occlusive.[35–37] Contrary evidence derives from studies showing that the demographic features of patients with multiple small-vessel occlusion are similar to those with proximal artery disease and that they lack genetic features found in idiopathic pulmonary hypertension.[105] Pulmonary hypertension developed within 2 years of a first objectively confirmed episode of pulmonary embolism in 2 of 135 Italian patients, an incidence of 1.5%.[106]

Pulmonary thrombosis occasionally causes pulmonary hypertension in conditions such as sickle cell disease,[107–110] paroxysmal nocturnal haematuria[111] and the Klippel–Trenaunay syndrome.[112–115] Splenectomy also appears to be a risk factor.[116] The morphological changes are then identical to those of multiple small thromboemboli but with plexiform lesions also described in some patients.[108,109] Secondary thrombosis is common in all forms of pulmonary hypertension and may make it difficult to distinguish thromboembolic pulmonary hypertension from other types complicated by thrombosis. If thromboembolic or thrombotic pulmonary hypertension can be recognised early enough, some mitigation of their progress can be achieved with anticoagulant drugs.

On rare occasions, emboli from malignant tumours obstruct the pulmonary circulation and cause pulmonary hypertension,[117–120] or excite a fibrocellular intimal proliferation that occludes small pulmonary arteries[121] while in some countries severe schistosomiasis is an important cause of embolic pulmonary hypertension. Schistosomal eggs block the lumen of the small pulmonary arteries, damage the wall to cause thrombosis and work their way through into the surrounding tissues where they excite a severe foreign-body inflammatory reaction. Proximal to the obstruction, changes indicative of severe pulmonary hypertension are found, including angiomatoid and possibly plexiform lesions.[60] The intravenous injection of drugs formulated for oral use is another embolic cause of pulmonary hypertension (see pp. 378 and 411).

Figure 8.2.14 Pulmonary venous hypertension. (A) In a patient with cardiomyopathy, small blood vessels show medial hypertrophy while in the same patient (B) pulmonary veins show intimal fibrosis. (B) Elastin van Gieson stain.

Figure 8.2.15 Pulmonary venous hypertension. In a case of mitral stenosis, a postmortem arteriogram shows marked pruning of the finer vessels in the lower lobe, the lobar difference being due to the venous hypertension being added to the hydrostatic forces entailed in our upright posture.

VENOUS PULMONARY HYPERTENSION

An increase of pressure in the pulmonary veins may result from mitral stenosis, prolonged left ventricular failure, fibrosing mediastinitis, or rarely, pulmonary veno-occlusive disease.[122]

Mitral stenosis

In mitral stenosis, the medial muscle of the pulmonary veins is hypertrophied, especially in the lower lobes, and there is a similar hypertrophy of the media on the arterial side of the capillaries (Fig. 8.2.14A).[123] In both arteries and veins there is also intimal sclerosis (Fig. 8.2.14B) and again the changes are worse in the lower lobes (Fig. 8.2.15). This is due to the added hydrostatic forces which result from

our upright posture.[123] In very severe cases there may be necrotising arteriopathy but this is unusual and plexiform lesions are not a feature of such passive pulmonary hypertension. The distinctive feature of passive pulmonary hypertension is the venous hypertrophy and sclerosis. However, in mitral stenosis the arterial changes do not merely reflect transmission of the raised left atrial pressure across the pulmonary capillary bed: pulmonary artery pressure rises disproportionately to the left atrial pressure, indicating that there is arterial constriction.[124] Pulmonary venous hypertension is also characterised by pulmonary oedema,[125,126] interstitial fibrosis[127] and haemosiderosis which together characterise the condition long known as 'brown induration of the lungs' (see Fig. 8.1.3, p. 405).

Pulmonary veno-occlusive disease (pulmonary occlusive venopathy)[128–135]

Pulmonary veno-occlusive disease is a rare disorder of unknown aetiology that is seldom diagnosed in life, and then usually by lung biopsy. However, the presence of Kerley B lines in the absence of any evidence of left atrial enlargement provides a valuable clue to the diagnosis in life.[130] As in true primary pulmonary hypertension, children and young adults are mainly affected but, unlike primary pulmonary hypertension, there is no female predominance: in children no predilection for either sex has been observed but in adults men are affected twice as often as women.[131] Familial cases are described.[136,137]

Figure 8.2.16 Pulmonary veno-occlusive disease. Two blood vessels are greatly narrowed by intimal fibrosis. The larger has distinct internal and external elastic laminae, as seen in pulmonary arteries, but the position of these blood vessels within an interlobular septum indicates that they are 'arterialised' pulmonary veins.

Aetiology

Pulmonary veno-occlusive disease is to be distinguished from pulmonary vein stenosis, which represents congenital atresia of the extrapulmonary veins (see p. 76). In pulmonary veno-occlusive disease the intra- or extrapulmonary veins are narrowed or obliterated by fibrous thickening of the intima. This is presumed to be postthrombotic but thrombosis is seldom seen. The cause of the fibrosis is unknown, except in a few cases. where factors such as chemotherapy, radiotherapy, bone marrow transplantation, renal transplantation, HIV infection, Felty's syndrome, systemic sclerosis, sickle cell disease and the antiphospholipid syndrome have been incriminated (Box 8.2.2). There is no recognised connection with the bush teas that cause hepatic veno-occlusive disease, despite the observation that related pyrollizidine alkaloids cause an arterioconstrictive form of pulmonary hypertension in experimental animals.[60] Very rarely, immune complexes are identified in the pulmonary vessels,[148] or there is a granulomatous pulmonary phlebitis[149,150] or the disease is seen in the setting of a generalised venulopathy.[151] An onset characterised by fever may suggest a viral aetiology but could equally reflect pulmonary infarction attributable to the disease. However, in a case believed to have been contracted in utero, the baby also had myocarditis and the mother was thought to have had a viral infection when pregnant.[152]

Pathology

The condition is characterised by obliterative sclerosis of pulmonary veins, either between the lungs and the heart or within the lungs themselves and therefore evident on lung biopsy. The venous obliteration causes venous hypertension, which in turn results in venous medial hypertrophy. This may be so extreme that the veins resemble arteries in structure, with internal and external elastic laminae, but the true nature of the affected vessel can still be recognised from its anatomical location in an interlobular septum, contrasting with the centriacinar position of the arteries alongside the airways (Fig. 8.2.16).The venous obstruction also results in marked pulmonary congestion and haemosisderosis. It also leads to the development of leashes of fine anastomotic vessels both around and within the occluded veins,[153] simulating the appearances of pulmonary capillary haemangiomatosis, if this is indeed a separate condition (see below). The venous obstruction also results in prolonged severe interstitial oedema, which in turn causes interstitial fibrosis (Fig. 8.2.17).[154] Attention to the veins will help the pathologist avoid the error of diagnosing idiopathic pulmonary fibrosis in such cases.

Figure 8.2.17 Pulmonary veno-occlusive disease. At necropsy the lungs show alternating areas of intense congestion and pallor, the latter due to interstitial fibrosis consequent upon severe interstitial oedema.

Sometimes it is the small intralobular veins that are diseased, either alone or in conjunction with larger veins.[155] These are difficult to recognise without elastin stains but there are often clues that they are occluded. Firstly there may be focal areas of intense capillary congestion within the affected lobules (Fig. 8.2.18),[128] a change that is practically pathognomonic of venular obstruction. Secondly, there may be so-called endogenous pneumoconiosis. This oddly termed process may be found whenever there is pulmonary haemosiderosis but is especially common in veno-occlusive disease. The haemosiderosis not only takes the form of iron-laden alveolar macrophages but encrusts the capillary basement membranes and venular elastic laminae, often with calcium being deposited there as well as iron. The heavily mineralised laminae are unduly rigid and break up to attract foreign-body giant cells (see Figs 8.3.23 and 8.3.24, p. 450). Not realising the significance of this unusual change, earlier workers referred to it as 'endogenous pneumoconiosis'.[156] More recently it has been termed mineralising pulmonary elastosis.[157] It is not confined to veno-occlusive disease but is very suggestive of this condition. It is also seen

Figure 8.2.18 Pulmonary veno-occlusive disease affecting small interlobular vessels and leading to focal areas of intense capillary engorgement. Venous occlusion is also evident (centre).

less frequently with other causes of pulmonary haemosiderosis, such as capillary haemangiomatosis (see below).[155]

Muscular pulmonary arteries show medial hypertrophy, and thrombosis may cause eccentric intimal thickening similar to that seen in thromboembolic pulmonary hypertension or on rare occasions may be the presenting feature.[158] It is debatable whether the arterial changes are entirely secondary, as implied by the name veno-occlusive disease, or represent a primary component of a wider process, in which case the name vaso-occlusive disease would be more appropriate.[133] Widespread small-vessel occlusion justifying the term vaso-occlusive disease is seen in the pulmonary hypertension associated with sickle cell disease (see p. 483) and the antiphospholipid syndrome,[147] where the occlusion is due respectively to sludging of deformed red cells and platelets.

Pulmonary capillary haemangiomatosis (pulmonary microvasculopathy)

Pulmonary capillary haemangiomatosis is a very rare condition that represents one of the more unusual patterns of pulmonary hypertension.[159–168] Its supposed neoplastic nature is questionable and it possibly represents an unusual manifestation of pulmonary veno-occlusive disease.[155,161] The term 'pulmonary microvasculopathy' is suitably non-committal aetiologically.[135]

Clinical features

Most patients are young adults (age range 14–71 years, mean 35 years) who present with dyspnoea and are found to be in cardiac failure. They may also complain of haemoptysis. Chest radiographs and computed tomography usually show pulmonary infiltrates or nodules, or pleural effusion. Radiological and hemodynamic findings are similar to those found in pulmonary veno-occlusive disease but differ from those identified with other causes of pulmonary hypertension.[169] The patient usually dies of right-sided heart failure within a few years; median survival from the first clinical manifestation is 3 years. The diagnosis is rarely established before death,[163] although focal lesions have been identified incidentally.[170,171] However, one patient diagnosed on biopsy went into complete remission when treated with

dioxycycline, an angiogenesis inhibitor.[172] In another patient, pulmonary capillary haemangiomatosis was associated with multiple pulmonary vascular malformations that formed part of hereditary haemorrhagic telangiectasia.[173]

Pathology

At autopsy the lungs appear firm and haemorrhagic. They may be affected diffusely or there may be well-circumscribed nodules, with the most severely affected areas found in the periphery of the lower lobes.[174] The characteristic histological finding is alveolar wall thickening by a proliferation of small, thin-walled, capillary-sized vessels (Fig. 8.2.19A–C), although in one case the vessels were much larger, measuring up to 180 μm in diameter.[175] The proliferating vessels also infiltrate the walls of larger blood vessels, particularly veins, and there is marked involvement of the interlobular septa. The veins are often obliterated whereas arteries are usually less severely involved. In the most severely affected areas nodules of new capillaries replace the lung parenchyma. The distribution of the proliferating capillaries is particularly well demonstrated by CD34 immunostaining (Fig. 8.2.19D).[155] Where the pulmonary architecture is better preserved, alveolar walls, which at low magnification appear congested, can be seen on close examination to consist of a double layer of capillaries.[161] The process may extend to involve the pleura. It may also invade the walls of bronchi to form intraluminal tufts of capillaries (Fig. 8.2.19C). Haemorrhage and congestion lead to haemosiderosis, with accumulation of haemosiderin-laden macrophages. Secondary hypertensive changes in the arteries include medial hypertrophy and intimal fibrosis.

Aetiology and differential diagnosis

In the first reported case, the endothelial cells of the proliferating vessels were atypical and the authors regarded the process as being neoplastic.[159] However, atypia has not been seen in other examples and the disease remains confined to the lungs and pleura. Its age distribution (14–71 years) renders hamartomatous growth unlikely but its development in three siblings suggests that it might have a genetic basis, possibly involving the release of as yet unidentified angiogenic factors.[162] Rarely, the condition appears to complicate severe passive pulmonary congestion.[176]

The distinction between pulmonary capillary haemangiomatosis and pulmonary veno-occlusive disease is a fine one, if it exists at all. The histological similarities are close and described differences are debatable.[155] The distinction is said to depend on the presence of infiltrating capillaries in the lung parenchyma and larger vessels, in contrast to fibroelastic obliteration of veins in veno-occlusive disease, but this may merely represent the establishment of more florid anastomoses bypassing occluded veins. Angiogenesis is a feature of pulmonary veno-occlusive disease[153] and pulmonary capillary haemangiomatosis may represent an exaggerated degree of such angiogenesis. Figure 8.2.20 outlines a proposed relationship between the two conditions.[155]

Capillary haemangiomatosis should not be confused with the separate condition of diffuse pulmonary haemangiomatosis, which is a form of vascular malformation and is described on page 632.

PULMONARY HYPERTENSION IN CONNECTIVE TISSUE DISEASE

Pulmonary disease of very varied type may develop in several connective tissue disorders (see Table 10.1, p. 472).[74,145,146,177–189]

Figure 8.2.19 Pulmonary capillary haemangiomatosis. (A) An area of alveolar wall thickening is seen. (B) At high power, the thickening is seen to be due to an irregular proliferation of alveolar capillaries. (C) In a separate case, the proliferating capillaries infiltrate the bronchiolar epithelium. (D) Immunostaining for CD34 highlights the capillary proliferation.

Pulmonary hypertension is one of the less common of these and when present may be secondary to another pulmonary manifestation of the connective tissue disorder, particularly interstitial fibrosis. Pulmonary hypertension secondary to parenchymal lung disease is considered above and this section deals only with the pulmonary hypertension that develops in patients with connective tissue disorders who do not have parenchymal lung disease.

Although the changes in any one connective disease are often said to be distinctive, on comparing them they obviously have much in common, not only with each other but also with those of primary pulmonary hypertension, at least in the early stages of that disease. However, an important difference from primary pulmonary hypertension is a relative rarity of plexiform or angiomatoid lesions in the connective tissue diseases.

The characteristic changes in pulmonary hypertension associated with connective tissue diseases are to be found mainly in small intralobular pulmonary arteries and chiefly affect the intima, although such media as extends into these small vessels is often hypertrophied. The intima is thickened by a concentric spindle cell proliferation, which resembles the many skins of an onion, or by the deposition of acellular collagenous material, often resulting in gross reduction or obliteration of the lumen (Fig. 8.2.21). Although described in several connective tissue disorders, this pattern of disease is particularly seen in systemic sclerosis, in which condition such changes are well described in systemic arteries.[177] The form of systemic sclerosis most likely to be associated with pulmonary hypertension is that known as the CREST syndrome (calcinosis, Raynaud's phenomenon, oesophageal dysfunction, sclerodactyly and telangiectasia). In some patients with pulmonary hypertension complicating systemic sclerosis histology shows the changes of pulmonary veno-occlusive disease, as described above (see also p. 476).[189]

Another change described in pulmonary hypertension associated with connective tissue disease is vasculitis.[190] It is likely that this represents a true vasculitis, probably of an immune nature, rather than the necrotising arteritis of plexogenic arteriopathy, but this is disputed.[178] A further association is veno-occlusion.[190] This is particularly seen in patients with the antiphospholipid syndrome, which may be idiopathic but is often associated with systemic lupus erythematosus

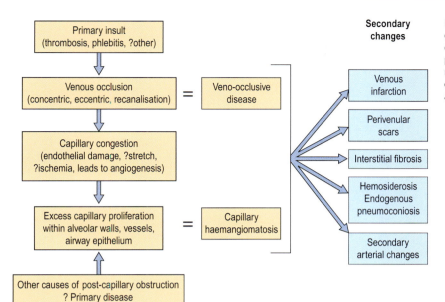

Figure 8.2.20 Proposed relationship of pulmonary capillary haemangiomatosis to pulmonary veno-occlusive disease. It is envisaged that in both conditions postcapillary obstruction leads to the excessive growth of new capillaries representing an attempt to bypass the obstruction. The primary insult is probably multifactorial and may be repetitive and of variable chronicity.[155]

Figure 8.2.21 Pulmonary arteries in two patients with the CREST variant of systemic sclerosis and severe pulmonary hypertension (see text for details). In one (A) the pulmonary arteries show marked 'onion-skinning' (circumferential intimal cell proliferation) while in the other (B) hyaline intimal fibrosis reduces the lumen to a thin slit.

or other connective tissue disorder.[147] In these patients lung biopsy shows platelet thrombi occluding small arteries and veins. The occlusion of small intralobular veins leads to secondary changes such as the patchy capillary congestion and haemosiderosis described above under pulmonary veno-occlusive disease.

EFFECTS OF PULMONARY HYPERTENSION

In long-standing pulmonary hypertension the larger pulmonary arteries may be dilated, and atheromatous plaques may be found in them at necropsy (Fig. 8.2.22).[191] Secondary thrombosis may supervene, occasionally resulting in pulmonary infarction. The dilatation may assume aneurysmal proportions and rupture is recorded, often in association with mucoid medial degeneration (cystic medial 'necrosis') and even dissection.[192–194] Some of the breathlessness associated with pulmonary hypertension may be due to aneurysmal dilatation of a major pulmonary artery pressing on the adjacent bronchus. Cholesterol granulomas have been described in the lungs of patients with pulmonary hypertension of varied aetiology,[195] but this is a rare finding.

Cor pulmonale

Irrespective of its pathogenesis, long-standing pulmonary hypertension leads to right heart strain and hypertrophy of the right ventricle (Fig. 8.2.23). For poorly understood reasons, the left ventricle also undergoes hypertrophy but not so markedly as the right.[196,197] Ultimately the hypertrophied right ventricle fails and passive venous congestion develops in the systemic circulation. If the pulmonary hypertension is caused by disease within the lung, the term 'cor pulmonale' may be used to denote the consequent right heart strain. Cor pulmonale is defined as 'hypertrophy of the right ventricle resulting from diseases affecting the function or structure of the lung, except when the pulmonary alterations are the result of diseases that primarily affect the left side of the heart or of congenital heart disease'.[198] Hypertrophy of the right ventricle can only be assessed accurately from its weight; thickness of the ventricular muscle is affected by dila-

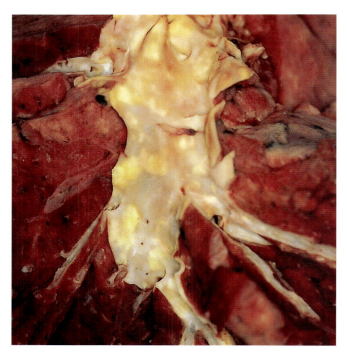

Figure 8.2.22 Atheroma of large pulmonary arteries, a change that is virtually confined to patients with pulmonary hypertension.

Figure 8.2.23 Cor pulmonale in a patient dying of pulmonary veno-occlusive disease. The dilated right ventricle is hypertrophied to such an extent that its thickness equals that of the left.

tation of the heart and is a poor index of hypertrophy.[197] To weigh the ventricles separately, the heart should be divided at the atrioventricular ring and the right ventricle trimmed away from the septum and left ventricle.[199] Normal values are right ventricle 65 g and left ventricle plus septum 185 g. Right ventricular hypertrophy is indicated by a right ventricular weight over 80 g or a ratio of the weights of the left ventricle plus septum to right ventricle of less than 2 : 1. This ratio normally lies between 2.3 : 1 and 3.3 : 1.

TREATMENT OF PULMONARY HYPERTENSION

Apart from the appropriate treatment of any recognisable cause of pulmonary hypertension, such as surgery for congenital heart disease, dietary modification, HIV treatment and anticoagulation, therapy is aimed at arterial dilatation for which an array of drugs has recently been developed. These include calcium channel blockers, prostacyclin (iloprost), endothelin receptor antagonists (bosentan, sitaxsentan, ambrisentan) and phosphodiesterase inhibitors (sildenafil). Lung and heart/lung transplantation present is a further options.

REFERENCES

1. Badesch DB, Champion HC, Sanchez MA, et al. Diagnosis and assessment of pulmonary arterial hypertension. J Am Coll Cardiol 2009;54: S55–S66.
2. Galie N, Hoepar MM, Humbert M, et al. Guidelines on the diagnosis and treatment of pulmonary hypertension. Eur Resp J 2009;34:1219–63.
3. Galie N, Hoepar MM, Humbert M, et al. Guidelines on the diagnosis and treatment of pulmonary hypertension. Eur Resp J 2009;30:2493–573.
4. Wagenvoort CA. Classifying pulmonary vascular disease. Chest 1973;64: 503–4.
5. Wagenvoort CA. Lung biopsy specimens in the evaluation of pulmonary vascular disease. Chest 1980;77:614–25.
6. Rubin LJ. Diagnosis and management of pulmonary arterial hypertension: ACCP evidence-based clinical practice guidelines. Chest 2004;126:7S–10S.

7. Simonneau G, Gali FN, Rubin LJ, et al. Clinical classification of pulmonary hypertension. Journal of the American College of Cardiology 2004;43:S5–S12.
8. Mooi WJ, Grunberg K. Histopathology of pulmonary hypertensive diseases. Current Diagnostic Pathology 2006;12:429–40.
9. Giaid A. Nitric oxide and endothelin-1 in pulmonary hypertension. Chest 1998;114:S208–S212.
10. Fernie JM, Lamb D. A new method for quantitating the medial component of pulmonary arteries. Arch Pathol Lab Med 1985;109:156–62.
11. Hattano S, Strasser T. Primary Pulmonary Hypertension. Geneva: World Health Organisation; 1975.

Plexogenic pulmonary arteriopathy

12. Wagenvoort CA. Plexogenic arteriopathy. Thorax 1994;49:S39–S45.
13. Wagenvoort CA, Wagenvoort N. Primary pulmonary hypertension. A pathologic

study of the lung vessels in 156 clinically diagnosed cases. Circulation 1970;42:1163–84.
14. Yamaki S, Wagenvoort CA. Comparison of primary plexogenic arteriopathy in adults and children. A morphological study in 40 patients. Br Heart J 1985;54:428–34.
15. Caslin AW, Heath D, Madden B, et al. The histopathology of 36 cases of plexogenic pulmonary arteriopathy. Histopathology 1990;16:9–16.
16. Smith P, Heath D. Electron microscopy of the plexiform lesion. Thorax 1979;34:177–86.
17. Balk AG, Dingemans KP, Wagenvoort CA. The ultrastructure of the various forms of pulmonary arterial intimal fibrosis. Virchows Arch A Pathol Anat Histopathol 1979;382:139–50.
18. Arciniegas E, Frid MG, Douglas IS, et al. Perspectives on endothelial-to-mesenchymal transition: potential contribution to vascular remodeling in

chronic pulmonary hypertension. Am J Physiol Lung Cell Mol Physiol 2007;293:L1–L8.

19. Asosingh K, Aldred MA, Vasanji A, et al. Circulating angiogenic precursors in idiopathic pulmonary arterial hypertension. Am J Pathol 2008;172:615–27.

20. Yaginuma G, Mohri H, Takahashi T. Distribution of arterial lesions and collateral pathways in the pulmonary hypertension of congenital heart disease: a computer aided reconstruction study. Thorax 1990;45:586–90.

21. Heath D, Edwards JE. The pathology of hypertensive pulmonary vascular disease. A description of six grades of structural changes in the pulmonary arteries with special reference to congenital cardiac septal defects. Circulation 1958;18:533–47.

22. Wagenvoort CA. Grading of pulmonary vascular lesions – a reappraisal. Histopathology 1981;5:595–8.

23. Jamison BM, Michel RP. Different distribution of plexiform lesions in primary and secondary pulmonary hypertension. Hum Pathol 1995;26:987–93.

24. Elliott FM, Reid L. Some new facts about the pulmonary artery and its branching pattern. Clin Radiol 1965;16:193–8.

25. Tuder RM, Groves B, Badesch DB, et al. Exuberant endothelial cell growth and elements of inflammation are present in plexiform lesions of pulmonary hypertension. Am J Pathol 1994;144:275–85.

26. Lee SD, Shroyer KR, Markham NE, et al. Monoclonal endothelial cell proliferation is present in primary but not secondary pulmonary hypertension. J Clin Invest 1998;101:927–34.

27. Tuder RM, Radisavljevic Z, Shroyer KR, et al. Monoclonal endothelial cells in appetite suppressant-associated pulmonary hypertension. Amer J Respir Crit Care Med 1998;158:1999–2001.

28. Pare PD, Chan-Yan C, Wass H, et al. Portal and pulmonary hypertension with microangiopathic hemolytic anemia. Am J Med 1983;74:1093–6.

29. Kay JM. Pulmonary vascular lesions in chronic thromboembolic pulmonary hypertension. Chest 1994;105:1619–20.

30. Wagenvoort CA, Mulder PGH. Thrombotic lesions in primary plexogenic arteriopathy – similar pathogenesis or complication? Chest 1993;103:844–9.

31. Wagenvoort CA, Wagenvoort N, Draulans-Noe Y. Reversibility of plexogenic pulmonary arteriopathy following banding of the pulmonary artery. J Thorac Cardiovasc Surg 1984;87:876–86.

32. Wagenvoort CA. Open lung biopsies in congenital heart disease for evaluation of pulmonary vascular disease. Predictive value with regard to corrective operability. Histopathology 1985;9:417–36.

33. Gorenflo M, Vogel M, Hetzer R, et al. Morphometric techniques in the evaluation of pulmonary vascular changes due to congenital heart disease. Pathol Res Pract 1996;192:107–16.

34. Haworth SG. Pulmonary vascular disease in ventricular septal defect: structural and functional correlations in lung biopsies from 85 patients, with outcome of intracardiac repair. J Pathol 1987;152:157–68.

35. Pietra GG, Edwards WD, Kay JM, et al. Histopathology of primary pulmonary hypertension. A qualitative and quantitative study of pulmonary blood vessels from 59 patients in the National Heart, Lung, and Blood Institute primary pulmonary hypertension registry. Circulation 1989;80:1198–206.

36. Loyd JE, Atkinson JB, Pietra GG, et al. Heterogeneity of pathologic lesions in familial primary pulmonary hypertension. Am Rev Respir Dis 1988;138:952–7.

37. Pietra GG. Histopathology of primary pulmonary hypertension. Chest 1994;105:S2–S6.

38. Rich S, Dantzker DR, Ayres SM, et al. Primary pulmonary hypertension. Ann Intern Med 1987;107:216–23.

39. Nichols WC, Koller DL, Slovis B, et al. Localization of the gene for familial primary pulmonary hypertension to chromosome 2q31-32. Nat Genet 1997;15:277–80.

40. Morse JH, Jones AC, Barst RJ, et al. Mapping of familial primary pulmonary hypertension locus (PPH1) to chromosome 2q31-q32. Circulation 1997;95:2603–6.

41. Loyd JE, Primm RK, Newman JH. Familial primary pulmonary hypertension: clinical patterns. Am Rev Respir Dis 1984;129:194–7.

42. Newman JH, Wheeler L, Lane KB, et al. Mutation in the gene for bone morphogenetic protein receptor II as a cause of primary pulmonary hypertension in a large kindred. N Engl J Med 2001;345:319–24.

43. Lane KB, Machado RD, Pauciulo MW, et al. Heterozygous germline mutations in BMPR2, encoding a TGF-beta receptor, cause familial primary pulmonary hypertension. The International PPH Consortium. Nature Gen 2000 20:81–4.

44. Rudarakanchana N, Trembath RC, Morrell NW. New insights into the pathogenesis and treatment of primary pulmonary hypertension. Thorax 2001;56:888–90.

45. Loyd JE. Genetics and gene expression in pulmonary hypertension. Chest 2002;121:46S–50S.

46. Eddahibi S, Morrell N, DOrtho MP, et al. Pathobiology of pulmonary arterial hypertension. Eur Resp J 2002;20:1559–72.

47. Trembath RC, Thomson JR, Machado RD, et al. Clinical and molecular genetic features of pulmonary hypertension in patients with hereditary hemorrhagic telangiectasia. N Engl J Med 2001;345:325–34.

48. Abdalla SA, Gallione CJ, Barst RJ, et al. Primary pulmonary hypertension in families with hereditary haemorrhagic telangiectasia. Eur Resp J 2004;23:373–7.

49. Zaiman A, Fijalkowska I, Hassoun PM, et al. One hundred years of research in the pathogenesis of pulmonary hypertension. Am J Respir Cell Mol Biol 2005;33:425–31.

50. Giaid A, Yanagisawa M, Langleben D, et al. Expression of endothelin-1 in the lungs of patients with pulmonary hypertension. N Engl J Med 1993;328:1732–9.

51. Giaid A, Saleh D. Reduced expression of endothelial nitric oxide synthase in the lungs of patients with pulmonary hypertension. N Engl J Med 1995;333:214–21.

52. Orte C, Polak JM, Haworth SG, et al. Expression of pulmonary vascular angiotensin-converting enzyme in primary and secondary plexiform pulmonary hypertension. J Pathol 2000;192:379–84.

53. Barberis MCP, Veronese S, Bauer D, et al. Immunocytochemical detection of progesterone receptors: a study in a patient with pulmonary primary hypertension. Chest 1995;107:869–72.

54. Heath D, Yacoub M, Gosney JR, et al. Pulmonary endocrine cells in hypertensive pulmonary vascular disease. Histopathology 1990;16:21–8.

55. Madden BP, Gosney J, Coghlan JG, et al. Pretransplant clinicopathological correlation in end-stage primary pulmonary hypertension. Eur Respir J 1994;7:672–8.

56. Gosney JR, Resl M. Pulmonary endocrine cells in plexogenic pulmonary arteriopathy associated with cirrhosis. Thorax 1995;50:92–3.

57. Theegarten D, Anhenn O, Aretz S, et al. Detection of *Chlamydia pneumoniae* in unexplained pulmonary hypertension. Eur Resp J 2002;19:192–4.

58. Chu JW, Kao PN, Faul JL, et al. High prevalence of autoimmune thyroid disease in pulmonary arterial hypertension. Chest 2002;122:1668–73.

59. McDonnell PJ, Toye PA, Hutchins GM. Primary pulmonary hypertension in cirrhosis: are they related? Am Rev Respir Dis 1983;127:437–41.

60. Harris P, Heath D. The Human Pulmonary Circulation. Its Form and Function in Health and Disease. 3rd ed. Edinburgh: Churchill Livingstone; 1986.

61. Budhiraja R, Hassoun PM. Portopulmonary hypertension – A tale of two circulations. Chest 2003;123:562–76.

62. Rydell R, Hoffbauer FW. Multiple pulmonary arteriovenous fistulas in

juvenile cirrhosis. Am J Med 1956;21:450–60.

63. Berthelot P, Walker JG, Sherlock S, et al. Arterial changes in the lungs in cirrhosis of the liver – lung spider nevi. N Engl J Med 1966;274:291–8.

64. Stanley NN, Williams AJ, Dewar CA, et al. Hypoxia and hydrothoraces in a case of liver cirrhosis: correlation of physiological, radiographic, scintigraphic, and pathological findings. Thorax 1977;32:457–71.

65. Lamps LW, Carson K, Bradley AL, et al. Pulmonary vascular morphological changes in cirrhotic patients undergoing liver transplantation. Liver Transpl Surg 1999;5:57–64.

66. Kay JM, Smith P, Heath D. Aminorex and the pulmonary circulation. Thorax 1971;26:262–70.

67. Douglas JG, Munro JF, Kitchin AH, et al. Pulmonary hypertension and fenfluramine. BMJ 1981;283:881–3.

68. McMurray J, Bloomfield P, Miller HC. Irreversible pulmonary hypertension after treatment with fenfluramine. BMJ 1986;292:239–40.

69. Abenhaim L, Moride Y, Brenot F, et al. Appetite-suppressant drugs and the risk of primary pulmonary hypertension. N Engl J Med 1996;335:609–16.

70. Delcroix M, Kurz X, Walckiers D, et al. High incidence of primary pulmonary hypertension associated with appetite suppressants in Belgium. Eur Resp J 1998;12:271–6.

71. Kay JM. Dietary pulmonary hypertension. Thorax 1994;49:S33–S38.

72. Speich R, Jenni R, Opravil M, et al. Primary pulmonary hypertension in HIV infection. Chest 1991;100: 1268–71.

73. Mette SA, Palevsky HI, Pietra GG, et al. Primary pulmonary hypertension in association with human immunodeficiency virus infection – a possible viral etiology for some forms of hypertensive pulmonary arteriopathy. Am Rev Respir Dis 1992;145:1196–200.

74. Cool CD, Kennedy D, Voelkel NF, et al. Pathogenesis and evolution of plexiform lesions in pulmonary hypertension associated with scleroderma and human immunodeficiency virus infection. Hum Pathol 1997;28:434–42.

75. Mehta NJ, Khan IA, Mehta RN, et al. HIV-related pulmonary hypertension – analytic review of 131 cases. Chest 2000;118:1133–41.

76. Orenstein JM, Preble OT, Kind P, et al. The relationship of serum alpha-interferon and ultrastructural markers in HIV-seropositive individuals. Ultrastruct Pathol 1987;11:673–9.

77. Wang X, Chai H, Lin PH, et al. Roles and mechanisms of human immunodeficiency virus protease inhibitor ritonavir and other anti-human immunodeficiency virus drugs

in endothelial dysfunction of porcine pulmonary arteries and human pulmonary artery endothelial cells. Am J Pathol 2009;174:771–81.

78. Mesa RA, Edell ES, Dunn WF, et al. Human immunodeficiency virus infection and pulmonary hypertension: two new cases and a review of 86 reported cases. Mayo Clin Proc 1998;73:37–45.

79. Laney AS, De Marco T, Peters JS, et al. Kaposi sarcoma-associated herpesvirus and primary and secondary pulmonary hypertension. Chest 2005;127:762–7.

Hypoxic pulmonary hypertension

80. Kato M, Staub NC. Response of small pulmonary arteries to unilobar hypoxia and hypercapnia. Circ Res 1966;19:426–39.

81. Nagasaka Y, Bhattacharya F, Nanjo S, et al. Micropuncture measurement of lung microvascular pressure profile during hypoxia in cats. Circ Res 1984;54: 90–5.

82. Kourembanas S, Bernfield M. Hypoxia and endothelial smooth muscle cell interactions in the lung. Am J Respir Cell Mol Biol 1994;11:373–4.

83. Brij SO, Peacock AJ. Cellular responses to hypoxia in the pulmonary circulation. Thorax 1998;53:1075–9.

84. Nakanishi K, Tajima F, Nakata Y, et al. Expression of endothelin-1 in rats developing hypobaric hypoxia-induced pulmonary hypertension. Lab Invest 1999;79:1347–57.

85. Wagenvoort CA, Wagenvoort N. Pulmonary venous changes in chronic hypoxia. Virchows Arch A Pathol Anat Histopathol 1976;372:51–6.

86. Smith P, Heath D, Williams D, et al. The earliest histopathological response to hypobaric hypoxia in rabbits in the Rifugio Torino (3370-m) on Monte Bianco. J Pathol 1993;170:485–91.

87. Hicken P, Heath D, Brewer D. The relation between the weight of the right ventricle and the percentage of abnormal air space in the lung in emphysema. J Pathol Bacteriol 1966;92:519–28.

88. Hicken P, Brewer D, Heath D. The relation between the weight of the right ventricle of the heart and the internal surface area and number of alveoli in the human lung in emphysema. J Pathol Bacteriol 1966;92:529–46.

89. Barbera JA, Peinado VI, Santos S. Pulmonary hypertension in chronic obstructive pulmonary disease. Eur Resp J 2003;21:892–905.

90. Hasleton PS, Heath D, Brewer DB. Hypertensive pulmonary vascular disease in states of chronic hypoxia. J Path Bact 1968;95:431–40.

91. Wilkinson M, Langhorne CA, Heath D, et al. A pathophysiological study of 10 cases of hypoxic cor pulmonale. Q J Med 1988;66:65–87.

92. Magee F, Wright JL, Wiggs BR, et al. Pulmonary vascular structure and function in chronic obstructive pulmonary disease. Thorax 1988;43:183–9.

93. Ahmed Q, Chung-Park M, Tomashefski JF. Cardiopulmonary pathology in patients with sleep apnea/obesity hypoventilation syndrome. Hum Pathol 1997;28: 264–9.

94. Weibel E. Die Entstehung der Langsmuskulatur in den Asten der *A bronchialis*. Zeitschrift fur Zellforschung 1958;47:440–68.

95. Wagenaar SJ, Wagenvoort CA. Experimental production of longitudinal smooth muscle cells in the intima of muscular arteries. Lab Invest 1978;39:370–4.

96. Wagenvoort CA, Keutel J, Mooi WJ, et al. Longitudinal smooth muscle in pulmonary arteries. Occurrence in congenital heart disease. Virchows Arch A Pathol Anat Histopathol 1984;404:265–74.

Pulmonary hypertension in diffuse parenchymal lung disease

97. Wagener OE, Roncoroni AJ, Barcat JA. Severe pulmonary hypertension with diffuse smooth muscle proliferation of the lungs. Pulmonary tuberous sclerosis? Chest 1989;95:234–7.

98. Kay JM, Kahana LM, Rihal C. Diffuse smooth muscle proliferation of the lungs with severe pulmonary hypertension. Hum Pathol 1996;27:969–74.

Embolic pulmonary hypertension

99. Wagenvoort CA. Pathology of pulmonary thromboembolism. Chest 1995;107:S10–S17.

100. Moser KM, Bloor CM. Pulmonary vascular lesions in chronic thromboembolic pulmonary hypertension – reply. Chest 1994;105:1620.

101. Wagenvoort CA, Mooi WJ. Biopsy pathology of the pulmonary vasculature. London: Chapman & Hall Medical; 1989.

102. Matsubara O, Yoshimura N, Tamura A, et al. Pathological features of the pulmonary artery in Takayasu arteritis. Heart Vessels 1992;(Suppl 7):18–25.

103. Fedullo PF, Rubin LJ, Kerr KM, et al. The natural history of acute and chronic thromboembolic disease: the search for the missing link. Eur Respir J 2000;15:435–7.

104. Egermayer P, Peacock AJ. Is pulmonary embolism a common cause of chronic pulmonary hypertension? Limitations of the embolic hypothesis. Eur Respir J 2000;15:440–8.

105. Suntharalingam J, Machado RD, Sharples LD, et al. Demographic features, BMPR2 status and outcomes in distal chronic thromboembolic pulmonary hypertension. Thorax 2007;62:617–22.

106. Becattini C, Agnelli G, Pesavento R, et al. Incidence of chronic thromboembolic pulmonary hypertension after a first episode of pulmonary embolism. Chest 2006;130:172–5.

107. Collins FS, Orringer EP. Pulmonary hypertension and cor pulmonale in the sickle hemoglobinopathies. Am J Med 1982;73:814–21.

108. Adedeji MO, Cespedes J, Allen K, et al. Pulmonary thrombotic arteriopathy in patients with sickle cell disease. Arch Pathol Lab Med 2001;125:1436–41.

109. Haque AK, Gokhale S, Rampy BA, et al. Pulmonary hypertension in sickle cell hemoglobinopathy: A clinicopathologic study of 20 cases. Hum Pathol 2002;33:1037–43.

110. Gladwin MT, Sachdev V, Jison ML, et al. Pulmonary hypertension as a risk factor for death in patients with sickle cell disease. N Engl J Med 2004;350: 886–95.

111. Heller PG, Grinberg AR, Lencioni M, et al. Pulmonary hypertension in paroxysmal nocturnal hemoglobinuria. Chest 1992;102:642–3.

112. Joshi M, Cole S, Knibbs D, et al. Pulmonary abnormalities in Klippel–Trenaunay syndrome – a histologic, ultrastructural, and immunocytochemical study. Chest 1992;102:1274–7.

113. Gianlupi A, Harper RW, Dwyre DM, et al. Recurrent pulmonary embolism associated with Klippel–Trenaunay–Weber syndrome. Chest 1999;115:1199–201.

114. Walder B, Kapelanski DP, Auger WR, et al. Successful pulmonary thromboendarterectomy in a patient with Klippel–Trenaunay syndrome. Chest 2000;117:1520–2.

115. Ulrich S, Fischler M, Walder B, et al. Klippel–Trenaunay syndrome with small vessel pulmonary arterial hypertension. Thorax 2005;60:971–3.

116. Jais X, Ioos V, Jardim C, et al. Splenectomy and chronic thromboembolic pulmonary hypertension. Thorax 2005;60:1031–4.

117. Bagshawe KD, Brooks WDW. Subacute pulmonary hypertension due to chorionepithelioma. Lancet 1959;1: 653–8.

118. He XW, Tang YH, Luo ZQ, et al. Subacute cor pulmonale due to tumor embolization to the lungs. Angiology 1989;40:11–7.

119. Snyder LS, Harmon KR, Estensen RD. Intravascular lymphomatosis (malignant angioendotheliomatosis) presenting as pulmonary hypertension. Chest 1989;96:1199–200.

120. Hibbert M, Braude S. Tumour microembolism presenting as 'primary pulmonary hypertension'. Thorax 1997;52:1016–7.

121. Sato Y, Marutsuka K, Asada Y, et al. Pulmonary tumor thrombotic microangiopathy. Pathol Int 1995;45:436–40.

Venous pulmonary hypertension

122. Chazova I, Robbins I, Loyd J, et al. Venous and arterial changes in pulmonary veno-occlusive disease, mitral stenosis and fibrosing mediastinitis. Eur Resp J 2000;15:116–22.

123. Harrison CV. The pathology of the pulmonary vessels in pulmonary hypertension. Br J Radiol 1958;31:217–26.

124. Goodwin JF. The nature of pulmonary hypertension. Br J Radiol 1958;31:174–88.

125. Heard BE, Steiner RE, Herdan A, et al. Oedema and fibrosis of the lungs in left ventricular failure. Br J Radiol 1968;41:161–71.

126. Grainger RG. Interstitial pulmonary oedema and its radiological diagnosis. A sign of pulmonary venous and capillary hypertension. Br J Radiol 1958;31:201–17.

127. Goyette EM, Farinacci CJ, Forsee JH, et al. The clinicopathologic correlation of lung biopsies in mitral stenosis. Am Heart J 1954;47:645–52.

128. Brewer DB, Humphreys DR. Primary pulmonary hypertension with obstructive venous lesions. Br Heart J 1960;22:445–8.

129. Carrington CB, Liebow AA. Pulmonary veno-occlusive disease. Hum Pathol 1970;1:322–4.

130. Liebow AA, Moser KM, Southgate MT. Clinical pathological conference; rapidly progressive dyspnoea in a teenage boy. JAMA 1973;223:1243–53.

131. Wagenvoort CA, Wagenvoort N. The pathology of pulmonary veno-occlusive disease. Virchows Arch A Pathol Anat Histopathol 1974;364:69–79.

132. Thadani U, Burrow C, Whitaker W, et al. Pulmonary veno-occlusive disease. Q J Med 1975;44:133–59.

133. Wagenvoort CA, Wagenvoort N, Takahashi T. Pulmonary veno-occlusive disease. Involvement of pulmonary arteries and review of the literature. Hum Pathol 1985;16:1033–41.

134. Mandel J, Mark EJ, Hales CA. Pulmonary veno-occlusive disease. Am J Respir Crit Care Med 2000;162:1964–73.

135. Pietra GG, Capron F, Stewart S, et al. Pathologic assessment of vasculopathies in pulmonary hypertension. J Am Coll Cardiol 2004;43:25S–32S.

136. Voordes CG, Kuipers JRG, Elema JD. Familial pulmonary veno-occlusive disease: a case report. Thorax 1977;32:763–6.

137. Davies P, Reid L. Pulmonary veno-occlusive disease in siblings: case reports and morphometric study. Hum Pathol 1982;13:922.

138. Lombard CM, Churg A, Winokur S. Pulmonary veno-occlusive disease following therapy for malignant neoplasms. Chest 1987;92:871–6.

139. Swift GL, Gibbs A, Campbell IA, et al. Pulmonary veno-occlusive disease and Hodgkin's lymphoma. Eur Respir J 1993;6:596–8.

140. Kramer MR, Estenne M, Berkman N, et al. Radiation-induced pulmonary veno-occlusive disease. Chest 1993;104: 1282–4.

141. Williams LM, Fussell S, Veith RW, et al. Pulmonary veno-occlusive disease in an adult following bone marrow transplantation: case report and review of the literature. Chest 1996;109: 1388–91.

142. Canny GJ, Arbus GS, Wilson GJ, et al. Fatal pulmonary hypertension following renal transplantation. Br J Dis Chest 1985;79:191–5.

143. Ruchelli ED, Nojadera G, Rutstein RM, et al. Pulmonary veno-occlusive disease – another vascular disorder associated with human immunodeficiency virus infection? Arch Pathol Lab Med 1994;118:664–6.

144. Escamilla R, Hermant C, Berjaud J, et al. Pulmonary veno-occlusive disease in a HIV-infected intravenous drug abuser. Eur Respir J 1995;8:1982–4.

145. Devereux G, Evans MJ, Kerr KM, et al. Pulmonary veno-occlusive disease complicating Felty's syndrome. Resp Med 1998;92:1089–91.

146. Morassut PA, Walley VM, Smith CD. Pulmonary veno-occlusive disease and the CREST variant of scleroderma. Can J Cardiol 1992;8:1055–8.

147. Levine JS, Branch DW, Rauch J. The antiphospholipid syndrome. N Engl J Med 2002;346:752–63.

148. Corrin B, Spencer H, Turner-Warwick M, et al. Pulmonary veno-occlusion – an immune complex disease? Virchows Arch A Pathol Anat Histopathol 1974;364:81–91.

149. Crissman JD, Koss M, Carson RP. Pulmonary veno-occlusive disease secondary to granulomatous venulitis. Am J Surg Pathol 1980;4:93–9.

150. Dwyer N, Smith R, Challis D, et al. Granulomatous angiitis leading to a pulmonary veno-occlusive disease-like picture. Eur Respir J 2009;33:666–9.

151. Liang MH, Stern S, Fortin PR, et al. Fatal pulmonary veno-occlusive disease secondary to a generalized venulopathy: a new syndrome presenting with facial swelling and pericardial tamponade. Arthritis Rheum 1991;34:228–33.

152. Wagenvoort CA, Losekoot G, Mulder E. Pulmonary veno-occlusive disease of presumably intrauterine origin. Thorax 1971;26:429–34.

153. Schraufnagel DE, Sekosan M, McGee T, et al. Human alveolar capillaries undergo angiogenesis in pulmonary veno-occlusive disease. Eur Respir J 1996;9:346–50.

154. Eppinger H. Die Permeabilitatspathologie als die Lehre vom Krankheitsbeginn. Vienna: Springer; 1949.

155. Lantuejoul S, Sheppard MN, Corrin B, et al. Pulmonary veno-occlusive disease and pulmonary capillary hemangiomatosis: a clinicopathologic

study of 35 cases. Am J Surg Pathol 2006;30:850–7.

156. Walford RI, Kaplan L. Pulmonary fibrosis and giant cell reaction to altered elastic tissue – endogenous pneumoconiosis. Arch Pathol Lab Med 1957;63:75–90.

157. Pai UH, McMahon J, Tomashefski JF. Mineralizing pulmonary elastosis in chronic cardiac failure – endogenous pneumoconiosis revisited. Am J Clin Pathol 1994;101:22–8.

158. Katz DS, Scalzetti EM, Katzenstein ALA, et al. Pulmonary veno-occlusive disease presenting with thrombosis of pulmonary arteries. Thorax 1995;50:699–700.

159. Wagenvoort CA, Beetstra A, Spijker J. Capillary haemangiomatosis of the lung. Histopathology 1978;2:401–6.

160. Heath D, Reid R. Invasive pulmonary haemangiomatosis. Br J Dis Chest 1985;79:284–94.

161. Tron V, Magee F, Wright JL, et al. Pulmonary capillary hemangiomatosis. Hum Pathol 1986;17:1144–50.

162. Langleben D, Heneghan JM, Batten AP, et al. Familial pulmonary capillary hemangiomatosis resulting in primary pulmonary hypertension. Ann Intern Med 1988;109:106–9.

163. Wagenaar SJSC, Mulder JJS, Wagenvoort CA, et al. Pulmonary capillary haemangiomatosis diagnosed during life. Histopathology 1989;14:209–24.

164. Faber CN, Yousem SA, Dauber JH, et al. Pulmonary capillary hemangiomatosis. A report of three cases and a review of the literature. Am Rev Respir Dis 1989;140:808–13.

165. Domingo C, Encabo B, Roig J, et al. Pulmonary capillary hemangiomatosis – report of a case and review of the literature. Respiration 1992;59:178–80.

166. Masur Y, Remberger K, Hoefer M. Pulmonary capillary hemangiomatosis as a rare cause of pulmonary hypertension. Pathol Res Pract 1996;192:290–5.

167. Ishii H, Iwabuchi K, Kameya T, et al. Pulmonary capillary haemangiomatosis. Histopathology 1996;29:275–8.

168. Unterborn J, Shepard JAO, Mark EJ, et al. A 45-year-old woman with exertional dyspnea, hemoptysis, and pulmonary nodules. Pulmonary-capillary hemangiomatosis. N Engl J Med 2000;343:1788–96.

169. Almagro P, Julia J, Sanjaume M, et al. Pulmonary capillary hemangiomatosis associated with primary pulmonary hypertension: report of 2 new cases and review of 35 cases from the literature. Medicine (Baltimore) 2002;81:417–24.

170. Havlik DM, Massie LW, Williams WL, et al. Pulmonary capillary hemangiomatosis-like foci – An autopsy study of 8 cases. Amer J Clin Pathol 2000;113:655–62.

171. Moritani S, Ichihara S, Seki Y, et al. Pulmonary capillary hemangiomatosis incidentally detected in a lobectomy specimen for a metastatic colon cancer. Pathology International 2006;56:350–7.

172. Ginns LC, Roberts DH, Mark EJ, et al. Pulmonary capillary hemangiomatosis with atypical endotheliomatosis – Successful antiangiogenic therapy with doxycycline. Chest 2003;124:2017–22.

173. Varnholt H, Kradin R. Pulmonary capillary hemangiomatosis arising in hereditary hemorrhagic telangiectasia. Hum Pathol 2004;35:266–8.

174. Erbersdobler A, Niendorf A. Multifocal distribution of pulmonary capillary haemangiomatosis. Histopathology 2002;40:88–91.

175. Whittaker JS, Pickering CAC, Heath D, et al. Pulmonary capillary haemangiomatosis. Diag Histopathol 1983;6:77–84.

176. Jing XF, Yokoi T, Nakamura Y, et al. Pulmonary capillary hemangiomatosis: A unique feature of congestive vasculopathy associated with hypertrophic cardiomyopathy. Arch Pathol Lab Med 1998;122:94–6.

Pulmonary hypertension in connective tissue disease

177. Gardner DL, Duthie JJR, Macleod J, et al. Pulmonary hypertension in rheumatoid arthritis: report of a case with intimal sclerosis of the pulmonary and digital arteries. Scot med J 1957;2:183–8.

178. Kay JM, Banik S. Unexplained pulmonary hypertension with pulmonary arteritis in rheumatoid disease. Br J Dis Chest 1977;71:53–9.

179. Young RH, Mark GJ. Pulmonary vascular changes in scleroderma. Am J Med 1978;64:998–1004.

180. Kobayashi H, Sano T, Li K, et al. Mixed connective tissue disease with fatal pulmonary hypertension. Acta Pathol Jpn 1982;32:1121–9.

181. Asherson RA, Mackworth-Young CG, Boey ML, et al. Pulmonary hypertension in systemic lupus erythematosus. BMJ 1983;287:1024–5.

182. Wakaki K, Koizumi F, Fukase M. Vascular lesions in systemic lupus erythematosus (SLE) with pulmonary hypertension. Acta Pathol Jpn 1984;34:593–604.

183. Wilson L, Tomita T, Braniecki M. Fatal pulmonary hypertension in identical twins with systemic lupus erythematosus. Hum Pathol 1991;22:295–7.

184. Sato T, Matsubara O, Tanaka Y, et al. Association of Sjögren's syndrome with pulmonary hypertension – report of two cases and review of the literature. Hum Pathol 1993;24:199–205.

185. Kishida Y, Kanai Y, Kuramochi S, et al. Pulmonary venooclusive disease in a patient with systemic lupus erythematosus. J Rheumatol 1993;20:2161–2.

186. Ribadeau-Dumas S, Tillie-Leblond I, Rose C, et al. Pulmonary hypertension associated with POEMS syndrome. Eur Respir J 1996;9:1760–2.

187. Pronk LC, Swaak AJG. Pulmonary hypertension in connective tissue disease. Rheumatology 1991;11:83–6.

188. Hoeper MM. Pulmonary hypertension in collagen vascular disease. Eur Resp J 2002;19:571–6.

189. Overbeek MJ, Vonk MC, Boonstra A, et al. Pulmonary arterial hypertension in limited cutaneous systemic sclerosis: a distinctive vasculopathy. Eur Respir J 2009;34:371–9.

190. Dorfmuller P, Humbert M, Perros F, et al. Fibrous remodeling of the pulmonary venous system in pulmonary arterial hypertension associated with connective tissue diseases. Human Pathology 2007;38:893–902.

Effects of pulmonary hypertension

191. Moore GW, Smith RRL, Hutchins GM. Pulmonary artery atherosclerosis. Correlation with systemic atherosclerosis and hypertensive pulmonary vascular disease. Arch Pathol Lab Med 1982;106:378–80.

192. Walley VM, Virmani R, Silver MD. Pulmonary arterial dissections and ruptures: to be considered in patients with pulmonary arterial hypertension presenting with cardiogenic shock or sudden death. Pathology 1990;22:1–4.

193. Coard KCM, Martin MP. Ruptured saccular pulmonary artery aneurysm associated with persistent ductus arteriosus. Arch Pathol Lab Med 1992;116:159–61.

194. Masuda S, Ishii T, Asuwa N, et al. Concurrent pulmonary arterial dissection and saccular aneurysm associated with primary pulmonary hypertension. Arch Pathol Lab Med 1996;120:309–12.

195. Glancy DL, Frazier PD, Roberts WC. Pulmonary parenchymal cholesterol-ester granulomas in patients with pulmonary hypertension. Am J Med 1968;45:198–210.

196. Kohama A, Tanouchi J, Hori M, et al. Pathologic involvement of the left ventricle in chronic cor pulmonale. Chest 1990;98:794–800.

197. Mitchell RS, Stanford RE, Silvers GW, et al. The right ventricle in chronic airway obstruction: a clinicopathologic study. Am Rev Respir Dis 1976;114:147–54.

198. World Health Organization. Chronic cor pulmonale: report of an expert committee. Circulation 1963;27:594–615.

199. Fulton RM, Hutchinson EC, Jones AM. Ventricular weight in cardiac hypertrophy. Br Heart J 1952;14:413–20.

8.3 Vasculitis and granulomatosis; haemorrhage and haemosiderosis

PULMONARY VASCULITIS AND GRANULOMATOSIS

This section deals with certain vasculitides in which the lungs are the sole or major site of involvement. In the Chapel Hill consensus classification they largely come in the small vessel category (Box 8.3.1),[1] and are frequently combined with granulomatosis. Forms of vasculitis and granulomatosis dealt with elsewhere include bronchocentric granulomatosis on page 464, allergic granulomatosis (Churg–Strauss syndrome) on page 465, lymphomatoid granulomatosis on page 664 and hypertensive arteritis on page 420. Most of the diseases considered here have an immune basis and are treated by immunosuppressive therapy. However, they share many morphological features with the infective granulomas and it is very important that an infective aetiology is excluded before treatment is commenced. To emphasise the importance of this, infective vasculitis will be considered first.

INFECTIVE AND EMBOLIC VASCULITIS

Infective vasculitis may be due to bacterial, fungal or parasitic infection of the vessel wall. Haematogenous *Pseudomonas* pneumonia is a good example as it is typically characterised by heavy bacterial colonisation of the arterial wall, which results in vasculitis, thrombosis and infarction (see Fig. 5.2.13, p. 187). Such arterial involvement is also seen on occasion in pulmonary tuberculosis, with inflammatory weakening of the vessel wall resulting in aneurysm formation (Rasmussen aneurysms).[2] Aneurysms caused by infected emboli (so-called mycotic aneurysms – a term used regardless of whether the infection is fungal or bacterial) are best known on the cerebral arteries but are occasionally encountered in the pulmonary circulation, the cause usually being infective endocarditis of the valves of the right side of the heart secondary to congenital disease or intravenous drug abuse (see Fig. 5.4.25B,C, p. 235).[3]

Drug addicts also develop granulomatous pulmonary arteritis because they inject substances intended for oral use. Many tablets include fillers such as talc, starch and cellulose, which impact on small pulmonary arteries causing foreign-body granulomas within and around the vessel (see Fig. 7.2.10, p. 379), with subsequent thrombosis.[4-7] A similar form of granulomatous arteritis is provoked by schistosome ova lodging in small pulmonary vessels but here, in addition to foreign-body giant cells, there may also be a necrotising arteritis, which is presumed to represent an immune response to the ova (see p. 254).[8]

WEGENER'S GRANULOMATOSIS

A triad combining necrotising granulomatous inflammation and vasculitis of the upper and lower airways with glomerulonephritis was initially described by Klinger,[9] and only later by Wegener,[10,11] but it was the eponymous term Wegener's granulomatosis that was popularised by Godman and Churg.[12] These workers redefined the triad as comprising: (1) granulomatosis of the upper and lower respiratory tracts; (2) generalised vasculitis; and (3) glomerulonephritis, thus recognising that the vasculitis has a wide distribution. So too does the granulomatosis but it is the respiratory tract that is most frequently affected (Table 8.3.1).[13] The glomerulonephritis was the major factor in the once high mortality of the disease but since cyclophosphamide became widely used in the 1960s the 5-year survival rate has improved from less than 10% to over 80%.[14] Limited forms of the disease, largely confined to the lungs, are dealt with below (p. 442).

Box 8.3.1 The Chapel Hill consensus classification of systemic vasculitis[1]

Large vessels

Giant cell arteritis	Typically involves the temporal arteries in patients older than 50. May involve the aorta. Pulmonary involvement rare
Takayasu's arteritis	Typically involves the aorta in patients younger than 50. May involve the major pulmonary arteries

Medium-sized vessels

Polyarteritis nodosa	Pulmonary involvement rare
Kawasaki disease	Children. Pulmonary involvement not described

Small vessels

Wegener's granulomatosis	Typically involves the respiratory tract
Churg–Strauss syndrome	Typically involves the respiratory tract
Microscopic polyangiitis	Typically involves the respiratory tract
Henoch–Schönlein purpura	Respiratory involvement unusual
Essential cryoglobulinaemic vasculitis	Respiratory involvement unusual
Cutaneous leukocytoclastic angiitis	Limited to the skin

Aetiology

The recognition of circulating antineutrophil cytoplasmic antibodies (ANCA) in Wegener's disease and related conditions provides considerable evidence that these diseases have an autoimmune basis.[15-17] ANCA titres correlate with disease activity and in vitro it has been shown that ANCA cause cytokine-primed neutrophils to degranulate, releasing lysosomal enzymes and toxic oxygen radicals. This mechanism probably underlies the 'pathergic' process envisaged by Fienberg, which is characterised in its early stages by granulomas centred on small collections of neutrophils.[18,19] ANCA binding causes primed neutrophils to adhere to endothelial surfaces, with neutrophil degranulation at this site accounting for the vasculitis.[17,20]

The cause of ANCA production is not fully understood but there is increasing evidence incriminating cross-reactivity with certain bacterial antigens. *Staphylococcus aureus* can often be recovered from the nose of patients with Wegener's granulomatosis, and by bronchoalveolar lavage when there is recrudesence of the disease,[21,22] while more recently the Gram-negative bacilli *Escherichia coli*, *Klebsiella pneumoniae* and *Proteus mirabilis* have attracted attention. These bacteria attach to host epithelia by adhesion molecules located at the tips of their fimbriae and cross-reactivity has been demonstrated between one of these molecules and a constituent of the neutrophil granule. Immunisation of laboratory rats with the fimbrial antigen resulted in the production of neutrophil autoantibodies and the development of crescentic glomerulonephritis and a haemorrhagic pulmonary vasculitis.[23,24]

As well as Wegener's granulomatosis, ANCAs are associated with the Churg–Strauss syndrome (see p. 465) and microscopic polyangiitis (see p. 445). Immune deposits are not readily identifiable in any of these conditions and they are therefore termed pauci-immune.

Clinical features[25]

Wegener's granulomatosis is a rare disease with a prevalence of about 3 per 100 000.[26] It affects men more than women and occurs at all ages. It generally presents with systemic features such as fever, weight loss, anaemia and arthralgia, combined with respiratory complaints such as nasal discharge and crusting, otitis media, cough, haemoptysis and chest pain. Rarer forms of presentation include acute pulmonary haemorrhage,[27-29] glomerulonephritis[14,30] and thromboembolism.[31] Saddle-nose deformity of the nose may occur and nasal destruction may be so great as to suggest lethal midline granuloma. Almost all patients have involvement of the lungs or upper respiratory tract but virtually any organ may be affected. A classic triad of pulmonary, upper respiratory tract and renal disease is described but is not always evident: it was encountered in only 56% of patients in one series.[32]

Table 8.3.1 Frequency of organ involvement in Wegener's granulomatosis, microscopic polyangiitis and Churg–Strauss syndrome[13]

	Wegener's granulomatosis (%)	Microscopic polyangiitis (%)	Churg–Strauss syndrome (%)
Lung	90	50	70
Upper respiratory tract	90	35	50
Kidney	80	90	45
Musculoskeletal	60	60	50
Skin	40	40	60
Neurological	50	30	70
Gastrointestinal	50	50	50

Radiological examination shows multiple lung masses resembling metastases or, if cavitating, abscesses. Eosinophilia is not a feature of the disease and if present should alert one to the possibility of Churg–Strauss granulomatosis (see p. 465). Fibroptic and aspiration biopsies are of limited use in the diagnosis of Wegener's granulomatosis but the identification of any one of the characteristic pathological features may suggest the diagnosis, provided that other processes such as infection have been ruled out. Serological tests, which are dealt with next, may also be helpful, but in many cases a surgical biopsy is required to establish the diagnosis.

Antineutrophil cytoplasmic antibodies

The recognition of circulating ANCA in Wegener's disease and related conditions represents a major advance in diagnosis.[15,16,20,33–35] There are at least two such antibodies, both of which are of IgG type. Under indirect immunofluorescent microscopy, one antibody gives centrally accentuated granular staining in the cytoplasm of neutrophils: the antigen here is a 29-kDa serine proteinase 3 and the antibody is known as cytoplasmic, c- or PR3-ANCA. The second antibody is recognised by perinuclear staining. It is directed principally against myeloperoxidase and is known as perinuclear, p- or MPO-ANCA (Fig. 8.3.1). However, atypical immunofluorescent patterns are sometimes encountered and more specific, solid-phase enzyme-linked immunoabsorbent assays (ELISAs) are preferred.[36] More recently a third ANCA has been identified, one that reacts with lysosomal membrane protein-2, which is contained in the same neutrophil granules that harbour MPO and PR3.[23]

There is considerable overlap in the histological features associated with c- and p-ANCAs,[34,37] but Wegener's granulomatosis shows a strong association with c-ANCA, the Churg–Strauss syndrome with p-ANCA and microscopic polyangiitis with either c- or p-ANCA (Table 8.3.2).[38] The specificity of c-ANCA for Wegener's granulomatosis is high, about 95% in the classic form of the disease and about 65% in the limited form. The rare false positives are encountered with diseases of the lung such as tuberculosis, lymphoma, human immunodeficiency virus (HIV) infection, various connective tissue disorders and thromboembolism.[39] The sensitivity varies with disease activity and this provides a useful means of monitoring treatment.[33,36,40]

Pathological features of the lung lesions[41–43]

At necropsy, multiple irregular but well-circumscribed masses of various size are seen in the lungs. They consist of grey indurated tissue surrounding a soft, friable, grey or haemorrhagic necrotic centre, which may cavitate (Fig. 8.3.2). There is often a fibrinous pleurisy or effusion. The large airways may be ulcerated, thickened by nodules of granulation tissue, or stenotic.[44,45]

Microscopically, the nodules show irregular areas of necrosis surrounded by inflammatory granulation tissue (Fig. 8.3.3). The outlines of necrotic vessels or other structures may be evident centrally and

Figure 8.3.1 Antineutrophil cytoplasmic antibodies (ANCA) demonstrated by fluorescent microscopy following the application of the patient's serum to test smears. (A) Cytoplasmic antibodies (c-ANCA); (B) perinuclear antibodies (p-ANCA). *(Courtesy of Dr G Valesini, Rome, Italy.)*

Figure 8.3.2 Wegener's granulomatosis. Numerous pale, cavitating masses replace the lung tissue, which elsewhere is haemorrhagic.

Table 8.3.2 Frequency of antineutrophil cytoplasmic antibody (ANCA) types in pauci-immune vasculitis[38]

ANCA type	Wegener's granulomatosis	Microscopic polyangiitis	Churg–Strauss syndrome
Cytoplasmic (PR-3)	75%	40%	10%
Perinuclear (MPO)	20%	50%	60%

Figure 8.3.3 Wegener's granulomatosis. (A) A central area of necrosis is bordered by granulation tissue that is infiltrated by numerous lymphocytes and plasma cells and an occasional multinucleate giant cell. (B) The necrotic debris is often notably haematoxyphilic due to neutrophilic debris.

Figure 8.3.4 Wegener's granulomatosis. Neutrophilic microabscesses bordered by a granulomatous reaction probably represent an early stage in the development of the larger irregular areas of necrotising granulomatosis.

Figure 8.3.5 Wegener's granulomatosis. (A) A pulmonary artery is involved by necrotising vasculitis. (B) Deficiencies in the external elastic lamina of this pulmonary artery indicate that it has been previously affected by necrotising vasculitis. Elastin van Gieson stain.

there is often extensive karyorrhexis resulting in the accumulation of fine haematoxyphilic nuclear dust (see Fig 8.3.3). The inflammatory infiltrate of the surrounding granulation tissue includes lymphocytes, which are predominantly T cells,[46] plasma cells, neutrophils and macrophages, the last often arranged in a palisade about the necrosis. Variable numbers of multinucleate foreign-body or Langhans giant cells may be seen, scattered individually or forming loose clusters, but seldom forming cohesive tuberculoid granulomas. Neutrophilic microabscesses form a further pattern of tissue necrosis and probably represent an early change (Fig. 8.3.4).[18,19] Eosinophils are seldom conspicuous, except in a rare eosinophilic variant of Wegener's granulomatosis[47] in which there is intense tissue eosinophilia within the inflammatory granulomatosis but not the eosinophilic pneumonia or the blood eosinophilia and asthma of the Churg–Strauss syndrome. The granulomatosis is fairly characteristic but the possibility of infection should always be kept in mind and stains for mycobacteria and fungi undertaken.

The necrotizing granulomatosis is accompanied by focal vasculitis that involves medium-sized or small arteries or veins, or capillaries (Fig. 8.3.5). Its primary nature is best appreciated in areas not involved

(A)

(B)

Figure 8.3.6 Bronchocentric injury in Wegener's granulomatosis. (A) A focus of necrosis is centred on a bronchiole. However, the necrosis is notably haematoxyphilic, raising the possibility of Wegener's granulomatosis. (B) An elastin stain shows destruction of a vessel wall adjacent to the necrotic area but more significant vasculitis was evident elsewhere in the lung well away from the granulomatosis. Positive cytoplasmic antineutrophil cytoplasmic antibodies (c-ANCA) provided further support for the diagnosis of Wegener's granulomatosis. *(Courtesy of Dr D Rassl, Papworth, UK.)*

Figure 8.3.7 Wegener's granulomatosis. The vasculitis is sometimes manifest as a capillaritis, which is evident as a neutrophilic infiltrate of the alveolar walls.

in the granulomatosis. Involved arteries and veins show transmural infiltration by neutrophils, lymphocytes, plasma cells and giant cells in varying proportions, and there is often fibrinoid necrosis. The vasculitis is sometimes granulomatous. Elastin stains are useful for demonstrating the partial loss of elastic laminae indicative of a previous necrotising vasculitis (see Fig. 8.3.5). The process is usually focal, involving only a segment of the vessel wall. Occasionally, the necrosis is strikingly bronchocentric (Fig. 8.3.6),[44] but vasculitis can also be identified. Capillaritis is manifest as a heavy neutrophil infiltrate of the alveolar septa (Fig. 8.3.7).[29] It may be leukocytoclastic and often leads to alveolar haemorrhage, which may obscure the inflammation

(Fig. 8.3.8). Previous haemorrhagic episodes are characterised by haemosiderosis.

Immunofluorescence microscopy for immunoglobulins and complement is either negative or very weakly positive, giving rise to the term 'pauci-immune'.

The vasculitis causes thrombosis and wedge-shaped areas of haemorrhagic infarction but it is unlikely that the extensive necrosis is ischaemic as small foci are seen in the earliest form of the disease[19] and larger necrotising lesions are seen away from foci of vasculitis.[48]

The lung between the lesions may show non-specific changes, including organising pneumonia, bronchiolitis, obstructive lipid pneumonia, haemorrhage and haemosiderosis, any of which may mask the characteristic lesions.[42,49] Also, the classic histological features may be considerably diminished if the biopsy is taken after the instigation of treatment.[50] Often, the pathologist is confronted with very small biopsy specimens from which the vasculitic lesions, formerly thought essential to the diagnosis, may be absent. However, foci of necrosis bordered by inflammatory granulation tissue with palisaded histiocytes at the interface are by themselves strongly suggestive – some would say diagnostic – of Wegener's granulomatosis.[19,51]

Extrapulmonary lesions

The same combination of necrotising granulomatous inflammation and vasculitis is seen in the upper respiratory tract[52–54] and skin[55,56] but biopsies may not show the full spectrum of changes. It is claimed that cutaneous biopsies characterised by leukocytoclastic vasculitis indicate a worse prognosis than those showing granulomatous inflammation.[56] The vascular lesions may be indistinguishable from those of classic polyarteritis nodosa. Such lesions may be present in the kidneys as well as the focal and segmental necrotising glomerulonephritis that forms part of the classic triad of lesions. The glomerulonephritis is characterised by fibrinoid necrosis of capillary loops and epithelial crescent formation (Fig. 8.3.9).[57]

Differential diagnosis (Table 8.3.3)

Granulomatous fungal and mycobacterial infection must always be considered in the differential diagnosis of Wegener's granulomatosis.

Figure 8.3.8 Wegener's granulomatosis resulting in diffuse pulmonary haemorrhage. (A) Gross appearances; (B) microscopy.

Well-formed granulomas favour infection (or sarcoidosis) but the histopathological appearances can be very similar and special stains, culture, serology or even molecular techniques may be necessary to identify infection. However, Wegener's granulomatosis entails a risk of opportunistic infection and both processes may be present. Tests for ANCA are helpful as these are negative in patients with infection (apart from very occasional patients with tuberculosis) or sarcoidosis.

Churg–Strauss granulomatosis shares some histopathological features with Wegener's granulomatosis but there is also marked tissue eosinophilia. The p-ANCA test is positive and c-ANCA negative, and there is usually asthma and blood eosinophilia. The pattern of organ involvement also differs (see Table 8.3.3).

Figure 8.3.9 Wegener's granulomatosis. Kidney showing the classic focal necrotising glomerulonephritis (right) and also necrotising arteritis (left).

Wegener's granulomatosis that is predominantly broncho-centric[44,45,58] has to be distinguished from bronchocentric granulomatosis (see p. 464), which is characterised by necrotising granulomatous inflammation centred on airways but lacks the vasculitis of Wegener's disease.

Wegener's granulomatosis that is centred on the pulmonary capillaries has to be distinguished from microscopic polyangiitis (see p. 445), a condition that lacks the distinctive necrotising granulomatosis and is characterised by either p- or c-ANCA.

Other entities that enter the differential diagnosis of Wegener's granulomatosis include lymphomatoid granulomatosis (see p. 664), which is distinguished by the presence of atypical lymphoid cells of B-cell phenotype within the infiltrate and a relative absence of destructive vasculitis, and rheumatoid nodules (see p. 473), which also lack a vasculitic component and show even more prominent palisading.

Limited forms of Wegener's granulomatosis

Wegener's granulomatosis does not always show the widespread distribution described above. Limited forms of the disease have been described.[18,59,60] These lack the upper respiratory and glomerular components but show the typical pulmonary lesions, which are sometimes solitary.[61] Alternatively, there may be only capillaritis with diffuse pulmonary haemorrhage.[62,63] One biopsy series of Wegener's granulomatosis comprised 48 cases of classic disease and 19 of the limited form.[42]

Limited Wegener's granulomatosis affects women more than men and has a much better prognosis than the classic disease.[60] About 30% of patients with limited Wegener's granulomatosis lack ANCA. As with the classic form of the disease, granulomatous infection figures prominently in the differential diagnosis. At one hospital, the application of simple stains for mycobacteria and fungi to 86 archival cases that had been filed as 'solitary necrotising granulomas' of the lung revealed an infectious aetiology in 75, presumably representing patients who had not received the appropriate treatment.[64]

Table 8.3.3 The differential diagnosis of pulmonary vasculitis and granulomatosis

	Vessels involved	ANCA type	Necrotising vasculitis	Parenchymal necrosis	Sarcoid granulomas	Palisaded granulomas	Blood eosinophilia	Asthma	Atypical cells
Polyarteritis nodosa	Small to medium systemic arteries	–	+	– (except infarction)	–	–	–	–	–
Microscopic polyangiitis	Capillaries	c=p	+	–	–	–	–	–	–
Wegener's granulomatois	Small arteries, veins and capillaries	c>p	+	+	–	+	–	–	–
Necrotising sarcoid granulomatosis	Small arteries and veins	–	+	+	+	–	–	–	–
Churg–Stauss syndrome	Small arteries and veins	p>c	+	+	–	+	+	+	–
Lymphomatoid granulomatosis	Small arteries and veins	–	– (infiltration)	+	–	–	–	–	+
Bronchocentric granulomatosis	None	–	–	+	±	+	+	+	–
Sarcoidosis	Veins and small arteries	–	–	–	+	–	–	–	–
Infective granuloma	Any involved in the inflammation	–	±	+	+	+	–	–	–
Rheumatoid nodule	Any near the granuloma	–	–	+	–	+	–	–	–

ANCA, antineutrophil cytoplasmic antibody.

CONDITIONS LINKING WEGENER'S GRANULOMATOSIS WITH SARCOIDOSIS AND OTHER DISORDERS

Vascular involvement is common in sarcoidosis (se p. 286 and Fig. 6.1.33) but is usually no more than an incidental histological finding rather than a component of a systemic vasculitic syndrome. However, the two conditions that are about to be described indicate that there is a spectrum of conditions between sarcoidosis and Wegener's granulomatosis. In their classic forms sarcoidosis and Wegener's granulomatosis are very different but these intermediate conditions demonstrate that there can be considerable overlap. Other unusual combinations are pulmonary vascular lesions in the so-called non-infectious granulomatous angiitis with a predilection for the nervous system[65] and temporal arteritis associated with Wegener's granulomatosis.[66,67] There are also occasional reports of Wegener's granulomatosis being associated with alpha-1 antitrypsin deficiency and bullous emphysema, both perhaps adversely affecting proteinase/antiproteinase balance in the lung.[68–70]

Necrotising sarcoid angiitis and granulomatosis

Necrotising sarcoid angiitis and granulomatosis combines the vasculitis and necrotising granulomatosis of Wegener's granulomatosis with numerous non-necrotising sarcoid granulomas.[71] Women are affected more than men and the age range is wide, with a mean of about 35 years.[72–77] Some patients are asymptomatic but most have non-specific respiratory symptoms accompanied by malaise.[77]

Chest radiographs usually show multiple nodules or masses measuring up to several centimetres in diameter, most numerous in the lower zones. Occasionally the lesions are unilateral or even single.[72,78] Diffuse infiltrates are also reported.[77] Cavitation is rare.

Evidence of extrapulmonary involvement is uncommon but hilar lymph node enlargement was a feature of more than half the patients in one series[73] and granulomas may be found in these nodes. Ocular and central nervous system involvement has also been reported[73,77,79–81] and in some patients the disease has been associated with dacro-adenitis and ulcerative colitis[82] or cutaneous involvement.[83] Generally however, the disease is confined to the lungs and the prognosis is good, with resolution occurring either spontaneously or following corticosteroid therapy.[76]

Figure 8.3.10 Necrotising sarcoid granulomatosis. The lung contains numerous non-necrotising epithelioid and giant cell granulomas and a necrotising arteritis is also evident.

Figure 8.3.11 Necrotising sarcoid granulomatosis. This low-power view shows non-necrotising sarcoid-like granulomas (right) in conjunction with a large area of necrosis (left).

Pathological features

The lesions form irregular areas of induration, which microscopically consist of confluent aggregates of epithelioid and giant cell granulomas with surrounding fibrosis and chronic inflammation (Fig. 8.3.10). The granulomas are identical to those seen in sarcoidosis and, as in sarcoidosis, they tend to follow lymphatic pathways in the bronchovascular bundles, the interlobular septa and the pleura, and may show a small central area of necrosis. However, there are also larger areas of coagulative necrosis (Fig. 8.3.11). Regression of the inflammation may leave the necrotic areas surrounded only by hyaline connective tissue. Various patterns of vasculitis may be seen, all involving both arteries or veins, and destroying the vessel wall to a varying extent. The vessels may show discrete granulomas, a more diffuse proliferation of giant cells and epithelioid macrophages, or merely lymphocyte and plasma cell infiltration (Figs 8.3.11 and 8.3.12). There may also be bronchial involvement, as in Wegener's granulomatosis.

Differential diagnosis

The differential diagnosis is chiefly from Wegener's granulomatosis and infection. The distinction from Wegener's is usually not difficult

Figure 8.3.12 Necrotising sarcoid granulomatosis. A pulmonary artery shows a granulomatous vasculitis.

because well-formed non-necrotising sarcoid granulomas are rarely a feature of Wegener's. Differentiation from infection may be more difficult and requires negative special stains and culture. Whether the condition is to be distinguished from sarcoid is a moot point that is considered next.

Aetiology

It has been suggested that necrotising sarcoid granulomatosis merely represents a variant of sarcoidosis in which mass lesions form, so-called nodular sarcoidosis.[73,84] This is supported by reports of raised levels of serum angiotensin-converting enzyme and selective migration of T-helper lymphocytes to the lung,[85] and by the development of the disease in one of a family with a strong history of sarcoidosis.[86] Furthermore, a granulomatous vasculitis is frequently seen in sarcoidosis.[87] However, the broad areas of necrosis seen in necrotising sarcoid granulomatosis are not a feature of classic sarcoidosis. In one case onset coincided with *Chlamydia pneumoniae* infection.[88]

Sarcoidosis combined with disseminated visceral giant cell angiitis

In contrast to necrotising sarcoid angiitis and granulomatosis, which, with the rare exceptions noted above, is confined to the lungs, occasional patients combine the features of sarcoidosis with those of disseminated visceral giant cell angiitis.[89-92] Such patients have disseminated necrotising granulomatosis, glomerulonephritis and systemic angiitis (the full spectrum of classic Wegener's granulomatosis) combined with typical sarcoid granulomas.

PULMONARY INVOLVEMENT IN OTHER FORMS OF SYSTEMIC VASCULITIS

Polyarteritis nodosa

When polyarteritis nodosa was first described in the nineteenth century it was stressed that it was a disease of the systemic circulation and that pulmonary involvement was unusual.[93] This has subsequently been borne out[94] but when a national survey of 'biopsy-proven' cases was conducted in 1957, roughly half were classified as being of 'respiratory type'.[95] However, the clinical details of these cases

Figure 8.3.13 Polyarteritis nodosa affecting pulmonary arteries, an unusual feature of this disease.

Figure 8.3.14 Microscopic polyangiitis represented by focal interstitial neutrophil accumulation.

include features such as nasal granulomatosis or eosinophilia and it is evident that they represent Wegener's granulomatosis or Churg–Strauss granulomatosis rather than polyarteritis nodosa. This demonstrates that the same vasculitis is seen in these three conditions. The term 'polyangiitis overlap syndrome' has accordingly been applied to any systemic vasculitis that shows features of two or more of the well-defined vasculitic syndromes: polyarteritis nodosa, Churg–Strauss syndrome, Wegener's granulomatosis, temporal arteritis, Takayasu's arteritis and Henoch–Schönlein purpura.[96,97]

On the occasions when polyarteritis nodosa does affect the lungs it is generally limited to the bronchial vessels but it occasionally involves the pulmonary circulation in the absence of features such as granulomatosis or eosinophilia or the presence of ANCAs that place it in one of the other categories of vasculitis (i.e. Wegener's and Churg–Strauss granulomatosis), resulting in necrotising inflammation of medium-sized muscular pulmonary arteries (Fig. 8.3.13).[98–99a] So-called microscopic polyarteritis nodosa affects capillaries, arterioles and venules and is accordingly better known as microscopic polyangiitis, under which title it is dealt with next.

Microscopic polyangiitis

Microscopic polyangiitis affects only the smallest blood vessels – arterioles, capillaries and venules – as opposed to the medium-sized arteries affected in polyarteritis nodosa. Most patients have glomerulonephritis and ANCA, which may be of either cytoplasmic or perinuclear type (see Table 8.3.2). About 50% of patients have pulmonary involvement and in about a third the upper respiratory tract is involved (see Table 8.3.1). Pulmonary involvement is generally characterised by lung haemorrhage; the granulomatosis of Wegener's disease is not a feature. Microscopic polyangiitis is the commonest cause of combined pulmonary and renal haemorrhagic failure (the pulmonary–renal syndrome). In the lungs it is manifest as a haemorrhagic capillaritis characterised by neutrophil infiltration of the alveolar walls, sometimes with diffuse alveolar damage (Fig. 8.3.14).[13,38,62,63,100–104] Cases in which the changes are limited to the lungs have been referred to as isolated pauci-immune pulmonary capillaritis.[105] One group reported on 17 patients with all the features of idiopathic pulmonary fibrosis but who also had ANCA, of whom seven developed microscopic polyangiitis.[106] Microscopic polyangiitis is touched upon again under diffuse pulmonary haemorrhage (see below).

Hypersensitivity vasculitis

The term 'hypersensitivity vasculitis' covers a variety of clinical conditions that are characterised pathologically by leukocytoclastic small-vessel disease. They include clinical syndromes such as Henoch–Schönlein purpura[107,108] and essential mixed cryoglobulinaemia.[109] These conditions typically involve sites such as the skin or the bowel and pulmonary manifestations are unusual.[96,110] They are thought to be due to deposition of immune complexes in vessel walls. The antigen may be exogenous, such as a drug or infective agent, or endogenous, as in some connective tissue diseases. Haemoptysis is the principal complaint in all the hypersensitivity vasculitides that involve the lungs and the pathology is assumed to be a capillaritis, as described above. The hypocomplementaemic urticarial vasculitis syndrome is sometimes associated with progressive airflow obstruction due to emphysema, possibly related to the release of proteolytic enzymes from the disrupted leukocytes (Fig. 8.3.15).[111]

Vasculitis in the connective tissue diseases

Capillaritis has been identified in some patients with systemic lupus erythematosus complicated by alveolar haemorrhage[112–117] (see p. 477), and necrotising pulmonary vasculitis in rare rheumatoid patients (Figs 8.3.16 and 8.3.17)[118–120] seen as either an autoimmune phenomenon or a component of plexogenic pulmonary hypertension.[121] Vasculitis is rare in the other connective diseases but is recorded as an apparently isolated phenomenon in a patient with anti-Jo-1 antibodies, which are usually associated with myositis.[35]

Giant cell arteritis

Giant cell arteritis of the lung principally occurs in three clinical settings: Takayasu's disease,[122–124] temporal arteritis[125,126] and disseminated visceral giant cell arteritis.[127,128] These conditions differ in the distribution of the lesions, the size of the arteries involved and the type of patient they affect rather than the pathological changes within the affected vessels.

Takayasu's disease is a giant cell arteritis that typically affects the arch of the aorta and its branches, leading to so-called pulseless disease. It occurs predominantly in young women and is commonest in Japan whereas temporal arteritis typically affects elderly men and the racial distribution is wide. Only 10% of patients with temporal

Figure 8.3.15 Hypocomplementaemic urticarial vasculitis syndrome associated with emphysema. (A) At low power, the main feature is panacinar emphysema. (B) At high power, capillaritis and focal small-vessel vasculitis are evident.

Figure 8.3.16 (A, B) Vasculitis in systemic lupus erythematosus. The lung shows both follicular bronchiolitis and small-vessel vasculitis. Mixed patterns of lung disease are often seen in connective tissue disorders. (B) Elastin van Gieson stain.

Figure 8.3.17 Pulmonary arteritis as a manifestation of rheumatoid disease.

arteritis have extracranial involvement and pulmonary involvement is very rare, whereas evidence of pulmonary artery involvement is present in up to 70% of patients with Takayasu's disease.[122,123] Disseminated visceral giant cell arteritis is very rare and involvement of the pulmonary arteries is usually overshadowed by disease of systemic arteries such as those supplying the myocardium. The age range is wide (infancy to old age) and the arteries affected are small muscular vessels whereas Takayasu's disease and temporal arteritis typically involve the large elastic arteries (Table 8.3.4).

Takayasu's disease is characterised by chronic giant cell inflammation of the affected arteries resulting in elastic tissue defects, eccentric intimal fibrosis or complete occlusion and recanalisation (Fig. 8.3.18).[129–131] Some of the stenosis is caused by cicatricial contracture, as indicated by the greatly reduced external diameter of the affected arteries.[131] Angiomatoid lesions (see p. 421) are also described, evidence that Takayasu's disease may cause pulmonary hypertension.[131]

Table 8.3.4 Giant cell arteritis involving the lungs

	Takayasu's disease	Temporal arteritis	Disseminated visceral giant cell arteritis
Age	Below 50 years	Over 50 years	Any age
Symptoms	Pulmonary infarction	Pulmonary infarction, headache, polymyalgia rheumatica	Sudden death, e.g. from myocardial infarction
Extrapulmonary distribution	Aorta and its major branches	Temporal artery	Coronary, renal, hepatic, pancreatic, gastric and mesenteric arteries
Pulmonary distribution	Large elastic arteries	Large elastic arteries	Small muscular arteries

Figure 8.3.19 Behçet's disease. Three aneurysms are seen arising from segmental branches of the lobar pulmonary artery. Rupture of one of these resulted in fatal haemorrhage. *(Courtesy of Dr B J Addis, formerly of Brompton, UK.)*

Figure 8.3.18 Takayasu's disease. This involvement of a medium-sized pulmonary artery represents peripheral extension of disease that principally affected a lobar artery and led to infarction of that lobe. Giant cells are very prominent amongst the inflammatory infiltrate. *(Courtesy of Dr Sj Sc Wagenaar, Utrecht, Netherlands.)*

This is partly attributable to pulmonary artery obstruction and partly to recanalisation by bronchial arteries establishing bronchopulmonary shunts.[131] More often, pulmonary Takayasu's disease is asymptomatic or mimics thromboembolic disease, sometimes resulting in infarction of a whole lung or lung lobe.[132–135]

Very rarely, giant cell arteritis is limited to the lesser circulation and categorisation then depends solely upon the age and sex of the patient, which is imprecise. Because pulmonary involvement is much commoner in Takayasu's disease than in temporal arteritis and because the pulmonary vessels affected are large elastic arteries it would be reasonable to regard isolated pulmonary disease as a manifestation of the Takayasu's disease, but if the patient were an elderly man this would be a counterargument. Few such patients have been reported.[132,133,135–139] Of five available for review by one author, three were women aged 25, 34 and 42 years, and two were men aged 33 and 66 years: only one was Japanese.[135]

Behçet's disease

Behçet's disease, which is also considered on page 479, is a form of systemic vasculitis associated with immune complex deposition.[140–142] It is particularly common in Japan and eastern Mediterranean countries and predominantly affects young men of HLA-B51 phenotype; the average age is 36 years and the male:female ratio 11.[143] The diagnostic criteria are oral ulceration and any two of genital ulceration, typical eye lesions (most commonly uveitis), pustular skin lesions and a positive pathergy test, this last consisting of a sterile pustule that develops 24–48 hours after a needle prick to the skin.[144]

Pulmonary lesions are rare and usually take the form of a necrotising vasculitis involving arteries, veins and capillaries of all sizes.[145,146] The lesions may be single or multiple. Small vessels usually show a leukocytoclastic vasculitis associated with deposition of IgA and complement, while larger vessels generally show a transmural, predominantly mononuclear, inflammatory infiltrate. Adventitial fibrosis may result in prominent perivascular cuffing while inflammatory destruction of the media leads to aneurysm formation (Fig. 8.3.19).[146–148] Computed tomography shows aneurysms, irregularities or sharp cut-offs of the pulmonary arteries.[143,149] Repeated haemoptysis is common and may be fatal.[150,151]

Pulmonary artery aneurysms are also a feature of the so-called Hughes–Stovin syndrome, which probably represents a variant of Behçet's disease.[146,149] It affects young males, in whom the aneurysms develop in association with recurrent episodes of peripheral venous thrombosis and a pyrexial illness. Blood cultures are negative and, although the oral and genital ulcers of Behçet's disease are lacking, pustular skin lesions may be present.[152–154] Occasionally, the bronchial arteries may be affected.[155]

PULMONARY HAEMORRHAGE AND HAEMOSIDEROSIS

This section will concentrate on diseases that result in widespread alveolar haemorrhage. However, it should be remembered that haemorrhage from localised lesions such as neoplasms and tuberculosis may be disseminated widely through the lower respiratory tract by aspiration.

Aetiology (Box 8.3.2)

Widespread leakage of blood into alveolar spaces may be caused by a bleeding diathesis, increased capillary pressure or capillary damage.

Increased pulmonary capillary pressure generally reflects pulmonary venous hypertension or occlusion of pulmonary veins, the principal causes of which are mitral stenosis, left atrial myxoma, mediastinal fibrosis, pulmonary veno-occlusive disease (see p. 427), lymphangioleiomyomatosis (see p. 293) and capillary haemangiomatosis (see p. 429). Arterial constriction tends to protect the pulmonary capillary bed from pressure surges but if patchy the capillaries in those areas of the lung in which there is little upstream constriction are subjected to inordinately high pressures and may suffer stress failure. This is probably the mechanism underlying the haemorrhagic oedema seen in acute mountain sickness (see pp. 379 and 402). Similar stress failure with resultant haemorrhage in highly trained racehorses and occasional athletes is touched upon on page 402 [ch. 8.1].

Diffuse capillary damage may be due to extraneous chemicals but is mainly autoimmune, representing small-vessel vasculitis.[13,62,63,100–105] Immune mechanisms fall into three categories: anti-basement membrane disease (Goodpasture's disease), immune complex-mediated injury and conditions characterised by ANCA (pauci-immune vasculitis). In all these categories the pulmonary haemorrhage may be combined with haematuria caused by glomerulonephritis. In one series of 40 cases in which lung haemorrhage was associated with glomerulonephritis 7 had anti-basement membrane disease, 22 had systemic vasculitis and 11 had neither basement membrane antibodies nor systemic vasculitis.[156] Anti-basement membrane disease, immune complex-mediated disease and pauci-immune vasculitis are considered separately below but together with idiopathic pulmonary haemosiderosis they share many clinical and pathological features and these aspects will be dealt with collectively. However, differences between these categories may be apparent on immunofluorescent or electron microscopy (Table 8.3.5) and it may therefore be worth ensuring that some biopsy material is appropriately preserved if diffuse pulmonary haemorrhage is suspected clinically or on frozen section.

Clinical features

The clinical features of diffuse pulmonary haemorrhage vary from massive life-threatening haemoptysis to recurrent or continuous slow leakage leading to tiredness from iron-deficiency anaemia. There is often concomitant haematuria and renal failure, forming a pulmonary–

renal syndrome.[157] Chest radiographs show widespread, ill-defined, transient opacities. Carbon monoxide transfer may appear to be increased but the gas is being taken up by blood sequestered in the air spaces rather than transferred to the circulation. Serological tests for ANCA, rheumatoid factor and antinuclear factor may give clues to the aetiology and help diagnostically.[62,63] Further diagnostic support is provided by the identification of haemosiderin-laden macrophages in sputum or lavage material,[158,159] but it should be noted that stains for iron may be positive in healthy smokers, foundry workers and patients with conditions as diverse as idiopathic pulmonary fibrosis, chronic bronchitis and carcinoma of the lung.[160] However, haemosiderin-laden macrophages are not a normal feature of the lung in infancy and if at autopsy the cause of an infant's death is not readily identified haemosiderin-laden macrophages should alert the pathologist to the possibility of an asphyxial death from overlying or smothering rather than the case being an example of the sudden infant death syndrome.[161,162]

Box 8.3.2 Causes of pulmonary haemorrhage and haemosiderosis

Localised

Tuberculosis, carcinoma, infarction, Wegener's granulomatosis

Diffuse

Generalised bleeding disorders

Capillary hypertension

Mitral stenosis, atrial myxoma, mediastinal fibrosis
Pulmonary veno-occlusive disease
Pulmonary lymphangioleiomyomatosis
Stress failure

Chemical injury

Silicone implants
Lymphography

Asphyxia

Autoimmune vascular disease

ANCA-associated capillaritis

Microscopic polyangiitis
Wegener's granulomatosis (capillaritis variety)

Antibasement membrane disease (Goodpasture's syndrome)

Immune complex-mediated vasculitis

Systemic lupus erythematosus
Rheumatoid disease
Behçet's disease
Henoch–Schönlein purpura
Coeliac disease
Dermatitis herpetiformis
Haemolytic anaemia
Cow's milk hypersensitivity
Trimellitic anhydride-induced
Naphthylene-1,5-diisocyanate-induced
Penicillamine-induced

Idiopathic pulmonary haemosiderosis

ANCA, antineutrophil cytoplasmic antibody.

Table 8.3.5 Immunohistochemical and ultrastructural abnormalities in the lung in various immune disorders and idiopathic pulmonary haemosiderosis

	Immunofluorescent pattern	Electron-dense deposits
Immune complex-mediated disease	Granular	Present
Goodpasture's (anti-basement membrane) disease	Diffuse	Absent
Neutrophil cytoplasmic antibody-mediated disease	Little or none (pauci-immune)	Absent
Idiopathic pulmonary haemorrhage	None	Absent

Figure 8.3.20 (A) Pulmonary haemorrhage and (B) haemosiderosis. In biopsy material haemorrhage is of uncertain significance as it could be operative but haemosiderosis provides firm evidence of previous bleeding.

Pathological features

Whatever the aetiology, biopsy shows a combination of alveolar haemorrhage and haemosiderosis (Fig. 8.3.20). The cause of the haemorrhage is often not evident histologically but there may be intense neutrophil infiltration of the alveolar walls representing capillaritis and rare cases show diffuse alveolar damage (see p. 136).[29,163]

The haemosiderin is largely contained within alveolar macrophages, which generally congregate in the centres of the acini. It is a brown, coarsely granular pigment that gives a strongly positive Prussian blue reaction with Perl's stain (Figs 8.3.20B and 8.3.21), in contrast to smoker's pigment, which is finely dispersed and gives a weaker Prussian blue reaction. Haemosiderin takes 2–3 days to develop after haemorrhage has occurred. It has been identified in tracheal macrophages 50 hours after acute pulmonary haemorrhage and in cultured macrophages 72 hours after the uptake of red blood cells.[164] A similar time course is reported in rats whose airways were injected with blood.[165,166]

In severe haemosiderosis there is also encrustation of the elastic laminae of small blood vessels and alveolar walls (Figs 8.3.21 and 8.3.22). Calcium is often added to the iron (Fig. 8.3.23), as in the Gamna–Gandy nodules that develop in haemorrhagic splenic infarcts. The mineralised elastic fibres tend to fragment and attract giant cells of foreign-body type, a process that has been quaintly termed 'endogenous pneumoconiosis' (Fig. 8.3.24).[168,169] Mild interstitial fibrosis and type II alveolar epithelial cell proliferation may also be seen.

Goodpasture's syndrome (anti-basement membrane disease)

The term 'Goodpasture's syndrome' was first applied to the association of pulmonary haemorrhage and glomerulonephritis in 1958,[170] nearly 40 years after Goodpasture's original report, which was written in the wake of the 1918–19 influenza pandemic with the primary object of discussing the aetiology of influenza.[171] The eponym is now reserved for those cases in which antibodies to glomerular or alveolar basement membrane can be demonstrated, and is often replaced by the term 'anti-basement membrane disease'. It is not clear what initiates the disease but it has been suggested that damage to basement membrane by external agents, such as viruses or chemicals, alters its antigenicity.[172] Some patients have both anti-basement membrane and

Figure 8.3.21 Pulmonary haemosiderosis giving a strongly positive Prussian blue reaction. The haemosiderin is largely contained within alveolar macrophages but also impregnates elastin in the walls of small pulmonary blood vessels. Perl's stain.

Figure 8.3.22 Electron microscopy shows that haemosiderin is preferentially deposited in the basement membrane and interstitial elastin tissue of the alveolar walls, sparing the collagen. Electron micrograph × 34 000. (Reproduced from Corrin et al. (1987)[167] by permission of the editor of the Journal of Pathology.)

Figure 8.3.23 Pulmonary haemosiderosis. Calcium is often added to the haemosiderin deposits and being basophilic is evident without special stains.

ANCA and here it is possible that the former arise because of immune complex-mediated damage to the basement membrane.[173]

Most patients with Goodpasture's syndrome are male. The mean age is about 20 years but the age range is wide and the disease has been reported in children.[174,175] Family clustering and associations

Figure 8.3.24 Pulmonary haemosiderosis. The heavily mineralised elastin fibres tend to fragment and attract foreign-body giant cells, giving an appearance that has been likened to pneumoconiosis, although here the minerals are endogenous.

with the major histocompatibity antigens HLA-DR2 and HLA-DQ have been reported.[176] Almost invariably, respiratory symptoms precede evidence of renal disease, sometimes by weeks or months.[177] Most patients have episodes of haemoptysis, although some develop anaemia, radiographic abnormalities and hypoxaemia without haemoptysis. Proteinuria, haematuria and renal failure indicate glomerular disease, which takes the form of a focal segmental glomerulonephritis with crescent formation. Immunofluorescent microscopy of biopsy material was initially used to demonstrate the antibodies but serological assays are now preferred, despite them not being completely sensitive.[178] Therapy involves immunosuppression and removal of antibodies by plasma exchange.[103,179]

Immunofluoresence microscopy shows that antibodies are deposited along basement membranes in both glomeruli and alveolar walls (Fig. 8.3.25 and Table 8.3.5).[180] In 90% of cases they can also be demonstrated in the serum[181] and the disease can be passively transferred to animals.[182] The severity of the disease is proportional to the antibody titre. Cross-reactivity between pulmonary and renal basement membranes has been demonstrated.[183] The antiglomerular basement membrane antibodies consist of a mixture of IgG subtypes[184] that react with a non-collagenous domain of the alpha3 chain of type IV collagen.[185,186] The alpha3 chain is restricted to sites such as the glomerular and alveolar basement membranes, in contrast to the ubiquitous alpha1 and alpha2 type IV chains. Antibody is deposited in a linear fashion along glomerular basement membranes, outlining the capillary loops, and similar linear fluorescence is seen in alveolar walls. In about two-thirds of cases immunoglobulin deposition is accompanied by complement deposition with a similar pattern.[187]

Electron microscopy (see Table 8.3.5) shows fragmentation of the basement membranes but not the dense deposits evident in immune complex-mediated disease.[188,189]

Figure 8.3.25 Goodpasture's syndrome. Immunofluorescent microscopy showing linear deposition of immunoglobulin in the glomerular (A) and alveolar (B) basement membranes. *(Courtesy of Dr A Paiva-Correia, formerly of Oporto, Portugal.)*

Antineutrophil cytoplasmic antibody-associated pulmonary haemorrhage

ANCAs are associated with pulmonary haemorrhage in conditions such as microscopic polyangiitis (including cases limited to the lungs, known as isolated pauci-immune pulmonary capillaritis, see p. 445),[38,62,63,100–105,105] Wegener's granulomatosis (see p. 438),[27–29,100,190,191] Churg–Strauss syndrome (see p. 465)[192] and systemic vasculitis.[115] In all these conditions immunofluoresence microscopy shows only a weak or negative ('pauci-immune') reaction and electron microscopy fails to demonstrate electron-dense deposits (see Table 8.3.5). Wegener's granulomatosis and the Churg–Strauss syndrome usually show necrotising granulomatosis and inflammation of medium-sized vessels but microscopic polyangiitis is limited to the smallest blood vessels and in the lung haemorrhage is the predominant lesion. Microscopic polyangiitis is the commonest cause of the pulmonary–renal syndrome.

Immune complex-mediated pulmonary haemorrhage

Immune complex deposition is the probable pathogenetic mechanism of diffuse pulmonary haemorrhage associated with conditions such as systemic lupus erythematosus,[113–117,193] Henoch–Schönlein purpura,[107,108] Behçet's disease,[145,194,195] rheumatoid disease,[119] cystic fibrosis[196] and some instances of isolated pulmonary haemorrhage.[105] Immune complex disease also appears to underlie occasional cases of pulmonary haemorrhage associated with penicillamine therapy[197] or exposure to epoxy resin paint powder containing the curing agent mellitic anhydride.[198,199] Diffuse pulmonary haemorrhage is also described in patients undergoing lymphangiography,[200,201] receiving silicone implants[202,203] or smoking cocaine[204] but the pathogenesis in these cases is not well understood.

The haemorrhage is usually due to pulmonary capillaritis, which may develop in isolation, together with larger pulmonary vessel disease or as part of a systemic vasculitis. Capillaritis may be difficult to recognise but periodic acid–silver methenamine staining helps in the identification of basement membrane abnormalities.[104] In well-established disease, neutrophils, nuclear debris, fibrin thrombi, fibrinoid necrosis, disruption of alveolar walls and fibrin lining alveoli may be seen.[29,115,116]

The association of immune complex-mediated glomerulonephritis and diffuse pulmonary haemorrhage is indistinguishable clinically from Goodpasture's syndrome. However, in contrast to Goodpasture's disease and idiopathic haemosiderosis, granular deposits of IgG may be demonstrated along alveolar walls[205] and electron-dense deposits in the capillary basement membrane (see Table 8.3.5).[205] Sometimes there is evidence of immune complex deposition in the kidney but not in the lung,[206–208] or immunostaining may be negative in both organs[207] despite the presence of circulating complexes[209] or vasculitis.[94]

Idiopathic pulmonary haemosiderosis

Pulmonary haemorrhage and haemosiderosis may occur without evidence of vasculitis, immune complex deposition, antiglomerular basement membrane antibodies or associated renal disease. If the other causes of pulmonary haemorrhage listed in Box 8.3.2 can be excluded the condition falls into the category of idiopathic pulmonary haemosiderosis.[210,211]

Epidemiology and clinical features

Idiopathic pulmonary haemosiderosis is predominantly a disease of children and young adults, usually occurring in the first three decades of life. The sex incidence is equal in children whereas in adults there is 2 : 1 male predominance.[212] Familial cases have been described.[213–215] The disease tends to be more severe in children: they develop severe iron deficiency and have episodes of massive pulmonary haemorrhage, which may prove fatal. A more prolonged course is seen in adults and overt haemorrhage is not an invariable feature in this age group.[158] Treatment with steroids and azathioprine is empirical and, because of the varying course of the disease, difficult to assess,[216] but immunosuppressive treatment has been successful in several cases.[217,218]

Aetiology

The cause of the disease is unknown but exposure to as yet unrecognised inhaled agents may play a role. Certain associations suggest that the disease has an immunological basis: these include coeliac disease, or at least a flattened jejunal mucosa,[219–223] dermatitis herpetiformis, autoimmune haemolytic anaemia,[224] thyrotoxicosis[225] and sensitivity to cow's milk, this last being seen in young children who have a positive skin test and serum precipitins to cows' milk, and who improve when cows' milk is removed from the diet.[226,227] An elevated serum IgA has also been noted in children with idiopathic pulmonary haemosiderosis.[228]

Pathological features

Bronchoalveolar lavage is the method of choice to confirm the alveolar bleeding, especially if this is occult.[229] The lavage fluid shows free red blood cells and phagocytosed erythrocytes within macrophages if there has been recent bleeding, and numerous haemosiderin-laden macrophages if the bleeding is old. Transbronchial biopsy can also show haemosiderosis but only open-lung biopsy can exclude other causes of diffuse alveolar haemorrhage.

The microscopic features are not specific, consisting merely of centriacinar collections of haemosiderin-laden macrophages, as described above. Interstitial fibrosis is sometimes regarded as being more characteristic of idiopathic pulmonary haemosiderosis than of other diseases which cause alveolar haemorrhage[230] but this is more likely to reflect the long duration of the disease than a specific process.

Immunostaining of the lung shows no evidence of immunoglobulin or complement deposition (see Table 8.3.5). Various ultrastructural features have been described but no consistent pattern has emerged and it is uncertain whether the changes represent a primary manifestation of the disease or are secondary to the haemorrhage.[167,231] The abnormalities described include focal defects in the vascular endothelium and its basement membrane, and are more severe in children than adults. The capillary basement membrane may show focal thickening, splitting with the accumulation of fibrillar material and duplication.[167] Non-specific abnormalities include damage to type I epithelial cells and regeneration of type II epithelial cells.

REFERENCES

1. Jennette JC, Falk RJ, Andrassy K, et al. Nomenclature of systemic vasculitides. Proposal of an international consensus conference. Arthritis Rheum 1994;37:187–92.

Infective and embolic vasculitis

2. Auerbach O. Pathology and pathogenesis of pulmonary arterial aneurysm in tuberculous cavities. Am Rev Tuberc 1939;39:99–115.

3. Morgan JM, Morgan AD, Addis BJ, et al. Fatal haemorrhage from mycotic aneurysms of the pulmonary artery. Thorax 1985;41:70–1.

4. Gross EM. Autopsy findings in drug addicts. Pathol Annu 1978;13: 35–67.

5. Tomashefski JF Jr, Hirsch CS. The pulmonary vascular lesions of intravenous drug abuse. Hum Pathol 1980;11: 133–45.

6. Tomashefski JF, Hirsch CS, Jolly PN. Microcrystalline cellulose pulmonary embolism and granulomatosis. Arch Pathol Lab Med 1981;105:89–93.

7. Rajs J, Harm T, Ormstad K. Postmortem findings of pulmonary lesions of older datum in intravenous drug addicts. A forensic–pathologic study. Virchows Arch A Pathol Anat Histopathol 1984;402:405–14.

8. Chaves E. The pathology of the arterial pulmonary vasculature in Manson's schistosomiasis. Dis Chest 1966;50: 72–7.

Wegener's granulomatosis

9. Klinger H. Grenzformen der periarteritis nodosa. Frankf Z Pathol 1931;42:455–80.

10. Wegener F. Uber generaliserte, septische Gefasserkrankungen. Verh Dtsch Ges Pathol 1936;29:202–10.

11. Wegener F. Uber eine eigenartiger rhinogene Granulomatose mit besonderer Beteiligung des Arterien Systems und der Nieren. Beitr Pathol Anat 1939;102: 36–68.

12. Godman GC, Churg J. Wegener's granulomatosis. Arch Pathol Lab Med 1954;58:533–53.

13. Jennette JC, Falk RJ. Small-vessel vasculitis. N Engl J Med 1997;337:1512–23.

14. Fauci AS, Haynes BF, Katz P, et al. Wegener's granulomatosis: prospective clinical and therapeutic experience with 85 patients for 21 years. Ann Intern Med 1983;98:76–85.

15. van der Woude FJ, Rasmussen N, Lobatto S, et al. Autoantibodies against neutrophils and monocytes: tool for diagnosis and marker for disease activity in Wegener's granulomatosis. Lancet 1985;i:425–9.

16. Ramirez G, Khamashta MA, Hughes GRV. The ANCA test: its clinical relevance. Ann Rheum Dis 1990;49:741–2.

17. Jennette JC, Falk RJ. Pathogenesis of the vascular and glomerular damage in ANCA-positive vasculitis. Nephrol Dial Transplant 1998;13:16–20.

18. Fienberg R. Pathergic granulomatosis. Am J Med 1955;19:829–31.

19. Mark EJ, Matsubara O, Tan-Liu N, et al. The pulmonary biopsy in the early diagnosis of Wegener's (pathergic) granulomatosis: a study based on 35 open lung biopsies from 67 patients. Hum Pathol 1988;19:1065–71.

20. Gomez-Puerta JA, Hernandez-Rodriguez J, Lopez-Soto A, et al. Antineutrophil cytoplasmic antibody-associated vasculitides and respiratory disease. Chest 2009;136:1101–11.

21. Popa ER, Stegeman CA, Kallenberg CG, et al. *Staphylococcus aureus* and Wegener's granulomatosis. Arthritis Res 2002;4:77–9.

22. Richter AG, Stockley RA, Harper L, et al. Pulmonary infection in Wegener granulomatosis and idiopathic pulmonary fibrosis. Thorax 2009;64:692–7.

23. Kain R, Exner M, Brandes R, et al. Molecular mimicry in pauci-immune focal necrotizing glomerulonephritis. Nat Med 2008;14:1088–96.

24. Gomez-Puerta JA, Bosch X. Anti-neutrophil cytoplasmic antibody pathogenesis in small-vessel vasculitis: an update. Am J Pathol 2009;175:1790–8.

25. Abdou NI, Kullman GJ, Hoffman GS, et al. Wegener's granulomatosis: survey of 701 patients in North America. Changes in outcome in the 1990s. Journal of Rheumatology 2002;29:309–16.

26. Duna GF, Galperin C, Hoffman GS. Wegener's granulomatosis. Rheum Dis Clin North Am 1995;21:949–86.

27. Travis WD, Carpenter HA, Lie JT. Diffuse pulmonary hemorrhage. An uncommon manifestation of Wegener's granulomatosis. Am J Surg Pathol 1987;11:702–8.

28. Myers JL, Katzenstein ALA. Wegener's granulomatosis presenting with massive pulmonary hemorrhage and capillaritis. Am J Surg Pathol 1987;11:895–8.

29. Yoshimura N, Matsubara O, Tamura A, et al. Wegener's granulomatosis – associated with diffuse pulmonary hemorrhage. Acta Pathol Jpn 1992;42:657–61.

30. Fauci AS, Wolff SM. Wegener's granulomatosis: studies in eighteen patients and a review of the literature. Medicine (Baltimore) 1973;52:535–61.

31. Allenbach Y, Seror R, Pagnoux C, et al. High frequency of venous thromboembolic events in Churg–Strauss syndrome, Wegener's granulomatosis and microscopic polyangiitis but not polyarteritis nodosa: a systematic retrospective study on 1130 patients. Ann Rheum Dis 2009;68:564–7.

32. DeRemee RA, McDonald TJ, Weiland LH. Wegener's granulomatosis and other vasculitides of the respiratory tract. Sem Respir Med 1989;10:109–90.

33. Nolle B, Specks U, Ludemann J, et al. Anticytoplasmic autoantibodies: their immunodiagnostic value in Wegener's granulomatosis. Ann Intern Med 1989;111:28–40.

34. Gal AA, Salinas FF, Staton GW. The clinical and pathological spectrum of antineutrophil cytoplasmic autoantibody-related pulmonary disease: a comparison

between perinuclear and cytoplasmic antineutrophil cytoplasmic autoantibodies. Arch Pathol Lab Med 1994;118:1209–14.

35. Brown I, Joyce C, Hogan PG, et al. Pulmonary vasculitis associated with anti-Jo-1 antibodies. Resp Med 1998;92:986–8.

36. Higgs CMB. Anti-neutrophil cytoplasmic antibodies. Respir Med 1992;86:367–9.

37. Gaudin PB, Askin FB, Falk RJ, et al. The pathologic spectrum of pulmonary lesions in patients with anti-neutrophil cytoplasmic autoantibodies specific for anti-proteinase 3 and anti-myeloperoxidase. Am J Clin Pathol 1995;104:7–16.

38. Jennette JC, Thomas DB, Falk RJ. Microscopic polyangiitis (microscopic polyarteritis). Semin Diagn Pathol 2001;18:3–13.

39. Gal AA. Antineutrophil cytoplasmic autoantibody in the absence of Wegener's granulomatosis or microscopic polyangiitis: Implications for the surgical pathologist – Reply. Modern Pathol 2002;15:1236–7.

40. Specks U, Wheatley CL, McDonald TJ, et al. Anticytoplasmic antibodies in the diagnosis and follow-up of Wegener's granulomatosis. Mayo Clin Proc 1989;64:28–38.

41. Yoskikawa Y, Watanabe T. Pulmonary lesions in Wegener's granulomatosis: a clinicopathologic study of 22 autopsy cases. Hum Pathol 1986;17:401–10.

42. Travis WD, Hoffman GS, Leavitt RY, et al. Surgical pathology of the lung in Wegener's granulomatosis – review of 87 open lung biopsies from 67 Patients. Am J Surg Pathol 1991;15:315–33.

43. Colby TV, Specks U. Wegener's granulomatosis in the 1990s – A pulmonary pathologist's perspective. In: Churg A, Katzenstein ALA, editors. The Lung. Current Concepts. Baltimore: Williams & Wilkins; 1993. p. 195–218.

44. Yousem SA. Bronchocentric injury in Wegener's granulomatosis – a report of five cases. Hum Pathol 1991;22:535–40.

45. Daum TE, Specks U, Colby TV, et al. Tracheobronchial involvement in Wegener's granulomatosis. Am J Respir Crit Care Med 1995;151:522–6.

46. Gephardt GN, Ahmed M, Tubbs RR. Pulmonary vasculitis (Wegener's granulomatosis). Study of T and B cell markers. Am J Med 1983;74:700–4.

47. Yousem SA, Lombard CM. The eosinophilic variant of Wegener's granulomatosis. Hum Pathol 1988;19:682–8.

48. Goulart RA, Mark EJ, Rosen S. Tumefactions as an extravascular manifestation of Wegener's granulomatosis. Am J Surg Pathol 1995;19:145–53.

49. Uner AH, Rozumslota B, Katzenstein ALA. Bronchiolitis obliterans-organizing pneumonia (BOOP)-like variant of Wegener's granulomatosis: a clinicopathologic study of 16 cases. Am J Surg Pathol 1996;20:794–801.

50. Mark EJ, Flieder DB, Matsubara O. Treated Wegener's granulomatosis: Distinctive pathological findings in the lungs of 20 patients and what they tell us about the natural history of the disease. Hum Pathol 1997;28:450–8.

51. Lombard CM, Duncan SR, Rizk NW, et al. The diagnosis of Wegener's granulomatosis from transbronchial biopsy specimens. Hum Pathol 1990;21:838–42.

52. Devaney KO, Travis WD, Hoffman GS, et al. Interpretation of head and neck biopsies in Wegener's granulomatosis. A pathologic study of 126 biopsies in 70 patients. Am J Surg Pathol 1990;14:555–64.

53. del Buono EA, Flint A. Diagnostic usefulness of nasal biopsy in Wegener's granulomatosis. Hum Pathol 1991;22:107–10.

54. Matsubara O, Yoshimura N, Doi Y, et al. Nasal biopsy in the early diagnosis of Wegener's (pathergic) granulomatosis – significance of palisading granuloma and leukocytoclastic vasculitis. Virchows Arch 1996;428:13–9.

55. Hu CH, O'Loughlin S, Winkelmann RK. Cutaneous manifestations of Wegener's granulomatosis. Arch Dermatol 1977;113:175–82.

56. Barksdale SK, Hallahan CW, Kerr GS, et al. Cutaneous pathology in Wegener's granulomatosis: a clinicopathologic study of 75 biopsies in 46 patients. Am J Surg Pathol 1995;19:161–72.

57. Weiss MA, Crissman JD. Renal biopsy findings in Wegener's granulomatosis: segmental necrotizing glomerulonephritis with glomerular thrombosis. Hum Pathol 1984;15:943–56.

58. Cordier J-F, Valeyre D, Guillevin L, et al. Pulmonary Wegener's granulomatosis: a clinical and imaging study of 77 cases. Chest 1990;97:906–12.

59. Carrington CB, Liebow AA. Limited forms of angiitis and granulomatosis of Wegener's type. Am J Med 1966;41:497–527.

60. Cassan SM, Coles DT, Harrison EG. The concept of limited forms of Wegener's granulomatosis. Am J Med 1970;49:366–79.

61. Katzenstein ALA, Locke WK. Solitary lung lesions in Wegener's granulomatosis: pathologic findings and clinical significance in 25 cases. Am J Surg Pathol 1995;19:545–52.

62. Bosch X, Lopez-Soto A, Mirapeix E, et al. Antineutrophil cytoplasmic autoantibody-associated alveolar capillaritis in patients presenting with pulmonary hemorrhage. Arch Pathol Lab Med 1994;118:517–22.

63. Schwarz MI, Brown KK. Small vessel vasculitis of the lung. Thorax 2000;55:502–10.

64. Ulbright TM, Katzenstein ALA. Solitary necrotizing granulomas of the lung. Am J Surg Pathol 1980;4:13–28.

65. Cravioto H, Feigin I. Noninfectious granulomatous angiitis with a predilection for the nervous system. Neurology 1959;9:599–609.

66. Nishino H, DeRemee RA, Rubino FA, et al. Wegener's granulomatosis associated with vasculitis of the temporal artery – report of five cases. Mayo Clin Proc 1993;68:115–21.

67. Zenone T, Souquet PJ, Bohas C, et al. Unusual manifestations of giant cell arteritis: pulmonary nodules, cough, conjunctivitis and otitis with deafness. Eur Respir J 1994;7:2252–4.

68. Barnett VT, Sekosan M, Khurshid A. Wegener's granulomatosis and alpha1-antitrypsin-deficiency emphysema: proteinase-related diseases. Chest 1999;116:253–5.

69. Mazodier P, Elzouki AN, Segelmark M, et al. Systemic necrotizing vasculitides in severe alpha1-antitrypsin deficiency. QJM 1996;89:599–611.

70. Mouly S, Brillet G, Stern M, et al. Pulmonary giant bulla in Wegener's granulomatosis. Scand J Rheumatol 2000;29:333–5.

Necrotising sarcoid angiitis and granulomatosis

71. Liebow AA. Pulmonary angiitis and granulomatosis. Am Rev Respir Dis 1973;108:1–18.

72. Saldana MJ. Necrotizing sarcoid granulomatosis: clinicopathologic observations in 24 patients. Lab Invest 1978;38:364 abstract.

73. Churg A, Carrington CB, Gupta R. Necrotizing sarcoid granulomatosis. Chest 1979;76:406–13.

74. Koss MN, Hochholzer L, Feigin DS, et al. Necrotizing sarcoid-like granulomatosis: clinical, pathologic and immunopathologic findings. Hum Pathol 1980;11:510–9.

75. Churg A. Pulmonary angiitis and granulomatosis revisited. Hum Pathol 1983;14:868–83.

76. Chittock DR, Joseph MG, Paterson NAM, et al. Necrotizing sarcoid granulomatosis with pleural involvement. Chest 1994;106:672–6.

77. Quaden C, Tillie-Leblond I, Delobbe A, et al. Necrotising sarcoid granulomatosis: clinical, functional, endoscopical and radiographical evaluations. Eur Respir J 2005;26:778–85.

78. Stephen JG, Braimbridge MV, Corrin B, et al. Necrotizing 'sarcoidal' angiitis and granulomatosis of the lung. Thorax 1976;31:356–60.

79. Beach RC, Corrin B, Scopes JW, et al. Necrotizing sarcoid granulomatosis with

neurologic lesions in a child. J Pediatr 1980;97:950–3.

80. Dykhuizen RS, Smith CC, Kennedy MM, et al. Necrotizing sarcoid granulomatosis with extrapulmonary involvement. Eur Respir J 1997;10:245–7.

81. Strickland-Marmol LB, Fessler RG, Rojiani AM. Necrotizing sarcoid granulomatosis mimicking an intracranial neoplasm: Clinicopathologic features and review of the literature. Modern Pathol 2000;13:909–13.

82. Legall F, Loeuillet L, Delaval P, et al. Necrotizing sarcoid granulomatosis with and without extrapulmonary involvement. Pathol Res Pract 1996;192:306–13.

83. Shirodaria CC, Nicholson AG, Hansell DM, et al. Lesson of the month – Necrotizing sarcoid granulomatosis with skin involvement. Histopathology 2003;43:91–3.

84. Popper HH, Klemen H, Colby TV, et al. Necrotizing sarcoid granulomatosis – is it different from nodular sarcoidosis? Pneumologie 2003;57:268–71.

85. Spiteri MA, Gledhill A, Campbell D, et al. Necrotizing sarcoid granulomatosis. Br J Dis Chest 1987;81:70–5.

86. Lazzarini LC, de Fatima do Amparo Teixeira M, Souza RR, et al. Necrotizing sarcoid granulomatosis in a family of patients with sarcoidosis reinforces the association between both entities. Respiration 2008;76:356–60.

87. Rosen Y, Moon S, Huang C-T, et al. Granulomatous pulmonary angiitis in sarcoidosis. Arch Pathol Lab Med 1977;101:170–4.

88. Tauber E, Wojnarowski C, Horcher E, et al. Necrotizing sarcoid granulomatosis in a 14-yr-old female. Eur Resp J 1999;13:703–5.

Sarcoidosis combined with disseminated visceral giant cell angiitis

89. Gartside IB. Granulomatous arteritis in a lesion resembling sarcoidosis. J Pathol Bacteriol 1944;56:61–6.

90. Marcussen N, Lund C. Combined sarcoidosis and disseminated visceral giant cell vasculitis. Pathol Res Pract 1989;184:325–30.

91. Shintaku M, Mase K, Ohtsuki H, et al. Generalized sarcoid-like granulomas with systemic angiitis, crescentic glomerulonephritis, and pulmonary hemorrhage. Arch Pathol Lab Med 1989;113:1295–8.

92. Lie JT. Combined sarcoidosis and disseminated visceral giant cell angiitis – a third opinion. Arch Pathol Lab Med 1991;115:210–1.

Polyarteritis nodosa

93. Kussmaul A, Maier M. Ueber eine bisher nicht besdriebane eigenthumleche Arteriomerkrankung (periarteritis nodosa) die mit morbus Briqhtii und rapid

fortschreitender allgemeiner, Muskallahmung einherght. Deutches Arch Klin Med 1866;1:484–518.

94. Thomashaw BM, Felton CP, Navarro C. Diffuse intrapulmonary haemorrhage, renal failure and a systemic vasculitis. Am J Med 1980;68:299–304.

95. Rose GA, Spencer H. Polyarteritis nodosa. Q J Med 1957;26:43–81.

96. Fauci AS, Haynes BF, Katz P. The spectrum of vasculitis: clinical, pathologic, immunologic and therapeutic considerations. Ann Intern Med 1978;89:660–76.

97. Leavitt RY, Fauci AS. Polyangiitis overlap syndrome. Classification and prospective clinical experience. Am J Med 1986;81:79–85.

98. Matsumoto T, Homma S, Okada M, et al. The lung in polyarteritis nodosa – a pathologic study of ten cases. Hum Pathol 1993;24:717–24.

99. Nick J, Tuder R, May R, et al. Polyarteritis nodosa with pulmonary vasculitis. Am J Respir Crit Care Med 1996;153:450–3.

99a. Naniwa T, Maeda T, Shimizu S, Ito R. Hepatitis B virus-related polyarteritis nodosa presenting with multiple lung nodules and cavitary lesions. Chest 2010;138:195–7.

Microscopic polyangiitis

100. Haworth SJ, Savage CD, Carr D, et al. Pulmonary haemorrhage complicating Wegener's granulomatosis and microscopic polyarteritis. BMJ 1985;290:1775–8.

101. Bosch X, Font J, Mirapeix E, et al. Antimyeloperoxidase autoantibody-associated necrotizing alveolar capillaritis. Am Rev Respir Dis 1992;146:1326–9.

102. Akikusa B, Kondo Y, Irabu N, et al. Six cases of microscopic polyarteritis exhibiting acute interstitial pneumonia. Pathol Int 1995;45:580–8.

103. Green RJ, Ruoss SJ, Kraft SA, et al. Pulmonary capillaritis and alveolar hemorrhage: update on diagnosis and management. Chest 1996;110:1305–16.

104. Akikusa B, Sato T, Ogawa M, et al. Necrotizing alveolar capillaritis in autopsy cases of microscopic polyangiitis: incidence, histopathogenesis, and relationship with systemic vasculitis. Arch Pathol Lab Med 1997;121:144–9.

105. Jennings CA, King TE, Tuder R, et al. Diffuse alveolar hemorrhage with underlying isolated, pauciimmune pulmonary capillaritis. Am J Respir Crit Care Med 1997;155:1101–9.

106. Foulon G, Delaval P, Valeyre D, et al. ANCA-associated lung fibrosis: Analysis of 17 patients. Respiratory Medicine 2008;102:1392–8.

Hypersensitivity vasculitis

107. Kathuria S, Chejfec G. Fatal pulmonary Henoch–Schönlein syndrome. Chest 1982;82:654–6.

108. Markus HS, Clark JV. Pulmonary haemorrhage in Henoch–Schönlein purpura. Thorax 1989;44:525–6.

109. Bombardieri S, Paoletti P, Ferro C, et al. Lung involvement in essential mixed cryoglobulinaemia. Am J Med 1979;66:749–56.

110. Dreisen RB. Pulmonary vasculitis. Clin Chest Med 1982;3:607–18.

111. Schwarz MI, Mortenson RL, Colby TV, et al. Pulmonary capillaritis. The association with progressive irreversible airflow limitation and hyperinflation. Am Rev Respir Dis 1993;148:507–11.

Connective tissue diseases

112. Kuhn C. Systemic lupus erythematosus in a patient with ultrastructural lesions of the pulmonary capillaries previously reported in the review as due to idiopathic pulmonary hemosiderosis. Am Rev Respir Dis 1972;106:931–2.

113. Churg A, Franklin W, Chan KL, et al. Pulmonary hemorrhage and immune-complex deposition in the lung. Complications in a patient with systemic lupus erythematosus. Arch Pathol Lab Med 1980;104:388–91.

114. Marino CT, Pertschuk LP. Pulmonary haemorrhage in systemic lupus erythematosus. Arch Intern Med 1981;141:201–3.

115. Mark EJ, Ramirez JF. Pulmonary capillaritis and hemorrhage in patients with systemic vasculitis. Arch Pathol Lab Med 1985;109:413–8.

116. Myers JL, Katzenstein ALA. Microangiitis in lupus-induced pulmonary haemorrhage. Am J Clin Pathol 1986;85:552–6.

117. Santos Ocampo AS, Mandell BF, Fessler BJ. Alveolar hemorrhage in systemic lupus erythematosus – Presentation and management. Chest 2000;118:1083–90.

118. Price TML, Skelton MO. Rheumatoid arthritis with lung lesions. Thorax 1956;11:234–40.

119. Lemley PE, Katz P. Rheumatoid-like arthritis presenting as idiopathic pulmonary hemosiderosis: a report and review of the literature. J Rheumatol 1986;13:954–7.

120. Baydur A, Mongan ES, Slager UT. Acute respiratory failure and pulmonary arteritis without parenchymal involvement. Demonstration in a patient with rheumatoid arthritis. Chest 1979;75:518–20.

121. Kay JM, Banik S. Unexplained pulmonary hypertension with pulmonary arteritis in rheumatoid disease. Br J Dis Chest 1977;71:53–9.

Giant cell arteritis

122. Kawai C, Ishikawa K, Kato M, et al. Pulmonary pulseless disease: pulmonary involvement in so-called Takayasu's disease. Chest 1978;73:651–7.

123. Yamada I, Shibuya H, Matsubara O, et al. Takayasu arteritis: angiographic findings with special reference to pulmonary arterial change. Am J Radiol 1992;159:263–9.

124. Johnston SL, Lock RJ, Gompels MM. Takayasu arteritis: a review. J Clin Pathol 2002;55:481–6.

125. Bradley JD, Pinals RS, Poston WM. Giant cell arteritis with pulmonary nodules. Am J Med 1984;77:135–40.

126. Doyle L, McWilliam L, Hasleton PS. Giant cell arteritis with pulmonary involvement. Br J Dis Chest 1988;82:88–92.

127. Lie JT. Disseminated visceral giant cell arteritis. Am J Clin Pathol 1978;69:299–305.

128. Kagata Y, Matsubara O, Ogata S, et al. Infantile disseminated visceral giant cell arteritis presenting as sudden infant death. Pathol Int 1999;49:226–30.

129. Rose AG, Halper J, Factor SM. Primary arteriopathy in Takayasu's disease. Arch Pathol Lab Med 1984;108:644–8.

130. Ladanyi M, Fraser RS. Pulmonary involvement in giant cell arteritis. Arch Pathol Lab Med 1987;111:1178–80.

131. Matsubara O, Yoshimura N, Tamura A, et al. Pathological features of the pulmonary artery in Takayasu arteritis. Heart Vessels 1992;(Suppl 7):18–25.

132. Wagenaar SS, Westermann CJJ, Corrin B. Giant cell arteritis limited to large elastic pulmonary arteries. Thorax 1981;36:876–7.

133. Wagenaar SS, van den Bosch JMM, Westermann CJJ, et al. Isolated granulomatous giant cell vasculitis of the pulmonary elastic arteries. Arch Pathol Lab Med 1986;110:962–4.

134. Kerr KM, Auger WR, Fedullo PF, et al. Large vessel pulmonary arteritis mimicking chronic thromboembolic disease. Am J Respir Crit Care Med 1995;152:367–73.

135. Lie JT. Isolated pulmonary Takayasu arteritis: clinicopathologic characteristics. Mod Pathol 1996;9:469–74.

136. Okubo S, Kunieda T, Ando M, et al. Idiopathic isolated pulmonary arteritis with chronic cor pulmonale. Chest 1988;94:665–6.

137. Masuda S, Ishii T, Asuwa N, et al. Isolated pulmonary giant cell vasculitis. Pathol Res Pract 1994;190:1095–100.

138. Lie JT. Pulmonary granulomatous (giant cell) vasculitides – commentary. Pathol Res Pract 1994;190:1101–2.

139. Brugiere O, Mal H, Sleiman C, et al. Isolated pulmonary arteries involvement in a patient with Takayasu's arteritis. Eur Resp J 1998;11:767–70.

Behçet's disease

140. Chajek T, Fainaru M. Behçet's disease. Report of 41 cases and a review of the literature. Medicine (Baltimore) 1975;54:179–96.

141. Witt C, John M, Martin H, et al. Behçet's syndrome with pulmonary involvement – combined therapy for endobronchial stenosis using neodym-YAG laser, balloon dilation and immunosuppression. Respiration 1996;63:195–8.

142. Abadoglu O, Osma E, Ucan ES, et al. Behçet's disease with pulmonary involvement, superior vena cava syndrome, chyloptysis and chylous ascites. Respir Med 1996;90:429–31.

143. Erkan F, Cavdar T. Pulmonary vasculitis in Behçet's disease. Am Rev Respir Dis 1992;146:232–9.

144. International Study Group for Behçet's disease. Criteria for diagnosis of Behcet's disease. Lancet 1990;335:1078–80.

145. Gamble CN, Wiesner KB, Shapiro RF, et al. The immune complex pathogenesis of glomerulonephritis and pulmonary vasculitis in Behçet's disease. Am J Med 1979;66:1031–9.

146. Slavin RF, de Groot WJ. Pathology of the lung in Behçet's disease: case report and review of the literature. Am J Surg Pathol 1981;5:779–88.

147. Lie JT. Cardiac and pulmonary manifestations of Behçet syndrome. Pathol Res Pract 1988;183:347–52.

148. Aktogu S, Erer OF, Urpek G, et al. Multiple pulmonary arterial aneurysms in Behçet's disease: Clinical and radiologic remission after cyclophosphamide and corticosteroid therapy. Respiration 2002;69:178–81.

149. Jerray M, Benzarti M, Rouatbi N. Possible Behçet's disease revealed by pulmonary aneurysms. Chest 1991;99:1282–4.

150. Raz I, Okon E, Chajek-Shaul T. Pulmonary manifestations in Behçet's syndrome. Chest 1989;95:585–9.

151. Demontpreville VT, Macchiarini P, Dartevelle PG, et al. Large bilateral pulmonary artery aneurysms in Behçet's disease: rupture of the contralateral lesion after aneurysmorrhaphy. Respiration 1996;63:49–51.

152. Hughes JP, Stovin PGI. Segmental pulmonary artery aneurysms with peripheral venous thrombosis. Br J Dis Chest 1959;53:19–27.

153. Kopp WL, Green RA. Pulmonary artery aneurysms with recurrent thrombophlebitis. The Hughes–Stovin syndrome. Ann Intern Med 1962;56:105–14.

154. Frater R, Beck W, Shire V. The syndrome of pulmonary vascular aneurysms, pulmonary artery thrombi and peripheral venous thrombi. J Thorac Cardiovasc Surg 1965;49:330–8.

155. Herb S, Hetzel M, Hetzel J, et al. An unusual case of Hughes–Stovin syndrome. Eur Resp J 1998;11:1191–3.

155a. Lara AR, Schwarz MI. Diffuse alveolar hemorrhage. Chest 2010;137:1164–71.

Pulmonary haemorrhage and haemosiderosis

156. Holdsworth S, Boyce N, Thomson NM, et al. The clinical spectrum of acute glomerulonephritis and lung haemorrhage (Goodpasture's syndrome). Q J Med 1985;55:75–86.

157. Young KR Jr. Pulmonary–renal syndromes. Clin Chest Med 1989;10:655–75.

158. Morgan PGM, Turner-Warwick M. Pulmonary haemosiderosis and pulmonary haemorrhage. Br J Dis Chest 1981;75:225–42.

159. Delassence A, Fleury-Feith J, Escudier E, et al. Alveolar hemorrhage – diagnostic criteria and results in 194 immunocompromised hosts. Am J Respir Crit Care Med 1995;151:157–63.

160. Corhay JL, Weber G, Bury T, et al. Iron content in human alveolar macrophages. Eur Respir J 1992;5:804–9.

161. Becroft DMO, Lockett BK. Intra-alveolar pulmonary siderophages in sudden infant death: A marker for previous imposed suffocation. Pathology 1997;29:60–3.

162. Yukawa N, Carter N, Rutty G, et al. Intra-alveolar haemorrhage in sudden infant death syndrome: a cause for concern? J Clin Pathol 1999;52:581–7.

163. Lombard CM, Colby TV, Elliott CG. Surgical pathology of the lung in anti-basement membrane antibody-associated Goodpasture's syndrome. Hum Pathol 1989;20:445–51.

164. Sherman JM, Winnie G, Thomassen MJ, et al. Time course of hemosiderin production and clearance by human pulmonary macrophages. Chest 1984;86:409–11.

165. Magarey FR. Experimental pulmonary haemosiderosis. J Pathol Bacteriol 1951;63:729–34.

166. Epstein CE, Elidemir O, Colasurdo GN, et al. Time course of hemosiderin production by alveolar macrophages in a murine model. Chest 2001;120:2013–20.

167. Corrin B, Jagusch M, Dewar A, et al. Fine structural changes in idiopathic pulmonary haemosiderosis. J Pathol 1987;153:249–56.

168. Walford RI, Kaplan L. Pulmonary fibrosis and giant cell reaction to altered elastic tissue – endogenous pneumoconiosis. Arch Pathol Lab Med 1957;63:75–90.

169. Pai UH, McMahon J, Tomashefski JF. Mineralizing pulmonary elastosis in chronic cardiac failure – endogenous pneumoconiosis revisited. Am J Clin Pathol 1994;101:22–8.

Goodpasture's syndrome

170. Stanton MC, Tange JD. Goodpasture's syndrome. Aust Ann Med 1958;7:132–49.

171. Goodpasture EW. The significance of certain pulmonary lesions in relation to the aetiology of influenza. Am J Med Sci 1919;158:863–70.

172. Markowitz AS, Battifora HA, Schwartz F, et al. Immunological aspects of Goodpasture's syndrome. Clin Exp Immunol 1968;3:585–91.

173. Fanburg BL, McLoud TC, Niles JL, et al. A 17-year-old girl with massive hemoptysis and acute oliguric renal failure – Goodpasture's syndrome, with ANCA and anti-GBM antibodies – Wegener's granulomatosis, involving lungs, kidneys, and spleen. N Engl J Med 1993;329:2019–26.

174. Ozsoylu S, Hisconmex G, Berkel I, et al. Goodpasture's syndrome. Pulmonary haemosiderosis with nephritis. Clin Pediatr (Phila) 1976;15:358–60.

175. Briggs WA, Johnson JP, Teichman S, et al. Antiglomerular basement membrane antibody mediated glomerulonephritis and Goodpasture's syndrome. Medicine (Baltimore) 1979;58:348–61.

176. Huey B, McCormick K, Capper J, et al. Associations of HLA-DR and HLA-DQ types with anti-GBM nephritis by sequence-specific oligonucleotide probe hybridization. Kidney Int 1993;44:307–12.

177. Tobler A, Schurch E, Altermatt HJ, et al. Anti-basement membrane antibody disease with severe pulmonary haemorrhage and normal renal function. Thorax 1991;46:68–9.

178. Serisier DJ, Wong RCW, Armstrong JG. Alveolar haemorrhage in anti-glomerular basement membrane disease without detectable antibodies by conventional assays. Thorax 2006;61:636–9.

179. Peters DK, Rees AJ, Lockwood CM, et al. Treatment and prognosis in antibasement membrane antibody mediated nephritis. Transplant Proc 1982;14:513–21.

180. Beechler CR, Enquist RW, Hunt KK, et al. Immunofluorescence of transbronchial biopsies in Goodpasture's syndrome. Am Rev Respir Dis 1980;121:869–72.

181. Wilson CB, Dixon FJ. Anti-glomerular basement membrane induced glomerulonephritis. Kidney Int 1973;3:74–89.

182. Lerner RA, Dixon FJ. The induction of acute glomerulonephritis in rabbits with soluble antigens isolated from normal homologous and autologous urine. J Immunol 1968;100:1277.

183. Koffler D, Sandson J, Carr R. Immunologic studies concerning the pulmonary lesions in Goodpasture's syndrome. Am J Pathol 1969;54:293–305.

184. Poskitt TR. Immunologic and electron microscopic studies in Goodpasture's syndrome. Am J Med 1970;49:250–7.

185. Wieslander J, Heinegard D. The involvement of type IV collagen in Goodpasture's syndrome. Ann N Y Acad Sci 1985;460:363–74.

186. Gunwar S, Bejarano PA, Kalluri R, et al. Alveolar basement membrane – molecular properties of the noncollagenous domain (hexamer) of collagen-IV and its reactivity with Goodpasture autoantibodies. Am J Respir Cell Mol Biol 1991;5:107–12.

187. Thomas HM, Irwin RS. Classification of diffuse intrapulmonary haemorrhage. Chest 1975;68:483–4.

188. Botting AJ, Brown Jr AL, Divertie MB. The pulmonary lesion in a patient with Goodpasture's syndrome, as studied with the electron microscope. Am J Clin Pathol 1964;42:387–94.

189. Donald KJ, Edwards RL, McEvoy JDS. Alveolar capillary basement membrane lesions in Goodpasture's syndrome and idiopathic pulmonary haemosiderosis. Am J Med 1975;59:642–9.

Antineutrophil cytoplasmic antibody-associated pulmonary haemorrhage

190. Stokes TC, McCann BG, Rees RT, et al. Acute fulminating intrapulmonary haemorrhage in Wegener's granulomatosis. Thorax 1982;37:315–6.

191. Travis WD, Colby TV, Lombard C, et al. A clinicopathologic study of 34 cases of diffuse pulmonary hemorrhage with lung biopsy confirmation. Am J Surg Pathol 1990;14:1112–25.

192. Clutterbuck EJ, Pusey CD. Severe alveolar haemorrhage in Churg–Strauss syndrome. Eur J Respir Dis 1987;71:158–63.

Immune complex-mediated pulmonary haemorrhage

193. Hughson MD, He Z, Henegar J, et al. Alveolar hemorrhage and renal microangiopathy in systemic lupus erythematosus – Immune complex small vascular injury with apoptosis. Arch Path Lab Med 2001;125:475–83.

194. Davies JD. Behcet's syndrome with haemoptysis and pulmonary lesions. J Pathol 1973;109:351–6.

195. Efthimiou J, Johnston C, Spiro SG, et al. Pulmonary disease in Behçet's syndrome. Q J Med 1986;58:259–80.

196. Finnegan MJ, Hinchcliffe J, Russell-Jones D, et al. Vasculitis complicating cystic fibrosis. Q J Med 1989;72:609–22.

197. Sternlieb I, Bennett B, Scheinberg IH. D-penicillamine induced Goodpasture's syndrome in Wilson's disease. Ann Intern Med 1975;82:673–6.

198. Ahmad D, Petterson R, Morgan WKC, et al. Pulmonary haemorrhage and haemolytic anaemia due to trimellitic anhydride. Lancet 1979;2:328–30.

199. Kaplan V, Baur X, Czuppon A, et al. Pulmonary hemorrhage due to inhalation of vapor containing pyromellitic dianhydride. Chest 1993;104:644–5.

200. Wiertz LM, Gagnon JH, Anthonisen NR. Intrapulmonary hemorrhage with anemia after lymphangiography. N Engl J Med 1971;285:1364–5.

201. Marglin SI, Castellino RA. Severe pulmonary haemorrhage following lymphography. Cancer 1979;43:482–3.

202. Chastre J, Brun P, Soler P, et al. Acute and latent pneumonitis after subcutaneous injections of silicone in transsexual men. Am Rev Respir Dis 1987;135:236–40.

203. Lai YF, Chao TY, Wong SL. Acute pneumonitis after subcutaneous injections of silicone for augmentation mammaplasty. Chest 1994;106:1152–5.

204. Murray RJ, Smialek JE, Golle M, et al. Pulmonary artery medial hypertrophy in cocaine users without foreign particle microembolization. Chest 1989;96:1050–3.

205. Eagen JW, Memoli VA, Roberts JL, et al. Pulmonary haemorrhage in systemic lupus erythematosus. Medicine (Baltimore) 1978;57:545–50.

206. Loughlin GM, Taussig LM, Murphy SA, et al. Immune complex-mediated glomerulonephritis and pulmonary haemorrhage simulating Goodpasture's syndrome. J Pediatr 1978;93:181–4.

207. Leatherman JW, Sibley RK, Davies SF. Diffuse intrapulmonary haemorrhage and glomerulonephritis unrelated to anti-glomerular basement antibody. Am J Med 1982;72:401–10.

208. Goldstein J, Weil J, Liel Y. Intrapulmonary haemorrhages and immune complex glomerulonephritis masquerading as Goodpasture's syndrome. Hum Pathol 1986;17:754–7.

209. Martinez JS, Kohler PF. Variant 'Goodpasture's Syndrome'? Ann Intern Med 1971;75:67–76.

Idiopathic pulmonary haemosiderosis

210. Turner-Warwick M, Dewar A. Pulmonary haemorrhage and pulmonary haemosiderosis. Clin Radiol 1982;33:361–70.

211. Milman N, Pedersen FM. Idiopathic pulmonary haemosiderosis. Epidemiology, pathogenic aspects and diagnosis. Respir Med 1998;92:902–7.

212. Soergel KH, Sommers SC. Idiopathic pulmonary hemosiderosis and related syndromes. Am J Med 1962;32:499–511.

213. Thaell JF, Greipp PR, Stubbs SE, et al. Idiopathic pulmonary hemosiderosis. Two cases in a family. Mayo Clin Proc 1978;53:113–8.

214. Breckenridge RL, Ross JS. Idiopathic pulmonary haemosiderosis: a report of familial occurrence. Chest 1979;75:636–9.

215. Beckerman RC, Taussig LM, Pinnas JL. Familial pulmonary hemosiderosis. Am J Dis Child 1979;133:609–11.

216. Saeed MM, Woo MS, MacLaughlin EF, et al. Prognosis in pediatric idiopathic pulmonary hemosiderosis. Chest 1999;116:721–5.

217. Byrd RB, Gracey DR. Immunosuppressive treatment of idiopathic pulmonary hemosiderosis. JAMA 1973;226:458–9.

218. Yeager H, Powell D, Weinberg RM, et al. Idiopathic pulmonary hemosiderosis.

Ultrastructural studies and response to azathioprine. Arch Intern Med 1976;136:1145–9.

219. Wright PH, Menzies IS, Pounder RE, et al. Adult idiopathic pulmonary haemosiderosis and coeliac disease. Q J Med 1981;197:95–102.

220. Wright PH, Buxton-Thomas M, Keeling PWN, et al. Adult idiopathic pulmonary hemosiderosis: a comparison of lung function changes and the distribution of pulmonary disease in patients with and without coeliac disease. Br J Dis Chest 1983;77:282–92.

221. Bouros D, Panagou P, Rokkas T, et al. Bronchoalveolar lavage findings in a young adult with idiopathic pulmonary haemosiderosis and coeliac disease. Eur Respir J 1994;7:1009–12.

222. Hammami S, Ghedira Besbes L, Hadded S, et al. Co-occurrence pulmonary haemosiderosis with coeliac disease in child. Respiratory Medicine 2008;102:935–6.

223. Hay JG, Turner-Warwick M. Pulmonary hemosiderosis, hemorrhagic syndromes and other rare infiltrative disorders. In: Murray JF, Nadel JA, editors. Textbook of Respiratory Medicine. Philadelphia: W.B. Saunders; 1988. p. 1501–14.

224. Rafferty JR, Cook MK. Idiopathic pulmonary haemosiderosis with autoimmune haemolytic anaemia. Br J Dis Chest 1984;78:282–5.

225. Bain SC, Bryan RL, Hawkins JB. Idiopathic pulmonary haemosiderosis and autoimmune thyrotoxicosis. Respir Med 1989;83:447–50.

226. Stafford HA, Polmar SHJ, Boat TF. Immunologic studies in cow's milk-induced pulmonary haemosiderosis. Pediatr Res 1977;11:898–903.

227. Cohen GA, Berman BA. Pulmonary hemosiderosis. Cutis 1985;35:106–9.

228. Valassy-Adam H, Rouska A, Karpouzas J, et al. Raised IgA in idiopathic pulmonary hemosiderosis. Arch Dis Child 1975;50:320–2.

229. Danel C, Israel-Biet D, Costabel U, et al. The clinical role of BAL in rare pulmonary diseases. Eur Respir Rev 1992;2:83–8.

230. Bradley JD. The pulmonary haemorrhage syndromes. Clin Chest Med 1982;3:593–605.

231. Irwin RS, Cottrell TS, Hsu KC, et al. Idiopathic pulmonary hemosiderosis: an electron microscopic and immunofluorescent study. Chest 1974;65:41–5.

Chapter | 9 |

Pulmonary eosinophilia

Pulmonary eosinophilia is a clinical term used to describe the association of radiographic lung opacities and blood eosinophilia.[1] Synonyms include 'pulmonary infiltrates with eosinophilia' and 'PIE syndrome'.[2] Some lung diseases that are characterised by an eosinophilic lung infiltrate are not associated with blood eosinophilia and are therefore dealt with elsewhere – eosinophilic granuloma (now termed Langerhans cell histiocytosis) on page 288 and reactive eosinophilic pleurisy on page 711. Other eosinophilic infiltrates are associated with blood eosinophilia but not with radiographic opacities, e.g. asthma. The eosinophilia–myalgia syndrome seen with the ingestion of certain tryptophan preparations may well have been considered in this chapter but is dealt with under drug reactions (see p. 389).

Pulmonary eosinophilia may be classified clinically, aetiologically or pathologically. Here the emphasis will be on pathology, but first the aetiology and pathogenesis will be outlined.

Aetiology

Aetiologically, pulmonary eosinophilia may be classified as cryptogenic or of known cause, the latter including allergy to fungi, parasites or drugs (Box 9.1).

Allergic aspergillosis is a common cause of pulmonary eosinophilia in the UK whereas infestation by metazoan parasites is commoner in communities in which these parasites are prevalent (Box 9.2). In some parts of the world filariasis is the cause: this is tropical pulmonary eosinophilia, which can be readily diagnosed from the patient's history of residence in the tropics, by the presence of extraordinarily high levels of both serum IgE and antifilarial antibodies, and by the dramatic therapeutic response to filaricides.[3–5] Pulmonary eosinophilia is also caused by a number of drugs, notably nitrofurantoin but occasionally sulphonamides and aspirin, amongst others (Box 9.3). Pulmonary eosinophilia may also be a manifestation of rheumatoid disaease.[6]

In other patients the cause of the pulmonary eosinophilia is not recognised: such cases are categorised as suffering from cryptogenic pulmonary eosinophilia.[7] A majority of these patients are atopic, giving a history of rhinitis or asthma.[8] There is a high level of activated helper T lymphocytes in their bronchoalveolar lavage fluid.[9] They also show a transient increase in circulating immune complexes.[10] The Churg–Strauss syndrome of allergic angiitis and granulomatosis may be regarded as a subset of cryptogenic pulmonary eosinophilia but the hypereosinophilic syndrome is quite distinct from all these reactive forms of eosinophilia and probably represents a leukoproliferative disorder.

Pathogenesis

The eosinophil leukocyte is central to the pathogenesis of all the diseases in this chapter. Eosinophil leukocytes are produced in the bone marrow under the control of cytokines secreted by type 2 helper lymphocytes, notably interleukin-5. Once released into the blood they normally remain there for 12–18 hours, maintaining a count of 50–250/μl. An absolute count is more meaningful than the percentage in a differential white blood cell count. They enter the tissues under the influence of chemotactic agents known as eotaxins,[11] of which three are now recognised. These agents are small proteins produced by a variety of cells, which in the lung include bronchial epithelial cells, smooth-muscle cells and fibroblasts, acting under the influence of interleukins derived from type 2 helper lymphocytes and mast cells (see Fig. 3.30, p. 115).[11–13]

©2010 Elsevier Ltd
DOI: 10.1016/B978-0-7020-3369-8.00009-4

Tissue eosinophilia does not necessarily correlate with blood eosinophilia even though the two usually go together: blood counts may dip as eosinophils flood the lung and then rise as the infiltrate resolves due to a lag in bone marrow response. Sputum and bronchoalveolar lavage counts reflect lung tissue eosinophilia better than blood counts but, like neutrophils, eosinophils appear to be washed out of the lung more easily than macrophages so that raised lavage counts are encountered in diseases such as idiopathic pulmonary fibrosis that are seldom characterised by any appreciable degree of tissue eosinophilia. Bronchoalveolar lavage eosinophils are usually expressed as a percentage of total cells recovered from the lungs, the normal being less than 3%. Eosinophils in sputum are generally expressed only in broad qualitative terms (e.g. 'small, moderate or large numbers'). When there is eosinophilic pneumonia, eosinophils are the predominant cell in both sputum and bronchoalveolar lavage fluid. They are represented at levels greatly in excess of those found in diseases such as idiopathic pulmonary fibrosis.

Biopsy is the only way to establish tissue eosinophilia with certainty but in practice a tissue diagnosis is often inferred from the clinical features coupled with sputum, blood and bronchoalveolar lavage findings. If a tissue diagnosis is deemed essential a transbronchial biopsy will generally suffice because most of the conditions causing pulmonary eosinophilia affect sufficiently large areas of the lung to be targeted successfully by the bronchoscopist. However, some forms of tissue eosinophilia are characterised by an associated vasculitis and it is unlikely that a transbronchial biopsy will identify this. Vasculitis is more likely to be revealed by thoracoscopic biopsy. Alternatively, it may be identified in more accessible tissue, such as skin or muscle.

Once in the tissues, eosinophils secrete a number of products, some of which counter the action of substances secreted by mast cells. Histaminase and aryl sulphatase, for example, respectively destroy histamine and the leukotriene complex formerly known as slow-reacting substance of anaphylaxis. Eosinophils also phagocytose immune complexes and mast cell granules, and tend to dampen reaginic hypersensitivity reactions. However, they also secrete substances such as reactive oxygen radicals, major basic protein and eosinophil cationic protein which, whilst helping to eliminate parasites, are also toxic to host cells (Fig. 9.1).[14–17] These eosinophil products are thought to be responsible for much of the tissue damage in the eosinophilic disorders about to be described. Activation of the cells involved in cryptogenic eosinophilic pneumonia is suggested by the demonstration that they express intercellular adhesion molecules, probably under the influence of the activated T lymphocytes referred to above.[18] Electron microscopy shows that released eosinophil granules are closely associated with degenerate and necrotic alveolar tissue.[19]

Corticosteroids act on eosinophils in a variety of ways.[20] They cause rapid eosinophil sequestration in peripheral blood vessels and inhibit their production in the bone marrow. They also reduce eosinophil survival by blocking lymphokines that inhibit eosinophil apoptosis. Eosinophil adherence and chemotaxis are also diminished by corticosteroids. In view of these many actions it is not surprising that corticosteroids are effective in treating many diseases characterised by eosinophilia.

SIMPLE PULMONARY EOSINOPHILIA

The Swiss physician Löffler described two conditions that were characterised by blood eosinophilia. One is the hypereosinophilic syndrome, which is dealt with below. The other is one that later came to be known as simple pulmonary eosinophilia.[21] Rarely a patient may

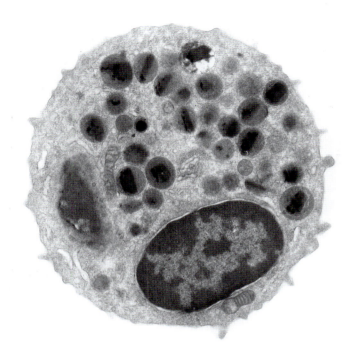

Figure 9.1 Electron micrograph of an eosinophil. A bilobed nucleus is surrounded by granules, many of which have a bar-shaped electron-dense core. The granule core consists of a basic protein whilst the surrounding matrix contains cationic protein, both of which are highly toxic.[14] *(Courtesy of Miss A Dewar, Brompton, UK.)*

Figure 9.2 Fatal cryptogenic eosinophilic pneumonia. Confluent areas of consolidation represent alveoli filled with eosinophils.

display features of both conditions.[22] The term 'Löffler's syndrome' is confusingly applied to both and therefore best avoided.

Simple pulmonary eosinophilia is characterised by migratory pulmonary opacities accompanied by blood eosinophilia and minimal or no pulmonary symptoms. Ascariasis was prevalent in Switzerland in Löffler's day and was probably the cause of the eosinophilia in his cases. Drug reactions are a more important cause today but many cases are unexplained. Löffler emphasised the benign transient nature of the condition. Corticosteroids are highly effective but are rarely required because the condition is usually self-limiting. However, an underlying cause such as parasitic infestation should always be considered. The lung is seldom biopsied but it may be presumed to show changes similar to those seen in chronic eosinophilic pneumonia.

CHRONIC EOSINOPHILIC PNEUMONIA

Chronic eosinophilic pneumonia is a serious condition which generally requires treatment with corticosteroids.[8,20,23–26] These usually prove efficacious but may have to be continued for many months, or even indefinitely, to prevent relapse. The disease is occasionally life-threatening. The peak incidence is in the fifth decade and females preponderate 2 : 1. There is often a history of atopic illnesses such as rhinitis or asthma and the condition is regarded as having an allergic basis. Any of the aetiological agents outlined above may be responsible, drugs, fungi or parasites, or the cause may not be identified.

Clinical features

The onset is insidious, with gradually worsening cough, dyspnoea, fever and weight loss. There is blood and sputum eosinophilia. However, blood and tissue eosinophil levels are not always elevated contemporaneously, the raised blood counts often having abated whilst eosinophils are still evident in the lung tissue. Bronchoalveolar lavage cell counts correlate better with the tissue findings, eosinophils being the predominant cell in lavage fluid from an involved segment.[13] The chest radiograph is distinctive, showing bilateral opacification that is peripheral and apical.[27] It has been likened to the plume of a volcano or the photographic negative of the perihilar shadowing of pulmonary oedema. This is mirrored by subpleural consolidation on high-resolution computed tomography.

Pathology

In the occasional case that comes to autopsy the lungs are found to be heavy and firm with irregular areas of pale consolidation (Fig. 9.2). Microscopically, eosinophils fill the alveoli and infiltrate the interstitium (Fig. 9.3).[8,23,28] The alveoli also contain a variable number of macrophages, some of which may be multinucleate (Fig. 9.4). The macrophages may outnumber the eosinophils to mimic the appearances of desquamative interstitial pneumonia (Fig. 9.5). Focal collections of eosinophils may undergo necrosis to form so-called eosinophil abscesses, which are sometimes attended by foreign-body-type giant cells engulfing eosinophilic debris (Fig. 9.6).[8] Sparse sarcoid-like granulomas are occasionally seen, and in rare cases are unduly prominent.[29] The eosinophil infiltrate may involve small blood vessels but necrotising vasculitis is not encountered: its presence would suggest Churg–Strauss allergic granulomatosis, which is dealt with below. Knowledge of treatment is important as eosinophils diminish with corticosteroid administration. Healing, whether occurring spontaneously or in response to such treatment, usually results in complete resolution but may be by repair, this resulting in alveolar fibrosis that is indistinguishable from any other organising pneumonia.[10,30]

Differential diagnosis

The location of the eosinophils in air spaces as well as in the interstitium helps to distinguish eosinophilic pneumonia from eosinophilic

Figure 9.3 Eosinophilic pneumonia. The alveoli contain many eosinophil polymorphonuclear leukocytes.

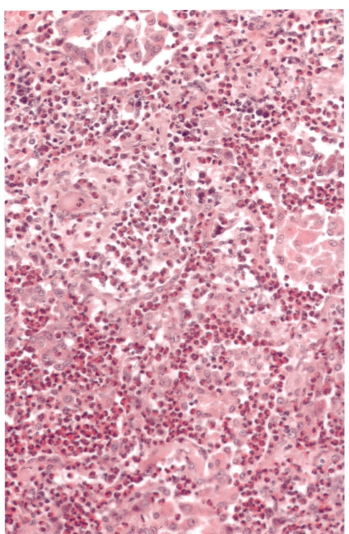

Figure 9.4 Eosinophilic pneumonia in which the alveoli are filled by both eosinophils and macrophages. *(Courtesy of Dr T Jelihovsky, Sydney, Australia.)*

granuloma (Langerhans cell histiocytosis), as do the presence of eosinophils in the blood, sputum and bronchoalveolar lavage fluid and a lack of Langerhans cells aggregation. Pneumothorax may provoke a reactive eosinophilic infiltrate but this is limited to the alveoli immediately beneath the pleura.

ACUTE EOSINOPHILIC PNEUMONIA

Clinical features

The term 'acute eosinophilic pneumonia' was introduced in 1989 for a condition characterised by the sudden onset of a febrile illness accompanied by myalagia, pleuritic pain and hypoxaemia.[31,32] Patients may be of any age and either sex.[33] Chest radiographs show extensive bilateral opacification and effusions.[27] Blood eosinophil counts are often normal but many eosinophils are found on bronchoalveolar lavage and pleural aspirates. A history of asthma is unusual but there may be one of allergic rhinitis.[34] Apart from the lavage and aspirate findings, the clinical features suggest severe infection or the acute respiratory distress syndrome. The condition is life-threatening but responds well to corticosteroids.

Aetiology

Most cases reported to date have been cryptogenic but a few appear to have represented drug reactions or have been associated with smoking.[35,36] In the latter case, disease onset has generally been within 1 month of the patient starting to smoke, restarting or substantially increasing the number of cigarettes smoked.[37]

Pathology

Acute eosinophilic pneumonia shows the features of diffuse alveolar damage in its exudative or organising phases, coupled with a heavy interstitial infiltrate and a lesser alveolar exudate of eosinophils.[38] In its exudative phase diffuse alveolar damage is characterised by hyaline membranes and in its organising phase by interstitial fibroblast proliferation, prominent alveolar epithelial regeneration and organising alveolar exudates (Fig. 9.7).

Figure 9.5 Eosinophilic pneumonia. There is moderate eosinophil exudation but these cells are outnumbered by alveolar macrophages.

Figure 9.7 Acute eosinophilic pneumonia. (A) The alveolar walls are expanded by oedema and a mixed inflammatory cell infiltrate, which includes eosinophils. The alveolar epithelium shows focal desquamation and there is prominent type II pneumocyte hyperplasia. (B) An eosinophilic microabscess (left centre) is highlighted in (C).

Figure 9.6 An eosinophilic 'abscess' consisting of agglutinated necrotic eosinophils attended by a giant cell granulomatous reaction.

Differential diagnosis

Acute eosinophilic pneumonia is more likely to be mistaken for diffuse alveolar damage than chronic eosinophilic pneumonia: therefore, whenever diffuse alveolar damage is being considered it is advisable to search for eosinophils, which may be focal in acute eosinophilic pneumonia. Chronic eosinophilic pneumonia lacks the features of diffuse alveolar damage seen in the acute condition and usually shows more eosinophils, which are often mixed with alveolar macrophages. The Churg–Strauss syndrome, which is described below, is also characterised by vasculitis, necrotising granulomatosis and asthma, features which are not seen in acute eosinophilic pneumonia.

BRONCHOCENTRIC GRANULOMATOSIS

Bronchocentric granulomatosis was first described in 1973 as a necrotising granulomatous inflammation of the airway walls and surrounding lung tissue.[39] It may be associated with asthma but this is not always the case.[40,41]

Clinical features and prognosis

In one series of 23 patients, the mean age was 22 years in the 10 asthmatic patients, and 50 years in the 13 non-asthmatics. The sex distribution was almost equal in both groups.[40] Asthmatics with bronchocentric granulomatosis complain of increased wheezing, cough, fever and occasionally haemoptysis. Blood eosinophilia and positive sputum culture for *Aspergillus* are commonly seen.[40] The non-asthmatic patients are a more heterogeneous group. They may be asymptomatic or present with an acute febrile illness and cough. Blood eosinophilia is uncommon in this group. Chest radiographic abnormalities are similar in the two groups and include solitary or multiple infiltrates or tumour-like masses and areas of atelectasis, usually involving the upper lobes.[27,40,42] Apart from fever and blood eosinophilia the condition is confined to the lungs. The prognosis is good. Corticosteroids generally result in rapid clinical and radiological resolution. Some patients recover without treatment.

Aetiology and pathological findings

Bronchocentric granulomatosis usually represents a type of allergic bronchopulmonary aspergillosis that affects more distal airways than mucoid impaction.[43-45] Medium or small bronchi, or even bronchioles, are affected rather than large central airways.[39,40,46,47] The condition is characterised by a necrotising granulomatous inflammation (Figs 9.8 and 9.9). This destroys much of the airway wall and results in necrotic debris occluding the lumen (see Fig. 5.4.18 on p. 231 and Figs 9.8 and 9.9). The inflammation usually includes many eosinophils, together with lymphocytes, plasma cells and prominent epithelioid cells, which often border the necrotic debris in a palisade pattern. That the process is bronchocentric may sometimes be recognisable only from its location alongside unaffected pulmonary arteries or by tracing its distribution in step sections. Often, just a remnant of respiratory epithelium indicates that the disease is centred on the airways. Sparse hyphae are generally to be found within mucous plugs occluding larger airways. Rarely, bronchocentric granulomatosis may complicate an aspergilloma.[48]

In other cases no allergen is ever identified: these cases differ from those caused by aspergillus in that there is no blood eosinophilia or history of asthma and eosinophils are sparse in the affected tissues, where plasma cells are predominate.[46] In other patients bronchocentric granulomatosis is associated with other pathogens,

Figure 9.8 Bronchocentric granulomatosis as a manifestation of allergic bronchopulmonary aspergillosis. The lesion was thought to be neoplastic until it was resected and dilated airways impacted with mucopurulent debris were identified.

Figure 9.9 Bronchocentric granulomatosis. Several areas of necrotising granulomatous inflammation are seen. They are situated alongside arteries, which are themselves largely spared, and an occasional remnant of respiratory epithelium confirms that they are centred on airways. In the absence of recognisable bronchial remnants the bronchocentricity of the lesion has to be inferred from its location next to a pulmonary artery.

such as *Echinococcus*, mycobacteria, *Blastomyces*, *Histoplasma* or *Mucor*.[49-52] Tuberculosis, histoplasmosis, blastomycosis and coccidioidomycosis may all show a histological process indistinguishable from bronchocentric granulomatosis and many cases of bronchocentric granulomatosis in non-asthmatic patients may represent unrecognized infections.[50] Atopy does not appear to be important in these cases but sometimes the patient is immunosuppressed.[51] Bronchocentric granulomatosis has also been reported in association with rheumatoid arthritis,[53-55] ankylosing spondylitis,[56] glomerulonephritis[57] and red cell aplasia.[58] It is also described beyond an obstructing bronchial carcinoma, the mechanism here being sustained non-allergic inflammation.[59,60] A bronchocentric form of Wegener's granulomatosis is distinguished from bronchocentric granulomatosis by its characteristic necrotising vasculitis.[61]

ALLERGIC ANGIITIS AND GRANULOMATOSIS (CHURG–STRAUSS SYNDROME)

Allergic angiitis and granulomatosis is a clinicopathological syndrome, consisting of asthma, eosinophilia, vasculitis and necrotising granulomas, that was first described in 1951 by Churg and Strauss.[62] Since then, several additional series have appeared.[63-65] The cause is unknown but the predominant clinical features implicate the respiratory tract as the portal of entry of an as yet unidentified antigen. The condition shares with Wegener's granulomatosis and microscopic polyangiitis an association with antineutrophil cytoplasmic antibodies (ANCAs), for which there is increasing evidence that cross-reactivity with certain bacterial antigens is responsible (see p. 438). There are rare reports of allergic angiitis and granulomatosis developing in patients with allergic bronchopulmonary mycoses[66,67] or diffuse panbronchiolitis.[68]

Clinical features

The majority of patients are atopic. They initially suffer from allergic rhinitis and then asthma. They next develop pulmonary infiltrates accompanied by blood eosinophilia (often exceeding $5 \times 10^9/l$) and finally enter a vasculitic phase.[63,65] Serum IgE levels may be increased during the vasculitic phase.[65] Many patients have systemic symptoms, such as fever and weight loss. Non-cavitating pulmonary infiltrates that may be diffuse and transient or massive and nodular, are generally found.[27] There may be eosinophilic pleural effusions. Myocardial or pericardial lesions are evident in about 50% of patients. Most deaths are associated with complications of cardiac involvement.[65] Many patients also have involvement of the skin, gastrointestinal tract, joints, muscles, nervous system or lower urinary tract[63]; thymic and laryngeal lesions have also been described.[69,70] Renal disease is usually mild and renal failure is rare. Antimyeloperoxidase antibodies (p-ANCA) are found in the majority of cases.[71,72] Unlike Wegener's granulomatosis, cytotoxic therapy is rarely indicated and corticosteroids usually provide effective treatment. The substitution of leukotriene antagonists for corticosteroids in the treatment of asthma appears to be unmasking previously unsuspected cases of Churg–Strauss syndrome[73,74]; the syndrome has also been recognised in asthmatic patients who have had their corticosteroid dosage reduced or who have been transferred from systemic to inhaled corticosteroids.[75]

The American College of Rheumatology has established six criteria, of which four must be fulfilled for a diagnosis of Churg–Strauss syndrome (Box 9.4). This yields a sensitivity of 85% and a specificity of 99.7%. Alternatively, three particular criteria (asthma, blood eosinophilia greater than 10% and a history of allergy other than

asthma or drug sensitivity) carried a sensitivity of 95% and a specificity of 99.2%.[76]

Figure 9.10 Allergic angiitis and granulomatosis (Churg–Strauss syndrome). Multiple confluent yellow nodules are seen while several airways show mucous plugging indicative of the underlying asthma.

Pathology

Three histological features accompany the asthma and blood eosinophilia: tissue eosinophilia, vasculitis and necrotising granulomatosis. These features are not necessarily seen together and in practice the diagnosis is usually made on clinical grounds with histological verification of perhaps just one of them. The likelihood of all three features being identified increases with the size and number of the biopsies and is greatest in autopsy material.

At autopsy or in an adequate biopsy soft yellow nodules may be seen on the cut surface of the lung (Fig. 9.10). These represent foci of eosinophilic pneumonia within which irregular areas of necrosis containing the debris of dead eosinophils and Charcot–Leyden crystals are often seen.

Granulomas may be numerous but more usually are infrequent and may not be readily identifiable in biopsy material. Early granulomas consist of small irregular clusters of giant cells and histiocytes, usually with a small central focus of densely eosinophilic necrosis. Epithelioid cells are not a feature and the granulomas lack the cohesion and lymphocytic rim typical of those seen in sarcoidosis. In larger granulomas the central necrotic area is surrounded by radially arranged palisading histiocytes and multinucleate cells (Fig. 9.11).

The vasculitis, which involves arteries, veins and even capillaries,[77] may be eosinophilic, neutrophilic or granulomatous[78] but usually

Figure 9.11 Allergic angiitis and granulomatosis (Churg–Strauss syndrome). A necrotising granuloma and prominent eosinophil infiltration are seen in the pericardium.

takes the form of focal necrosis of vessel walls associated with perivascular and transmural infiltration by eosinophils (Fig. 9.12). Capillary involvement may cause alveolar haemorrhage.[79] If the vasculitis is neutrophilic the appearances are similar to those of poly-arteritis nodosa[80] and the diagnosis of allergic granulomatosis has to depend upon extravascular features. Affected vessels may be obliterated by fibrous tissue. Electron-dense deposits,[77] IgE[63] and IgM[65] have all been reported in the vascular basement membrane.

Other changes in the lungs include those of asthma, as described on page 109 (Figs 9.10 and 9.13). Extrapulmonary lesions show vasculitis and necrotising granulomatosis with prominent tissue eosinophilia, as in the lungs (Fig. 9.14).

Differential diagnosis

The relationship of the Churg–Strauss syndrome to other forms of vasculitis, hypereosinophilia and granulomatosis has been the subject of much debate.[65,81–83] Strictly speaking, the eponym should be reserved for cases in which all the criteria are present: asthma, eosinophilia, vasculitis and necrotising granulomatosis, but Churg and Strauss[62] considered the combination of marked tissue eosinophilia and granulomatosis to be pathognomonic. All their patients were asthmatic. Patients with the histological features of the Churg–Strauss syndrome but lacking a history of asthma and blood eosinophilia have been variously regarded as suffering from an eosinophilic variant of Wegener's granulomatosis[83] or atypical forms of the Churg–Strauss syndrome.[69,84] At various stages in the course of the Churg–Strauss syndrome patients may fulfil the criteria for the hypereosinophilic syndrome (see below) or simple pulmonary eosinophilia, as described above.

The differences between Churg–Strauss syndrome and Wegener's granulomatosis are both clinical and pathological. Asthma and blood eosinophilia are not features of Wegener's granulomatosis whilst the destructive upper respiratory tract lesions of this condition are not present in the Churg–Strauss syndrome. The pulmonary lesions are generally less extensively necrotic in the Churg–Strauss syndrome than in Wegener's granulomatosis. Tissue eosinophilia is found in an eosinophilic variant of Wegener's granulomatosis[83] but is usually limited to the chronic inflammatory granulation tissue that surrounds areas of necrosis rather than flooding air spaces as in the eosinophilic pneumonia of the Churg–Strauss syndrome. The pathological changes

Figure 9.12 Allergic angiitis and granulomatosis (Churg–Strauss syndrome). The vasculitis predominantly involves medium-sized and small pulmonary arteries (A and B), but may also involve pulmonary capillaries (C).

Figure 9.13 Allergic angiitis and granulomatosis (Churg–Strauss syndrome). On the left there is an area of geographic necrosis, within which foci of vasculitis can be seen while on the right there is a bronchus plugged by mucus, reflecting the patient's underlying asthma.

Figure 9.14 Allergic angiitis and granulomatosis (Churg–Strauss syndrome). A muscle biopsy shows necrotising vasculitis and eosinophilia.

in the kidney may be similar in the two diseases but they are rarely progressive in the Churg–Strauss syndrome and cause only mild impairment of function. Lastly, the p-ANCA test tends to be positive in the Churg–Strauss syndrome and c-ANCA negative, the reverse of what is found in Wegener's granulomatosis. The Churg–Strauss syndrome, Wegener's granulomatosis and microscopic polyangiitis are compared in Table 8.3.1 (see p. 441).

HYPEREOSINOPHILIC SYNDROME

The term 'hypereosinophilic syndrome' was introduced in 1968 for what had previously been known as Löffler's syndrome, one of two conditions named after the Swiss physician who first described them.[22,85] The other is simple pulmonary eosinophilia, which is

Table 9.1 Systemic involvement in hypereosinophilic syndrome[89]

Cardiovascular	58%
Cutaneous	56%
Neurological	54%
Pulmonary	49%
Splenic	43%
Hepatic	30%
Ocular	23%
Gastrointestinal	23%

described above. This one represents a rare and often fatal systemic disease of uncertain aetiology that is regarded by many as representing a leukoproliferative disorder.[86] The disease is marked by sustained overproduction of eosinophils (blood eosinophils in excess of $1.5 \times 10^9/l$ for longer than 6 months) and widespread organ damage.[87] It affects adults in the third and fourth decades and men outnumber women by 7 to 1.[88] Many organs are involved (Table 9.1), those with cardiac or central nervous system involvement having a particularly poor prognosis.[89] Vascular involvement is generally described as being thrombotic or haemorrhagic rather than vasculitic.

Aetiology

The proposed leukoproliferative basis of the hypereosinophilic syndrome is supported by the identification of monoclonal cell populations. Conventional cytogenetic analysis is often normal but a cryptic interstitial deletion of chromosome 4 resulting in the formation of an *FIP1L1-PDGFRA* fusion gene has led to the recognition that many patients who would previously have been regarded as having the hypereosinophilic syndrome actually have chronic eosinophilic leukaemia.[90,91] In other patients with hypereosinophilia there is a clonal proliferation of type 2 helper lymphocytes (Th2, CD4 cells).[86,92] Th2 cells produce cytokines implicated in eosinophil proliferation and activation, notably interleukin-5. The consequent eosinophil activation results in the release of cytotoxic factors such as major basic protein and eosinophil cationic protein that are probably responsible for much of the tissue damage encountered in the syndrome. In rare cases, lymphoma or leukaemia cells overproduce interleukin-5, and consequently hypereosinophilia.

Clinical features

The clinical picture is generally dominated by cardiovascular or neurological features. Vascular disease is characterised by an early thrombotic phase followed by fibrosis and cardiac involvement by dysrhythmia, valvular incompetence, and ultimately heart failure. Neurological disease is characterised by intellectual impairment, a variety of localising signs and peripheral neuropathy. The commonest respiratory symptom is a non-productive cough: asthma is rare. Pleural effusions are common but are generally transudates attributable to cardiac failure; they rarely contain eosinophils. Interstitial pulmonary infiltrates are detected in about a quarter of cases and these may progress to the adult respiratory distress syndrome.[93] Computed tomography findings include small pulmonary nodules with or without a halo of ground-glass attenuation and focal areas of ground-glass attenuation which are mainly peripheral.[27,94] Many patients with pulmonary involvement respond to corticosteroids but cytotoxic drugs have been deemed necessary in severe cases.[93]

Pathology

Pulmonary involvement is characterised by a heavy infiltrate of mature eosinophils and consolidation of the air spaces by the same cells, often with small foci of necrosis. There may be many Charcot–Leyden crystals, as with any heavy eosinophil infiltrate. Thus, in the lungs the pathological features of the hypereosinophilic syndrome are identical to those of eosinophilic pneumonia (see above). Secondary changes include widespread thrombosis and infarction.

REFERENCES

1. Crofton JW, Livingstone JL, Oswald NC, et al. Pulmonary eosinophilia. Thorax 1952;7:1–35.
2. Reeder WH, Goodrich BE. Pulmonary infiltration with eosinophilia (PIE syndrome). Ann Intern Med 1952;36:1217–40.
3. Danaraj TJ, Pacheco G, Shanmugaratnam K, et al. The etiology and pathology of eosinophilic lung (tropical eosinophilia). Am J Trop Med Hyg 1966;15:183–9.
4. Udwadia FE. Tropical eosinophilia – a review. Respir Med 1993;87:17–21.
5. Ong RKC, Doyle RL. Tropical pulmonary eosinophilia. Chest 1998;113:1673–9.
6. Norman D, Piecyk M, Roberts DH. Eosinophilic pneumonia as an initial manifestation of rheumatoid arthritis. Chest 2004;126:993–5.
7. McCarthy DS, Pepys J. Cryptogenic pulmonary eosinophilias. Clin Allergy 1973;3:339–51.
8. Liebow AA, Carrington CB. The eosinophilic pneumonias. Medicine (Baltimore) 1969;48:251–85.
9. Albera C, Ghio P, Solidoro P, et al. Activated and memory alveolar T-lymphocytes in idiopathic eosinophilic pneumonia. Eur Respir J 1995;8:1281–5.
10. Miyagawa Y, Nagata N, Shigematsu N. Clinicopathological study of migratory lung infiltrates. Thorax 1991;46:233–8.
11. Conroy DM, Williams TJ. Eotaxin and the attraction of eosinophils to the asthmatic lung. Respir Res 2001;2:150–6.
12. Mukae H, Kadota J, Kohno S, et al. Increase of activated T-cells in BAL fluid of Japanese patients with bronchiolitis obliterans organizing pneumonia and chronic eosinophilic pneumonia. Chest 1995;108:123–8.
13. Kita H, Sur S, Hunt LW, et al. Cytokine production at the site of disease in chronic eosinophilic pneumonitis. Am J Respir Crit Care Med 1996;153:1437–41.
14. Peters MS, Rodriguez M, Gleich GJ. Localization of human eosinophil granule major basic protein, eosinophil cationic protein, and eosinophil-derived neurotoxin by immunoelectron microscopy. Lab Invest 1986;54:656–62.
15. Plager DA, Loegering DA, Tang J, et al. Eosinophil Proteins: Human eosinophil granule major basic protein homolog: biochemical, genetic and immunochemical aspects. Respiratory Medicine 2000;94:1011–2.
16. Ackerman SJ, Swaminathan GJ, Leonidas DD, et al. Eosinophil Proteins: Structural biology of Charcot–Leyden crystal protein (Galectin-10): new insights into an old protein. Respiratory Medicine 2000;94:1014–6.
17. Venge P. Eosinophil Proteins: Eosinophil granule proteins as markers of eosinophil activity in vivo. Respiratory Medicine 2000;94:1016–7.
18. Azuma M, Nakamura Y, Sano T, et al. Adhesion molecule expression on eosinophils in idiopathic eosinophilic pneumonia. Eur Respir J 1996;9:2494–500.
19. Saitoh K, Shindo N, Toh Y, et al. Electron microscopic study of chronic eosinophilic pneumonia. Pathol Int 1996;46:855–61.
20. Allen JN, Davis WB. Eosinophilic lung diseases. Am J Respir Crit Care Med 1994;150:1423–38.

Simple pulmonary eosinophilia

21. Löffler W. Zur Differential-Diagnose der Lungeninfiltrierungen II. Uber fluchtige Succedan-Infiltrate (mit Eosinophilie). Beitr Z Klin D Tuberk 1932;79:368–92.
22. Brink AJ, Weber HW. Fibroplastic parietal endocarditis with eosinophilia. Loffler's endocarditis. Am J Med 1963;34:52–70.

Chronic eosinophilic pneumonia

23. Carrington CB, Addington WW, Goff AM, et al. Chronic eosinophilic pneumonia. N Engl J Med 1969;280:788–98.
24. Jederlinic PJ, Sicilian L, Gaensler EA. Chronic eosinophilic pneumonia: a report of 19 cases and a review of the literature. Medicine (Baltimore) 1988;67:154–62.
25. Naughton M, Fahy J, FitzGerald MX. Chronic eosinophilic pneumonia – a long-term follow-up of 12 patients. Chest 1993;103:162–5.
26. Hayakawa H, Sato A, Toyoshima M, et al. A clinical study of idiopathic eosinophilic pneumonia. Chest 1994;105:1462–6.
27. Jeong YJ, Kim KI, Seo IJ, et al. Eosinophilic lung diseases: a clinical, radiologic, and pathologic overview. Radiographics 2007;27:617–37.
28. Baggenstoss AH, Bayley EC, Lindberg DON. Loffler's syndrome. Report of a case with pathologic examination of lungs. Proc Mayo Clin 1946;21:457–65.
29. Shijubo N, Fujishima T, Morita S, et al. Idiopathic chronic eosinophilic pneumonia associated with noncaseating epithelioid granulomas. Eur Respir J 1995;8:327–30.
30. Yoshida K, Shijubo N, Koba H, et al. Chronic eosinophilic pneumonia progressing to lung fibrosis. Eur Respir J 1994;7:1541–4.

Acute eosinophilic pneumonia

31. Allen JN, Pacht ER, Gadek JE, et al. Acute eosinophilic pneumonia as a reversible cause of noninfectious respiratory failure. N Engl J Med 1989;321:569–74.
32. Badesch DB, King TE, Schwarz MI. Acute eosinophilic pneumonia: a hypersensitivity pneumonia? Am Rev Respir Dis 1989;139:249–52.
33. Alp H, Daum RS, Abrahams C, et al. Acute eosinophilic pneumonia: a cause of reversible, severe, noninfectious respiratory failure. J Pediatr 1998;132:540–3.
34. King MA, Pope-Harman AL, Allen JN, et al. Acute eosinophilic pneumonia: radiologic and clinical features. Radiology 1997;203:715–9.
35. Shintani H, Fujimura M, Yasui M, et al. Acute eosinophilic pneumonia caused by cigarette smoking. Intern Med 2000;39:66–8.
36. Al Saieg N, Moammar O, Kartan R. Flavored cigar smoking induces acute eosinophilic pneumonia. Chest 2007;131:1234–7.
37. Uchiyama H, Suda T, Nakamura Y, et al. Alterations in smoking habits are associated with acute eosinophilic pneumonia. Chest 2008;133:1174–80.
38. Tazelaar HD, Linz LJ, Colby TV, et al. Acute eosinophilic pneumonia: histopathologic findings in nine patients. Am J Respir Crit Care Med 1997;155:296–302.

Bronchocentric granulomatosis

39. Liebow AA. Pulmonary angiitis and granulomatosis. Am Rev Respir Dis 1973;108:1–18.
40. Katzenstein ALA, Liebow AA, Friedman PJ. Bronchocentric granulomatosis, mucoid impaction and hypersensitivity reaction to fungi. Am Rev Respir Dis 1975;111:497–537.

41. Koss MN, Robinson RG, Hochholzer L. Bronchocentric granulomatosis. Hum Pathol 1981;12:632–8.
42. Robinson RB, Wehunt WD, Tsou E, et al. Bronchocentric granulomatosis: roentgenographic manifestations. Am Rev Respir Dis 1982;125:751–6.
43. Hanson G, Flod N, Wells I, et al. Bronchocentric granulomatosis: a complication of allergic bronchopulmonary aspergillosis. J Allergy Clin Immunol 1977;59:83–90.
44. Bosken CH, Myers JL, Greenberger PA, et al. Pathologic features of allergic bronchopulmonary aspergillosis. Am J Surg Pathol 1988;12:216–22.
45. Sulavik SB. Bronchocentric granulomatosis and allergic bronchopulmonary aspergillosis. Clin Chest Med 1988;9:609–21.
46. Koss MN, Robinson RG, Hochholzer L. Bronchocentric granulomatosis. Hum Pathol 1981;12:632–8.
47. Saldana MJ. Bronchocentric granulomatosis: clinicopathologic observations in 17 patients. Lab Invest 1979;40:281–2.
48. Makker H, McConnochie K, Gibbs AR. Postirradiation pulmonary fibrosis complicated by aspergilloma and bronchocentric granulomatosis. Thorax 1989;44:676–7.
49. Den Hertog RW, Wagenaar SJSC, Westermann CJJ. Bronchocentric granulomatosis and pulmonary echinococcosis. Am Rev Respir Dis 1982;126:344–7.
50. Myers JL, Katzenstein ALA. Granulomatous infection mimicking bronchocentric granulomatosis. Am J Surg Pathol 1986;10:317–22.
51. Tazelaar HD, Baird AM, Mill M, et al. Bronchocentric mycosis occurring in transplant recipients. Chest 1989;96:92–5.
52. Maguire GP, Lee M, Rosen Y, et al. Pulmonary tuberculosis and bronchocentric granulomatosis. Chest 1986;89:606–8.
53. Berendsen HH, Hofstee N, Kapsenberg PD, et al. Bronchocentric granulomatosis associated with rheumatoid arthritis. Chest 1983;5:831–2.
54. Bonafede RP, Benatar SR. Bronchocentric granulomatosis and rheumatoid arthritis. Br J Dis Chest 1987;81:197–201.
55. Hellems SO, Kanner RE, Renzetti AD. Bronchocentric granulomatosis associated with rheumatoid arthritis. Chest 1983;5:831–2.
56. Rohatgi PK, Turrisi BC. Bronchocentric granulomatosis and ankylosing spondylitis. Thorax 1984;39:317–8.
57. Warren J, Pitchenik AE, Saldana MJ. Bronchocentric granulomatosis with glomerulonephritis. Chest 1985;125:751–6.
58. Martinez-Lopez MA, Pena JM, Quiralte J, et al. Bronchocentric granulomatosis associated with pure red cell aplasia and lymphadenopathy. Thorax 1992;47:131–3.
59. Clee MD, Lamb D, Clark RA. Bronchocentric granulomatosis: a review and thoughts on pathogenesis. Br J Dis Chest 1983;77:227–34.
60. Houser SL, Mark EJ. Bronchocentric granulomatosis with mucus impaction due to bronchogenic carcinoma – An association with clinical relevance. Arch Pathol Lab Med 2000;124:1168–71.
61. Yousem SA. Bronchocentric injury in Wegener's granulomatosis – a report of five cases. Hum Pathol 1991;22:535–40.

Allergic angiitis and granulomatosis (Churg–Strauss syndrome)

62. Churg J, Strauss L. Allergic granulomatosis, allergic angiitis and periarteritis nodosa. Am J Pathol 1951;27:277–301.
63. Chumbley LC, Harrison EG, DeRemee RA. Allergic granulomatosis and angiitis (Churg–Strauss syndrome). Mayo Clin Proc 1977;52:477–84.
64. Koss MN, Antonovych T, Hochholzer L. Allergic granulomatosis (Churg–Strauss syndrome): pulmonary and renal morphological findings. Am J Surg Pathol 1981;5:21–8.
65. Lanham JC, Elkon KB, Pusey CD, et al. Systemic vasculitis with asthma and eosinophilia; a clinical approach to the Churg–Strauss syndrome. Medicine (Baltimore) 1984;63:65–81.
66. Stephens M, Reynolds S, Gibbs AR, et al. Allergic bronchopulmonary aspergillosis progressing to allergic granulomatosis and angiitis (Churg–Strauss syndrome). Am Rev Respir Dis 1988;137:1226–8.
67. Matsumoto H, Niimi A, Suzuki K, et al. Allergic granulomatous angiitis (Churg–Strauss syndrome) associated with allergic bronchopulmonary candidiasis. Respiration 2000;67:577–9.
68. Sasaki A, Hasegawa M, Nakazato Y, et al. Allergic granulomatosis and angiitis (Churg–Strauss syndrome). Report of an autopsy case in a nonasthmatic patient. Acta Pathol Jpn 1988;38:781–8.
69. Jessurun J, Azevedo M, Saldana M. Allergic angiitis and granulomatosis (Churg–Strauss syndrome): report of a case with massive thymic involvement in a non-asthmatic patient. Hum Pathol 1986;17:637–9.
70. Al-Ammar AY, Yasin SS, Al-Muhsen SZ, et al. A laryngeal presentation of Churg-Strauss syndrome in childhood. Ann Saudi Med 2009;29:142–5.
71. Gaskin G, Ryan JJ, Rees AJ, et al. Anti-myeloperoxidase antibodies in vasculitis: relationship to ANCA and clinical diagnosis. APMIS 1990;98:33.
72. Tervaert JWC, Elema JD, Kallenberg CGM. Clinical and histopathological association of 29kD-ANCA and MPO-ANCA. APMIS 1990;98:35.
73. Wechsler ME, Finn D, Gunawardena D, et al. Churg-Strauss syndrome in patients receiving montelukast as treatment for asthma. Chest 2000;117:708–13.
74. Solans R, Bosch JA, Selva A, et al. Montelukast and Churg–Strauss syndrome. Thorax 2002;57:183–5.
75. LeGall C, Pham S, Vignes S, et al. Inhaled corticosteroids and Churg–Strauss syndrome: a report of five cases. Eur Resp J 2000 MAY;15(5):978-981 2000;15:978–81.
76. Masi AT, Hunder GG, Lie JT, et al. The American College of Rheumatology 1990 criteria for the classification of Churg–Strauss syndrome (allergic granulomatosis and angiitis). Arthritis Rheum 1990;33:1094–100.
77. Lichtig C, Ludatscher R, Eisenberg E, et al. Small blood vessel disease in allergic granulomatous angiitis (Churg–Strauss syndrome). J Clin Pathol 1989;42:1001–2.
78. Clausen KP, Bronstein H. Granulomatous pulmonary arteritis. A hypereosinophilic syndrome. Am J Clin Pathol 1974;62:82–7.
79. Clutterbuck EJ, Pusey CD. Severe alveolar haemorrhage in Churg-Strauss syndrome. Eur J Respir Dis 1987;71:158–63.
80. Rose GA, Spencer H. Polyarteritis nodosa. Q J Med 1957;26:43–81.
81. Dreisen RB. Pulmonary vasculitis. Clin Chest Med 1982;3:607–18.
82. Katzenstein ALA. Diagnostic features and differential diagnosis of Churg–Strauss syndrome in the lung – A review. Am J Clin Pathol 2000;114:767–72.
83. Yousem SA, Lombard CM. The eosinophilic variant of Wegener's granulomatosis. Hum Pathol 1988;19:682–8.
84. Lipworth BJ, Slater DN, Corrin B, et al. Allergic granulomatosis without asthma: a rare 'forme fruste' of the Churg-Strauss syndrome. Respir Med 1989;83:249–50.

Hypereosinophilic syndrome

85. Hardy WR, Anderson RE. The hypereosinophilic syndrome. Ann Intern Med 1968;68:1220–9.
86. Schwartz RS. The hypereosinophilic syndrome and the biology of cancer. N Engl J Med 2003;348:1199–200.
87. Chusid MJ, Dale DC, West BC, et al. The hypereosinophilic syndrome: analysis of fourteen cases with review of the literature. Medicine 1975;54:1–27.
88. Spry CJE, Davies J, Tai PC, et al. Clinical features of fifteen patients with the hypereosinophilic syndrome. Q J Med 1983;205:1–22.
89. Weller PF, Bubley GJ. The idiopathic hypereosinophilic syndrome. Blood 1994;83:2759–79.
90. Cools J, DeAngelo DJ, Gotlib J, et al. A tyrosine kinase created by fusion of the PDGFRA and FIP1L1 genes as a therapeutic target of imatinib in idiopathic hypereosinophilic syndrome. N Engl J Med 2003;348:1201–14.
91. Bain BJ. Relationship between idiopathic hypereosinophilic syndrome, eosinophilic

leukemia, and systemic mastocytosis. Am J Hematol 2004;77:82–5.

92. Cogan E, Schandené L, Crusiaux A, et al. Brief report: clonal proliferation of type 2 helper T-cells in a man with the hypereosinophilic syndrome. N Engl J Med 1994;330:535–8.

93. Winn RE, Kollef MH, Meyer JI. Pulmonary involvement in the hypereosinophilic syndrome. Chest 1994;105:656–60.

94. Kang EY, Shim JJ, Kim JS, et al. Pulmonary involvement of idiopathic hypereosinophilic syndrome: CT findings in five patients. J Comput Assist Tomogr 1997;21: 612–5.

Chapter |10|

Pulmonary manifestations of systemic disease

©2010 Elsevier Ltd
DOI: 10.1016/B978-0-7020-3369-8.00010-0

Some systemic diseases particularly affect the lungs but are dealt with exclusively in other chapters: examples of these include sarcoidosis (p. 283), vasculitis and granulomatosis (p. 437) and Langerhans cell histiocytosis (p. 288). Other diseases often affect the lungs in isolation and are described in full elsewhere but as they also form part of systemic illnesses they also have to be referred to here: examples of these include interstitial pneumonia, which is associated with many of the systemic connective tissue disorders. Drug reactions are usually systemic, but are dealt with separately on pages 383–391.

CONNECTIVE TISSUE DISEASES

The connective tissue diseases form a heterogeneous group of immunologically mediated disorders that share certain characteristics, notably inflammation of synovial and serosal membranes, connective tissue and blood vessels in various tissues. The lung is often involved in this group of diseases, probably because of its abundant connective tissue and vasculature. Pulmonary associations of connective tissue diseases include abnormalities of airways, alveoli, pulmonary blood vessels, pleura and chest wall, any of which may precede, accompany or follow the onset of the systemic disease (Table 10.1). Many of the pulmonary associations of connective tissue diseases also occur in isolation, although often accompanied by serological markers. A prime example is interstitial pulmonary fibrosis but it is notable that, in contrast to the idiopathic form of the disease, the histological pattern is more often that of non-specific interstitial pneumonia (NSIP) than usual interstitial pneumonia (UIP).[1-5] Also, its progression is often slower and its prognosis correspondingly better.[6-8] The few patients with connective tissue diseases who show a UIP pattern have fewer fibroblastic foci and a correspondingly better prognosis than patients with idiopathic interstitial pneumonia and UIP.[9,10]

Table 10.1 Respiratory associations of acquired connective tissue disorders

	Airways	Alveoli	Pulmonary vessels	Pleura	Diaphragm and chest wall
Rheumatoid arthritis (see also Box 10.1)	Bronchitis Bronchiectasis Follicular bronchiolitis Constrictive bronchiolitis	Pneumonia Interstitial pneumonia (NSIP or, rarely, UIP or LIP) Rheumatoid nodules	Hypertension Vasculitis	Pleurisy Empyema	
Systemic lupus erythematosus		Interstitial pneumonia (DAD or rarely NSIP, UIP or OP)	Hypertension Thrombosis Vasculitis Haemorrhage	Pleurisy	'Shrinking lungs' with high diaphragms
Systemic sclerosis		Interstitial pneumonia (NSIP or rarely UIP, OP, DAD or LIP) Aspiration pneumonia	Haemorrhage		'Hidebound' chest
Sjögren's syndrome	'Sicca' features	Interstitial pneumonia (NSIP or LIP, rarely UIP, OP or DAD) Lymphoma		Pleurisy	
Dermatomyositis and polymyositis		Aspiration pneumonia Interstitial pneumonia (NSIP or OP, rarely UIP, DAD)			Myositis
Ankylosing spondylitis		Upper-lobe fibrosis			Costovertebral restriction
Behçet's syndrome	Stenosis Ulceration		Arteritis Aneurysms		
Relapsing polychondritis	Stenosis				
Rheumatic fever		DAD	Vasculitis		Pleurisy Diaphragmatic paralysis

NSIP, non-specific interstitial pneumonia; UIP, usual interstitial pneumonia; LIP, lymphoid interstitial pneumonia; OP, organising pneumonia; DAD, diffuse alveolar damage.

The histological features of connective tissue diseases need to be separated from the effects of therapy, including drug reactions and opportunistic infections, as well as any coexistent disease processes not directly associated with the connective tissue disease. This may be difficult as, in most cases, the histological patterns found in the lung are rarely specific for a particular connective tissue disease. Detailed clinicopathological correlation is therefore essential.[7]

A further association of lung disease and various connective tissue disorders is seen with the pneumoconioses, particularly silicosis. There is a well-recognised association between silicosis and disorders such as systemic sclerosis and rheumatoid disease.[11–13] It is doubtful whether the relationship is causal but the one seems to aggravate the other and may lead to its earlier development. For example, the presence of dust results in rheumatoid lesions in the lungs being particularly florid (see pp. 335 and 341 [Caplan's syndrome]).

Rheumatoid disease

It was the association of pulmonary fibrosis with rheumatoid arthritis that first drew attention to the fact that this disease is not confined to the joints, and led to the use of the term 'rheumatoid disease' (rather than arthritis) to indicate the generalised nature of the disorder.[14] It is now recognised that rheumatoid disease has many pleuro-pulmonary manifestations (see Table 10.1 and Box 10.1), some of which are dealt with in the appropriate chapters.

Although rheumatoid disease is commoner in women, pulmonary complications are more frequent in men, possibly reflecting the prevalence of smoking, which may increase pulmonary vascular permeability and aggravate the inflammatory process in the lung. As with many connective tissue disorders, the pulmonary manifestations of rheumatoid disease may precede other clinical or serological evidence of the disease, although in most cases there are other features, such as arthritis, subcutaneous nodules, digital vasculitis and positive serology.

Pleurisy[15–18]

Pleural effusion is the commonest respiratory manifestation of rheumatoid disease. The effusion is often small and asymptomatic but it may be large and bilateral and cause pleuritic pain, fever and breathlessness. It is an exudate rather than a transudate (see p. 709). Most rheumatoid pleural effusions resolve spontaneously. Biopsy usually shows non-specific chronic inflammation of the pleura but multiple rheumatoid nodules or a linear granulomatous process showing prominent palisading of histiocytes may replace the mesothelium, in which case epithelioid histiocytes recognisable in the pleural aspirate may permit a cytological diagnosis (see Fig. 13.7, p. 714).[15,19]

Empyema

Patients with rheumatoid disease are prone to infections[20] and occasionally a pleural effusion in a rheumatoid patient is found to be purulent. Occasionally there is pyopneumothorax,[21,22] probably due to rupture into the pleural cavity of a pleural or subpleural rheumatoid nodule.

Rheumatoid nodules

Nodules identical to those found in the subcutis of patients with rheumatoid disease occasionally develop in the substance of the lung or the trachea.[23–26] They may be the only manifestation of rheumatoid disease, developing before there is any arthritis or seroconversion.[23] Thus, they may herald generalised disease. As they may develop in any part of the body, the occasional involvement of the major airways should occasion no surprise.[25]

Box 10.1 Respiratory abnormalities in rheumatoid disease

Cricoarytenoid arthritis
Pleurisy
Empyema
Necrobiotic nodules
Non-specific interstitial pneumonia
Usual interstitial pneumonia
Organising pneumonia
Lymphocytic interstitial pneumonia
Diffuse alveolar damage
Apical fibrosis
Bronchitis
Bronchiectasis
Bronchocentric granulomatosis
Follicular bronchiolitis
Constrictive bronchiolitis
Diffuse panbronchiolitis
Pulmonary hypertension
Pulmonary vasculitis
Pulmonary drug toxicity
Carcinoma of the lung
Lymphoma of the lung
Pulmonary involvement in systemic amyloidosis

The nodules in the lungs may be recurrent or appear first in one lung and then the other. They may be solitary or multiple and may enlarge, remain static or shrink to an insignificant scar. Resolution is usually by absorption but occasionally a nodule cavitates and discharges its necrotic contents through an airway. Erosion of both an airway and the pleura establishes a bronchopleural fistula, and perhaps pyopneumothorax.[21,22] Direct involvement of the pleura by rheumatoid nodules is considered on page 714.

Patients with rheumatoid nodules may present with haemoptysis, or chest pain if there is pleural involvement, or they may have no symptoms. The radiographic findings may be suspected of representing malignant disease. Rheumatoid nodules have a tendency to develop in the subpleural regions of the upper and mid zones.[24] They are round and typically measure up to 3 cm across but larger nodules are sometimes found, particularly when synergistic factors such as mine dust are also present (see Caplan's syndrome, p. 341).[27] As elsewhere, the nodules have a necrotic centre of finely granular eosinophilic debris surrounded by a capsule of chronic inflammatory granulation tissue (Fig. 10.1A). The boundary between dead and viable tissue is marked by a characteristic palisade of radially oriented macrophages (Fig. 10.1B). The inflammatory cells include a small number of giant cells as well as plentiful lymphocytes and plasma cells. Fungal colonisation is a rare complication of rheumatoid nodules.[28]

The differential diagnosis is principally from infection and Wegener's granulomatosis (see Table 8.3.3, p. 443). The satellite granulomas seen in tuberculosis are not a feature of rheumatoid nodules, and special stains for mycobacteria and fungi give negative results. However, staining for these organisms should always be undertaken if there is any doubt about the diagnosis. Less common infective granulomas that enter the differential diagnosis include syphilis and dirofilariasis, the former requiring serological investigation and the latter step sections to identify fragments of the worm (see pp. 216 and 258 respectively). In Wegener's granulomatosis there is also vasculitis whereas blood vessels near rheumatoid nodules show intimal fibrosis and a cuff of lymphocytes, but not a true vasculitis.

Figure 10.1 A pulmonary rheumatoid nodule. (A) The nodule consists of a necrotic centre surrounded by a thick fibrous capsule and an intervening inflammatory zone. (B) As in the subcutaneous nodules of rheumatoid disease, a palisade of radially oriented macrophages borders the central necrosis.

Interstitial pneumonia

Clinically overt pulmonary parenchymal disease in the form of interstitial pneumonia is reported in approximately 5% of patients with rheumatoid arthritis but the figure rises to 19% when patients without respiratory symptoms are studied by high-resolution computed tomography (HRCT).[29] All seven patterns of interstitial pneumonia described in the consensus classification (see p. 264) have been described, with UIP, NSIP and organising pneumonia being especially frequent, and often seen in association with follicular bronchiolitis.[5,8,10,30–34] The available data on prognosis are contradictory: some groups have reported that the prognosis of these patterns in rheumatoid disease corresponds to that seen in their idiopathic counterparts while others claim that it is better when they are associated with connective tissue disease.[8–10,31,34]

Apical fibrosis

Occasional patients with rheumatoid disease develop cavitating upper-lobe fibrosis similar to that described in ankylosing spondylitis (see below).[35–37]

Bronchial disease

Bronchitis and bronchiectasis are commoner in patients with rheumatoid arthritis than in matched controls[38,39] and occasional rheumatoid patients develop bronchocentric granulomatosis.[40] High resolution computed tomography (HRCT) has permitted the recognition of airway disease in a high proportion of patients with rheumatoid arthritis.[41]

Follicular bronchiolitis

Rheumatoid disease is characterised by widespread lymphoid hyperplasia. This is best seen in lymph nodes but the bronchopulmonary lymphoid tissue is also involved in this process, resulting in the development of lymphoid follicles alongside the bronchioles, a process termed follicular bronchiolitis (Fig. 10.2).[42,43] Patients complain of breathlessness with cough, fever or recurrent pneumonia. They have bilateral reticulonodular radiographic opacities and lung function tests show an obstructive, restrictive or combined defect. When follicular bronchiolitis accompanies an interstitial pneumonia it suggests that the latter is part of a systemic connective tissue disorder.[10]

Figure 10.2 Follicular bronchiolitis as a manifestation of rheumatoid disease. Several lymphoid follicles are seen, particularly bordering the central bronchiole.

Figure 10.3 Constrictive obliterative bronchiolitis in a patient with rheumatoid disease. The mucosa of the bronchiole seen to the left is thickened by granulation tissue so that the airway lumen is reduced to a pinpoint.

Constrictive bronchiolitis obliterans

Rare patients with rheumatoid disease and other connective tissue disorders develop a bronchiolar disorder that is of considerably greater clinical consequence than follicular bronchiolitis, one that is characterised by a severe ventilatory disturbance that often proves fatal. This is the constrictive form of obliterative bronchiolitis (Fig. 10.3).[44–46] The primary lesion appears to involve continuing auto-immune damage to the respiratory epithelium. This is replaced by granulation tissue, which is laid down in a circumferential pattern and gradually narrows and finally obliterates the airway lumen. It has been suggested that the process is a consequence of penicillamine[47,48] or gold[49] antirheumatoid therapy rather than a direct result of the connective tissue disease but as rheumatoid patients who have not received these drugs have also developed constrictive obliterative bronchiolitis this appears unlikely. Furthermore, constrictive obliterative bronchiolitis has not been reported in patients treated with peni-cillamine for disorders such as Wilson's disease and primary biliary cirrhosis. Alternatively, it has been suggested that the bronchiolitis

may have an infective basis. However, the obliterative process has the constrictive pattern seen when there is constant attrition of the respiratory epithelium rather than the proliferative intraluminal form of the disease seen after brief viral or chemical injury (see p. 121). It is notable that a case of obliterative bronchiolitis attributed to the domestic inhalation of a common cleansing agent concerned a patient with rheumatoid disease and that the airway obliteration was of the constrictive variety,[50] suggesting that the process was the result of continuing injury rather than an isolated episode of fume inhalation.

Diffuse panbronchiolitis

This disease, which is described on page 124, is also recorded in association with rheumatoid arthritis.[51,52]

Pulmonary hypertension

Pulmonary hypertension is occasionally reported in rheumatoid disease. The vascular changes are described as showing advanced fibroelastic intimal proliferation that obliterates the lumen of small arteries, either in isolation[53,54] or in combination with pulmonary arteritis.[55] The dilatation lesions of plexogenic arteriopathy are not observed.[53–55]

Pulmonary vasculitis

Digital vasculitis is a common manifestation of rheumatoid disease and identical changes are occasionally encountered in the pulmonary vasculature (see Fig. 8.3.17, p. 446).[55–57] It is likely that this represents a true vasculitis, probably of an immune nature, rather than the necrotising arteritis of plexogenic arteriopathy, although this is disputed.[55]

Pulmonary drug toxicity

Adverse pulmonary effects may be caused by drugs used in the treatment of rheumatoid disease. For example, aspirin and other non-steroidal anti-inflammatory drugs may cause asthma and eosinophilic pneumonia while gold and penicillamine may exert a cytotoxic effect resulting in diffuse alveolar damage and pulmonary fibrosis. Similarly, methotrexate may result in varying patterns of interstitial pneumonia.[58]

Pulmonary eosinophilia

As well as representing a reaction to the drugs used to treat rheumatoid disease, eosinophilic pneumonia may be a manifestation of the rheumatoid process itself.[59]

Pulmonary malignancy

Both carcinoma and lymphoma occasionally arise at the edge of a rheumatoid nodule.[60–62]

Rheumatic fever

Rheumatic fever is now rare in developed countries but remains common in many parts of the world. It involves serosal surfaces and often results in pleurisy, which is generally manifest as a sterile exudative effusion. Less commonly, there is a fibrinous alveolar exudate, organisation of which results in Masson bodies, hyaline membrane formation, chronic interstitial pneumonia or a focal necro-tising process involving alveoli and pulmonary blood vessels.[63–66]

Figure 10.4 Pulmonary fibrosis as a manifestation of systemic sclerosis. (A) The fibrosis is seen as a subpleural band of pallor, chiefly affecting the base and posterior of the lung. (B) Microscopy shows non-specific interstitial pneumonia. (C) Malignant change may complicate the fibrosis. Here there is both non-specific interstitial pneumonia and adenocarcinoma.

Systemic sclerosis

Systemic sclerosis (also known as scleroderma) is a multisystem disease that is subclassified according to the degree of skin involvement as diffuse or limited cutaneous. The former is associated with a greater degree of visceral disease and carries a worse prognosis. The limited cutaneous form is more often associated with the CREST syndrome (calcinosis cutis, Raynaud's phenomenon, oesophageal dysfunction, sclerodactyly and telangiectasia) and has a better prognosis, although it is the form that is more often associated with pulmonary hypertension.[67] Parenchymal pulmonary involvement in systemic sclerosis may take the form of interstitial pneumonia[3,7,68] or diffuse alveolar haemorrhage,[69,70] whilst oesophageal involvement may result in aspiration pneumonia and centriacinar fibrosis.[71] Constrictive bronchiolitis is also reported[72,73] and there is an increased risk of lung cancer, particularly adenocarcinoma, which is often of lepidic (bronchioloalveolar) pattern.[74,75]

Interstitial pneumonia

Interstitial pneumonia is the commonest pulmonary manifestation of systemic sclerosis (Fig. 10.4), the prevalence at autopsy being approximately 70%.[76,77] However, many of these cases have subclinical involvement[78] and the prognosis is better than in idiopathic interstitial pneumonia.[7,79–81] NSIP is the commonest pattern, accounting for 55–77% of cases.[2–4,8,82] The second commonest pattern is UIP but the adverse prognosis associated with this pattern in idiopathic disease is not so marked.[3,4,10,82] This may be related to differences in neutrophil numbers and degranulation in the lung.[83] Other histological patterns seen in systemic sclerosis include desquamative interstitial pneumonia and respiratory bronchiolitis although, it is likely that these patterns are related to smoking more than systemic sclerosis.[72,84] Organising pneumonia has been reported in occasional patients,[85] as has diffuse alveolar damage.[33,70,86] Sarcoid granulomas have also been noted but whether they relate to systemic sclerosis or are incidental is unknown.[3,87]

Pulmonary hypertension

In some patients with systemic sclerosis the lung parenchyma is unremarkable but there are marked vascular changes. These patients have severe pulmonary hypertension and are mainly those with the CREST variant of systemic sclerosis (see above).[67] Pathologically there is generally myxoid thickening of the wall of small pulmonary arteries, usually involving intimal fibroblasts arranged circumferentially in an 'onion skin' pattern (see Fig. 8.2.21, p. 431); the appearances are similar to those described in the kidney in systemic sclerosis.[88,89] There is also adventitial fibrosis[90] but plexiform lesions are not seen.[88,91] In other patients with the CREST variant of systemic sclerosis pulmonary hypertension is caused by veno-occlusive disease.[91–93]

Pulmonary hypertension is also recorded in the POEMS syndrome,[94,95] a rare variant of plasma cell dyscrasia with multisystem features. The name POEMS is an acronym for its principal features, polyneuropathy, organomegaly, endocrinopathy, M protein and skin changes that resemble scleroderma. It is noteworthy that in the POEMS syndrome there is overproduction of the endothelial cell-specific mitogen and potent angiogenic peptide vascular endothelial growth factor,[95] which has also been reported in the plexiform lesions of other patients with pulmonary hypertension.[96] Other pulmonary manifestations of the POEMS syndrome include restrictive lung disease, respiratory muscle weakness, diminished diffusing capacity and pleural effusions.[97]

Systemic lupus erythematosus

Systemic lupus erythematosus (SLE) is a chronic multisystem disorder associated with antinuclear autoantibodies and immune complex deposition. Women of child-bearing age are most commonly affected, the female-to-male ratio being approximately eight. Particularly common manifestations include arthropathy, skin lesions, renal disease and serositis. There are also several pleuropulmonary manifestations,[98] in addition to which reactions to drugs such as methotrexate and cyclophosphamide used to treat SLE may affect the lungs. Respiratory disease is commoner in SLE than in any other connective tissue disease but the prognosis is more dependent upon renal than pleuropulmonary involvement.

Pleural disease

Pleuritis, seen either as a dry fibrinous exudate or an exudative effusion, is the commonest respiratory manifestation of SLE. The effusion contains neutrophils, lymphocytes, lupus erythematosus cells and antinuclear factor in high titre, and shows positive nuclear immunofluorescence.

Parenchymal disease

Although parenchymal disease is less common than pleural involvement, it is more serious. Acute lupus pneumonitis is characterised by diffuse alveolar damage or, less commonly, by pulmonary haemorrhage or cryptogenic organising pneumonia.[99–102] Infection, which is common because of the use of immunosuppressive drugs, needs to be excluded in such acute cases.[103] In survivors, healing may be by resolution but more commonly leaves the lungs permanently scarred. Chronic pulmonary injury is rarer in SLE than in rheumatoid disease and systemic sclerosis[104] but both UIP and NSIP have been reported,[99] and, more rarely, organising pneumonia,[101,102] amyloidosis[106] and lymphoid interstitial pneumonia (LIP).[107] Renal involvement may lead to uraemic pulmonary oedema. Some patients with SLE are severely breathless and radiologically appear to have small lungs; the term 'shrinking lungs' is often applied to these cases but this is misleading as the fault lies in the respiratory muscles, which show myopathic changes, rather than in the lungs.[108] Dyspnoea has been attributed to the tight skin about the chest but the cutaneous changes rarely affect respiratory function.

Pulmonary vascular disease

Pulmonary vascular disease in SLE may be secondary to systemic venous thrombosis (pulmonary thromboembolism), or widespread thrombosis may affect the pulmonary as well as the systemic circulation while diffuse alveolar haemorrhage and haemosiderosis are well-recognised complications of SLE.[100,109–113] Pulmonary thrombosis, infarction and haemorrhage have been linked to the presence of circulating phospholipid antibody (also known as cardiolipin or lupus anticoagulant) in the antiphospholipid syndrome (see p. 489).[114] Thrombosis may underlie the pulmonary hypertension that has been reported in association with SLE,[114–119] or the pathogenesis of the hypertension may involve vasospasm, which is suggested by the frequent association of Raynaud's phenomenon with pulmonary hypertension in SLE.[115] As in systemic sclerosis, the dilatation lesions of plexogenic arteriopathy are seldom observed.[116,117,119] Pulmonary veno-occlusive disease, probably due to organisation of widespread venular thrombosis, has also been described in SLE.[120]

Other patients with SLE have pulmonary vasculitis or capillaritis with evidence of immune complex deposition.[99,121–125] The capillaritis may be complicated by diffuse alveolar haemorrhage[109–112] or haemosiderosis.[113] Tubuloreticular endothelial cell inclusions, once thought to be specific for SLE but later identified in AIDS and other conditions, are probably non-specific indicators of cell damage, possibly mediated by interferon.[126]

Malignant change

Rare examples of pulmonary lymphoma are recorded in SLE.[127,128]

Polymyositis and dermatomyositis

These inflammatory disorders of skin and skeletal muscle affect women more frequently than men and have a peak onset in the sixth decade. The most common pleuropulmonary complication of these diseases is aspiration pneumonia due to a depressed cough reflex and weakness of pharyngeal and intercostal muscles and the diaphragm, which may result in ventilatory failure.[129]

Interstitial pneumonia

Patients with myositis may develop interstitial pneumonia, the incidence of this complication being less than 10% in patients with polymyositis[130] but in the region of 41–67% in dermatomyositis.[129,131,132] Patients with polymyositis and antibodies against histidyl-tRNA synthetase (Jo-1) also have a high incidence of interstitial lung disease.[133–136] The commonest histological pattern is NSIP (see p. 276), which is often mixed with a component of organising pneumonia.[1,134,137,138] Other patterns of interstitial lung disease that have been associated with myositis include DAD, UIP and, rarely, alveolar proteinosis.[137,137a]

Pulmonary vascular disease

Pulmonary vasculitis has also been reported in patients with polymyositis and the anti-Jo-1 syndrome.[134,136,139] Antibodies against endothelial cells may underlie the capillaritis and resultant pulmonary haemorrhage that have been described in a few patients with dermatomyositis.[139,140]

Pulmonary malignancy

Dermatomyositis is often a complication of malignant disease and so may be secondary to bronchopulmonary carcinoma. Pulmonary lymphoma has also been described in association with dermatomyositis.[141]

Mixed connective tissue disease

Mixed connective tissue disease is characterised by overlapping features of other connective tissue disorders, notably SLE, systemic sclerosis and polymyositis, in association with high titres of an antinuclear antibody that gives a speckled pattern of immunofluorescence.[142] The frequency of pulmonary involvement has ranged from 25 to 85%, the commonest form being interstitial pneumonia, followed by pleuritis, pulmonary hypertension, vasculitis and diffuse alveolar damage.[33,143–147] Pulmonary hypertension is especially seen when features of systemic sclerosis are prominent but the pathological features are those of plexogenic arteriopathy rather than the myxoid intimal thickening seen in systemic sclerosis.[148]

Ankylosing spondylitis

Ankylosing spondylitis typically affects the spine of young men with an HLA-B27 haplotype. Pulmonary associations include apical fibrosis. This develops in 1–2% of patients with ankylosing spondylitis, typically many years after the onset of the joint disease.[149,150] Whereas the spinal lesions typically appear early in adult life, it is not until the fifth decade or so that pulmonary disease develops, often being discovered incidentally on chest radiographs. Initially, the changes may be unilateral but they have often become bilateral if cough or dyspnoea first draws attention to pulmonary involvement. As the disease progresses, cystic changes develop and the appearances resemble those of tuberculosis, but mycobacteria do not appear to play a causal role. However, like all cavities in the lungs, those of ankylosing spondylitis are liable to secondary saprophytic infection by *Aspergillus* species or colonisation by opportunistic mycobacteria.[151]

At necropsy, there is bilateral apical fibrosis (Fig. 10.5), which may be associated with bronchiectasis and bulla formation. Secondary infection may be found but generally microscopy shows only fibrosis and lymphocytic infiltration. The process is not granulomatous and the aetiology is unknown. The changes cannot be attributed to the irradiation that was formerly used to treat ankylosing spondylitis as this was confined to the spine and the pulmonary changes may develop without such therapy. Occasionally, identical changes are found in association with rheumatoid disease[35] or with psoriatic spondylitis.[152]

Sicca syndrome and Sjögren's syndrome

Bronchial disease

The sicca syndrome of dry eyes and dry mouth, due respectively to keratoconjunctivitis sicca and xerostomia, may be combined with one of the connective tissue disorders, usually rheumatoid disease, to form Sjögren's syndrome. The dryness of the eyes and mouth is due to inflammatory destruction of the lacrimal and salivary glands. The same process may extend into the lower respiratory tract to destroy the tracheobronchial glands and lead to dryness of the trachea and bronchi.[153–156] Airway clearance is impaired and bronchitis, bronchiectasis, bronchiolitis and pneumonia may develop. The

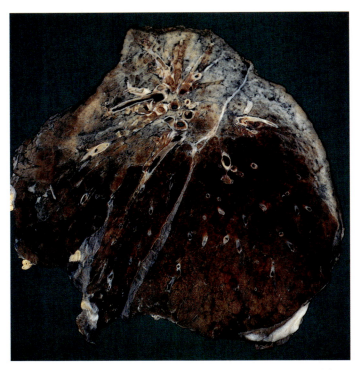

Figure 10.5 Gross apical fibrosis in a patient with ankylosing spondylitis.

destruction of the glands is of unknown cause. In both sicca and the full Sjögren's syndrome, the glands show a heavy lymphoid infiltrate with destruction of the secretory acini (Fig. 10.6).[157] Further extensions of the sicca syndrome are encapsulated in the term TASS syndrome (thyroiditis, Addison's disease, Sjögren's and sarcoidosis).[158] The association with rheumatoid disease, thyroiditis and Addison's disease suggests an autoimmune aetiology. The immunoparesis associated with human immunodeficiency virus infection is also reported in the sicca syndrome.[159]

Parenchymal disease

Parenchymal disease occurs in both primary and secondary Sjögren's disease but is more common in the latter, where it often reflects the pulmonary manifestations of the associated connective tissue disease. Parenchymal disease includes amyloidosis and the formation of bullae (Fig. 10.7).[160–164] Interstitial pneumonia of NSIP pattern is the commonest manifestation of primary Sjögren's disease.[165] Pulmonary hypertension, LIP, UIP and organising pneumonia are also reported.[165–172]

Pulmonary lymphoma

Primary pulmonary lymphoma has been reported in Sjögren's syndrome, usually marginal zone non-Hodgkin's lymphomas of the mucosa-associated lymphoid tissue.[173–175]

Relapsing polychondritis

Relapsing polychondritis is a rare systemic disorder affecting connective tissues with a high content of glycosaminoglycans, notably cartilage, the aorta, the sclera and cornea.[176–180] It is associated with rheumatoid arthritis in about 20% of cases. Autoantibodies to cartilage and type III collagen are sometimes found[181] and there

Figure 10.6 Sjögren's syndrome. The bronchial glands show an intense lymphoid infiltrate.

may be vasculitis, glomerulonephritis, rheumatoid disease, Sjögren's syndrome, SLE or other autoimmune disease.[180,182,183]

Constitutional symptoms are common while involvement of the pinnae and nasal cartilage leads to crumpled ears and a saddle-nose deformity.[178,179] Involvement of the lower respiratory tract is uncommon, especially in isolation, but may result in life-threatening tracheobronchial narrowing (see p. 95).[184–186]

Histologically, there is erosion of the edges of the affected cartilages by a dense lymphocytic, plasma cell and giant cell infiltrate (see Fig. 3.4, p. 95). Immunoglobulins and complement components have been demonstrated at the chondrofibrous junction.[187] Resolution of the inflammation, which may be spontaneous, may leave a deformed cartilage showing fibrosis and metachromasia of its ground substance.[186]

Behçet's syndrome and Hughes–Stovin syndrome

Behçet's syndrome combines recurrent orogenital ulceration with a variety of systemic disorders. A family history is sometimes obtained and the disease is associated with HLA-B51, suggesting that it has a genetic basis. Pulmonary involvement occurs in up to 8% of cases, most commonly as multiple pulmonary artery aneurysms due to a necrotising arteritis (see Fig. 8.3.19, p. 447).[188] Arteries of any size may be affected. Leakage or rupture of the aneurysms causes pulmonary haemorrhage, which may be fatal. Alternatively, the arteritis may

Figure 10.7 Sjögren's syndrome. (A) The lung shows amyloidosis, lymphoid hyperplasia and air space destruction. (B) High-resolution computed tomography scan showing cystic destruction and peripheral nodules, the latter probably reflecting the focal amyloid deposition.

result in widespread pulmonary thrombosis.[189] Other respiratory manifestations include pulmonary embolism, pleurisy, pulmonary fibrosis, bronchial ulceration and stenosis, and chyloptysis.[188,190–197] The Hughes–Stovin syndrome of haemoptysis due to pulmonary artery aneurysms probably represents a limited form of Behçet's syndrome.[198–200]

Figure 10.8 Ehlers–Danlos syndrome. (A) Fibrous scars, shown red in this van Gieson stain, are probably the result of spontaneous tearing of the lung. (B) Fibrous pseudotumours may represent a development of the same process.

Cutis laxa

Cutis laxa is a rare hereditary disease of connective tissue in which the skin lacks its normal elasticity and hangs in folds like the dewlaps of a bloodhound. It may be associated with dissection of the aorta and pulmonary emphysema.[201]

Ehlers–Danlos syndrome

Ehlers–Danlos syndrome is another hereditary defect of connective tissue, one caused by mutation of the gene that encodes the chains of type III procollagen. There are 10 recognised subtypes, with corresponding clinical heterogeneity. The syndrome is generally characterised by soft, hyperextensible skin and hyperextensibility of the joints. Visceral abnormalities include fragility of blood vessels with consequent haemorrhage, hernias, visceral rupture, mitral valve prolapse and premature rupture of the membranes in pregnancy. Respiratory complications include tracheobronchomegaly, pulmonary laceration with subsequent haemorrhage, cystic change, fibrous pseudotumours that frequently show osseous metaplasia (Fig. 10.8), pneumothoraces and haemothorax.[202–205] Occasionally some of these respiratory features are seen in isolation. Ehlers–Danlos syndrome

and cutis laxa have both been associated with Mounier–Kuhn's and Klippel–Trenaunay syndromes (see pp. 163 and 482).

Pseudoxanthoma elasticum

Pseudoxanthoma elasticum is a further generalised connective tissue disorder that has its principal manifestations in the skin but may involve the lung. As in other tissues the pulmonary elastic tissue is damaged and the site of dystrophic calcification.[206]

Marfan's syndrome

Marfan's syndrome is a further hereditary disorder of connective tissue. It is an autosomal disorder caused by mutation of the gene encoding fibrillin-1, which is a major component of the microfibrillar part of elastin.[207] Dysregulation of transforming growth factor-β (TGF-β) signalling due to mutations in the TGF-β genes has also been implicated in certain patients with Marfan's syndrome.[208] Patients with Marfan's syndrome are of a tall, thin build and have arachnodactyly, a high arched palate, pectus excavatum, scoliosis, flat feet, dislocation of the lens, aortic incompetence, dissection of the aorta and mitral valve prolapse. Pulmonary complications of the connective tissue fragility include recurrent pneumothoraces and emphysema.[209–211]

Hypertrophic pulmonary osteoarthropathy

Hypertrophic pulmonary osteoarthropathy is characterised by digital clubbing associated with arthropathy and periostitis that mainly affects the distal long bones in a symmetrical manner and causes painful swelling of the ankles, wrists, knees and elbows. Scans show abundant periosteal new bone. The condition is mainly associated with primary carcinoma of the lung, of which it may be the presenting feature. The tumour is usually peripheral and may be of any cell type but is rarely small cell. The numerous other associations include bronchopulmonary carcinoid, carcinoma of the oesophagus, thymus and thyroid, thoracic lymphoma, localised fibrous tumour of the pleura, leiomyoma of the oesophagus, pleuropulmonary sepsis, cystic fibrosis, sarcoidosis, cyanotic congenital heart disease, thyrotoxicosis and inflammatory bowel disease. The aetiology is obscure. Vagal stimulation, hormonal and immune mechanisms have all been suggested while the digital clubbing has been attributed to the release of growth factors following the impaction of platelet aggregates in distal blood vessels.

VASCULAR DISEASE

Cardiovascular disease often leads to cardiac hypertrophy and if this is severe it may affect the lungs. For example, the enlarged heart may come to occupy a significant proportion of the thoracic space, restricting lung volume, or an enlarged left atrium may compress the oesophagus, causing swallowing difficulties and so promoting aspiration pneumonia. In infancy the bronchi are narrow and still quite pliable and are therefore liable to be compressed at certain points if the pulmonary arteries are distended, as in acyanotic congenital cardiac disease, resulting in absorption collapse (Fig. 10.9).[212] Congenital heart disease may have profound effects upon the pulmonary circulation, as may failure of the left ventricle and mitral stenosis; these conditions are considered in Chapters 2 and 8.1 respectively. Pulmonary hypertension secondary to disorders of the heart and systemic vasculature is dealt with in Chapter 8.2 and vasculitis in Chapter 8.3.

Figure 10.9 The major airways and thoracic arteries viewed from in front with the latter in dotted outline demonstrating the sites where the bronchi and arteries are in particularly close proximity and the narrow, pliable bronchi of infants are liable to be compressed if the pulmonary arteries are distended. 1. The superior aspect of the left bronchus (LB) is compressed where it is crossed by a distended left pulmonary artery. 2. The posterior aspect of the left upper-lobe bronchus (LUB) is compressed as the left pulmonary artery hooks around it. 3. The lateral side of the junction of the intermediate (IB) and right middle-lobe (RMB) bronchi is compressed by the right lower-lobe artery. 4. A distended left pulmonary artery pushes the aorta (A) medially and upwards against the left lateral aspect of the trachea (T) to accentuate the normal indentation of the trachea by the aorta. *(Reproduced from Stanger et al. (1969)[212] by permission of the editor of Pediatrics.)*

Figure 10.10 Left pulmonary artery sling syndrome. In comparison with the normal arrangement shown on the left, the left pulmonary artery passes to the right and then backwards over the origin of the right main bronchus before crossing to the left side behind the trachea just above its bifurcation and in front of the oesophagus. The arrow indicates the course of the left pulmonary artery. *(Reproduced from Brewis RAL, Corrin B, Geddes DM et al. (eds) Respiratory Medicine, 2nd edn. London: Saunders, 1995, with permission.)*

Anomalies of the great vessels compressing the trachea

Four vascular anomalies are liable to compress the trachea. These are the left pulmonary artery sling syndrome and three varieties of vascular ring.

The left pulmonary artery sling syndrome

In this syndrome,[213] the left pulmonary artery crosses to the right in front of the trachea, curls around it above the origin of the right main bronchus and runs to the left between the trachea and the oesophagus (Fig. 10.10). The lower trachea is liable to be compressed, causing stridor or wheeze.

Vascular rings

Certain congenital anomalies of the great vessels result in a ring of arteries surrounding and possibly compressing the trachea. Three conditions are liable to do this:

1. a double aortic arch in which the ring is formed by the heart to the front, the twin arches to either side and the common descending aorta behind
2. an anomalous right subclavian artery. Here the ring consists of the heart to the front, the aortic arch to the left, an anomalous right subclavian artery behind and a ductus (or ligamentum)

arteriosus connecting the anomalous right subclavian artery to the right pulmonary artery to the right

3. a right-sided aortic arch with an anomalous left subclavian artery. This is the mirror image of the above and here the vascular ring is formed by the heart in front, the aortic arch to the right, an anomalous left subclavian artery behind and a ductus (or ligamentum) arteriosus connecting the left subclavian artery to the left pulmonary artery to the left (Fig. 10.11).[214]

It will be noted that in two of these conditions there is a right-sided aortic arch. This can be identified radiologically and in a child thought to have corticosteroid-resistant asthma is a valuable indication that the true cause of the child's wheezing is a vascular ring compressing the trachea.[215]

Hereditary haemorrhagic telangiectasia (Osler–Weber–Rendu disease)

Hereditary haemorrhagic telangiectasia is an autosomal-dominant condition characterised by multiple telangiectases in the skin and mucous membranes, often resulting in distressing and sometimes life-threatening haemorrhage.[216–218] Epistaxis and gastrointestinal haemorrhage are common manifestations while there may be haemoptysis, haematuria and iron-deficiency anaemia. Viscera such as the lungs, liver and brain may also be involved. The telangiectases connect arteries and veins, bypassing the normal resistance vessels so that they are subject to arterial pressure.[219] They act as arteriovenous fistulae and increase cardiac output. About 15% of patients have large pulmonary arteriovenous fistulae (see p. 76).[220] These permit paradoxical embolisation with the danger of infarction and abscesses in sites such as the brain.

Genetic mutations have been identified at three loci involving cell surface receptors for TGF-β. Two, which are located at 9q33-34 and 3p22 and respectively encode for endogline and ALK1, are found in families in whom pulmonary arteriovenous fistulae are common.[221–223] The third mutation, which is less common, has been mapped to the long arm of chromosome 12.[224] This mutation is associated with primary (plexogenic) pulmonary hypertension rather than pulmonary arteriovenous fistulae.[224–226] Thus, two mechanisms underlie the development of pulmonary hypertension in hereditary haemorrhagic telangiectasia: there may be either high-output left-sided cardiac failure or primary pulmonary vasoconstriction.[227]

Figure 10.11 Right-sided aortic arch with anomalous left subclavian artery. In this condition a vascular ring is formed by the heart in front, the aortic arch (AA) to the right, an anomalous left subclavian artery (ALS) behind and a left ductus arteriosus (LD) connecting the left subclavian artery to the left pulmonary artery to the left. Arrows indicate aortic flow; DA, descending aorta; PT, pulmonary trunk; RCC, right common carotid artery; LCC, left common carotid artery; RS, right subclavian artery. *(Reproduced from Stewart et al. (1966)[214] with permission from the* American Journal of Roentgenology.*)*

Klippel–Trenaunay syndrome

This is a congenital disorder characterised by a triad of cutaneous vascular lesions, venous abnormalities of the extremities and soft-tissue or bony hypertrophy. Venous thromboembolism is a common complication, sometimes leading to pulmonary hypertension and right heart failure.[228–231] Occasionally, there are also pulmonary angiomas.

Idiopathic arterial calcification of infancy

In this condition there is calcification of the arterial internal elastic laminae, generally involving systemic vessels but also pulmonary arteries on occasion.[232] Affected babies usually die in infancy and the diagnosis is often made at autopsy. Medium-sized arteries are rigid and as well as showing calcification of the internal elastic lamina they are often obliterated by secondary thrombosis and fibrosis.

Blue rubber bleb disease

Blue rubber bleb disease is characterised by cavernous haemangiomas involving the skin and gastrointestinal tract. Rarely the lesions extend into the trachea and bronchi where they are seen as discrete bluish mucosal nodules.[233]

Box 10.2 Renal disease associated with pulmonary haemorrhage

With anti-GBM antibody
Goodpasture's syndrome

Without anti-GBM antibody
Without systemic disease
Glomerulonephritis
Penicillamine-associated disease

With connective tissue disorders
Systemic lupus erythematosus
Systemic sclerosis
Rheumatoid disease
Mixed connective tissue disease

With systemic vasculitis
Wegener's granulomatosis
Polyangiitis overlap syndrome
Henoch–Schönlein purpura
Behçet's disease

GBM, glomerular basement membrane.

Yellow-nail syndrome

This syndrome is characterised by lymphatic hypoplasia, lymphoedema, chylous effusions and yellow discoloration of the nails. It is described more fully on page 709.

Aortic fistula

Fistulas between the aorta and the tracheobronchial tree may complicate previous thoracic vascular surgery, aortic aneurysm, bacterial aortitis or radiation therapy. They often present as recurrent episodes of haemoptysis but the initial event may be a catastrophic flooding of the airways.[234]

RENAL DISEASE

A combination of haematuria and pulmonary haemorrhage (or haemosiderosis) is seen in a variety of pulmonary–renal syndromes (Box 10.2).

Microalbuminuria is a risk marker for thromboembolism, probably because it reflects generalised endothelial dysfunction.[235]

Renal failure

The commonest respiratory conditions encountered in renal failure are infection and pulmonary oedema. The latter is often described as 'uraemic lung' but is indistinguishable from pulmonary oedema of other cause, described in full on page 401. Several mechanisms may contribute to the development of pulmonary oedema in renal failure. They include fluid retention; hypertensive left ventricular failure secondary to chronic glomerulonephritis, chronic pyelonephritis and polycystic renal disease; and hypoproteinaemia, which is a prominent feature of the nephrotic syndrome.[236] Cytotoxic factors may also operate.[237] Pleural effusion may develop for the same reasons.

Renal failure may be complicated by secondary hyperparathyroidism, leading to absorption of bone and a secondary rise in serum calcium levels. This may be followed by metastatic calcification, in which the lungs are amongst the most commonly affected organs (see below). Pulmonary hypertension is also reported in chronic renal failure, affecting 29% of such patients in one study; its etiology is poorly understood but it appears to be unrelated to secondary hyperparathyroidism or pulmonary vascular calcification.[238]

The treatment of renal failure introduces further respiratory hazards. The immunosuppression involved in renal transplantation is associated with azathioprine-associated interstitial pneumonitis, opportunistic infection and posttransplantation lymphoproliferative disease, while dialysis has its own detrimental effects on lung function. Peritoneal dialysis entails a reduction in diaphragmatic excursions so that a low vital capacity and hypoxaemia are regularly seen with this form of dialysis. Haemodialysis may be accompanied by hypoxaemia, probably because the filters employed activate complement and lead to the sequestration of neutrophils in the pulmonary capillaries, as in shock (see Figs 4.20 and 4.21, p. 144).

Autosomal-dominant polycystic kidney disease

The association of bronchiectasis with this renal disorder is described on page 65.

Familial Fanconi syndrome (renal tubular acidosis)

An unexplained association of bilateral diffuse pleural fibrosis has been described in two siblings with renal tubular acidosis.[239]

BLOOD DISORDERS

Attention here will be concentrated on the respiratory associations of diseases that are essentially haematological, although it may be noted that any lung disease liable to impair oxygenation of the blood may give rise to secondary polycythaemia while the paraneoplastic syndromes associated with lung tumours include conditions such as red cell aplasia.[240] Lymphoproliferative disease is dealt with in Chapter 12.4.

Anaemia

Anaemia from any cause is liable to give rise to breathlessness because of impaired oxygen transport, even when cardiorespiratory function is normal. More specific is an association of autoimmune haemolytic anaemia with idiopathic pulmonary fibrosis.[241]

Hypercoaguability

Hypercoaguability of the blood gives rise to pulmonary thromboembolism, pulmonary thrombosis and pulmonary infarction, conditions that are accordingly seen in association with polycythaemia,[242] thrombocythaemia,[242] myelomatosis, macroglobulinaemia,[243] cryoglobulinaemia,[244] cryofibrinogenaemia,[245] the antiphospholipid syndrome (see p. 489),[246–249] the hypereosinophilic syndrome (see p. 467) and haemoglobinopathies such as sickle cell disease,[250–255] spherocytosis,[256] thalassaemia[258,259] and paroxysmal nocturnal haemoglob-

inuria.[260] The thrombosis and subsequent organisation may be widespread and lead to pulmonary hypertension of the pattern seen in thromboembolic disease (see p. 404).[260]

Sickle cell disease

Sickle cell disease is a serious haemolytic disorder caused by homozygosity for haemoglobin S. The sickle cell trait is its milder heterozygous counterpart in which there is both haemoglobin S and A. The gene is found in Africa and Mediterranean countries. Whenever oxygen tension drops, haemoglobin S is liable to alter its molecular shape and deform the red blood cell, causing haemolysis and thrombosis. Infarction is widespread and may involve the lungs. Two major clinical forms of pulmonary involvement are recognised: an acute chest syndrome and sickle cell chronic lung disease. Acute chest syndrome is characterised by fever, chest pain and the appearance of new radiographic opacities. It represents an acute pulmonary vaso-occlusive crisis leading to acute right ventricular failure and sometimes death. Histologically, this may mimic veno-occlusive disease by causing patchy congestion through capillary sludging of the abnormal red blood cells (Fig. 10.12). Exchange transfusion has been shown to be effective.[261] Chronic lung disease on the other hand is manifest as radiographic infiltrates, impaired pulmonary function and, in its most severe form, pulmonary hypertension.[262–264] The pulmonary hypertension is due to pulmonary thrombosis (Fig. 10.13).[250–255] In severe cases there is plexogenic arteriopathy.[265,266] Veins as well as arteries thrombose and, when the venous thrombus organises, the appearances are similar to those seen in veno-occlusive disease. Rarely, pneumococcal septicaemia is also seen in sickle cell disease, possibly because of the splenic infarction that occurs in this condition. Fatal bone marrow embolism is a further occasional complication of sickle cell disease.[259,267]

Thalassaemia

Thalassaemia is another serious haemoglobinopathy, in this case caused by persistence of fetal haemoglobin because of a genetic inability to form adult haemoglobin A. Again there is haemolysis coupled with hypercoaguability of the blood, leading to thrombosis and infarction. Pulmonary hypertension may develop but is not as common as in sickle cell disease.[258] Haemosiderin deposition is a prominent pulmonary change and may lead to interstitial fibrosis.[258,259,268,269] Hypoxaemia is often noted in thalassaemia; this is possibly due to arteriovenous anastomoses in the form of 'spider naevi' that have been demonstrated in the periphery of the lung by postmortem injection techniques in thalassaemia patients that also have cirrhosis, which is a further complication of this disease.[258] Such anastomoses are recorded in the lungs of other patients with liver disease (see below). Mixed sickle cell thalassaemia has led to fatal bone marrow embolism.[259]

Myeloproliferative disease

Myeloproliferative disease may extend from the bone marrow to the lung, generally involving the pulmonary interstitium. Pulmonary involvement in myelofibrosis is seen as interstitial fibrosis accompanied by foci of extramedullary haemopoiesis.[270–272] In rare cases there is also air space and vascular involvement leading to pulmonary haemorrhage and pulmonary hypertension.[242,273] Thus, in diseases such as polycythaemia and thrombocythaemia, pulmonary hypertension may be the result of either thromboembolism or plugging of pulmonary blood vessels by haemopoietic cells.[242] Leukaemic processes also infiltrate the interstitial compartment of the

Figure 10.13 Sickle cell disease. A pulmonary artery shows recanalisation, following thrombosis.

Figure 10.12 Sickle cell disease. (A) In a patient who died of an acute vaso-occlusive crisis the lungs show differential congestion similar to that seen in veno-occlusive disease but here due to sludging of the abnormal red blood cells (B) rather than postcapillary obstruction.

Figure 10.14 Chronic granulomatous disease. A collection of neutrophils is surrounded by epithelioid and giant cells and beyond that chronic inflammatory granulation tissue. Eosinophils are prominent throughout. *(Courtesy of Dr K Dhaene, Ghent, Belgium.)*

lung, but generally as a terminal event[274]: before the lungs are directly involved they are liable to be the seat of opportunistic infection. Alveolar lipóproteinosis is also described (see p. 316). Pulmonary fibrosis is recorded in occasional patients with human T-cell lymphotropic virus type I-associated myelopathy[275] and leukaemia.[276] The pulmonary effects of treating leukaemia with cytotoxic drugs and by bone marrow transplantation are discussed on page 668.

Chronic granulomatous disease

Chronic granulomatous disease is characterised by opportunistic infections, both bacterial and fungal, with *Staphyloccus aureus*, *Nocardia* and *Aspergillus* species being particularly implicated.[277,278] It is due to a genetic disorder that impairs the production of oxygen metabolites by neutrophils, eosinophils and macrophages. Over 400 gene defects are recognised, involving both mutations and inactivating recombinations. They are all recessive and may be either X-linked or autosomal.

Phagocytic cells lack nicotinamide adenine dinucleotide phosphate (NADPH) oxidase and ingested microbes are therefore not killed following phagocytosis. Abscesses develop throughout the body in the first year of life, and the lung is only one of many organs affected. Within the lung, the granulomatosis may affect the lung parenchyma or be centred on the airways.[279,280] Often a balance is arrived at whereby viable microbes survive within granulomas composed of lymphocytes and yellow-brown, foamy macrophages centred on collections of neutrophils and eosinophils (Fig. 10.14).

Sea-blue histiocytosis

Sea-blue histiocytosis takes its name from the appearance of macrophages laden with cytoplasmic granules of this colour in Giemsa-stained preparations. In haematoxylin and eosin-stained sections the macrophages have an abundant pale, granular cytoplasm. Such cells are seen in Niemann–Pick disease (see below) and occasionally within the pulmonary interstitium and air spaces in a variety of acquired haematological disorders, including myelofibrosis.[281]

Mastocytosis

Mastocytosis is a rare disease of uncertain aetiology, characterised by infiltration and proliferation of mast cells in the skin (urticaria pigmentosa), bone marrow, gastrointestinal tract and lymph nodes. Pulmonary mast cell infiltration is particularly rare.[282]

IgG₄-related systemic sclerosing disease

The term 'IgG4-related systemic sclerosing disease' has been applied to lymphoproliferative lesions found in various sites throughout the body in association with high serum levels of IgG₄.[283–285c] The lesions contain abundant IgG₄-positive cells, generally accompanying exuberant fibrous tissue, which progresses to dense hyalinosis. Idiopathic retroperitoneal fibrosis and sclerosing pancreatitis are archetypal examples. The lungs have been involved in some cases of multisystem disease[286,287] and in a few instances pulmonary pseudotumours (plasma cell granulomas) have represented the sole evidence of hyper-IgG₄ disease.[288,289] Such patients have ranged from 42 to 78 years in age and shown an equal sex distribution. Several were asymptomatic at presentation. Imaging varies from ill-defined infiltrative lesions to nodular or multifocal opacities. Histology shows varying degrees of fibrosis with intense infiltration by lymphocytes, plasma cells, scattered neutrophils and occasional aggregates of eosinophils (Fig. 10.15A). Obliterative venulitis and obliterative arteritis (mimicking lymphomatoid granulomatosis) are common and there is sometimes a stenosing peribronchiolar infiltrate (see Fig. 10.15B, C). Immunohistochemistry shows polyclonality and many IgG₄-positive plasma cells, identification of which distinguishes the condition from its principal mimics, lymphatoid granulomatosis and NSIP. Most patients have been treated surgically but it is becoming apparent that the condition responds well to systemic corticosteroids.[288,290] The cases that have been classified as plasma cell granuloma or inflammatory pseudotumour need to be distinguished from inflammatory myofibroblastic tumour, a further condition to which these terms have been applied but which is now considered to be neoplastic (see p. 620). The distinction may be difficult as inflammatory myofibroblastic tumours also contain IgG₄-positive plasma cells, as do conditions such as Rosai–Dorfman disease.[291] The precise relationship of the IgG₄-related sclerosing disease to various lung disorders requires further elucidation.

Splenectomy

Splenectomy results in lowered immunity, particularly to pneumococcal infection. Many patients who have lost their spleen have died of pneumococcal pneumonia or septicaemia and all who have undergone this operation should be offered pneumococcal immunisation. Splenectomy also appears to be a risk factor for chronic thromboembolic pulmonary hypertension.[292]

Figure 10.15 IgG₄ disease. (A) Lung biopsy showing bronchiolocentric and subpleural consolidation. (B) The infiltrate narrows the airway lumen. (C) The infiltrate mainly consists of plasma cells, many of which stain for IgG₄.

ALIMENTARY TRACT DISORDERS

Disorders of the upper alimentary tract

A variety of upper alimentary tract disorders may be associated with pulmonary disease, chiefly the consequence of aspiration of ingested material or of alimentary tract secretions (Box 10.3). The patient may be unaware of such aspiration. Otherwise asymptomatic gastro-oesophageal reflux has been associated with several respiratory disorders.[293] Complications of aspiration include chronic cough, asthma, recurrent infections, aspiration pneumonia, abscess, empyema, bronchiectasis, exogenous lipid pneumonia, Mendelson's syndrome (see p. 145) and chronic interstitial pneumonia and fibrosis.

Coeliac disease

In coeliac disease there is villous atrophy in the small intestine because of allergy to dietary gluten. Some patients with coeliac disease experience respiratory problems and it is likely that these are also based on hypersensitivity. Of particular interest are allergy to avian protein and pulmonary haemosiderosis.

When it was discovered that some patients with coeliac disease and respiratory symptoms had serum antibodies against avian antigens,[294] it was naturally assumed that they also had bird fancier's lung, a form of extrinsic allergic alveolitis (see p. 279). However, further investigations showed that the antigen concerned was a globulin and that this was not found in bird droppings, unlike the avian albumin responsible for bird fancier's lung.[295] The source of the allergen is believed to be egg yolk and the allergy probably stems from the ingestion of hens' eggs rather than the inhalation of bird droppings. Attempts to establish a link between coeliac disease and other forms of extrinsic allergic alveolitis such as farmer's lung[296] have proved inconclusive. The relationship of the antibodies against avian globulin to the patients' respiratory disease is unclear. Increased lung permeability and reduced gas transfer suggest that there is an alveolitis, but most histological investigations have been limited to transbronchial biopsies. These are reported to show peribronchiolar fibrosis and chronic inflammation.[297] Radiology has identified bronchiectasis in one coeliac patient.[298]

The second area of interest in coeliac disease is pulmonary haemosiderosis.

Some patients diagnosed as having idiopathic pulmonary haemosiderosis are found to be suffering from malabsorption associated with jejunal villous atrophy, and some of them improve on removing gluten from the diet.[299–302] The association appears to be more than coincidental but its basis is unclear.

Table 10.2 **Respiratory associations of inflammatory bowel disease**

	Ulcerative colitis	Crohn's disease
Bronchitis[304–310,331,332]	+	+
Granulomatous bronchitis/bronchiolitis[308,323]	–	+
Bronchiectasis[304,310–312,324,331,332]	+	+
Bronchial stenosis[306]	+	+
Bronchiolitis[314]	+	+
Organising pneumonia[315]	+	+
Interstitial pneumonia[314,316–318]	+	+
Pulmonary eosinophilia (drug-related)[325]	+	+
Pyogenic nodules[309]	+	–
Necrotising granulomata[327]	+	+
Amyloidosis[319]	–	+
Apical fibrosis[320]	+	–
Thromboembolism	+	+
Hypoproteinaemic oedema[321]	–	+
Pleurisy	+	+
Antineutrophil cytoplasmic antibody[322]	+	–

Inflammatory bowel disease

Pulmonary abnormalities are being increasingly recognised in association with inflammatory bowel disease, both ulcerative colitis and Crohn's disease, but particularly the former.[303] A wide variety of pulmonary associations has now been described (Table 10.2).[304–327] Furthermore, it is possible that some patients have subclinical lung involvement as bronchoalveolar lavage has shown lymphocytosis in Crohn's disease patients who are free of pulmonary symptoms.[328,329] Similarly, lung function studies have shown that about 20% of patients with active bowel disease have a reduced diffusing capacity.[330] In a minority of cases the lung disease precedes that in the bowel.[309] Lung disease has also developed many years after the colon has been totally removed.

The commonest respiratory association of inflammatory bowel disease is inflammation of the airways.[304–311,331,332] There is a productive cough yet the patient is usually a non-smoker.[331] Biopsy shows either severe non-specific chronic inflammation[332] or non-necrotising tuberculoid granulomas (Fig. 10.16).[308,325,326,333] The appearances have been likened to those in the bowel and it is possible that the gut and the lung are both affected because they share common antigens. Progression of the bronchitis to bronchiectasis[304,310,311,324,331,332] and tracheobronchial stenosis[306] has been reported, and occasionally the airway disease causes acute respiratory failure.[334] When inflammatory bowel disease was sought in patients with large-airways disease the prevalence was found to be four times higher than expected.[335]

Many of these associations listed in Table 10.2 have been reported in patients under treatment with salazine-type drugs but, except for pulmonary eosinophilia, they are all recorded in patients who were not under treatment. However, drug effects need to be excluded

Figure 10.16 Necrotising granulomatous lung disease associated with (A) ulcerative colitis and (B) Crohn's disease.

before attributing pulmonary symptoms to the inflammatory bowel disease.

Whipple's disease

Whipple's disease[333] is a rare disorder that was for long considered to be a storage disorder of uncertain aetiology but is now known to represent infection by the bacilliform bacterium *Tropheryma whippelii*.[339–341] Patients usually give a long history of polyarthritis and insidious weight loss due to malabsorption, which later results in anaemia and diarrhoea.[342] Diagnosis is usually by jejunal biopsy, which shows heavy mucosal infiltration by macrophages distended by diastase-resistant periodic acid–Schiff-positive material. Electron microscopy shows that the macrophages contain large numbers of bacilli, which may be identified as *T. whippelii* by immunohistochemistry.[341,343] Few inflammatory cells are seen. It is postulated that a cytopathic effect of *T. whippelii* to plasma cells contributes to the bacilli evading the local immune response.[341,344,345] The condition usually responds to antibiotic treatment.[346–348]

The changes may extend to lymph nodes and other viscera, including the lungs.[346–350] Respiratory symptoms such as breathlessness, cough and pleuritic pain may precede the diarrhoea, and, rarely, pulmonary disease may be detected in the absence of intestinal features.[347] Radiographs show pleural thickening and effusion and patchy pulmonary opacification. Some patients suffer from pulmo-

nary hypertension, possibly due to *T. whippelii* colonizing the pulmonary arteries.[348,351]

Lung biopsy shows nodular collections of foam cells surrounding the centriacinar bronchioles and arteries and thickening the interlobular septa and pleura. As in the intestine, the foam cells stain strongly with diastase-controlled periodic acid–Schiff reagents and electron microscopy shows that they contain numerous bacilli.[346]

Pneumatosis coli

In this condition there are numerous gas-filled cysts beneath the mucosa of the colon. It has been associated with emphysema and was once thought to be due to interstitial emphysema tracking through the mediastinal and retroperitoneal tissues. However, it is now considered that the gas is produced locally by intestinal bacteria and that the association with emphysema is not a causal one.

Hepatic disease

Pulmonary vascular disease

A number of abnormalities of the pulmonary blood vessels may be found in association with cirrhosis.[352] It is suspected that vasoactive substances that are normally metabolised in the liver and thereby prevented from reaching the lungs do so through the portosystemic anastomoses that develop in cirrhosis. Pulmonary hypertension of the plexogenic variety (see p. 424) is a particularly serious but rare complication of cirrhosis associated with portal hypertension.[353–357] Hypoxaemia is a commoner finding, often referred to as the hepatopulmonary syndrome.[358] Although pulmonary arteriovenous anastomoses ('spider naevi') have been demonstrated in such patients,[258,359–361] they are uncommon and a more likely explanation of the syndrome is that the normal vasoconstrictive response of the lungs to hypoxia is inhibited, with consequent ventilation/perfusion mismatching (see p. 22).[362–364]

Ascites and pleural effusion

Ascites is common in cirrhosis because of portal hypertension and hypoproteinaemia and, if the effusion is large, lung volumes are reduced, resulting in breathlessness. In many patients this is aggravated by a concomitant right-sided pleural effusion, which is attributable to the pressure difference between the pleural and peritoneal cavities drawing fluid into the thorax through diaphragmatic defects.

Primary biliary cirrhosis

The pathological basis of this liver disease is a granulomatous destruction of intrahepatic bile ducts and it is therefore noteworthy that there are reports of pulmonary or multiorgan granulomas similar to those of sarcoidosis in association with the condition.[366–368] Other biopsy studies have demonstrated a non-granulomatous lymphocytic infiltrate of either the alveoli[369,370] or the airways.[371] Sjögren's syndrome, the pulmonary manifestations of which are described earlier in this chapter, has also been reported in association with primary biliary cirrhosis.[372] Interstitial pneumonia is largely confined to those patients with primary biliary cirrhosis who also have another autoimmune disease, such as systemic sclerosis.[370,373] It is possible that many patients with primary biliary cirrhosis have subclinical lung disease as they have been shown to have a pulmonary lymphocytosis by bronchoalveolar lavage.[374]

Hepatitis

The incidence of hepatitis C virus infection appears to be raised in idiopathic pulmonary fibrosis, leading to speculation that the association is causal, although not necessarily direct.[375] Autoimmune factors are prominent in several forms of hepatitis and some patients with chronic active hepatitis and non-organ-specific autoantibodies also develop interstitial pneumonia.[241,376] Bronchiectasis,[377] LIP[378] and pulmonary haemorrhage[379] have also been reported in association with autoimmune hepatitis on occasion.

α_1-Antitrypsin deficiency

This genetic disorder may cause panacinar emphysema (see p. 103) or cirrhosis. The coexistence of the two conditions in affected patients is recorded, but is rare.[380]

Liver abscess

Pyogenic or amoebic abscesses in the liver are prone to spread through the diaphragm to cause right-sided pleurisy, pneumonia, lung abscess or hepatobronchial fistula.

Pancreatic disease

The inflammation involved in acute pancreatitis may spread through the diaphragm to cause left-sided, or rarely bilateral, pleurisy. Acute pancreatitis of severe degree causes shock and the clinical and pathological features of this condition may develop (respectively, adult respiratory distress syndrome and diffuse alveolar damage).[381,382] The pancreas and the lungs may both be involved in IgG$_4$ systemic sclerosing disease, described above.[291]

NEUROMUSCULAR DISEASE

Neuromuscular diseases secondary to non-metastatic bronchopulmonary neoplasia (the paraneoplastic neuromuscular syndromes) are considered on page 544 and this section will be limited to the pulmonary manifestations of neuromuscular disease. Neuromuscular disease of varying aetiology may promote pulmonary infection by impairing the cough reflex and weakening respiration. Also, there is a danger of aspiration if swallowing is affected.

'Neurogenic' pulmonary oedema

'Neurogenic' pulmonary oedema is a well-recognised feature of cerebral damage, especially that due to trauma and subarachnoid haemorrhage. Its pathogenesis is thought to involve widespread adrenergic vasoconstriction resulting in marked systemic hypertension.[383–385] Fluid then shifts from the systemic circulation to the relatively more compliant pulmonary circulation, with a resultant outpouring of fluid into the lung.

Tuberous sclerosis

Tuberous sclerosis is a genetic disorder characterised by hamartomas in multiple tissues. The classic form of the disease is a dominant hereditary condition caused by mutation of a gene known as TSC1, which is situated on the long arm of chromosome 9q34. The brain, skin and kidney are chiefly affected. Pulmonary lymphangioleio-

myomatosis (see p. 293) is clinically evident in only 2.3% of these patients[386] but accounts for 10% of deaths.[387] However, radiological scans show clinically silent lung cysts suggestive of lymphangioleiomyomatosis in 34–39%.[388,389] In an another form of tuberous sclerosis, which is attributable to mutation of a gene known as TSC2 located on the short arm of chromosome 16p13.3, more severe lymphangioleiomyomatosis develops and is responsible for most deaths. This form of tuberous sclerosis is not hereditary and is often termed the sporadic form of pulmonary lymphangioleiomyomatosis. Neither the TSC1 nor the TSC2 gene is carried on a sex chromosome and, indeed, tuberous sclerosis typically affects both sexes but, with very few exceptions, whenever there is lymphangioleiomyomatosis the patient is female, and sexually mature. This is attributed to the lesional cells bearing receptors responsive to normal levels of oestrogen and progesterone. The protein products of the TSC1 and TSC2 genes are respectively known as hamartin and tuberin. They dimerise to form a coiled complex that plays a pivotal role in the phosphoinositide signalling pathway, functioning as an inhibitor of cell growth, proliferation and differentiation. It is not surprising therefore that mutation of either gene results in increased cell growth.[390] Pulmonary lymphangioleiomyomatosis is described in full on p. 293.

An even rarer pulmonary manifestation of tuberous sclerosis is the multifocal micronodular type II pneumocyte hyperplasia described on page 701. This lesion may be seen alone or in association with pulmonary lymphangioleiomyomatosis but has not been described in patients who do not have the classic (TSC1) form of tuberous sclerosis. Aneurysms of systemic arteries are a rare feature of tuberous sclerosis and occasionally affect a pulmonary artery.[391]

Angiomyolipomas of the kidney, retroperitoneum and liver are a further feature of tuberous sclerosis and are found in about half the women with lymphangioleiomyomatosis.[392] A few examples have been reported in the lungs (see p. 630), one in a patient with tuberous sclerosis but not lymphangioleiomyomatosis.[393] Renal angiomyolipomas are commoner in women and those associated with tuberous sclerosis often have progesterone receptors, suggesting that hormonal factors are important in their pathogenesis, as in lymphangioleiomyomatosis.[394] The benign clear cell tumour of the lung described on page 625 may also develop in patients with tuberous sclerosis.[395] The constituent cells of lymphangioleiomyomatosis, angiomyolipoma and benign clear cell tumour of the lung share an unusual mixed phenotype in that they express both smooth-muscle and melanocyte markers. It is suggested that they derive from certain 'perivascular epithelioid cells' and their resultant lesions have therefore been collectively termed PEComas.[396,397]

Neurofibromatosis

Neurofibromatosis is a common disorder of dysregulated tissue growth secondary to mutations of the tumour suppressor gene NF1. One of its many manifestations is pulmonary hypertension, which has a plexogenic pattern, indicating prolonged vasoconstriction (see p. 420).[398] Neurofibromatosis is occasionally associated with interstitial lung disease described as pulmonary fibrosis indistinguishable pathologically from the variety (idiopathic pulmonary fibrosis).[399–403] However, these reports antedate current concepts of disease patterns in interstitial pneumonia and, although they describe fibrocystic disease, the appearances are not those of UIP. A review of 156 patients with neurofibromatosis found little evidence to support an association with parenchymal lung disease and the authors suggested that previous reports may have, in part, represented the effects of smoking.[404] The thoracic neurofibromas of von Recklinghausen's disease and their obstructive complications are dealt with on page 640.

METABOLIC AND ENDOCRINE DISORDERS

Obesity

Obesity restricts ventilation by the fat splinting the chest wall and buttressing the underside of the diaphragm. This increases the work of breathing and contributes to the common symptom of breathlessness, which may be present at rest but is accentuated by the effort of moving an overweight body. In the supine position gas exchange is compromised in the lower lobes, resulting in relative hypoxaemia in the inferior pulmonary veins.[405] Not surprisingly therefore, poor lung function is found in the metabolic syndrome, a complex disorder in which obesity is combined with elevated triglycerides, hypertension, hyperglycaemia and insulin resistance.[405a,b]

A few grossly obese patients have a severely disturbed sleep pattern due to repeated episodes of nocturnal apnoea, attributable to neck fat compressing the pharyngeal airway. The resultant daytime somnolence is well illustrated by the fat messenger boy Joe described by Charles Dickens in his *Pickwick Papers*, hence the term 'pickwickian syndrome' (see p. 93). Further respiratory diseases linked to obesity include chronic obstructive pulmonary disease, asthma, thromboembolism and aspiration pneumonia.[406,407]

A retrospective autopsy study of 76 obese patients showed a greater occurrence of diabetes mellitus, systemic hypertension, pulmonary oedema, haemorrhage and pulmonary hypertensive changes than a control group. Cardiomegaly with biventricular hypertrophy was found in all obese patients and 72% showed evidence of pulmonary venous hypertension, in 50%. Eight had thrombosed or recanalised pulmonary blood vessels but none showed vascular necrosis or plexiform lesions. The authors attributed the pulmonary venous hypertension to hypoxia and left ventricular dysfunction.[408]

Antiphospholipid syndrome

The antiphospholipid syndrome, first described in 1983,[114,408a] is a systemic autoimmune disorder characterised by venous, arterial and capillary thrombosis and raised titres of antiphospholipid antibodies. It usually occurs in isolation but may be associated with other autoimmune diseases, especially systemic lupus erythematosus (SLE). Up to a third of patients with SLE develop secondary antiphospholipid syndrome. Young women are mainly affected, the mean age at diagnosis being 34 (standard deviation 13) years and the male:female ratio being 1:3.5 for primary disease and 1:7 when the syndrome is secondary to SLE.

The clinical features of the antiphospholipid syndrome are diverse as the disease may affect any system. The pulmonary effects include venous thromboembolism, pulmonary hypertension, microvascular thrombosis (possibly resulting in veno-occlusive disease) and alveolar haemorrhage.[120,246–249,408b] Extrapulmonary features include recurrent fetal loss, pre-eclampsia, transient ischaemic attacks, stroke, non-bacterial thrombotic endocarditis, myocardial infarction, renal infarction and microangiopathy. Treatment depends mainly upon anticoagulation.

Hypercalcaemia and metastatic calcification

The causes of hypercalcaemia include hyperparathyroidism, skeletal metastases, tumours secreting a parathormone-like peptide, sarcoidosis and hypervitaminosis D (Box 10.4). In sarcoidosis the epithelioid cells of the granulomas participate in a number of metabolic activities, including the final hydroxylation and hence activation of vitamin D,[409] thereby accounting for the hypercalcaemia that is so

frequently found in this condition.[410–412] Activation of vitamin D normally takes place in the kidneys and renal failure may be complicated by secondary hyperparathyroidism, again leading to hypercalcaemia and metastatic calcification. Metastatic calcification involving viscera takes the form of whitlockite ($(CaMg)_3(PO_4)_2$), whereas in the soft tissues it is deposited as hydroxyapatite ($(Ca_{10}(PO_4)_6(OH)_2)$).

The lungs, kidneys and stomach are particularly likely to be involved in metastatic calcification. Virchow suggested that this was because all these organs excrete acid and are therefore slightly alkaline.[413] In line with this is the observation that metastatic calcification may be localised to lung tissue beyond an obstructed pulmonary artery, the increased ventilation–perfusion ratio there raising the pH.[414] Basement membranes and elastic fibres are favoured sites of calcium deposition and the walls of blood vessels and alveoli are therefore particularly affected by metastatic calcification.[413,415–417] In severe cases every alveolar wall is delicately impregnated. The calcium is recognisable in routine sections due to its affinity for haematoxylin (Fig. 10.17), but if only a little is present the diagnosis may be confirmed by von Kossa's stain. Not surprisingly, the permeability of the alveolar walls may be increased; some patients with severe pulmonary involvement have died of massive pulmonary oedema.[418] Organisation of such protein-rich oedema fluid may explain the alveolar fibrosis that sometimes accompanies metastatic calcification. In rare cases the calcification is confined to the airway mucosa.[419]

Systemic amyloidosis

Amyloidosis of the lower respiratory tract may develop as part of generalised amyloidosis or in isolation. The isolated form is dealt with on page 696 and this section deals only with involvement of the lungs in systemic amyloidosis. Pathological evidence of pulmonary involvement is common in all forms of systemic amyloidosis, including the rare familial and senile (cardiac) forms[420–426a] and the α_2-microglobulin-derived amyloidosis that sometimes complicates long-term haemodialysis.[423,427] Despite this multiplicity of amyloid types evident pathologically, most patients with respiratory symptoms attributable to systemic amyloidosis have primary or myeloma-associated disease. The amyloid is therefore of the light-chain (AL) type. This is also true of amyloidosis confined to the lungs. The distinction of localised from systemic amyloidosis is clinically important. The two forms are distinguished by their organ distribution, as revealed by cardiac echocardiography and serum amyloid protein scintigraphy, screening for plasma cell dyscrasias and biopsy.

In primary systemic amyloidosis there is usually a fine diffuse interstitial deposition. Multifocal nodules may develop but the mass lesions of localised amyloid are not seen. Microscopy shows a widespread delicate thickening of the alveolar and vascular walls by an eosinophilic, amorphous deposit (Fig. 10.18). Larger pulmonary vessels are also involved, in similar fashion to systemic vessels. Electron microscopy shows that the amyloid is preferentially deposited in the alveolar epithelial and endothelial basement membranes.[425] On occasion there may be prominent pleural involve-

---

> **Box 10.4 The causes of hypercalcaemia**
>
> Hyperparathyroidism
> Skeletal metastases
> Neoplastic parathormone-like activity
> Sarcoidosis
> Hypervitaminosis D

Figure 10.17 Metastatic calcification in a patient with hypercalcaemia. Heavy deposition of calcium salts renders the alveolar walls basophilic.

ment.[428] The alveolar wall thickening is liable to be mistaken for interstitial fibrosis but the inflammatory component that usually accompanies such scarring is not a feature and a Congo red stain should quickly lead to the correct diagnosis. The potassium permanganate/Congo red reaction conforms to the amyloid being of the AL type (derived from immunoglobulin)[421] and this is supported by immunohistochemistry.[429,430] If what appears to be amyloid fails to stain as such, it might represent pulmonary involvement in light-chain deposition disease, which is considered on page 698.[431] Multifocal nodules of amyloid may stimulate the foreign-body giant cell reaction that is more characteristic of localised bronchopulmonary amyloidosis (see p. 696).

The severity of the pulmonary involvement generally parallels that in the heart but to a lesser degree.[421] It is often an incidental postmortem finding in patients known to have amyloid elsewhere but it may impair gas transfer and only be discovered when lung biopsy is undertaken to investigate the cause of abnormal blood gases or, rarely, dyspnoea. Pulmonary blood vessels are particularly involved and rarely this may be so severe as to cause pulmonary hypertension.[432,433]

In secondary (AA-type) amyloidosis, pulmonary involvement is generally limited to blood vessels and bronchial glands: alveolar walls are not affected and there is seldom any clinical evidence of lung disease.[420]

Figure 10.18 Systemic amyloidosis. (A) The alveolar walls are slightly thickened by a diffuse interstitial deposition of amyloid. (B) The media of a pulmonary artery shows deposition of amyloid.

Figure 10.19 Fabry's disease as an example of a lipidosis. Electron microscopy shows numerous large osmiophilic lamellar inclusions.

Figure 10.20 Gaucher's disease. The alveoli are filled by macrophages which have a swollen eosinophilic cytoplasm.

Storage disorders

The storage disorders comprise a wide variety of rare congenital defects. They often involve specific lysosomal enzymes, in which case they are generally manifest by the accumulation of the enzyme's substrate and deficiency of its reaction product. They are best known by the chemical character of the substrate and are often grouped under terms such as lipidoses, mucopolysaccharidoses and glycogenoses. The excess substrate is stored in the reticuloendothelial system and hepatosplenomegaly is a common feature of many storage diseases. The lungs contain many cells of the histiocyte series and pulmonary involvement is therefore commonly found postmortem. It is seldom troublesome in life but may cause significant morbidity, for example in adults with Niemann–Pick disease type B, in which case whole-lung lavage may be successful.[434] In the lungs there is an increase in both alveolar and interstitial macrophages, the cytoplasm of which is swollen due to the accumulation of the indigestible lysosomal substrate, which in the lipidoses is generally evident on electron microscopy as membrane-bound inclusions of osmiophilic, lamellar material (Fig. 10.19). In the mucopolysaccharidoses the macrophage cytoplasm is weakly haematoxyphil, and in cystine storage disease free crystals can be identified if an alcoholic fixative and polarisers are used.

Gaucher's disease

This lipidosis is characterised by an accumulation of glucosylceramide.[435–439] The alveolar macrophage cytoplasm may be foamy or finely granular and eosinophilic and the appearances may mimic those of desquamative interstitial pneumonia (Fig. 10.20).[434,440,441]

Fabry's disease

In this lipidosis periodic acid–Schiff-positive laminated inclusion bodies of β-galactoside are found in endothelial cells, alveolar epithelial cells and bronchial muscle,[443] sometimes narrowing the airways.[444] Their ultrastructural features are illustrated in Figure 10.19.

Niemann–Pick's disease

This lipidosis is characterised by an accumulation of sphingomyelin and cholesterol lipidosis.[434,441,442,445,446] The macrophage cytoplasm is foamy and the features are those of endogenous lipid pneumonia. The process also involves ciliated cells but spares the alveolar lining cells (Fig. 10.21).

Ceroidosis and the Hermansky–Pudlak syndrome

The storage disorders seldom affect the lungs in isolation but very occasionally conspicuous pulmonary lipidosis is associated with insignificant systemic involvement. This is seen particularly in patients with malignant cachexia who develop ceroidosis.[447,448] In these cases the swollen macrophages contain much brown ceroid pigment. The histological appearances simulate those of haemosiderosis but stains for iron and ceroid readily distinguish these two conditions.

In contrast to isolated pulmonary involvement, the Hermansky–Pudlak syndrome is characterised by generalised ceroid storage, which is associated with albinism and platelet dysfunction resulting in a bleeding diathesis.[449,450] This familial condition, largely confined to Dutch and Puerto Rican patients, is of interest to pulmonologists because it is sometimes associated with chronic interstitial pneumonitis and fibrosis with honeycombing (Fig. 10.22). The changes are widespread and lack the basal and subpleural predilection seen in idiopathic pulmonary fibrosis. The fibrosis is maximal around respiratory bronchioles and is accompanied by florid foamy swelling of type II pneumocytes.[450–457] The ceroid accumulation is thought to reflect lipid peroxidation, with oxygen radical release during this process being responsible for the pulmonary fibrosis. Identification of the ceroid from its autofluorescent properties in urinary sediment or buccal scrapings aids the diagnosis.

Morquio's disease

Morquio's disease represents a further storage disorder that is occasionally responsible for respiratory disability. It is due to a deficiency of galactosamine-6-sulphatase, which leads to a build-up of keratin sulphate. Deposits of this substance may obstruct the upper airways or impair movement of the chest wall.[458]

Xanthogranulomatosis

This condition is characterised by focal collections of foamy macrophages rich in cholesterol and other lipids. Such deposits are found

Figure 10.21 Niemann–Pick disease. (A) The alveoli are filled by macrophages which have a swollen foamy cytoplasm and some of the macrophages show Touton-type giant cell formation. The appearances are those of a florid endogenous lipid pneumonia. (B) Bronchiolar epithelial cells also have a foamy cytoplasm, in contrast to the type II alveolar lining cells seen in (A), which do not.

in the lung in diabetes mellitus and generalised xanthomatosis.[459] Cholesterol pneumonitis is considered further on page 319.

Alkane lipogranulomatosis

Certain indigestible waxes found in the skin of apples and other foodstuffs are absorbed unaltered. The amounts are usually trivial and of no importance but persons consuming inordinate amounts of such foodstuffs are liable to have these alkane waxes deposited in their tissues. One French farmer, for example, was estimated to have consumed 5 tons of apples. He was found to have lipogranulomatous nodules throughout his lungs while being investigated for angina, and after he died of coronary disease similar deposits were identified in many other organs, including the liver, spleen, adrenal glands and lymph nodes.[460] Mass spectrometry showed the lipid to consist of straight-line saturated aliphatic hydrocarbons (n-alkanes) with the

formula $C_{29}H_{60}$ or $C_{31}H_{64}$. Histologically the deposits resemble cholesterol granulomas as they take the form of acicular crystals being engulfed by macrophages and foreign-body giant cells (Fig. 10.23).

Erdheim–Chester disease

Erdheim–Chester disease is a rare form of generalised histiocytosis that is chiefly characterised by fibrosis and foam cell infiltration of the bone marrow resulting in osteosclerosis, particularly of the long bones of the legs.[461–463] Clonality has been reported.[464]

The sexes are affected equally and the mean age at presentation is in the sixth decade. Pulmonary involvement is characterised by dyspnoea of insidious onset or, rarely, acute respiratory failure. Pulmonary function tests show restricted lung volumes. Imaging shows diffuse thickening of the interlobular septa and pleurae with centriacinar nodules.

Microscopically, a fibrosing infiltrate of foamy CD68-positive reticular cells thickens the interlobular septa, pleura and bronchovascular bundles but spares the alveolar tissue (Fig. 10.24).[465–469] Grouping of the cells may simulate granulomatous disease.[466]

Diabetes insipidus and pulmonary fibrosis are features that Erdheim–Chester disease shares with Langerhans cell histiocytosis,[463,470,471] and occasionally the two diseases are associated.[465] However, in Erdheim–Chester disease the infiltrate fails to react for the Langerhans cell marker CD1a. The osteosclerotic lesions of Erdheim–Chester disease also differ from the osteolysis seen in Langerhans cell histiocytosis. Pulmonary involvement generally augers a poor prognosis,[467,468] although one case showed a response to immunosuppressive therapy.[472]

Rosai–Dorfman disease

Rosai–Dorfman disease, which is also known as sinus histiocytosis with massive lymphadenopathy, represents a rare idiopathic, non-neoplastic proliferation of histiocytes that typically affects children and young adults.[473] It is primarily a disease of lymph nodes, particularly those in the neck, but extranodal sites are involved in about a third of cases and the lungs are affected in about 2% of these. Pulmonary involvement is thus particularly rare but solitary or multiple masses may affect the airways or lungs, or there may be diffuse pulmonary or pleural infiltration.[473–477a] The basic fault appears to be hypersecretion of macrophage colony-stimulating factor leading to monocyte chemotaxis and differentiation, but the underlying cause is unknown.

Histologically, lymph node sinuses are distended by large numbers of histiocytes while pulmonary involvement is characterised by replacement or infiltration of the tissues by these cells. The histiocytes have oval nuclei with dispersed chromatin and one or more nucleoli, and abundant palely staining eosinophilic cytoplasm which reacts for S-100, CD31 and CD68, but not CD1a. Plasma cells and lymphocytes are also seen, with the latter often invading the histiocytes by a process known as emperipolesis. The plasma cells may react strongly for IgG₄.[477a] The differential diagnosis includes Langerhans cell histiocytosis, Erdheim–Chester disease, Hodgkin's lymphoma, Gaucher's disease, IgG₄ systemic sclerosing disease and mycobacterial infection. Negative staining for CD1a helps to exclude Langerhans cell histiocytosis, while the eosinophils seen in that condition are not a feature of Rosai–Dorfman disease, nor is the characteristic osteosclerosis of long bones that is seen in Erdheim–Chester disease, and none of these other diseases shows the lymphocyte emperipolesis that is characteristic of Rosai–Dorfman disease.

Cases in which the disease is limited to the lymph nodes usually resolve spontaneously but systemic disease carries a worse prognosis

Figure 10.22 Hermansky–Pudlak syndrome. (A) There is widespread interstitial fibrosis and inflammation resembling non-specific interstitial pneumonia. (B) Higher magnification shows marked vacuolation of the type II pneumocytes (top left) with the interstitial accumulation of pale histiocytes, occasionally containing golden brown pigment.

Figure 10.23 Alkane lipogranulomatosis. The granulomas consist of macrophages and foreign-body giant cells surrounding alkane crystals, which are acicular and resemble those of cholesterol. *(Courtesy of Dr Duboucher, Paris, France.)*

Figure 10.24 Erdheim–Chester disease. (A) There is prominent fibrous thickening of the interlobular septa. *(Courtesy of Dr M Kambouchner, Paris, France.)* (B) At high power, histiocytes and eosinophils are seen. *(Courtesy of Dr T Ashcroft, Newcastle-upon-Tyne, UK.)*

and may prove fatal despite surgery or radiotherapy. Chemotherapy is ineffective.

Acromegaly

The lungs share in the general visceromegaly seen in acromegaly. Being a disease of adult life, they are affected after development is complete and for this reason the lung enlargement represents an increase in alveolar size rather than number. Acromegalic enlargement of the tongue and laryngeal tissues may cause upper-airway obstruction, and pulmonary venous hypertension may stem from acromegalic cardiomyopathy.

Thyroid disease

A retrosternal goitre may compress the trachea, thyrotoxicosis may result in pulmonary hypertension secondary to high-output cardiac failure[478] and myxoedema may be associated with pericardial and pleural transudates[479] related to the perivascular deposits of amorphous, eosinophilic material that have been described in this disease.[480]

Diabetes mellitus

Lung function is impaired in diabetes mellitus because of autonomic neuropathy and pulmonary microangiopathy. The former is probably responsible for diminished ventilatory responses to hypoxaemia and hypercapnia, and the latter for a mild reduction in diffusing capacity and pulmonary capillary blood volume.[481,482] Changes within the lungs develop independently of those attributable to diabetes in other organs.

No dramatic morphological changes are evident in the lungs in diabetes but microangiopathy similar to that observed elsewhere in the body has been reported – principally thickening of the alveolar capillary and epithelial basement membranes.[483–487] Micronodular fibrosis of alveolar walls is a rarely reported phenomenon.[488] Occasional perivascular xanthogranulomatous deposits have also been identified.[459]

Similar basement membrane and connective tissue alterations have been described in laboratory animals rendered diabetic with alloxan or streptozotocin,[489–493] together with impairment of lung growth in young animals[49]: insulin treatment prevented all these changes.

Diabetes mellitus predisposes to infection and confers an increased risk of bronchitis, bronchiectasis, pneumonia, pulmonary tuberculosis and fungal lung disease.

Hypovitaminosis A

Vitamin A is essential to the integrity of the respiratory mucosa. Deficiency leads to squamous metaplasia.[494] This has led to proposals that hypovitaminosis A is a cofactor promoting the development of lung cancer. Extensive trials of vitamin A and carotene supplementation have consequently been conducted, but these have failed to show that these dietary measures have any effect on the incidence of lung cancer.[495,496]

SKIN DISEASE

Cutaneous manifestations of malignant lung disease

Apart from skin metastases and infections of the skin secondary to impaired host defence consequent upon disseminated cancer, there are several skin conditions that, although not malignant themselves, are sometimes associated with systemic cancer, including bronchopulmonary carcinoma. They include the cutaneous consequences of thrombophlebitis migrans (one of Trousseau's signs), dermatomyositis, acanthosis nigricans, arsenical keratoses and several non-metastatic endocrinopathies that elicit changes in the skin, for example, ectopic adrenocorticotrophic hormone secretion and acromegaly.[497,498] Lastly, nicotine staining of the fingers should alert the physician to the increased danger of cancer and other lung diseases caused by smoking.

Skin disease associated with non-malignant lung disease

Psoriasis may be associated with spondylitis, including that of the ankylosing variety, which is sometimes associated with apical lung fibrosis.[152] *Pemphigoid* of the sclerosing variety, also known as benign mucous membrane pemphigoid, rarely extends below the larynx but has caused fatal tracheobronchial obstruction.[499] Necrotising tracheobronchitis has also complicated paraneoplastic *pemphigus*,[500] and pustules similar to those seen in the skin in *acute febrile neutrophilic dermatosis (Sweet's syndrome)* have been described in the bronchial mucosa and lung in patients with this disease.[501–503] Pulmonary manifestations of *pyoderma gangrenosa* are rare but multiple nodules showing aseptic necrosis are recorded,[504] similar to those occasionally seen in the lungs in inflammatory bowel disease (see above).[309] *Cutis laxa* and *Ehlers–Danlos syndrome* sometimes involve the lungs, as described on page 482. Other diseases manifest in both the skin and lungs, which are also described elsewhere, include *tuberous sclerosis* (p. 488), various *vasculitides* (p. 437), *systemic sclerosis* (p. 476), *rheumatoid disease* (p. 473), *Langerhans cell histiocytosis* (p. 288), *sarcoidosis* (p. 283) and the *Birt–Hogg–Dubé* syndrome, which is described next. *Erythema multiforme* may be a manifestation of sarcoidosis or changing immunity to tuberculosis and a variety of *infections* may be common to the skin and lungs. Lastly, *drug reactions* developing during the treatment of many lung diseases may be first evident in the skin.

Birt–Hogg–Dubé syndrome

This rare familial condition is characterised by multiple benign skin tumours, a variety of renal tumours and pulmonary cysts.[505] The mutant gene is an autosomal dominant that has been mapped to 17p12q11.2 and the normal gene product, which is possibly a tumour suppressor, has been named folliculin after the cutaneous fibrofolliculomas that characterise the syndrome.[506] The pulmonary cysts generally measure no more than a few millimetres in diameter but they are thin-walled and liable to rupture into the pleural cavity, resulting in pneumothorax, often in adult life. This appears to be the only clinical effect of the lung cysts of any consequence and indeed may be the only manifestation of the mutation as this abnormality has now been identified in patients with familial pneumothorax who do not have the skin lesions and renal tumours of the complete syndrome,[507–509] in which case the non-apical location of the cysts may suggest the diagnosis.[510] Histology shows that the cysts are closely associated with the peripheral interlobular septa, often at a septopleural junction. They are lined by cuboidal epithelium resting on delicate connective tissue, devoid of muscle (Fig. 10.25).[510,511] Significant mortality attaches to the syndrome, chiefly due to the development of renal cell carcinoma and for this reason annual abdominal computed tomography scans are recommended.

Figure 10.25 Birt–Hogg–Dubé syndrome. Microscopy shows a small cyst that is intimately involved with an interlobular septum, although immunocytochemistry shows that it is lined by epithelial cells and represents an expanded air space. *(Cytokeratin immunostain courtesy of Dr K Hiroshima, Chiba, Japan.)*

GYNAECOLOGICAL AND OBSTETRIC CONDITIONS

Meigs' syndrome

Meigs' syndrome consists of a pleural effusion associated with ascites and a pelvic neoplasm, removal of which results in resolution of both effusions.[512,513] The ascitic fluid is thought to spread to the pleural space through small apertures in the diaphragm. The effusion is right-sided in 70% of cases, bilateral in 20% and left-sided in 10%. The pelvic tumour is usually an ovarian fibroma but ovarian cysts and uterine fibroids have also been responsible.[514]

Pregnancy

Increased levels of progesterone result in an increased respiratory drive from the early weeks of pregnancy while in the third trimester the mechanical effects of the enlarging uterus may cause breathlessness. Successful deliveries have been achieved despite severe lung disease but pulmonary hypertension may deteriorate during pregnancy. Accelerated lung transplant rejection is also recorded during pregnancy.[515] Complications of pregnancy that may have an adverse affect on the lungs include uterine haemorrhage and infection, either of which may result in 'shock lung', and eclampsia, which is sometimes associated with pulmonary oedema.[516,517] The incidence of thromboembolism is also increased in pregnancy. Embolism of amniotic fluid, trophoblast and decidua is considered on page 410.

Thoracic endometriosis

Thoracic endometriosis generally affects the pleura and subpleural lung tissue but occasionally the process appears to be entirely intrapulmonary.[518] The mechanisms underlying pleural and pulmonary endometriosis differ but proffered explanations are not entirely satisfactory. Pleural deposits may represent serosal metaplasia or be due

Figure 10.26 Pleural endometriosis comprising both endometrial glands and endometrial stroma. *(Courtesy of Dr M Neyra, Lyons, France.)*

to transdiaphragmatic spread of pelvic endometriosis, whereas embolism is the probable explanation of the parenchymal lesions. The clinical effects of pleural and pulmonary endometriosis also differ, except that either may first be identified coincidentally as an asymptomatic tumour.

Pleural endometriosis is usually characterised by catamenial pneumothorax,[519–521] and occasionally by catamenial haemothorax,[522] both of which are almost always limited to the right side. Serosal metaplasia is a possible explanation but many cases have pelvic endometriosis, congenital diaphragmatic perforations and multiple endometriotic implants on both the visceral and the parietal pleura and in these, transdiaphragmatic spread of pelvic endometriosis seems likely. The almost universal limitation of the disease to the right side is attributed to diaphragmatic fenestrations preponderating on that side.[523] Pneumothorax secondary to pneumoperitoneum, and haemothorax secondary to haemoperitoneum are also largely limited to the right, as is the pleural effusion of Meigs' syndrome (see above).[523] Many small diaphragmatic fenestrae must go unnoticed but a complicating factor is that some diaphragmatic perforations may be secondary to endometriotic implants.[523]

Intrapulmonary endometriosis is even rarer than the pleural variety.[524–526] It is typically characterised by catamenial haemoptysis, affects either or both lungs and is seldom associated with pelvic endometriosis.[526] On the other hand, there is a strong association with gynaecological surgery,[526] suggesting that blood-borne endometrial seeding of the lung following uterine instrumentation or parturition is responsible. This is supported by animal experiments in which intravenously injected endometrial tissue migrated from pulmonary blood vessels into the lung substance where it remained viable and underwent cyclic change.[527]

Whatever its pathogenesis, thoracic endometriosis is similar in its age distribution (23–45 years) and pathological appearance to that encountered more commonly elsewhere. CT findings include irregular opacities, nodular lesions, cystic change and bulla formation.[528,529] Magnetic resonance imaging is also useful as it highlights changes related to bleeding.[530] Grossly, lesions may be single or multifocal,

well circumscribed or infiltrative, nodular, cystic or nodulocystic. Rarely the disease may be predominantly endobronchial.[530,531] The heterotopic tissue consists of both stroma and glands and reproduces the appearances of normal endometrium in every way (Fig. 10.26). Decidual change takes place in pregnancy[532,533] and cyclic haemorrhagic disruption, with consequent haemosiderosis, may obscure the nature of the tissue, in which case immunocytochemistry may be used to demonstrate oestrogen and progesterone receptors and in the stromal component CD10.[534] The ectopic tissue also responds to steroid derivatives that suppress gonadotrophin release[526] and this has proved successful therapeutically.[518,535] Others prefer local surgical resection to avoid the side-effects of hormonal therapy.[536] Pleural abrasion is reported to be superior to hormonal treatment in the management of pneumothorax.[535]

REFERENCES

Connective tissue diseases

1. Douglas WW, Tazelaar HD, Hartman TE, et al. Polymyositis-dermatomyositis-associated interstitial lung disease. Amer J Respir Crit Care Med 2001;164:1182–5.

2. Fujita J, Yoshinouchi T, Ohtsuki Y, et al. Non-specific interstitial pneumonia as pulmonary involvement of systemic sclerosis. Ann Rheum Dis 2001;60:281–3.

3. Bouros D, Wells AU, Nicholson AG, et al. Histopathologic subsets of fibrosing alveolitis in patients with systemic sclerosis and their relationship to outcome. Amer J Respir Crit Care Med 2002;165:1581–6.

4. Kim DS, Yoo B, Lee JS, et al. The major histopathologic pattern of pulmonary fibrosis in scleroderma is nonspecific interstitial pneumonia. Sarcoidosis Vasc Diffuse Lung Dis 2002;19:121–7.

5. Kitaichi M, Nagai SIIYS. Pulmonary pathology in association with connective tissue disorders. Current Diagnostic Pathology 2004;10:291–303.

6. Agusti C, Xaubet A, Roca J, et al. Interstitial pulmonary fibrosis with and without associated collagen vascular disease – results of a two year follow up. Thorax 1992;47:1035–40.

7. Homma Y, Ohtsuka Y, Tanimura K, et al. Can interstitial pneumonia as the sole presentation of collagen vascular diseases be differentiated from idiopathic interstitial pneumonia? Respiration 1995;62:243–51.

8. Tansey D, Wells AU, Colby TV, et al. Variations in histological patterns of interstitial pneumonia between connective tissue disorders and their relationship to prognosis. Histopathology 2004;44:585–96.

9. Flaherty KR Colby TV, Travis WD, et al. Fibroblastic foci in usual interstitial pneumonia – Idiopathic versus collagen vascular disease. Amer J Respir Crit Care Med 2003;167:1410–5.

10. Song JW, Do KH, Kim MY, et al. Pathologic and radiologic differences between idiopathic and collagen vascular disease-related usual interstitial pneumonia. Chest 2009;136:23–30.

11. Erasmus LD. Scleroderma in gold-miners on the Witwatersrand with particular reference to pulmonary manifestations. S Afr J Lab Clin Med 1957;3:209–31.

12. Scheule RK, Holian A. Mini-review – immunologic aspects of pneumoconiosis. Exp Lung Res 1991;17:661–85.

13. Beckett W, Abraham J, Becklake M, et al. Adverse effects of crystalline silica exposure. Amer J Respir Crit Care Med 1997;155:761–8.

14. Ellman P, Ball RE. "Rheumatoid disease" with joint and pulmonary manifestations. BMJ 1948;2:816.

15. Ellman P, Cudkowicz L, Elwood JS. Widespread serous membrane involvement by rheumatoid nodules. J Clin Pathol 1954;7:239–44.

16. MacFarlane JD, Dieppe PA, Rigden BG, et al. Pulmonary and pleural disease in rheumatoid disease. Br J Dis Chest 1978;72:288–300.

17. Engel U, Aru A, Francis D. Rheumatoid pleurisy. Acta Path Microbiol Immunol 1986;94:53–6.

18. Anderson RJ, Hansen KK, Kuzo RS, et al. A 38-year-old woman with chronic rheumatoid arthritis and a new pleural effusion – rheumatoid pleuritis. N Engl J Med 1994;331:1642–7.

19. Nosanchuk JS, Naylor B. A unique cytologic picture in pleural fluid from patients with rheumatoid arthritis. Am J Clin Pathol 1968;50:330–5.

20. Walker WC. Pulmonary infections and rheumatoid arthritis. Q J Med 1967;36:239–51.

21. Hindle W, Yates DAH. Pyopneumothorax complicating rheumatoid lung disease. Ann Rheum Dis 1965;24:57–60.

22. Davies D. Pyopneumothorax in rheumatoid lung disease. Thorax 1966;21:230–5.

23. Eraut D, Evans J, Caplin M. Pulmonary necrobiotic nodules without rheumatoid arthritis. Br J Dis Chest 1978;72:301–6.

24. Walters MN-I, Ojeda VJ. Pleuropulmonary necrobiotic rheumatoid nodules. A review and clinicopathological study of six patients. Med J Aust 1986;144:648–51.

25. Ip MSM, Wong MP, Wong KL. Rheumatoid nodules in the trachea. Chest 1993;103:301–3.

26. White DA, Mark EJ, Kradin RL, et al. A 53-year-old woman with arthritis and pulmonary nodules – rheumatoid lung disease with rheumatoid nodules, pleuritis, and interstitial fibrosis. New Engl J Med 2001;344:997–1004.

27. Gough J, Rivers D, Seal RME. Pathological studies of modified pneumoconiosis in coal-miners with rheumatoid arthritis (Caplan's syndrome). Thorax 1955;10:9–18.

28. Cavazza A, Paci M, Turrini E, et al. Fungus colonisation of pulmonary rheumatoid nodule. J Clin Pathol 2003;56:636–7.

29. Dawson JK, Fewins HE, Desmond J, et al. Fibrosing alveolitis in patients with rheumatoid arthritis as assessed by high resolution computed tomography, chest radiography, and pulmonary function tests. Thorax 2001;56:622–7.

30. Dixon ASTJ, Ball J. Honeycomb lung and chronic rheumatoid arthritis. Ann Rheum Dis 1957;16:241–5.

31. Lee HK, Kim DS, Yoo B, et al. Histopathologic Pattern and Clinical Features of Rheumatoid Arthritis-Associated Interstitial Lung Disease. Chest 2005;127:2019–27.

32. Reference removed in text.

33. Parambil JG, Myers JL, Ryu JH. Diffuse alveolar damage: uncommon manifestation of pulmonary involvement

in patients with connective tissue diseases. Chest 2006;130:553–8.

34. Kim EJ, Collard HR, King TE. Rheumatoid arthritis-associated interstitial lung disease. Chest 2009;136:1397–405.

35. Petrie GR, Bloomfield P, Grant IWB, et al. Upper lobe fibrosis and cavitation in rheumatoid disease. Br J Dis Chest 1980;74:263–7.

36. MacFarlane JD, Francken CK, Van Leeuwen AW. Progressive cavitating pulmonary changes in rheumatoid arthritis. Ann Rheum Dis 1984;43:98–101.

37. Cheung CY, Chan HP, Kurshner I. Apical fibrocavitary lesions of the lung in rheumatoid arthritis. Am J Med 1986;81:741–6.

38. Takanami I, Imamuma T, Yamamoto Y, et al. Bronchiectasis complicating rheumatoid arthritis. Respir Med 1995;89:453–4.

39. Despaux J, Manzoni P, Toussirot E, et al. Prospective study of the prevalence of bronchiectasis in rheumatoid arthritis using high-resolution computed tomography. Rev Rhum Engl Ed 1998;65:453–61.

40. Bonafede RP, Benatar SR. Bronchocentric granulomatosis and rheumatoid arthritis. Br J Dis Chest 1987;81:197–201.

41. Perez T, Remy Jardin M, Cortet B. Airways involvement in rheumatoid arthritis: Clinical, functional, and HRCT findings. Am J Respir Crit Care Med 1998;157:1658–65.

42. Yousem SA, Colby TV, Carrington CB. Follicular bronchitis/bronchiolitis. Hum Pathol 1985;16:700–6.

43. Fortoul TI, Cano Valle F, Oliva E, et al. Follicular bronchiolitis in association with connective tissue diseases. Lung 1985;163:305–14.

44. Geddes DM, Corrin B, Brewerton DA, et al. Progressive airway obliteration in adults and its association with rheumatoid disease. Q J Med 1977;46:427–44.

45. Hakala M, Paakko P, Sutinen S, et al. Association of bronchiolitis with connective tissue disorders. Ann Rheum Dis 1986;45:656–62.

46. Devouassoux G, Cottin V, Liote H, et al. Characterisation of severe obliterative bronchiolitis in rheumatoid arthritis. Eur Respir J 2009;33:1053–61.

47. Epler GR, Snider GL, Gaensler EA, et al. Bronchiolitis and bronchitis in connective tissue disease. A possible relationship to the use of penicillamine. JAMA 1979;242:528–32.

48. Boehler A, Vogt P, Speich R, et al. Bronchiolitis obliterans in a patient with localized scleroderma treated with D-penicillamine. Eur Respir J 1996;9:1317–9.

49. Schwartzman KJ, Bowie DM, Yeadon C, et al. Constrictive bronchiolitis obliterans following gold therapy for psoriatic arthritis. Eur Respir J 1995;8:2191–3.

50. Murphy DMF, Fairman RP, Lapp NL, et al. Severe airway disease due to inhalation of fumes from cleansing agents. Chest 1976;69:372–6.

51. Sugiyama Y, Saitoh K, Kano S, et al. An autopsy case of diffuse panbronchiolitis accompanying rheumatoid arthritis. Respir Med 1996;90:175–7.

52. Homma S, Kawabata M, Kishi K, et al. Diffuse panbronchiolitis in rheumatoid arthritis. Eur Resp J 1998;12:444–52.

53. Gardner DL, Duthie JJR, Macleod J, et al. Pulmonary hypertension in rheumatoid arthritis: report of a case with intimal sclerosis of the pulmonary and digital arteries. Scot med J 1957;2:183–8.

54. Balagopal VP, DaCosta P, Greenstone MA. Fatal pulmonary hypertension and rheumatoid vasculitis. Eur Respir J 1995;8:331–3.

55. Kay JM, Banik S. Unexplained pulmonary hypertension with pulmonary arteritis in rheumatoid disease. Br J Dis Chest 1977;71:53–9.

56. Price TML, Skelton MO. Rheumatoid arthritis with lung lesions. Thorax 1956;11:234–40.

57. Baydur A, Mongan ES, Slager UT. Acute respiratory failure and pulmonary arteritis without parenchymal involvement. Demonstration in a patient with rheumatoid arthritis. Chest 1979;75:518–20.

58. Imokawa S, Colby TV, Leslie KO, et al. Methotrexate pneumonitis: review of the literature and histopathological findings in nine patients. Eur Resp J 2000;15:373–81.

59. Norman D, Piecyk M, Roberts DH. Eosinophilic pneumonia as an initial manifestation of rheumatoid arthritis. Chest 2004;126:993–5.

60. Baruch AC, Steinbronn K, Sobonya R. Pulmonary adenocarcinomas associated with rheumatoid nodules: a case report and review of the literature. Arch Pathol Lab Med 2005;129:104–6.

61. Mellemkjaer L, Linet MS, Gridley G, et al. Rheumatoid arthritis and cancer risk. Eur J Cancer 1996;32A:1753–7.

62. Nicholson AG, Wotherspoon AC, Jones AL, et al. Pulmonary B-cell non-Hodgkin's lymphoma associated with autoimmune disorders: a clinicopathological review of six cases. Eur Respir J 1996;9:2022–5.

63. Paul JR. Pleural and pulmonary lesions in rheumatic fever. Medicine (Baltimore) 1928;7:383–410.

64. Masson P, Riopelle JL, Martin P. Poumon rheumatismal. Ann Anat Path 1937;14:359–82.

65. Neuberger KT, Geever EF, Rutledge EK. Rheumatic pneumonia. Arch Pathol 1944;37:1–15.

66. Grunow WA, Esterly JR. Rheumatic pneumonitis. Chest 1972;61:298–301.

67. Stupi AM, Steen VD, Owens GR, et al. Pulmonary hypertension in the CREST syndrome variant of systemic sclerosis. Arthritis Rheum 1986;29:515–24.

68. Harrison NK, Myers AR, Corrin B, et al. Structural features of interstitial lung disease in systemic sclerosis. Am Rev Respir Dis 1991;144:706–13.

69. Griffin MT, Robb JD, Martin JR. Diffuse alveolar haemorrhage associated with progressive systemic sclerosis. Thorax 1990;45:903–4.

70. Nishi K, Myou S, Ooka T, et al. Diffuse cutaneous systemic sclerosis associated with pan-serositis, disseminated intravascular coagulation, and diffuse alveolar haemorrhage. Respir Med 1994;88:471–3.

71. de Souza RB, Borges CT, Capelozzi VL, et al. Centrilobular fibrosis: an underrecognized pattern in systemic sclerosis. Respiration 2009;77:389–97.

72. Yousem SA. The pulmonary pathologic manifestations of the CREST syndrome. Human Pathology 1990;21:467.

73. Tzeng DZ, Leslie KO, Shelton D, et al. Unusual dyspnea in a woman with CREST syndrome. Chest 2008;133:286–90.

74. Rosenthal AK, McLaughlin JK, Linet MS, et al. Scleroderma and malignancy: an epidemiological study. Ann Rheum Dis 1993;52:531–3.

75. Yang Y, Fujita J, Tokuda M, et al. Lung cancer associated with several connective tissue diseases: with a review of literature. Rheumatol Int 2001;21:106–11.

76. D'Angelo WA, Fries JF, Masi AT, et al. Pathologic observations in systemic sclerosis scleroderma: a study of fifty-eight autopsy cases and fifty-eight matched controls. Am J Med 1969;46:428–40.

77. Wiedemann HP, Matthay RA. Pulmonary manifestations of the collagen vascular diseases. Clin Chest Med 1989;10:677–722.

78. Harrison NK, Glanville AR, Strickland B, et al. Pulmonary involvement in systemic sclerosis: the detection of early changes by thin section CT scan, bronchoalveolar lavage and 99mTc-DTPA clearance. Respir Med 1989;83:403–14.

79. Chan TYK, Hansell DM, Rubens MB, et al. Cryptogenic fibrosing alveolitis and the fibrosing alveolitis of systemic sclerosis: morphological differences on computed tomographic scans. Thorax 1997;52:265–70.

80. Wells AU, Cullinan P, Hansell DM, et al. Fibrosing alveolitis associated with systemic sclerosis has a better prognosis than lone cryptogenic fibrosing alveolitis. Am J Respir Crit Care Med 1994;149:1583–90.

81. Wells AU, Hansell DM, Rubens MB, et al. Fibrosing alveolitis in systemic sclerosis: indices of lung function in relation to extent of disease on computed tomography. Arthritis Rheum 1997;40:1229–36.

82. Fischer A, Swigris JJ, Groshong SD, et al. Clinically significant interstitial lung disease in limited scleroderma: histopathology, clinical features, and survival. Chest 2008;134:601–5.

83. Cailes JB, O'Connor C, Pantelidis P, et al. Neutrophil activation in fibrosing alveolitis: a comparison of lone cryptogenic fibrosing alveolitis and systemic sclerosis. Eur Respir J 1996;9:992–9.

84. Moon J, Dubois RM, Colby TV, et al. Clinical significance of respiratory bronchiolitis on open lung biopsy and its relationship to smoking related interstitial lung disease. Thorax 1999;54:1009–14.

85. Bridges AJ, Hsu KC, Dias-Arias AA, et al. Bronchiolitis obliterans organizing pneumonia and scleroderma. J Rheumatol 1992;19:1136–40.

86. Muir TE, Tazelaar HD, Colby TV, et al. Organizing diffuse alveolar damage associated with progressive systemic sclerosis. Mayo Clin Proc 1997;72:639–42.

87. Biasi D, Caramaschi P, Carletto A, et al. Localized scleroderma associated with sarcoidosis. Clin Exp Rheumatol 1998;16:761–2.

88. Young RH, Mark GJ. Pulmonary vascular changes in scleroderma. Am J Med 1978;64:998–1004.

89. Landzberg MJ, Ko J, King ME, et al. A 38-year-old woman with increasing pulmonary hypertension after delivery – scleroderma overlap syndrome with pulmonary vasculopathy and malignant pulmonary hypertension accelerated during puerperium. N Engl J Med 1999;340:455–64.

90. Cool CD, Groshong SD, Oakey J, et al. Pulmonary hypertension: cellular and molecular mechanisms. Chest 2005;128:565S–571.

91. Overbeek MJ, Vonk MC, Boonstra A, et al. Pulmonary arterial hypertension in limited cutaneous systemic sclerosis: a distinctive vasculopathy. Eur Respir J 2009;34:371–9.

92. Morassut PA, Walley VM, Smith CD. Pulmonary veno-occlusive disease and the CREST variant of scleroderma. Can J Cardiol 1992;8:1055–8.

93. Dorfmuller P, Humbert M, Perros F, et al. Fibrous remodeling of the pulmonary venous system in pulmonary arterial hypertension associated with connective tissue diseases. Human Pathology 2007;38:893–902.

94. Ribadeau-Dumas S, Tillie-Leblond I, Rose C, et al. Pulmonary hypertension associated with POEMS syndrome. Eur Respir J 1996;9:1760–2.

95. Lesprit P, Godeau B, Authier FJ, et al. Pulmonary hypertension in POEMS syndrome: A new feature mediated by cytokines. Amer J Respir Crit Care Med 1998;157:907–11.

96. Hirose S, Hosoda Y, Furuya S, et al. Expression of vascular endothelial growth factor and its receptors correlates closely with formation of the plexiform lesion in human pulmonary hypertension. Pathol Int 2000;50:472–9.

97. Allam JS, Kennedy CC, Aksamit TR, et al. Pulmonary manifestations in patients with POEMS syndrome: a retrospective review of 137 patients. Chest 2008;133:969–74.

98. Keane MP, Lynch JP. Pleuropulmonary manifestations of systemic lupus erythematosus. Thorax 2000;55:159–66.

99. Miller LR, Greenberg SD, McLarty JW. Lupus lung. Chest 1985;88:265–9.

100. Matthay RA, Schwarz MI, Petty TL, et al. Pulmonary manifestations of systemic lupus erythematosus: review of twelve cases of acute lupus pneumonitis. Medicine (Baltimore) 1974;54:397–408.

101. Gammon RB, Bridges TA, Alnezir H, et al. Bronchiolitis obliterans organizing pneumonia associated with systemic lupus erythematosus. Chest 1992;102:1171–4.

102. Mana F, Mets T, Vincken W, et al. The association of bronchiolitis obliterans organizing pneumonia, systemic lupus erythematosus, and Hunner's cystitis. Chest 1993;104:642–4.

103. Kim WU, Kim SI, Yoo WH, et al. Adult respiratory distress syndrome in systemic lupus erythematosus: causes and prognostic factors: a single center, retrospective study. Lupus 1999;8:552–7.

104. Murin S, Wiedemann HP, Matthay RA. Pulmonary manifestations of systemic lupus erythematosus. Clin Chest Med 1998;19:641–65, viii.

105. Attanoos RL, Goddard H, Gibbs AR. Mesothelioma-binding antibodies: thrombomodulin, OV 632 and HBME-1 and their use in the diagnosis of malignant mesothelioma. Histopathology 1996;29:209–15.

106. Marenco JL, Sanchez-Burson J, Ruiz CJ, et al. Pulmonary amyloidosis and unusual lung involvement in SLE. Clin Rheumatol 1994;13:525–7.

107. Yood RA, Steigman DM, Gill LR. Lymphocytic interstitial pneumonitis in a patient with systemic lupus erythematosus. Lupus 1995;4:161–3.

108. Gibson GJ, Edmonds JP, Hughes GRV. Diaphragm function and lung involvement in systemic lupus erythematosus. Am J Med 1977;63:926–32.

109. Marino CT, Pertschuk LP. Pulmonary haemorrhage in systemic lupus erythematosus. Arch Intern Med 1981;141:201–3.

110. Myers JL, Katzenstein AL. Microangiitis in lupus-induced pulmonary haemorrhage. Am J Clin Pathol 1986;85:552–6.

111. Santos Ocampo AS, Mandell BF, Fessler BJ. Alveolar hemorrhage in systemic lupus erythematosus – presentation and management. Chest 2000;118:1083–90.

112. Hughson MD, He Z, Henegar J, et al. Alveolar hemorrhage and renal microangiopathy in systemic lupus erythematosus – Immune complex small vascular injury with apoptosis. Arch Pathol Lab Med 2001;125:475–83.

113. Kuhn C. Systemic lupus erythematosus in a patient with ultrastructural lesions of the pulmonary capillaries previously reported in the review as due to idiopathic pulmonary hemosiderosis. Am Rev Respir Dis 1972;106:931–2.

114. Boey ML, Colaco CB, Gharavi AE, et al. Thrombosis in systemic lupus erythematosus: striking association with the presence of circulating lupus anticoagulant. BMJ 1983;287:1021–3.

115. Asherson RA, Mackworth-Young CG, Boey ML, et al. Pulmonary hypertension in systemic lupus erythematosus. BMJ 1983;287:1024–5.

116. Wakaki K, Koizumi F, Fukase M. Vascular lesions in systemic lupus erythematosus (SLE) with pulmonary hypertension. Acta Pathol Jpn 1984;34:593–604.

117. Wilson L, Tomita T, Braniecki M. Fatal pulmonary hypertension in identical twins with systemic lupus erythematosus. Hum Pathol 1991;22:295–7.

118. Nair SS, Askari AD, Popelka CG, et al. Pulmonary hypertension and systemic lupus erythematosus. Arch Intern Med 1980;140:109–11.

119. Yokoi T, Tomita T, Fukaya M, et al. Pulmonary hypertension associated with systemic lupus erythematosus: Predominantly thrombotic arteriopathy accompanied by plexiform lesions. Arch Pathol Lab Med 1998;122:467–70.

120. Kishida Y, Kanai Y, Kuramochi S, et al. Pulmonary venoocclusive disease in a patient with systemic lupus erythematosus. J Rheumatol 1993;20:2161–2.

121. Olsen EGJ, Lever JV. Pulmonary changes in systemic lupus erythematosus. Br J Dis Chest 1972;66:71–7.

122. Fayemi AO. Pulmonary vascular disease in systemic lupus erythematosus. Am J Clin Pathol 1976;65:284–90.

123. Churg A, Franklin W, Chan KL, et al. Pulmonary hemorrhage and immune-complex deposition in the lung. Complications in a patient with systemic lupus erythematosus. Arch Pathol Lab Med 1980;104:388–91.

124. Gross M, Esterly JR, Earle RH. Pulmonary alterations in systemic lupus erythematosus. Am Rev Respir Dis 1972;105:572–7.

125. Brown JH, Doherty CC, Allen DC, et al. Fatal cardiac failure due to myocardial microthrombi in systemic lupus erythematosus. BMJ 1988;296:1505.

126. Hammar SP, Winterbauer RH, Bockus D, et al. Endothelial cell damage and tubuloreticular structures in interstitial lung disease associated with collagen vascular disease and viral pneumonia. Am Rev Respir Dis 1983;127:77–84.

127. Yum M, Ziegler J, Walker P, et al. Pseudolymphoma of the lung in a patient with systemic lupus erythematosus. Am J Med 1979;66:172.

128. Dux S, Pitlik S, Rosenfeld JB, et al. Localised visceral immunocytoma associated with serological findings suggesting systemic lupus erythematosus. BMJ 1984;288:898–9.

129. Lakhanpal S, Lie JT, Conn DL, et al. Pulmonary disease in polymyositis and dermatomyositis: a clinico-pathological analysis of 65 autopsy cases. Ann Rheum Dis 1987;46:23–9.

130. Salmeron G, Greenberg SD, Lidsky MD. Polymyositis and diffuse interstitial lung disease. A review of the pulmonary histopathologic findings. Arch Intern Med 1981;141:1005–10.

131. Takizawa H, Shiga J, Moroi Y, et al. Interstitial lung disease in dermatomyositis: clinicopathological study. J Rheumatol 1987;14:102–7.

132. Fathi M, Dastmalchi M, Rasmussen E, et al. Interstitial lung disease, a common manifestation of newly diagnosed polymyositis and dermatomyositis. Ann Rheum Dis 2004;63:297–301.

133. Bernstein RM, Morgan SH, Chapman J, et al. Anti-Jo-1 antibody: a marker for myositis with interstitial lung disease. BMJ 1984;289:151–2.

134. Chan WM, Ip M, Lau CS, et al. Anti-Jo-1 syndrome presenting as cryptogenic organizing pneumonia. Respir Med 1995;89:639–41.

135. Kiely JL, Donohoe P, Bresnihan B, et al. Pulmonary fibrosis in polymyositis with the Jo-1 syndrome: an unusual mode of presentation. Resp Med 1998;92:1167–9.

136. Brown I, Joyce C, Hogan PG, et al. Pulmonary vasculitis associated with anti-Jo-1 antibodies. Resp Med 1998;92:986–8.

137. Tazelaar HD, Viggiano RW, Pickersgill J, et al. Interstitial lung disease in polymyositis and dermatomyositis. Am Rev Respir Dis 1990;141:727–33.

137a. Yousem SA, Gibson K, Kaminski N, Oddis CV, Ascherman DP. The pulmonary histopathologic manifestations of the anti-Jo-l tRNA synthetase syndrome. Mod Pathol 2010 Jun;23(6):874–80.

138. Cottin V, ThivoletBejui F, ReynaudGaubert M, et al. Interstitial lung disease in amyopathic dermatomyositis and polymyositis. Eur Resp J 2003;22:245–50.

139. Schwarz MI, Sutarik JM, Nick JA, et al. Pulmonary capillaritis and diffuse alveolar hemorrhage – a primary manifestation of polymyositis. Am J Respir Crit Care Med 1995;151:2037–40.

140. Cervera R, Ramirez G, Fernandez-Sola J, et al. Antibodies to endothelial cells in dermatomyositis: association with interstitial lung disease. BMJ 1991;302:880–1.

141. Kamel OW, van de Rijn M, Lebrun DP, et al. Lymphoid neoplasms in patients with rheumatoid arthritis and dermatomyositis: frequency of Epstein–Barr virus and other features associated with immunosuppression. Hum Pathol 1994;25:638–43.

142. Sharp GS, Irvin WS, Tan EM, et al. Mixed connective tissue disease: an apparently distinct rheumatic disease syndrome associated with a specific antibody to an extractable nuclear antigen (ENA). Am J Med 1972;52:148–59.

143. Bennett RM, O'Connell DJ. Mixed connective tissue disease: a clinicopathologic study of 20 cases. Sem Arthritis Rheum 1980;10:25–51.

144. Kobayashi H, Sano T, Li K, et al. Mixed connective tissue disease with fatal pulmonary hypertension. Acta Pathol Jpn 1982;32:1121–9.

145. Sullivan WD, Hurst DJ, Harmon CE, et al. A prospective evaluation emphasizing pulmonary involvement in patients with mixed connective tissue disease. Medicine (Baltimore) 1984;63:92–102.

146. Prakash UBS, Luthra HS, Divertie MB. Intrathoracic manifestations in mixed connective tissue disease. Mayo Clin Proc 1985;60:813–21.

147. Lazarus DS, Mark EJ, McLoud TC. A 46-year old woman with dermatomyositis, increasing pulmonary insufficiency, and terminal right ventricular failure – mixed connective-tissue disease, with diffuse alveolar damage, interstitial pneumonitis, pulmonary hypertension, epicarditis, esophageal fibrosis, and sclerodactyly. N Engl J Med 1995;333:369–77.

148. Wiener-Kronish JP, Solinger AM, Warnock ML, et al. Severe pulmonary involvement in mixed connective tissue disease. Am Rev Respir Dis 1981;124:499–503.

149. Rosenow EC, Strimlan CV, Muhm JR, et al. Pleuropulmonary manifestations of ankylosing spondylitis. Mayo Clin Proc 1977;52:641–9.

150. Davies D. Ankylosing spondylitis and lung fibrosis. Q J Med 1972;41:395–417.

151. Levy H, Hurwitz MD, Strimling M, et al. Ankylosing spondylitis lung disease and *Mycobacterium scrofulaceum* Br J Dis Chest 1988;82:84–7.

152. Guzman LR, Gall EP, Pitt M, et al. Psoriatic spondylitis. Association with advanced nongranulomatous upper lobe pulmonary fibrosis. JAMA 1978;239:1416–7.

153. Ellman P, Weber FP, Goodier TEW. A contribution to the pathology of Sjögren's disease. Q J Med 1951;20:33–42.

154. Bucher UG, Reid L. Sjögren's syndrome – report of a fatal case with pulmonary and renal lesions. Br J Dis Chest 1959;53:237–52.

155. Bloch KJ, Buchanan WW, Wohl MJ, et al. Sjögren's syndrome. A clinical, pathological, and serological study of sixty-two cases. Medicine (Baltimore) 1965;44:187–231.

156. Constantopoulos SH, Papdimitrious CS, Moutsopoulos HM. Respiratory manifestations in primary Sjögren's syndrome. Chest 1985;88:226–9.

157. Amin K, Ludviksdottir D, Janson C, et al. Inflammation and structural changes in the airways of patients with primary Sjögren's syndrome. Resp Med 2001;95:904–10.

158. Deheinzelin D, de Carvalho CR, Tomazini ME, et al. Association of Sjögren's syndrome and sarcoidosis. Report of a case. Sarcoidosis 1988;5:68–70.

159. Itescu S, Brancato LJ, Winchester R. A sicca syndrome in HIV infection: association with HLA-DR5 and CD8 lymphocytosis. Lancet 1989;ii:466–8.

160. Inase N, Usui Y, Tachi H, et al. Sjögren's syndrome with bronchial gland involvement and multiple bullae. Respiration 1990;57:286–8.

161. Bonner H, Ennis RS, Geelhoed GW, et al. Lymphoid infiltration and amyloidosis of lung in Sjögren's syndrome. Arch Pathol Lab Med 1973;95:42–4.

162. Kobayashi H, Matsuoka R, Kitamura S, et al. Sjögren's syndrome with multiple bullae and pulmonary nodular amyloidosis. Chest 1988;94:438–40.

163. Desai SR, Nicholson AG, Stewart S, et al. Benign pulmonary lymphocytic infiltration and amyloidosis: computed tomographic and pathologic features in three cases. J Thorac Imaging 1997;12:215–20.

164. Harris RS, Mark EJ. A 42-year-old man with multiple pulmonary cysts and recurrent respiratory infections. Sjögren's syndrome involving the lungs, with follicular bronchiolitis, air trapping with cyst formation, and deposition of amyloid-like material. N Engl J Med 2001;344:1701–8.

165. Yamadori I, Fujita J, Bandoh S, et al. Nonspecific interstitial pneumonia as pulmonary involvement of primary Sjögren's syndrome. Rheumatol Int 2002;22:89–92.

166. Sato T, Matsubara O, Tanaka Y, et al. Association of Sjögren's syndrome with pulmonary hypertension – report of two cases and review of the literature. Hum Pathol 1993;24:199–205.

167. Sowa JM. The association of Sjögren's syndrome and primary pulmonary hypertension. Hum Pathol 1993;24:1035.

168. Kadota J, Kusano S, Kawakami K, et al. Usual interstitial pneumonia associated with primary Sjögren's syndrome. Chest 1995;108:1756–8.

169. Deheinzelin D, Capelozzi VL, Kairalla RA, et al. Interstitial lung disease in primary Sjögren's syndrome – clinical-pathological evaluation and response to treatment. Am J Respir Crit Care Med 1996;154:794–9.

170. Deheinzelin D, Capelozzi VL, Kairalla RA, et al. Interstitial lung disease in primary

Sjögren's syndrome. Clinical–pathological evaluation and response to treatment. Am J Respir Crit Care Med 1996;154: 794–9.

171. Gardiner P, Ward C, Allison A, et al. Pleuropulmonary abnormalities in primary Sjögren's syndrome. J Rheumatol 1993;20:831–7.

172. Parambil JG, Myers JL, Lindell RM, et al. Interstitial lung disease in primary Sjögren syndrome. Chest 2006;130:1489–95.

173. Schuurman H-J, Gooszen HCH, Tan IWN, et al. Low-grade lymphoma of immature T-cell phenotype in a case of lymphocytic interstitial pneumonia and Sjögren's syndrome. Histopathology 1987;11:1193–204.

174. Mariette X. Lymphomas in patients with Sjögren's syndrome: review of the literature and physiopathologic hypothesis. Leuk Lymphoma 1999;33:93–9.

175. Kojima M, Nakamura S, Ban S, et al. Primary pulmonary low-grade marginal zone B-cell lymphoma of mucosa-associated lymphoid tissue type with prominent hyalinosis. A case report. Pathol Res Pract 2002;198:685–8.

176. Pearson CM. Cline HM, Newcomer VD. Relapsing polychondritis. N Engl J Med 1960;263:51–8.

177. Verity MA, Larson WM, Madden SC. Relapsing polychondritis. Report of two necropsied cases with histochemical investigation of the cartilage lesion. Am J Pathol 1963;42:251–69.

178. Kaye RL, Sones DA. Relapsing polychondritis. Clinical and pathological features in 14 cases. Ann Intern Med 1964;60:653–64.

179. Hughes RAC, Berry CL, Seifert M, et al. Relapsing polychondritis. Three cases with a clinico-pathological study and literature review. Q J Med 1972;41:363–80.

180. McAdam LP, O'Hanlan MA, Bluestone R, et al. Relapsing polychondritis: prospective study of 23 patients and a review of the literature. Medicine (Baltimore) 1976;55:193–215.

181. Ebringer R, Rook G, Swana GT, et al. Autoantibodies to cartilage and type II collagen in relapsing polychondritis and other rheumatic diseases. Ann Rheum Dis 1979;40:473–9.

182. Somers G, Potvliege P. Relapsing polychondritis: relation to periarteritis nodosa. BMJ 1978;2:603–4.

183. Neild GH, Cameron JS, Lessof MH, et al. Relapsing polychondritis with crescentic glomerulonephritis. BMJ 1978;1: 743–5.

184. Higgenbottam T, Dixon J. Chondritis associated with fatal intramural bronchial fibrosis. Thorax 1979;34:563–4.

185. Rogerson ME, Higgins EM, Godfrey RC. Tracheal stenosis due to relapsing polychondritis in rheumatoid arthritis. Thorax 1987;42:905–6.

186. Sheffield E, Corrin B. Fatal bronchial stenosis due to isolated relapsing chondritis. Histopathology 1992;20: 442–3.

187. Valenzuela R, Cooperrider PA, Gogate P, et al. Relapsing polychondritis. Immunomicroscospic findings in cartilage of ear biopsy specimens. Hum Pathol 1980;11:19–22.

188. Uzun O, Akpolat T, Erkan L. Pulmonary vasculitis in Behçet disease: A Cumulative Analysis. Chest 2005;127:2243–53.

189. Uzun O, Erkan L, Akpolat I, et al. Pulmonary involvement in Behçet's disease. Respiration 2008;75:310–21.

190. Chajek T, Fainaru M. Behçet's disease. Report of 41 cases and a review of the literature. Medicine (Baltimore) 1975;54:179–96.

191. Slavin RE, de Groot WJ. Pathology of the lung in Behçet's disease: case report and review of the literature. Am J Surg Pathol 1981;5:779–88.

192. Efthimiou J, Johnston C, Spiro SG, et al. Pulmonary disease in Behçet's syndrome. Q J Med 1986;58:259–80.

193. Lie JT. Cardiac and pulmonary manifestations of Behçet syndrome. Pathol Res Pract 1988;183:347–52.

194. Demontpreville VT, Macchiarini P, Dartevelle PG, et al. Large bilateral pulmonary artery aneurysms in Behçet's disease: rupture of the contralateral lesion after aneurysmorrhaphy. Respiration 1996;63:49–51.

195. Witt C, John M, Martin H, et al. Behçet's syndrome with pulmonary involvement – combined therapy for endobronchial stenosis using neodym-YAG laser, balloon dilation and immunosuppression. Respiration 1996;63:195–8.

196. Erkan F, Gul A, Tasali E. Pulmonary manifestations of Behçet's disease. Thorax 2001;56:572–8.

197. Aktogu S, Erer OF, Urpek G, et al. Multiple pulmonary arterial aneurysms in Behçet's disease: Clinical and radiologic remission after cyclophosphamide and corticosteroid therapy. Respiration 2002;69:178–81.

198. Hughes JP, Stovin PGI. Segmental pulmonary artery aneurysms with peripheral venous thrombosis. Br J Dis Chest 1959;53:19–27.

199. Kopp WL, Green RA. Pulmonary artery aneurysms with recurrent thrombophlebitis. The Hughes–Stovin syndrome. Ann Intern Med 1962;56:105–14.

200. Jerray M, Benzarti M, Rouatbi N. Possible Behçet's disease revealed by pulmonary aneurysms. Chest 1991;99:1282–4.

201. Corbett E, Glaisyer H, Chan C, et al. Congenital cutis laxa with a dominant inheritance and early onset emphysema. Thorax 1994;49:836–7.

202. Ayres JG, Pope FM, Reidy JF, et al. Abnormalities of the lungs and thoracic

cage in the Ehlers–Danlos syndrome. Thorax 1985;40:300–5.

203. Corrin B, Simpson CGB, Fisher C. Fibrous pseudotumours and cyst formation in the lungs in Ehlers–Danlos syndrome. Histopathology 1990;17:478–9.

204. Watanabe A, Kawabata Y, Okada O, et al. Ehlers–Danlos syndrome type IV with few extrathoracic findings: a newly recognized point mutation in the COL3A1 gene. Eur Resp J 2002;19:195–8.

205. Kawabata Y, Watanabe A, Yamaguchi S, et al. Pleuropulmonary pathology of vascular Ehlers–Danlos syndrome: Spontaneous laceration, haematoma, and fibrous nodules. Histopathology 2010;56:944–50.

206. Jackson A, Loh C-L. Pulmonary calcification and elastic tissue damage in pseudoxanthoma elasticum. Histopathology 1980;4:607–11.

207. Maslen CL, Glanville RW. The molecular basis of Marfan syndrome. DNA Cell Biol 1993;12:561–72.

208. Mizuguchi T, Matsumoto N. Recent progress in genetics of Marfan syndrome and Marfan-associated disorders. J Hum Genet 2007;52:1–12.

209. Sharma BK, Talukdar B, Kapoor R. Cystic lung in Marfan's syndrome. Thorax 1989;44:978–9.

210. Yellin A, Shiner RJ, Lieberman Y. Familial multiple bilateral pneumothorax associated with Marfan syndrome. Chest 1991;100:577–8.

211. Rigante D, Segni G, Bush A. Persistent spontaneous pneumothorax in an adolescent with Marfan's syndrome and pulmonary bullous dysplasia. Respiration 2001;68:621–4.

Vascular disease

212. Stanger P, Lucas RV, Jr., Edwards JE. Anatomic factors causing respiratory distress in acyanotic congenital cardiac disease. Special reference to bronchial obstruction. Pediatrics 1969;43:760–9.

213. Cohen SR, Landing BH. Tracheostenosis and bronchial anomalies associated with pulmonary artery sling. Ann Otol Rhinol Laryngol 1976;85:1.

214. Stewart JR, Kincaid OW, Titus JL. Right aortic arch: plain film diagnosis and significance. Am J Respir Crit Care Med 1966;97:377–89.

215. Stoica SC, Lockowandt U, Coulden R, et al. Double aortic arch masquerading as asthma for thirty years. Respiration 2002;69:92–5.

216. Dines DE, Arms RA, Bernatz PE, et al. Pulmonary arteriovenous fistulas. Mayo Clin Proc 1974;49:460–5.

217. Hughes JMB. Intrapulmonary shunts: coils to transplantation. J R Coll Physicians Lond 1994;28:247–53.

218. Shovlin CL, Letarte M. Hereditary haemorrhagic telangiectasia and

pulmonary arteriovenous malformations: issues in clinical management and review of pathogenic mechanisms. Thorax 1999;54:714–29.

219. Braverman IM, Keh A, Jacobson BS. Ultrastructure and three-dimensional organization of the telangiectases of hereditary hemorrhagic telangiectasia. J Invest Dermatol 1990;95:422–7.

220. Hodgson CH, Burchell HB, Good CA, et al. Hereditary hemorrhagic telagiectasia and pulmonary arteriovenous fistula. Survey of a large family. N Eng J Med 1959;261:625–36.

221. McAllister KA, Lennon F, Bowles-Biesecker B, et al. Genetic heterogeneity in hereditary haemorrhagic telangiectasia: possible correlation with clinical phenotype. J Med Genet 1994;31:927–32.

222. McAllister KA, Grogg KM, Johnson DW, et al. Endoglin, a TGF-beta binding protein of endothelial cells, is the gene for hereditary haemorrhagic telangiectasia type 1. Nat Genet 1994;8:345–51.

223. Mahmoud M, Borthwick GM, Hislop AA, et al. Endoglin and activin receptor-like-kinase 1 are co-expressed in the distal vessels of the lung: implications for two familial vascular dysplasias, HHT and PAH. Lab Invest 2008;89:15–25.

224. Vincent P, Plauchu H, Hazan J, et al. A third locus for hereditary haemorrhagic telangiectasia maps to chromosome 12q. Hum Mol Genet 1995;4:945–9.

225. Trell E, Johansson BW, Linell F, et al. Familial pulmonary hypertension and multiple abnormalities of large systemic arteries in Osler's disease. Am J Med 1972;53:50–63.

226. Trembath RC, Thomson JR, Machado RD, et al. Clinical and molecular genetic features of pulmonary hypertension in patients with hereditary hemorrhagic telangiectasia. N Engl J Med 2001;345:325–34.

227. Faughnan ME, Granton JT, Young LH. The pulmonary vascular complications of hereditary haemorrhagic telangiectasia. Eur Respir J 2009;33:1186–94.

228. Joshi M, Cole S, Knibbs D, et al. Pulmonary abnormalities in Klippel–Trenaunay syndrome – a histologic, ultrastructural, and immunocytochemical study. Chest 1992;102:1274–7.

229. Gianlupi A, Harper RW, Dwyre DM, et al. Recurrent pulmonary embolism associated with Klippel–Trenaunay–Weber syndrome. Chest 1999;115:1199–201.

230. Walder B, Kapelanski DP, Auger WR, et al. Successful pulmonary thromboendarterectomy in a patient with Klippel–Trenaunay syndrome. Chest 2000;117:1520–2.

231. Ulrich S, Fischler M, Walder B, et al. Klippel–Trenaunay syndrome with small vessel pulmonary arterial hypertension. Thorax 2005;60:971–3.

232. Morton R. Idiopathic arterial calcification in infancy. Histopathology 1978;2:423–32.

233. Gilbey LK, Girod CE. Blue rubber bleb nevus syndrome – Endobronchial involvement presenting as chronic cough. Chest 2003;124:760–3.

234. Allende DS, Rodriguez ER, Tan CD. Aortotracheal fistula secondary to bacterial aortitis. Arch Pathol Lab Med 2009;133:983–6.

Renal disease

235. Mahmoodi BK, Gansevoort RT, Veeger NJ, et al. Microalbuminuria and risk of venous thromboembolism. JAMA 2009;301:1790–7.

236. Rocker GM, Morgan AG, Pearson D, et al. Pulmonary vascular permeability to transferrin in the pulmonary oedema of renal failure. Thorax 1987;42:620–3.

237. Crosbie WA, Snowden S, Parsons V. Changes in lung capillary permeability in renal failure. BMJ 1972;4:388–90.

238. Amin M, Fawzy A, Hamid MA, et al. Pulmonary hypertension in patients with chronic renal failure – Role of parathyroid hormone and pulmonary artery calcifications. Chest 2003;124:2093–7.

239. Hayes JP, Wiggins J, Ward K, et al. Familial cryptogenic fibrosing pleuritis with Fanconi's syndrome (renal tubular acidosis): a new syndrome. Chest 1995;107:576–8.

Blood disorders

240. Entwistle CC, Fentem PH, Jacobs A. Red-cell aplasia with carcinoma of the bronchus. BMJ 1964;2:1504–6.

241. Williams AJ, Marsh J, Stableforth DE. Cryptogenic fibrosing alveolitis, chronic active hepatitis and autoimmune haemolytic anaemia in the same patient. Br J Dis Chest 1985;79:200–3.

242. Guilpain P, Montani D, Damaj G, et al. Pulmonary hypertension associated with myeloproliferative disorders: a retrospective study of ten cases. Respiration 2008;76:295–302.

243. Rausch PG, Herion JC. Pulmonary manifestations of Waldenström's macroglobulinaemia. Am J Hematol 1980;9:201–9.

244. Bombardieri S, Paoletti P, Ferri C, et al. Lung involvement in mixed cryoglobulinaemia. Am J Med 1979;66:748–56.

245. Nash JW, Ross P, Crowson AN, et al. The histopathologic spectrum of cryofibrinogenemia in four anatomic sites – Skin, lung, muscle, and kidney. Amer J Clin Pathol 2003;119:114–22.

246. Lai YP, Kuo PH, Wu HD, et al. A patient with haemoptysis, rapidly changing pulmonary infiltrates and left flank pain – primary antiphospholipid syndrome with pulmonary infarction, pulmonary

haemorrhage and left adrenal haemorrhage. Eur Respir J 1996;9:2184–7.

247. Pilling J, Cutaia M. The antiphospholipid antibody syndrome – A vascular disease with pulmonary manifestations. Chest 1997;112:1451–3.

248. Kerr JE, Poe R, Kramer Z. Antiphospholipid antibody syndrome presenting as a refractory noninflammatory pulmonary vasculopathy. Chest 1997;112:1707–10.

249. Greaves M. Antiphospholipid syndrome. J Clin Pathol 1997;50:973–4.

250. Heath D, Thompson IM. Bronchopulmonary anastomoses in sickle cell anaemia. Thorax 1969;24:232–8.

251. Oppenehimer EH, Esterly JR. Pulmonary changes in sickle cell disease. Am Rev Respir Dis 1971;103:858–9.

252. Collins FS, Orringer EP. Pulmonary hypertension and cor pulmonale in the sickle hemoglobinopathies. Am J Med 1982;73:814–21.

253. Athanasou NA, Hatton C, McGee JO, et al. Vascular occlusion and infarction in sickle cell crisis and the sickle chest syndrome. J Clin Pathol 1985;38:659–64.

254. Gray A, Anionwu EN, Davies SC, et al. Patterns of mortality in sickle cell disease in the United Kingdom. J Clin Pathol 1991;44:459–63.

255. Weil JV, Castro O, Malik AB, et al. Pathogenesis of lung disease in sickle hemoglobinopathies. Am Rev Respir Dis 1993;148:249–56.

256. Verresen D, Debacker W, Vanmeerbeeck J, et al. Spherocytosis and pulmonary hypertension: coincidental occurrence or causal relationship? Eur Respir J 1991;4:629–31.

258. Landing BH, Nadorra R, Hyman CB, et al. Pulmonary lesions of thalassemia major. In: Rosenberg HS, Bernstein J, editors. Respiratory and Alimentary Tract Diseases. Volume 11 Perspectives in Pediatric Pathology. Basel: Karger; 1987. p. 82–96.

259. Zaidi Y, Sivakumaran M, Graham C, et al. Fatal bone marrow embolism in a patient with sickle cell beta(+) thalassaemia. J Clin Pathol 1996;49:774–5.

260. Heller PG, Grinberg AR, Lencioni M, et al. Pulmonary hypertension in paroxysmal nocturnal hemoglobinuria. Chest 1992;102:642–3.

261. Emre U, Miller ST, Gutierez M, et al. Effect of transfusion in acute chest syndrome of sickle cell disease. J Pediatr 1995;127:901–4.

262. Siddiqui AK, Ahmed S. Pulmonary manifestations of sickle cell disease. Postgrad Med J 2003;79:384–90.

263. Gladwin MT, Sachdev V, Jison ML, et al. Pulmonary hypertension as a risk factor for death in patients with sickle cell disease. New Eng J Med 2004;350:886–95.

264. Aliyu ZY, Kato GJ, Taylor J, et al. Sickle cell disease and pulmonary hypertension in

Africa: a global perspective and review of epidemiology, pathophysiology, and management. Am J Hematol 2008;83:63–70.

265. Adedeji MO, Cespedes J, Allen K, et al. Pulmonary thrombotic arteriopathy in patients with sickle cell disease. Arch Pathol Lab Med 2001;125:1436–41.

266. Haque AK, Gokhale S, Rampy BA, et al. Pulmonary hypertension in sickle cell hemoglobinopathy: A clinicopathologic study of 20 cases. Hum Pathol 2002;33:1037–43.

267. McMahon LEC, Mark EJ, Shepard JAO. A 22-year-old man with a sickle cell crisis and sudden death – Sickle cell anemia. N Engl J Med 1997;337:1293–301.

268. Aessopos A, Stamatelos G, Skoumas V, et al. Pulmonary hypertension and right heart failure in patients with beta-thalassemia intermedia. Chest 1995;107:50–3.

269. Tai DYH, Wang YT, Lou J, et al. Lungs in thalassaemia major patients receiving regular transfusion. Eur Respir J 1996;9:1389–94.

270. Asakura S, Colby TV. Agnogenic myeloid metaplasia with extramedullary hematopoiesis and fibrosis in the lung – report of two cases. Chest 1994;105:1866–8.

271. Yusen RD, Kollef MH. Acute respiratory failure due to extramedullary hematopoiesis. Chest 1995;108:1170–2.

272. Coyne JD, Burton IE. Interstitial pneumonitis due to extramedullary haematopoiesis (EMH) in agnogenic myeloid metaplasia. Histopathology 1999;34:275–6.

273. Ozbudak IH, Shilo K, Hale S, et al. Alveolar airspace and pulmonary artery involvement by extramedullary hematopoiesis: a unique manifestation of myelofibrosis. Arch Pathol Lab Med 2008;132:99–103.

274. Doran HM, Sheppard MN, Collins PW, et al. Pathology of the lung in leukaemia and lymphoma – a study of 87 autopsies. Histopathology 1991;18:211–9.

275. Couderc LJ, Rain B, Desgranges C. Pulmonary fibrosis in association with human T cell lymphotropic virus type 1 (HTLV-1) infection. Respir Med 2000;94:1010.

276. Yoshioka R, Yamaguchi K, Yoshinaga T, et al. Pulmonary complications in patients with adult T-cell leukemia. Cancer 1985;55:2491–4.

277. Moskaluk CA, Pogrebniak HW, Pass HI, et al. Surgical pathology of the lung in chronic granulomatous disease. Am J Clin Pathol 1994;102:684–91.

278. Del GI, Iori AP, Mengarelli A, et al. Allogeneic stem cell transplant from HLA-identical sibling for chronic granulomatous disease and review of the literature. Ann Hematol 2003;82:189–92.

279. Moltyaner Y, Geerts WH, Chamberlain DW, et al. Underlying chronic granulomatous disease in a patient with bronchocentric granulomatosis. Thorax 2003;58:1096–8.

280. Levine S, Smith VV, Malone M, et al. Histopathological features of chronic granulomatous disease (CGD) in childhood. Histopathology 2005;47:508–16.

281. Yamauchi K, Shimamura K. Pulmonary fibrosis and sea-blue histiocyte infiltration in a patient with primary myelofibrosis. Eur Respir J 1995;8:1620–3.

282. Schmidt M, Dercken C, Loke O, et al. Pulmonary manifestation of systemic mast cell disease. Eur Resp J 2000;15:623–5.

283. Neild GH, Rodriguez-Justo M, Wall C, et al. Hyper-IgG$_4$ disease: report and characterisation of a new disease. BMC Med 2006;4:23.

284. Kojima M, Sipos B, Klapper W, et al. Autoimmune pancreatitis: frequency, IgG$_4$ expression, and clonality of T and B cells. Am J Surg Pathol 2007;31:521–8.

285. Zen Y, Fujii T, Sato Y, et al. Pathological classification of hepatic inflammatory pseudotumor with respect to IgG$_4$-related disease. Mod Pathol 2007;20:884–94.

285a. Dhobale S, Bedetti C, Killian P, et al. IgG$_4$ related sclerosing disease with multiple organ involvements and response to corticosteroid treatment. J Clin Rheumatol 2009;15:354–7.

285b. Zen Y, Inoue D, Kitao A, et al. IgG$_4$-related lung and pleural disease: a clinicopathologic study of 21 cases. Am J Surg Pathol 2009;33:1886–93.

285c. Shrestha B, Sekiguchi H, Colby TV, et al. Distinctive pulmonary histopathology with increased IgG$_4$-positive plasma cells in patients with autoimmune pancreatitis: Report of 6 and 12 cases with similar histopathology. Am J Surg Pathol 2009;33:1450–62.

286. Hirano K, Kawabe T, Komatsu Y, et al. High-rate pulmonary involvement in autoimmune pancreatitis. Intern Med J 2006;36:58–61.

287. Hamed G, Tsushima K, Yasuo M, et al. Inflammatory lesions of the lung, submandibular gland, bile duct and prostate in a patient with IgG$_4$-associated multifocal systemic fibrosclerosis. Respirology 2007;12:455–7.

288. Zen Y, Kitagawa S, Minato H, et al. IgG$_4$-positive plasma cells in inflammatory pseudotumor (plasma cell granuloma) of the lung. Hum Pathol 2005;36:710–7.

289. Yamashita K, Haga H, Kobashi Y, et al. Lung involvement in IgG$_4$-related lymphoplasmacytic vasculitis and interstitial fibrosis: report of 3 cases and review of the literature. Am J Surg Pathol 2008;32:1620–6.

290. Bateman AC, Deheragoda MG. IgG$_4$-related systemic sclerosing disease – an emerging and under-diagnosed condition. Histopathology 2009;55:373–83.

291. Reference removed in text.

292. Jais X, Ioos V, Jardim C, et al. Splenectomy and chronic thromboembolic pulmonary hypertension. Thorax 2005;60:1131–4.

Alimentary tract disorders

293. Allen CJ, Newhouse MT. Gastroesophageal reflux and chronic respiratory disease. Am Rev Respir Dis 1984;129:645–7.

294. Berrill WT, Fitzpatrick PF, Macleod WM, et al. Bird-fancier's lung and jejunal villous atrophy. Lancet 1975;2:1006–8.

295. Faux JA, Hendrick DJ, Amand F. Precipitins to different avian serum antigens in bird fanciers' lung and coeliac disease. Clin Allergy 1978;8:101–8.

296. Robinson TJ. Coeliac disease with farmers' lung. Br Med J 1976;1:745–6.

297. Edwards C, Williams A, Asquith P. Bronchopulmonary disease in coeliac patients. J Clin Pathol 1985;38 361–7.

298. Mahadeva R, Flower C, Shneerson J. Bronchiectasis in association with coeliac disease. Thorax 1998;53:527–9.

299. Wright PH, Menzies IS, Pounder RE, et al. Adult idiopathic pulmonary haemosiderosis and coeliac disease. Q J Med 1981;197:95–102.

300. Wright PH, Buxton-Thomas M, Keeling PWN, et al. Adult idiopathic pulmonary hemosiderosis: a comparison of lung function changes and the distribution of pulmonary disease in patients with and without coeliac disease. Br J Dis Chest 1983;77:282–92.

301. Bouros D, Panagou P, Rokkas T, et al. Bronchoalveolar lavage findings in a young adult with idiopathic pulmonary haemosiderosis and coeliac disease. Eur Respir J 1994;7:1009–12.

302. Hammami S, Ghedira Besbes L, Hadded S, et al. Co-occurrence pulmonary haemosiderosis with coeliac disease in child. Respiratory Medicine 2008;102:935–6.

303. Black H, Mendoza M, Murin S. Thoracic manifestations of inflammatory bowel disease. Chest 2007;131:524–32.

304. Butland RJA, Cole P, Citron KM, et al. Chronic bronchial suppuration and inflammatory bowel disease. Q J Med 1981;50:63–75.

305. Wilcox P, Miller R, Miller G, et al. Airway involvement in ulcerative colitis. Chest 1987;92:18–21.

306. Rickli H, Fretz C, Hoffman M, et al. Severe inflammatory upper airway stenosis in ulcerative colitis. Eur Respir J 1994;7:1899–902.

307. Vasishta S, Wood JB, McGinty F. Ulcerative tracheobronchitis years after colectomy for ulcerative colitis. Chest 1994;106:1279–81.

308. Lemann M, Messing B, D'Agay F, et al. Crohn's disease with respiratory tract involvement. Gut 1987;28:1669–72.

309. Camus P, Piard F, Ashcroft T, et al. The lung in inflammatory bowel disease. Medicine 1993;72:151–83.

310. Gibb WRG, Dhillon DP, Zilkha KJ, et al. Bronchiectasis with ulcerative colitis and myelopathy. Thorax 1987;42:155–6.

311. Higenbottam T, Cochrane GM, Clark TJH, et al. Bronchial disease in ulcerative colitis. Thorax 1980;35:581–5.

312. Eaton TE, Lambie N, Wells AU. Bronchiectasis following colectomy for Crohn's disease. Thorax 1998;53:529–31.

313. Spira A, Grossman R, Balter M. Large airway disease associated with inflammatory bowel disease. Chest 1998;113:1723–6.

314. Kayser K, Probst F, Gabius HJ, et al. Are there characteristic alterations of lung tissue associated with Crohn's disease? Pathol Res Pract 1990;186:485–90.

315. Swinburne CR, Jackson GJ, Cobden I, et al. Bronchiolitis obliterans organising pneumonia in a patient with ulcerative colitis. Thorax 1988;43:735–6.

316. Shneerson JM. Steroid-responsive alveolitis associated with ulcerative colitis. Chest 1992;101:585–6.

317. Dawson A, Gibbs AR, Anderson G. An unusual perilobular pattern of pulmonary interstitial fibrosis associated with Crohn's disease. Histopathology 1993;23:553–6.

318. Hotermans G, Benard A, Guenanen H, et al. Nongranulomatous interstitial lung disease in Crohn's disease. Eur Respir J 1996;9:380–2.

319. Beer TW, Edwards CW. Pulmonary nodules due to reactive systemic amyloidosis (AA) in Crohn's disease. Thorax 1993;48:1287–8.

320. Meadway J, Hills EA. Ulcerative colitis, colitic spondylitis and associated apical pulmonary fibrosis. Proc R Soc Med 1974;67:324–5.

321. Bradshaw MJ, Harvey RF, Burns-Cox CJ. Crohn's disease presenting as recurrent pulmonary edema. BMJ 1981;ii: 1437–8.

322. Hardarson S, Labrecque DR, Mitros FA, et al. Antineutrophil cytoplasmic antibody in inflammatory bowel and hepatobiliary diseases – high prevalence in ulcerative colitis, primary sclerosing cholangitis, and autoimmune hepatitis. Am J Clin Pathol 1993;99:277–81.

323. Vandenplas O, Casel S, Delos M, et al. Granulomatous bronchiolitis associated with Crohn's disease. Amer J Respir Crit Care Med 1998;158:1676–9.

324. Cohen M, Sahn SA. Bronchiectasis in systemic diseases. Chest 1999;116:1063–74.

325. Faller M, Gasser B, Massard G, et al. Pulmonary migratory infiltrates and pachypleuritis in a patient with Crohn's disease. Respiration 2000;67:459–63.

326. Casey MB, Tazelaar HD, Myers JL, et al. Noninfectious lung pathology in patients with Crohn's disease. Am J Surg Pathol 2003;27:213–9.

327. Shulimzon T, Rozenman J, Perelman M, et al. Necrotizing granulomata in the lung

preceding colonic involvement in 2 patients with Crohn's disease. Respiration 2007;74:698–702.

328. Wallert B, Colombel JF, Tonnel AB, et al. Evidence of lymphocyte alveolitis in Crohn's disease. Chest 1985;87:363–7.

329. Bonniere P, Wallaert B, Cortot A, et al. Latent pulmonary involvement in Crohn's disease: biological, functional, bronchoalveolar lavage and scintigraphic studies. Gut 1986;27:919–25.

330. Tzanakis N, Bouros D, Samiou M, et al. Lung function in patients with inflammatory bowel disease. Respir Med 1998;92:516–22.

331. Moles KW, Varghese G, Hayes JR. Pulmonary involvement in ulcerative colitis. Br J Dis Chest 1988;82:79–83.

332. Kraft SC, Earle RH, Roesler M, et al. Unexplained bronchopulmonary disease with inflammatory bowel disease. Arch Intern Med 1976;136:454–9.

333. Trow TK, Morris DG, Miller CR, et al. Granulomatous bronchiolitis of Crohn's disease successfully treated with inhaled budesonide. Thorax 2009;64:546–7.

334. Lamblin C, Copin MC, Billaut C, et al. Acute respiratory failure due to tracheobronchial involvement in Crohn's disease. Eur Respir J 1996;9:2176–8.

335. Raj AA, Birring SS, Green R, et al. Prevalence of inflammatory bowel disease in patients with airways disease. Respir Med 2008;102:780–5.

336. Golpe R, Mateos A, PerezValcarcel J, et al. Multiple pulmonary nodules in a patient with Crohn's disease. Respiration 2003;70:306–9.

337. Isenberg JI, Goldstein H, Korn AS, et al. Pulmonary vasculitis – an uncommon complication of ulcerative colitis. N Engl J Med 1968;279:1376–7.

338. Whipple GH. A hitherto undescribed disease characterised anatomically by deposits of fat and fatty acids in the intestinal and mesenteric lymphatic tissues. Bull Johns Hopkins Hospital 1907;18:382.

339. Bayless TM, Knox DL. Whipple's disease: a multisystemic infection. N Engl J Med 1979;300:920–1.

340. Relman DA, Schmidt TM, MacDermott RP, et al. Identification of the uncultured bacillus of Whipple's disease. N Engl J Med 1992;327:293–301.

341. Eck M, Kreipe H, Harmsen D, et al. Invasion and destruction of mucosal plasma cells by *Tropheryma whippelii*. Hum Pathol 1997;28:1424–8.

342. Fleming JL, Weisner RH, Shorter RG. Whipple's disease: clinical, biochemical, and histopathologic features and assessment of treatment in 29 patients. Mayo Clin Proc 1988;63:539–51.

343. Baisden BL, Lepidi H, Raoult D, et al. Diagnosis of Whipple disease by immunohistochemical analysis: a sensitive and specific method for the detection of

Tropheryma whipplei (the Whipple bacillus) in paraffin-embedded tissue. Am J Clin Pathol 2002;118:742–8.

344. Marth T, Schneider T. Whipple disease. Curr Opin Gastroenterol 2008;24: 141–8.

345. Schneider T, Moos V, Loddenkemper C, et al. Whipple's disease: new aspects of pathogenesis and treatment. Lancet Infect Dis 2008;8:179–90.

346. Winberg CD, Rose ME, Rappaport H. Whipple's disease of the lung. Am J Med 1978;65:873–80.

347. Kelly CA, Egan M, Rawlinson J. Whipple's disease presenting with lung involvement. Thorax 1996;51:343–4.

348. Riemer H, Hainz R, Stain C, et al. Severe pulmonary hypertension reversed by antibiotics in a patient with Whipple's disease. Thorax 1997;52:1014–5.

349. Symmons DPM, Shepherd AN, Boardman PL, et al. Pulmonary manifestations of Whipple's disease. Q J Med 1985;56:497–504.

350. MacDermott RP, Shepard JAO, GraemeCook FM, et al. A 59-year-old man with anorexia, weight loss, and a mediastinal mass – Whipple's disease involving the small intestine and mesenteric and mediastinal lymph nodes. N Engl J Med 1997;337:1612–9.

351. James TN, Bulkley BH. Whipple bacilli within the tunica media of pulmonary arteries. Chest 1984;86:454–8.

352. Herve P, Lebrec D, Brenot F, et al. Pulmonary vascular disorders in portal hypertension. Eur Resp J 1998;11:1153–66.

353. Mantz FA, Craige E. Portal axis thrombosis with spontaneous portacaval shunt and resultant cor pulmonale. Arch Pathol 1951;52:91–7.

354. McDonnell PJ, Toye PA, Hutchins GM. Primary pulmonary hypertension in cirrhosis: are they related? Am Rev Respir Dis 1983;127:437–41.

355. Lockhart A. Pulmonary arterial hypertension in portal hypertension. Clin Gastroenterol 1985;14:123–38.

356. Robalina BD, Moodie DS. Association between primary pulmonary hypertension and portal hypertension: analysis of its pathophysiology and clinical laboratory and hemodynamic manifestations. J Am Coll Cardiol 1991;17II:492–8.

357. Rodriguez-Roisin R, Krowka MJ, Herve P, et al. Pulmonary–hepatic vascular disorders (PHD). Eur Respir J 2004;24:861–80.

358. Stratakos G, Malagari K, Broutzos E, et al. Dyspnoea and cyanosis in a cirrhotic patient – diagnosis: hepatopulmonary syndrome with diffuse (Type I) intrapulmonary vascular dilatations. Eur Resp J 2002;19:780–3.

359. Rydell R, Hoffbauer FW. Multiple pulmonary arteriovenous fistulas in juvenile cirrhosis. Am J Med 1956;21:450–60.

360. Berthelot P, Walker JG, Sherlock S, et al. Arterial changes in the lungs in cirrhosis of the liver – lung spider nevi. N Engl J Med 1966;274:291–8.

361. Stanley NN, Williams AJ, Dewar CA, et al. Hypoxia and hydrothoraces in a case of liver cirrhosis: correlation of physiological, radiographic, scintigraphic, and pathological findings. Thorax 1977;32:457–71.

362. Andrivet P, Cadranel J, Housset B, et al. Mechanism of impaired arterial oxygenation in patients with liver cirrhosis and severe respiratory insufficiency. Chest 1993;103:500–7.

363. Rodriguez-Roisin R, Roca J, Agusti AG, et al. Gas exchange and pulmonary vascular reactivity in patients with liver cirrhosis. Am Rev Respir Dis 1987;135:1085–92.

364. Krowka MJ, Cortese DA. Hepatopulmonary syndrome – current concepts in diagnostic and therapeutic considerations. Chest 1994;105:1528–37.

366. Stanley NN, Fox RA, Whimster WF, et al. Primary biliary cirrhosis or sarcoidosis – or both. N Engl J Med 1972;287:1282–4.

367. Fagan EA, Moore-Gillon JC, Turner-Warwick M. Multiorgan granulomas and mitochondrial antibodies. N Engl J Med 1983;308:572–5.

368. Hughes P, McGavin CR. Sarcoidosis and primary biliary cirrhosis with co-existing myositis. Thorax 1997;52:201–2.

369. Weissman E, Becker N. Interstitial lung disease in primary biliary cirrhosis. Am J Med Sci 1983;285:21–7.

370. Wallace JG, Tong MJ, Ueki BH, et al. Pulmonary involvement in primary biliary cirrhosis. J Clin Gastroenterol 1987;9:431–5.

371. Chatte G, Streichenberger N, Boillot O, et al. Lymphocytic bronchitis/bronchiolitis in a patient with primary biliary cirrhosis. Eur Respir J 1995;8:176–9.

372. Tsianos EV, Hoofnagle JH, Fox PC, et al. Sjögren's syndrome in patients with primary biliary cirrhosis. Hepatology 1990;11:730–4.

373. Golding PL, Smith M, Williams R. Multisystem involvement in chronic liver disease: studies on the incidence and pathogenesis. Am J Med 1973;55:772–82.

374. Johnson MA, Spiteri MA, Epstein U, et al. Subclinical alveolitis in patients with primary biliary cirrhosis. Eur Respir J 1988;1:246p.

375. Meliconi R, Andreone P, Fasano L, et al. Incidence of hepatitis C virus infection in Italian patients with idiopathic pulmonary fibrosis. Thorax 1996;51:315–7.

376. Turner-Warwick M. Fibrosing alveolitis and chronic liver disease. Q J Med 1968;37:133.

377. Kayser K, Paul K, Feist D. et al. Alteration of the lung parenchyma associated with autoimmune hepatitis. Virchows Arch A Pathol Anat Histopathol 1991;419:153–7.

378. Helman CA, Keeton GR, Benatar SR. Lymphoid interstitial pneumonia with associated chronic active hepatitis and renal tubular acidosis. Am Rev Respir Dis 1977;115:161–4.

379. Kagalwalla AF, Rahman A, Taleb A, et al. Pulmonary hemorrhage in association with autoimmune chronic active hepatitis. Chest 1993;103:634–6.

380. Glasgow JFG, Lynch MJ, Herez A, et al. Alpha-1 antitrypsin deficiency in association with both cirrhosis and chronic obstructive lung disease in two sibs. Am J Med 1973;54:181.

381. Bachofen M, Weibel ER. Basic pattern of tissue repair in human lungs following unspecific injury. Chest 1974;65:14s–9s.

382. Greer SE, Burchard KW. Acute pancreatitis and critical illness. Chest 2009;136:1413–9.

Neuromuscular disease

383. Editorial. Neurogenic pulmonary oedema. Lancet 1985;1:1430–1.

384. Wray NP, Nicotra MB. Pathogenesis of neurogenic pulmonary oedema. Am Rev Respir Dis 1978;118:783–6.

385. Carlson RW, Schaeffer RC, Michaels SG, et al. Pulmonary oedema following intracranial haemorrhage. Chest 1979;75:731–4.

386. Castro M, Shepherd CW, Gomez MR, et al. Pulmonary tuberous sclerosis. Chest 1995;107:189–95.

387. Shepherd CW, Gomez MR, Lie JT, et al. Causes of death in patients with tuberous sclerosis. Mayo Clin Proc 1991;66:792–6.

388. Franz DN, Brody A, Meyer C, et al. Mutational and radiographic analysis of pulmonary disease consistent with lymphangioleiomyomatosis and micronodular pneumocyte hyperplasia in women with tuberous sclerosis. Am J Respir Crit Care Med 2001;164:661–8.

389. Moss J, Avila NA, Barnes PM, et al. Prevalence and clinical characteristics of lymphangioleiomyomatosis (LAM) in patients with tuberous sclerosis complex. Am J Respir Crit Care Med 2001;164:669–71.

390. Chorianopoulos D, Stratakos G. Lymphangioleiomyomatosis and tuberous sclerosis complex. Lung 2008;186:197–207.

391. Burrows NJ, Johnson SR. Pulmonary artery aneurysm and tuberous sclerosis. Thorax 2004;59:86.

392. Chu SC, Horiba K, Usuki J, et al. Comprehensive evaluation of 35 patients with lymphangioleiomyomatosis. Chest 1999;115:1041–52.

393. Wu K, Tazelaar HD. Pulmonary angiomyolipoma and multifocal micronodular pneumocyte hyperplasia associated with tuberous sclerosis. Hum Pathol 1999;30:1266–8.

394. Henske EP, Ao X, Short MP, et al. Frequent progesterone receptor immunoreactivity in tuberous sclerosis-associated renal angiomyolipomas. Modern Pathol 1998;11:665–8.

395. Flieder DB, Travis WD. Clear cell 'Sugar' tumor of the lung: Association with lymphangioleiomyomatosis and multifocal micronodular pneumocyte hyperplasia in a patient with tuberous sclerosis. Am J Surg Pathol 1997;21:1242–7.

396. Bonetti F, Pea M, Martignoni G, et al. Clear cell ('sugar') tumor of the lung is a lesion strictly related to angiomyolipoma – the concept of a family of lesions characterized by the presence of the perivascular epithelioid cells (PEC). Pathology 1995;26:230–6.

397. Folpe AL, Kwiatkowski DJ. Perivascular epithelioid cell neoplasms: pathology and pathogenesis. Human Pathology 2010;41:1–15.

398. Stewart DR, Cogan JD, Kramer MR, et al. Is pulmonary arterial hypertension in neurofibromatosis type 1 secondary to a plexogenic arteriopathy? Chest 2007;132:798–808.

399. Davies PDB. Diffuse pulmonary involvement in von Recklinghausen's disease: a new syndrome. Thorax 1963;18:198.

400. Israel-Asselain R, Chebat J, Sors C, et al. Diffuse interstitial pulmonary fibrosis in a mother and son with von Recklinghausen's disease. Thorax 1965;20:153–7.

401. Massaro D, Katz S. Fibrosing alveolitis: its occurrence, roentgenographic, and pathologic features in von Recklinghausen's neurofibromatosis. Am Rev Respir Dis 1966;93:934–42.

402. Webb WR, Goodman PC. Fibrosing alveolitis in patients with neurofibromatosis. Radiology 1977;122:289–93.

403. De Scheerder I, Elinck W, Van Renterghem D, et al. Desquamative interstitial pneumonia and scar cancer of the lung complicating generalised neurofibromatosis. Eur J Respir Dis 1984;65:623–6.

404. Ryu JH, Parambil JG, McGrann PS, et al. Lack of evidence for an association between neurofibromatosis and pulmonary fibrosis. Chest 2005;128:2381–6.

Metabolic and endocrine disorders

405. Yamane T, Date T, Tokuda M, et al. Hypoxemia in inferior pulmonary veins in supine position is dependent on obesity. Am J Respir Crit Care Med 2008;178:295–9.

405a. Rogliani P, Curradi G, Mura M, et al. Metabolic syndrome and risk of pulmonary involvement. Respiratory Medicine 2010;104:47–51

405b. Paek YJ, Jung KS, Hwang YI, et al. Association between low pulmonary function and metabolic risk factors in

Korean adults: the Korean National Health and Nutrition Survey. Metabolism 2010;In Press

406. McClean KM, Kee F, Young IS, et al. Obesity and the lung: 1. Epidemiology. Thorax 2008:63:649–54.

407. Sin DD, Sutherland ER. Obesity and the lung: 4. Obesity and asthma. Thorax 2008;63:1018–23.

408. Haque AK, Gadre S, Taylor J, et al. Pulmonary and cardiovascular complications of obesity: an autopsy study of 76 obese subjects. Arch Pathol Lab Med 2008;132:1397–404.

408a. Hughes GR. Thrombosis, abortion, cerebral disease, and the lupus anticoagulant. Br Med J (Clin Res Ed) 1983;287:1088–89.

408b. Espinosa G, Cervera R, Font J, et al. The lung in the antiphospholipid syndrome. Ann Rheum Dis 2002;61:195–8.

409. Adams JS, Sharma OP, Glacad MA, et al. Metabolism of 25-hydroxyvitamin D_3 by cultured pulmonary alveolar macrophages in sarcoidosis. J Clin Invest 1983;72:1856–60.

410. Bell NH, Stern PH, Pantzer E, et al. Evidence that increased circulating 1-alpha, 25-dihydroxyvitamin D is the probable cause of abnormal calcium metabolism in sarcoidosis. J Clin Invest 1979;64:218–25.

411. Papapoulos SE, Frahjer LJ, Sandler LM, et al. 1,25-dihydroxycholecalciferol in the pathogenesis of the hypercalcemia of sarcoidosis. Lancet 1979;ii:627–30.

412. Sharma OP. Vitamin D, calcium, and sarcoidosis. Chest 1996;109:535–9.

413. Virchow R. Kalk-Metastasen. Virchows Arch A Pathol Anat Histopathol 1855;8:103–13.

414. Bloodworth J, Tomashefski JF. Localised pulmonary metastatic calcification associated with pulmonary artery obstruction. Thorax 1992;47:174–8.

415. Mulligan RM. Metastatic calcification. Arch Pathol 1947;43:177–230.

416. Kaltreider HB, Baum GL, Bogaty G, et al. So-called "metastatic" calcification of the lung. Am J Med 1969;46:189–96.

417. Hartman TE, Muller NL, Primack SL, et al. Metastatic pulmonary calcification in patients with hypercalcaemia. AJR 1994;162:799–802.

418. Holmes F, Harlan J, Felt S, et al. Pulmonary oedema in hypercalcaemic crisis. Lancet 1974;1:311–2.

419. Wright J, Jones E. Diffuse calcification of the airways. Modern Pathol 2001;14:717–9.

420. Celli BR, Rubinow A, Cohen AS, et al. Patterns of pulmonary involvement in systemic amyloidosis. Chest 1978;74:543–7.

421. Smith RRL, Hutchins GM, Moore GW, et al. Type and distribution of pulmonary parenchymal and vascular amyloid: correlation with cardiac amyloidosis. Am J Med 1979;66:96–104.

422. Ishi T, Hosoda Y, Ikegami N, et al. Senile amyloid deposition. J Pathol 1983;139:1–22.

423. Theaker JM, Raine AEG, Rainey AJ, et al. Systemic amyloidosis of β_2-microglobulin type: a complication of long term haemodialysis. J Clin Pathol 1987;40:1247–51.

424. Planes C, Kleinknecht D, Brauner M, et al. Diffuse interstitial lung disease due to AA amyloidosis. Thorax 1992;47:323–4.

425. Cordier JF, Loire R, Brune J. Amyloidosis of the lower respiratory tract. Chest 1986;90:827–31.

426. Utz JP, Swensen SJ, Gertz MA. Pulmonary amyloidosis. The Mayo Clinic experience from 1980 to 1993. Ann Intern Med 1996;124:407–13.

426a. Roden AC, Aubry MC, Zhang K, et al. Nodular senile pulmonary amyloidosis: a unique case confirmed by immunohistochemistry, mass spectrometry, and genetic study. Human Pathology 2010 Jul;41(7):1040–7.

427. Gal R, Korzets A, Schwartz A, et al. Systemic distribution of beta(2)-microglobulin-derived amyloidosis in patients who undergo long-term hemodialysis – report of seven cases and review of the literature. Arch Pathol Lab Med 1994;118:718–21.

428. Kavuru MS, Adamo JP, Ahmad M, et al. Amyloidosis and pleural disease. Chest 1990;98:20–3.

429. Gillmore JD, Hawkins PN. Amyloidosis and the respiratory tract. Thorax 1999;54:444–51.

430. Shah PL, Gillmore JD, Copley SJ, et al. The importance of complete screening for amyloid fibril type and systemic disease in patients with amyloidosis in the respiratory tract. Sarcoidosis Vasc Diffuse Lung Dis 2002;19:134–42.

431. Kijner CH, Yousem SA. Systemic light chain deposition disease presenting as multiple pulmonary nodules. A case report and review of the literature. Am J Surg Pathol 1988;12:405–13.

432. Shiue ST, McNally DP. Pulmonary hypertension from prominent vascular involvement in diffuse amyloidosis. Arch Intern Med 1988;148:687–9.

433. Johnson WJ, Lie JT. Pulmonary hypertension and familial Mediterranean fever – a previously unrecognized association. Mayo Clin Proc 1991;66:919–25.

434. Nicholson AG, Wells AU, Hooper J, et al. Successful treatment of endogenous lipoid pneumonia due to Niemann–Pick type B disease with whole-lung lavage. Amer J Respir Crit Care Med 2002;165:128–31.

435. Wolsen AH. Pulmonary findings in Gaucher's disease. AJR 1975;123:712–5.

436. Schneider EL, Epstein CJ, Kaback MJ, et al. Severe pulmonary involvement in adult Gaucher's disease: report of three cases and review of the literature. Am J Med 1977;63:475–80.

437. Smith RRL, Hutchins GM, Sack GH, et al. Unusual cardiac, renal and pulmonary involvement in Gaucher's disease. Interstitial glucocerebroside accumulation, pulmonary hypertension and fatal bone marrow embolization. Am J Med 1978;65:352–9.

438. Morimura Y, Hojo H, Abe M, et al. Gaucher's disease, type i (adult type), with massive involvement of the kidneys and lungs. Virchows Arch 1994;425:537–40.

439. Santamaria F, Parenti G, Guidi G, et al. Pulmonary manifestations of Gaucher disease: an increased risk for L444P homozygotes? Am J Respir Crit Care Med 1998;157:985–9.

440. Amir G, Ron N. Pulmonary pathology in Gaucher's disease. Hum Pathol 1999;30:666–70.

441. Minai OA, Sullivan EJ, Stoller JK. Pulmonary involvement in Niemann–Pick disease: Case report and literature review. Resp Med 2000;94:1241–51.

442. Elleder M, Houstkova H, Zeman J, et al. Pulmonary storage with emphysema as a sign of Niemann–Pick type C2 disease (Second complementation group). Report of a case. Virchows Archiv 2001;439:206–11.

443. Smith P, Heath D, Rodgers B, et al. Pulmonary vasculature in Fabry's disease. Histopathology 1991;19:567–9.

444. Brown LK, Miller A, Bhuptani A, et al. Pulmonary involvement in Fabry disease. Amer J Respir Crit Care Med 1997;155:1004–10.

445. Niggemann B, Rebien W, Rahn W, et al. Asymptomatic pulmonary involvement in two children with Niemann–Pick disease type B. Respiration 1994;61:55–7.

446. Nicholson AG, Florio R, Hansell DM, et al. Pulmonary involvement by Niemann–Pick disease. A report of six cases. Histopathology 2006;48:596–603.

447. Takahashi K, Hakozaki H, Kojima M. Idiopathic pulmonary ceroidosis. Acta Pathol Jpn 1978;28:301–11.

448. Sastre J, Renedo G, Mangado NG, et al. Pulmonary ceroidosis. Chest 1987;91:281–3.

449. Hermansky F, Pudlak P. Albinism associated with hemorrhagic diathesis and unusual pigmented cells in the bone marrow: report of two cases with histochemical studies. Blood 1959;14:162–9.

450. Gahl WA, Brantly M, Kaiser Kupfer MI, et al. Genetic defects and clinical characteristics of patients with a form of oculocutaneous albinism (Hermansky–Pudlak syndrome). N Engl J Med 1998;338:1258–64.

451. Garay SM, Gardella JE, Fazzini EP, et al. Hermansky–Pudlak syndrome. Pulmonary manifestations of a ceroid storage disorder. Am J Med 1979;66:737–47.

452. Luisetti M, Fiocca R, Pozzi E, et al. The Hermansky–Pudlak syndrome. A case with macrophage–neutrophil alveolitis. Eur J Respir Dis 1986;68:301–5.

453. Shinella RA, Greco MA, Garay SM. Hermansky–Pudlak syndrome: a clinicopathologic study. Hum Pathol 1985;16:366–76.

454. White DA, Walker Smith GJ, Cooper JAD, et al. Hermansky–Pudlak syndrome and interstitial lung disease: a report of a case with lavage findings. Am Rev Respir Dis 1984;130:138–41.

455. Reynolds SP, Davies BH, Gibbs AR. Diffuse pulmonary fibrosis and the Hermansky–Pudlak syndrome: clinical course and postmortem findings. Thorax 1994;49:617–8.

456. Wockel W, Sultz J. Diffuse pulmonary fibrosis and Hermansky–Pudlak syndrome. Thorax 1995;50:591.

457. Nakatani Y, Nakamura N, Sano J, et al. Interstitial pneumonia in Hermansky–Pudlak syndrome: significance of florid foamy swelling/degeneration (giant lamellar body degeneration) of type-2 pneumocytes. Virchows Archiv 2000;437:304–13.

458. Walker PP, Rose E, Williams JG. Upper airways abnormalities and tracheal problems in Morquio's disease. Thorax 2003;58:458–9.

459. Reinila A. Perivascular xanthogranulomatosis in the lungs of diabetic patients. Arch Pathol Lab Med 1976;100:542–3.

460. Duboucher C, Escamilla R, Rocchiccioli F, et al. Pulmonary lipogranulomatosis due to excessive consumption of apples. Chest 1986;90:611–2.

461. Rosier RN, Rosenberg AE, Hornicek FJ. A 41-year-old man with multiple bony lesions and adjacent soft-tissue masses – Erdheim–Chester disease involving multiple bones, with pathologic fractures and soft-tissue masses. N Engl J Med 2000;342:875–83.

462. AlQuran S, Reith J, Bradley J, et al. Erdheim–Chester disease: Case report, PCR-based analysis of clonality, and review of literature. Modern Pathol 2002;15:666–72.

463. Veyssier-Belot C, Cacoub P, Caparros-Lefebvre D, et al. Erdheim–Chester disease. Clinical and radiologic characteristics of 59 cases. Medicine (Baltimore) 1996;75:157–69.

464. Chetritt J, Paradis V, Dargere D, et al. Chester–Erdheim disease: A neoplastic disorder. Hum Pathol 1999;30:1093–6.

465. Kambouchner M, Colby TV, Domenge C, et al. Erdheim–Chester disease with prominent pulmonary involvement associated with eosinophilic granuloma of mandibular bone. Histopathology 1997;30:353–8.

466. Devouassoux G, Lantuejoul S, Chatelain P, et al. Erdheim–Chester disease: A primary macrophage cell disorder. Am J Respir Crit Care Med 1998;157:650–3.

467. Egan AJM, Boardman LA, Tazelaar HD, et al. Erdheim–Chester disease – clinical, radiologic, and histopathologic findings in five patients with interstitial lung disease. Am J Surg Pathol 1999;23:17–26.

468. Rush WL, Andriko JAW, GalateauSalle F, et al. Pulmonary pathology of Erdheim–Chester disease. Modern Pathol 2000;13:747–54.

469. Allen TC, Chevez-Barrios P, Shetlar DJ, et al. Pulmonary and ophthalmic involvement with Erdheim–Chester disease: a case report and review of the literature. Arch Pathol Lab Med 2004;128:1428–31.

470. Brower AC, Worsham GF, Dudley AH. Erdheim–Chester disease: a distinct lipoidosis or part of the spectrum of histiocytosis? Radiology 1984;151:35–8.

471. Athanasou NA, Barbatis C. Erdheim–Chester disease with epiphyseal and systemic disease. J Clin Pathol 1993;46:481–2.

472. Bourke SC, Nicholson AG, Gibson GJ. Erdheim–Chester disease: pulmonary infiltration responding to cyclophosphamide and prednisolone. Thorax 2003;58:1004–5.

473. Foucar E, Rosai J, Dorfman R. Sinus histiocytosis with massive lymphadenopathy (Rosai–Dorfman disease): review of the entity. Semin Diagn Pathol 1990;7:19–73.

474. Wright DH, Richards DB. Sinus histiocytosis with massive lymphadenopathy (Rosai–Dorfman disease): report of a case with widespread nodal and extra nodal dissemination. Histopathology 1981;5:697–709.

475. Buchino JJ, Byrd RP, Kmetz DR. Disseminated sinus histiocytosis with massive lymphadenopathy: its pathologic aspects. Arch Pathol Lab Med 1982;106:13–6.

476. Ohori NP, Yu J, Landreneau RJ, et al. Rosai–Dorfman disease of the pleura: a rare extranodal presentation. Hum Pathol 2003;34:1210–1.

477. Ali A, Mackay D. Rosai–Dorfman disease of the lung. Thorax 2009;64:908–9.

477a. Cartin-Ceba R, Golbin JM, Yi ES, et al. Intrathoracic manifestations of Rosai-Dorfman disease. Resp Med 2010;104:1344–49.

478. Marvisi M, Brianti M, Marani G, et al. Hyperthyroidism and pulmonary hypertension. Resp Med 2002;96:215–20.

479. Gottehrer A, Roa J, Stanford GG, et al. Hypothyroidism and pleural effusion. Chest 1990;98:1130–2.

480. Naeye RL. Capillary and venous lesions in myxedema. Lab Invest 1963;12:465–70.

481. Sandler M, Bunn AE, Stewart RI. Cross-section study of pulmonary function in patients with insulin-dependent diabetes mellitus. Am Rev Respir Dis 1987;135:223–9.

482. Guazzi M, Brambilla R, DeVita S, et al. Diabetes worsens pulmonary diffusion in heart failure, and insulin counteracts this effect. Am J Respir Crit Care Med 2002;166:978–82.

483. Vracko R, Thorning D, Huang TW. Basal lamina of alveolar epithelium and capillaries: quantitative changes with aging and diabetes mellitus. Am Rev Respir Dis 1979;120:973–83.

484. Sandler M. Is the lung a target organ in diabetes mellitus? Arch Intern Med 1990;150:1385–8.

485. Watanabe K, Senju S, Toyoshima H, et al. Thickness of the basement membrane of bronchial epithelial cells in lung diseases as determined by transbronchial biopsy. Resp Med 1997;91:406–10.

486. Weynand B, Jonckheere A, Frans A, et al. Diabetes mellitus induces a thickening of the pulmonary basal lamina. Respiration 1999;66:14–9.

487. Minette P, Buysschaert M, Rahier J, et al. Pulmonary gas exchange in life-long nonsmoking patients with diabetes mellitus. Respiration 1999;66:20–4.

488. Farina J, Furio V, Fernandezacenero MJ, et al. Nodular fibrosis of the lung in diabetes mellitus. Virchows Arch 1995;427:61–3.

489. Sugahara K, Ushijima K, Morioka T, et al. Studies of the lung in diabetes mellitus. I. Ultrastructural studies of the lungs in alloxan-induced diabetic rats. Virchows Arch A Pathol Anat Histopathol 1981;390:313–24.

490. Kida K, Utsuyama M, Thurlbeck WM. Changes in lung morphologic features and elasticity caused by streptozotocin-induced diabetes mellitus in growing rats. Am Rev Respir Dis 1983;128:125–31.

491. Ofulue AF, Kida K, Thurlbeck WM. Experimental diabetes and the lung. I. Changes in growth, morphometry, and biochemistry. Am Rev Respir Dis 1988;137:162–6.

492. Ofulue AF, Thurlbeck WM. Experimental diabetes and the lung. II. In vivo connective tissue metabolism. Am Rev Respir Dis 1988;138:284–9.

493. Popov D, Simionescu M. Alterations of lung structure in experimental diabetes, and diabetes associated with hyperlipidaemia in hamsters. Eur Resp J 1997;10:1850–8.

494. Shields PA, Jeffery PK. The combined effects of vitamin A-deficiency and cigarette smoke on rat tracheal epithelium. Br J Exp Pathol 1987;68:705–17.

495. Hennekens CH, Buring JE, Manson JE, et al. Lack of effect of long-term supplementation with beta carotene on the incidence of malignant neoplasms and cardiovascular disease. N Engl J Med 1996;334:1145–9.

496. Omenn GS, Goodman GE, Thornquist MD, et al. Effects of a combination of beta

carotene and vitamin A on lung cancer and cardiovascular disease. N Engl J Med 1996;334:1150–5.

Skin disease

497. Pipkin CA, Lio PA. Cutaneous manifestations of internal malignancies: an overview. Dermatol Clin 2008;26:1–15, vii.

498. Moore RL, Devere TS. Epidermal manifestations of internal malignancy. Dermatol Clin 2008;26:17–29, vii.

499. de Carvalho CRR, Amato MBP, da Silva LMMF, et al. Obstructive respiratory failure in cicatricial pemphigoid. Thorax 1989;44:601–2.

500. Osmanski JP, Fraire AE, Schaefer OP. Necrotizing tracheobronchitis with progressive airflow obstruction associated with paraneoplastic pemphigus. Chest 1997;112:1704–7.

501. Takimoto CH, Warnock M, Golden JA. Sweet's syndrome with lung involvement. Am Rev Respir Dis 1991;143:177–9.

502. Lazarus AA, McMillan M, Miramadi A. Pulmonary involvement in Sweet's syndrome (acute febrile neutrophilic dermatosis). Preleukemic and leukemic phases of acute myelogenous leukemia. Chest 1986;90:922–4.

503. Thurnheer R, Stammberger U, Hailemariam S, et al. Bronchial manifestation of acute febrile neutrophilic dermatosis (Sweet's syndrome). Eur Resp J 1998;11:978–80.

504. Kruger S, Piroth W, Takyi BA, et al. Multiple aseptic pulmonary nodules with central necrosis in association with pyoderma gangrenosum. Chest 2001;119:977–8.

505. Birt AR, Hogg GR, Dube WJ. Hereditary multiple fibrofolliculomas with trichodiscomas and acrochordons. Arch Dermatol 1977;113:1674–7.

506. Khoo SK, Bradley M, Wong FK, et al. Birt–Hogg–Dube syndrome: mapping of a novel hereditary neoplasia gene to chromosome 17p12-q11.2. Oncogene 2001;20:5239–42.

507. Painter JN, Tapanainen H, Somer M, et al. A 4-bp deletion in the Birt–Hogg–Dube gene (FLCN) causes dominantly inherited spontaneous pneumothorax. Am J Hum Genet 2005;76:522–7.

508. Graham RB, Nolasco M, Peterlin B, et al. Nonsense mutations in folliculin presenting as isolated familial spontaneous pneumothorax in adults. Am J Respir Crit Care Med 2005;172:39–44.

509. Sundaram S, Tasker AD, Morrell NW. Familial spontaneous pneumothorax and lung cysts due to a Folliculin exon 10 mutation. Eur Respir J 2009;33:1510–2.

510. Butnor KJ, Guinee DG, Jr. Pleuropulmonary pathology of Birt–Hogg–Dube syndrome. Am J Surg Pathol 2006;30:395–9.

511. Koga S, Furuya M, Takahashi Y, et al. Lung cysts in Birt–Hogg–Dube syndrome: histopathological characteristics and aberrant sequence repeats. Pathol Int 2009;59:720–8.

Gynaecological and obstetric conditions

512. Meigs JV, Cass JW. Fibroma of the ovary with ascites and hydrothorax. Am J Obstet Gynecol 1937;33:249–67.

513. Meigs JV. Fibroma of the ovary with ascites and hydrothorax – Meigs' syndrome. Am J Obstet Gynecol 1954;67:962.

514. Meigs JV. Pelvic tumours other than fibromas of the ovary with ascites and hydrothorax. Obstet Gynecol 1954;3:471.

515. Parry D, Hextall A, Robinson VP, et al. Pregnancy following a single lung transplant. Thorax 1996;51:1162–4.

516. Phelan JP. Pulmonary edema in obstetrics. Obstet Gynecol Clin North Am 1991;18:319–31.

517. Sibai BM, Mabie WC. Hemodynamics of preeclampsia. Clin Perinatol 1991;18:727–47.

518. Flieder DB, Moran CA, Travis WD, et al. Pleuro-pulmonary endometriosis and pulmonary ectopic deciduosis: A clinicopathologic and immunohistochemical study of 10 cases with emphasis on diagnostic pitfalls. Hum Pathol 1998;29:1495–503.

519. Maurer RR, Schall JA, Mendex FLJ. Chronic recurring spontaneous pneumothorax due to endometriosis of the diaphragm. JAMA 1972;168:2012–4.

520. Stern H, Toole A, Merino M. Catamenial pneumothorax. Chest 1980;78:480–2.

521. Alifano M, Roth T, Broet SC, et al. Catamenial pneumothorax – A prospective study. 124 ed. 2003. 1004-1008.

522. Wilkins SB, Bell-Thompson J, Tyras DH. Hemothorax associated with endometriosis. J Thorac Cardiovasc Surg 1985;89:636–8.

523. Slasky BS, Siewers RD, Lecky JW, et al. Catamenial pneumothorax: the roles of diaphragmatic defects and endometriosis. AJR 1982;138:639–43.

524. Jelihovsky T, Grant AF. Endometriosis of the lung. A case report and brief review of the literature. Thorax 1968;23:434–7.

525. Di Palo S, Mari G, Castoldi R, et al. Endometriosis of the lung. Respir Med 1989;83:255–8.

526. Bateman ED, Morrison SC. Catamenial haemoptysis from endobronchial endometriosis – a case report and review of previously reported cases. Respir Med 1990;84:157–61.

527. Hobbs JE, Bortnick R. Endometriosis of the lung: an experimental and clinical study. Am J Obstet Gynecol 1940;40:832–43.

528. Kiyan E, Kilicaslan Z, Caglar E, et al. An unusual radiographic finding in pulmonary parenchymal endometriosis. Acta Radiol 2002;43:164–6.

529. Orriols R, Munoz X, Alvarez A, et al. Chest CT scanning: utility in lung endometriosis. Respir Med 1998;92:876–7.

530. Cassina PC, Hauser M, Kacl G, et al. Catamenial hemoptysis. Diagnosis with MRI. Chest 1997;111:1447–50.

531. Kuo PH, Wang HC, Liaw YS, et al. Bronchoscopic and angiographic findings in tracheobronchial endometriosis. Thorax 1996;51:1060–1.

532. Park WW. The occurrence of decidual tissue within the lung: report of a case. J Pathol Bacteriol 1954;67:563–70.

533. Cameron HM, Park WW. Decidual tissue within the lung. J Obstet Gynaec Brit Commonw 1965;72:748–52.

534. Groisman GM, Meir A. CD10 is helpful in detecting occult or inconspicuous endometrial stromal cells in cases of presumptive endometriosis. Arch Pathol Lab Med 2003;127:1003–6.

535. Joseph J, Sahn SA. Thoracic endometriosis syndrome: new observations from an analysis of 110 cases. Am J Med 1996;100:164–70.

536. Inoue T, Kurokawa Y, Kaiwa Y, et al. Video-assisted thoracoscopic surgery for catamenial hemoptysis. Chest 2001;120:655–8.

Chapter

Lung transplantation

Revised by Margaret Burke and Alexandra Rice

Human lung transplantation was first performed in 1963 but few patients survived and the operation was largely abandoned until the advent of ciclosporin and the development of combined heart and lung transplantation nearly 20 years later. Today over 30 000 lung transplants have been performed and the procedure is firmly established amongst the therapeutic options available for patients with severe lung disease.[1] Donor shortage is the main factor limiting its application and this drives the search for new strategies to increase the number of lungs available for transplantation. These include the use of live donors, easing of donor selection criteria and ex vivo techniques to recondition lungs of marginal viability.[2,3] About 2% of lung transplants are repeat operations, performed because of graft failure. Patients receiving lung transplants have ranged from infants to the elderly, with the peak age being about 50 years. The principal conditions treated by lung transplantation in adults have been chronic obstructive pulmonary disease/emphysema (36%), idiopathic pulmonary fibrosis (21%), cystic fibrosis (16%), α_1-antitrypsin deficiency (7%) and primary pulmonary hypertension (4%). The remainder include sarcoidosis, lymphangioleiomyomatosis, connective tissue disease and, rarely, lung cancer.[4] The commonest indication for lung transplantation in adolescents is cystic fibrosis and in children congenital heart disease.[5]

TYPES OF LUNG TRANSPLANT

Combined heart and lung transplantation, which was first performed in 1981, was followed by single-lung transplantation, then double-lung transplantation, and lastly sequential bilateral lung transplantation. The combined operation requires total cardiopulmonary bypass and if successful carries a risk of accelerated coronary atheroma and problems resulting from cardiac denervation. However, it is relatively simple technically, maintains coronary–tracheobronchial arterial anastomoses that help the tracheal anastomosis to heal, and is particularly suitable when both heart and lungs are damaged, as in pulmonary hypertension. In cystic fibrosis, it is necessary to replace both lungs to avoid the risk of spillover infection. Double-lung transplantation is a complex procedure but was initially used in emphysema because it was feared that with single-lung transplantation the native diseased lung would be preferentially ventilated. This proved not to be the case and single-lung transplantation is now widely used for both severe emphysema and pulmonary fibrosis. It is the commonest procedure, the simplest to perform, is associated with the fewest postoperative complications, requires the least amount of donor tissue and enables the greatest number of recipients to benefit from a single donor.[6]

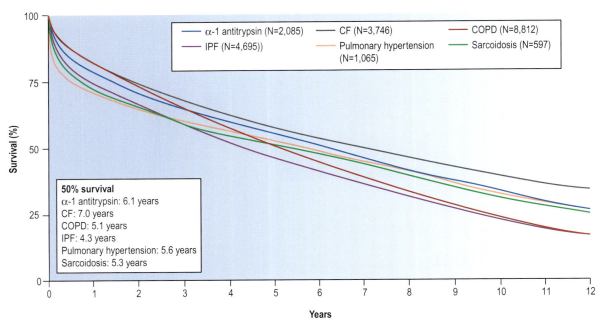

Figure 11.1 Adult lung transplantation: actuarial survival by diagnosis.[4] CF, cystic fibrosis; COPD, chronic obstructive pulmonary disease; IPF, idiopathic pulmonary fibrosis; PH, pulmonary hypertension.

Except for bronchial artery revascularisation, which is undertaken in only a few centres, no attempt is made to reanastomose the severed tracheal or bronchial blood vessels and nerves in any of these operations, or the lymphatics, which are also severed if the heart is not included. Loss of these structures promotes postoperative haemorrhage, breakdown of the tracheal or bronchial anastomosis, a reduction in the cough reflex and pulmonary oedema. A further aspect of lung transplantation is that some lymphatic tissue is inevitably included in the allograft, entailing a risk of graft-versus-host disease. This is greatest when the whole mediastinum is transferred, as in combined heart and lung transplantation, but in practice it is a rare complication.

The mortality associated with lung transplantation is constantly diminishing as techniques and immunosuppression improve. In 2009 the International Society of Heart–Lung Transplantation reported survival rates of 79%, 52% and 29% at 1, 5 and 10 years respectively for lung transplantation and 64%, 41% and 26% at the same periods for combined heart–lung transplantation (Fig. 11.1).[4] In the first postoperative month mortality is chiefly due to sepsis, haemorrhage and poor lung preservation. After the first month the principal causes of death are infection and rejection in the form of obliterative bronchiolitis.

RECIPIENT SELECTION

Lung transplantation is an operation of last resort. There are insufficient donors and patients are unlikely to be considered unless other measures have failed and their short-term prognosis is otherwise poor. The presence of uncontrolled systemic disease precludes consideration and good renal and hepatic function is essential, particularly in view of immunosuppressant drug toxicity. This is particularly important in α_1-antitrypsin deficiency and cystic fibrosis, both of which may affect the liver directly. Any infection that cannot be eliminated, either before or by the operation, is likely to disseminate postoperatively because of the immunosuppression and therefore militates against successful transplantation. An aspergilloma is a contraindication to any form of lung transplantation as its attempted removal inevitably leads to seeding of the pleural cavity and mediastinum. Previous thoracic surgery may make it difficult to operate and the possibility of a future lung transplant should therefore be borne in mind when considering the best treatment for conditions such as pneumothorax. Left ventricular function should be normal or near normal, although treatable coronary artery disease is not an absolute contraindication. Ventilator support prior to transplantation is a significant risk factor.[7] Pulmonary neoplasia is generally regarded as a contraindication because of its early dissemination but bronchioloalveolar carcinoma (now termed adenocarcinoma-in-situ) is often limited to the lungs and double-lung transplantation has been employed to treat this form of lung cancer.[8] Contraindications of less importance include age over 65 years and body mass index over 30.

In the USA, priority is given to those patients with rapidly progressive conditions such as idiopathic pulmonary fibrosis and who are in most need of a lung transplant. This is achieved with a numerical scoring system that takes into account the probability and duration of survival without a transplant as compared to that following transplantation. The system, which was introduced in 2005, has resulted in increased numbers of patients with idiopathic pulmonary fibrosis receiving transplants and a decrease in both waiting-list mortality and waiting-list time.[9,10] However, a high score predicts increased morbidity and mortality following transplantation, reflecting the poor clinical condition of many of the patients transplanted.[11,12] Such a system has yet to be widely adopted: in the UK organs are currently allocated on the basis of proximity and time on the waiting list.

DONOR MATCHING

The selection and management of donors and preservation of the harvested lung are crucial to reducing the impact of brainstem death on the lung and minimising reimplantation injury. Brainstem death leads to adrenergic systemic hypertension, which results in fluid shifting to the lesser circulation and neurogenic pulmonary oedema. Such injury is part of a generalised release of cytokines and other inflammatory mediators that damage many organs, including the lungs, where it may compound the other causes of injury, so that only about 20% of donated cadaver lungs can be used.[13]

Current donor selection criteria include age less than 65 years, ABO compatability, a clear chest X-ray, no airway mucosal inflammation at bronchoscopy and no history of lung contusion, severe chest trauma, previous cardiopulmonary surgery or aspiration.[14] Donor sero-positivity for cytomegalovirus is dangerous in a seronegative recipient.[7] Persistent hepatitis B and C antigenaemia and human immunodeficiency virus infection are further contraindications. However mild asthma and smoking do not adversely affect outcome.[15] Physiotherapy, bronchial toilet, prophylactic antibiotics as required and monitoring of blood gases and pulmonary wedge pressure are all important in managing a potential donor. Harvested lungs are best stored inflated, cooled and flushed through the pulmonary artery with Euro-Collins solution. Ischaemia is tolerated for up to 8 hours.[14] Donor–recipient matching includes an approximate similarity in chest size, although volume reduction surgery may circumvent this if there is a significant mismatch. One lobe of an adult's lung may be used to replace a whole lung of a child.[16] Tissue transplanted into a child grows at a normal rate.[17]

Potential recipients are screened for donor-specific lymphocytotoxic antibodies against a panel of HLA-A, -B and -DR antigens.[17a] The result is considered positive if the recipient's serum reacts to more than 10% of the HLA antigens in the panel, in which case donor-specific T- and B-lymphocytotoxic antibody cross-matching is required. A positive result here contraindicates transplantation from that donor as it is associated with accelerated graft rejection.[18]

IMMUNOSUPPRESSION

The recipient's immunity is suppressed with a combination of ciclosporin, azathiaprine and precnisolone with backup provided by immunosuppressive drugs such as tacrolimus, mycophenolate mofetil, everolimus and sirolimus. All these drugs have side-effects, notably renal, hepatic and bone marrow toxicity and an increased risk of neoplasia. Antithymocyte globulin is now seldom used and cyclophosphamide and plasmaphoresis are reserved for use in antibody-mediated rejection. Low-dose Septrin is administered prophylactically against *Pneumocystis* infection.

RECIPIENT MONITORING

Frequent monitoring of the lung transplant recipient is essential in the first 6 months after transplantation when the risk of the main complications, acute rejection and infection, is greatest. Recipients undergo frequent clinical review and bronchoscopy is undertaken in response to symptoms, radiographic changes, unexplained fever or a sudden deterioration in lung function. Both bronchoalveolar lavage and transbronchial biopsy are generally performed. Lavage is particularly useful for detecting infection while transbronchial lung biopsy, despite a false-negative rate of about 20%, is the mainstay in the diagnosis of allograft rejection. Some centres schedule their biopsies whereas others only biopsy as symptoms dictate. Rejection of the heart in combined heart and lung transplant recipients is rare and

> ### Box 11.1 The role of the histopathologist in lung transplantation
>
> Diagnosis of the underlying disease before transplantation
> Examination of the explanted lung to verify the diagnosis and identify any other diseases
> Examination of any unused donor tissue
> Biopsy assessment of posttransplant complications
> Postmortem examination
>
> As well as contributing to the outcome of the transplantation, the histopathologist is well placed to undertake collaborative research.

endomyocardial biopsies provide an unreliable guide to pulmonary rejection.

ROLE OF THE HISTOPATHOLOGIST

Histopathology plays a major role in assessing the postoperative complications of transplantation, but can contribute more than this to the management of transplant recipients, both before and after the operation (Box 11.1).[19,20] An accurate preoperative diagnosis is important because histopathological reassessment of the potential recipient may affect the choice of transplantation procedure and identify conditions treatable by other means or that need to be eradicated before transplantation is undertaken. It may also predict the presence of systemic disease and the likelihood of the original disease recurring in the allograft, or detect malignant disease, which apart from bronchioloalveolar carcinoma (now adenocarcinoma-in-situ) is an absolute contraindication to transplantation. Explanted lungs should also be examined, and without delay, in case they show unsuspected diseases such as tuberculosis, sarcoidosis or malignancy that may be active elsewhere in the recipient.[21] A major discrepancy between the pre-transplant diagnosis and that apparent on examining the explant has been reported in up to 10% of cases.[22] Similarly, if only one donor lung is used, the other should be examined as this may identify unsuspected infection or other disease that is likely also to be present in the graft. Thus, histopathologists should not be concerned solely in assessing complications, but this is undoubtedly their major role and the rest of this chapter will be largely confined to this aspect of transplantation.

COMPLICATIONS

To assess complications, at least five pieces of alveolated lung should be examined at a minimum of three levels each, using connective tissue and fungal stains in addition to haematoxylin and eosin. Because sequential sampling is common, the possibility of observed abnormalities being due to previous biopsies always has to be considered. It is also important to remember that some patterns of lung injury are non-specific. For example, diffuse alveolar damage may reflect severe reperfusion injury, infection or acute rejection. It may require special stains for infective agents and a consideration of the timing of events to distinguish these causes. There may be both rejection and infection and as their histological features overlap the biopsy findings should always be interpreted in the light of the clinical and radiological features, previous biopsy findings and results of current microbiological and serological investigations. The principal complications are listed in Box 11.2 and will now be considered.

Box 11.2 Complications of lung transplantation

- Postoperative
  - Haemorrhage and other surgical complications
  - Reimplantation syndrome
  - Diffuse alveolar damage
- Early and late airway complications
  - Anastomotic dehiscence, granulation tissue overgrowth
  - Bronchial stenosis, chondromalacia, ectasia
- Rejection
- Infection
- Neoplasia
- Posttransplantation lymphoproliferative disorders
- Graft-versus-host disease
- Recurrence of the underlying disease
- Drug effects

Perioperative allograft injury

Even if the operation goes well and there are no surgical complications, the early postoperative period is often marked by a temporary period of dyspnoea. Chest radiographs at this time often show hilar opacification and if biopsy is undertaken this generally shows pulmonary oedema accompanied by a mild neutrophil exudate (Fig. 11.2).[23] These changes, termed reimplantation injury, are variously attributed to deterioration of the graft, surgical trauma, ischaemia, severance of the pulmonary lymphatics and the release of free radicals and chemokines from neutrophils interacting with the graft endothelium damaged by ischaemia.[24] They usually appear within 48 hours and peak at day 4, slowly settling as lymphatics regenerate and lung drainage is re-established.

More severe changes include those of diffuse alveolar damage, to which the term 'primary graft failure' has been applied.[25] This may represent a reimplantation response, rejection or infection or occur for no obvious cause. The risk factors include those relating to the donor (advanced age, smoking history, prolonged ventilation and duration of ischaemia), the recipient (transplantation for pulmonary hypertension and pulmonary fibrosis) and the operation (cardiopulmonary bypass and excessive use of blood products).[26] Primary graft failure may progress to parenchymal fibrosis. It is associated with reduced survival at 1 year.[27]

Airway infection promoted by slow recovery of mucociliary clearance may also complicate the early postoperative period,[28,29] while alveolar proteinosis and an unusual neutrophil-rich pattern of mixed interstitial pneumonitis have also been described.[30,31]

Complications involving the airway anastomosis

Apart from the combined heart–lung procedure, lung transplantation inevitably involves severance of the tracheobronchial blood supply so that the donor airway receives only retrograde pulmonary arterial blood until new bronchial arterial anastomoses develop. It is not surprising therefore that poor healing at the airway anastomosis has been a serious complication, although bronchial artery revascularisation, performed at a few centres at the time of transplantation, have rendered it less common.[32,33] The anastomosis is also subject to infection until the surface epithelium heals and mucociliary clearance recovers.[29] Denervation contributes to the risk of infection by eliminating the cough reflex and promoting aspiration.[34] Dehiscence of the airway anastomosis is a devastating early complication, but one that

Figure 11.2 Reimplantation injury presenting as (A) hazy shadowing of left donor lung 3 days after single-lung transplantation for emphysema; (B) biopsy shows focal interstitial oedema, subacute inflammation, pneumocyte hyperplasia and aggregates of alveolar macrophages.

is fortunately now rare. More common is the development of exuberant granulation tissue. This may seriously narrow the airway and require endoscopic removal or cryotherapy.[35] Late airway complications include stenosis and bronchomalacia (Figs 11.3 and 11.4), requiring the insertion of stents.[36]

Complications involving the vascular anastomosis

Postoperative obstruction of the pulmonary artery anastomosis is rare but kinking may occur when the vessels are long. This usually develops in the first week. It may be diagnosed by ventilation/perfusion scan or arteriography. Venous obstruction may also develop early after transplantation, especially when size mismatch leads to torsion of a small donor lung on its vascular pedicle. The result may be thrombosis of one or more of the pulmonary veins with infarction of the corresponding lobe (Fig. 11.5).[37–39] Systemic embolisation may also occur if the thrombus extends into the left atrium and fragments. Diagnosis is by transoesophageal echocardiography.[38,40] Early

Figure 11.3 Tracheal stencsis following double-lung transplantation.

Figure 11.4 Bronchomalacia. There is erosion of the limiting plate of the bronchial cartilage.

Figure 11.5 (A) Thrombosis of pulmonary vein to left lower lobe following torsion of the vascular pedicle resulting in (B) infarction of the entire lower lobe.

recognition of this potentially catastrophic complication is essential if early surgical intervention with salvage of the graft (and patient) is to be achieved.

Rejection

The mechanisms underlying lung allograft rejection are not fully understood but the process is probably initiated by T-cell recognition of histocompatibility antigens on the surface of donor cells.[41] The brunt of the rejection damage is on the blood vessels and airways, presumably reflecting the increased expression of histocompatibility antigens by the pulmonary vascular endothelium and airway epithelium that has been shown to follow transplantation.[41] Incompatibility is followed by the activation and sequestration of platelets, neutrophils and macrophages within the pulmonary capillaries, the release of reactive oxygen species and inflammatory cytokines, and increased expression of endothelin and inducible nitric oxide synthase.[42–44] The rejection process probably involves both antibody and cell-mediated immune mechanisms but the extent to which these each contribute varies: hyperacute rejection is generally regarded as being antibody-mediated whereas acute and chronic rejection are thought to be predominantly cell-mediated.

Hyperacute allograft rejection

Hyperacute rejection occurs within 48 hours of transplantation and is caused by the reaction of preformed antibodies to donor endothelial cells. It is characterised by marked congestion and oedema, resulting in the production of copious frothy blood-stained fluid from the bronchial orifice of the allograft. Risk factors include multiple blood transfusions, pregnancy, surgery and previous transplantation, any of which necessitates donor-specific pretransplant T- and B-lymphocytotoxic antibody cross-matching (see above).

Microscopy shows marked pulmonary congestion and oedema, alveolar haemorrhage, vascular thrombosis, neutrophil infiltration, endothelial and epithelial damage, and ultimately diffuse alveolar damage (Fig. 11.6). The diagnosis is confirmed by the detection by immunofluorescence of C4d complement split product (as a marker of complement activation) and IgG deposition on endothelium,

along vessel walls and in alveolar spaces, and by a strongly positive IgG-mediated lymphocytotoxic reaction to donor T and/or B lymphocytes.[46,47]

Acute allograft rejection

Acute rejection is characterised clinically by dyspnoea, fever, hypoxaemia and pleuropulmonary opacification (Fig. 11.7). It is most frequent in the first postoperative year, typically developing within a few months of the operation but sometimes within a few weeks or several years later.

Acute and chronic rejection are classified and graded according to internationally agreed histological criteria (Box 11.3).[48] Acute rejection may be centred on the blood vessels or the airways but predominantly affects the former and the surrounding lung parenchyma. The vascular changes (class A) are treated separately from those involving the airways (class B) because the latter may also reflect chronic infection, ischaemia, aspiration or chronic rejection.[28,34,49,50]

Histologically, the vascular changes are characterised by an infiltrate of variable intensity comprising small lymphocytes, plasma cells, histiocytes and occasional neutrophils surrounding small blood vessels and infiltrating the adjacent alveolar interstitium. They are graded as minimal (grade A1) if they can hardly be discerned without high magnification and mild (grade A2) if they are just evident at low magnification and consist of an infiltrate that includes large activated lymphocytes with pyroninophilic cytoplasm and angulated nuclei. Neutrophils and eosinophils are also seen and there is infiltration of the vascular intima (lymphocytic intimitis or endothelialitis). Endothelial cells show hyperplasia. Moderate acute rejection (grade A3) is characterised by extension of the infiltrate into the alveolar interstitium, while in severe (grade A4) acute rejection, which is usually fatal, the infiltrate is widespread and accompanied by haemorrhagic oedema, increased numbers of alveolar macrophages, fibrinous exudates, hyaline membranes and destructive changes typical of

Figure 11.6 Hyperacute rejection. Neutrophils engorge the blood vessels and have passed into the alveolar interstitium and lumen. The patient died during the operation. Panel-reactive antibodies were positive and a donor-specific lymphocytotoxic cross-match was strongly positive for T and B lymphocytes.

Figure 11.7 Chest radiograph in acute rejection showing opacification of the lower zone of the right lung, which was transplanted because of emphysema.

Box 11.3 **Revised working formulation for the classification and grading of pulmonary allograft rejection**[48]

A Acute rejection

   Grade 0 None

         1 Minimal

         2 Mild

         3 Moderate

         4 Severe

B Airway inflammation – lymphocytic bronchitis/bronchiolitis

   Grade 0 None

   1R Low-grade

   2R High-grade

   BX Ungradable (sampling problems, infection, tangential sectioning)

A and B may coexist, as may C and D

C Chronic airway rejection – bronchiolitis obliterans

   0 Absent

   1 Present

D Chronic vascular rejection – accelerated graft vascular sclerosis

Figure 11.8 Acute parenchymal rejection. (A) Grade A1 (minimal) changes are not discernible at low magnification but high power shows a sparse perivascular lymphoid infiltrate. (B) Grade A2 (mild) shows a more marked infiltrate but this is still restricted to the vessels and the alveolar septa are spared. (C) Grade A3 (moderate) acute rejection showing spread of the infiltrate into surrounding alveolar septa. (D) Grade A4 (severe) acute rejection is characterised by diffuse alveolar damage and a dense perivascular lymphoid infiltrate.

Figure 11.9 Immunohistology of acute lung allograft rejection. The perivascular infiltrate stained by haematoxylin and eosin in (A) expresses the T-cell marker CD3 (B) and the proliferation marker Kiel-67 (C) while class II HLA-DR antigens are strongly expressed by alveolar epithelium and macrophages (D).

diffuse alveolar damage (Fig. 11.8). Grade A3 and A4 rejection may also be associated with organising pneumonia.[49,51–53] With successful suppression of the rejection, follow-up biopsies show a reduction in the infiltrate (termed resolving rejection/lower grade) and a change in its makeup to a mixture of small lymphocytes and haemosiderin-laden macrophages (termed resolved rejection or grade A0).[54]

Immunohistochemistry shows that the majority of the lymphoid cells are CD8-suppressor lymphocytes (Fig. 11.9).[55] They are often pyroninophilic and may express the lymphocyte activation antigen CD30 and the proliferation antigen Ki-67. B lymphocytes are usually sparse; larger numbers may reflect rejection based on humoral rather than cellular mechanisms and therefore predict a poor response to the usual cell-based immunosuppressive regimes.[56] However, their presence should also prompt consideration of other entities such as eosinophilic pneumonia, fungal infection and lymphoproliferative disease.[57,58] The vascular endothelium and alveolar epithelium both show upregulation of class II HLA (HLA-DR) antigens.[41]

Although perivascular lymphoid cell infiltration is the hallmark of acute rejection, similar infiltrates may be seen in patients with infections and other conditions for which augmented immunosuppression is inappropriate. For this reason acute rejection should only be diag-

nosed and graded in the absence of infection.[48] The opportunistic infections may be viral, particularly herpes simplex and cytomegalovirus, the distinctive inclusions of which may be modified by prior antiviral treatment and therefore difficult to identify (Fig. 11.10).[59] However, the infiltrates of a viral infection are generally more extensive and the pattern is predominantly that of an interstitial pneumonitis with secondary involvement of vessels.[59] Perivascular lymphoid infiltrates may also be seen in *Pneumocystis jirovecii* pneumonia.[60] and in other fungal and bacterial infections, necessitating special stains, and in difficult cases immunocytochemistry and in situ hybridisation.[61,62] Eosinophilic pneumonia is an uncommon manifestation of graft rejection and, before accepting it as such, infection by organisms such as *Aspergillus* should be excluded.[63,64] A predominantly neutrophilic infiltrate, necrosis and granuloma formation all favour infection rather than rejection.

Acute rejection should also be distinguished from the ischaemia–reperfusion injury described above and from the lymphoproliferative disorders described below.[58] Ischaemia–reperfusion injury lacks the perivascular and interstitial infiltration of rejection while a polymorphous, perivascular infiltrate of B and T lymphocytes with a predominance of the latter favours rejection rather than lympho-

Figure 11.10 Fragmented cytomegalovirus inclusions after treatment with ganciclovir.

Figure 11.11 Acute airway rejection (lymphocytic bronchiolitis). (A) Grade B1 acute rejection is characterised by occasional small lymphocytes infiltrating the bronchiolar epithelium and lamina propria. (B) Grade B3 acute airway rejection shows extensive infiltration and obliteration of bronchiolar epithelium by lymphocytes.

proliferative disease, which is characterised by a monomorphous infiltrate of large B lymphocytes.[57] Mass lesions also favour lymphoproliferative disease or infection rather than rejection. Recurrence in the allograft of diseases such as sarcoidosis and Langerhans cell histiocytosis may also be misinterpreted as acute rejection if their characteristic features are not well represented.

Airway inflammation in the form of lymphocytic bronchiolitis is the other major pattern of acute rejection. Evidence that it represents rejection includes its progression to chronic rejection (bronchiolitis obliterans) and frequent response to augmented immunosuppression.[65] It may accompany or succeed the perivascular infiltrates described above or be seen alone, but it most frequently follows the vascular changes.[28,50] Airway inflammation may be graded in the same way as the perivascular infiltration but in practice the small size of the biopsies generally precludes the precision required for this. The changes range from sparse airway cuffing by small lymphoid cells (grade B1R) to diffuse infiltration of the lamina propria and epithelium by medium and large lymphoid cells and epithelial apoptosis (grade B2R) (Fig. 11.11). In severe cases the lymphoid infiltrate is particularly dense and there is ulceration and fibrino-purulent exudation. The importance of large-airway inflammation in rejection is unclear as it is more often secondary to infection. Grading of airway inflammation is therefore currently restricted to the bronchioles.

The differential diagnosis of airway inflammation includes the presence of bronchus-associated lymphoid tissue of donor origin, low-grade infection and the consequences of aspiration. Bronchus-associated lymphoid tissue is distinguished by it comprising aggregates of B lymphocytes, sometimes with admixed anthracotic macrophages, in contrast to the T-cell-rich infiltrates of rejection. Prominent neutrophil or eosinophil infiltration is suggestive of infection or aspiration. However, it is important to note that airway or parenchymal infection, notably by cytomegalovirus, may accompany rejection.[66]

Chronic allograft rejection

Chronic rejection of the transplanted lung is marked by progressive breathlessness, cough, which is often productive, fever and a decline in lung function.[67] The changes, which can be monitored by spirometry and imaging (Fig. 11.12), are centred on the bronchioles (class C) and blood vessels (class D).

The histological features are those of constrictive bronchiolitis obliterans. Typically there is concentric or eccentric hyaline fibrous thickening of the bronchiolar submucosa, encroaching on the airway lumen and eventually resulting in total occlusion (Fig. 11.13).[68–71] The changes may be subtle, in which case an elastin stain can be invaluable in identifying the fibrosed bronchioles. Residual bronchiolar epithelium may show squamous metaplasia and there is usually disruption of the muscle coat. The process may be active (i.e. associated with lymphocytic bronchiolitis) or inactive (consisting of dense fibrous scarring with minimal or no inflammation), although this is of no prognostic significance and does not predict response to treatment. The infiltrating cells are T lymphocytes.[72] The process is patchy and therefore not always evident in small biopsies,[73,74] but its presence may be suggested by obstructive features such as the accumulation of foamy macrophages in distal air spaces. In the current classification constrictive bronchiolitis is simply recorded as being present (C1) or absent (C0).

The recognition of bronchiolitis obliterans is the key discriminator between acute and chronic rejection. The adjacent lung may also show

Figure 11.12 Computed tomography scan appearances in bronchiolitis obliterans syndrome. (A) The inspiratory image shows mild generalised hyperinflation with bronchial dilatation and wall thickening while (B) the expiratory image shows irregular dark areas of focal air-trapping.

Figure 11.13 The histological spectrum of chronic airway rejection (bronchiolitis obliterans). (A) Partial occlusion of a bronchiole by plaque-like submucosal fibrous tissue with sparse chronic inflammation. (B) An incomplete ring of smooth muscle provides the only evidence that this focal pulmonary scar represents an obliterated bronchiole.

evidence of concomitant acute rejection (Fig. 11.14). Most patients with bronchiolitis obliterans also have bronchiectasis (Fig. 11.15), which probably results from a combination of factors, including rejection, infection and denervation. Concomitant acute airway inflammation suggests postobstructive infection.

Unfortunately, sampling error renders the diagnosis of bronchiolitis obliterans unreliable on small biopsies and its identification generally depends upon recognition of a bronchiolitis obliterans syndrome. This is defined as 'graft deterioration due to progressive airways disease for which there is no other cause'.[75,76] The principal role of transbronchial lung biopsy is therefore to exclude treatable causes of deterioration in lung function.

Bronchiolitis obliterans is seldom seen within 6 months of the operation and, while its incidence diminishes after 1–2 years, it affects 50% of recipients by 5 years.[73] Risk factors include earlier rejection episodes and histocompatibility mismatch,[57,70,77,78] supporting the view that it represents a late manifestation of rejection[50,79] with an immunological pathogenesis analogous to that occurring in rheumatoid and graft-versus-host disease (see p. 121).[80–83] The development

of de novo anti-HLA antibodies following transplantation is also associated with an increased incidence of bronchiolitis obliterans, suggesting that humoral rejection may play a role.[84,85] Gastro-oesophageal reflux and chronic airway infection may also contribute to the development of obliterative bronchiolitis.[86–88] Other causes include cytomegalovirus infection,[28,59,77,89,90] community-acquired viral infection[91,92] and ischaemia.[93] Finally, it has been suggested that some early cases, characterised by acute inflammation on biopsy and lavage (in the absence of infection), respond well to azithromycin therapy (so-called neutrophilic reversible allograft dysfunction).[94–96]

The pathogenesis of the obliterative fibrosis has yet to be fully elucidated, but it is intriguing that some of the cells that participate in the fibrosis are derived from circulating fibroblast precursors of recipient bone marrow origin.[97] There is also evidence suggesting a role for epithelial–mesenchymal transition in the sclerosing process.[98,99]

Chronic rejection may also involve the pulmonary vasculature, resulting in fibrointimal sclerosis of arteries and veins analogous to that occurring in the coronary arteries of heart and heart–lung allografts (Fig. 11.16).[100–103] This uncommon complication may be active or inactive and may be seen in association with obliterative bronchi-

Figure 11.14 Concomitant acute and chronic rejection. Acute rejection is evidenced by a perivascular lymphoid infiltrate while a bronchiole totally obstructed by fibrous tissue is indicative of chronic rejection.

Figure 11.16 Chronic vascular rejection. (a) Active chronic rejection affecting a muscular artery. (b) A pulmonary artery showing severe intimal fibrosis, the appearances of inactive alveolar infection.

Figure 11.15 Radiological and macroscopic appearances of chronic airway rejection complicated by bronchiectasis. *(Courtesy of Dr H Tazelaar, Rochester, Minnesota, USA)*

olitis, which would then dominate the clinical picture. Sclerosis of small vessels may also represent chronic rejection but is generally disregarded as it may also follow ischaemia, acute rejection, non-rejection-related pulmonary inflammation and non-specific donor-related factors.

Antibody-mediated rejection

Hyperacute rejection is the archetypal form of antibody-mediated rejection, in which preformed antibodies cross-react with graft antigens resulting in fulminant rejection. However, it is known from renal and cardiac transplantation that a less acute form of antibody-mediated rejection, may occur. The criteria for diagnosing this include the presence of de novo donor-specific antibodies, clinical allograft dysfunction, histological features of antibody-mediated rejection and the deposition of complement protein C4d, a stable biproduct of complement C4d activation, on capillary endothelium.[104,104a] The role of antibody-mediated rejection in lung allograft rejection is far from clear but there are reports of lung transplant patients with many of the features of antibody-mediated rejection being treated successfully with plasmapheresis and intravenous immunoglobulin.[105–111] While it has been suggested that capillaritis may represent antibody-mediated rejection,[109,112,113] there is currently no consensus on what histological features define the condition in the lung.[114] Furthermore C4d deposition may be seen in lungs with primary graft failure and infection,[115,116] limiting its use as a marker of rejection remains to be elucidated. Recent work has revealed complex interactions between components of the complement system, platelets and endothelial cells as well as evidence suggesting an influence of complement on T and B lymphocyte function.[104a,114] Endothelial activation appears to play a central role in the development of antibody-mediated rejection and further work may provide more specific and sensitive markers of this serious complication of lung transplantation humoral rejection.

Upper-lobe fibrosis

Progressive upper-lobe fibrosis has occasionally been described after lung transplantation. Imaging shows interlobular septal thickening and ground-glass change, progressing to traction bronchiectasis and honeycombing. Biopsy shows non-specific inflammation and fibrosis.[117] Further research is required to determine whether this provisional clinicopathological entity is related to rejection or other factors.

Figure 11.17 Cytomegalovirus antigenaemia. Positive immunohistochemical staining of peripheral blood leukocytes for cytomegalovirus pp65 antigen.

Infection

Infection is a major hazard for the immunosuppressed recipient of a lung allograft.[118] It is often multiple and may affect the native lung and other organs as well as the allograft. Its recognition in the lungs largely depends upon the microbiological examination of bronchoalveolar lavage fluid but the addition of transbronchial lung biopsy increases the detection rate.[119] Problems in biopsy interpretation include distinguishing rejection from infection, which is compounded by the atypical host response of the immunosuppressed patient. Distinguishing colonisation, subclinical infection and clinically significant disease may also be difficult. The pathology of pulmonary infection is described in Chapter 5 but the special circumstances associated with transplantation warrant further comment on some infective agents here.

Viruses

Cytomegalovirus infection of a seronegative recipient, transmitted by blood transfusion or the graft, increases the incidence of rejection, probably by promoting the expression of the major histocompatibility antigens in the alveolar epithelium.[41,120,121] The recognition of clinically significant disease (as opposed to mere carriage of the virus) is based upon identification of blood cytomegalovirus pp65 antigen,[122,123] biopsy evidence of interstitial pneumonitis and bronchiolitis[124] (Fig. 11.17) and the detection of the virus. The latter often requires immunohistochemistry or molecular techniques such as the polymerase chain reaction because in the early stages of infection typical viral inclusions are often sparse (Fig. 11.18). Only in the later stages are there numerous intranuclear and cytoplasmic inclusions (Fig. 11.19). Other patterns of cytomegalovirus disease include poorly formed granulomas, diffuse alveolar damage and mass lesions simulating a tumour.[125] Viral prophylaxis may result in fragmented inclusions and an acute neutrophilic pneumonitis (see Fig. 11.10).

Infection by herpes simplex virus is infrequent in lung allograft recipients but may cause necrotising tracheobronchitis and pneumonia in these patients.[126] Similarly, infection by influenza and respiratory syncytial viruses may cause significant morbidity and contribute to the development of bronchiolitis obliterans.[92,127] Other viral

Figure 11.18 Early cytomegalovirus pneumonitis. (A) Focal acute interstitial pneumonitis with several possible cytomegaloviral inclusions, (B) confirmed by immunohistochemistry.

Figure 11.19 Severe cytomegalovirus pneumonitis in a cytomegalovirus-negative recipient of a cytomegalovirus-positive lung.

Figure 11.20 Fatal chickenpox pneumonitis. Foci of necrosis are surrounded by extensive alveolar haemorrhage.

infections of note in transplant patients include pulmonary and systemic infection by varicella-zoster (Fig. 11.20).

Community-acquired respiratory viruses such as rhinovirus, enterovirus, coronavirus, respiratory syncytial virus, parainfluenza virus, influenza A and B and adenovirus infect up to 57% of lung transplant recipients. The severity varies from mild upper respiratory tract disease to severe pneumonia complicated by bacterial or fungal superinfection. Some studies have linked such infection with the onset of acute and chronic rejection. Features on biopsy are often of a non-specific interstitial pneumonitis. Occasionally, a specific viral cytopathic effect may be seen on biopsy, such as with adenovirus (see p. 161), but usually viral culture is required to identify the organism. Molecular techniques applied to lavage material greatly enhance the sensitivity and specificity of viral diagnosis.

Bacteria

Opportunistic mycobacteria originating in either the donor or recipient infect lung allograft recipients on rare occasions, or merely colonise the graft without causing disease.[128–130] Other bacterial infections of these patients include nocardiosis and *Legionella* pneumonia.

Fungi

Pneumocystis jirovecii pneumonia is rare in lung transplantation because of chemoprophylaxis; the reported incidence is less than 1%.[20] It mostly follows the immunosuppression being increased because of acute rejection.[131] The histological patterns include a predominantly lymphoplasmacytic interstitial pneumonitis with scanty exudate, and a granulomatous pneumonitis. The fungal cysts are sparse and the classic foamy alveolar exudate is rarely encountered. The perivascular component of the lymphoplasmacytic pattern resembles that of acute rejection, hence the mandatory use of silver staining techniques for all transbronchial lung allograft biopsies and the routine screening of all bronchoalveolar lavage specimens using immunocytochemistry or the polymerase chain reaction.[132]

Other fungi that infect lung allograft patients include *Candida* and *Aspergillus*. These agents may merely colonise the airways[133] or cause ulcerative tracheobronchitis, dehiscence of the anastomosis, bronchocentric granulomatosis, cavitating pneumonia, mediastinitis and multiple haematogenous abscesses.[134–137]

Toxoplasmosis

Infection of the lung allograft by *Toxoplasma gondii* is rare, having been largely eliminated in seronegative solid-organ transplant recipients given a positive organ by prophylaxis with pyrimethamine. It usually occurs as part of systemic infection following graft mismatch.[138] Identification of the organism in biopsy material may be difficult as the cysts of *T. gondii* are sparse and extracellular tachyzoites may be mistaken for haematoxyphil debris (see Fig. 5.5.1, p. 252). The diagnosis may be confirmed by immunohistochemistry or by the polymerase chain reaction applied to tissue, body fluids or peripheral blood.[139]

Aspiration

Gastro-oesophageal reflux and aspiration are fairly common following lung transplantation and are being increasingly recognised as risk factors for the development of obliterative bronchiolitis through repeated episodes of epithelial injury.[86,140–142] The histological features are generally those of non-specific active chronic inflammation, although a foreign-body giant cell reaction to aspirated material occasionally allows a definitive diagnosis (see Fig. 5.2.16, p. 190). Bronchoalveolar lavage studies suggest that it is the aspiration of bile salts rather than gastric acid that is related to the subsequent development of obliterative bronchiolitis.[88]

Neoplasia

After rejection, neoplasia is the most significant factor limiting long-term survival in solid-organ transplantation.[7,143] It ranges in incidence from 6% to 11%.[144,145] The tumours may arise de novo or be inadvertently introduced within the allograft. They are often particularly aggressive. Predisposing factors in addition to immunosuppression include ultraviolet irradiation and activation of oncogenic viruses such as Epstein–Barr virus, papillomavirus and herpesvirus. Molecular techniques have shown that those tumours apparently arising de novo may be of donor rather than recipient origin.[146]

The most frequently encountered de novo tumours include the posttransplantation lymphoproliferative disorders dealt with see and cutaneous tumours, notably squamous carcinoma, preceded by premalignant skin lesions, which are often multiple. The carcinomas frequently metastasise and may contain papillomavirus.[143,147] Intraepithelial neoplasia and squamous carcinomas of the uterine cervix, vulva and perineum, also associated with human papillomavirus infection, may occur. Other tumours reputed to occur with greater frequency than in the general population include carcinomas of the kidney,[148] hepatobiliary tract and lung,[118,149] the last of these often presenting at an advanced stage and being of donor origin.[146] Cytological specimens of the bronchi often show epithelial atypia but this is more often reactive than malignant.[150]

Other tumours seen more commonly in lung transplant recipients than the general population include Kaposi's sarcoma[151] and low-grade leiomyosarcoma.[152,153] Between 3% and 7% of single-lung transplant recipients develop bronchogenic carcinoma within their native lung. This may reflect the large number of transplants performed for smoking-related diseases such as emphysema and idiopathic pulmonary fibrosis.[154] The role of immunosuppression in the development of these tumours is unclear but it is notable that they behave aggressively.

Posttransplantation lymphoproliferative disorders

A spectrum of lymphoproliferative disorders may complicate transplantation of many organs, including the lungs.[155–158]

Immunosuppression would appear to underlie this escape from normal control as similar disease is seen in other conditions characterised by profound immunosuppression – the acquired immunodeficiency syndrome (AIDS), for example. Epstein–Barr virus is suspected of playing a part in the causation of these lesions, having been identified in many of them by immunostaining and the application of molecular probes.[159-161] The incidence of lymphoproliferative disease is higher in recipients who are sero-negative for Epstein–Barr virus before the operation,[162] suggesting that the viral infection is primary rather than representing reinfection or reactivation of latent disease.[159] The virus is detectable more often with early than late disease. A notable feature is that the lesions are potentially reversible once immunosuppression is reduced.[157,163]

Posttransplantation lymphoproliferative disorders have been described in association with virtually all currently used immunosuppressive agents and are thought to result from uncontrolled proliferation of Epstein–Barr virus-immortalised B cells due to loss of cytotoxic T-cell control.[160,164] As with most solid-organ transplants, the lymphoproliferation usually involves cells of recipient origin, in contrast to bone marrow transplantation where the lymphoproliferative disorders generally involve cells of donor origin.[165-170] Nevertheless they often first present in the allograft itself.

Risk factors include the type of transplant, young age, multiple rejection episodes, multiagent immunosuppression, anti-T-cell therapy and pretransplant Epstein–Barr virus sero-negativity.[162,166] The interval between lung transplantation and the development of the lymphoproliferative process is generally short (median time 7 months), as is the median time to death (5 months).[161]

The incidence of posttransplantation lymphoproliferative disorders ranges from about 1% with bone marrow and kidney transplants to nearly 10% with lung and heart–lung and 17% with intestine.[167] This is thought to reflect the relatively higher levels of immunosuppression required for lung and intestinal transplantation.

Posttransplantation lymphoproliferative disease may involve the lung in isolation or as part of disseminated disease.[158,159,161] The lungs may also be involved by posttransplantation lymphoproliferative disease in recipients of other solid-organ transplants.[171,172] The disease may be asymptomatic or cause cough, fever and malaise. Radiographs may show diffuse infiltrates or single or multiple nodules. High serum levels of Epstein–Barr virus DNA predict the development of posttransplant lymphoproliferative disease. Tissue should be examined for Epstein–Barr virus by immunocytochemistry or in situ hybridisation, cell phenotype and immunoglobulin clonality, and the lesion classified according to the scheme advocated by the World Health Organization (Box 11.4).[173] Clinical suspicion of posttransplantation lymphoproliferative disease should be conveyed to the pathologist so that some tissue can be snap-frozen for appropriate molecular studies. Synchronous and metachronous lesions should all be investigated as variations in clonality and morphology occur both within an individual lesion and between simultaneous or subsequent lesions. Difficulties encountered in diagnosis, especially on core biopsies, stem from the small size of the sample, crush artefact and extensive necrosis caused by angioinvasion. The differential diagnosis includes infections such as cytomegalovirus and *Pneumocystis*, inflammation caused by previous biopsies, the presence of bronchus-associated lymphoid tissue and, in the transplanted lung, acute allograft rejection and, rarely, graft-versus-host disease.

The chief pulmonary manifestations of posttransplantation lymphoproliferative disease are lymphoid hyperplasia, lymphoid interstitial pneumonia and the full spectrum of lymphomas,[159,173] all of which are described in Chapter 12.4. They predominantly involve B lymphocytes whereas T lymphocytes predominate in the infiltrates that characterise rejection.[158] High-grade lymphomas often show angioinvasion and extensive necrosis, thereby resembling lymphomatoid

---

Box 11.4 World Health Organization classification of posttransplantation lymphoproliferative disorders (PTLD)[173]

1. Early lesions
Reactive plasmacytic hyperplasia
Infectious mononucleosis-like lesion

2. PTLD – polymorphic
Polyclonal (rare)
Monoclonal

3. PTLD – monomorphic (classify according to lymphoma they resemble)
B-cell neoplasms
Diffuse large B-cell lymphoma
Burkitt lymphoma
Plasma cell myeloma
Plasmacytoma-like lesion
Other

T-cell neoplasms
Peripheral T-cell lymphoma, not otherwise categorised
Hepatosplenic T-cell lymphoma
Other

4. Classic Hodgkin lymphoma-type PTLD

---

granulomatosis. Early lesions may be rich in mature plasma cells or show changes suggestive of infectious mononucleosis. Polymorphous infiltrates often include plasmacytoid cells (Fig. 11.21). Monomorphous infiltrates may consist of transformed blasts, centroblast-like, centrocyte-like cells or immunoblasts showing a high proliferation index (Fig. 11.22). Single-cell necrosis is common. Histiocytes and T lymphocytes often cuff the lesion and infiltrate the bronchiolar epithelium while the uninvolved lung may show patchy organising pneumonia. Immunoglobulin clonality is variable. Early lesions tend to be polyclonal. Monomorphous lesions are usually monoclonal while polymorphous lesions may be either polyclonal or monoclonal.[167,174]

A reduction of immunosuppression and treatment with antiviral agents usually leads to rapid resolution[159] but relapse is frequent and may require radiation treatment or chemotherapy. Newer, less toxic treatments such as cytotoxic T-lymphocyte infusions, interferon-α and antibodies to B cells (anti-CD20; Rituximab) are now available.[175-177]

Graft-versus-host disease

The transplanted lung or heart–lung block contains a significant amount of lymphoid tissue and on rare occasions a rash, colitis, pancytopenia and liver dysfunction may suggest that graft-versus-host disease has developed.[178-181] The identification of donor lymphocytes in the blood and bronchoalveolar lavage fluid of such patients supports this possibility. Graft-versus-host disease tends to develop in the early postoperative period. It may be severe but is fortunately rare and usually responds to increased immunosuppression. The graft-versus-host disease of bone marrow transplantation may cause constrictive obliterative bronchiolitis that is indistinguishable from that seen in lung rejection[81,82,182,183] but of course in lung transplantation the donor lung is spared this complication.

Biopsy diagnosis is generally dependent upon the histological appearances in the skin rather than the lung. The diagnosis may be

Figure 11.21 Pulmonary posttransplantation lymphoproliferative disorder (polymorphous, lymphoplasmacytoid). (A) Plasma cells, plasmacytoid cells and medium-sized lymphocytes surround an alveolar duct. (B) CD79a-positivity shows that the infiltrate is of B-cell origin.

confirmed by demonstrating donor and recipient chimerism on HLA typing of peripheral blood lymphocytes and bronchoalveolar lavage fluid.

Recurrent disease in the allograft

The systemic effects of underlying diseases such as cystic fibrosis may have a significant impact on recovery but only recurrence in the allograft will be considered here.

The aetiology of many diseases treated by lung transplantation is imperfectly understood but our knowledge of them has been broadened by their behaviour following transplantation. Some of these diseases are prone to recur in the new lungs whereas others are not. Of particular interest is the finding that lungs transplanted into patients with cystic fibrosis do not appear to develop the basic defect of membrane transport that underlies this disease.[184,185] It is also

notable that whereas asthma appears to be cured by lung transplantation, it may also be transferred by transplanting the lungs of asthmatic donors to non-atopic patients.[186] Sarcoidosis has recurred in the graft in up to 60% of cases[187–189] but is seldom of clinical significance.[189] Other diseases that have recurred in the graft include emphysema in an α_1-antitrypsin-deficient recipient,[190] the giant cell interstitial pneumonia of hard-metal workers,[191] desquamative interstitial pneumonia,[192,193] panbronchiolitis,[194] alveolar proteinosis,[195] Langerhans cell histiocytosis[196–198] and lymphangioleiomyomatosis.[199–201] This last disease is almost entirely confined to women and it is notable that the donors of some lungs affected by recurrent disease were men; the recurrent smooth-muscle proliferation is of recipient origin,[202,203] as are the immune cells that contribute to recurrent sarcoidosis.[204] Recurrent bronchioloalveolar cell carcinoma has been shown to have originated in the recipient and the recurrence to have taken place despite both lungs having been replaced and there being no evidence of extrapulmonary involvement.[205] Idiopathic pulmonary fibrosis and emphysema are examples of diseases that have not yet been reported to recur in transplanted lungs.

Drug injury

Some of the immunosuppressive drugs used to maintain a transplant may harm other organs. For example, ciclosporin may cause renal damage and rhabdomyolysis while azathioprine may damage the liver and bone marrow. Several patterns of lung disease have been described in the recipients of lung and other organ transplants following treatment with sirolimus: these include lymphocytic interstitial pneumonia, organising pneumonia, diffuse alveolar haemorrhage and pulmonary haemorrhage.[206–208] Sirolimus is also contraindicated postoperatively as it may cause dehiscence of the bronchial anastomosis. Amiodarone may be used to treat atrial fibrillation, which is a common postoperative complication, and rare cases of amiodarone lung have been reported in transplant recipients.

FUTURE PROSPECTS

With increasing numbers of patients awaiting lung transplantation and a limited donor pool, the pressure on transplant centres is immense. Advances in the medical treatment of those pulmonary conditions for which patients are often transplanted (such as cystic fibrosis, pulmonary hypertension and fibrosing lung disease) will reduce demand on transplant services but new strategies are required. Those being explored include attempts to improve the condition of borderline lungs, the use of mechanical assist devices, xenotransplantation and the construction of new lungs by bioengineering.

So far the only strategy to enter the clinical arena is reconditioning ex vivo, whereby the condition of borderline donor lungs is improved by mechanical ventilation and perfusion in a specially designed circuit.[209–211] Stem cell therapy may also prove of benefit in reconditioning borderline lungs.

While mechanical assist devices have a well-established role in end-stage heart failure, the use of such devices to support patients awaiting lung transplantation is limited. Extracorporeal membrane oxygenation has been used successfully as a short-term bridge to transplantation in some patients, but the development of a portable artificial lung for longer support outside hospital is still awaited. Pulmonary xenotransplantation is an area of active research, with several groups exploring the use of porcine lungs.

Figure 11.22 Pulmonary posttransplantation lymphoproliferative disorder (monomorphous, large B-cell lymphoma). (A) Large pleomorphic lymphoid cells, some with immunoblastic features, show angiocentricity. (B) Some of the lymphoid cells infiltrating the vessel wall show immunoblastic features. (C) CD20-positivity shows that the infiltrate is of B-cell origin. (D) In situ hybridisation for Epstein–Barr virus-encoded RNA shows strong nuclear positivity. *(D courtesy of Dr JA Thomas, London, UK.)*

REFERENCES

1. Hertz MI, Aurora P, Christie JD, et al. Scientific Registry of the International Society for Heart and Lung Transplantation: introduction to the 2009 Annual Reports. J Heart Lung Transplant 2009;28:989–92.

2. Starnes VA, Bowdish ME, Woo MS, et al. A decade of living lobar lung transplantation: recipient outcomes. J Thorac Cardiovasc Surg 2004;127:114–22.

3. Van Raemdonck DE, Verleden GM, Coosemans W, et al. Increasing the donor pool. European Respiratory Society, Lausanne, Switzerland; 2009. p. 104–27.

4. Christie JD, Edwards LB, Aurora P, et al. The Registry of the International Society for Heart and Lung Transplantation: Twenty-sixth Official Adult Lung and Heart–Lung Transplantation Report-2009. J Heart Lung Transplant 2009;28:1031–49.

5. Aurora P, Edwards LB, Christie JD, et al. Registry of the International Society for Heart and Lung Transplantation: Twelfth Official Pediatric Lung and Heart/Lung Transplantation Report-2009. J Heart Lung Transplant 2009;28:1023–30.

Types of lung transplant

6. Keating D, Levvey B, Kotsimbos T, et al. Lung transplantation in pulmonary fibrosis: challenging early outcomes counterbalanced by surprisingly good outcomes beyond 15 years. Transplant Proc 2009;41:289–91.

Recipient selection

7. Trulock EP, Edwards LB, Taylor DO, et al. The Registry of the International Society for Heart and Lung Transplantation: twenty-first official adult heart transplant report – 2004. J Heart Lung Transplant 2004;23:804–15.

8. Zorn GL, McGiffin DC, Young KR, et al. Pulmonary transplantation for advanced bronchioloalveolar carcinoma. J Thorac Cardiovasc Surg 2003;125:45–8.

9. Levine SM. Angel LF. Is the lung allocation score working? A qualified yes. Chest 2009;135:890–2.

10. Osaki S, Maloney JD, Meyer KC, et al. The impact of the lung allocation scoring system at the single national Veterans Affairs Hospital lung transplantation

program. Eur J Cardiothorac Surg 2009;36:497–501.

11. Russo MJ, Iribarne A, Hong KN, et al. High lung allocation score is associated with increased morbidity and mortality following transplantation. Chest 2009;137.651–7.

12. Weiss ES, Allen JG, Merlo CA, et al. Lung allocation score predicts survival in lung transplantation patients with pulmonary fibrosis. Ann Thorac Surg 2009;88:1757–64.

Donor matching

13. Pratschke J, Wilhelm MJ, Kusaka M, et al. Brain death and its influence on donor organ quality and outcome after transplantation. Transplantation 1999;67:343–8.

14. Dark J. Single and bilateral lung transplantation. In: Banner NR, Polak JM, Yacoub M, editors. Lung Transplantation. Cambridge, UK: Cambridge University Press; 2003. p. 132–40.

15. Oto T, Griffiths A, Levvey B, et al. Donor history of asthma is not a contraindication to lung transplantation: 12-year single-center experience. J Heart Lung Transplant 2004;23:309–16.

16. Keating DT, Marasco SF, Negri J, et al. Long-term outcomes of cadaveric lobar lung transplantation: Helping to maximize resources. J Heart Lung Transplant 2010;29:434–44.

17. Cohen AH, Mallory GB, Ross K, et al. Growth of lungs after transplantation in infants and in children younger than 3 years of age. Amer J Respir Crit Care Med 1999;159:1747–51.

17a. Carter V. My approach to cardiothoracic transplantation and the role of the histocompatibility and immunogenetics laboratory in a rapidly developing field. J Clin Pathol 2010;63:189–93.

18. Scornik JC, Zander DS, Baz MA, et al. Susceptibility of lung transplants to preformed donor-specific HLA antibodies as detected by flow cytometry. Transplantation 1999;68:1542–6.

Role of the histopathologist

19. Wallace WAH, Bellamy COC, Rassl DM, et al. Transplant histopathology for the general histopathologist. Histopathology 2003;43:313–22.

20. Burke M. Transplant pathology. In: Banner NR, Polak JM, Yacoub M, editors. Lung Transplantation. Cambridge, UK: Cambridge University Press; 2005. p. 294–325.

21. Stewart S, McNeil K, Nashef SA, et al. Audit of referral and explant diagnoses in lung transplantation: a pathologic study of lungs removed for parenchymal disease. J Heart Lung Transplant 1995;14:1173–86.

22. Calabrese F, Alessandrini L, Loy M, et al. Comparison between referral diagnosis of patients requiring transplantation and pathologic diagnosis of native lungs. J Heart Lung Transplant 2009;28:1135–40.

Complications

23. Khan SU, Salloum J, Odonovan PB, et al. Acute pulmonary edema after lung transplantation – the pulmonary reimplantation response. Chest 1999;116:187–94.

24. Ng CSH, Wan S, Yim APC. Pulmonary ischaemia–reperfusion injury: role of apoptosis. Eur Respir J 2005;25: 356–63.

25. Zenati M, Yousem SA, Dowling RD. Primary graft failure following pulmonary transplantation. Transplantation 1990;50:165–7.

26. Lee JC, Christie JD. Primary graft dysfunction. Proc Am Thorac Soc 2009;6:39–46.

27. Gammie JS, Stukus DR, Pham SM, et al. Effect of ischemic time on survival in clinical lung transplantation. Ann Thorac Surg 1999;68:2015–9.

28. Ohori NP, Iacono AT, Grgurich WF, et al. Significance of acute bronchitis/ bronchiolitis in the lung transplant recipient. Am J Surg Pathol 1994;18:1192–204.

29. Rivero DHRF, Lorenzi G, Pazetti R, et al. Effects of bronchial transection and reanastomosis on mucociliary system. Chest 2001;119:1510–15.

30. Yousem SA. Alveolar lipoproteinosis in lung allograft recipients. Hum Pathol 1997;28:1383–6.

31. McDonald JW, Keller CA, Ramos RR, et al. Mixed (neutrophil-rich) interstitial pneumonitis in biopsy specimens of lung allografts: a clinicopathologic evaluation. Chest 1998;113:117–23.

32. Kshettry VR, Kroshus TJ, Hertz MI, et al. Early and late complications after lung transplantation: incidence and management. Ann Thorac Surg 1997;63:1576–83.

33. Norgaard MA, Andersen CB, Pettersson G. Does bronchial artery revascularization influence results concerning bronchiolitis obliterans syndrome and/or obliterative bronchiolitis after lung transplantation? Eur J Cardiothorac Surg 1998;14:311–8.

34. Yousem SA, Paradis IL, Dauber JA, et al. Large airway inflammation in heart–lung transplant recipients – its significance and prognostic implications. Transplantation 1990;49:654–6.

35. Maiwand MO, Zehr KJ, Dyke CM, et al. The role of cryotherapy for airway complications after lung and heart–lung transplantation. Eur J Cardiothorac Surg 1997;12:549–54.

36. Yousem SA, Dauber JH, Griffith BP. Bronchial cartilage alterations in lung transplantation. Chest 1990;98:1121–4.

37. Schulman LL, Anandarangam T, Leibowitz DW, et al. Four-year prospective study of pulmonary venous thrombosis after lung transplantation. J Am Soc Echocardiogr 2001;14:806–12.

38. Fadel BM, Abdulbaki K, Nambiar V, et al. Dual thrombosis of the pulmonary arterial and venous anastomotic sites after single lung transplantation: role of transesophageal echocardiography in diagnosis and management. J Am Soc Echocardiogr 2007;20:438–12.

39. Uhlmann EJ, Dunitz JM, Fiol ME. Pulmonary vein thrombosis after lung transplantation presenting as stroke. J Heart Lung Transplant 2009;28:209–10.

40. Gonzalez-Fernandez C, Gonzalez-Castro A, Rodriguez-Borregan JC, et al. Pulmonary venous obstruction after lung transplantation. Diagnostic advantages of transesophageal echocardiography. Clin Transplant 2009;23:975–80.

41. Taylor PM, Rose M, Yacoub MH. Expression of class I and class II MHC antigens in normal and transplanted human lung. Transplant. Proc 1989;21:451–2.

42. Karamsetty MR, Klinger JR. NO: More than just a vasodilator in lung transplantation. Amer J Respir Cell Molec Biol 2002;26:1–5.

43. Mason NA, Springall DR, Pomerance A, et al. Expression of inducible nitric oxide synthase and formation of peroxynitrite in posttransplant obliterative bronchiolitis. J Heart Lung Transplant 1998;17: 710–4.

44. Gabbay E, Haydn WE, Orsida B, et al. In stable lung transplant recipients, exhaled nitric oxide levels positively correlate with airway neutrophilia and bronchial epithelial iNOS. Am J Respir Crit Care Med 1999;160:2093–9.

46. Choi JK, Kearns J, Palevsky HI, et al. Hyperacute rejection of a pulmonary allograft. Immediate clinical and pathologic findings. Am J Respir Crit Care Med 1999;160:1015–8.

47. Bittner HB, Dunitz J, Hertz M, et al. Hyperacute rejection in single lung transplantation – case report of successful management by means of plasmapheresis and antithymocyte globulin treatment. Transplantation 2001;71:649–51.

48. Stewart S, Fishbein MC, Snell GI, et al. Revision of the 1996 working formulation for the standardization of nomenclature in the diagnosis of lung rejection. J Heart Lung Transplant 2007;26:1223–8.

49. Yousem SA, Duncan SR, Griffith BP. Interstitial and airspace granulation tissue reactions in lung transplant recipients. Am J Surg Pathol 1992;16:877–84.

50. Yousem SA. Lymphocytic bronchitis/ bronchiolitis in lung allograft recipients. Am J Surg Pathol 1993;17:491–6.

51. Hasleton PS, Woodcock AA, Yonan N, et al. Should cryptogenic organizing pneumonia be included in the classification of pulmonary allograft rejection? J Heart Lung Transplant 1996;15:1268–9.

52. Gabbay E, Dark JH, Ashcroft T, et al. Cryptogenic organizing pneumonia is an important cause of graft dysfunction and should be included in the classification of pulmonary allograft rejection. J Heart Lung Transplant 1998;17:230–1.

53. Chaparro C, Maurer JR, Chamberlain DW, et al. Role of open lung biopsy for diagnosis in lung transplant recipients: ten-year experience. Ann Thorac Surg 1995;59:928–32.

54. Clelland CA, Higenbottam TW, Stewart S, et al. The histological changes in transbronchial biopsy after treatment of acute lung rejection in heart–lung transplants. J Pathol 1990;161:105–12.

55. de Blic J, Peuchmaur M, Carnot F, et al. Rejection in lung transplantation – an immunohistochemical study of transbronchial biopsies. Transplantation 1992;54:639–44.

56. Yousem SA, Martin T, Paradis IL, et al. Can immunohistological analysis of transbronchial biopsy specimens predict responder status in early acute rejection of lung allografts? Hum Pathol 1994;25:525–9.

57. Rosendale B, Yousem SA. Discrimination of Epstein–Barr virus-related posttransplant lymphoproliferations from acute rejection in lung allograft recipients. Arch Pathol Lab Med 1995;119:418–23.

58. Longchampt E, Achkar A, Tissier F, et al. Coexistence of acute cellular rejection and lymphoproliferative disorder in a lung transplant patient. Arch Pathol Lab Med 2001;125:1500–2.

59. Nakhleh RE, Bolman RM III, Henke CA, et al. Lung transplant pathology. A comparative study of pulmonary acute rejection and cytomegaloviral infection. Am J Surg Pathol 1991;15:1197–201.

60. Tazelaar HD. Perivascular inflammation in pulmonary infections: implications for the diagnosis of lung rejection. J Heart Lung Transplant 1991;10:437–41.

61. Niedobitek G, Finn T, Herbst H, et al. Detection of cytomegalovirus by in-situ hybridisation and histochemistry using a monoclonal antibody CCH2: a comparison of methods. J Clin Pathol 1988;41:1005–9.

62. Weiss LM, Movahed LA, Berry GJ, et al. In situ hybridization studies for viral nucleic acids in heart and lung allograft biopsies. Am J Clin Pathol 1990;93:675–9.

63. Yousem SA. Graft eosinophilia in lung transplantation. Hum Pathol 1992;23:1172–7.

64. Gerhardt SG, Tuder RM, Girgis RE, et al. Pulmonary eosinophilia following lung transplantation for sarcoidosis in two patients. Chest 2003;123:629–32.

65. Husain AN, Siddiqui MT, Holmes EW, et al. Analysis of risk factors for the development of bronchiolitis obliterans syndrome. Am J Respir Crit Care Med 1999;159:829–33.

66. Sibley RK, Berry GJ, Tazelaar HD, et al. The role of transbronchial biopsies in the management of lung transplant recipients. J Heart Lung Transplant 1993;12:308–24.

67. Scott JP, Peters SG, McDougall JC, et al. Posttransplantation physiologic features of the lung and obliterative bronchiolitis. Mayo Clin Proc 1997;72:170–4.

68. Burke CM, Theodore J, Dawkins KD, et al. Post-transplant obliterative bronchiolitis and other late lung sequelae in human heart–lung transplantation. Chest 1984;86:824–9.

69. Yousem SA, Burke CM, Billingham ME. Pathologic pulmonary alterations in long-term human heart–lung transplantation. Hum Pathol 1985;16:911–23.

70. Kramer MR. Bronchiolitis obliterans following heart–lung and lung transplantation. Respir Med 1994;88:9–15.

71. Cagle PT, Brown RW, Frost A, et al. Diagnosis of chronic lung transplant rejection by transbronchial biopsy. Mod Pathol 1995;8:137–42.

72. Milne DS, Gascoigne A, Wilkes J, et al. The immunohistopathology of obliterative bronchiolitis following lung transplantation. Transplantation 1992;54:748–50.

73. Kramer MR, Stoehr C, Whang JL, et al. The diagnosis of obliterative bronchiolitis following heart–lung and lung transplantations: low yield of transbronchial lung biopsy. J Heart Lung Transplant 1993;12:675–81.

74. Pomerance A, Madden B, Burke MM, et al. Transbronchial biopsy in heart and lung transplantation: clinicopathologic correlations. J Heart Lung Transplant 1995;14:761–73.

75. Estenne M, Maurer JR, Boehler A, et al. Bronchiolitis obliterans syndrome 2001: an update of the diagnostic criteria. J Heart Lung Transplant 2002;21:297–310.

76. Ramsey R, Hachem RR, Chakinala MM, et al. The predictive value of bronchiolitis obliterans syndrome stage 0-p. Am J Respir Crit Care Med 2004;169:468–72.

77. Heng D, Sharples LD, McNeil K, et al. Bronchiolitis obliterans syndrome: incidence, natural history, prognosis, and risk factors. J Heart Lung Transplant 1998;17:1255–63.

78. Boehler A, Estenne M. Post-transplant bronchiolitis obliterans. Eur Resp J 2003;22:1007–18.

79. Clelland C, Higenbottam T, Otulana B, et al. Histologic prognostic indicators for the lung allografts of heart–lung transplants. J Heart Transplant 1990;9:177–85.

80. Geddes DM, Corrin B, Brewerton DA, et al. Progressive airway obliteration in adults and its association with rheumatoid disease. Q J Med 1977;46:427–44.

81. Urbanski SJ, Kossakowska AE, Curtis J, et al. Idiopathic small airways pathology in patients with graft-versus-host disease following allogeneic bone marrow transplantation. Am J Surg Pathol 1987;11:965–71.

82. Epler GR. Bronchiolitis obliterans and airway obstruction associated with graft-versus-host disease. Clin Chest Med 1988;9:551–6.

83. Yousem SA. The histological spectrum of pulmonary graft versus host disease in bone marrow transplant recipients. Hum Pathol 1995;26:668–75.

84. Palmer SM, Davis RD, Hadjiliadis D, et al. Development of an antibody specific to major histocompatibility antigens detectable by flow cytometry after lung transplant is associated with bronchiolitis obliterans syndrome. Transplantation 2002;74:799–804.

85. Rose ML. De novo production of antibodies after heart or lung transplantation should be regarded as an early warning system. J Heart Lung Transplant 2004;23:385–95.

86. King BJ, Iyer H, Leidi AA, et al. Gastroesophageal reflux in bronchiolitis obliterans syndrome: a new perspective. J Heart Lung Transplant 2009;28:870–5.

87. D'Ovidio F, Mura M, Tsang M, et al. Bile acid aspiration and the development of bronchiolitis obliterans after lung transplantation. J Thorac Cardiovasc Surg 2005;129:1144–52.

88. Blondeau K, Mertens V, Vanaudenaerde BA, et al. Gastro-oesophageal reflux and gastric aspiration in lung transplant patients with or without chronic rejection. Eur Respir J 2008;31:707–13.

89. Kroshus TJ, Kshettry VR, Savik K, et al. Risk factors for the development of bronchiolitis obliterans syndrome after lung transplantation. J Thorac Cardiovasc Surg 1997;114:195–202.

90. Koskinen PK, Kallio EA, Bruggeman CA, et al. Cytomegalovirus infection enhances experimental obliterative bronchiolitis in rat tracheal allografts. Amer J Respir Crit Care Med 1997;155:2078–88.

91. Billings JL, Hertz MI, Savik K, et al. Respiratory viruses and chronic rejection in lung transplant recipients. J Heart Lung Transplant 2002;21:559–66.

92. Khalifah AP, Hachem RR, Chakinala MM, et al. Respiratory viral infections are a distinct risk for bronchiolitis obliterans syndrome and death. Am J Respir Crit Care Med 2004;170:181–7.

93. Luckraz H, Goddard M, McNeil K, et al. Microvascular changes in small airways predispose to obliterative bronchiolitis after lung transplantation. J Heart Lung Transplant 2004;23:527–31.

94. Verleden GM, Vos R, De Vleeschauwer SI, et al. Obliterative bronchiolitis following lung transplantation: from old to new concepts? Transpl Int 2009;22:771–9.

95. Verleden GM, Dupont LJ. Azithromycin therapy for patients with bronchiolitis obliterans syndrome after lung

transplantation. Transplantation 2004;77:1465–7.

96. Vanaudenaerde BM, Meyts I, Vos R, et al. A dichotomy in bronchiolitis obliterans syndrome after lung transplantation revealed by azithromycin therapy. Eur Respir J 2008;32:832–43.

97. Brocker V, Langer F, Fellous TG, et al. Fibroblasts of recipient origin contribute to bronchiolitis obliterans in human lung transplants. Am J Respir Crit Care Med 2006;173:1276–82.

98. Guarino M, Tosoni A, Nebuloni M. Direct contribution of epithelium to organ fibrosis: epithelial–mesenchymal transition. Human Pathology 2009;40:1365–76.

99. Hodge S, Holmes M, Banerjee B, et al. Posttransplant bronchiolitis obliterans syndrome is associated with bronchial epithelial to mesenchymal transition. Am J Transplant 2009;9:727–33.

100. Yousem SA, Paradis IL, Dauber JH, et al. Pulmonary arteriosclerosis in long-term human heart–lung transplant recipients. Transplantation 1989;47:564–9.

101. Pucci A, Forbes RD, Berry GJ, et al. Accelerated posttransplant coronary arteriosclerosis in combined heart–lung transplantation. Transplant Proc 1991;23:1228–9.

102. Hasleton PS, Brooks NH. Severe pulmonary vascular change in patients dying from right ventricular failure after heart transplantation. Thorax 1995;50:210–2.

103. Chaparro C, Maurer JR, Chamberlain DW, et al. Role of open lung biopsy for diagnosis in lung transplant recipients: ten-year experience. Ann Thorac Surg 1995;59:928–32.

104. Takemoto SK, Zeevi A, Feng S, et al. National conference to assess antibody-mediated rejection in solid organ transplantation. Am J Transplant 2004;4:1033–41.

104a. Murata K, Baldwin WM. Mechanisms of complement activation, C4d deposition and their contribution to the pathogenesis of antibody-mediated rejection. Transplantation Reviews 2009;23:139–50.

105. Miller GG, Destarac L, Zeevi A, et al. Acute humoral rejection of human lung allografts and elevation of C4d in bronchoalveolar lavage fluid. Am J Transplant 2004;4:1323–30.

106. Ionescu DN, Girnita AL, Zeevi A, et al. C4d deposition in lung allografts is associated with circulating anti-HLA alloantibody. Transpl Immunol 2005;15:63–8.

107. Girnita AL, McCurry KR, Zeevi A. Increased lung allograft failure in patients with HLA-specific antibody. Clin Transpl 2007;231–9.

108. Girnita AL, McCurry KR, Yousem SA, et al. Antibody-mediated rejection in lung transplantation: case reports. Clin Transpl 2006;508–10.

109. Badesch DB, Zamora M, Fullerton D, et al. Pulmonary capillaritis: a possible histologic form of acute pulmonary allograft rejection. J Heart Lung Transplant 1998;17:415–22.

110. Astor TL, Weill D, Cool C, et al. Pulmonary capillaritis in lung transplant recipients: treatment and effect on allograft function. J Heart Lung Transplant 2005;24:2091–7.

111. Morrell MR, Patterson GA, Trulock EP, et al. Acute antibody-mediated rejection after lung transplantation. J Heart Lung Transplant 2009;28:96–100.

112. Astor TL, Galantowicz M, Phillips A, et al. Pulmonary capillaritis as a manifestation of acute humoral allograft rejection following infant lung transplantation. Am J Transplant 2009;9:409–12.

113. Magro CM, Deng A, Pope-Harman A, et al. Humorally mediated posttransplantation septal capillary injury syndrome as a common form of pulmonary allograft rejection: a hypothesis. Transplantation 2002;74:1273–80.

114. Chang AT, Platt JL. The role of antibodies in transplantation. Transplantation Reviews 2009;23:191–8.

115. Wallace WD, Reed EF, Ross D, et al. C4d staining of pulmonary allograft biopsies: an immunoperoxidase study. J Heart Lung Transplant 2005;24:1565–70.

116. Westall GP, Snell GI, McLean C, et al. C3d and C4d deposition early after lung transplantation. J Heart Lung Transplant 2008;27:722–8.

117. Pakhale SS, Hadjiliadis D, Howell DN, et al. Upper lobe fibrosis: a novel manifestation of chronic allograft dysfunction in lung transplantation. J Heart Lung Transplant 2005;24:1260–8.

118. Kotloff RM, Ahya VN. Medical complications of lung transplantation. Eur Resp J 2004;23:334–42.

119. Guilinger RA, Paradis IL, Dauber JH, et al. The importance of bronchoscopy with transbronchial biopsy and bronchoalveolar lavage in the management of lung transplant recipients. Am J Respir Crit Care Med 1995;152:2037–43.

120. Arbustini E, Morbini P, Grasso M, et al. Human cytomegalovirus early infection, acute rejection, and major histocompatibility class II expression in transplanted lung. Molecular, immunocytochemical, and histopathologic investigations. Transplantation 1996;61:418–27.

121. You XM, Steinmuller C, Wagner TO, et al. Enhancement of cytomegalovirus infection and acute rejection after allogeneic lung transplantation in the rat: virus-induced expression of major histocompatibility complex class II antigens. J Heart Lung Transplant 1996;15:1108–19.

122. Egan JJ, Barber L, Lomax J, et al. Detection of human cytomegalovirus antigenaemia: a rapid diagnostic technique for predicting cytomegalovirus infection/pneumonitis in lung and heart transplant recipients. Thorax 1995;50:9–13.

123. Tikkanen J, Lemstrom K, Halme M, et al. Cytological monitoring of peripheral blood, bronchoalveolar lavage fluid, and transbronchial biopsy specimens during acute rejection and cytomegalovirus infection in lung and heart–lung allograft recipients. Clin Transplant 2001;15:77–88.

124. Fend F, Prior C, Margreiter R, et al. Cytomegalovirus pneumonitis in heart–lung transplant recipients: histopathology and clinicopathologic considerations. Hum Pathol 1990;21:918–26.

125. Allen TC, Bag R, Zander DS, et al. Cytomegalovirus infection masquerading as carcinoma in a lung transplant patient. Arch Pathol Lab Med 2005;129:e1-3.

126. Smyth RL, Higenbottam TW, Scott JP, et al. Herpes simplex virus infection in heart–lung transplant recipients. Transplantation 1990;49:735–9.

127. Vilchez R, McCurry K, Dauber J, et al. Influenza and parainfluenza respiratory viral infection requiring admission in adult lung transplant recipients. Transplantation 2002;73:1075–8.

128. Dromer C, Nashef SA, Velly JF, et al. Tuberculosis in transplanted lungs. J Heart Lung Transplant 1993;12:924–7.

129. Tazelaar HD, Baird AM, Mill M, et al. Bronchocentric mycosis occurring in transplant recipients. Chest 1989;96:92–5.

130. Kesten S, Chaparro C. Mycobacterial infections in lung transplant recipients. Chest 1999;115:741–5.

131. Gryzan S, Paradis IL, Zeevi A, et al. Unexpectedly high incidence of *Pneumocystis carinii* infection after heart–lung transplantation. Implications for lung defense and allograft survival. Am Rev Respir Dis 1988;137:1268–74.

132. Wakefield AE, Miller RF, Guiver LA, et al. Granulomatous *Pneumocystis carinii* pneumonia: DNA amplification studies on bronchoscopic alveolar lavage samples. J Clin Pathol 1994;47:664–6.

133. Cahill BC, Hibbs JR, Savik K, et al. *Aspergillus* airway colonization and invasive disease after lung transplantation. Chest 1997;112:1160–4.

134. Skerrett SJ, Martin TR. Alveolar macrophage activation in experimental legionellosis. J Immunol 1991;147:337–45.

135. Kramer MR, Denning DW, Marshall SE, et al. Ulcerative tracheobronchitis after lung transplantation – a new form of invasive aspergillosis. Am Rev Respir Dis 1991;144:552–6.

136. Egan JJ, Yonan N, Carroll KB, et al. Allergic bronchopulmonary aspergillosis in lung allograft recipients. Eur Respir J 1996;9:169–71.

137. Mehrad B, Paciocco G, Martinez FJ, et al. Spectrum of *Aspergillus* infection in lung

transplant recipients – Case series and review of the literature. Chest 2001;119:169–75.

138. Wreghitt TG, Hakim M, Gray JJ, et al. Toxoplasmosis in heart and heart and lung transplant recipients. J Clin Pathol 1989;42:194–9.

139. Holliman R, Johnson J, Savva D, et al. Diagnosis of toxoplasma infection in cardiac transplant recipients using the polymerase chain reaction. J Clin Pathol 1992;45:931–2.

140. Vos R, Blondeau K, Vanaudenaerde BM, et al. Airway colonization and gastric aspiration after lung transplantation: do birds of a feather flock together? J Heart Lung Transplant 2008;27:843–9.

141. Robertson AG, Griffin SM, Murphy DM, et al. Targeting allograft injury and inflammation in the management of post-lung transplant bronchiolitis obliterans syndrome. Am J Transplant 2009;9:1272–8.

142. Hadjiliadis D, Duane DR, Steele MP, et al. Gastroesophageal reflux disease in lung transplant recipients. Clin Transplant 2003;17:363–8.

143. Penn I. Occurrence of cancers in immunosuppressed organ transplant recipients. Clin Transpl 1998;147–58.

144. Mihalov ML, Gattuso P, Abraham K, et al. Incidence of post-transplant malignancy among 674 solid-organ-transplant recipients at a single center. Clin Transplant 1996;10:248–55.

145. Rinaldi M, Pellegrini C, D'Armini AM, et al. Neoplastic disease after heart transplantation: single center experience. Eur J Cardiothorac Surg 2001;19:696–701.

146. DeSoyza AG, Dark JH, Parums DV, et al. Donor-acquired small cell lung cancer following pulmonary transplantation. Chest 2001;120:1030–1.

147. Harwood CA, Surentheran T, McGregor JM, et al. Human papillomavirus infection and non-melanoma skin cancer in immunosuppressed and immunocompetent individuals. J Med Virol 2000;61:289–97.

148. Torbenson M, Wang J, Nichols L, et al. Renal cortical neoplasms in long term survivors of solid organ transplantation. Transplantation 2000;69:864–8.

149. Anyanwu AC, Townsend ER, Banner NR, et al. Primary lung carcinoma after heart or lung transplantation: management and outcome. J Thorac Cardiovasc Surg 2002;124:1190–7.

150. Ohori NP. Epithelial cell atypia in bronchoalveolar lavage specimens from lung transplant recipients. Amer J Clin Pathol 1999;112:204–10.

151. Sleiman C, Mal H, Roue C, et al. Bronchial Kaposi's sarcoma after single lung transplantation. Eur Respir J 1997;10:1181–3.

152. Flint A, Lynch JP, Martinez FJ, et al. Pulmonary smooth muscle proliferation occurring after lung transplantation. Chest 1997;112:283–4.

153. Somers CR, Tesoriero AA, Hartland E, et al. Multiple leiomyosarcomas of both donor and recipient origin arising in a heart–lung transplant patient. Am J Surg Pathol 1998;22:1423–8.

154. Mathew J, Kratzke RA. Lung cancer and lung transplantation: a review. J Thorac Oncol 2009;4:753–60.

155. Swerdlow SH. Post-transplant lymphoproliferative disorders: a morphologic, phenotypic and genotypic spectrum of disease. Histopathology 1992;20:373–85.

156. Craig FE, Gulley ML, Banks PM. Posttransplantation lymphoproliferative disorders. Am J Clin Pathol 1993;99:265–76.

157. Swerdlow SH. Post-transplant lymphoproliferative disorders: a working classification. Current Diagnostic Pathology 1997;4:28–35.

158. Reams D, McAdams HP, Howell DN, et al. Posttransplant lymphoproliferative disorder – Incidence, presentation, and response to treatment in lung transplant recipients. Chest 2003;124:1242–9.

159. Yousem SA, Randhawa P, Locker J, et al. Posttransplant lymphoproliferative disorders in heart–lung transplant recipients: primary presentation in the allograft. Hum Pathol 1989;20:361–9.

160. Delecluse HJ, Kremmer E, Rouault JP, et al. The expression of Epstein–Barr virus latent proteins is related to the pathological features of post-transplant lymphoproliferative disorders. Am J Pathol 1995;146:1113–20.

161. Ramalingam P, Rybicki L, Smith MD, et al. Posttransplant lymphoproliferative disorders in lung transplant patients: The Cleveland Clinic experience. Modern Pathol 2002;15:647–56.

162. Aris RM, Maia DM, Neuringer IP, et al. Post-transplantation lymphoproliferative disorder in the Epstein–Barr virus-naive lung transplant recipient. Amer J Respir Crit Care Med 1996;154:1712–7.

163. Starzl TE, Nalesnik MA, Porter KA, et al. Reversibility of lymphomas and lymphoproliferative lesions developing under cyclosporin-steroid therapy. Lancet 1984;1:583–7.

164. Thomas JA, Crawford DH, Burke M. Clinicopathologic implications of Epstein–Barr virus related B cell lymphoma in immunocompromised patients. J Clin Pathol 1995;48:287–90.

165. Peterson MR, Emery SC, Yung GL, et al. Epstein–Barr virus-associated posttransplantation lymphoproliferative disorder following lung transplantation is more commonly of host origin. Arch Pathol Lab Med 2006;130:176–80.

166. Swerdlow AJ, Higgins CD, Hunt BJ, et al. Risk of lymphoid neoplasia after cardiothoracic transplantation. a cohort study of the relation to Epstein–Barr virus. Transplantation 2000;69:897–904.

167. Nalesnik MA, Jaffe R, Starzl TE, et al. The pathology of posttransplant lymphoproliferative disorders occurring in the setting of cyclosporine A-prednisone immunosuppression. Am J Pathol 1988;133:173–92.

168. Weissmann DJ, Ferry JA, Harris NL, et al. Posttransplantation lymphoproliferative disorders in solid organ recipients are predominantly aggressive tumors of host origin. Am J Clin Pathol 1995;103:748–55.

169. Chadburn A, Suciufoca N, Cesarman E, et al. Post-transplantation lymphoproliferative disorders arising in solid organ transplant recipients are usually of recipient origin. Am J Pathol 1995;147:1862–70.

170. Spiro IJ, Yandell DW, Li C, et al. Brief report: lymphoma of donor origin occurring in the porta hepatis of a transplanted liver. N Engl J Med 1993;329:27–9.

171. Ohori NP, Whisnant RE, Nalesnik MA, et al. Primary pleural effusion posttransplant lymphoproliferative disorder: Distinction from secondary involvement and effusion lymphoma. Diagn Cytopathol 2001;25:50–3.

172. Halkos ME, Miller JI, Mann KP, et al. Thoracic presentations of posttransplant lymphoproliferative disorders. Chest 2004;126:2013–20.

173. Swerdlow SH, Campo E, Harris N, et al. WHO Classification of Tumours of Haemopoietic and Lymphoid Tissues. 4th ed. Lyons, France: IARC Press; 2008.

174. Knowles DM, Cesarman E, Chadburn A, et al. Correlative morphologic and molecular genetic analysis demonstrates three distinct categories of posttransplantation lymphoproliferative disorders. Blood 1995;85:552–65.

175. Swinnen LJ. Organ transplant-related lymphoma. Curr Treat Options Oncol 2001;2:301–8.

176. Milpied N, Vasseur B, Parquet N, et al. Humanized anti-CD20 monoclonal antibody (Rituximab) in post transplant B-lymphoproliferative disorder: a retrospective analysis on 32 patients. Ann Oncol 2000;11:113–6.

177. Knoop C, Kentos A, Remmelink M, et al. Post-transplant lymphoproliferative disorders after lung transplantation: first-line treatment with rituximab may induce complete remission. Clin Transplant 2006;20:179–87.

178. Chau EM, Lee J, Yew WW, et al. Mediastinal irradiation for graft-versus-host disease in a heart–lung transplant recipient. J Heart Lung Transplant 1997;16:974–9.

179. Smith DM, Agura ED, Ausloos K, et al. Graft-vs-host disease as a complication of lung transplantation. J Heart Lung Transplant 2006;25:1175–7.

180. Assi MA, Pulido JS, Peters SG, et al. Graft-vs.-host disease in lung and other solid organ transplant recipients. Clin Transplant 2007;21:1–6.

181. Worel N, Bojic A, Binder M, et al. Catastrophic graft-versus-host disease after lung transplantation proven by PCR-based chimerism analysis. Transpl Int 2008;21:1098–101.

182. Roca J, Granena A, Rodriguez-Roisin R, et al. Fatal airway disease in an adult with chronic graft-versus-host disease. Thorax 1982;37:77–8.

183. Ralph DD, Springmeyer SC, Sullivan KM, et al. Rapidly progressive air-flow obstruction in marrow transplant recipients. Possible association between obliterative bronchiolitis and chronic graft-versus-host disease. Am Rev Respir Dis 1984;129:641–4.

184. Alton EWFW, Khagani A, Taylor RFH, et al. Effect of heart–lung transplantation on airway potential difference in patients with and without cystic fibrosis. Eur Respir J 1991;4:5–9.

185. Tsang VT, Alton EWFW, Hodson ME, et al. In vitro bioelectric properties of bronchial epithelium from transplanted lungs in recipients with cystic fibrosis. Thorax 1993;48:1006–11.

186. Corris PA, Dark JH. Aetiology of asthma – lessons from lung transplantation. Lancet 1993;341:1369–71.

187. Kazerooni EA, Jackson C, Cascade PN. Sarcoidosis: recurrence of primary disease in transplanted lungs. Radiology 1994;192:461–4.

188. Martinez FJ, Orens JB, Deeb M, et al. Recurrence of sarcoidosis following bilateral allogeneic lung transplantation. Chest 1994;106:1597–9.

189. Walker S, Mikhail G, Banner N, et al. Medium term results of lung transplantation for end stage pulmonary sarcoidosis. Thorax 1998;53:281–4.

190. Mal H, Guignabert C, Thabut G, et al. Recurrence of pulmonary emphysema in an α_1 proteinase inhibitor-deficient lung transplant recipient. Am J Respir Crit Care Med 2004;170:811–4.

191. Frost AE, Keller CA, Brown RW, et al. Giant cell interstitial pneumonitis – disease recurrence in the transplanted lung. Am Rev Respir Dis 1993;148:1401–4.

192. King MB, Jessurun J, Hertz MI. Recurrence of desquamative interstitial pneumonia after lung transplantation. Amer J Respir Crit Care Med 1997;156:2003–5.

193. Verleden GM, Sels F, VanRaemdonck D, et al. Possible recurrence of desquamative interstitial pneumonitis in a single lung transplant recipient. Eur Resp J 1998;11:971–4.

194. Baz MA, Kussin PS, Vantrigt P, et al. Recurrence of diffuse panbronchiolitis after lung transplantation. Am J Respir Crit Care Med 1995;151:895–8.

195. Parker LA, Novotny DB. Recurrent alveolar proteinosis following double lung transplantation. Chest 1997;111:1457–8.

196. Etienne B, Bertocchi M, Gamondes JP, et al. Relapsing pulmonary Langerhans cell histiocytosis after lung transplantation. Amer J Respir Crit Care Med 1998;157:288–91.

197. Habib SB, Congleton J, Carr D, et al. Recipient Langerhans cell histiocytosis recurring following bilateral lung transplantation. Thorax 1998;53:323–5.

198. Gabbay E, Dark JH, Ashcroft T, et al. Recurrence of Langerhans' cell granulomatosis following lung transplantation. Thorax 1998;53:326–7.

199. Nine JS, Yousem SA, Paradis IL, et al. Lymphangioleiomyomatosis recurrence after lung transplantation. J Heart Lung Transplant 1994;13:714–9.

200. O'Brien JD, Lium JH, Parosa JF et al. Lymphangiomyomatosis recurrence in the allograft after single-lung transplantation. Am J Respir Crit Care Med 1995;151:2033–6.

201. Bittmann I, Dose TB, Muller C, et al. Lymphangioleiomyomatosis: Recurrence after single lung transplantation. Hum Pathol 1997;28:1420–3.

202. Carsillo T, Astrinidis A, Henske EP. Mutations in the tuberous sclerosis complex gene TSC2 are a cause of sporadic pulmonary lymphangioleiomyomatosis. Proc Natl Acad Sci U S A 2000;97:6085–90.

203. Bittmann I, Rolf B, Amann G, et al. Recurrence of lymphangioleiomyomatosis after single lung transplantation: New insights into pathogenesis. Hum Pathol 2003;34:95–8.

204. Milman N, Andersen CB, Burton CM, et al. Recurrent sarcoid granulomas in a transplanted lung derive from recipient immune cells. Eur Respir J 2005;26:549–52.

205. Garver RI, Zorn GL, Wu X, et al. Recurrence of bronchioloalveolar carcinoma in transplanted lungs. N Engl J Med 1999;340:1071–4.

206. Pham PT, Pham PC, Danovitch GM, et al. Sirolimus-associated pulmonary toxicity. Transplantation 2004;77:1215–20.

207. Garrean S, Massad MG, Tshibaka M, et al. Sirolimus-associated interstitial pneumonitis in solid organ transplant recipients. Clinical Transplantation 2005;19:698–703.

208. Hamour IM, Mittal TK, Bell AD, et al. Reversible sirolimus-associated pneumonitis after heart transplantation. J Heart Lung Transplant 2006;25:241–4.

Future prospects

209. Steen S, Ingemansson R, Eriksson L, et al. First human transplantation of a nonacceptable donor lung after reconditioning ex vivo. Ann Thorac Surg 2007;83:2191–4.

210. Ingemansson R, Eyjolfsson A, Mared L, et al. Clinical transplantation of initially rejected donor lungs after reconditioning ex vivo. Ann Thorac Surg 2009;87:255–60.

211. Pego-Fernandes PM, de Medeiros IL, Mariani AW, et al. Ex vivo lung perfusion: initial Brazilian experience. J Bras Pneumol 2009;35:1107–11.

Chapter |12|

Tumours

12.1   Carcinoma of the lung

INCIDENCE AND MORTALITY

The last 100 years have seen the incidence of lung cancer transformed from it being an almost unknown disease to it far outstripping all other forms of cancer as a cause of death in many western countries. The death rate from lung cancer exceeds 60 per 100 000 in Great Britain and is close to this in many developed countries. In British men, it is responsible for about 35% of cancer deaths, and about 8% of all deaths, whilst in women it now rivals breast cancer as the major cause of cancer mortality. In many developed countries the incidence in men has levelled off and in some it has started to decline, but in women it is still rising,[1] the lag being almost totally due to women taking to smoking later than men. The male-to-female ratio was nearly equal in England and Wales at the end of the nineteenth century but climbed to 6 by 1951.[2] Now it is again verging on equality as deaths in men decline slightly and deaths in women rise at a rate comparable to that seen in men in the first half of the twentieth century. Furthermore, for a given level of smoking women are at higher risk of developing lung cancer than men.[3-5] A higher level of aromatic DNA adducts (indicating DNA damage) is reported in the lungs of female smokers.[6]

Many developing countries have a relatively low incidence of lung cancer but are beginning to see the rises already experienced elsewhere

©2010 Elsevier Ltd
DOI: 10.1016/B978-0-7020-3369-8.00012-4

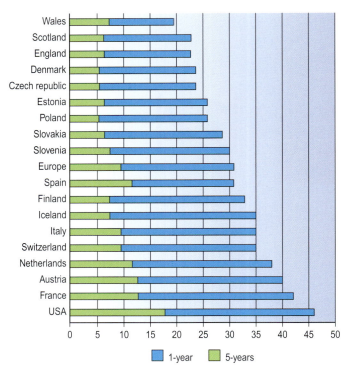

Figure 12.1.1 National 1-year and 5-year survival rates (%) from lung cancer in men. Rates in women are slightly better but broadly similar.[10,11]

as the inhabitants take to smoking in increasing numbers. There are also substantial racial differences in susceptibility to the carcinogenic effect of cigarette smoke. For example, at any level of smoking black Americans have a risk of lung cancer 1.8 times greater than that of their white compatriots.[3] It is likely that in the twenty-first century there will be a significant shift in the geographical distribution of lung cancer.

Lung cancer is largely a disease of later life. In patients younger than 40 years of age there is a lower male-to-female ratio and a higher proportion of adenocarcinoma but as in the elderly cigarette smoking is the most important cause.[7] The tumour is very rare in children but occasional cases are encountered.[8]

Lung cancer carries a very poor prognosis. Surgical survival figures may reach 46% (and nearly 60% for T1N0M0 tumours)[9] but they are based on a highly selected group of patients. Spread of the tumour often results in it being inoperable at presentation while many patients with lung cancer also have coexistent chronic obstructive lung disease that renders them unfit for surgery. Overall 5-year survival rates vary from 6% to 14%, the variation being mainly attributable to national differences in access to specialist care (Fig. 12.1.1).[10–12] Note also has to be taken of the significant number of patients who suffer recurrence more than five years after apparent eradication of their tumour; 11% in one study.[12a]

AETIOLOGY

There is convincing evidence that cigarette smoking is by far the most important cause of lung cancer. This is based mainly on sound epidemiological studies, supplemented by pathological findings. Other factors have been identified but these are considerably less important than cigarette smoking.

Smoking

The evidence linking cigarette smoking and lung cancer was first established in the early 1950s when the smoking habits of large groups of patients with lung cancer were compared with those of matched controls. These provided clear evidence that the majority of patients with carcinoma of the lung were heavy cigarette smokers and that the incidence of the disease in non-smokers was low.[13–15] Later prospective studies, in which the incidence of lung cancer was determined over a long period of time in large groups of people with different smoking habits, were even more conclusive. One of the best known of these studies was carried out in the UK on a group of 40 000 doctors. In 1951, each completed a questionnaire asking for details of their smoking habits. By 1964 there was ample evidence of a clear link between cigarette smoking and deaths from lung cancer.[16,17] Similar studies were carried out in the USA with identical conclusions.[18,19] These studies established that the risk of lung cancer is increased in smokers compared with non-smokers by a factor of 10. Pipe smokers and cigar smokers have a significantly lower incidence than cigarette smokers, probably due to them not inhaling their smoke to the same degree.[20] The risk increases with the number of cigarettes smoked and is proportional to the length of time a person has smoked, being greatest in those who commenced at an early age.[18] The term 'pack years' is often used to quantify this combination of risk factors, '1 pack year' equating to 20 cigarettes per day for 1 year or 40 per day for 6 months. In those who stop smoking, the risk begins to decline immediately but it takes about 15 years for the risk in ex-smokers to approach that of non-smokers.[16] The incidence of lung cancer is increased in those with other smoking-related diseases, such as chronic bronchitis.[21]

The risk of lung cancer is reduced by switching to filter tip and low-tar cigarettes,[22] and from cigarettes to cigars or pipes.[23] However, it is suggested that the switch to low-tar cigarettes has led smokers to inhale more deeply and thereby contributed to the increased incidence of peripheral tumours.[24] There is no clear evidence that French cigarettes, which contain air-cured tobacco, are any safer than those made of flue-cured tobacco, but the resultant smoke is more alkaline and the contained nicotine can be absorbed from the mouth. Consequently, fewer French than British cigarette smokers admit to inhaling their smoke and this may contribute to the observed lower incidence of lung cancer in France than the UK, but there are other differences between the two countries: dietary differences are mentioned below.

Passive smoking, which is exposure to the cigarette smoke exhaled by others and the smoke emitted by their smouldering cigarettes (referred to as mainstream and sidestream smoke respectively), carries a small risk of lung cancer.[25,26] Compared with a non-smoker, the increased risk of lung cancer is generally quoted as a percentage for a passive smoker but so-many-fold for an active smoker, the respective figures being in the order of 25% and 13-fold (which equate to 1.25-fold versus 13-fold). A comparison of nicotine metabolite levels suggests that passive smoking entails an exposure equivalent of up to 1 cigarette a day. It is estimated that passive smoking accounts for one extra death from lung cancer or heart disease for every 10 000.

Numerous carcinogens have been identified in cigarette smoke. The more important ones are listed in Box 12.1.1. Many of them are thought to act by binding to DNA. Of particular note are the polycyclic hydrocarbons found in the neutral fraction of the particulate phase and the nitrosamines of the basic fraction. The former has been linked to squamous cell carcinoma and the latter to adenocarcinoma.[27] There appears to be genetic susceptibility to the carcinogenic effects of these chemicals, which is possibly based on differences in the amounts of activating enzymes in the lung, many of which are P450 cytochromes.[28]

Direct evidence of the effects of cigarette smoke on bronchial epithelium is provided by pathological studies, which demonstrate a close association between metaplasia and atypia and the number of cigarettes smoked.[29,30] Long-term animal experiments have been difficult to institute but have provided further supportive evidence of the link between tobacco smoke and lung cancer.[31,32]

Cigarette smoking predisposes to pulmonary carcinoma of all the major histological types, but the link is strongest with squamous cell and small cell carcinoma, which generally arise in central airways, and weakest with adenocarcinoma, which is commoner in the periphery of the lung.[33,34]

Environmental carcinogens

As with constituents of cigarette smoke, many inhaled chemicals are not hazardous as such but are transformed to reactive intermediates within the lungs by enzymes such as N-acetyl transferase, glutathione-S-transferase and members of the P450 family. After allowing for differences in smoking habits it is found that the risk of lung cancer is higher in urban areas than in rural areas, suggesting a role for general atmospheric pollution.[35,36] Major atmospheric pollutants include polycyclic hydrocarbons from the combustion of fossil fuels. Domestic coal fires were formerly the prime source of polycyclic hydrocarbons in the UK and it was estimated that in the 1950s air pollution accounted for about 10% of lung cancer in men.[37] Since that time coal fires have been eliminated in most major conurbations and concentrations of benzpyrene have fallen dramatically. The main source in the UK, as in many countries, is now motor vehicle exhaust and particular attention is being paid to diesel smoke. Some epidemiological studies have identified an increased risk of lung cancer in occupational groups having heavy exposure to diesel exhaust, notably one that examined American maintenance workers exposed to fumes from diesel locomotives.[38] A review by an international agency concluded that there was evidence that diesel engine exhaust was carcinogenic in experimental animals and that there was limited support for this in humans.[39] There appears to be only a weak link between urban nitrogen oxide and sulphur dioxide pollution and lung cancer.[40]

Ionising radiation

One of the earliest examples of occupational lung cancer is provided by the miners of the Erzgebirge ('ore mountains'), which separate Saxony from the Czech Republic. For four centuries ore from these mountains has proved a rich source of many metals – silver, copper, lead, cobalt, bismuth, iron and, recently, uranium. For much of this time, miners in Schneeberg on the Saxony side and Joachimstal on the Czech side suffered from a fatal respiratory disease – *Bergkrankheit* – that was recognised as lung cancer in the late nineteenth century. It is estimated that as many as 50% of the miners died from this cause; the average time from starting work in the mines to the development of a tumour was about 17 years. The overall risk of developing lung cancer was about 30 times that of the general population and repeated widowhood was commonplace. The lung cancer is attributable to the miners being exposed to very high levels of ionising radiation in the form of radon gas that is emitted from the rock face and when inhaled subjects the respiratory epithelium to α-irradiation.

Similar increases in lung cancer incidence were seen in North American miners exposed to radon and its daughter products[41,42] and such exposure probably accounts for the increased incidence seen in English haematite miners.[43] The increase involves both squamous cell carcinoma and small cell carcinoma, but particularly the latter.[44,45] Cigarette smoking is an important cofactor . The increased risk is 67 times greater in heavy smokers exposed to heavy doses of irradiation than in non-smokers with comparable radiation exposure, indicating a multiplicative effect, as seen with asbestos.[46,47]

Radon levels may also reach dangerous levels within the home; the degree of danger depends on the character of the underlying rock.[48,49] It is difficult to prevent radon seeping into buildings and easier to instal solid floors over a radon sump that can be exhausted to the exterior. Many countries have policies to control indoor radon, usually focusing on buildings where radon levels exceed a certain level, although there is evidence that in some countries it would be cost-effective if basic preventive measures were required for all new homes.[50]

There is also an increased incidence of lung carcinoma in patients given therapeutic irradiation, for example to the spine for ankylosing spondylitis[51] and to the breast for mammary carcinoma.[52,53] Survivors of the Hiroshima and Nagasaki nuclear bombings were also at increased risk of lung cancer.[54,55]

Asbestos

An association between exposure to asbestos and carcinoma of the lung was first demonstrated conclusively in 1955.[56] As with mesothelioma, the association is stronger with amphibole asbestos than chrysotile, but with all forms of asbestos much higher levels of exposure are required to produce carcinoma than mesothelioma. All histological types are involved but the proportion of adenocarcinoma is increased.[57-59] Cigarette smoking is an important cofactor. In a study of 17 800 asbestos workers the risk in smokers was 14 times that in non-smokers.[60] Table 7.1.7 (p. 349) provides further data on this, showing that the lung cancer risk for workers heavily exposed to asbestos is 5 times that of unexposed persons whatever their smoking status, while the risk for smokers is 11 times that of non-smokers whether they are exposed to asbestos or not. As a consequence, the lung cancer incidence among smokers exposed to asbestos is 53 times higher than that among unexposed non-smokers – a multiplicative rather than additive effect.[61] The risk diminishes in those who cease smoking. A practical preventive point arising from this is that most of the excess risk can be abolished by eliminating or decreasing exposure to either asbestos or cigarette smoke. Also, it suggests that asbestos acts as a promoting agent rather than a primary carcinogen. The vexed question of whether asbestos causes lung cancer in the absence of asbestosis is considered on page 349. Asbestos fibre burdens are generally low in lungs resected because of cancer, indicating that asbestos is not a major cause of lung cancer in the general population.[62,63]

Known carcinogens (group 1)

Arsenic
Asbestos
Bis(chloromethyl)ether
Chromium, hexavalent
Nickel and nickel compounds
Polycyclic aromatic compounds
Radon
Vinyl chloride

Probable carcinogens (group 2A)

Acrylonitrile
Beryllium
Cadmium
Formaldehyde

Possible carcinogens (group 2B)

Acetaldehyde
Manmade fibres
Silica
Welding fumes

Other industrial chemicals

Apart from asbestos and ionising radiation, six other agents encountered in industry are accepted pulmonary carcinogens: arsenic, chloromethyl ethers, chromium, nickel, polyaromatic hydrocarbons and vinyl chloride. Many others, including cadmium, formaldehyde and dioxin, are suspected of having a similar effect (Box 12.1.2).[64] Cigarette smoking is often an additional factor.[65]

Workers in the coal gas industry exposed to polyaromatic hydrocarbons have a lung cancer risk twice that of the general population,[66] and lung cancer has also been associated with a range of metal-refining and smelting processes: nickel, chromium, arsenic and cadmium have all been incriminated.[67,68] In the 1930s a higher incidence was reported amongst workers at the Clydach nickel refinery in south Wales. Changes in the process later resulted in a reduction of the risk but the hazard remains in several other nickel refineries.[69] Exposure to both nickel and cadmium was related to lung cancer in workers in a battery plant.[70] Poorly soluble hexavalent chromium pigments cause lung cancer but very soluble chromium compounds are comparatively safe.[71,72]

Arsenic and its compounds are associated with skin and lung carcinomas, an increased incidence being found in people administered arsenic therapeutically, in vineyard workers involved in spraying arsenical insecticides, and in copper smelters exposed to arsenic.[73] Arsenic may also be responsible for an increased risk of lung cancer identified in antimony workers.[74] It is also anticipated that the next decade will witness widespread arsenic-induced cancer in Bengal and Bangladesh following the provision of water free of bacterial contamination by extraction from shallow aquifers. Up to 10 million shallow tube wells have been dug and it is estimated that 1 million of these are heavily contaminated with naturally occurring arsenic released by anaereobic metal-reducing bacteria.[75] At least 100 000 cases of arsenic-induced skin growths have been identified and it seems inevitable that cancer of the skin and respiratory tract will follow.

Exposure to the alkylating agent chloromethyl methyl ether, which is used as a cross-linking agent in ion exchange resins and as an intermediate in the production of organic chemicals, carries an increased risk of lung cancer, particularly if there is contamination with bis(chloromethyl) ether.[76] Small-cell carcinoma is particularly increased.[77]

Epidemiological studies have also incriminated silica exposure as a risk factor for lung cancer, and as with asbestos there is uncertainty as to whether the risk is due to high silica levels alone or to the fibrotic process.[78] Claims for compensation are therefore more likely to succeed if silicosis as well as carcinoma can be demonstrated.

Diet

Many of the differences in disease incidence seen between Mediterranean and northern European countries have been ascribed to diet, especially the differing intake of antioxidants. Dietary differences are probably important in regard to cardiovascular disease but may also affect cancer incidence. Many cigarette smokers have therefore gleefully increased their consumption of red wine on evidence that is to date at best equivocal.[79]

Vitamin A deficiency leads to squamous metaplasia of mucosal surfaces, dryness of the skin, eyes and mouth, and to an increased susceptibility to cancer.[80] Cigarette smoke augments the metaplastic action of vitamin A deficiency in rats,[81] whilst in humans low vitamin A intake leads to an increased incidence of lung cancer in smokers.[82] Folate is another dietary component that protects against squamous metaplasia.[83] Diets high in carotenoid-rich fruits and vegetables are associated with a reduced risk of lung cancer, as are high serum levels of vitamin E and beta-carotene, but long-term dietary supplementation with these substances either had no effect or resulted in a slightly higher incidence of lung cancer in male smokers.[84–86]

Pulmonary fibrosis

Idiopathic pulmonary fibrosis is associated with a 14-fold increased incidence of lung cancer,[87–89] similar to that noted above in asbestosis.[60] In both these diseases, the tumours are of all histological types and they arise more frequently in the periphery of the lower lobes where the fibrosis is most marked.[90,91] Although the original publications suggested that adenocarcinoma was the most common histological type, it is now believed that the cell-type distribution is similar to that in the general population.[58] Sarcoidosis has been reported to convey an increased risk of lung cancer in some studies[92,93] but not in others.[94]

In contrast to these forms of diffuse pulmonary fibrosis, the role of localised scars in the development of lung cancer is now questioned. Many adenocarcinomas show pronounced pleural puckering due to central scarring (see Fig. 12.1.23, p. 554) and have often been assumed to represent 'scar cancers', meaning that the scar preceded and predisposed to the cancer. However, it is often impossible to tell whether the tumour developed in a pre-existing scar, and can therefore be designated a true scar cancer, or whether the central scar is secondary to the tumour.[95] Nevertheless, there is considerable evidence, both radiological and pathological, supporting the view that the scar is the product of the tumour rather than the reverse. Relevant radiological observations[96] include the following:

- a scar is not usually evident in previous radiographs
- as peripheral tumours develop they may shrink in size despite involving a greater proportion of the affected lobe
- initially soft opacities often become more opaque centrally
- adjacent airways and blood vessels increasingly converge on the tumour.

Pathological observations[97–101] supporting the view that central scars are usually a product of the tumour rather than the reverse include the following:

- the size of the scar generally matches that of the tumour
- similar scars develop in extrapulmonary metastases
- similar scars are found in the pulmonary metastases of other adenocarcinomas
- psammoma bodies derived from the carcinoma may be found deep within the central scar
- the scars often show a predominance of myofibroblasts and type III collagen
- elastin stains often show that the central scar is formed on an area of collapse consequent upon airway or arterial obstruction by the tumour.

Irrespective of whether the scar or the tumour comes first, central scarring in a pulmonary adenocaricoma is an adverse prognostic indicator, being associated with increased vascular and pleural invasion and lymph node metastasis.[97,102]

Viruses

Viral oncogenes participate in carcinogenesis by the RNA of the viral genome being transcribed into the DNA genome of the host by the enzyme reverse transcriptase. The DNA sequences transcribed by viral oncogenes are virtually identical to sequences in the cellular DNA of most animal species and presumably have the same potential for affecting malignant growth as cellular oncogenes. Viruses have been suggested in the past as being related to the development of some lung cancers, and the application of molecular probes has given some impetus to such investigations. Papillomavirus of types 6 and 11 is commonly found in tracheobronchial papillomatosis and in the rare papillary squamous carcinomas that complicate papillomatosis[103] while type 18 has been identified in a small proportion of the more common non-papillary squamous cell carcinomas of the bronchus.[104] Particularly notable is an exceptionally high rate of human papillomavirus 16- and 18-positive lung cancers in non-smoking Taiwanese women.[105] Epstein–Barr virus has been shown to be associated with bronchopulmonary as well as nasopharyngeal lymphoepitheliomas but with only occasional lung tumours of the more common histological types.[106,107] There is an increased incidence of lung cancer in acquired immunodeficiency syndrome (AIDS) but this is not thought to be directly attributable to the human immunodeficiency virus.[108]

Heredity

The great majority of smokers reaching old age do not die of lung cancer, suggesting that individuals differ greatly in the way they metabolise xenobiotic substances.[109] These differences are presumably inborn. Genetic differences could influence the risk of cancer in several ways.[110] They could affect the enzymatic elimination or activation of carcinogens,[111,112] or the expression of oncogenes or tumour suppressor genes (see below). Epidemiological studies have shown an excess of lung cancer in close relatives, identifying an approximately twofold-increased risk of lung cancer in those with a family history of the disease.[113–115] Various genes conferring increased susceptibility to lung cancer have now been identified.[116,117] Those located on chromosomes 6 and 15 are particularly notable, chromosome 15 being the site of the nicotinic acetylcholine receptor gene cluster. The susceptibility these genes confer appears to be unrelated to smoking status or propensity to smoke tobacco.[118] The role of genetic factors in the development of lung cancer is dealt with more extensively below, under pathogenesis.

Malformations

The cystic type 1 congenital pulmonary airway malformation is often accompanied by focal mucous cell hyperplasia that occasionally undergoes malignant transformation, usually to a mucinous adenocarcinoma of predominantly lepidic pattern (see p. 59), but the common hamartoma (see p. 626) is not a precursor of bronchopulmonary carcinoma.[119–121]

PATHOGENESIS

Premalignant changes evident morphologically

Carcinoma of the lung largely arises from the epithelial cells lining the air spaces. The few carcinomas that develop in the bronchial glands are dealt with in the next chapter. The next chapter also considers diffuse neuroendocrine hyperplasia as a precursor of tumourlets and carcinoids (but not of small cell carcinoma). Attention here is confined to the precursors of squamous cell carcinoma and adenocarcinoma. No precursor of small cell carcinoma has been identified.

Four main cell types make up the surface epithelium of the bronchi – basal, mucous, neuroendocrine and ciliated – and only the last of these appear to be end cells. The others are all capable of division and thus have malignant potential. Clara cells and type II pneumocytes are the respective stem cells of the bronchioles and the alveoli and are found in some adenocarcinomas of the lung.

Squamous metaplasia and dysplasia

The regenerative capability of bronchial epithelial cells has been extensively studied. Hyperplasia of the surviving basal cells is an early regenerative event that is followed by the development of a stratified squamous epithelium.[122] Further differentiation into mucous cells and thence ciliated cells follows but mucous differentiation is dependent upon the availability of vitamin A.[81,123] The application of carcinogens such as benz-pyrene, asbestos or nitrosamines results in the proliferation of bronchial neuroendocrine cells, which may undergo squamous metaplasia.[124–126] It is clear therefore that basal, mucous, neuroendocrine and metaplastic squamous cells are closely related and readily transform one to another. This marked metaplastic potential of the bronchial epithelium provides no support for facile suppositions regarding the histogenesis of particular types of lung carcinoma from particular precursor cells.

The sequence of hyperplasia–metaplasia–dysplasia–carcinoma-in-situ–invasive carcinoma (Fig. 12.1.2) is well documented in human airways[127–129] and a grading system, which details the histological features evident in the surface epithelium, has been introduced (Table 12.1.1).[130] Changes are also found in the mucosal blood vessels. Several groups have described hyperplastic capillary loops in close apposition to dysplastic epithelium, giving rise to the term 'angiogenic squamous dysplasia'.[131] The vascular changes can be detected by fluorescence bronchoscopy, suggesting that it may be possible to eradicate the lesions before they become invasive.[132]

Uranium miners in the USA provided cytopathologists with the opportunity of studying the gradual evolution of bronchial carcinoma. Periodic sputum examination showed squamous metaplasia followed by gradually increasing cellular atypia in those miners who later developed invasive carcinoma of either squamous or small cell type. Atypical cells could be identified in the sputum for many years prior to the development of invasive tumours: on average, dysplastic changes lasted 8 years and carcinoma-in-situ a further 4 years

Figure 12.1.2 Smokers' bronchi showing (A) basal cell hyperplasia (left) and squamous metaplasia (right), (B) squamous dysplasia and (C) carcinoma in situ (right).

before there was invasion (Table 12.1.2).[127] Isolated foci of in situ squamous cell carcinoma amenable to limited surgical procedures are occasionally identified[133] but at presentation invasion has generally supervened.

Further evidence of dysplasia preceding carcinoma came from a large autopsy study in which the whole bronchial tree was examined in a series of patients dying of lung cancer.[29] This showed widespread premalignant changes involving mucosa that appeared macroscopi-

cally normal, including foci of carcinoma-in-situ and occasional microinvasive cancers distant from the main tumour.

Foci of hyperplasia, metaplasia and dysplasia are also frequently seen adjacent to invasive tumours in surgical specimens,[134] and similar changes have been described in experimental dogs exposed to cigarette smoke.[31] Full-thickness squamous metaplasia is not necessary before atypical features are seen in the proliferating basal cells; dysplasia may be present beneath an intact surface layer of columnar cells.[29] The transition from normal bronchial epithelium to squamous epithelium is usually abrupt. Atypical epithelium may extend deeply into bronchial glands replacing duct and acinar lining cells, resulting in appearances that mimic microinvasive carcinoma, but the basement membrane as yet remains intact.

The risk of squamous metaplasia and dysplasia progressing to invasion has been assessed by following patients with these lesions by periodic bronchoscopy. One study extending for up to 7 years put the risk at 4% for squamous metaplasia, 9% for low-grade dysplasia and 32% for high-grade dysplasia.[135] Another extending over a similar period found that low-grade dysplasia did not progress at all but that the risk of progression in severe dysplasia/carcinoma-in-situ was 17%.[136]

In view of the extent of these premalignant changes, it is not surprising that there is a high incidence of double or second primary lung cancers.[137,137a] Even triple primary tumours are described.[138] Using standard criteria of a double primary growth, namely involvement of different lobes, or different histological types, or a time interval over 3 years,[139] it has been shown that 4% of lung cancer patients have more than one lung tumour at presentation and that a further 6% develop a second primary lung growth later.[137,137a] The patients most at risk of developing lung cancer are therefore those who have had one in the past. These patients might therefore be worth following up particularly frequently.

Patients with squamous dysplasia or carcinoma-in-situ may be asymptomatic or present with cough and haemoptysis. However, it is often difficult to know how much their cough is due to the dysplastic change rather than other smoking-related diseases such as chronic bronchitis. The epithelial changes are focal, usually developing at the bifurcations of segmental bronchi and subsequently extending proximally and distally. They are sometimes evident as a grey plaque but are not always visible to the bronchoscopist, particularly when routine white light is used. Autofluorescence bronchoscopy is more sensitive.[140] Treatment is problematical because the lesions are frequently multiple. Patients are therefore often followed up by serial bronchoscopy until early invasion is apparent when the lesion may be treated by local ablation or surgical resection.[141]

Atypical adenomatous hyperplasia and adenocarcinoma-in-situ

The hyperplasia–dysplasia–neoplasia sequence is again encountered in the periphery of the lung, where it is important in the development of non-mucinous adenocarcinomas,[142,143] particularly when there is diffuse pulmonary fibrosis.[87–89] More recently it has been recognised that focal alveolar hyperplasia in the absence of fibrosis is an important precursor of pulmonary adenocarcinoma, evolving through a stage of adenocarcinoma-in-situ to invasive adenocarcinoma. The hyperplasia phase is generally known as atypical adenomatous hyperplasia,[144–147] although in the past it has also been termed bronchioloalveolar cell adenoma.[148,149] Adenocarcinoma-in-situ is a new term that replaces the older one of bronchioloalveolar cell carcinoma.[150]

Remarkably, foci of atypical adenomatous hyperplasia are quite commonly found when sought in lungs resected for cancer, yet they have evidently lain undiscovered by generations of pathologists

Table 12.1.1 Morphology of squamous dysplasia and carcinoma-in-situ[130]

Abnormality	Thickness	Cell size	Maturation/orientation	Nuclei
Mild dysplasia	Mildly increased	Mildly increased Mild anisocytosis and pleomorphism	Continuous progression of maturation Basilar zone expanded with cellular crowding in lower third Distinct intermediate (prickle cell) zone present Superficial flattening of epithelial cells	Mild variation of N/C ratio Finely granular chromatin Minimal angulation Nucleoli inconspicuous or absent Nuclei vertically oriented in lower third Mitoses absent or very rare
Moderate dysplasia	Moderately increased	Mildly increased Moderate anisocytosis and pleomorphism	Partial progression of maturation Basilar zone expanded with cellular crowding in lower two-thirds Intermediate zone confined to upper third of epithelium Superficial flattening of epithelial cells	Moderate variation of N/C ratio Finely granular chromatin Nuclear angulations, grooves, lobulations Nucleoli inconspicuous or absent Nuclei vertically oriented in lower two-thirds Mitotic figures present in lower third
Severe dysplasia	Markedly increased	Markedly increased May show marked anisocytosis and pleomorphism	Little progression of maturation from base to luminal surface Basilar zone expanded with cellular crowding well into upper third Intermediate zone greatly attenuated Superficial flattening of epithelial cells	N/C ratio often high and variable Chromatin coarse and uneven Nuclear angulations and folding prominent Nucleoli frequently present and conspicuous Nuclei vertically oriented in lower two-thirds Mitotic figures present in lower two-thirds
Carcinoma-in-situ	May or may not be increased	May be markedly increased May show marked anisocytosis and pleomorphism	No progression of maturation from base to luminal surface Basilar zone expanded with cellular crowding throughout epithelium Intermediate zone absent Surface flattening only of most superficial cells	N/C ratio often high and variable Chromatin coarse and uneven Nuclear angulations and folding prominent No consistent orientation of nuclei in relation to epithelial surface Mitotic figures present through full thickness

N/C, nuclear to cytoplasmic.

Table 12.1.2 Evolution of invasive squamous cell carcinoma in American uranium miners followed by periodic sputum examination[127]

	Average age at onset (range)	Average duration (years)
Mild atypia	48 years (38–59)	2.89
Moderate atypia	51 years (34–67)	3.23
Marked atypia	55 years (38–70)	2.23
Carcinoma-in-situ	57 years (37–70)	4.04
Invasive carcinoma	61 years	

dealing with such specimens. Admittedly, they are generally small and easily overlooked. Their identification is facilitated by immersion in Bouin's solution.[151] They represent foci of hyperplastic type II alveolar epithelial cells or bronchiolar Clara cells. Autopsy studies of cases free of lung cancer have identified focal adenomatous hyperplasia in 3–6%,[152,153] while in lungs resected for cancer atypical adenomatous hyperplasia has been reported in up to 50% of cases, with the highest figures coming from Japan.[148,151,154–157] The tumour that atypical

adenomatous hyperplasia most often accompanies is a non-mucinous adenocarcinoma, but it is sometimes a large cell or squamous cell carcinoma.[157] Multiple foci of atypical adenomatous hyperplasia may be found, particularly in association with multiple adenocarcinomas. Molecular studies show that individual lesions differ in their genetic make-up, establishing that they are independent of each other and of any accompanying carcinoma and do not represent micrometastases of the latter.[158]

Atypical adenomatous hyperplasia is a focal lesion, generally less than 5 mm in diameter, in which the alveoli are lined by cuboidal to low columnar cells (Fig. 12.1.3), which have the ultrastructural features of type II pneumocytes and Clara cells. Ciliated and mucous cells are not a feature.[130,159] The interstitium may show some fibrosis but this is generally mild. Atypical adenomatous hyperplasia is distinguished from adenocarcinoma-in-situ by its size (generally less than 5 mm whereas most carcinomas exceed 10 mm), gaps between the epithelial cells as opposed to a continuous cell line and the cells being cuboidal rather than columnar (Table 12.1.3). They have dense chromatin, prominent nucleoli and sparse cytoplasm. Mitoses are rarely evident but varying degrees of atypia are observed[146,160] and the familiar hyperplasia–dysplasia–neoplasia sequence is easily envisaged. Morphometry,[161,162] argyrophilic nucleolar organiser counts,[163] DNA status,[162,163] loss of heterozygosity[164] and the identification of a range of oncogenes within the atypical lesions[145,161,165–170] provide further support for this form of hyperplasia being premalignant. The demonstration of monoclonality suggests that it is neoplastic[144,171] and

Table 12.1.3 Atypical adenomatous hyperplasia, peribronchiolar metaplasia (lambertosis, see p. 121) and adenocarcinoma-in-situ (formerly non-mucinous bronchioloalveolar cell carcinoma)

	Atypical adenomatous hyperplasia	Peribronchiolar metaplasia (lambertosis)	Adenocarcinoma-in-situ
Size	<5 mm	<5 mm	>10 mm
Cell shape	Cuboidal	Columnar	Columnar or cuboidal
Intercellular gaps	Present	Absent	Absent
Fibrosis	Mild	Moderate	Mild
Cilia	Absent	Present	Absent
Nuclear atypia	Present	Absent	Present

Figure 12.1.3 A focus of atypical adenomatous hyperplasia identified in a random section of lung excised because of carcinoma.

Figure 12.1.4 Adenocarcinoma-in-situ, formerly bronchioloalveolar carcinoma. The tumour cells grow along the alveolar walls without disrupting them in a so-called lepidic (scale-like) fashion. There is no evidence of invasive activity.

it is now widely regarded as being the precursor of most peripheral adenocarcinomas. Nevertheless, the presence of multiple foci of atypical adenomatous hyperplasia does not appear to be related to patient survival.[149,155] Patients without cancer who are found to harbour this lesion should be kept under surveillance: further intervention is not warranted.

As mentioned above, adenocarcinoma-in-situ is a new term that replaces bronchioloalveolar carcinoma.[156] Its new name reflects better

its non-invasive nature. The lesional cells grow along the alveolar walls without destroying them (Fig. 12.1.4), a pattern of growth known as lepidic, meaning scale-like (as in the scales of a fish). Two forms of bronchioloalveolar carcinoma have traditionally been described, mucinous and non-mucinous, but it is now recognised that the mucinous variety almost always shows some invasive activity. Adenocarcinoma-in-situ is therefore almost always non-mucinous while the great majority of tumours formerly classified as mucinous bronchioloalveolar carcinoma are now termed mucinous adenocarcinoma of predominantly lepidic pattern. The latter is accordingly described later on page 554. Only non-mucinous adenocarcinoma-in-situ will be described here.

Non-mucinous adenocarcinom-in-situ predominates in smokers and is usually evident radiologically as a ground-glass opacity. It consists of Clara cells or type II pneumocytes, often in combination (Fig. 12.1.5).[172,173] The Clara cells have a narrow base and a bulbous apex, resulting in a characteristic 'hobnail' pattern. On occasion it can be difficult to distinguish the tumour from reactive hyperplasia but a tall columnar cell shape, cellular crowding, cytological atypia and papillary infolding all favour malignancy. The presence of cilia does not exclude malignancy,[174] but renders it unlikely. Immunocytochemistry and molecular studies emphasise the differences between non-

Figure 12.1.5 Adenocarcinoma-in-situ. (A) In this field the tumour cells are cuboidal and largely comprise type II pneumocytes whereas hobnail or peg-shaped Clara cells predominate in (B).

Figure 12.1.6 Bronchial carcinogenesis is a multistep process characterised by the gradual accumulation of genetic and molecular abnormalities. *(Redrawn from a diagram provided by Prof S Lantuejoul, Grenoble, France.)*

mucinous adenocarcinoma-in-situ and mucinous adenocarcinoma of predominantly lepidic pattern.[175] Non-mucinous adenocarcinoma-in-situ expresses the pulmonary marker thyroid transcription factor (TTF-1) but fails to stain with the colonic marker cytokeratin 20 whereas the reverse is found with mucinous adenocarcinoma of predominantly lepidic pattern.[176–179] Also, non-mucinous adenocarcinoma-in-situ often displays mutation of the epidermal growth factor receptor (*EGFR*) gene whereas mucinous adenocarcinoma of predominantly lepidic pattern shows K-*ras* but not *EGFR* when a mutation is present.[180]

Invasive activity excludes a diagnosis of adenocarcinoma-in-situ but it can be difficult to recognise early invasion, particularly when there is alveolar collapse. The distinction is important because patients with adenocarcinoma-in-situ show 100% 5-year survival whereas invasion implies metastatic potential.[181] Microinvasion, defined as invasion no greater than 5 mm, carries a prognosis intermediate between that of adenocarcinoma-in-situ and adenocarcinoma containing invasive areas greater than 5 mm across.[182,183] Collapse is recognised by the lining cells being similar to those in non-collapsed areas and the spaces being regularly distributed, whereas with invasive tumour the acini vary in size and their lining cells are irregular. Solid nests or

single cells also favour invasion.[184] The presence of intraluminal macrophages implies continuity between the malignant cells and surrounding alveolar spaces, favouring non-invasive growth. Conversely, basement membrane stains, such as those recognising type IV collagen, facilitate the identification of invasion.[182,185,186] They also demonstrate that the epithelial basement membrane is usually destroyed when there is central fibrosis.[187] Not surprisingly, therefore, it has been shown that prominent central scarring as opposed to simple collapse is an adverse prognostic feature in small peripheral lung cancers.[97,102,181,188] The terms Noguchi types A–C have come into use: type A is an in-situ adenocarcinoma that shows no collapse, type B an in-situ adenocarcinoma that shows collapse and type C an acinar adenocarcinoma in which invasion is detected within a central scar. It is envisaged that these represent successive stages in the evolution of a peripheral adenocarcinoma.

The multifocal micronodular hyperplasia of type II pneumocytes reported in tuberous sclerosis (see p. 701) is not recognised as being premalignant.

An infectious disease of sheep known as jaagsiekte, droning sickness or pulmonary adenomatosis closely resembles human adenocarcinoma-in-situ[189] but the two are considered to be separate diseases. A report of a protein immunologically related to the jaagsiekte sheep retrovirus in some human lung carcinomas[190] has not been supported by subsequent molecular investigations.[191]

Genetic factors in the development of lung cancer

That the morphological changes described above are truly premalignant is supported by the demonstration that they show genetic abnormalities similar to those found in adjacent invasive cancer.[192,193] They reflect a multistep accumulation of genetic abnormalities, the number of which gradually increases as dysplasia progresses (Fig. 12.1.6).[128,194–196] The earliest molecular changes may be detected before any abnormality is evident at the microscopic level. Mutations involving a single gene are generally insufficient to cause cancer. Successive mutations affecting 10–20 different genes are required before malignant change is eventually established.[197] Molecular techniques therefore enable the identification of premalignant change in tissues that may be normal histologically.[198–202] Some of the earliest genetic changes involve loci on chromosomes 3p and 9p.[203,204] Inactivation of the *p17* gene is also an early event, whereas mutations involving the K-*ras* and *p53* genes occur late in the sequence of genetic alterations.[196,205] These genetic changes promote malignant transformation in a variety of ways, including enhanced cell growth by means of oncogene activation, inactivation of tumour suppressor genes, inhibition of apoptosis, altered DNA repair leading to cellular immortalization and the promotion of angiogenesis.[196] Important growth factors that have been implicated in lung cancer are listed in Box 12.1.3. They are obviously important to the prognosis of lung cancer and are touched upon again under that heading on page 573.

Oncogene activation

Oncogenes include those identified in viruses (v-*onc* genes), the possible role of which in pulmonary carcinogenesis is touched upon above, and the cellular oncogenes (c-*onc* genes), which control normal cell growth and differentiation and have the potential to influence tumour behaviour. In contrast to tumour suppressor genes, which are dealt with next, oncogenes are generally dominant and mutation of only one allele is therefore sufficient to promote undue cell growth. The activity of growth factors is largely dependent on oncogenes because these involve receptors on the cell surface concerned in signal transduction.

Some of the oncogenes involved in lung cancer belong to the epidermal growth factor receptor family, *EGFR*1 (*HER1*), *EGFR2* (*HER2/neu, c-erbB2*), *HER3* and *HER4*. They act as transmembrane tyrosine kinase (TK) receptors, so promoting TKs, enzymes that regulate the activity of other proteins and which have been implicated in the development of many cancers. They are most commonly situated on chromosomes 19 and 21 and their presence predicts TK inhibitor response.[206] They are targeted by the small-molecule TK inhibitors, such as gefitinib and erlotinib, and by monoclonal antibodies such as cetuximab and trastuzumab (Herceptin, which counters HER2).[206–210] *EGFR* genes are especially overexpressed in papillary adenocarcinomas, particularly those arising in East Asian female non-smokers.[210–212] Other *EGFR* mutations are associated with drug resistance. *EGFR* mutations occur early in tumour development with increased copy number being a late event.[213]

A structural homology between certain growth factor receptors and oncogenes probably underlies the autocrine activity evinced by certain tumours, in which the tumour secretes substances that induce self-

proliferation. Gastrin-releasing peptide (human bombesin) is one of the best-known autocrine factors and is particularly involved in the remarkably rapid growth of small cell carcinomas.[214] The gastrin-releasing peptide receptor gene appears to be activated by cigarette smoke and, being located on the X chromosome, is more strongly expressed in women than men,[215] possibly contributing to the greater female susceptibility to tobacco-induced lung cancer noted above.[4]

Other oncogenes important in pulmonary carcinogenesis include members of the *ras* and *myc* gene families, especially K-*ras* and c-*myc*. Activating point mutations of *ras* genes result in an aberrant p21 membrane-associated protein that continuously transduces an inappropriate growth signal. K-*ras* is mutated in 30% of pulmonary adenocarcinomas,[216] and particularly in smokers with mucinous adenocarcinomas.[180,212,217] It is recorded in the precursor lesion atypical alveolar hyperplasia that is described above. K-*ras* mutation is therefore a good candidate for the early detection of lung cancer as it should be detectable in bronchioloalveolar cells shed in sputum or recovered by lavage. K-*ras* and *EGFR* mutations are mutually exclusive, the former being involved mainly in smokers' tumours and the latter mainly in non-smokers' adenocarcinomas.[210] Furthermore, K-*ras* mutation is possibly responsible for resistance to cisplatin and the TK inhibitors referred to above. In adenocarcinoma, a pathway involving K-*ras* appears to be predominant in western smokers whereas the *EGFR* pathway appears to be more important in East Asian female non-smokers.[210,211]

Myc oncogenes encode for cell cycle-specific nuclear phosphoproteins and thereby control cell growth and differentiation. Their amplification accounts for *myc* protein accumulation in 20% of small cell carcinomas and 10% of non-small cell carcinomas. *Myc* gene amplification is found particularly in patients with recurrent tumour.[218–220] Conversely, *myc* genes are seldom amplified in carcinomas from patients who have not undergone treatment and thus appear to be associated with tumour progression rather than initiation. Some drug regimens result in *myc* amplification more than others.

Fusion genes have long been recognised as being important in certain haematological malignancies and sarcomas but have not been thought to play a major role in epithelial tumours. Recently however the fusion gene *EML4-ALK* has been identified in non-small cell lung cancer as an alternative promoter of TK activity, thus opening up the possibility of further TK inhibitors being developed.[221] The *EML4-ALK* gene has been found in about 5–10% of lung cancers, mainly adenocarcinomas in younger non-smokers.[222–224] *BRAF* gene mutations are also seen in a minority of non-small cell lung cancers, again mainly adenocarcinomas.[225,226] The Akt/mammalian (mTOR) pathway is frequently activated in human cancers and plays an important role in small cell lung cancer biology.[227]

Further genes involved in malignant change include the human homologue of the *Drosophila* neurogenic gene *hASH1*, which promotes the growth of small cell carcinoma, large cell neuroendocrine carcinoma and some atypical carcinoids,[228] and members of the Forkhead box (Fox) family, dysregulation of which has been demonstrated in squamous cell carcinomas of the lung, particularly those of a more malignant nature.[229]

Tumour suppressor genes

In contrast to oncogenes, tumour suppressor genes are generally recessive and mutation of both alleles is therefore required for their inactivation. The first mutation results in heterozygosity, which has little effect because the mutant gene is recessive, whereas mutation of the other allele involves complete loss of the gene. The second mutation can be detected following suitable amplification, for example by the polymerase chain reaction, as a single band on gel electrophoresis, a change that is often termed 'loss of heterozygosity'. Tumour suppressor genes (antioncogenes) are believed to play an important role in the pathogenesis of lung cancer because deletions or mutations of certain chromosomes are frequently found, notably chromosomes 3p, 13q and 17p.[230–232] 13q is the site of the retinoblastoma gene, 17p the *p53* gene and 3p the FHIT (fragile histidine triad) antioncogene. 3p deletion is particularly common in small cell carcinoma and 13q and 17p deletion in non-small cell carcinoma.[233–235] FHIT deletion is one of the earliest mutations and p53 deletion one of the last in the bronchial cancer gene sequence but loss of the FHIT antioncogene is relatively late in the atypical adenomatous hyperplasia–adenocarcinoma-in-situ–invasive peripheral adenocarcinoma sequence.[168] Mutation of the *EGFR* is also increasingly found in the development of peripheral invasive adenocarcinomas from atypical adenomatous hyperplasia.[169,236] Mutation of p53 is the commonest genetic alteration in human cancer and occurs in over half of lung cancers; p53 is normally responsible for apoptosis and abnormalities of this gene are thought to permit unchecked cell proliferation. The normal p53 protein product is generally undetectable due to a short half-life but mutations frequently extend this so that the protein accumulates and can be detected imunocytochemically. Accumulation of p53 protein product has been associated with an adverse prognosis in lung cancer and may provide a marker for early diagnosis of premalignant states.[237]

The retinoblastoma gene (*Rb*) is the main effector of G1 arrest, which is mediated by p53 and utilised in the repair of DNA damage. Rb protein expression is lost in 80% of small cell lung cancer and in 15% of non-small cell lung cancer, but is not found in preinvasive lesions.[238] Inactivation of Rb is often due to methylation of p16 or overexpression of cyclin D1.

Bax and *bcl*-2 (B-cell lymphoma-2) are further genes involved in apoptosis, which is promoted by the former and blocked by the latter. The *bcl*-2 gene is overexpressed in preinvasive lesions, a variable number of non-small cell carcinomas of the lung,[239–241] most small cell carcinomas and a variety of other lung tumours showing neuroendocrine differentiation, thereby permitting unchecked cell division.[242,243] A high *bcl*-2:*bax* ratio generally accompanies mutation of the p53 tumour suppressor gene.[243]

Cellular immortalisation

Telomerase is an enzyme that adds nucleotide repeats to the ends (telomeres) of chromosomes to compensate for the nucleotide losses that occur with each round of DNA replication.[244–247] Normal somatic cells show no telomerase activity and stop dividing when their telomeres are sufficiently shortened. Telomerase can be detected in most lung cancers and is frequently found in bronchial epithelium showing premalignant change. The indefinite proliferation of cancer cells probably owes much to their telomerase activity.

Vascular endothelium growth factor and other autocrine factors

Angiogenesis is an important process in the dissemination of invasive growths and the autocrine production of vascular endothelium growth factor by such lung tumours is therefore important in pulmonary carcinogenesis.[248,249] Other autocrine factors secreted by certain lung tumours include epidermal growth factor (the genetic control of which is considered above), gastrin-releasing peptide, transferrin, insulin-like growth factor and endothelin (Table 12.1.4).[214,250–254]

Table 12.1.4 Molecular markers associated with lung cancer

Gene mutation	Chromosome involved	Type of mutation
Proto-oncogene activation		
K-ras, Ha-ras, N-ras	12p	Point mutation
EGFR-2 (Her-2/neu, c-erb-B2) Ki-ras, Ha-ras, N-ras	17q	Translocation
c-myc, L-myc, N-myc c-erb-B2 (Her-2/neu) (epidermal growth factor receptor gene)	8	Translocation
bcl-2 c-myc, L-myc, N-myc	14–18	Translocation
Tumour suppressor gene inactivation		
FHIT (fragile histidine triad gene)	3p	Deletion
Retinoblastoma gene	13q	Point mutation
p53	17p	Deletion
Telomerase activation		

Screening for lung cancer

Lung cancer fulfils many of the criteria necessary for a successful screening programme. The condition is common, the population at risk is well known and premalignant changes can be detected cheaply (by sputum cytology). Unfortunately the premalignant changes cannot be easily eradicated: there is no bronchopulmonary equivalent of a uterine cone biopsy. Nor does screening for early invasive growths by a combination of sputum cytology and radiography appear to reduce mortality.[255–257] The relative failure of surgery, radical radiotherapy and preventive screening programmes is partly explained by backward extrapolations of observed tumour size doubling times, which suggest that malignant change takes place years before a tumour is first detectable clinically (Table 12.1.5).[258] Nevertheless, sparked by the advances in molecular pathology described above and refinements in high-resolution computed tomography, there has been a renewal of interest in early detection.[255] For example, it appears that p53 immunohistochemistry may assist in the identification of preneoplastic lesions,[192] the detection of *p16*^{INK4a} inactivation in sputum may identify smokers at increased risk of developing lung cancer,[259,260] and low-dose computed tomography (CT) screening trials are proving more sensitive in detecting small peripheral tumours.[261–266] Wedge resection rather than lobectomy is undertaken for these small asymptomatic lesions, with good results, particularly for those showing ground-glass opacification, which is characteristic of adenocarcinoma-in-situ and minimally invasive adenocarcinoma of lepidic pattern.[267–270] Nevertheless, evidence-based reviews do not support general CT screening,[256,257] possibly because it identifies many unimportant abnormalities and leads to unnecessary surgery (see asymptomatic solitary pulmonary nodule, below).

Table 12.1.5 Natural history of lung cancer[258]

Cell type	Volume doubling time (days)	Years from malignant change to the tumour reaching	
		1 cm (diagnosis)	10 cm (death)
Squamous cell carcinoma	88	8.4	9.6
Adenocarcinoma	161	15.4	17.6
Large cell carcinoma	86	8.2	9.4
Small cell carcinoma	29	2.8	3.2

SITE OF ORIGIN AND SPREAD

As might be expected from the relative size of the two lungs, slightly more carcinomas arise on the right than the left. There is also a slight preponderance in the upper lobes. Historically, most carcinomas arose in large central bronchi (Fig. 12.1.7) but increasing numbers now develop in the periphery of the lung so that whereas the ratio of central to peripheral tumours was formerly 2:1, it now approaches equality.[271–274] This change has been accompanied by one involving the histological types of bronchopulmonary carcinoma, particularly squamous cell carcinoma (see Fig. 12.1.18, p. 550).

Within the conductive airways, carcinoma arises particularly at bifurcations where inhaled particles tend to impinge and mucociliary clearance is delayed (Fig. 12.1.8 and see Fig. 1.18, p. 13)[275–277] It is probably because the trachea lacks side branches that primary carcinoma of the trachea is rare.[278] The few tumours that arise in the trachea are generally of salivary gland type or carcinoids.[279]

Dissemination of the tumour is chiefly along lymphatic routes, at least initially. Blood spread usually follows. Metastases in hilar and mediastinal lymph nodes, and perhaps beyond, have often developed by the time symptoms first cause the patient to seek attention. Retrograde spread within the lung may lead to widespread lymphatic permeation, resulting in so-called lymphangitis carcinomatosa, which is described in Chapter 12.6, as are other routes of tumour spread within the lung. Further tumour growth and dissemination give rise to a variety of clinical effects, which will now be described.

CLINICAL EFFECTS

Most lung cancers are diagnosed because the patient presents with symptoms: less than 15% are discovered by chance, usually during the course of radiological investigations performed for other purposes, such as routine preoperative assessment, the investigation of chest injuries, the detection of metastases of other tumours or life insurance.

An asymptomatic solitary pulmonary nodule ('coin lesion')

The traditional management of an asymptomatic patient found to have a solitary, well-circumscribed pulmonary opacity has been based

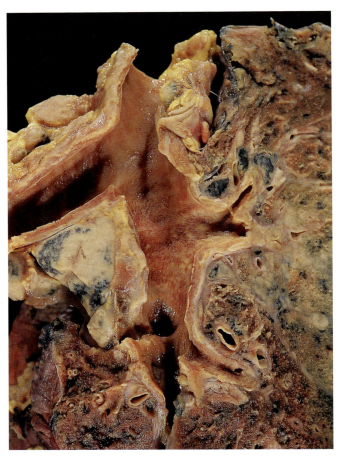

Figure 12.1.7 Carcinoma involving the right main and intermediate bronchi. Note the slight roughening of the bronchial mucosa and the invasion of adjacent hilar lymph nodes. *(Courtesy of Dr GA Russell, Tunbridge Wells, UK.)*

on the supposition that the lesion is malignant until proved otherwise. However, improvements in imaging have led to the realisation that small asymptomatic nodules are very common. Up to 51% of smokers older than 49 years have pulmonary nodules and the great majority of these prove to be benign (99% of those no greater than 4 mm diameter). It is therefore now recommended that nodules measuring 8 mm or less should be merely kept under surveillance.[280] In nodules larger than 8 mm, central calcification and a slow growth rate suggest that the lesion is benign whereas fine linear strands radiating from the edge of the nodule, cavitation and air bronchograms favour the converse, but these features are not wholly reliable.[281] Not infrequently all investigations short of thoracotomy fail to provide a diagnosis and the lesion is biopsied or resected. While it may well prove to be fungal in the USA, an echinococcal cyst in the Orient, and tuberculosis worldwide, a malignant tumour is often the cause (71% in a New Zealand series).[282] Metastases account for about 20% of such malignancies but this figure rises to nearly 50% in patients with an extrapulmonary cancer.[283]

Local effects

Central tumours are prone to obstruct the larger airways (Fig. 12.1.9), leading to pulmonary collapse, infection and 'endogenous lipid pneumonia' (see p. 315). This results in cough, dyspnoea, pain and fever.

Figure 12.1.8 Mucociliary clearance is impaired at bronchial branching points, as shown in this drawing of a rat's airways following the experimental insufflation of carbon, shown here in dark red. *(Reproduced from Iravani and van As (1972)[275] with permission of the editor of* Journal of Pathology.*)*

Figure 12.1.10 Carcinoma of the bronchus with extensive pulmonary and pleural extension. *(Courtesy of W Edwards, Gordon Museum, Guy's Hospital, London, UK.)*

Figure 12.1.9 Squamous cell carcinoma arising in a central bronchus. The tumour has grown in a largely endobronchial manner within the intermediate and right lower-lobe bronchi, obstructing the lumen and causing distal bronchiectasis in the lower lobe and obstructive pneumonia in the middle lobe.

Haemoptysis caused by ulceration of the tumour is another common symptom but is not usually severe. However, many peripheral tumours reach a substantial size and metastasise before causing any symptoms at all. Cavitation is often evident radiologically, particularly with squamous cell carcinomas, whilst the radiographic features of mucinous adenocarcinoma of predominantly lepidic pattern often simulate those of pneumonic consolidation. Patients being treated for pneumonia should therefore be observed until there is complete roentgenographic resolution. Any pneumonia that does not resolve within 4 weeks should be evaluated further to exclude carcinoma. The expectoration of large amounts of watery or mucoid sputum (bronchorrhoea) is occasionally encountered in patients harbouring adenocarcinoma-in-situ or mucinous adenocarcinomas of predominantly lepidic pattern.

Intrathoracic spread

Direct spread may cause pleural or chest wall pain whilst either pleural involvement or poststenotic bronchopneumonia may cause pleural effusion, which if neoplastic is characteristically haemorrhagic (Fig. 12.1.10).

Apical tumours are prone to invade the ribs, the brachial plexus and the cervical part of the sympathetic system (Fig. 12.1.11), causing pain in the shoulder and the ulnar side of the arm, atrophy of the hand muscles, Horner's syndrome (ptosis, constricted pupil, enophthalmos and decreased ipsilateral facial sweating), bone destruction and an apical radiographic opacity. This syndrome was first described by Hare in 1838,[284] but is generally named after Pancoast who described it afresh a century later[285]; the term 'superior sulcus syndrome' is also used.[285,286] Most tumours that cause Pancoast's syndrome are squamous cell carcinomas.

Figure 12.1.11 Pancoast tumour. A tumour in the apex of the left lung has invaded the ribs, the cervical sympathetic chain and the brachial plexus.

Hoarseness due to involvement of the left recurrent laryngeal nerve as it loops around the aorta is another characteristic neurological complication of bronchopulmonary carcinoma. Diaphragmatic paralysis may be caused by involvement of the phrenic nerves, particularly on the right where the phrenic nerve passes close to the hilum of the lung.

Superior vena caval obstruction may be caused by compression and infiltration of the vein by either the primary tumour or metastases in superior mediastinal lymph nodes (Fig. 12.1.12). Small cell carcinoma is particularly likely to present in this way, with massive mediastinal nodes and a small or even undetectable primary tumour. Hilar lymph node metastases may also cause bronchial narrowing and its sequelae. Any lung tumour that extends into the pericardium or oesophagus (Fig. 12.1.13) is likely to cause cardiac tamponade or dysphagia respectively, but invasion of the heart itself is unusual.

Extrathoracic spread

Many patients with carcinoma of the lung eventually develop cervical or abdominal lymph node involvement whilst about a third present with distant metastases, which may obviously lead to a wide variety of symptoms. These include general features such as loss of appetite, fatigue and loss of weight, and local effects that depend on the site involved. Blood-borne metastases of lung carcinoma occur most often in the liver, adrenal glands, brain, skeleton and kidneys; in many countries the commonest cerebral tumour of adults is metastatic carcinoma of the lung. The pattern of metastases varies with the histological type (Table 12.1.6).[287]

Paraneoplastic manifestations

Paraneoplastic syndromes are non-metastatic disorders of distant organs. They develop in 10–20% of cases of lung cancer. Some of the better-established paraneoplastic syndromes are listed in Box 12.1.4.

Neuromuscular paraneoplastic syndromes include the carcinomatous neuromyopathies, a term that covers a variety of encephalopathies, myelopathies, peripheral neuropathies and myopathies.[288,289] Polymyositis and dermatomyositis come within the myopathies and up to 30% of patients with these diseases have an underlying neoplasm.[290] Carcinomatous neuropathy and the myasthenia gravis-like Eaton–Lambert syndrome are particularly associated with small cell

Figure 12.1.12 Superior vena caval compression by mediastinal tumour. (A) Cross-section of the mediastinum viewed from above at the level of the aortic arch showing compression of the superior vena cava by metastatic small cell carcinoma. The compressed vein is situated to the right of the ascending aorta and in front of the carbon-pigmented pretracheal lymph node. (B) In life the patient had shown distension of veins over the front of the chest.

Figure 12.1.13 (A) Anterior and (B) posterior views of a squamous cell carcinoma of the left main bronchus that metastasised to subcarinal lymph nodes and thence invaded the oesophagus which has been opened from behind to show the tumour.

lung cancer.[291] The Eaton–Lambert myasthenic syndrome is a disorder of acetylcholine production at neuromuscular junctions in which an autoantibody directed against determinants on the tumour cell membrane cross-reacts with components of the nerve terminal.[292] Autoantibodies directed against a neuronal or muscle cell antigen underlie many carcinomatous neuromyopathies.[293] These syndromes are not related to the size or duration of the tumour and may develop months before the tumour becomes apparent.

Inappropriate or ectopic hormone secretion is responsible for another important group of paraneoplastic syndromes. It is most often associated with small cell carcinoma. Common examples include the secretion of adrenocorticotrophic hormone and antidiuretic hormone by the tumour.[294] Antidiuretic hormone is raised in the serum of 30–40% of patients with small cell carcinoma but the clinical syndrome of severe hyponatraemia, hypo-osmolality of the serum and continued urinary sodium excretion is recognised in only 5–10%.[295] Excess antidiuretic hormone is sometimes found with non-neoplastic lung disease but here it is pituitary in origin rather than ectopic.

Severe clinical symptoms due to adrenocorticotrophic hormone production are seen in 3–7% of patients with small cell carcinoma. The classic features of Cushing's syndrome (Fig. 12.1.14) are unusual but glucose intolerance and hypokalaemic alkalosis are often severe and hyperpigmentation is usually pronounced.[296]

Less common is the production of atrial natriuretic peptide and vasopressin[297] or the kinins responsible for the carcinoid syndrome.[298] Rare peptide syndromes include hypoglycaemia, hyperpigmentation and hypercalcaemia. Cancer-associated hypercalcaemia is usually due to bone metastases but occasionally occurs without metastatic disease, when it is generally mediated by parathyroid-related protein which increases both bone resorption and renal tubular re-absorption of calcium: serum parathyroid hormone levels are characteristically low or unmeasurable in these cases. The lung tumour most commonly associated with such hypercalcaemia is squamous cell carcinoma.[299] Gynaecomastia and testicular atrophy are occasionally encountered, again with squamous cell carcinoma. Adenocarcinoma of the lung is occasionally responsible for elevated serum levels of amylase.[300] Elevated levels of human chorionic gonadotrophin, α-fetoprotein and other trophoblast markers are sometimes associated with a variety of non-small cell carcinomas of the lung,[301] but notably ones resembling hepatocellular carcinoma ('hepatoid carcinoma of the lung').[302]

Table 12.1.6 Metastatic patterns of lung cancer at autopsy (%) in patients dying of lung cancer[287]

	Squamous cell	Adenocarcinoma	Large cell	Small cell
Hilar/mediastinal nodes	77	80	84	96
Pleura	34	60	67	34
Chest wall	20	20	20	13
Limited to thorax	46	18	14	4
Liver	25	41	48	74
Adrenals	23	50	59	55
Bone	20	36	30	37
Abdominal nodes	10	23	30	29
Central nervous system	Not stated	37	25	29

Box 12.1.4 Paraneoplastic syndromes associated with lung cancer

Neuromuscular

Polymyositis
Myasthenic syndrome
Sensory motor neuropathy
Encephalopathy
Myelopathy
Cerebellar degeneration
Psychosis
Dementia

Endocrine

Cushing's syndrome
Inappropriate ADH secretion
Hypercalcaemia
Carcinoid syndrome
Gynaecomastia
Hyperglycaemia
Hypoglycaemia
Galactorrhoea
Growth hormone excess
Secretion of TSH
Calcitonin secretion

Cardiovascular

Superficial thrombophlebitis (Trousseau's syndrome)
Thrombosis
Marantic endocarditis

Musculoskeletal and cutaneous

Hypertrophic osteoarthropathy
Clubbing
Dermatomyositis
Acanthosis nigricans
Pruritus
Urticaria
Erythema multiforme
Hyperpigmentation

Haematological

Haemolytic anaemia
Red cell aplasia
Polycythaemia
Thrombocytopenic purpura
Thrombocytosis
Dysproteinaemia
Eosinophilia
Leukoerythroblastic reaction including thrombocytopenia

Others

Nephrotic syndrome
Hyperuricaemia
Amyloidosis
Secretion of alkaline phosphatae
Secretion of immunoglobulin A

ADH, antidiuretic hormone; TSH, thyroid-stimulating hormone.

Figure 12.1.14 Cushingoid obesity and facial hirsutism due to inappropriate production of adrenocorticotrophic hormone in a patient with small cell carcinoma of the bronchus.

Common haematological abnormalities include the anaemia of chronic disease and thrombocytosis. As with many other cancers, there may be activation of the coagulation cascade resulting in venous thrombosis and thromboembolism or disseminated intravascular coagulation.[303] Cardiovascular syndromes also include non-bacterial thrombotic (marantic) endocarditis, the vegetations of which may embolise and cause transient ischaemia. Less commonly, carcinoma of the lung releases haemopoietic growth or chemotactic factors, resulting in either blood or local tissue eosinophilia[304] or neutrophilia.[305–307]

Other associated disorders include finger clubbing and pulmonary hypertrophic osteoarthropathy (Fig. 12.1.15), acanthosis nigricans and scleroderma, while lung tumour antigens may result in immune complex glomerulonephritis and vasculitis.[308–311]

DIAGNOSTIC PROCEDURES FOR OBTAINING TUMOUR MATERIAL

The main methods of obtaining material for the pathological diagnosis of lung cancer are sputum collection, bronchoscopy and transthoracic needle aspiration, supplemented as required by tissue

Figure 12.1.15 (A) Finger clubbing and (B) hypertrophic pulmonary osteoarthropathy affecting the tibia and fibula in a patient with squamous cell carcinoma of the lung. Arrows indicate periosteal new bone formation. *(Courtesy of Professor M Hodson and Dr I Kerr, Brompton, UK.)*

Figure 12.1.16 Squamous metaplasia seen over an infiltrating small cell carcinoma. Superficial sampling could lead to erroneous cell typing.

obtained at thoracotomy, or on biopsies or aspirates of distant metastases. Thoracotomy is now generally video-assisted. Mediastinal sampling is important in cancer staging as well as diagnosis but the traditional techniques of mediastinoscopy and mediastinotomy are now giving way to ultrasound-guided transtracheal, transbronchial and transoesophageal needle aspiration.[311a-c]

If necessary, sputum production can be induced by the inhalation of a saline spray. When cancer is present, the detection rate after four good specimens of sputum, obtained on waking and after cleaning the mouth, is about 85%.[312] Poor-quality specimens result in this figure being considerably lower. A freshly fixed smear stained with Papanicolaou's stain, haematoxylin and eosin or other stain of choice may be examined, or sputum may be collected for several days in a container of alcohol, and the specimen then smeared or blocked for the preparation of paraffin sections. Alternatively, the sputum may first be homogenised.[313] Cytological typing of lung tumours is possible in most cases[314] and is often superior to histological typing.[315]

Cytological specimens may also be obtained at bronchoscopy, by washing, brushing or increasingly by transbronchial fine-needle aspiration[316-318] The combination of cytology and biopsy has been shown to be cost-effective.[319] Brushing many branches increases the detection rate and can identify the site of an occult carcinoma.[320] When the tumour is located peripherally and cannot be visualised by bronchoscopy, selective bronchial lavage can be useful.[321] As noted above, transbronchial needle aspiration of enlarged mediastinal lymph nodes is now often performed under ultrasound guidance. It has the advantage of combining diagnosis and staging in a single procedure.[311a-c,318,322,323]

The flexible fibreoptic bronchoscope has greatly facilitated bronchopulmonary biopsy. The specimens are small but many can be taken. It is reported that four biopsies are sufficient to ensure the diagnosis of central tumours but that six may be required if the tumour is peripheral.[324] Typing is relatively easy if the tumour is well differentiated but it can be difficult to type poorly differentiated tumours in these small specimens. For this reason the term 'undifferentiated non-small cell carcinoma – not otherweise specified' is

widely used when specimens are small; large cell carcinoma is only diagnosed when the tumour can be widely sampled and differentiation excluded.[325-328] With the limited treatment options available in the twentieth century this categorisation was quite adequate but the advent of drugs based on molecular features is now placing greater demands upon the pathologist, as discussed in subsequent sections. The degree of differentiation varies greatly from one part of a tumour to another and adequate grading of lung tumours is never possible on biopsy specimens. Surface abnormalities may not reflect the cell type of an underlying tumour and caution is needed if the biopsy is unduly superficial. For instance, small cell carcinoma may be covered by atypical metaplastic epithelium or even squamous carcinoma-in-situ and if the invasive tumour is not sampled an erroneous report may be issued (Fig. 12.1.16).[329]

Transcutaneous fine-needle aspiration is useful for peripheral growths. It requires fluoroscopic control and the radiologist greatly appreciates the attendance of a laboratory worker in the radiology suite to attend to the rapid fixation of material for cytology and on-the-spot verification that the specimen is adequate. However, with the introduction of spring-loaded wide-bore (18-gauge) needles, excellent specimens sufficient for histology are now obtained, negating the need for laboratory personnel in the radiology department (see p. 753).

HISTOLOGICAL TYPING

The histological typing of lung cancer has long been subject to debate. This is partly due to the heterogeneity many lung tumours display.[330] Many are of mixed cell type[331-335] or their cell type changes on treatment,[336] thus supporting Willis's unitary view that all pulmonary carcinomas arise from a common stem cell that has the potential to differentiate along various pathways.[337] On the other hand, the different tumour types clearly differ in their clinical behaviour and response to treatment, so histological typing is of considerable clinical importance. Unfortunately, the small size of fibreoptic bronchoscopic biopsy specimens imposes considerable problems in the accurate typing of lung tumours.

The classification adopted here is based upon that advocated by the World Health Organization (WHO) (Table 12.1.7).[130] This was last revised in 2004, since when weaknesses in the subtyping of adeno-

Table 12.1.7 The 2004 World Health Organization histological classification of malignant epithelial tumours of lung[130]

Squamous cell carcinoma	
Variants:	Papillary
	Clear cell
	Small cell
	Basaloid
Small cell carcinoma	
Variant:	Combined
Adenocarcinoma	
Mixed adenocarcinoma	
Acinar adenocarcinoma	
Papillary adenocarcinoma	
Bronchioloalveolar carcinoma	
Solid adenocarcinoma with mucus formation	
Variants:	Fetal adenocarcinoma
	Mucinous ('colloid') carcinoma
	Mucinous cystadenocarcinoma
	Signet ring adenocarcinoma
	Clear cell adenocarcinoma
Large cell carcinoma	
Variants:	Large cell neuroendocrine carcinoma
	Basaloid carcinoma
	Lymphoepithelioma-like carcinoma
	Clear cell carcinoma
	Large cell carcinoma with rhabdoid phenotype
	Adenosquamous carcinoma
	Sarcomatoid carcinoma
	Pleomorphic carcinoma
	Spindle cell carcinoma
	Giant cell carcinoma
	Carcinosarcoma
	Pulmonary blastoma
Carcinoid tumour	
	Typical carcinoid
	Atypical carcinoid
Salivary gland tumours	
	Mucoepidermoid carcinoma
	Adenoid cystic carcinoma
	Epithelial-myoepithelial carcinoma

The adenocarcinoma section has undergone modification – see Box 12.1.5, p. 556.

carcinoma have become apparent and modifications in this area have been suggested. One of these has been referred to above, namely the transference of bronchioloalveolar cell carcinoma from the frankly malignant to the premalignant category and its rebirth there as adenocarcinoma-in-situ. Other modifications will be considered in the adenocarcinoma section.

The WHO classification depends solely upon light microscopy and consequently has the advantage that it can be used by histopathologists everywhere. However, electron microscopy (Table 12.1.8) and immunohistochemistry can undoubtedly sharpen the histological diagnosis on occasion and with the introduction of new drugs based upon molecular changes information on these is being increasingly demanded.[330,338–344] Molecular studies are increasingly being required

in relation to the anti-TK drugs, but these supplement rather than supplant histology. Surgical pathology remains important and is both cheaper and faster than molecular characterisation. At the moment therefore the likely clinical response to the new drugs is often inferred from the histology. This is not wholly reliable but efforts are under way to refine the histological characteristics by applying panels of antibodies capable of dividing non-small cell carcinomas into various clusters in which one particular histological pattern generally predominates.[345]

The relative frequency of the various histological types varies according to the type of material examined (Table 12.1.9)[57,273,287,312,346–353] and thus depends upon the site and metastatic potential of the tumour. Surgical series include more peripheral tumours than bron-

Table 12.1.8 Histological typing of 75 lung cancers before and after the application of electron microscopy[330]

Histological type by light microscopy	Histological type by light and electron microscopy	
Squamous cell carcinoma (n = 37)		
	Pure squamous cell	9
	Squamous cell and adenocarcinoma	6
	Squamous cell and small cell carcinoma	11
	Squamous cell and adeno- and small cell carcinoma	11
Adenocarcinoma (n = 26)		
	Pure adenocarcinoma	7
	Adeno- and squamous cell carcinoma	5
	Adeno- and small cell carcinoma	8
	Adeno- and squamous cell and small cell carcinoma	6
Small cell carcinoma (n = 3)		
	Pure small cell carcinoma	2
	Small cell and squamous and adenocarcinoma	1
Large cell carcinoma (n = 9)		
	Pure large cell carcinoma	0
	Adenocarcinoma	7
	Squamous cell carcinoma	2

Table 12.1.9 Frequency (%) of histological subtypes of lung carcinoma by source of specimen[57,273,287,312,346–353]

	Biopsy/cytology	Surgery	Autopsy
Squamous cell	46	59	36
Small cell	16	3	21
Adenocarcinoma	22	28	26
Large cell	16	10	17

stronger with centrally situated tumours such as squamous and small cell carcinomas than with tumours such as large cell and adenocarcinomas that are commoner in the periphery of the lung but this is changing with changes in cigarette manufacture.[273,363,364] Asbestos is particularly associated with adenocarcinoma[57–59,365] whilst irradiation and chloromethyl ether are both particularly associated with small cell carcinoma.[77] It has also been claimed that polyaromatic hydrocarbons, arsenic, chromates and nickel are all associated with squamous cell carcinoma but this is not well substantiated.[77]

In considering trends in the proportions of the various histological types, it should be borne in mind that the criteria for histological classification of lung carcinomas have changed.[366] Thus, the 1981 revision of the WHO classification is possibly relevant to some reports that adenocarcinoma is on the increase, because the revision recommended that solid tumours showing mucin secretion should be categorised as adenocarcinoma, rather than large cell carcinoma, as previously. However, quite apart from this, there appears to be a genuine increase in the proportion of adenocarcinomas[273,355–357,367–369] This is seen in both men and women but is more marked among women.[356] It presumably reflects the increased popularity of low-tar and filter-tipped cigarettes[364] and the increasing proportion of female smokers. This change in the proportions of the various histological types appears to be accompanied by a change in their distribution within the lung so that the historical predominace of adenocarcinomas in the periphery and squamous cell carcinomas in the central region is now less distinct.[274]

choscopic studies whilst those tumours that disseminate early are more numerous in autopsy series. Figures derived from large surveys provide the most reliable information but even these vary with time as smoking patterns change. There are also geographical differences. Squamous cell carcinoma has been the commonest type in many countries but adenocarcinoma is increasing in frequency and is now the commonest in many American and Japanese series.[354–357] Figures also vary according to the detail put into the pathological examination. If mucous stains are neglected many poorly differentiated adenocarcinomas will be classified as undifferentiated large cell carcinoma, whilst if electron microscopy is used the undifferentiated category is eliminated altogether and adenosquamous carcinoma becomes the commonest (Fig. 12.1.17).[358,359] There may also be considerable interobserver variability: one group of pathologists reached agreement on 72% of small cell carcinomas, 56% of adenocarcinomas, 48% of squamous cell carcinomas and only 5% of large-cell carcinomas.[360] However, less interobserver variation is reported in other studies.[325,361,362]

Many pulmonary carcinogens are associated with particular histological types of lung cancer. The association with smoking has been

SQUAMOUS CELL CARCINOMA

Squamous cell carcinoma has classically been regarded as a tumour of the central bronchi but there has been a reduction in the number of central tumours and peripheral examples are now just as common (Fig. 12.1.18).[24] The cut surface is often granular or friable and large tumours frequently cavitate because of central necrosis (Fig. 12.1.19). Hilar lymph nodes are often directly invaded. Metastasis occurs later than with the other histological types of bronchopulmonary carcinoma.

Histological appearances

Squamous cell carcinomas form irregular nests and strands of tumour cells separated by varying amounts of fibrous stroma. The tumour cells have large irregular nuclei, clumped chromatin and nucleoli of varying size. Stratification is often evident but by itself this is considered inadequate evidence of squamous differentiation as it is also seen in

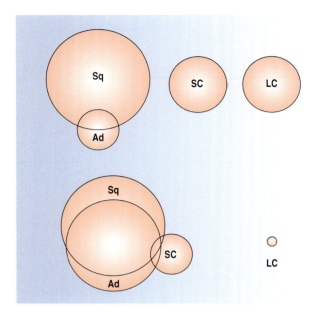

Figure 12.1.17 Types of lung carcinoma: frequency assessed by light microscopy (top) and electron microscopy (bottom). Sq, squamous cell carcinoma; Ad, adenocarcinoma; SC, small cell carcinoma; LC, large cell carcinoma. Adenosquamous carcinoma is represented by the overlapping Sq and Ad circles. For the electron microscopist adenosquamous carcinoma is the commonest pattern, large cell carcinoma is very rare, small cell carcinoma is less distinct and rare tumours showing tripartite differentiation are recognised.

occasional poorly differentiated adenocarcinomas. Categorisation of a pulmonary carcinoma as squamous cell requires evidence of either keratinisation or intercellular bridging.[130] Well-differentiated squamous cell carcinomas show prominent keratinisation throughout whereas poorly differentiated tumours require careful scrutiny to identify keratinisation or intercellular bridging. Grading is of prognostic value but this is best confined to resection specimens as there is often considerable variation within a tumour: small biopsies are inadequate for tumour grading.

Keratinisation may involve single tumour cells but is easier to recognise when it forms concentrically laminated squamous 'pearls' (Fig. 12.1.20). Individually keratinised cells are rounded and have slightly refractile eosinophilic cytoplasm. Their nuclei may be pyknotic or show karyolysis, but all these features are seen in any apoptotic tumour cell. To be confident that cytoplasmic eosinophilia represents keratinisation it is necessary to concentrate on cells with viable nuclei. Intercellular bridging is another marker of squamous differentiation. The bridges (or 'prickles') represent desmosomal cell junctions that are evident at the light microscopic level only because artefactual cell shrinkage results in the junctions being stretched across intercellular spaces, where they are seen as regularly spaced thin cytoplasmic threads (Fig. 12.1.21).

Central necrosis is often evident within groups of squamous carcinoma cells, often sharply demarcated from the viable tumour cells. Squamous debris may elicit a foreign-body giant cell reaction. Alternatively, the necrotic debris may be absorbed, leaving a space that could be misinterpreted as evidence of glandular differentiation. At the growing edge of the tumour alveoli may be destroyed or invaded.[370] Some squamous cell carcinomas show oncocytic change, due to large

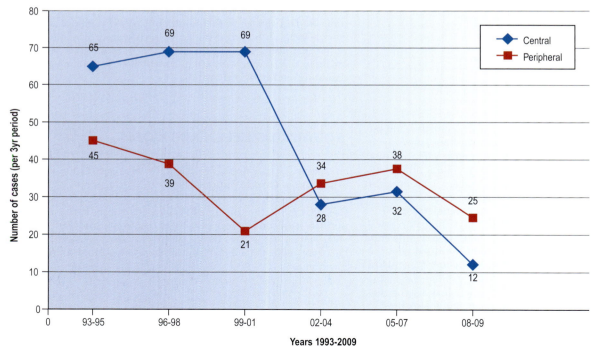

Figure 12.1.18 Central versus peripheral location of bronchopulmonary squamous cell carcinomas resected at the Royal Brompton Hospital 1993–2009. There has been a marked reduction in the number of central tumours over this period.

Figure 12.1.20 Well-differentiated squamous cell carcinoma of the bronchus showing stratification and two keratin 'pearls'.

Figure 12.1.19 Two carcinomas of the lung, both squamous cell in type and both showing central cavitation. They are in different lobes, thereby fulfilling one of the criteria for double primary tumours.

Figure 12.1.21 (A) Well-differentiated squamous cell carcinoma showing well-developed 'prickles' connecting the tumour cells and representing desmosomes highlighted by artefactual cell shrinkage. (B) Electron micrograph of the desmosomes, without shrinkage artefact. *(B courtesy of Professor W Mooi, Amsterdam, Netherlands.)*

numbers of mitochondria within the cytoplasm. Osteocartilaginous stromal metaplasia is a further rare feature.[371] Rarely, squamous carcinomas of the lung have a distinctly adenoid structure and correspond to those more frequently encountered in the skin, where they are termed adenoacanthoma or adenoid or pseudovascular (pseudo-angiosarcomatous) squamous cell carcinoma.[372] Pilomatricoma-like differentiation is particularly rare.[373]

The WHO classification recognises four variants of squamous cell carcinoma – papillary, clear cell, small cell and basaloid.[130] The papillary variant (Fig. 12.1.22A) is well differentiated and most examples are endobronchial. Often there is no evidence of stromal invasion,

in which case they are better classified as carcinoma-in-situ with papillary architecture or even solitary squamous papilloma with dysplasia.[374] Most of these tumours are T1N0 and have a 5-year survival of over 60%.[375] Examples of the papillary variant developing in the periphery of the lung may show an alveolar filling pattern.[24]

In the clear cell variant (Fig. 12.1.22B) small foci of clear cell change are seen in what is otherwise evidently a squamous cell carcinoma. Such foci are commonly seen but seldom predominate.[376] Pure clear cell carcinomas are classified as a variant of large cell carcinoma and are described under that heading below. Focal clear cell change in a squamous cell carcinoma is of no prognostic significance.

Figure 12.1.22 Variants of squamous cell carcinoma. (A) The papillary variant. Papillae clothed by well-differentiated squamous cell carcinoma protrude into the bronchial lumen. (B) In the clear cell variant the tumour cell cytoplasm appears empty. (C) The small cell variant. Although the tumour cells are small (bottom) they lack the characteristic nuclear features of a small cell carcinoma and keratinisation is present in the upper half of the field. (D) The basaloid variant. Groups of tumour cells show peripheral palisading while the individual tumour cells are cuboidal or fusiform, and have scanty cytoplasm and hyperchromatic nuclei devoid of prominent nucleoli. Squamoid elements were present elsewhere in tumour.

The small cell variant (Fig. 12.1.22C) is a poorly differentiated squamous cell carcinoma in which the cells are small but retain the nuclear characteristics of a non-small cell carcinoma and show focal squamous differentiation. Thus, it is composed of cells that bear a resemblance to small cell carcinoma in that they are small, but their nuclei are vesicular and contain evident nucleoli, lacking the 'salt and pepper' chromatin pattern of small cell carcinoma. It is to be distinguished from the combined variant of small cell carcinoma described below.[377] The prognosis is that of a poorly differentiated squamous cell carcinoma.

The basaloid variant (Fig. 12.1.22D) of squamous cell carcinoma is characterised by foci resembling basal cell carcinoma of the skin in that there is peripheral palisading and the tumour cells are small and have hyperchromatic nuclei. Tumours with such features throughout (basaloid carcinomas) are classified as a variant of large cell carcinoma. The basaloid variant of squamous cell carcinoma shows an even closer resemblance to certain tumours of the upper aerodigestive tract that have been termed basaloid squamous cell carcinoma, and indeed this name has been applied on occasion to this bronchial tumour.[378] Some studies have shown that the basaloid variant of squamous cell carcinoma carries a worse prognosis than other poorly differentiated squamous cell carcinomas in stage I and II disease,[379–381] whilst others have failed to confirm this.[382]

Immunohistochemistry

Squamous cell carcinomas of the lung stain strongly for low-molecular-weight cytokeratins, and in the better-differentiated tumours high-

Table 12.1.10 Immunophenotypic characterisation of carcinoma of the lung

Cell type	Usual immunophenotype
Squamous cell carcinoma (including the basaloid variants of both squamous cell carcinoma and large cell carcinoma)	CK5+ve, CK7−ve > +ve, TTF-1−ve, CD56−ve
Most adenocarcinomas and large cell carcinomas (including sarcomatoid carcinoma)	CK5−ve, CK7+ve, TTF-1+ve,[a] CD56−ve
Small cell carcinoma and large cell neuroendocrine carcinoma	CK5−ve, CK7+ve, TTF-1+ve, CD56+ve

CK, cytokeratin; TTF-1, thyroid transcription factor-1.

[a]Mucinous tumours give variable results with TTF-1 (see text).

molecular-weight cytokeratins and carcinoembryonic antigen are also found.[383] There may also be focal staining for epithelial membrane antigen. Many squamous cell carcinomas stain for a variety of trophoblast markers[301,384–386] and high sensitivity and specificity are reported for desmoglein-3.[387] Negative reactions are usually obtained for TTF-1 and the neuroendocrine marker CD56 (Table 12.1.10). The *p63* gene, a member of the *p53* family, may be demonstrated by immunohistochemistry in squamous cell carcinomas of many organs, including those arising in the lungs, and *p63* is proving useful in assigning poorly differentiated non-small carcinomas to the squamous cell category when treatment with the TK inhibitor gefitinib is being considered, a squamous phenotype being a contraindication to this drug.[388,389]

Electron microscopy

Electron microscopy generally shows a wealth of tonofibrils, many of which converge on desmosomes and extend into the intercellular bridges (see Fig. 12.1.21). The cytoplasm otherwise contains relatively few organelles. Keratinisation is marked by increased numbers of tonofibrils, sometimes in a perinuclear arrangement. Thickening of the cell membrane by the deposition of small granules on its inner surface[390] appears to render the membrane impermeable and is followed by cytoplasmic shrinkage, pyknosis of the nucleus and ultimately cell death.

Differential diagnosis

There is seldom any difficulty in recognising squamous cell carcinoma but both histopathologists and cytopathologists need to beware of misinterpreting regenerative atypical squamous metaplasia. Quite alarming, but reversible, changes may be seen bordering a necrotising process in the lung, such as a tuberculous cavity, an infarct or Wegener's granulomatosis, or in the bronchus if a recent biopsy site is again sampled.[122] Irradiation, cytotoxic therapy or even previous instrumentation may also give rise to false-positive cytology results. Prolonged tracheal intubation may cause necrosis with extension of regenerative metaplasia into the submucosal glands, a process known as necrotising sialometaplasia (see pp. 97 and 696), which also needs to be distinguished from invasive carcinoma.[391,392]

ADENOCARCINOMA

In many parts of the world adenocarcinoma of the lung shows an increase in its incidence that cannot be ascribed solely to changes in histological typing.[273,354,355,357,368] This may be connected with the increasing number of women who smoke, for women appear to have a propensity to develop carcinoma of this particular histological pattern,[367] but the major factor is probably the increasing popularity of filter-tipped cigarettes, the carcinogens of which are thought to penetrate more deeply into the lungs. However, although most patients with pulmonary adenocarcinoma are elderly cigarette smokers, there is a higher proportion of adenocarcinoma in non-smokers[393] and the young.[394]

Most adenocarcinomas of the lung arise in the periphery of the lung, in what has been called the terminal respiratory unit. This comprises a terminal bronchiole and the respiratory bronchioles, alveolar ducts and alveoli derived therefrom. In a Japanese study less than 3% of adenocarcinomas arose in large central bronchi,[395] whereas this figure was over 13% in a British series.[396] It has been suggested that a simple division into central and peripheral would be better than histological subtyping, firstly because of histological heterogeneity and secondly because location has prognostic relevance, the central growths having the worse outlook.[396] Molecular studies demonstrating different mutations support the classification of pulmonary adenocarcinoma into bronchial and peripheral subtypes.[158,397]

Central adenocarcinomas often show polypoid endobronchial growth whereas peripheral adenocarcinomas often show central scarring with indrawing of the overlying pleura (Fig. 12.1.23). Central cavitation is not as common as with squamous cell carcinomas. Occasionally peripheral adenocarcinomas spread out over the pleura, thereby mimicking mesothelioma (so-called pseudomesotheliomatous carcinoma of the lung[398]). The bronchioloalveolar pattern of adenocarcinoma has its own distinctive gross appearances and is dealt with separately, under its new name adenocarcinoma-in-situ (see p. 536).

Histological appearances

The WHO classification of lung tumours (see Table 12.1.7) recognises five subtypes of adenocarcinoma (acinar, papillary, bronchioloalveolar, solid with mucin production and mixed) together with several rarer variants (fetal, colloid, mucinous cystadenocarcinoma, signet ring and clear cell).[130] It was last updated in 2004, since when others have proposed the addition of several further growth patterns – papillary with a prominent morular component,[399] micropapillary,[400] secretory endometrioid-like,[401] adenocarcinoma with massive lymphocyte infiltration,[402] basaloid[403] and those showing enteric differentiation.[404–406] These proposals, together with reservations concerning the value of recognising a mixed subtype, have led the International Association for the Study of Lung Cancer (IASLC), American Thoracic Society (ATS) and European Respiratory Society (ERS) to recommend modifications to the WHO classification in several respects (Box 12.1.5). The mixed subtype combines any of the other patterns, frequently exhibiting a lepidic, papillary or tubulopapillary architecture at its periphery and an acinar or solid pattern centrally (Fig. 12.1.24A). It makes up about 90% of cases and this predominance is one of the weaknesses of the WHO classification, leading to recommendations for abandoning it and classifying adenocarcinoma of the lung according to the predominant pattern (Box 12.1.5).[150] Such classification has been shown to correlate with both prognosis and the presence of mutations of genes such as *EGFR* and *K-ras*.[211] IASLC/ATS/ERS also recommend: (1) recognition of a mini-

Figure 12.1.23 (A, B) A peripheral adenocarcinoma of the lung showing a central pigmented scar and indrawing of the overlying pleura.

cell carcinomas and large cell carcinomas as a result of central necrosis and absorption. Remnants of entrapped alveoli may also be mistaken for glandular differentiation.[408]

The term 'lepidic pattern' (scale-like) is recommended for those areas where tumour cells grow along the alveolar walls without destroying them (see Figs 12.1.4A and 12.1.24A). It supplants the term 'bronchioloalveolar pattern' and is applied to non-invasive areas of a tumour that elsewhere shows evidence of invasive growth (as opposed to adenocarcinoma-in-situ, which shows non-invasive growth throughout).

In the papillary pattern (Fig. 12.1.24C), the tumour cells are again cuboidal or columnar and may again contain mucin but here they generally cover complex secondary and tertiary papillary structures with fibrovascular cores.[409]

In the micropapillary pattern (Fig. 12.1.24D) the minature papillae lack stromal cores and free cell clusters lie within the alveoli, often filling these spaces.[400,410–414] This pattern is associated with early lymph node metastasis and hence a relatively poor prognosis.

The solid pattern (Fig. 12.1.24E, F) is represented by sheets of polygonal cells devoid of intercellular bridges but containing large vesicular nuclei, prominent nucleoli and moderately abundant cytoplasm in which droplets of mucin may be demonstrated by appropriate methods. A little mucin may be present in squamous cell carcinoma, carcinoid or small cell lung carcinoma and only when a tumour that would otherwise be classified as a large cell carcinoma contains substantial numbers of mucin-positive cells (at least 5 per 2 high-power fields) is it categorised as an adenocarcinoma of solid pattern.

The fetal pattern of adenocarcinoma takes its name from a fanciful resemblance to fetal lung in the pseudoglandular stage of development (see Fig. 2.3, p. 41). However, it also resembles normal endometrium. Both these likenesses are spurious but have led to the introduction of two alternative names, pulmonary endodermal tumour resembling fetal lung and pulmonary adenocarcinoma with endometrioid features.[415–417,421] The term 'fetal pattern' is used in both the WHO and IASLC classifications, where it is described as a variant of adenocarcinoma. Low- and high-grade types are distinguished, dependent on the degree of pleomorphism.[418] The age range is wide but high-grade tumours tend to affect the elderly and low-grade ones the middle-aged.[418] Tumours of this pattern are generally parenchymal growths but endobronchial examples have been described.[419,420] Histologically, they are characterised by complex glandular structures lined by columnar cells with glycogen-rich clear cytoplasm separated by sparse fibromyxoid stroma (Fig. 12.1.25). In places the epithelial cells form solid squamoid collections that have been termed morulae. Immunocytochemistry shows focal neuroendocrine differentiation in the morulae.[419] Also in the morulae, the nuclei are often clear, the chromatin forming a thin peripheral rim due to the central accumulation of biotin.[421,422] Biotin is an essential cofactor for several enzymes but is normally found in the cytoplasm rather than the nucleus. However, biotin is stored in the nuclei of endometrial epithelial cells in pregnancy and in endometrioid ovarian carcinoma, supporting this tumour's alternative name of pulmonary endometrioid adenocarcinoma. Morular cells that express neuroendocrine markers and have optically clear, biotin-rich nuclei also show accumulation of ß-catenin, a component of cell junctions that also acts as a transcriptional activator of the ß-catenin gene, a feature that well-differentiated fetal adenocarcinoma shares with pulmonary blastoma as well as endometrioid adenocarcinoma of the female genital tract.[423,424] Unlike metastatic endometrioid adenocarcinoma of the female genital tract, fetal adenocarcinoma of the lung is usually positive for cytokeratin 7 and TTF-1.

Mucinous adenocarcinomas display a wide variety of patterns. In addition to the predominantly acinar, papillary, lepidic and solid patterns described above, they may be of signet ring cell, colloid or

mally invasive category of adnocarcinoma; (2) recognition of acinar, papillary, micropapillary, lepidic and solid predominance as the major patterns of adenocarcinoma; (3) separate grouping of mucinous carcinomas; and (4) changes to the less common variants of adenocarcinoma, including the elimination of clear cell and signet ring cell carcinomas as distinct types of lung tumour. Of the five major patterns, lepidic predominance appears to signify a lesser degree of malignancy than acinar and papillary, which are in turn less malignant than micropapillary and solid.

Minimally invasive adenocarcinoma usually measures 2 cm or less and is of predominantly non-mucinous lepidic pattern. It shows less than 5 mm of invasion at any one point. If multiple areas of micro-invasive areas are found, the largest invasive area should be measured, i.e. the size of invasion is not the summation of all such foci. The justification for recognising this pattern of adenocarcinoma is that, although invasive, its prognosis is the same as or close to that of adenocarcinoma-in-situ.[183,407]

The acinar pattern of adenocarcinoma is characterised by a proliferation of glandular structures in the form of acini and tubules (Fig. 12.1.24A, B). The lining tumour cells are typically cuboidal or columnar with moderately abundant cytoplasm that may contain mucin. The tubules of an acinar adenocarcinoma have to be distinguished from the pseudoglandular structures that may develop in squamous

Figure 12.1.24 Principal patterns of adenocarcinoma. (A) Mixed acinar (left) and lepidic (right). (B) Acinar. (C) Papillary. (D) Micropapillary, in which clusters of tumour cells form small papillary structures that lack stromal cores. (E, F) Solid with mucus formation. (F, di-periodic acid–Schiff stain.)

Box 12.1.5 **Changes to the World Health Organization histological classification of pulmonary adenocarcinoma proposed by the International Association for the Study of Lung Cancer (IASLC)[150] in conjunction with the American Thoracic Society (ATS) and European Respiratory Society (ERS)**

1. Preinvasive
   a. Atypical adenomatous hyperplasia
   b. Adenocarcinoma-in-situ (formerly bronchioloalveolar cell carcinoma)[a]
2. Minimally invasive (a lepidic predominant carcinoma with ≤5 mm invasion)
3. Invasive
   a. Lepidic predominant[b]
   b. Acinar predominant[b]
   c. Papillary predominant[b]
   d. Micropapillary predominant[b]
   e. Solid predominant[b]

Variant: Mucinous adenocarcinoma (includes most tumours formerly classified as mucinous bronchioloalvolar carcinoma)[a]

Variant: Mucinous cystadenocarcinoma

Variant: Colloid carcinoma

Variant: Fetal

Variant: Enteric

[a]The great majority of adenocarcinomas-in-situ are non-mucinous. Mucinous adenocarcinomas that are entirely non-invasive are exceptionally rare. Most tumours formerly classified as mucinous bronchioloalveolar carcinoma show some invasion and are included in the mucinous adenocarcinoma variant of invasive adenocarcinoma. This variant may be subclassified according to the predominant pattern (lepidic, acinar, papillary, micropapillary and solid) in the same way as the non-mucinous adenocarcinomas. Most mucinous bronchioloalveolar carcinomas are now termed mucinous adenocarcinoma showing lepidic predominance.

[b]Most adenocarcinomas are of mixed pattern, hence categorisation according to the predominant pattern. It is recommended that the pathologist should list all the patterns present and roughly estimate the proportion of the tumour formed of each using 5% increments, e.g. lepidic 45%, acinar 35%, papillary 20%, ensuring that the proportions total 100%.

Note: Signet ring cell and clear cell are no longer recognised as distinct subtypes as their characteristic features may be seen in many of the other patterns.

Figure 12.1.25 Well-differentiated adenocarcinoma resembling fetal lung. Note the clear cytoplasm, which is due to glycogen accumulation.

cystic pattern and sometimes resemble adenocarcinomas of the bowel.[404–406] Except for the mucinous cystadenocarcinoma they carry a worse prognosis than their non-mucinous counterparts, regardless of histological pattern.[425,426]

The predominantly lepidic pattern of mucinous adenocarcinoma encompasses the former bronchioloalveolar carcinoma of mucinous type as well as mucinous adenocarcinomas of mixed pattern in which lepidic growth predominates. The tumour cells are relatively monomorphic, show little atypia and produce large amounts of mucin, which may lead to bronchorrhoea. The tumour is often multifocal or affects the lung diffusely. The lung structure is maintained and, when a whole lobe is involved, the appearances may simulate those of lobar pneumonia, particularly the mucinous variety produced by *Klebsiella* species (Fig. 12.1.26). Deposits of similar tumour may involve the other lung but even when the disease is bilateral the mediastinal lymph nodes are frequently free of growth. This has led to speculation that the multicentricity represents aerogenous dissemination rather

than multifocal origin. A sparsity of intercellular junctions that would minimise cellular cohesion and promote such aerial metastasis has been noted on electron microscopy.[427] Molecular studies show that the multifocal lesions are monoclonal and thus support them being metastatic.[428] A lepidic growth pattern is also seen on occasion in the pulmonary metastases of adenocarcinomas arising in other sites, especially the pancreas, stomach, colon, breast and ovary.[429,430] The distinction of primary and metastatic adenocarcinomas is considered in Chapter 12.6 (see p. 688).

A 'signet ring cell' pattern is not included in the new IASLC classification of adenocarcinoma but still requires a description. It displays more mucin than the solid variety but the tumour cells are similarly arranged in poorly differentiated sheets. In contrast to the small droplets of mucin seen in the solid variety, a large vacuole of mucin distends the cell and indents the nucleus so much that it forms a crescent at the edge of the cell (Fig. 12.1.27). The appearances are similar to those seen in tumours of the same name in the stomach and elsewhere but there is no evidence of a primary tumour in these sites and reactions compatible with a pulmonary origin are obtained. For example, TTF-1 and cytokeratin 7 are positive and cytokeratin 20 is negative.[431–436] Carcinoma of the lung in which a signet ring cell configuration forms

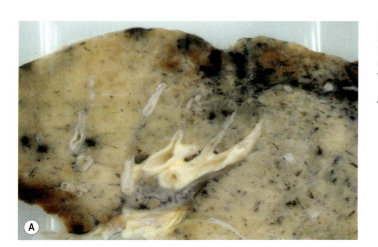

Figure 12.1.26 Mucinous adenocarcinoma of lepidic pattern. (A) The lung is consolidated throughout; the gross appearances mimic those of lobar pneumonia. *(Courtesy of Dr JW Seo, Seoul, Korea.)* (B) The consolidation is due to mucus filling the alveoli. (C) Mucous cells line the alveolar walls without destroying them.

Figure 12.1.27 Signet ring cell carcinoma. A primary pulmonary adenocarcinoma of signet ring cell morphology, mimicking metastatic gastric carcinoma.

Figure 12.1.28 Colloid carcinoma. Small groups of tumour cells lie free within their abundant mucous secretion.

at least 50% of the tumour is reported to have a particularly poor prognosis.[435] Others report a poor prognosis if signet ring cells merely exceed 5%.[437] An association with the *EML4-ALK* fusion gene has been reported.[224]

The 'colloid' pattern of mucinous adenocarcinoma is similar to the tumour of the same name in the gastrointestinal tract.[438] It affects the middle-aged or elderly of either sex. The mucoid nature of the tumour is evident upon macroscopic examination of the cut surface. Microscopically, tumour cells with large vesicular nuclei, prominent nucleoli and moderately abundant cytoplasm float free within copious amounts of mucin that fill and often distend alveoli. Growth along the alveolar walls is often deficient (Fig. 12.1.28). Colloid carcinoma lacks the capsule of a mucinous cystadenocarcinoma and the pools of tumour cell-bearing mucin frequently spill over into neighbouring air spaces that are not themselves lined by neoplastic cells. Variable reactions are reported for cytokeratins 7 and 20.[439]

Mucinous cystadenocarcinoma is particularly rare. It occurs in patients who are middle-aged or elderly and of either sex, shows a wide range of behaviour and is often of only borderline malignancy.[440–442] Some examples have shown no evidence of malignancy whatsoever and have been termed cystadenoma.[443,444] Some have seeded out on to the pleura in a manner reminiscent of pseudomyxoma peritonei produced by comparable tumours of the appendix or ovary.[445] Cytological atypia and microglandular solid areas may suggest malignancy but there is seldom any evidence of invasive activity. Most can be excised in their entirety and do not recur. The tumour is typically peripheral, well demarcated, cystic and either unilocular or multilocular. It is filled with mucus and microscopically is lined by stratified mucous cells, which are sometimes thrown into folds. Its capsule distinguishes it from colloid carcinoma.

Adenocarcinoma of enteric pattern reproduces in the lung morphological features indistinguishable from those of the common pattern of colorectal carcinoma.[404] Some report that its immunohistological characteristics are also those of colorectal cancer[405] whereas others find that they differ.[406]

Immunohistochemistry

Adenocarcinomas of the lung express a wide range of cytokeratins, but not 5 and 6, which are characteristic of squamous cell carcinomas and

epithelioid mesotheliomas, and 20, which is found more frequently in intestinal carcinomas (see Table 12.1.10). They also generally stain for carcinoembryonic antigen, BerEP4, AUA1, epithelial membrane antigen and vimentin. TTF-1[446] is a relatively sensitive and specific marker of pulmonary adenocarcinomas but variable results are reported with mucinous lung tumours.[439] Mucinous adenocarcinoma of predominantly lepidic pattern generally fails to react with TTF-1 but gives positive results for intestinal markers such as CDX2, CK20 and MUC-2. Mucinous adenocarcinomas described as being composed of goblet rather than signet ring cells may display a similar intestinal pattern or react for both intestinal and lung markers. It is suggested that such tumours arise in bronchial rather than bronchiolar cells.[436,439] The neuroendocrine markers chromogranin and neuron-specific enolase can be demonstrated in some pulmonary adenocarcinomas but CD56 is generally negative. Trophoblastic markers can often be demonstrated, as in other non-small cell carcinomas of the lung.[301,386]

Electron microscopy

The heterogeneity of adenocarcinoma of the lung noted above is again evident when these tumours are examined by electron microscopy.[426,447] Some reflect the embryological derivation of the lower respiratory tract from the primitive foregut by showing the microvillous core rootlets and glycocalyceal bodies that are better known in intestinal carcinomas,[404,448,449] whilst many are composed of cells rich in cytoplasmic organelles that indicate active mucin synthesis and storage. The mucin granules vary in size and electron density and tend to coalesce into large vacuoles. Sometimes the secretory product is amylase rather than mucin and the cytoplasm contains large zymogen-like granules.[300] Occasionally, neuroendocrine granules are seen, indicating dual differentiation.[300] Many adenocarcinomas are composed of cells resembling type II pneumocytes[450] or Clara cells[173] while in some adenocarcinomas, type II pneumocytes may be seen alongside mucous or Clara cells, and occasionally overlying a basal layer of myoepithelial cells.[451] Various types of nuclear inclusion are described, the commonest being granular and staining for surfactant apoprotein,[452] while others consist of tubular structures derived from the nuclear envelope.[453]

Molecular features

Specific oncogene mutations have been identified in approximately 60% of pulmonary adenocarcinomas, the commonest involving *EGFR* and K-*ras*. Others include *BRAF*, *PIK3CA*, *ERBB2* and *EML4-ALK*.[454] *EGFR* and K-*ras* are mutually exclusive, indicating that they represent separate carcinogenic pathways.[210] *EGFR* mutation is reported in up to 50% of adenocarcinomas in Asian cohorts and 10–15% outside Asia, particularly in those tumours with a prominent lepidic or papillary pattern, and of non-mucinous type.[180] Such tumours are most likely to respond to TK inhibitors and are found particularly in Far Eastern women who have never smoked.[455] There is no strong association between K-*ras* mutation and any histological subtype[211] but an association between the *EML4-ALK* fusion gene and signet ring morphology has been reported.[224].

Differential diagnosis

The pulmonary metastases of adenocarcinomas of other organs are sometimes histologically indistinguishable from primary lung adenocarcinomas, so that in practice the diagnosis of primary adenocarcinoma of the lung should not be made before the patient has been screened for a primary tumour elsewhere and immunocytochemical markers have been sought, notably TTF-1 as a marker of primary lung

Figure 12.1.29 Small cell carcinoma that recurred after chemotherapy, extended widely within the thorax and metastasised widely.

Figure 12.1.30 Small cell carcinoma. Nuclear moulding is clearly evident in this sputum sample.

adenocarcinoma, and markers that are available for an increasing range of other adenocarcinomas, e.g. thyroid and prostate. It is particularly important that the metastases of adenocarcinomas that are amenable to hormonal manipulation or chemotherapy are identified. The distinction of primary and secondary adenocarcinomas is considered in detail on page 688.

SMALL CELL CARCINOMA

Small cell carcinoma generally arises in major airways (Fig. 12.1.29), grows rapidly, metastasises early and initially at least is sensitive to platinum-based chemotherapy. Untreated patients survive on average less than 3 months. With treatment, the patient usually dies with widely disseminated disease within 1–2 years: long-term disease-free survival is seen in only a minority of patients treated with chemotherapy.[456] Until recently oncologists have staged the tumour only as being 'limited' or 'extensive', believing that it has always disseminated by the time it is clinically manifest. However, surgery has been successful in early cases[457–460] and, although these cases are highly selected, it is now recommended that small cell carcinoma be staged in the same way as other lung tumours.[150,461,462] Although small cell carcinomas are generally central tumours, rare cases present as a peripheral nodule and it is these that have the best chances of successful surgical eradication.

Histological subtypes

In the 1981 WHO classification,[463] small cell carcinoma was divided into oat cell, intermediate cell and combined subtypes but this did not prove to be of prognostic significance.[464–466] The differences between the oat cell and the intermediate cell types are imprecise and probably artefactual. Classic oat cell carcinoma is most often observed in traumatised biopsies or poorly preserved autopsy material, whereas in well-preserved surgical material the intermediate cell type is seen almost exclusively. Accordingly, a recommendation that the terms oat cell and intermediate cell be abandoned[467] has been adopted in the current WHO classification, only the combined variant being retained (see Table 12.1.7).[130] The combined subtype, which is reported to comprise between 3 and 28% of the total, is characterised by the presence of squamous cell carcinoma, adenocarcinoma or large cell carcinoma in addition to small cell carcinoma, combinations that are generally easy to recognise.[468,469]

Histological appearances

Small cell carcinomas consist of closely packed small or medium-sized round or elongated cells, arranged in nests or strands or scattered singly within a scanty stroma.[470,471] The edge of the tumour is ill defined and lacks a capsule. Extensive necrosis is commonly seen. Mitoses are numerous and the nuclei of adjacent tumour cells characteristically press on one another, a feature termed nuclear moulding, which is especially prominent in cytological specimens (Fig. 12.1.30).[472] Rosettes of radially arranged tumour cells may be formed and genuine lumina may also be present, sometimes containing a little mucin.

Classic oat cells, which, as explained above, are probably artefactual, have dense pyknotic nuclei and very sparse cytoplasm. Well-preserved tumour cells are slightly larger, have a discernible but still small amount of cytoplasm and a nucleus with a finely divided chromatin pattern (Fig. 12.1.31). Nucleoli are inconspicuous in paraffin sections but may be quite striking in plastic sections. These nuclear characteristics are more important than cell size in separating small cell carcinoma from large cell carcinoma.[472–474] Some small cell carcinomas show scattered tumour cells with hyperchromatic giant nuclei.[469] This phenomenon can also be seen in other lung tumour types, and is especially common in tumours that have responded well to radiotherapy or chemotherapy.[475] A partial change to non-small cell

Figure 12.1.31 Small cell carcinoma. The tumour cells have little cytoplasm and finely dispersed nuclear chromatin. Nucleoli are not readily evident.

Figure 12.1.32 DNA deposition in vessel walls (Azzopardi effect) is seen in highly cellular necrotic tumours such as this small cell carcinoma.

Table 12.1.11 Comparison of small cell carcinoma and large cell carcinoma, other than on cell size

	Small cell carcinoma	Large cell carcinoma
Cell shape	Fusiform	Polygonal
Nuclear/cytoplasmic ratio	High	Low
Chromatin	Fine	Coarse
Nucleoli	Indistinct	Prominent
DNA staining of vessels	Frequent	Rare

histology during the course of the disease is encountered in about a fifth of patients.[476]

Haematoxyphil, Feulgen-positive nucleoprotein derived from degenerate tumour cells may be deposited in the walls of stromal blood vessels (so-called Azzopardi[470] effect – Fig. 12.1.32) but this feature is also found in other cellular tumours, such as lymphoma, seminoma and even other types of lung carcinoma. In biopsy specimens, the tumour cells are often crushed so that long strands and masses of haematoxyphil material are seen. This finding should prompt a careful search for viable, non-traumatised tumour cells. By itself it does not justify a diagnosis of small cell lung carcinoma because other tumours, such as lymphomas, and also inflammatory infiltrates, may show the same crush artifact.

In bronchial biopsies, the tumour cells are often seen beneath an intact surface epithelium that shows atypical squamous metaplasia (see Fig. 12.1.16), which is possibly due to the secretion of growth factors by the tumour.[329] Superficial sampling limited to this surface change may lead to erroneous histological classification and hence the wrong treatment: it is essential that invasive tumour be examined. On the other hand, there may be infiltration of the overlying epithelium by small groups of tumour cells, similar to that seen in Paget's disease of the nipple.

Differential diagnosis

Small cell carcinoma is liable to be mistaken for large cell carcinoma if attention is concentrated on cell size and the presence of discernible amounts of cytoplasm but these two tumours are generally separable on their nuclear characteristics: the finely divided, evenly dispersed chromatin of a small cell carcinoma contrasts greatly with the clumped chromatin and prominent nucleolus set in an otherwise vesicular nucleus of a large cell carcinoma (Table 12.1.11). Lymphocytes, either reactive or neoplastic, may also be mistaken for small cell carcinoma, especially if the tissue is traumatised: however, the carcinoma cells are larger than reactive lymphocytes and may be distinguished from lymphoma cells by immunocytochemistry, using antibodies against leukocytes (CD45) and cytokeratin. Some squamous cell and adeno-carcinomas are composed of small tumour cells but these lack the nuclear features of small cell carcinoma and show no immunohisto-chemical or ultrastructural evidence of neuroendocrine differentia-tion. Wider sampling generally reveals their true nature. If adequate, non-traumatised tissue is provided, small cell carcinomas are rela-tively easily distinguished from other histological types,[477] but problematical cases are certainly not rare,[478,478a] particularly in small bronchial biopsies.[325] This is one of the areas where immuno-histochemistry, electron microscopy[479] and image analysis[480] may prove to be important.

Figure 12.1.33 Small cell carcinoma. Electron microscopy demonstrates the presence of dense-core neuroendocrine granules. *(Courtesy of Professor W Mooi, Amsterdam, Netherlands.)*

Electron microscopy

Ultrastructurally, small cell lung carcinomas usually show neuroendocrine differentiation, the hallmark of which is the presence of small cytoplasmic granules.[481,482] These granules are round and have a central homogeneously electron-dense core that is separated from an outer membrane by a thin electron-lucent halo (Fig. 12.1.33). They measure 50–200 nm and are often concentrated near the cell membrane. The granules may be difficult to find, there being far fewer than in carcinoid tumours. They have to be distinguished from bristle-coated vesicles, small lysosomes and small exocrine granules. Bristle-coated vesicles have a fuzzy surrounding membrane whilst lysosomes and exocrine granules lack the halo separating the central core from the outer membrane. Exocrine granules are also usually more pleomorphic, and are concentrated near intercellular lumina lined by microvilli.

A minority of carcinomas of apparent small cell morphology show undoubted ultrastructural evidence of squamous or mucous cell differentiation, alone or in combination with neuroendocrine features.[377,479,483–485] Of 46 small cell carcinomas examined by electron microscopy, 22 proved to be neuroendocrine, 6 were squamous cell, 2 were mucous and 16 were not categorised.[486] However, these ultrastructural variations do not appear to be reflected in clinical behaviour or response to chemotherapy.[487] Conversely, a variety of non-small cell carcinomas are sometimes found to contain dense-core granules on electron microscopy.[488]

Immunocytochemistry

In line with their epithelial nature, a range of cytokeratins may be demonstrated in small cell lung carcinoma,[489] generally with a paranuclear dot-like distribution due to the formation of filament whorls.[490] Similarly, most small cell carcinomas express TTF-1 (see Table 12.1.10).[491] Immunohistochemistry has been widely used in attempts to distinguish small cell and non-small cell lung carcinoma but, to date, no completely satisfactory marker of neuroendocrine differentiation is available. At present, chromogranin A, synaptophysin, CD56 and *N*-cadherin probably represent the best com-

promise between specificity and sensitivity[492–496] and the first three of these fortunately retain their immunoreactivity when there is crush artefact.[495] Chromogranin A is a fairly specific protein component of endocrine granules but is usually difficult to detect because small cell lung carcinomas are only sparsely granulated. In situ hybridisation may be useful here for it demonstrates high levels of chromogranin A mRNA in these tumours.[497] CD56 detects the neural cell adhesion molecule and is very sensitive but lacks specificity.[498,499] The enzyme neuron-specific enolase and the neural protein PGP 9.5 are not granule-associated, and are positive in many small cell carcinomas, but are of low specificity. Leu-7, a surface antigen present on human natural killer cells and neuroendocrine cells,[500] is also of low specificity. In contrast to these neuroendocrine markers, CD44 is reported to be expressed only by non-small cell carcinomas.[501] Despite their distinct morphological appearances the minor components of combined small cell carcinomas generally express the same neuroendocrine markers as the more abundant small cell component.[502]

Cytogenetics and molecular pathology

Small cell carcinoma shows a high incidence of chromosomal deletions. Several chromosomes are involved but 3p, 13q and 17p are affected particularly frequently, respectively resulting in loss of the tumour suppressor genes FHIT, Rb and p53.[230–232,238,243,503] Conversely, the *myc* oncogene is overexpressed in many small cell carcinomas, but particularly in those that have recurred after treatment.[218,219]

LARGE CELL CARCINOMA

Large cell carcinomas of the lung are aggressive tumours[504] distinguished by an absence of differentiation when examined by light microscopy. The tumour cells are arranged in monotonous fields and individually are distinguished from small cell carcinoma by a variety of cytological features, of which size is one of the least and nuclear detail one of the most important (see Table 12.1.11): they generally have a moderate amount of cytoplasm, chromatin that is clumped at the periphery of the nucleus and a prominent nucleolus (Fig. 12.1.34).[472–474]

Immunocytochemistry shows that these tumours often express both cytokeratin and vimentin. Electron microscopy usually reveals evidence of squamous or glandular differentiation, or rarely, neuroendocrine features, or even a combination of the these (see Fig. 12.1.18 and Table 12.1.7).[359,505] Thus, large cell carcinoma is not a distinct entity, but rather a collection of very poorly differentiated epithelial tumours. The subtyping of large cell carcinoma by these special techniques[338,339] was of no clinical significance when the only therapeutic options were chemotherapy (for small cell carcinoma) and surgery (for the other types). A diagnosis of 'non-small cell carcinoma – not otherwise specified' then sufficed. Indeed, this was advocated to avoid having to amend a biopsy diagnosis of large cell carcinoma when the resection specimen showed squamous or glandular differentiation.[325,327] In the present era this is no longer adequate. New drugs aimed at correcting specific mutations require more specific characterisation and ideally this is provided by molecular techniques. However, there is some correlation between histological type and oncogene mutation and it may therefore be worth stretching the usual histological parameters. For example, stratification is accepted as evidence of squamous differentiation in carcinoma of the cervix uteri, oesophagus and skin, but so far not the lung. In the same vein, the histological typing of an undifferentiated non-small carcinoma could be sharpened by the application of supplementary histological techniques. Thus, it is suggested that an undifferentiated non-small

Figure 12.1.34 Large cell carcinoma. The tumour is undifferentiated and consists of cells with appreciable amounts of cytoplasm and nuclei that show coarse chromatin clumping and prominent nucleoli.

Figure 12.1.35 Clear cell variant of large cell carcinoma. The tumour is composed solely of undifferentiated large tumour cells with clear cytoplasm.

cell carcinoma that stains for mucin and TTF-1 but not for CK5/6, 34BE12 and p63 is probably of adenocarcinoma lineage whereas the reverse pattern favours squamous cell carcinoma.[506,507] Molecular characterisation is the ideal but even then histology is important, in particular to ensure that the results of molecular analysis reflect viable tumour and not areas of necrosis, stromal tissue, tumour capsule or reactive tissue. Often, the initial biopsy will not be large enough to permit these ancillary techniques and further sampling may be necessary.[328] Examples of the new drugs that require better tumour characterisation include pemetrexed, which is not effective in squamous cell carcinoma,[507a] bevacizumab, which is liable to cause life-threatening hemorrhage in squamous cell carcinoma[342] and the EGFR-directed TK inhibitors erlotinib and gefitinib, which work best in adenocarcinomas.[342,344]

Five variants of large cell carcinoma are recognised: clear cell, neuroendocrine, basaloid, lymphoepithelioma-like and rhabdoid. In the clear cell variant most of the tumour cells have a pale, watery cytoplasm, usually due to the presence of glycogen (Fig. 12.1.35).[376,508] Early series[509] included those that owed their clear cytoplasm to mucus but today such tumours would be classified as adenocarcinomas, despite their lack of glandular differentiation. The term 'clear cell

carcinoma' is now restricted to tumours that give negative mucous stains. They show no evidence of squamous or glandular differentiation on light microscopy but either may be detected by electron microscopy.[508] Focal clear cell change is sometimes seen in squamous cell carcinomas and adenocarcinomas but this is considered insufficient to justify a diagnosis of clear cell carcinoma. The nuclei may show little atypicality, in which case the distinction from benign clear cell tumour of the lung (see p. 625) may be difficult. However, the thin-walled sinusoidal blood vessels of a benign clear cell tumour are not evident in clear cell carcinoma. Metastatic renal carcinoma is perhaps a more likely alternative, one that would be supported by the presence of sudanophilic fat within the cytoplasm of tumour cells; however, fat stains are not possible if the material has all been embedded in paraffin, and in these circumstances recourse to renal imaging is probably the best option.[510] If mucin stains are positive, metastatic renal carcinoma, primary clear cell carcinoma and benign clear cell tumour can all be excluded.

Some large cell carcinomas display neuroendocrine features and are appropriately termed 'large cell neuroendocrine carcinoma'. Their diagnosis is based on recognition of both neuroendocrine morphology and the immunohistochemical demonstration of at least one specific neuroendocrine marker. As in any large cell carcinoma, the cells have moderate amounts of cytoplasm and nuclei that show peripheral clumping of chromatin and a prominent nucleolus, features that distinguish all large cell carcinomas from small cell carcinoma.[511] There is much mitotic activity and extensive necrosis. However, it is soon noticed that the tumour has an organoid pattern with its cells arranged in cords or well-demarcated groups showing rosette formation or peripheral palisading (Fig. 12.1.36). Some of these features are also seen in carcinoid tumours and the relationship to carcinoid is strengthened by shared immunocytochemical, ultrastructural and molecular features of neuroendocrine differentiation, such as the presence of chromogranin, synaptophysin or CD56, or their gene expression, and scanty dense-core granules evident on electron microscopy.[254,493,512–514] Despite this commonality, there are major differences between carcinoids and the high-grade neuroendocrine carcinomas, both small cell and large cell, which are summarised

Figure 12.1.36 Large cell neuroendocrine carcinoma. (A) There is peripheral palisading reminiscent of a carcinoid tumour but the tumour also exhibits much more extensive necrosis than is seen in an atypical carcinoid. (B) Immunoperoxidase staining for chromogranin is positive.

Table 12.1.12 Comparison of neuroendocrine large cell carcinoma and atypical carcinoid

	Neuroendocrine large cell carcinoma	Atypical carcinoid
Histological pattern	Large well-circumscribed cell groups with peripheral palisading	Small cell groups usually in a trabecular or mosaic pattern
Cell size	Large	Medium
Mitoses	10 or more/10 high-power fields	More than 2/10 and up to 10/10 high-power fields
Nuclear/cytoplasmic ratio	Low	Moderate
Chromatin	Coarse	Fine
Nucleoli	Prominent	Indistinct
Necrosis	Large areas	Usually confined to the centres of the cell groups
Atypia	Prominent	Moderate
Neuroendocrine stains	Necessary (positive)	Optional (positive)

in Table 12.2.1 on page 599. Genetic differences between small cell and large cell neuroendocrine carcinoma exist[515,516] but many characteristics are shared: both neuroendocrine carcinomas show an inverted *Bcl-2/Bax* ratio, *p53* mutation, deletions on chromosomes 3p and 17p and *Rb* inactivation.[238,243,503]

Occasionally, a conventional squamous cell carcinoma, adenocarcinoma or large cell carcinoma is encountered that is found to express neuroendocrine markers by immunohistochemistry. Such tumours are termed non-small cell carcinoma with neuroendocrine features.[130,517] Neuroendocrine differentiation can be demonstrated by electron microscopy or immunohistochemistry in 10–15% of non-small cell carcinomas of the lung despite an absence of morphological neuroendocrine features.[513,517–520]

The differential diagnosis of large cell neuroendocrine carcinoma includes atypical carcinoid tumour (Table 12.1.12) but the organoid pattern of that tumour is not so well developed in large cell neuroendocrine carcinoma and the degree of atypia, mitotic activity and necrosis all far exceeds those seen in an atypical carcinoid. A criterion recommended for distinguishing atypical carcinoid from large cell neuroendocrine carcinoma is mitotic number, atypical carcinoid having fewer than 10 mitoses per 10 high-power fields and large cell carcinoma 10 or more (if 1 high-power field = an area of 0.2 mm²).[512] Most large cell neuroendocrine carcinomas show considerably more

mitotic activity than this: the average number of mitoses per 10 high-power fields is in the order of 75. Large 'geographic' areas of necrosis characterise large cell neuroendocrine carcinoma whereas in atypical carcinoid necrosis is generally confined to the centres of individual cell groups. Small cell carcinoma also enters into the differential diagnosis of large cell neuroendocrine carcinoma;[478a] here reliance has to be placed upon the different nuclear characteristics, the fine granularity of the small cell carcinoma's chromatin differing from the clumped chromatin and prominent nucleoli of neuroendocrine large cell carcinoma.

In general, large cell neuroendocrine carcinomas are tumours of middle-aged or elderly cigarette smokers that arise in central bronchi. Despite the morphological evidence of neuroendocrine differentiation, ectopic hormone secretion is not a feature. The clinical significance of large cell neuroendocrine carcinoma and non-small cell carcinoma with neuroendocrine differentiation has yet to be fully evaluated but recognition of these tumours is of potential therapeutic significance for their undoubted neuroendocrine nature links them to classic small cell carcinoma and it would be important if their metastases were similarly sensitive to chemotherapy. Unfortunately, reports regarding their chemosensitivity are contradictory.[488,512,521–527] Some advise that these tumours behave like small cell carcinoma[528] and respond to the platinum-based regimens used for small cell carcinoma,[527] others that they are more aggressive than ordinary large cell carcinomas,[514,520,529–531] and yet others that neuroendocrine expression in large cell carcinoma is of no prognostic significance,[532–537] or even that it confers longer survival.[526,538] The presence of neuroendocrine markers in pulmonary adenocarcinoma is reported to be associated with increased sensitivity to chemotherapy,[519,521,524,525,534] and to be an independent favourable prognostic factor in chemotherapy-treated non-small cell lung carcinoma,[526] leading to suggestions that this treatment may be considered for those non-small cell carcinomas

Figure 12.1.37 Basaloid carcinoma. The tumour shows an exophytic endobrobronchial pattern of growth.

that express neuroendocrine features and are inoperable.[520,532] Other reports discount neuroendocrine differentiation detected only by immunostaining as being of no prognostic importance.[539] However, as yet there have been no large-scale, prospective, controlled trials of small cell chemotherapy for this subgroup of large cell carcinomas or for other non-small cell carcinomas showing neuroendocrine differentiation. Furthermore, the clinical importance of neuroendocrine differentiation may diminish if a current trend towards treating all inoperable lung carcinomas with aggressive chemotherapy continues.

Basaloid carcinoma[24,379,380,382,540–543] is a relatively rare variant of large cell carcinoma, forming only about 3% of all non-small cell carcinomas of the lung. Patients with this tumour do not differ from those with other large cell carcinomas in age, smoking history, clinical presentation or pattern of relapse.[379,380,382,540] However, they are reputed to fare badly compared with large cell carcinoma in general,[379–381,540] although this is disputed.[382]

The tumour is usually centrally located and often shows an exophytic, endobronchial pattern of growth and a well-defined edge (Fig. 12.1.37). Carcinoma-in-situ can often be recognised in the adjacent or distant bronchial epithelium. Histologically, basaloid carcinoma displays a lobular or anastomosing trabecular pattern with peripheral palisading. The tumour cells are small, cuboidal or fusiform with scanty cytoplasm and a hyperchromatic nucleus devoid of prominent nucleoli, as in the basaloid variant of squamous cell carcinoma portrayed in Figure 12.1.22D. Mitoses are frequent (over 25 per 10 high-power fields) and there is often centrilobular comedo-like necrosis. The stroma may show abundant hyaline basement membrane-like material, myxoid change or, rarely, chondroid or osseous metaplasia. There is no squamous differentiation: if it is present the tumour is classified as a basaloid variant of squamous cell carcinoma (see p. 549). Basaloid carcinoma expresses high-molecular-weight cytokeratins typical of bronchial basal cells (cytokeratins 1, 5, 6 and 14) but

not the low-molecular-weight cytokeratins (4, 10 and 11) that are more typical of cornifying squamous epithelium, nor the TTF-1 expressed by most adenocarcinomas and small cell carcinomas of the lung.[541] Like other non-small cell carcinomas, a small proportion (<10%) of tumour cells may express neuroendocrine markers. The 34βE12 monoclonal antibody against cytokeratins 1, 5, 10 and 14 is positive in basaloid (and squamous cell) carcinoma but not in neuroendocrine tumours of any category. Basaloid carcinoma is liable to be confused with small cell carcinoma, large cell neuroendocrine carcinoma and poorly differentiated squamous cell carcinoma, but none of these has the full constellation of features listed above.

'Lymphoepithelial carcinoma' is a term usually applied to a type of nasopharyngeal carcinoma that shows prominent lymphoid infiltration but tumours of this pattern have also been described in a number of other sites, including the lung, where they are regarded as a variant of large cell carcinoma.[106,544–548] As with the nasopharyngeal tumours, pulmonary lymphoepithelial carcinoma mainly affects Asians, in whom it is associated with the Epstein–Barr virus (Fig. 12.1.38). Most of the few lymphoepithelial carcinomas of the lung reported in non-Asian patients do not contain Epstein–Barr virus,[549,550] suggesting that the presence of this agent may be an epiphenomenon. However, Epstein–Barr virus was not found in any other form of lung cancer in a Hong Kong laboratory reporting pulmonary lymphoepithelial carcinomas associated with this virus.[545] Pulmonary lymphoepithelial carcinoma is also associated with the *bcl*-2 oncogene, chemosensitivity and a better survival rate than other large cell carcinomas of the lung.[546,547,551]

Pulmonary lymphoepithelial carcinoma affects adults of all ages and the sexes are affected equally. There is no strong association with cigarette smoking.[546] The tumour usually forms a solitary, discrete, subpleural nodule that is amenable to surgery. Major bronchi are not usually affected but the tumour may replace the lining of small bronchi. It generally has a soft fleshy appearance on its cut surface. Microscopy shows sheets of large cells with vesicular nuclei and prominent nucleoli, mixed with numerous lymphocytes and plasma cells, and, occasionally, granulomas (see Fig. 12.1.38). Thymoma of mixed cellularity may be suggested but lymphoepithelial carcinoma contains CD4- or CD8-positive lymphocytes and the less mature lymphocytes of CD1a phenotype encountered in thymoma are not identified. The lymphoid infiltrate may be so prominent as to suggest lymphoma, from which it is distinguished by the immunocytochemical demonstration of cytokeratin.

Rhabdoid carcinoma is a further rare variant of large cell carcinoma characterised by the presence of a hyaline eosinophilic globule indenting the nucleus.[552] The globule represents a tangle of intermediate filaments, both vimentin and cytokeratins (Fig. 12.1.39).[553,554] Rhabdoid foci are also found in lung tumours showing varying lines of differentiation, where they are thought to represent areas of dedifferentiation.[555,556] Not surprisingly, therefore, rhabdoid tumours appear to carry a poor prognosis, although numbers of analysed cases are small.[557,558]

ADENOSQUAMOUS CARCINOMA

Many non-small cell carcinomas of the lung show ultrastructural evidence of both squamous and glandular differentiation but the diagnosis of adenosquamous carcinoma is reserved for tumours that show both squamous and adenocarcinomatous differentiation on light microscopy (Fig. 12.1.40).[559–562] These are rare but the exact incidence is uncertain because until recently there were no agreed criteria as to how much of the minor component should be present: however, the current WHO classification[130] stipulates at least 10%.

Figure 12.1.38 Lymphoepithelial carcinoma. (A) The tumour is an undifferentiated large cell carcinoma that shows a heavy lymphoid infiltrate. (B) Cytokeratin (MNF116) and (C) lymphocyte (CD3) staining distinguishes the two components of the tumour. (D) EBERS *in situ* hybridisation demonstrates the Epstein–Barr virus.

Figure 12.1.39 Rhabdoid variant of large cell carcinoma. Large cell carcinoma cells show indentation of nuclei by a hyaline eosinophilic globule.

Figure 12.1.40 Adenosquamous carcinoma. The tumour shows evidence of both squamous and glandular differentiation, with each component making up more than 10% of the whole.

Alveoli entrapped within squamous carcinomas may be mistaken for tumour acini[408] but their lining cells are smaller and more uniform than those lining tumour acini.

Clinically and macroscopically, adenosquamous carcinomas resemble adenocarcinomas.[563] They are often peripheral tumours that metastasise widely, often showing the same intermingling of the two components in the metastases as in the primary tumour. The prognosis is poor, worse than for either pure squamous cell carcinoma or pure adenocarcinoma.[561,562]

SARCOMATOID CARCINOMA

Occasional carcinomas show foci of malignant spindle or giant cells, suggesting that the tumour is composed of a mixture of carcinoma and sarcoma. Such tumours were formerly thought to result from the merging of separate carcinomas and sarcomas (so-called collision tumours), or were considered to represent carcinomas merely exhibiting exuberant stromal growth. The current view is that they represent carcinomas showing connective tissue differentiation. This is an extension of the widely accepted concept of tumour heterogeneity used to explain tumours of mixed epithelial phenotype, such as adenosquamous carcinoma and the combined subgroup of small cell carcinoma. What appears to be a sarcomatous element may seem to stream from an obvious epithelial element (Fig. 12.1.41) and there is now considerable electron microscopic and immunohistochemical evidence that tumours that appear to be of mixed epithelial and connective tissue phenotype, or composed only of what appears histologically to be sarcoma, are entirely epithelial.[564-566] Molecular studies are in accord with this, showing identical mutations in the spindle cells and more obviously in the epithelial components.[567,568] Epithelial–mesenchymal transition is controlled by various transcription factors, several of which have been shown to be upregulated in sarcomatoid carcinomas of the head and neck.[569] The term 'sarcomatoid carcinoma' is therefore appropriate and could well supplant older terms such as carcinosarcoma and pulmonary blastoma. The latter are inaccurate but are retained in the WHO classification for historic reasons.

Some sarcomatoid carcinomas consist entirely of spindle or giant cells and for these the terms spindle cell carcinoma and giant cell carcinoma are appropriate. Spindle cell carcinoma was formerly classed as a variant of squamous cell carcinoma but it is now appreciated that spindle cell change may be found in any type of non-small cell carcinoma (Fig. 12.1.43), including giant cell carcinoma. This has led to the introduction of the term 'pleomorphic carcinoma' for a tumour that combines spindle and/or giant cell carcinoma with any of the more usual patterns of non-small cell carcinoma.[570] Occasionally there is an even greater degree of connective tissue differentiation so that bone, cartilage or muscle is formed. The WHO classification retains the inaccurate term 'carcinosarcoma' for sarcomatoid carcinomas containing such heterologous elements, although it recognises them as being basically epithelial in nature. In one form of carcinosarcoma the neoplastic glands and stroma have an embryonic appearance so that the tumour bears a spurious resemblance to fetal lung in its canalicular phase of development: the traditional (but inaccurate) term 'pulmonary blastoma' is retained for this pattern in the WHO classification.[130] In one of the largest series of sarcomatoid carcinomas, 58 cases were classified as pleomorphic carcinoma, 10 as spindle cell carcinoma, 3 as giant cell carcinoma, 3 as carcinosarcoma and 1 as pulmonary blastoma.[571]

An alternative classification to that advocated by WHO recognises only monophasic and biphasic sarcomatoid carcinomas, with the latter subdivided into homologous and heterologous varieties.[572,573] A monophasic sarcomatoid carcinoma is one in which the epithelial

Figure 12.1.41 Sarcomatoid carcinoma. The tumour consists of squamous and spindle cells, the latter obviously derived from the adjacent squamous cell carcinoma. Both components gave a strongly positive immunoreaction for cytokeratin.

nature of the tumour is only recognisable by the application of immunohistochemistry to demonstrate cytokeratin or other epithelial markers. It thus corresponds to both spindle cell and giant cell carcinoma. Biphasic sarcomatoid carcinoma combines an obvious epithelial component (e.g. glandular or squamous cell carcinoma) with a malignant stroma (spindle cell or giant cell). If the stroma shows chondroid, osseous or myogenic differentiation the tumour is classified as a heterologous biphasic sarcomatoid carcinoma (corresponding to carcinosarcoma and blastoma); if not, it is termed a homologous biphasic sarcomatoid carcinoma (corresponding to pleomorphic carcinoma). This classification has the merit of being understood by those unversed in the historic development of our understanding of lung tumours. It is also familiar to general histopathologists because it is applied to similar tumours that are encountered in the upper aerodigestive and genitourinary systems. The two classifications are compared in Table 12.1.13.

Sarcomatoid carcinomas are rare, accounting for about only 1% of all lung malignancies.[570,571] Patients are usually elderly and have been heavy smokers.[571] They typically give a short history, yet have bulky tumours. The prognosis is generally poor.[573] Even tumours that appear

Table 12.1.13 Sarcomatoid carcinoma. Corresponding terminology used by Wick and colleagues[572,573] and the World Health Organization[130]

Wick et al.	World Health Organization
Monophasic	Spindle cell
	Giant cell
Biphasic	
Homologous	Pleomorphic carcinoma
Heterologous	Blastoma

Figure 12.1.43 Giant cell carcinoma. The tumour cells are poorly cohesive and there is a rich polymorph infiltrate. Multinucleate tumour giant cells are evident.

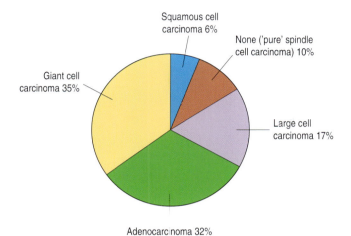

Squamous cell carcinoma 6%

None ('pure' spindle cell carcinoma) 10%

Giant cell carcinoma 35%

Large cell carcinoma 17%

Adenocarcinoma 32%

Figure 12.1.42 Frequency of patterns found to be associated with spindle cell carcinoma, illustrating the diversity that led to the introduction of the term 'pleomorphic carcinoma'.[570]

to be operable have a worse[571] or similar[574] prognosis to large cell carcinoma of the lung, which is itself poor.

Signs and symptoms are related to tumour localisation. Haemoptysis, fever due to recurrent pneumonia, cough and progressive dyspnoea are common with endobronchial lesions. Peripheral tumours may be asymptomatic and only discovered incidentally on chest radiography, but most eventually cause pleuritic pain.

Spindle cell carcinoma is a non-small cell carcinoma that consists only of spindle-shaped tumour cells (Fig. 12.1.42). It is a rare tumour but is nevertheless the commonest spindle cell malignancy appear to be in the lung. When encountering a tumour of such pattern one should therefore think of spindle cell carcinoma before considering a diagnosis of primary pulmonary sarcoma. It is distinguished from sarcoma by its expression of epithelial markers such as cytokeratin, epithelial membrane antigen and carcinoembryonic antigen.[565,575] Difficulty may be encountered in distinguishing spindle cell carcinoma from synovial sarcoma because they both express epithelial markers but synovial sarcoma also expresses the *bcl*-2 oncogene and shows t(X;18)(p11.2;q11.2) translocation. When there is pleural involvement it is particularly difficult to distinguish spindle cell carcinoma from sarcomatoid mesothelioma. Pankeratin, calretinin and thrombomodulin are frequently expressed in both, while neither commonly expresses cytokeratin 5/6 or WT1, but some difference is reported for smooth-muscle actin (positive in 60% of sarcomatoid mesotheliomas compared with only 10% of sarcomatoid carcinomas).[576] Inflammatory sarcomatoid carcinoma is an unusual variant

of spindle cell carcinoma that closely mimics an inflammatory myofibroblastic tumour. It shows a proliferation of cytologically bland neoplastic spindle cells in a myxoid background while lymphocytes and plasma cells surround or infiltrate the tumour. However, a dearth of neutrophils, eosinophils and foam cells together with small foci of necrosis and invasion of bronchi and blood vessels all favour sarcomatoid carcinoma.

Giant cell carcinoma is a non-small cell carcinoma composed of very large cells that are frequently multinucleate. The many nuclei are large, pleomorphic and often multilobed. The mitotic rate is high. The tumour cells are poorly cohesive and show a marked tendency to dissociate from each other (Fig. 12.1.43).[577,578] There is generally a rich inflammatory infiltrate, usually of neutrophils, which frequently invade the tumour cells.[305] This phenomenon was initially thought to represent phagocytosis by the tumour cells,[579] but more probably reflects emperipolesis[580] (active penetration of the leukocytes into the tumour cells, in contrast to passive engulfment). The inflammation is not necessarily associated with necrosis and is seen in metastases as well as the primary growth. Neutrophil sequestration within the tumour may be associated with peripheral granulocytosis and even a leukaemoid reaction. The granulocytosis is not dependent upon bone marrow metastases. An unidentified chemoattractant is presumably responsible for both the granulocytosis and the sequestration of neutrophils within the tumour.[305] The phenomenon is also seen in the inflammatory sarcomatoid carcinoma, mentioned above. The tumour cells often coexpress cytokeratin, vimentin, carcinoembryonic antigen and TTF-1. By electron microscopy aggregates of paranuclear filaments may be seen but otherwise the tumour cells possess few tonofibrils and are very poorly differentiated. Only very occasional desmosomes are identified, which is in accordance with the poor cohesiveness of the tumour cells.[581] The differential diagnosis of giant cell carcinoma includes not only other types of lung carcinoma, but also primary and metastatic malignant fibrous histiocytoma, pleomorphic rhabdomyosarcoma, metastatic adrenocortical carcinoma and other pleomorphic malignant tumours, most of which can be distinguished by their own distinctive markers.

Pleomorphic carcinoma is a poorly differentiated non-small cell carcinoma in which spindle cell carcinoma and/or giant cell carcinoma form at least 10% of what would otherwise be a pure squamous cell, adeno- or large cell carcinoma (Fig. 12.1.44), or a carcinoma consisting only of spindle and giant cells.[570,582] Immunostaining for epithelial markers to exclude sarcoma may be undertaken if

Figure 12.1.44 Pleomorphic carcinoma consisting of a mixture of glandular and spindle cell growth.

Figure 12.1.45 Carcinosarcoma (biphasic sarcomatoid carcinoma with heterologous elements). (A) An excised carcinosarcoma showing largely exophytic growth. (B) Microscopy shows a mixture of squamous and spindle cell carcinoma, the latter exhibiting chondroid differentiation.

the tumour lacks an obvious epithelial component. In these circumstances distinction from a mesothelioma of sarcomatoid pattern is particularly difficult for the sarcomatoid component of the carcinoma may express mesothelial markers such as podoplanin and calretinin.[583] Pseudoangiosarcomatous carcinoma is a variety of pleomorphic carcinoma in which squamous cell carcinoma is accompanied by an angiosarcomatoid component showing anastomosing channels lined by anaplastic cells focally aggregated in pseudopapillae. The channels contain erythrocytes and occasionally form 'blood lakes', thus simulating an angiosarcoma. However, the lining cells express epithelial rather than endothelial markers and represent the pulmonary counterpart of pseudovascular adenoid squamous cell carcinoma that one may see in other organs. Distinction from pleuropulmonary angiosarcoma is based on the carcinoma's lack of atypical endothelial cells, negative immunostaining for vascular markers and the presence of at least focal areas of squamous cell carcinoma.

Carcinosarcomas (heterologous type of biphasic sarcomatoid carcinomas) are malignant tumours that contain both epithelial and connective tissue elements, with the latter showing heterologous differentiation into bone, cartilage or smooth muscle. They are similar to those described in the upper aerodigestive tract, the urogenital organs and other sites as carcinosarcomas, biphasic sarcomatoid carcinomas or malignant mixed müllerian tumours. The first description of pulmonary carcinosarcoma is attributed to Kika in 1908.[584] Immunocytochemistry and electron microscopy (see below) support the view that carcinosarcoma is basically an epithelial tumour that shows varying degrees of mesenchymal differentiation. In line with this, molecular studies have shown that the epithelial and sarcomatoid components have a common genome.[568,585] Further support derives from experiments involving the transplantation of human lung carcinomas into inbred mice, in which environment the epithelial neoplasms showed connective tissue differentiation.[586]

Pulmonary carcinosarcomas occur in the same type of patient as the more common forms of lung cancer, namely elderly or middle-aged cigarette smokers, and carry a similarly poor prognosis.[587,588] The male:female ratio is about 7 with a mean and median age 65 years.[589] Two-thirds arise in the walls of large airways and form polypoid endobronchial lesions (Fig. 12.1.45A, B)[590] but some grow into large intrapulmonary masses that may invade the chest wall.[591] Central

tumours cause cough, haemoptysis and recurrent chest infection whereas peripheral lesions may be asymptomatic until they reach the pleura and give rise to effusion or pleurisy.

By definition these tumours are biphasic, composed of an intimate mixture of epithelial and connective tissue (Fig. 12.1.45C). The demarcation between the two may be sharp or poorly defined. The most frequent epithelial element is squamous cell carcinoma, followed by adenocarcinoma, large cell carcinoma, small cell carcinoma and carcinoid tumour but glandular differentiation is commoner in the rarer peripheral growths (Table 12.1.14).[591,592] The connective tissue component usually consists of undifferentiated spindle cells in which there are foci of malignant osteoid, cartilage, striated muscle or fat.[565,587,588,593,594] These connective tissue elements are clearly malignant, in contrast to the osteocartilaginous stromal metaplasia that is recorded in occasional squamous cell carcinomas.[371] Such differentiation may be sparse, rendering the distinction from spindle cell carcinoma and undifferentiated sarcoma difficult. Furthermore, the relative proportions of carcinoma and sarcoma vary considerably: it should therefore be borne in mind that sarcomas of the lung are very rare and before making such a diagnosis the lesion should be sampled widely to exclude the possibility that the tumour is a carcinosarcoma of predominantly sarcomatous pattern, particularly if it has the characteristic endobronchial growth pattern of a central carcinosarcoma.

Table 12.1.14 Pathological features of 46 cases of carcinosarcoma[591]

	Endobronchial (*n* = 32)	Peripheral (*n* = 14)
Epithelial component	Squamous 29 (91%)	Squamous 6 (43%)
	Glandular 3 (9%)	Glandular 7 (50%)
		Other 1 (7%)
Mesenchymal component	Undifferentiated spindle cell 26 (81%)	Undifferentiated spindle cell 11 (79%)
	Differentiated 6 (19%)	Differentiated 3 (21%)

Differentiated includes chondrosarcoma and rhabdomyosarcoma.

The malignant epithelial cells frequently express cytokeratin, epithelial membrane antigen, carcinoembryonic antigen and TTF-1, and the mesenchymal cells vimentin, but any of these markers may be found in either component.[565,566,595–597] Electron microscopy may also show epithelial features such as desmosomes in the spindle cell component, further emphasising the close relation between carcinosarcoma and spindle cell carcinoma.[565,566]

The metastases of a carcinosarcoma may consist of carcinoma or sarcoma or both.[595,598] If the epithelial component is glandular, pleural involvement may lead to confusion with a mesothelioma of mixed pattern but the identification of mucus and carcinoembryonic antigen excludes mesothelioma.[593]

The term 'pulmonary blastoma' was coined by Spencer[599] in 1961, superseding Barnard's earlier one of embryoma of lung.[600,601] At that time it was thought that the peripheral part of the lung was of mesenchymal origin and Spencer considered pulmonary blastomas to be analogous to nephroblastomas in that both their epithelial and mesenchymal components were derived from a common mesodermal blastema. The embryological basis for this concept is now known to be false (see p. 40). Occasional reports of tumours intermediate in structure between blastoma and carcinosarcoma[598,602–604] suggest that blastomas are related to carcinosarcomas,[565] and hence to spindle cell carcinomas. It has been suggested that the well-differentiated fetal adenocarcinoma represents one-sided epithelial development of a pulmonary blastoma, but this is unconvincing and it is therefore considered with other adenocarcinomas on page 554. Pleuropulmonary blastoma, a purely connective tissue tumour of the young that is described on page 623, is now considered to represent the true blastoma of the lung.

Pulmonary blastoma is a rare tumour that affects males three times more commonly than females. It may occur at any age from childhood to the ninth decade with the mean age being about 40 years, earlier than that of carcinosarcoma but considerably later than blastomas of other organs. Blastomas may reach a considerable size before cough, haemoptysis or chest pain causes the patient to seek attention, or they may be discovered incidentally by radiography. Pulmonary blastomas vary greatly in their behaviour but the prognosis is generally unfavourable: the overall 5-year survival is only 16%.[605]

Pulmonary blastomas are generally peripheral growths and often form large well-demarcated masses with foci of cystic change and haemorrhage (Fig. 12.1.46). However, up to a quarter are similar to carcinosarcomas in forming polypoid endobronchial tumours.[605,606] Microscopically, they are biphasic tumours composed of branching epithelial tubules or cords set in an undifferentiated stroma. The latter is formed of loosely arranged polygonal cells which have fairly

Figure 12.1.46 Pulmonary blastoma. A 20-cm partly necrotic and haemorrhagic tumour occupies much of the lower lobe. *(Courtesy of Dr PF Roberts, formerly of Norwich, UK.)*

uniform, small, dark, oval or spindle-shaped nuclei and scanty cytoplasm (Fig. 12.1.47): both components are malignant and either or both may be seen in the metastases. The mesenchymal cells tend to be arranged more compactly around the epithelial tubules, which are lined by cuboidal or columnar cells with clear glycogen-rich cytoplasm; the appearances closely resemble first-trimester fetal lung, hence the term blastoma.[599,607,608] The stromal component shows focal differentiation into cartilage, bone, fat and smooth or striated muscle in up to 25% of cases (see Fig. 12.1.47C).[606,609] In some tumours the epithelial element shows squamous differentiation. Other examples have had melanomatous,[610] small cell carcinoma[611] or yolk sac components.[612] Transition to carcinosarcoma is also described.[598,602–604]

Figure 12.1.47 Pulmonary blastoma. (A) The tumour consists of malignant epithelial elements, resembling those seen in fetal lung, set in a sarcomatous stroma. (B) High power shows epithelial tubules within a dense blastomatous stroma. (C) Elsewhere the malignant stroma shows chondroid differentiation.

Immunohistochemistry and electron microscopy support the view that pulmonary blastomas are true mixed tumours: epithelial markers are confined to the epithelial elements and connective tissue markers to the stromal component.[565,607–609,613–616] However, the features they share with carcinosarcoma indicate that they represent a further type of sarcomatoid carcinoma.

PROGNOSTIC FACTORS

Staging: the role of the pathologist

The appalling prognosis of carcinoma of the lung has already been touched upon, when it was noted that the best overall 5-year survival rates are no better than 14% (see Fig. 12.1.1, p. 532). This poor outlook is due to a combination of late presentation, early metastasis and a poor sustained response to chemotherapy. Surgeons can achieve 5-year survival rates of 50%, but only by being extremely rigorous in assessing operability and thereby excluding many patients (up to 80%).[9] Staging is therefore extremely important in both treatment and prognosis. Some believe it to be the only significant predictor of survival.[617]

An early step in the spread of a carcinoma is the transition from in situ to invasive growth, recognition of which can sometimes be difficult, in which case staining for constituents of the epithelial basement membrane such as laminin and type IV collagen can be helpful.[618] Similarly the integrity of lymphatic and capillary endothelium can be investigated with antibodies to factor VIII-related antigen, *Ulex europeus*, CD31 and CD34.

The accurate assessment of metastasis requires histology and a variety of tissues suspected of harbouring metastatic tumour may be submitted to the laboratory for this purpose. Mediastinal lymph nodes are now more often sampled by ultrasound-guided transbronchial or transoesophageal needle aspiration than mediastinoscopy or mediastinotomy.[317,619] They are usually targeted because they are enlarged, although histology shows that the correlation between size and involvement by tumour is poor.[620,621] However, positron emission tomography has led to more accurate targeting of involved areas. If the tumour is known to be a small cell carcinoma, bone marrow may be aspirated. The histological detection of micrometastases in these tissues may be helped by the use of epithelial or neuroendocrine markers.[622,623] Molecular techniques have also been used for this purpose.[624] However, the clinical impact of applying these special techniques is questionable.[625,626]

After surgery, pathological staging provides a useful adjunct to the clinical assessment of tumour size and lymph node involvement.[627] Protocols for the examination of specimens from patients with lung cancer have been drawn up by several institutions. Whichever is followed the resection specimen should be dissected and sampled in such a way that, apart from ensuring adequate typing of the tumour, all questions pertaining to the pathological tumour stage can be answered. As a routine, the bronchial resection margin, the peribronchial lymph nodes within the lung, the hilar lymph nodes, the resection margins of the large vessels and the pleura nearest to the tumour should be sampled. Lung tissue away from the tumour should also be sampled to detect occult spread and for the assessment of conditions such as asbestosis that might have led to the development of the tumour. Any further nodules should also be examined. The full pathological TNM classification is shown in Table 12.1.15, regional lymph node nomenclature in Box 12.1.6, stage grouping in Table 12.1.16 and the effect of stage in Figure 12.1.48.[628–632]

Carcinoma-in-situ at the bronchial resection margin carries a risk of stump recurrence and is often assessed by frozen section before

Table 12.1.15 The 2009 (7th edition) lung cancer staging system: definitions of the descriptors[631,632]

Descriptors	Definitions
T	**Primary tumour**
T0	No primary tumour
T1	Tumour ≤3 cm in greatest dimension, surrounded by lung or visceral pleura, not more proximal than the lobar bronchus
T1a	Tumour ≤2 cm in greatest dimension
T1b	Tumour >2 but ≤3 cm in greatest dimension
T2	Tumour >3 but ≤7 cm in greatest dimension or tumour with any of the following: invades visceral pleura, involves main bronchus ≥2 cm distal to the carina, atelectasis/obstructive pneumonia extending to hilum but not involving the entire lung
T2a	Tumour >3 but ≤5 cm in greatest dimension
T2b	Tumour >5 but ≤7 cm in greatest dimension
T3	Tumour >7 cm or directly invading chest wall, diaphragm, phrenic nerve, mediastinal pleura or parietal pericardium or tumour in the main bronchus <2 cm distal to the carina or atelectasis/obstructive pneumonitis of entire lung or separate tumour nodules in the same lobe
T4	Tumour of any size with invasion of heart, great vessels, trachea, recurrent laryngeal nerve, oesophagus, vertebral body or carina; or separate tumour nodules in a different ipsilateral lobe
N	**Regional lymph nodes**
N0	No regional node metastasis
N1	Metastasis in ipsilateral peribronchial and/or perihilar lymph nodes and intrapulmonary nodes, including involvement by direct extension
N2	Metastasis in ipsilateral mediastinal and/or subcarinal lymph nodes
N3	Metastasis in contralateral mediastinal, contralateral hilar, ipsilateral or contralateral scalene or supraclavicular lymph nodes
M	**Distant metastasis**
M0	No distant metastasis
M1a	Separate tumour nodules in a contralateral lobe or tumour with pleural nodules or malignant pleural dissemination
M1b	Distant metastasis
Special situations	
TX, NX, MX	T, N or M status not able to be assessed
Tis	Focus of in situ cancer
T1	Superficial spreading tumour of any size but confined to the wall of the trachea or mainstem bronchus

surgery is completed.[633] If the tumour is close to, but not obviously through, the pleura, an elastin stain is useful to delineate the deep margin of the pleura.[634,635] Penetration of the outer visceral pleural elastic layer is regarded as the minimum criterion of penetration (Fig. 12.1.49).[636] A classification of the extent of pleural invasion is shown in Table 12.1.17.[637]

Staging becomes problematical when a lobectomy specimen contains two carcinomas of the same histological pattern.[638] If they are independent growths they may both be T1 but, if one is considered to be a metastasis of the other this advances the stage to T3. Similarly,

tumours of the same pattern in separate lobes might be either independent M0 growths or represent a single M1 tumour. It is now recommended that such tumours in the same lung be classed T4, but M1a if both lungs are affected. Molecular techniques have been applied in such cases. One such study found that discordant and concordant genotypic profiles exist in morphologically similar synchronous adenocarcinomas of the lung.[639] In two other studies genomic profiling contradicted the clinicopathological stage in 4 of 22 cases and 3 of 6 cases repectively.[640,641] In practice, patients with such T4 or M1 tumours are generally treated surgically and have

N2 lymph nodes

Superior mediastinal lymph nodes

1. Highest mediastinal
2. Upper paratracheal
3. Pre- and retrotracheal
4. Lower paratracheal

Aortic lymph nodes

5. Subaortic
6. Paraaortic (ascending aorta or phrenic)

Inferior mediastinal lymph nodes

7. Subcarinal
8. Paraoesophageal (below the carina)
9. Pulmonary ligament

N1 lymph nodes

10. Hilar
11. Interlobar
12. Lobar
13. Segmental
14. Subsegmental

Above the highest mediastinal nodes and unnumbered are the scalene and supraclavicular lymph nodes, involvement of which categorises the tumour as N3, and above these the cervical lymph nodes involvement of which categorises the tumour as M1.

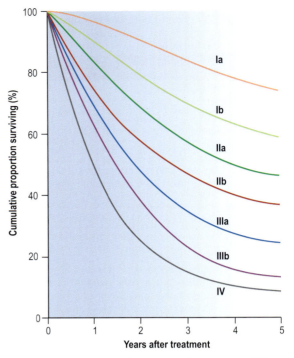

Figure 12.1.48 Survival of patients with carcinoma of the lung according to pathological stage: cumulative proportion (%) surviving up to 5 years after treatment. *(Data from the International Union Against Cancer[632].)*

Table 12.1.16 Stage grouping and survival of pTNM subsets after treatment for lung cancer[631,632]

Stage grouping	pTNM subset	Deaths/ total	5-year survival (%)	Median survival (months)
Ia	T1 N0 M0	1168/3566	73	119
Ib	T2a N0 M0	1450/3100	58	81
IIa	T1 N1 M0 or T2a N1 M0 or T2b N0 M0	1485/2579	46	49
IIb	T2b N1 M0 or T3 N0 M0	1502/2252	36	31
IIIa	T1 N2 M0 or T2 N2 M0 or T3 N1 M0 or T3 N2 M0 or T4 N0 M0 or T4 N1 M0	2896/3792	24	22
IIIb	T1 N3 M0 or T2 N3 M0 or T3 N3 M0 or T4 N2 M0 or T4 N3 M0	263/297	9	13
IV	Any T Any N M1	224/256	12	17

better outcomes than lung cancer patients with tumours designated T4 on the basis of invasion of mediastinal structures or M1 because of extrapulmonary metastases.

Large inoperable tumours may be reduced to an operable size by chemotherapy or irradiation, a process known as neoadjuvant therapy.[642] The extent of these changes should be incorporated in the pathologist's report of the resection specimen. Successful neoadjuvant therapy results in haemorrhagic necrosis of the tumour. The necrosis is generally bordered by chronic inflammatory granulation tissue in which foamy macrophages, foreign-body giant cells and cholesterol crystal clefts may be seen. Alternatively, the tumour site may show only a fibrous scar of non-specific appearance. Occasionally, the tumour appears quite viable but is of a less malignant pattern than was seen in the preoperative biopsy. For example, only adenocarcinoma-in-situ may be found postoperatively in a patient whose preoperative biopsy showed invasive tumour.[643] Similar changes may be encountered in pulmonary metastases (see p. 686).

The pathologist should attempt to identify and sample lymph nodes at the hilum of the resection specimen, involvement of these taking the tumour stage to N1. The laboratory will usually receive several separate specimens of higher lymph node stations, all numbered according to the internationally approved classification shown in Box 12.1.6.[631,632] The assessment of these will decide whether stage N2 has been reached. It is usually sufficient for the pathologist to record the presence or absence of tumour in each of these. Some surgeons wish to know whether the lymph node capsule has been breached but the higher nodes are often received piecemeal. There is some evidence that direct spread to N1 nodes has a better prognosis than metastatic spread to these nodes[644] and, similarly, that intrapulmonary N1 lymph node involvement is better than extrapulmonary N1 disease.[645]

Histological type and grade

Bearing in mind that stage is far more important than any other prognostic factor,[617] histological type, subtype and grade cannot be considered to have a major impact, but all have some relevance to prognosis.[361,646–651] In regard to tumour typing, interobserver variability is reported to be small[325,362] but grading is more subjective. The worst histological type, small cell carcinoma, has a 5-year survival rate of only 4% (Fig. 12.1.50).[652] Many oncologists regard all small cell carcinomas as inoperable and only divide them according to whether spread is limited or extensive but it is now recommended that these tumours be fully staged by the TNM system. Adenocarcinoma is recognised as having more metastatic potential than squamous cell carcinoma and with this cell type it is worth extending pre-operative screening procedures for metastases to include the brain. Within adenocarcinoma, mucin-forming varieties are recognised to be the more aggressive.[426] Histological typing is also important in regard to treatment; small cell carcinoma generally is considered the only type that responds to chemotherapy, if only temporarily. However, the neoadjuvant chemotherapy for non-small cell carcinoma shows that these tumours are also chemosensitive,[642] albeit to a lesser extent than small cell carcinoma. Considerable attention is being paid today to the implications of neuroendocrine differentiation in non-small cell carcinomas, in particular to the possibility that such differentiation may be associated with the chemosensitivity shown by small cell carcinoma: the limited evidence for this is discussed under large cell neuroendocrine carcinoma (see p. 563).[537,539]

Other prognostic factors

As well as tumour stage, histological type and grade, various other factors, listed in Box 12.1.7, have been reported to carry prognostic significance, albeit rather limited.[97,102,214,248–254,525,653–694] However, reports tend to be conflicting. Furthermore, this discordance is compounded by the heterogeneity of lung tumours, which is found to apply to the results of these more sophisticated investigations as much as to simple histological typing. Therefore, if it were planned to introduce any of these techniques into routine laboratory practice quite extensive standardised sampling of the tumour would be required.[695,696]

Oncogene expression also appears to be linked to prognosis.[697–699] Not all groups have found a positive correlation,[700–702] but expression of the *ras* oncogene in lung tumours is widely reported to auger a poor prognosis.[703–706] Similar findings are reported in respect of *Her2/neu*

Figure 12.1.49 Pleural penetration. Elastin stains clarify the relation of a peripheral growth to the pleura. (A) This pulmonary carcinoma (right) abuts but does not penetrate the outer elastin layer of the visceral pleura whereas in (B) another carcinoma broaches this elastin layer.

Table 12.1.17 Classification of visceral pleural invasion[637]

PL0	Tumour located within the lung parenchyma or only superficially invading in the pleural connective tissue, but not beyond the elastic layer of the visceral pleura
PL1	Tumour invades the visceral pleura beyond the elastic layer
PL2	Tumour invades to visceral pleural surface
PL3	Tumour invades the parietal pleura or the chest wall

Correlation between PL and T status: T1 = PL0; T2 = PL1 or PL2; T3 = PL3.

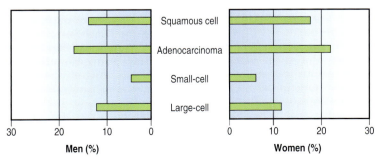

Figure 12.1.50 Five-year-survival rates (%) of lung cancer according to histological type.[652]

(*EGFR2*, *c-erbB2*).[707] Mutations of genes that control cell growth and apoptosis, such as *p53*, *RB* and *bcl-2*, are found in many lung neoplasms,[663,705,708–713] with obvious implications for the growth of the tumour. For example, squamous cell carcinomas of the lung expressing the Forkhead box M1 (FoxM1) transcription factor are poorly differentiated, metastasise earlier and have more malignant potential than other tumours of this type.[229] Furthermore, genetic abnormalities enhancing tumour growth may be induced by the very chemotherapy aimed at eliminating the tumour. For example, amplification of c-*myc* is more often present in small cell carcinomas from patients who have relapsed after chemotherapy than in newly diagnosed patients; patients in relapse who showed amplification had shorter survivals than those who did not.[714]

Drug resistance is a major problem in chemotherapy, and one that is compounded by the observation that tumours that acquire resistance to one drug often simultaneously become resistant to a variety of other structurally unrelated drugs. Such multidrug resistance is under genetic control. The genes responsible encode glycoproteins in the cell membrane that eliminate various drugs from the cell and can be detected immunocytochemically.[715–717] Pemetrexed is effective only in carcinomas showing non-squamous histology and the presence of ERCC1 protein in tumour cells implies resistance to *cis*-platinum-based therapy. *EGFR*-targeted TK inhibitors show better response in patients with certain mutations (exons 19 and 21) whilst there are other mutations that confer resistance (exon 20).

One mechanism whereby aberrant gene expression may be linked to tumour aggressiveness is overelaboration of growth factors. Endothelin, for example, is a growth factor that has been demonstrated in large amounts in squamous cell and adenocarcinoma of the lung,[253] and transforming growth factor beta-1 is reported to be a prognostic factor for pulmonary adenocarcinoma.[718] Over 30 other growth factors are known to be synthesised by small cell lung cancer.[719] Some growth factors, notably gastrin-releasing peptide (human bombesin), evince autocrine activity by stimulating the proliferation of the cancer cells that produce them.[720,721] A further mechanism by which faulty genetic regulation may influence tumour growth is in the production of receptors for specific growth factors. An example of this is the strong expression of *EGFR* demonstrated in pulmonary squamous cell carcinoma.[722]

As well as the control of these recognised oncogenes, the total genetic make-up of a tumour may be mapped by microarrays and by comparing these results with the subsequent course and response to treatment in large series it may be possible to predict how subsequent tumours are likely to behave.[723,724] This is leading to molecular classifications of tumours, the clinical importance of which is likely to rival that of histological category. As yet, however, it is not known whether tumours are genetically homogeneous so that a sample can be used to predict the behaviour of the whole.[328]

DEVELOPMENTS IN TREATMENT

The traditional treatment of lung cancer is threefold: surgery for those patients whose tumours appear to be operable after extensive staging, aggressive chemotherapy for most small cell carcinomas (typically with etoposide and cisplatin), and palliative or radical chemotherapy and/or radiotherapy for inoperable non-small carcinoma. Neoadjuvant chemotherapy extends this by reducing the extent of the tumour to operable proportions, so providing curative treatment to patients formerly offered only palliation.[642] Postoperative (adjuvant) chemotherapy also improves survival.[725] New chemotherapeutic drugs are constantly being introduced and aggressive chemotherapy is being increasingly offered to patients with inoperable non-small cell carcinoma.[726,727] However, acting as they do against all dividing cells, healthy as well as cancerous, side-effects generally limit their dose. Fortunately, totally new anticancer treatments that act more specifically are being introduced.[343,723,728] A favourable feature is that some are far less toxic. These tend to retard tumour growth rather than kill cancer cells, leading to disease stabilisation rather than regression, but they often act synergistically with conventional chemotherapeutic agents.

Many of these new agents act by modifying transduction pathways important in the continued growth of cancer cells.[729] They include antibodies against both growth factor receptors on the surface of the tumour cell and small-molecule inhibitors of the receptor's cytoplasmic domain.[730] TK activation is an important growth signal for lung cancer[731] and members of the epidermal growth factor family such as *HER2/neu*, which act as TK receptors, are targeted by the monoclonal antibodies cetuximab and trastuzumab and the small-molecule TK inhibitors gefitinib and erlotinib. In combination with conventional chemotherapy, gefitinib is proving particularly effective in prolonging survival from lung cancers that express the appropriate gene mutation.[206–210,344,732–736] Conversely, mutation of K-*ras*, which encodes downstream of epidermal growth factor, and high ERCC1 expression are associated with resistance to TK inhibitors.[737,738] Genetic markers of sensitivity to specific cytotoxic agents are proving useful in guaging the likelihood of response to traditional chemotherapy. Examples include ERCC1 and BRCA1 for platinum, RRM1 for gemcitabine and thymidilate synthase for antifolates (such as pemetrexed).[739,740] Trials of chemotherapy targeting those patients with lung cancers containing *ELM4-ALK* gene rearrangement are also in progress.[229]

The rapamycin derivative RAD001 (Everolimus) is effective in inhibiting the Akt/mammalian target of rapamycin (mTOR) pathway, which is frequently activated in small cell lung cancer, and following the demonstration that it inhibits the growth of cell lines of small cell lung cancer, is likely to progress to clinical trials.[227]

REFERENCES

Incidence and mortality

1. La Vecchia C, Bosetti C, Lucchini F, et al. Cancer mortality in Europe, 2000–2004, and an overview of trends since 1975. Ann Oncol 2010;21:1323–60.

2. Doll R. Bronchial carcinoma: incidence and aetiology. BMJ 1953;2:521–7.

3. Harris RE, Zang EA, Anderson JI, et al. Race and sex differences in lung cancer risk associated with cigarette smoking. Int J Epidemiol 1993;22:592–9.

4. Zang EA, Wynder EL. Differences in lung cancer risk between men and women: examination of the evidence. J Natl Cancer Inst 1996;88:183–92.

5. Patel JD, Bach PB, Kris MG. Lung cancer in US women: a contemporary epidemic. JAMA 2004;291:1763–8.

6. Ryberg D, Hewer A, Phillips DH, et al. Different susceptibility to smoking-induced DNA damage among male and female lung cancer patients. Cancer Res 1994;54:5801–3.

7. Lienert T, Serke M, Schonfeld N, et al. Lung cancer in young females. Eur Resp J 2000;16:986–90.

8. Hartman GE, Shochat SJ. Primary pulmonary neoplasms of childhood: a review. Ann Thorac Surg 1983;36:108–19.

9. Strand TE, Rostad H, Moller B, et al. Survival after resection for primary lung cancer: a population based study of 3211 resected patients. Thorax 2006;61:710–5.

10. Sant M, Aareleid T, Berrino F, et al. EUROCARE-3: survival of cancer patients diagnosed 1990–1994 – results and commentary. Ann Oncol 2003;14:v61–118.

11. SEER Cancer Statistics Review, 1975–2003. Bethesda, Maryland, USA: National Cancer Institute; 2006.

12. National Cancer Institute. Surveillance, Epidemiology and End Results Programme 1975–2005. Bethesda, Maryland, USA; 2008.

12a. Maeda R, Yoshida J, Hishida T, et al. Late recurrence of non-small cell lung cancer more than 5 years after complete resection. Chest 2010;138:145–50.

Aetiology

13. Doll R, Hill AB. Smoking and carcinoma of the lung : preliminary report. BMJ 1950;2:1071–81.

14. Wynder EL, Graham EA. Tobacco smoking as a possible etiologic factor in bronchogenic carcinoma. A study of six hundred and eighty four proved cases. JAMA 1950;143:329–36.

15. Doll R, Hill AB. A study of the aetiology of carcinoma of the lung. BMJ 1952;2:1271–86.

16. Doll R, Hill AB. Mortality in relation to smoking: ten years' observations of British doctors. BMJ 1964;1:1399–410.

17. Doll R, Hill AB. Mortality in relation to smoking: ten years' observations of British doctors. BMJ 1964;1:1460–7.

18. Kahn HA. The Dorn study of smoking and mortality among US veterans: a report on eight and one half years of observation. In: Haenszel W, editor. Natl Cancer Inst Mongr No 19. Bethesda, Maryland, USA; 1966. p. 1–25.

19. United States Public Health Service. The health consequences of smoking – cancer. Rockville, Maryland: Department of Health and Human Services, Office on Smoking and Health; 1982.

20. Lange P, Nyboe J, Appleyard M, et al. Relationship of the type of tobacco and inhalation pattern to pulmonary and total mortality. Eur Respir J 1992;5:1111–17.

21. Skillrud DM, Offord KP, Miller RD. Higher risk of lung cancer in chronic obstructive pulmonary disease. A prospective, matched, controlled study. Ann Intern Med 1986;105:503–7.

22. Wynder EL, Stellman SD. Impact of long-term filter cigarette usage on lung and larynx cancer risk: a case-control study. J Natl Cancer Inst 1979;62:471.

23. Wald NJ, Watt HC. Prospective study of effect of switching from cigarettes to pipes or cigars on mortality from three smoking related diseases (see comments). BMJ 1997;314:1860–3.

24. Funai K, Yokose T, Ishii G, et al. Clinicopathologic characteristics of peripheral squamous cell carcinoma of the lung. Amer J Surg Pathol 2003;27:978–84.

25. US Environmental Protection Agency. Respiratory health effects of passive smoking: lung cancer and other disorders. Washington: National Cancer Institute; 1993.

26. International Agency for Research on Cancer. Tobacco smoking and involuntary smoking. Lyons: IARC; 2004.

27. Hecht S. Tobacco smoke carcinogens and lung cancer. J Nat Cancer Inst 1999;91:1194–210.

28. Murray GI. The role of cytochrome P450 in tumour development and progression and its potential in therapy. J Pathol 2000;192:419–26.

29. Auerbach O, Stout AP, Hammond EC, et al. Changes in bronchial epithelium in relation to cigarette smoking and in relation to lung cancer. N Engl J Med 1961;265:253–67.

30. Peters EJ, Morice R, Benner SE, et al. Squamous metaplasia of the bronchial mucosa and its relationship to smoking. Chest 1993;103:1429–32.

31. Auerbach O, Hammond EC, Kirman D, et al. Histologic changes in bronchial tubes of cigarette smoking dogs. Cancer 1967;20:2055–66.

32. Auerbach O, Hammond EC, Kirman D, et al. Effects of cigarette smoking on dogs. II Pulmonary neoplasms. Arch Env Health 1970;21:754–68.

33. Kreyberg L. Histological lung cancer types: a morphological and biological correlation. Acta Path Microbiol Scand 1962;157:1–93.

34. Morabia A, Wynder EL. Cigarette smoking and lung cancer cell types. Cancer 1991;68:2074–8.

35. Dockery DW, Pope CA, Xu XP, et al. An association between air pollution and mortality in 6 United States cities. N Engl J Med 1993;329:1753–9.

36. Jakobsson R, Gustavsson P, Lundberg I. Increased risk of lung cancer among male professional drivers in urban but not rural areas of Sweden. Occup Environ Med 1997;54:189–93.

37. Cederlof R, Doll R, Fowler B, et al. Air pollution and cancer risk assessment. Methodology and epidemiological evidence. European Health Perspect 1978;22:1–12.

38. Gershick E, Schenker MB, Munoz A. A retrospective cohort study of lung cancer and diesel exhaust exposure in railroad workers. Am Rev Respir Dis 1988;137:820–5.

39. International Agency for Research on Cancer. Diesel and engine exhausts and some nitroarenes. Lyons: IARC; 1989.

40. Nafstad P, Haheim LL, Oftedal B, et al. Lung cancer and air pollution: a 27 year follow up of 16 209 Norwegian men. Thorax 2003;58:1071–6.

41. Sui GJ, Scott R. Relationship of radioactive radon daughters and cigarette smoking in the genesis of lung cancer in uranium miners. Cancer 1988;62:1402–8.

42. Kusiak RA, Ritchie AC, Muller J, et al. Mortality from lung cancer in Ontario uranium miners. Br J Ind Med 1993;50:920–8.

43. Boyd JT, Doll R, Faulds JS, et al. Cancer of the lung in iron ore (haematite) miners. Br J Ind Med 1970;27:97–105.

44. Saccomanno G, Archer VE, Auerbach O, et al. Histologic types of lung cancer among uranium miners. Cancer 1971;27:515–23.

45. Horacek J, Placek V, Sevc J. Histologic types of bronchogenic cancer in relation to different conditions of radiation exposure. Cancer 1977;40:832–5.

46. Archer VE, Wagoner JK, Lundin FE. Uranium mining and cigarette smoking effects on man. J Occup Med 1973;15:204–11.

47. Archer VE, Gillam JD, Wagoner JK. Respiratory disease mortality among uranium miners. Ann N Y Acad Sci 1976;271:280–93.

48. Darby S, Whitley E, Silcocks P, et al. Risk of lung cancer associated with residential radon exposure in south-west England: a case-control study (see comments). Br J Cancer 1998;78:394–408.

49. Darby S, Hill D, Auvinen A, et al. Radon in homes and risk of lung cancer: collaborative analysis of individual data from 13 European case-control studies. BMJ 2005;330:223.

50. Gray A, Read S, McGale P, et al. Lung cancer deaths from indoor radon and the cost effectiveness and potential of policies to reduce them. BMJ 2009;338:a3110.

51. Court-Brown WM, Doll R. Mortality from cancer and other causes after radiotherapy for ankylosing spondylitis. BMJ 1965;2:1327–32.

52. Neugut AI, Murray T, Santos J, et al. Increased risk of lung cancer after breast cancer radiation therapy in cigarette smokers. Cancer 1994;73:1615–20.

53. Deutsch M, Land SR, Begovic M, et al. The incidence of lung carcinoma after surgery for breast carcinoma with and without postoperative radiotherapy. Results of National Surgical Adjuvant Breast and Bowel Project (NSABP) clinical trials B-04 and B-06. Cancer 2003;98:1362–8.

54. Cihak RW, Ishimaru T, Steer A, et al. Lung cancer at autopsy in A-bomb survivors and controls, Hiroshima and Nagasaki 1961–1970. Cancer 1974;33:1580–8.

55. Ishimaru T, Cihak RW, Land CE, et al. Lung cancer at autopsy in A-bomb survivors and controls, Hiroshima and Nagasaki 1961–1970. II Smoking, occupation and A-bomb exposure. Cancer 1975;36:1723–8.

56. Doll R. Mortality from lung cancer in asbestos workers. Br J Ind Med 1955;12:81–6.

57. Whitwell F, Newhouse ML, Bennett DR. A study of the histological cell types of lung cancer in workers suffering from asbestosis in the United Kingdom. Br J Ind Med 1974;31:298–303.

58. Churg A. Lung cancer cell type and asbestos exposure. JAMA 1985;253:2984–5.

59. Raffn E, Lynge E, Korsgaard B. Incidence of lung cancer by histological type among asbestos cement workers in Denmark. Br J Ind Med 1993;50:85–9.

60. Selikoff IJ, Hammond EC, Churg J. Asbestos exposure, smoking and neoplasia. JAMA 1968;204:104–12.

61. Hammond EC, Selikoff IJ, Seidman H. Asbestos exposure, cigarette smoking and death rates. Ann N Y Acad Sci 1979;330:473–90.

62. Martischnig KM, Newell DJ, Barnsley WC, et al. Unsuspected exposure to asbestos and bronchogenic carcinoma. BMJ 1977;1:746–9.

63. Wright CM, Bowman RV, Tan ME, et al. Lung asbestos content in lungs resected for primary lung cancer. J Thorac Oncol 2008;3:569–76.

64. International Agency for Research on Cancer. An evaluation of carcinogenic risk to humans. Overall evaluation of carcinogenicity: an updating of IARC monographs vols 1–42. Supplement 7. Lyons: IARC; 1987.

65. Andersen A, Berge SR, Engeland A, et al. Exposure to nickel compounds and smoking in relation to incidence of lung and nasal cancer among nickel refinery workers. Occup Environ Med 1996;53:708–13.

66. Doll R, Vessey MP, Beasley RWR. Mortality of gasworkers – final report of a prospective study. Br J Ind Med 1972;29:394–406.

67. Enterline PE, Marsh GM. Cancer among workers exposed to arsenic and other substances in a copper smelter. Am J Epidemiol 1982;116:895–911.

68. Ades AE, Kazantzis G. Lung cancer in a non-ferrous smelter: the role of cadmium. Br J Ind Med 1988;45:435–42.

69. Sunderman FW, Morgan LG, Andersen A, et al. Histopathology of sinonasal and lung cancers in nickel refinery workers. Ann Clin Lab Sci 1989;19:44–9.

70. Sorohan T, Waterhouse JAH. Mortality study of nickel cadmium battery workers by the method of repression models in life tables. Br J Ind Med 1983;40:293–300.

71. Abe S, Ohsaki Y, Kimura K, et al. Chromate lung cancer with special reference to its cell type and relation to the manufacturing process. Cancer 1982;49:783–7.

72. Davies JM, Easton DF, Bidstrup PL. Mortality from respiratory cancer and other causes in United Kingdom chromate production workers. Br J Ind Med 1991;48:299–313.

73. Enterline PE, Day R, Marsh GM. Cancers related to exposure to arsenic at a copper smelter. Occup Environ Med 1995;52:28–32.

74. Jones RD. Survey of antimony workers: mortality 1961–1992. Occup Environ Med 1994;51:772–6.

75. Islam FS, Gault AG, Boothman C, et al. Role of metal-reducing bacteria in arsenic release from Bengal delta sediments. Nature 2004;430:68–71.

76. Weiss W, Moser RL, Auerbach O. Lung cancer in chloromethyl ether workers. Am Rev Respir Dis 1979;120:1031–7.

77. Churg A. Lung cancer cell type and occupational exposure. In: Samet JM, editor. Epidemiology of lung cancer. New York: Marcel Dekker, Inc.; 1994. p. 413–36.

78. Goldsmith DF. Silica exposure and pulmonary cancer. In: Samet JM, editor. Epidemiology of Lung Cancer. New York: Marcel Dekker, Inc; 1994. p. 245–98.

79. Koo LC. Diet and lung cancer 20+ years later: More questions than answers? Int J Cancer 1997;22–9.

80. Wald N, Idle M, Boreham J, et al. Low serum vitamin A and subsequent risk of cancer. Lancet 1980;ii:813–15.

81. Shields PA, Jeffery PK. The combined effects of vitamin A-deficiency and cigarette smoke on rat tracheal epithelium. Br J Exp Pathol 1987;68:705–17.

82. Mettlin C, Graham S, Swanson MJ. Vitamin A and lung cancer. J Natl Cancer Inst 1979;62:1435–8.

83. Kamei T, Kohno T, Ohwada H, et al. Experimental study of the therapeutic effects of folate, vitamin-A, and vitamin-B$_{12}$ on squamous metaplasia of the bronchial epithelium. Cancer 1993;71:2477–83.

84. The alpha-tocopherol BCCPSG. The effect of vitamin E and beta carotene on the incidence of lung cancer and other cancers in male smokers. N Engl J Med 1994;330:1029–35.

85. Hennekens CH, Buring JE, Manson JE, et al. Lack of effect of long-term supplementation with beta carotene on the incidence of malignant neoplasms and cardiovascular disease. N Engl J Med 1996;334:1145–9.

86. Omenn GS, Goodman GE, Thornquist MD, et al. Effects of a combination of beta carotene and vitamin A on lung cancer and cardiovascular disease. N Engl J Med 1996;334:1150–5.

87. Turner-Warwick M, Lebowitz M, Burrows B, et al. Cryptogenic fibrosing alveolitis and lung cancer. Thorax 1980;35:496–9.

88. Hubbard R, Venn A, Lewis S, et al. Lung cancer and cryptogenic fibrosing alveolitis – A population- based cohort study. Am J Respir Crit Care Med 2000;161:5–8.

89. Park J, Kim DS, Shim TS, et al. Lung cancer in patients with idiopathic pulmonary fibrosis. Eur Resp J 2001;17:1216–19.

90. Mizushima Y, Kobayashi M. Clinical characteristics of synchronous multiple lung cancer associated with idiopathic pulmonary fibrosis: a review of Japanese cases. Chest 1995;108:1272–7.

91. Hironaka M, Fukayama M. Pulmonary fibrosis and lung carcinoma: A comparative study of metaplastic epithelia in honeycombed areas of usual interstitial pneumonia with or without lung carcinoma. Pathol Int 1999;49:1060–6.

92. Askling J, Grunewald J, Eklund A, et al. Increased risk for cancer following sarcoidosis. Am J Respir Crit Care Med 1999;160:1668–72.

93. Bouros D, Hatzakis K, Labrakis H, et al. Association of malignancy with diseases causing interstitial pulmonary changes. Chest 2002;121:1278–89.

94. Seersholm N, Vestbo J, Viskum K. Risk of malignant neoplasms in patients with pulmonary sarcoidosis. Thorax 1997;52:892–4.

95. Bakris GL, Mulopulos GP, Korchik R, et al. Pulmonary scar carcinoma. A

clinicopathologic analysis. Cancer 1983;52:493–7.

96. Suzuki A. Growth characteristics of peripheral type adenocarcinoma of the lung in terms of roentgenological findings. In: Shimosato Y, Melamed MR, Nettesheim P, editors. Morphogenesis of Lung Cancer. Boca Raton: CRC Press; 1982. p. 91–110.

97. Shimosato Y, Hashimoto T, Kodama T, et al. Prognostic implication of fibrotic focus (scar) in small peripheral lung cancers. Am J Surg Pathol 1980;4: 365–73.

98. Barsky SH, Huang SJ, Bhuta S. The extracellular matrix of pulmonary scar carcinomas is suggestive of a desmoplastic origin. Am J Pathol 1986;124:412–19.

99. Madri JA, Carter D. Scar cancers of the lung: origin and significance. Hum Pathol 1984;15:625–31.

100. Kung ITM, Lui IOl, Loke SL, et al. Pulmonary scar cancer. A pathologic reappraisal. Am J Surg Pathol 1985;9:391–400.

101. Kolin A, Koutoulakis A. Role of arterial occlusion in pulmonary scar cancers. Hum Pathol 1988;19:1161–7.

102. Goldstein NS, Mani A, Chmielewski G, et al. Prognostic factors in T1 N0 M0 adenocarcinomas and bronchioloalveolar carcinomas of the lung. Am J Clin Pathol 1999;112:391–402.

103. Xu H, Lu DW, El Mofty SK, et al. Metachronous squamous cell carcinomas evolving from independent oropharyngeal and pulmonary squamous papillomas: association with human papillomavirus 11 and lack of aberrant p53, Rb, and p16 protein expression. Hum Pathol 2004;35:1419–22.

104. Bohlmeyer T, Le TN, Shroyer AL, et al. Detection of human papillomavirus in squamous cell carcinomas of the lung by polymerase chain reaction. Am J Respir Cell Molec Biol 1998;18:265–9.

105. Cheng YW, Chiou HL, Sheu GT, et al. The association of human papillomavirus 16/18 infection with lung cancer among nonsmoking Taiwanese women. Cancer Res 2001;61:2799–803.

106. Chan JKC, Hui PK, Tsang WYW, et al. Primary lymphoepithelioma-like carcinoma of the lung – a clinicopathologic study of 11 cases. Cancer 1995;76:413–22.

107. Conway EJ, Hudnall SD, Lazarides A, et al. Absence of evidence for an etiologic role for Epstein–Barr virus in neoplasms of the lung and pleura. Mod Pathol 1996;9:491–5.

108. Bazoes A, Bower M, Powles T. Smoke and mirrors: HIV-related lung cancer. Curr Opin Oncol 2008;20:529–33.

109. Smyth JF. Cancer genetics and cell and molecular biology: is this the way forward? Chest 1996;109:S125–9.

110. Schwartz AG. Genetic predisposition to lung cancer. Chest 2004;125:86S–9S.

111. Ayesh R, Idle JR, Ritchie JC, et al. Metabolic oxidation phenotypes as markers for susceptibility to lung cancer. Nature 1984;312:169–70.

112. Philpot RM. Modulation of the pulmonary cytochrome-p450 system as a factor in pulmonary-selective toxic responses – fact and fiction. Am J Respir Cell Mol Biol 1993;9:347–9.

113. Shaw GL, Falk RT, Pickle LW, et al. Lung cancer risk associated with cancer in relatives. J Clin Epidemiol 1991;44:429–37.

114. Ambrosone CB, Rao U, Michalek AM, et al. Lung cancer histologic types and family history of cancer – analysis of histologic subtypes of 872 patients with primary lung cancer. Cancer 1993;72:1192–8.

115. Nitadori J, Inoue M, Iwasaki M, et al. Association between lung cancer incidence and family history of lung cancer: data from a large-scale population-based cohort study, the JPHC study. Chest 2006;130:968–75.

116. Bailey-Wilson JE, Amos CI, Pinney SM, et al. A major lung cancer susceptibility locus maps to chromosome 6q23–25. Am J Hum Genet 2004;75:460–74.

117. Thorgeirsson TE, Geller F, Sulem P, et al. A variant associated with nicotine dependence, lung cancer and peripheral arterial disease. Nature 2008;452:638–42.

118. Hung RJ, McKay JD, Gaborieau V, et al. A susceptibility locus for lung cancer maps to nicotinic acetylcholine receptor subunit genes on 15q25. Nature 2008;452:633–7.

119. Ota H, Langston C, Honda T, et al. Histochemical analysis of mucous cells of congenital adenomatoid malformation of the lung: Insights into the carcinogenesis of pulmonary adenocarcinoma expressing gastric mucins. Am J Clin Pathol 1998;110:450–5.

120. Stacher E, Ullmann R, Halbwedl I, et al. Atypical goblet cell hyperplasia in congenital cystic adenomatoid malformation as a possible preneoplasia for pulmonary adenocarcinoma in childhood: a genetic analysis*1. Human Pathology 2004;35:565–70.

121. Lantuejoul S, Nicholson AG, Sartori G, et al. Mucinous cells in type 1 pulmonary congenital cystic adenomatoid malformation as mucinous bronchioloalveolar carcinoma precursors. Am J Surg Pathol 2007;31:961–9.

Pathogenesis

122. Chandraratnam EA, Henderson DW, Meredith DJ, et al. Regenerative atypical squamous metaplasia in fibreoptic bronchial biopsy sites – a lesion liable to misinterpretation as carcinoma on rebiopsy-report of 5 cases. Pathology 1987;19:419–24.

123. Ayers MM, Jeffery PK. Proliferation and differentiation in mammalian airway epithelium. Eur Respir J 1988;1:58–80.

124. Chopra DP, Cooney RA. Histogenesis of benzo(a)pyrene-induced lesions in tracheal explants. Virchows Arch B Cell Pathol 1985;48:299–315.

125. Johnson NF, Wagner JC, Wills HA. Endocrine cell proliferation in the rat lung following asbestos exposure. Lung 1980;158:221–8.

126. Reznik-Schuller H. Sequential morphologic alterations in the bronchial epithelium of Syrian golden hamsters during N-nitrosomorpholine-induced pulmonary tumorigenesis. Am J Pathol 1977;89:59–66.

127. Saccomanno G, Archer VE, Auerbach O, et al. Development of carcinoma of the lung as reflected in exfoliated cells. Cancer 1974;33:256–70.

128. Hirsch FR, Franklin WA, Gazdar AF, et al. Early detection of lung cancer: clinical perspectives of recent advances in biology and radiology. Clin Cancer Res 2001;7:5–22.

129. Franklin WA. Premalignant Evolution of Lung Cancer: Gilles F. Filley Lecture. Chest 2004;125:90S–94S.

130. World Health Organization. Tumours of the lung, pleura, thymus and heart. Lyons: IARC Press; 2004.

131. Keith RL, Miller YE, Gemmill RM, et al. Angiogenic squamous dysplasia in bronchi of individuals at high risk for lung cancer. Clin Cancer Res 2000;6:1616–25.

132. Shibuya K, Hoshino H, Chiyo M, et al. Subepithelial vascular patterns in bronchial dysplasias using a high magnification bronchovideoscope. Thorax 2002;57:902–7.

133. Nagamoto N, Saito Y, Sato M, et al. Clinicopathological analysis of 19 cases of isolated carcinoma insitu of the bronchus. Am J Surg Pathol 1993;17:1234–43.

134. Solomon MD, Greenberg SD, Spjut HJ. Morphology of bronchial epithelium adjacent to adenocarcinoma of the lung. Mod Pathol 1990;3:684–7.

135. Breuer RH, Pasic A, Smit EF, et al. The natural course of preneoplastic lesions in bronchial epithelium. Clin Cancer Res 2005;11:537–43.

136. Jeremy GP, Banerjee AK, Read CA, et al. Surveillance for the detection of early lung cancer in patients with bronchial dysplasia. Thorax 2007;62:43–50.

137. van Bodegom PC, Wagenaar SjSc, Corrin B, et al. Second primary lung cancer: importance of long term follow up. Thorax 1989;44:788–93.

137a. Carey FA, Donnell SC, Walker WS, et al. Synchronous primary lung cancers: prevalence in surgical material and clinical implications. Thorax 1993;48:344–6.

138. Okada M, Tsubota N, Yoshimura M, et al. Simultaneous occurrence of three primary lung cancers. Chest 1994;105:631–2.

139. Martini N, Melamed MR. Multiple primary lung cancers. J Thorac Cardiovasc Surg 1975;70:606–12.

140. Banerjee AK, Rabbitts PH, George J. Lung cancer center dot 3: Fluorescence bronchoscopy: clinical dilemmas and research opportunities. Thorax 2003;58:266–71.

141. Kennedy TC, McWilliams A, Edell E, et al. Bronchial intraepithelial neoplasia/early central airways lung cancer: ACCP evidence-based clinical practice guidelines (2nd Edition). Chest 2007;132:221S–33S.

142. Raeburn C, Spencer H. A study of the origin and development of lung cancer. Thorax 1953;8:1–10.

143. Spencer H, Raeburn C. Atypical proliferation of bronchiolar epithelium. J Path Bact 1954;67:187–93.

144. Nakayama H, Noguchi M, Tsuchiya R, et al. Clonal growth of atypical adenomatous hyperplasia of the lung: cytofluorometric analysis of nuclear DNA content. Mod Pathol 1990;3: 314–20.

145. Kerr KM, Carey FA, King G, et al. Atypical alveolar hyperplasia: relationship with pulmonary adenocarcinoma, p53, and c-erbB-2 expression. J Pathol 1994;174:249–56.

146. Rao SK, Fraire AE. Alveolar cell hyperplasia in association with adenocarcinoma of lung. Mod Pathol 1995;8:165–9.

147. Chapman AD, Kerr KM. The association between atypical adenomatous hyperplasia and primary lung cancer. Br J Cancer 2000;83:632–6.

148. Miller RR. Bronchioloalveolar cell adenomas. Am J Surg Pathol 1990;14:904–12.

149. Logan PM, Miller RR, Evans K, et al. Bronchogenic carcinoma and coexistent bronchioloalveolar cell adenomas: assessment of radiologic detection and follow-up in 28 patients. Chest 1996;109:713–17.

150. Travis WD, Brambilla E, Noguchi M, Nicholson AG, Geisinger KR, Yatabe Y, et al. IASLC/ATS/ERS International multidisciplinary classification of lung adenocarcinoma. Journal of Thoracic Oncology, in press.

151. Miller RR, Nelems B, Evans KG, et al. Glandular neoplasia of the lung. A proposed analogy to colonic tumors. Cancer 1988;61:1009–14.

152. Sterner DJ, Mori M, Roggli VL, et al. Prevalence of pulmonary atypical alveolar cell hyperplasia in an autopsy population: a study of 100 cases. Mod Pathol 1997;10:469–73.

153. Yokose T, Doi M, Tanno K, et al. Atypical adenomatous hyperplasia of the lung in autopsy cases. Lung Cancer 2001;33:155–61.

154. Weng SY, Tsuchiya E, Kasuga T, et al. Incidence of atypical bronchioloalveolar cell hyperplasia of the lung – relation to histological subtypes of lung cancer. Virchows Arch A Pathol Anat Histopathol 1992;420:463–71.

155. Suzuki K, Nagai K, Yoshida J, et al. The prognosis of resected lung carcinoma associated with atypical adenomatous hyperplasia: A comparison of the prognosis of well-differentiated adenocarcinoma associated with atypical adenomatous hyperplasia and intrapulmonary metastasis. Cancer 1997;79:1521–6.

156. Nakahara R, Yokose T, Nagai K, et al. Atypical adenomatous hyperplasia of the lung: a clinicopathological study of 118 cases including cases with multiple atypical adenomatous hyperplasia. 56 ed. 2001. 302–5.

157. Koga T, Hashimoto S, Sugio K, et al. Lung adenocarcinoma with bronchioloalveolar carcinoma component is frequently associated with foci of high-grade atypical adenomatous hyperplasia. Amer J Clin Pathol 2002;117:464–70.

158. Cooper CA, Carey FA, Bubb VJ, et al. The pattern of K-ras mutation in pulmonary adenocarcinoma defines a new pathway of tumour development in the human lung. J Pathol 1997;181:401–4.

159. Mori M, Rao SK, Popper HH, et al. Atypical adenomatous hyperplasia of the lung: A probable forerunner in the development of adenocarcinoma of the lung. Modern Pathol 2001;14:72–84.

160. Mori M, Chiba R, Takahashi T. Atypical adenomatous hyperplasia of the lung and its differentiation from adenocarcinoma – characterization of atypical cells by morphometry and multivariate cluster analysis. Cancer 1993;72:2331–40.

161. Kitamura H, Kameda Y, Nakamura N, et al. Atypical adenomatous hyperplasia and bronchoalveolar lung carcinoma: analysis by morphometry and the expressions of p53 and carcinoembryonic antigen. Am J Surg Pathol 1996;20:553–62.

162. Yokozaki M, Kodama T, Yokose T, et al. Differentiation of atypical adenomatous hyperplasia and adenocarcinoma of the lung by use of DNA ploidy and morphometric analysis. Mod Pathol 1996;9:1156–64.

163. Nakanishi K, Hiroi S, Kawai T, et al. Argyrophilic nucleolar-organizer region counts and DNA status in bronchioloalveolar epithelial hyperplasia and adenocarcinoma of the lung. Hum Pathol 1998;29:235–9.

164. Takamochi K, Ogura T, Suzuki K, et al. Loss of heterozygosity on chromosomes 9q and 16p in atypical adenomatous hyperplasia concomitant with adenocarcinoma of the lung. Amer J Pathol 2001;159:1941–8.

165. Ohshima S, Shimizu Y, Takahama M. Detection of c-ki-ras gene mutation in paraffin sections of adenocarcinoma and atypical bronchioloalveolar cell hyperplasia of human lung. Virchows Arch 1994;424:129–34.

166. Kurasono Y, Ito T, Kameda Y, et al. Expression of cyclin D1, retinoblastoma gene protein, and p16 MTS1 protein in atypical adenomatous hyperplasia and adenocarcinoma of the lung – An immunohistochemical analysis. Virchows Archiv 1998;432:207–15.

167. Kitamura H, Kameda Y, Ito T, et al. Atypical adenomatous hyperplasia of the lung – Implications for the pathogenesis of peripheral lung adenocarcinoma. Am J Clin Pathol 1999;111:610–22.

168. Kerr KM, MacKenzie SJ, Ramasami S, et al. Expression of Fhit, cell adhesion molecules and matrix metalloproteinases in atypical adenomatous hyperplasia and pulmonary adenocarcinoma. J Pathol 2004;203: 638–44.

169. Blons H, Cote JF, Le Corre D, et al. Epidermal growth factor receptor mutation in lung cancer are linked to bronchioloalveolar differentiation. Am J Surg Pathol 2006;30:1309–15.

170. Wu M, Orta L, Gil J, et al. Immunohistochemical detection of XIAP and p63 in adenomatous hyperplasia, atypical adenomatous hyperplasia, bronchioloalveolar carcinoma and well-differentiated adenocarcinoma. Mod Pathol 2008;21:553–8.

171. Niho S, Yokose T, Suzuki K, et al. Monoclonality of atypical adenomatous hyperplasia of the lung. Amer J Pathol 1999;154:249–54.

172. Clayton F. Bronchioloalveolar carcinomas. Cell types, patterns of growth, and prognostic correlates. Cancer 1986;57:1555–64.

173. Ogata T, Endo K. Clara cell granules of peripheral lung cancers. Cancer 1984;54:1635–44.

174. Nakamura S, Koshikawa T, Sato T, et al. Extremely well differentiated papillary adenocarcinoma of the lung with prominent cilia formation. Acta Pathol Jpn 1992;42:745–50.

175. Garfield DH, Cadranel J, West HL. Bronchioloalveolar carcinoma: the case for two diseases. Clin Lung Cancer 2008;9:24–9.

176. Goldstein NS, Thomas M. Mucinous and nonmucinous bronchioloalveolar adenocarcinomas have distinct staining patterns with thyroid transcription factor and cytokeratin 20 antibodies. Amer J Clin Pathol 2001;116:319–25.

177. Lau SK, Desrochers MJ, Luthringer DJ. Expression of thyroid transcription factor-1, cytokeratin 7, and cytokeratin 20 in bronchioloalveolar carcinomas: an immunohistochemical evaluation of 67 cases. Modern Pathol 2002;15: 538–42.

178. Simsir A, Wei XJ, Yee H, et al. Differential expression of cytokeratins 7 and 20 and thyroid transcription factor-1 in bronchioloalveolar carcinoma – An immunohistochemical study in fine-needle aspiration biopsy specimens. Am J Clin Pathol 2004;121:350–7.

179. Saad RS, Liu YL, Han H, et al. Prognostic significance of thyroid transcription factor-1 expression in both early-stage conventional adenocarcinoma and bronchioloalveolar carcinoma of the lung. Hum Pathol 2004;35:3–7.

180. Finberg KE, Sequist LV, Joshi VA, et al. Mucinous differentiation correlates with absence of EGFR mutation and presence of KRAS mutation in lung adenocarcinomas with bronchioloalveolar features. J Mol Diagn 2007;9:320–6.

181. Noguchi M, Morikawa A, Kawasaki M, et al. Small adenocarcinoma of the lung: histologic characteristics and prognosis. Cancer 1995;75:2844–52.

182. Terasaki H, Niki T, Matsuno Y, et al. Lung adenocarcinoma with mixed bronchioloalveolar and invasive components – clinicopathological features, subclassification by extent of invasive foci, and immunohistochemical characterization. Am J Surg Pathol 2003;27:937–51.

183. Borczuk AC, Qian F, Kazeros A, et al. Invasive size is an independent predictor of survival in pulmonary adenocarcinoma. Am J Surg Pathol 2009;33:462–9.

184. Yousem SA, Beasley MB. Bronchioloalveolar carcinoma: a review of current concepts and evolving issues. Arch Pathol Lab Med 2007;131:1027–32.

185. Nakano K, Iyama K, Mori T, et al. Loss of alveolar basement membrane type IV collagen alpha 3, alpha 4, and alpha 5 chains in bronchioloalveolar carcinoma of the lung. J Pathol 2001;194:420–7.

186. Kumaki F, Matsui K, Kawai T, et al. Expression of matrix metalloproteinases in invasive pulmonary adenocarcinoma with bronchioloalveolar component and atypical adenomatous hyperplasia. Am J Pathol 2001;159:2125–35.

187. Ohori NP, Yousem SA, Griffin J, et al. Comparison of extracellular matrix antigens in subtypes of bronchioloalveolar carcinoma and conventional pulmonary adenocarcinoma – an immunohistochemical study. Am J Surg Pathol 1992;16:675–86.

188. Suzuki K, Yokose T, Yoshida J, et al. Prognostic significance of the size of central fibrosis in peripheral adenocarcinoma of the lung. Ann Thorac Surg 2000;69:893–7.

189. Platt JA, Kraipowich N, Villafane F, et al. Alveolar type II cells expressing jaagsiekte sheep retrovirus capsid protein and surfactant proteins are the predominant neoplastic cell type in ovine pulmonary adenocarcinoma. Vet Pathol 2002;39:341–52.

190. DelasHeras M, Barsky SH, Hasleton P, et al. Evidence for a protein related immunologically to the jaagsiekte sheep retrovirus in some human lung tumours. Eur Resp J 2000;16:330–2.

191. Yousem SA, Finkelstein SD, Swalsky PA, et al. Absence of jaagsiekte sheep retrovirus DNA and RNA in bronchioloalveolar and conventional human pulmonary adenocarcinoma by PCR and RT-PCR analysis. Hum Pathol 2001;32:1039–42.

192. Ponticiello A, Barra E, Giani U, et al. p53 immunohistochemistry can identify bronchial dysplastic lesions proceeding to lung cancer: a prospective study. Eur Resp J 2000;15:547–52.

193. SanzOrtega J, Saez MC, Sierra E, et al. 3p21, 5q21, and 9p21 allelic deletions are frequently found in normal bronchial cells adjacent to non-small-cell lung cancer, while they are unusual in patients with no evidence of malignancy. J Pathol 2001;195:429–34.

194. Jeanmart M, Lantuejoul S, Fievet F, et al. Value of immunohistochemical markers in preinvasive bronchial lesions in risk assessment of lung cancer. Clin Cancer Res 2003;9:2195–203.

195. Brambilla C, Fievet F, Jeanmart M, et al. Early detection of lung cancer: role of biomarkers. Eur Respir J Suppl 2003;39:36s–44s.

196. Lantuejoul S, Salameire D, Salon C, et al. Pulmonary preneoplasia – sequential molecular carcinogenetic events. Histopathology 2009;54:43–54.

197. Park IW, Wistuba II, Maitra A, et al. Multiple clonal abnormalities in the bronchial epithelium of patients with lung cancer. J Natl Cancer Inst 1999;91:1863–8.

198. Hirano T, Franzen B, Kato H, et al. Genesis of squamous cell lung carcinoma – sequential changes of proliferation, DNA ploidy and p53 expression. Am J Pathol 1994;144:296–302.

199. Kitamura H, Kameda Y, Nakamura N, et al. Proliferative potential and p53 overexpression in precursor and early stage lesions of bronchioloalveolar lung carcinoma. Am J Pathol 1995;146:876–87.

200. Walker C, Robertson LJ, Myskow MW, et al. p53 expression in normal and dysplastic bronchial epithelium and in lung carcinomas. Br J Cancer 1994;70:297–303.

201. Boers JE, Tenvelde GPM, Thunnissen FBJM. P53 in squamous metaplasia: a marker for risk of respiratory tract carcinoma. Am J Respir Crit Care Med 1996;153:411–16.

202. Hayashi H, Miyamoto H, Ito T, et al. Analysis of p21(Waf1/Cip1) expression in normal, premalignant, and malignant cells during the development of human lung adenocarcinoma. Am J Pathol 1997;151:461–70.

203. Hung J, Kishimoto Y, Sugio K, et al. Allele-specific chromosome 3p deletions occur at an early stage in the pathogenesis of lung carcinoma [published erratum appears in JAMA 1995;273:1908]. JAMA 1995;273:558–63.

204. Kishimoto Y, Sugio K, Hung JY, et al. Allele-specific loss in chromosome 9p loci in preoplastic lesions accompanying non-small-cell lung cancers. J Natl Cancer Inst 1995;87:1224–9.

205. Dessy E, Rossi E, Berenzi A, et al. Chromosome 9 instability and alterations of p16 gene in squamous cell carcinoma of the lung and in adjacent normal bronchi: FISH and immunohistochemical study. Histopathology 2008;52:475–82.

206. Pao W, Miller VA. Epidermal growth factor receptor mutations, small-molecule kinase inhibitors, and non-small-cell lung cancer: current knowledge and future directions. J Clin Oncol 2005;23:2556–68.

207. Lynch TJ, Bell DW, Sordella R, et al. Activating mutations in the epidermal growth factor receptor underlying responsiveness of non-small-cell lung cancer to gefitinib. N Engl J Med 2004;350:2129–39.

208. Cappuzzo F, Hirsch FR, Rossi E, et al. Epidermal growth factor receptor gene and protein and gefitinib sensitivity in non-small-cell lung cancer. J Natl Cancer Inst 2005;97:643–55.

209. Cappuzzo F, Toschi L, Domenichini I, et al. HER3 genomic gain and sensitivity to gefitinib in advanced non-small-cell lung cancer patients. Br J Cancer 2005;93:1334–40.

210. Marchetti A, Martella C, Felicioni L, et al. EGFR mutations in non-small-cell lung cancer: analysis of a large series of cases and development of a rapid and sensitive method for diagnostic screening with potential implications on pharmacologic treatment. J Clin Oncol 2005;23:857–65.

211. Motoi N, Szoke J, Riely GJ, et al. Lung adenocarcinoma: modification of the 2004 WHO mixed subtype to include the major histologic subtype suggests correlations between papillary and micropapillary adenocarcinoma subtypes, EGFR mutations and gene expression analysis. Am J Surg Pathol 2008;32:810–27.

212. Dacic S, Shuai Y, Yousem S, et al. Clinicopathological predictors of EGFR/KRAS mutational status in primary lung adenocarcinomas. Mod Pathol 2009;23:159–68.

213. Soh J, Toyooka S, Ichihara S, et al. Sequential molecular changes during multistage pathogenesis of small peripheral adenocarcinomas of the lung. J Thorac Oncol 2008;3:340–7.

214. Hamid Q, Addis BJ, Springall DR, et al. Expression of the C-terminal peptide of human pro-bombesin in 361 lung endocrine tumours, a reliable marker and possible prognostic indicator for small cell carcinoma. Virchows Arch A Pathol Anat Histopathol 1987;411:185–92.

215. Shriver SP, Bourdeau HA, Gubish CT, et al. Sex-specific expression of gastrin-releasing peptide receptor: relationship to smoking history and risk of lung cancer. J Natl Cancer Inst 2000;92:24–33.

216. Westra WH, Slebos RJC, Offerhaus GJA, et al. K-ras oncogene activation in lung adenocarcinomas from former smokers – evidence that k-ras mutations are an early

and irreversible event in the development of adenocarcinoma of the lung. Cancer 1993;72:432–8.

217. Marchetti A, Buttitta F, Pellegrini S, et al. Bronchioloalveolar lung carcinomas: k-ras mutations are constant events in the mucinous subtype. J Pathol 1996;179:254–9.

218. Nau MM, Brooks BJ, Carney DN, et al. Human small-cell lung cancers show amplification and expression of the N-myc gene. Proc Natl Acad Sci USA 1986;83:1092–6.

219. Scott GM, Jones IG. A study of myc-related gene expression in small cell lung cancer by in situ hybridization. Am J Pathol 1988;132:13–7.

220. Gazdar AF. Oncogenes, antioncogenes and growth factors in the pathogenesis of small cell lung cancer (SCLC). Proceedings Second International Conference on Small Cell Lung Cancer 1990;23–5.

221. Soda M, Choi YL, Enomoto M, et al. Identification of the transforming EML4-ALK fusion gene in non-small-cell lung cancer. Nature 2007;448:561–6.

222. Inamura K, Takeuchi K, Togashi Y, et al. EML4-ALK lung cancers are characterized by rare other mutations, a TTF-1 cell lineage, an acinar histology, and young onset. Mod Pathol 2009;22:508–15.

223. Boland JM, Erdogan S, Vasmatzis G, et al. Anaplastic lymphoma kinase immunoreactivity correlates with ALK gene rearrangement and transcriptional up-regulation in non-small cell lung carcinomas. Hum Pathol 2009;40:1152–8.

224. Shaw AT, Yeap BY, Mino-Kenudson M, et al. Clinical features and outcome of patients with non-small-cell lung cancer who harbor EML4-ALK. J Clin Oncol 2009;27:4247–53.

225. Brose MS, Volpe P, Feldman M, et al. BRAF and RAS mutations in human lung cancer and melanoma. Cancer Res 2002;62:6997–7000.

226. Yousem SA, Nikiforova M, Nikiforov Y. The histopathology of BRAF-V600E-mutated lung adenocarcinoma. Am J Surg Pathol 2008;32:1317–21.

227. Marinov M, Ziogas A, Pardo OE, et al. AKT/mTOR pathway activation and BCL-2 family proteins modulate the sensitivity of human small cell lung cancer cells to RAD001. Clin Cancer Res 2009;15:1277–87.

228. Jiang SX, Kameya T, Asamura H, et al. hASH1 expression is closely correlated with endocrine phenotype and differentiation extent in pulmonary neuroendocrine tumors. Mod Pathol 2004;17:222–9.

229. Yang DK, Son CH, Lee SK, et al. Forkhead box M1 expression in pulmonary squamous cell carcinoma: correlation with clinicopathologic features and its prognostic significance. Hum Pathol 2009;40:464–70.

230. Kok K, Osinga J, Carritt B, et al. Deletion of a DNA sequence at the chromosomal region 3p21 in all major types of lung cancer. Nature 1987;330:578–81.

231. Yokota J, Wada M, Shimosato Y, et al. Loss of heterozygosity on chromosomes 3, 13, and 17 in small-cell carcinoma and on chromosome 3 in adenocarcinoma of the lung. Proc Natl Acad Sci USA 1987;84:9252–6.

232. Lehman TA, Bennett WP, Metcalf RA, et al. p53 mutations, ras mutations, and p53 – heat shock 70 protein complexes in human lung carcinoma cell lines. Cancer Res 1991;51:4090–6.

233. Whang-Peng J, Bunn PA Jr, Kao-Shan CS, et al. A nonrandom chromosomal abnormality, del 3p(14–23), in human small cell lung cancer (SCLC). Cancer Genet Cytogenet 1982;6:119–34.

234. Caamano J, Ruggeri B, Momiki S, et al. Detection of p53 in primary lung tumors and nonsmall cell lung carcinoma cell lines. Am J Pathol 1991;139:839–45.

235. Barbareschi M, Girlando S, Mauri FA, et al. Tumour suppressor gene products, proliferation, and differentiation markers in lung neuroendocrine neoplasms. J Pathol 1992;166:343–50.

236. Yoshida Y, Shibata T, Kokubu A, et al. Mutations of the epidermal growth factor receptor gene in atypical adenomatous hyperplasia and bronchioloalveolar carcinoma of the lung. Lung Cancer 2005;50:1–8.

237. Klein N, Vignaud JM, Sadmi M, et al. Squamous metaplasia expression of proto-oncogenes and p-53 in lung cancer patients. Lab Invest 1993;68:26–32.

238. Beasley MB, Lantuejoul S, Abbondanzo S, et al. The P16/cyclin D1/Rb pathway in neuroendocrine tumors of the lung. Hum Pathol 2003;34:136–42.

239. Pezzella F, Turley H, Kuzu I, et al. bcl-2 protein in non-small-cell lung carcinoma. N Engl J Med 1993;329:690–4.

240. Walker C, Robertson L, Myskow M, et al. Expression of the BCL-2 protein in normal and dysplastic bronchial epithelium and in lung carcinomas. Br J Cancer 1995;72:164–9.

241. Rao SK, Krishna M, Woda BA, et al. Immunohistochemical detection of bcl-2 protein in adenocarcinoma and non-neoplastic cellular compartments of the lung. Mod Pathol 1996;9:555–9.

242. Jiang SX, Kameya T, Sato Y, et al. Bcl-2 protein expression in lung cancer and close correlation with neuroendocrine differentiation. Am J Pathol 1996;148:837–46.

243. Brambilla E, Negoescu A, Gazzeri S, et al. Apoptosis-related factors p53, Bcl(2), and Bax in neuroendocrine lung tumors. Am J Pathol 1996;149:1941–52.

244. Hiyama K, Hiyama E, Ishioka S, et al. Telomerase activity in small-cell and non-small-cell lung cancers. J Natl Cancer Inst 1995;87:895–902.

245. Albanell J, Lonardo F, Rusch V, et al. High telomerase activity in primary lung cancers: association with increased cell proliferation rates and advanced pathologic stage. J Natl Cancer Inst 1997;89:1609–15.

246. Arinaga M, Shimizu S, Gotoh K, et al. Expression of human telomerase subunit genes in primary lung cancer and its clinical significance. Ann Thorac Surg 2000;70:401–5.

247. Brambilla E, Lantuejoul S. Telomerase activation in adenocarcinoma-bronchioloalveolar carcinoma. Eur Respir J 2006;27:1079–81.

248. Lantuejoul S, Constantin B, Drabkin H, et al. Expression of VEGF, semaphorin SEMA3F, and their common receptors neuropilins NP1 and NP2 in preinvasive bronchial lesions, lung tumours, and cell lines. J Pathol 2003;200:336–47.

249. Donnem T, Al Saad S, Al Shibli K, et al. Inverse prognostic impact of angiogenic marker expression in tumor cells versus stromal cells in non small cell lung cancer. Clin Cancer Res 2007;13:6649–57.

250. Nakashini Y, Mulshine JL, Kasprzyk PG, et al. Insulin-like growth factor-1 can mediate autocrine proliferation of human small cell lung cancer cell lines. J Clin Invest 1988;82:354–9.

251. Vostrejs M, Moran PL, Seligman PA. Transferrin synthesis by small cell lung cancer acts as an autocrine regulator of cellular proliferation. J Clin Invest 1988;82:331–9.

252. Hamid Q, Bishop A, Springall D, et al. Detection of human pro-bombesin mRNA in neuroendocrine (small cell) carcinoma of the lung. Cancer 1989;63:266–71.

253. Giaid A, Hamid QA, Springall DR, et al. Detection of endothelin immunoreactivity and mRNA in pulmonary tumours. J Pathol 1990;162:15–22.

254. Hamid QA, Corrin B, Dewar A, et al. Expression of gastrin-releasing peptide (human bombesin) gene in large cell undifferentiated carcinoma of the lung. J Pathol 1990;161:145–51.

255. Bach PB, Kelley MJ, Tate RC, et al. Screening for lung cancer – A review of the current literature. Chest 2003;123:72S–82S.

256. Manser RL, Irving LB, Byrnes G, et al. Screening for lung cancer: a systematic review and meta-analysis of controlled trials. Thorax 2003;58:784–9.

257. Bach PB, Silvestri GA, Hanger M, et al. Screening for lung cancer: ACCP evidence-based clinical practice guidelines (2nd edition). Chest 2007;132:69S–77S.

258. Geddes DM. The natural history of lung cancer: a review based on rates of tumour growth. Br J Dis Chest 1979;73:1–17.

259. Belinsky SA, Palmisano WA, Gilliland FD, et al. Aberrant promoter methylation in bronchial epithelium and sputum from current and former smokers. Cancer Res 2002;62:2370–7.

260. Palmisano WA, Divine KK, Saccomanno G, et al. Predicting lung cancer by detecting aberrant promoter methylation in sputum. Cancer Res 2000;60:5954–8.

261. Simpson NK, Johnson CC, Ogden SL, et al. Recruitment strategies in the Prostate, Lung, Colorectal and Ovarian (PLCO) Cancer Screening Trial: the first six years. Control Clin Trials 2000;21:356S–78S.

262. Henschke CI, Naidich DP, Yankelevitz DF, et al. Early lung cancer action project: initial findings on repeat screenings. Cancer 2001;92:153–9.

263. Henschke CI, Yankelevitz DF, Mirtcheva R, et al. CT screening for lung cancer: frequency and significance of part-solid and nonsolid nodules. Am J Roentgenol 2002;178:1053–7.

264. Henschke CI, Yankelevitz DF, McCauley D, et al. CT screening for lung cancer. Cancer Chemother Biol Response Modif 2002;20:665–76.

265. Sagawa M, Nakayama T, Tsukada H, et al. The efficacy of lung cancer screening conducted in 1990s: four case-control studies in Japan. Lung Cancer 2003;41:29–36.

266. Bach PB, Niewoehner DE, Black WC. Screening for lung cancer: the guidelines. Chest 2003;123:83S–8S.

267. Yamato Y, Tsuchida M, Watanabe T, et al. Early results of a prospective study of limited resection for bronchioloalveolar adenocarcinoma of the lung. The Annals of Thoracic Surgery 2001;71:971–4.

268. Kodama K, Higashiyama M, Yokouchi H, et al. Prognostic value of ground-glass opacity found in small lung adenocarcinoma on high-resolution CT scanning. Lung Cancer 2001;33:17–25.

269. Watanabe Si, Watanabe T, Arai K, et al. Results of wedge resection for focal bronchioloalveolar carcinoma showing pure ground-glass attenuation on computed tomography. The Annals of Thoracic Surgery 2002;73:1071–5.

270. Suzuki K, Asamura H, Kusumoto M, et al. 'Early' peripheral lung cancer: prognostic significance of ground glass opacity on thin-section computed tomographic scan. The Annals of Thoracic Surgery 2002;74:1635–9.

Site of origin and spread

271. Walter JB, Pryce DM. The site of origin of lung cancer and its relation to histological type. Thorax 1955;10:107–26.

272. Kerr IH. Radiological assessment. Recent Results Cancer Res 1984;92:30–42.

273. Auerbach O, Garfinkel L. The changing pattern of lung carcinoma. Cancer 1991;68:1973–7.

274. Quinn D, Gianlupi A, Broste S. The changing radiographic presentation of bronchogenic carcinoma with reference to cell types. Chest 1996;110:1474–9.

275. Iravani J, van As A. Mucus transport in the tracheobronchial tree of normal and bronchitic rats. J Pathol 1972;106:81–93.

276. Hilding AC. Ciliary streaming in the bronchial tree and the time element in carcinogenesis. N Engl J Med 1957;256:634–40.

277. Churg A, Vedal S. Carinal and tubular airway particle concentrations in the large airways of non-smokers in the general population: evidence for high particle concentration at airway carinas. Occup Environ Med 1996;53:553–8.

278. Salm R. Primary carcinoma of the trachea: a review. Br J Dis Chest 1964;58:61–72.

279. Gelder CM, Hetzel MR. Primary tracheal tumours – a national survey. Thorax 1993;48:688–92.

Clinical effects

280. MacMahon H, Austin JH, Gamsu G, et al. Guidelines for management of small pulmonary nodules detected on CT scans: a statement from the Fleischner Society. Radiology 2005;237:395–400.

281. Edey AJ, Hansell DM. Incidentally detected small pulmonary nodules on CT. Clin Radiol 2009;64:872–84.

282. Baldwin DR, Eaton T, Kolbe J, et al. Management of solitary pulmonary nodules: how do thoracic computed tomography and guided fine needle biopsy influence clinical decisions? Thorax 2002;57:817–22.

283. Khokhar S, Vickers A, Moore MS, et al. Significance of non-calcified pulmonary nodules in patients with extrapulmonary cancers. Thorax 2006;61:331–6.

284. Hare ES. Tumour involving certain nerves. London Medical Gazette 1838;23:16.

285. Pancoast HK. Superior pulmonary sulcus tumor: tumor characterized by pain, Horner's syndrome, destruction of bone and atrophy of hand muscles. JAMA 1932;99:1391–6.

286. Arcasoy SM, Jett JR. Current concept: Superior pulmonary sulcus tumors and Pancoast's syndrome. N Engl J Med 1997;337:1370–6.

287. Matthews MJ. Problems in morphology and behavior of bronchopulmonary malignant disease. In: Israel L, Chahinain P, editors. Lung cancer natural history, prognosis and therapy. New York: Academic Press; 1976. p. 23–62.

288. Gomm SA, Thatcher N, Barber PV, et al. A clinicopathological study of the paraneoplastic neuromuscular syndromes associated with lung cancer. Q J Med 1990;75:577–95.

289. Antoine JC, Mosnier JF, Absi L, et al. Carcinoma associated paraneoplastic peripheral neuropathies in patients with and without anti-onconeural antibodies. J Neurol Neurosurg Psychiatry 1999;67:7–14.

290. Bohan A, Peter JB. Polymyositis and dermatomyositis. N Engl J Med 1975;293:344–7.

291. Lambert–Eaton myasthenic syndrome. Semin Immunol 1985;8:129–40.

292. Kiers L, Altermatt HJ, Lennon VA. Paraneoplastic anti-neuronal nuclear IgG autoantibodies (type-I) localize antigen in small cell lung carcinoma. Mayo Clin Proc 1991;66:1209–16.

293. Grunwald GB, Klein R, Simmonds M, et al. Autoimmune basis for visual paraneoplastic syndrome in patients with small cell lung cancer. Lancet 1985;i:658–61.

294. Levine RJ, Metz SA. A classification of ectopic hormone-producing tumors. Ann N Y Acad Sci 1974;230:533–46.

295. De Troyer A, Demaner JC. Clinical, biological and pathogenic features of the syndrome of inappropriate secretion of ADH. Q J Med 1976;45:521–31.

296. Imura H, Matsukura S, Yamamoto H. Studies on ectopic ACTH-producing tumors. Cancer 1975;35:1430–7.

297. Campling BG, Sarda IR, Baer KA, et al. Secretion of atrial natriuretic peptide and vasopressin by small cell lung cancer. Cancer 1995;75:2442–51.

298. Salyer DC, Eggleston JC. Oat cell carcinoma of the bronchus and the carcinoid syndrome. Arch Pathol 1975;99:513–15.

299. Davidson LA, Black M, Carey FA, et al. Lung tumours immunoreactive for parathyroid hormone related peptide: analysis of serum calcium levels and tumour type. J Pathol 1996;178:398–401.

300. Yoshida Y, Mori M, Sonoda T, et al. Ultrastructural, immunohistochemical and biochemical studies on amylase and ACTH producing lung cancer. Virchows Arch A Pathol Anat Histopathol 1985;408:163–72.

301. Boucher LD, Yoneda K. The expression of trophoblastic cell markers by lung carcinomas. Hum Pathol 1995;26:1201–6.

302. Hiroshima K, Iyoda A, Toyozaki T, et al. Alpha-fetoprotein-producing lung carcinoma: report of three cases. Pathol Int 2002;52:46–53.

303. Carrier M, Le GG, Wells PS, et al. Systematic review: the Trousseau syndrome revisited: should we screen extensively for cancer in patients with venous thromboembolism? Ann Intern Med 2008;149:323–33.

304. Sawyers CL, Golde DW, Quan S, et al. Production of granulocyte-macrophage colony-stimulating factor in two patients with lung cancer, leukocytosis, and eosinophilia. Cancer 1992;69:1342–6.

305. Johnson RL, Donnell RM. Diffuse granulocytic infiltration of giant cell carcinoma of the lung: a distinctive histologic finding with clinical significance. Lab Invest 1979;40:262.

306. Ascensao JL, Oken MM, Ewing SL, et al. Leukocytosis and large cell lung cancer. A frequent association. Cancer 1987;60:903–5.

307. Adachi N, Yamaguchi K, Morikawa T, et al. Constitutive production of multiple colony-stimulating factors in patients with lung cancer associated with neutrophilia. Br J Cancer 1994;69:125–9.

308. Boon ES, Vrij AA, Nieuwhof C, et al. Small cell lung cancer with paraneoplastic nephrotic syndrome. Eur Respir J 1994;7:1192–3.

309. Ponge T, Boutoille D, Moreau A, et al. Systemic vasculitis in a patient with small-cell neuroendocrine bronchial cancer. Eur Resp J 1998;12:1228–9.

310. Pipkin CA, Lio PA. Cutaneous manifestations of internal malignancies: an overview. Dermatol Clin 2008;26: 1–15, vii.

311. Moore RL, Devere TS. Epidermal manifestations of internal malignancy. Dermatol Clin 2008;26:17–29, vii.

311a. Shah PL, Singh S, Bower M, et al. The role of transbronchial fine needle aspiration in an integrated care pathway for the assessment of patients with suspected lung cancer. J Thorac Oncol 2006;1:324–7.

311b. Wallace WAH, Monaghan HM, Salter DM, et al. Endobronchial ultrasound guided fine-needle aspiration and liquid-based thin-layer cytology. J Clin Pathol 2007;60:388–91.

311c. Natu S, Hoffman J, Siddiqui M, et al. The role of endobronchial ultrasound guided transbronchial needle aspiration cytology in the investigation of mediastinal lymphadenopathy and masses, the North Tees experience. J Clin Pathol 2010;63:445–51.

Diagnostic procedures for obtaining tumour material

312. Oswald NC, Hinson KFW, Canti G, et al. The diagnosis of primary lung cancer with special reference to sputum cytology. Thorax 1971;26:623–31.

313. Tang CS, Tang CMC, Lau YY, et al. Sensitivity of sputum cytology after homogenization with dithiothreitol in lung cancer detection – two years of experience. Acta Cytol 1995;39:1137–40.

314. Evans DMD, Shelley G. Respiratory cytodiagnosis: study in observer variation and its relation to quality of material. Thorax 1982;37:259–63.

315. Mennemeyer R, Hammar SP, Bauermeister DE, et al. Cytologic, histologic and electron microscopic correlations in poorly differentiated primary lung carcinoma. Study of 43 cases. Acta Cytol 1979;23:297–302.

316. Reichenberger F, Weber J, Tamm M, et al. The value of transbronchial needle aspiration in the diagnosis of peripheral pulmonary lesions. Chest 1999;116:704–8.

317. Hermens FHW, VanEngelenburg TCA, Visser FJ, et al. Diagnostic yield of transbronchial histology needle aspiration in patients with mediastinal lymph node enlargement. Respiration 2003;70:631–5.

318. Shah PL, Singh S, Bower M, et al. The role of transbronchial fine needle aspiration in an integrated care pathway for the assessment of patients with suspected lung cancer. J Thorac Oncol 2006;1:324–7.

319. Govert JA, Kopita JM, Matchar D, et al. Cost-effectiveness of collecting routine cytologic specimens during fiberoptic bronchoscopy for endoscopically visible lung tumor. Chest 1996;109:451–6.

320. Sato M, Saito Y, Nagamoto N, et al. Diagnostic value of differential brushing of all branches of the bronchi in patients with sputum positive or suspected positive for lung cancer. Acta Cytol 1993;37:879–83.

321. Pirozynski M. Bronchoalveolar lavage in the diagnosis of peripheral, primary lung cancer. Chest 1992;102:372–4.

322. Bilaceroglu S, Cagirici U, Gunel O, et al. Comparison of rigid and flexible transbronchial needle aspiration in the staging of bronchogenic carcinoma. Respiration 1998;65:441–9.

323. Chin R, McCain TW, Lucia MA, et al. Transbronchial needle aspiration in diagnosing and staging lung cancer – How many aspirates are needed? Amer J Respir Crit Care Med 2002;166:377–81.

324. Popovich J, Kvale PA, Eichenhorn MS, et al. Diagnostic accuracy of multiple biopsies from flexible fiberoptic bronchoscopy. A comparison of central versus peripheral carcinoma. Am Rev Respir Dis 1982;125:521–3.

325. Thomas JSJ, Lamb D, Ashcroft T, et al. How reliable is the diagnosis of lung cancer using small biopsy specimens? Report of a UKCCCR lung cancer working party. Thorax 1993;48:1135–9.

326. Chuang MT, Marchevsky A, Teirstein A, et al. Diagnosis of lung cancer by fibreoptic bronchoscopy: problems in the histological classification of non-small carcinomas. Thorax 1984;39:175–8.

327. Edwards SL, Roberts C, McKean ME, et al. Preoperative histological classification of primary lung cancer: accuracy of diagnosis and use of the non-small cell category. J Clin Pathol 2000;53:537–40.

328. Wallace WA. The challenge of classifying poorly differentiated tumours in the lung. Histopathology 2009;54:28–42.

329. Yoneda K, Boucher LD. Bronchial epithelial changes associated with small cell carcinoma of the lung. Hum Pathol 1993;24:1180–3.

Histological typing

330. Dunnill MS, Gatter KC. Cellular heterogeneity in lung cancer. Histopathology 1986;10:461–75.

331. Walter JB, Pryce DM. The frequency of differentiation in oat-cell carcinoma of the lung. J Pathol Bacteriol 1960;80:121–5.

332. Yesner R. The dynamic histopathologic spectrum of lung cancer. Yale J Biol Med 1981;54:447–56.

333. Roggli VL, Vollmer RT, Greenberg SD, et al. Lung cancer heterogeneity: a blinded and randomized study of 100 consecutive cases. Hum Pathol 1985;16:569–79.

334. Bombi JA, Martinez A, Ramirez J, et al. Ultrastructural and molecular heterogeneity in non-small cell lung carcinomas: Study of 110 cases and review of the literature. Ultrastruct Pathol 2002;26:211–18.

335. Fellegara G, D'Adda T, Pilato F, et al. Genetics of a combined lung small cell carcinoma and large cell neuroendocrine carcinoma with adenocarcinoma. Virchows Archiv 2008;453:107–15.

336. Begin P, Sahai S, Wang N-S. Giant cell formation in small cell carcinoma of the lung. Cancer 1983;52:1875–9.

337. Willis RA. Pathology of Tumours. 4th ed. London: Butterworths; 1967.

338. Horie A, Ohta M. Ultrastructural features of large cell carcinoma of the lung with reference to the prognosis of patients. Hum Pathol 1981;12:423–32.

339. Albain KS, True LD, Golomb HM, et al. Large cell carcinoma of the lung. Ultrastructural differentiation and clinicopathologic correlations. Cancer 1985;56:1618–23.

340. Mooi WJ, van Zandwijk N, Dingemans KP, et al. The 'grey area' between small cell and non-small cell lung carcinomas: light and electron microscopy versus clinical data in 14 cases. J Pathol 1986;149:49–54.

341. Johansson L. Histopathologic classification of lung cancer: Relevance of cytokeratin and TTF-1 immunophenotyping. Ann Diagn Pathol 2004;8:259–67.

342. Johnson DH, Fehrenbacher L, Novotny WF, et al. Randomized phase II trial comparing bevacizumab plus carboplatin and paclitaxel with carboplatin and paclitaxel alone in previously untreated locally advanced or metastatic non-small-cell lung cancer. J Clin Oncol 2004;22:2184–91.

343. Scagliotti GV, Germonpre P, Bosquee L, et al. A randomized phase II study of bortezomib and pemetrexed, in combination or alone, in patients with previously treated advanced non-small-cell lung cancer. Lung Cancer 2009;68:420–6.

344. Mok TS, Wu YL, Thongprasert S, et al. Gefitinib or carboplatin-paclitaxel in pulmonary adenocarcinoma. N Engl J Med 2009;361:947–57.

345. Ring BZ, Seitz RS, Beck RA, et al. A novel five-antibody immunohistochemical test for subclassification of lung carcinoma. Mod Pathol 2009;22:1032–43.

346. Yesner R, Gerstl B, Auerbach O. Application of the World Health Organization classification of lung carcinoma to biopsy material. Ann Thorac Surg 1965;1:33–45.

347. Kannerstein M, Churg J. Pathology of carcinoma of the lung associated with asbestos exposure. Cancer 1972;30:14–21.

348. Mountain CF, Carr DT, Anderson WAD. A system for the clinical staging of lung cancer. Am J Roentgenol 1974;120:130–8.

349. Feinstein AR, Gelfman NA, Yesner RA. The diverse effects of histopathology on manifestations and outcome of lung cancer. Chest 1974;66:225–9.

350. Matthews MJ, Gordon PR. Morphology of pulmonary and pleural malignancies. In: Strauss MJ, editor. Lung cancer: clinical diagnosis and treatment. New York: Grune and Stratton; 1977. p. 49–69.

351. Huhti E, Sutinen S, Reinila A, et al. Lung cancer in a defined geographical area: history and histological types. Thorax 1980;35:660–7.

352. Johnston WW. Histologic and cytologic patterns of lung cancer in 2580 men and women over a 15-year period. Acta Cytol 1987;32:163–8.

353. Edinburgh Lung Cancer Group. Patients presenting with lung cancer in South East Scotland. Thorax 1987;42:853–7.

354. Valaitis J, Warren S, Gamble D. Increasing incidence of adenocarcinoma of the lung. Cancer 1981;47:1042–6.

355. Barsky SH, Cameron R, Osann KE, et al. Rising incidence of bronchioloalveolar lung carcinoma and its unique clinicopathologic features. Cancer 1994;73:1163–70.

356. Zheng TZ, Holford TR, Boyle P, et al. Time trend and the age-period-cohort effect on the incidence of histologic types of lung cancer in Connecticut, 1960–1989. Cancer 1994;74:1556–67.

357. Travis WD, Travis LB, Devesa SS. Lung cancer. Cancer 1995;75:191–202.

358. McDowell EM, McLaughlin JS, Merenyl DK, et al. The respiratory epithelium. V. Histogenesis of lung carcinomas in the human. J Natl Cancer Inst 1978;61:587–606.

359. Carter N, Nelson F, Gosney JR. Ultrastructural heterogeneity in undifferentiated bronchial carcinoma. J Pathol 1993;171:53–7.

360. Keehn R, Auerbach O, Nambu S, et al. Reproducibility of major diagnoses in a binational study of lung cancer in uranium miners and atomic bomb survivors. Am J Clin Pathol 1994;101:478–82.

361. Sorensen JB, Hirsch FR, Gazdar A, et al. Interobserver variability in histopathologic subtyping and grading of pulmonary adenocarcinoma. Cancer 1993;71:2971–6.

362. Burnett RA, Howatson SR, Lang S, et al. Observer variability in histopathological reporting of non-small cell lung carcinoma on bronchial biopsy specimens. J Clin Pathol 1996;49:130–3.

363. Barbone F, Bovenzi M, Cavallieri F, et al. Cigarette smoking and histologic type of lung cancer in men. Chest 1997;112:1474–9.

364. Stellman SD, Muscat JE, Thompson S, et al. Risk of squamous cell carcinoma and adenocarcinoma of the lung in relation to lifetime filter cigarette smoking. Cancer 1997;80:382–8.

365. Coutts II, Gilson JC, Kerr IH, et al. Mortality in cases of asbestosis diagnosed by a pneumoconiosis medical panel. Thorax 1987;42:111–16.

366. Caldwell CJ, Berry CL. Is the incidence of primary adenocarcinoma of the lung increasing? Virchows Arch 1996;429:359–63.

367. Vincent RG, Pickren JW, Lane WW. The changing histopathology of lung cancer: a review of 1682 cases. Cancer 1977;39:1647–55.

368. Lam KY, Fu KH, Wong MP, et al. Significant changes in the distribution of histologic types of lung cancer in Hong-Kong. Pathology 1993;25:103–5.

369. Levi F, Franceschi S, LaVecchia C, et al. Lung carcinoma trends by histologic type in Vaud and Neuchatel, Switzerland, 1974–1994. Cancer 1997;79:906–14.

Squamous cell carcinoma

370. Yousem SA. Peripheral squamous cell carcinoma of lung: patterns of growth with particular focus on airspace filling. Human Pathology 2009;40:861–7.

371. Flanagan P, McCracken AW, Cross RMP. Squamous carcinoma of the lung with osteocartilaginous stroma. J Clin Pathol 1965;18:403–7.

372. Nappi O, Swanson PE, Wick MR. Pseudovascular adenoid squamous cell carcinoma of the lung: clinicopathologic study of three cases and comparison with true pleuropulmonary angiosarcoma. Hum Pathol 1994;25:373–8.

373. GarciaEscudero A, NavarroBustos G, JuradoEscamez P, et al. Primary squamous cell carcinoma of the lung with pilomatricoma-like features. Histopathology 2002;40:201–2.

374. Flieder DB, Koss MN, Nicholson A, et al. Solitary pulmonary papillomas in adults: A clinicopathologic and in situ hybridization study of 14 cases combined with 27 cases in the literature. Am J Surg Pathol 1998;22:1328–42.

375. Dulmet-Brender E, Jaubert F, Huchon G. Exophytic endobronchial epidermoid carcinoma. Cancer 1986;57:1358–64.

376. Katzenstein A-L, Prioleau PG, Askin FB. The histologic spectrum and significance of clear-cell change in lung carcinoma. Cancer 1980;45:943–7.

377. Churg A, Johnston WH, Stulbarg M. Small cell squamous and mixed small cell squamous-small cell anaplastic carcinomas of the lung. Am J Surg Pathol 1980;4:255–63.

378. Lin O, Harkin TJ, Jagirdar J. Basaloid-squamous cell carcinoma of the bronchus: report of a case with review of the literature. Arch Pathol Lab Med 1995;119:1167–70.

379. Brambilla E, Moro D, Veale D, et al. Basal cell (basaloid) carcinoma of the lung – a new morphologic and phenotypic entity with separate prognostic significance. Hum Pathol 1992;23:993–1003.

380. Moro D, Brichon PY, Brambilla E, et al. Basaloid bronchial carcinoma – a histologic group with a poor prognosis. Cancer 1994;73:2734–9.

381. Moro-Sibilot D, Lantuejoul S, Diab S, et al. Lung carcinomas with a basaloid pattern: a study of 90 cases focusing on their poor prognosis. Eur Respir J 2008;31:854–9.

382. Kim DJ, Kim KD, Shin DH, et al. Basaloid carcinoma of the lung: a really dismal histologic variant? Ann Thorac Surg 2003;76:1833–7.

383. Said JW, Nash G, Banks-Schlegel S, et al. Keratin in human lung tumors. Patterns of localization of different-molecular-weight keratin proteins. Am J Pathol 1983;113:27–31.

384. Wilson TS, McDowell EM, McIntire R, et al. Elaboration of human chorionic gonadotropin by lung tumors. Arch Pathol Lab Med 1981;105:169–73.

385. Miyake M, Ito M, Mitsuoka A, et al. Alpha-fetoprotein and human chorionic gonadotropin-producing lung cancer. Cancer 1987;59:227–32.

386. Dirnhofer S, Freund M, Rogatsch H, et al. Selective expression of trophoblastic hormones by lung carcinoma: Neurendocrine tumors exclusively produce human chorionic gonadotropin alpha-subunit (HCG alpha). Hum Pathol 2000;31:966–72.

387. Savci-Heijink CD, Kosari F, Aubry MC, et al. The role of desmoglein-3 in the diagnosis of squamous cell carcinoma of the lung. Am J Pathol 2009;174: 1629–37.

388. Wu M, Wang B, Gil J, et al. p63 and TTF-1 immunostaining. A useful marker panel for distinguishing small cell carcinoma of lung from poorly differentiated squamous cell carcinoma of lung. Am J Clin Pathol 2003;119:696–702.

389. Kargi A, Gurel D, Tuna B. The diagnostic value of TTF-1, CK 5/6, and p63 immunostaining in classification of lung carcinomas. Appl Immunohistochem Mol Morphol 2007;15:415–20.

390. Dingemans KP, Mooi WJ. Ultrastructure of squamous cell carcinoma of the lung. Pathol Annu 1984;19:249–73.

391. Romagosa V, Bella MR, Truchero C, et al. Necrotizing sialometaplasia (adenometaplasia) of the trachea. Histopathology 1992;21:280–2.

392. Littman CD. Necrotizing sialometaplasia (adenometaplasia) of the trachea. Histopathology 1993;22:298–9.

Adenocarcinoma

393. Zang EA, Wynder EL. Cumulative tar exposure – a new index for estimating lung cancer risk among cigarette smokers. Cancer 1992;70:69–76.

394. Bourke W, Milstein D, Giura R, et al. Lung cancer in young adults. Chest 1992;102:1723–9.

395. Kodama T, Shimosato Y, Kameya T. Histology and ultrastructure of bronchogenic and bronchial gland adenocarcinomas (including adenoid cystic and mucoepidermoid carcinomas) in relation to histogenesis. In: Shimosato Y, Melamed MR, Nettesheim P, editors. Morphogenesis of Lung Cancer. Boca Raton, Florida: CRC Press; 1982. p. 147–66.

396. Edwards CW. Pulmonary adenocarcinoma: review of 106 cases and proposed new classification. J Clin Pathol 1987;40:125–35.

397. Yatabe Y, Kosaka T, Takahashi T, et al. EGFR mutation is specific for terminal respiratory unit type adenocarcinoma. Am J Surg Pathol 2005;29:633–9.

398. Harwood TR, Gracey DR, Yokoo H. Pseudomesotheliomatous carcinoma of the lung – a variant of peripheral lung cancer. Am J Clin Pathol 1976;65: 159–67.

399. Moran CA, Jagirdar J, Suster S. Papillary lung carcinoma with prominent 'morular' component. Am J Clin Pathol 2004;122:106–9.

400. Amin MB, Tamboli P, Merchant SH, et al. Micropapillary component in lung adenocarcinoma – A distinctive histologic feature with possible prognostic significance. Am J Surg Pathol 2002;26:358–64.

401. Steinhauer JR, Moran CA, Suster S. 'Secretory endometrioid-like' adenocarcinoma of the lung. Histopathology 2005;47:219–20.

402. Tsuta K, Ishii G, Kim E, et al. Primary lung adenocarcinoma with massive lymphocyte infiltration. Am J Clin Pathol 2005;123:547–52.

403. Marci V, Volante M, Cappia S, et al. Basaloid adenocarcinoma. A new variant of pulmonary adenocarcinoma. Virchows Arch 2007;451:729–36.

404. Tsao MS, Fraser RS. Primary pulmonary adenocarcinoma with enteric differentiation. Cancer 1991;68:1754–7.

405. Inamura K, Satoh Y, Okumura S, et al. Pulmonary adenocarcinomas with enteric differentiation: histologic and immunohistochemical characteristics compared with metastatic colorectal cancers and usual pulmonary adenocarcinomas. Am J Surg Pathol 2005;29:660–5.

406. Yousem SA. Pulmonary intestinal-type adenocarcinoma does not show enteric differentiation by immunohistochemical study. Mod Pathol 2005;18:816–21.

407. Yim J, Zhu LC, Chiriboga L, et al. Histologic features are important prognostic indicators in early stages lung adenocarcinomas. Mod Pathol 2007;20:233–41.

408. Alvarez-Fernandez E. Alveolar trapping in pulmonary carcinomas. Diag Histopathol 1982;5:59–64.

409. Silver SA, Askin FB. True papillary carcinoma of the lung: a distinct clinicopathologic entity. Am J Surg Pathol 1997;21:43–51.

410. Miyoshi T, Satoh Y, Okumura S, et al. Early-stage lung adenocarcinomas with a micropapillary pattern, a distinct pathologic marker for a significantly poor prognosis. Amer J Surg Pathol 2003;27:101–9.

411. Roh MS, Lee JI, Choi PJ, et al. Relationship between micropapillary component and micrometastasis in the regional lymph nodes of patients with stage I lung adenocarcinoma. Histopathology 2004;45:580–6.

412. Makimoto Y, Nabeshima K, Iwasaki H, et al. Micropapillary pattern: a distinct pathological marker to subclassify tumours with a significantly poor prognosis within small peripheral lung adenocarcinoma (</=20 mm) with mixed bronchioloalveolar and invasive subtypes (Noguchi's type C tumours). Histopathology 2005;46:677–84.

413. Kamiya K, Hayashi Y, Douguchi J, et al. Histopathological features and prognostic significance of the micropapillary pattern in lung adenocarcinoma. Mod Pathol 2008;21:992–1001.

414. De Oliveira Duarte Achcar R, Nikiforova MN, Yousem SA. Micropapillary lung adenocarcinoma. Am J Clini Pathol 2009;131:694–700.

415. Kradin RL, Young RH, Dickerson GR, et al. Pulmonary blastoma with argyrophil cells and lacking sarcomatous features (pulmonary endodermal tumour resembling fetal lung). Am J Surg Pathol 1982;6:165–72.

416. Kodama T, Shimosato Y, Watanabe S, et al. Six cases of well-differentiated adenocarcinoma simulating fetal lung tubules in pseudoglandular stage: comparison with pulmonary blastoma. Am J Surg Pathol 1984;8:735–44.

417. Nakatani Y, Dickersin GR, Mark EJ. Pulmonary endodermal tumor resembling fetal lung – a clinicopathologic study of five cases with immunohistochemical and ultrastructural characterization. Hum Pathol 1990;21:1097–107.

418. Nakatani Y, Kitamura H, Inayama Y, et al. Pulmonary adenocarcinomas of the fetal lung type: A clinicopathologic study indicating differences in histology, epidemiology, and natural history of low-grade and high-grade forms. Am J Surg Pathol 1998;22:399–411.

419. Mardini G, Pai U, Chavez AM, et al. Endobronchial adenocarcinoma with endometrioid features and prominent neuroendocrine differentiation – a variant of fetal adenocarcinoma. Cancer 1994;73:1383–9.

420. Babycos PB, Daroca PJ. Polypoid pulmonary endodermal tumor resembling fetal lung: report of a case. Mod Pathol 1995;8:303–6.

421. Nakatani Y, Kitamura H, Inayama Y, et al. Pulmonary endodermal tumor resembling fetal lung – the optically clear nucleus is rich in biotin. Am J Surg Pathol 1994;18:637–42.

422. Yang P, Morizumi H, Sano T, et al. Pulmonary blastoma: an ultrastructural and immunohistochemical study with special reference to nuclear filament aggregation. Ultrastruct Pathol 1995;19:501–9.

423. Sekine S, Shibata T, Matsuno Y, et al. Beta-catenin mutations in pulmonary blastomas: association with morule formation. J Pathol 2003;200:214–21.

424. Makishi S, Kinjo T, Sawada S, et al. Morules and morule-like features associated with carcinomas in various organs: report with immunohistochemical and molecular studies. J Clin Pathol 2006;59:95–100.

425. Herrera GA, Alexander B, DeMoraes HP. Ultrastructural subtypes of pulmonary adenocarcinoma. A correlation with patient survival. Chest 1983;84:581–6.

426. Herrera GA, Turbat-Herrera EA, Alexander CB. Ultrastructural heterogeneity of pulmonary scar adenocarcinomas: correlation with patients' survival. Ultrastruct Pathol 1988;12:265–77.

427. Kodama T, Kameya T, Shimosato Y, et al. Cell incohesiveness and pattern of extension in a rare case of bronchioloalveolar carcinoma. Ultrastruct Pathol 1980;1:177–88.

428. Holst VA, Finkelstein S, Yousem SA. Bronchioloalveolar adenocarcinoma of lung: Monoclonal origin for multifocal disease. Am J Surg Pathol 1998;22:1343–50.

429. Hewer TF. The metastatic origin of alveolar cell tumour of the lung. J Pathol Bacteriol 1961;81:323–30.

430. Rosenblatt MB, Lisa JR, Collier F. Primary and metastatic bronchiolo-alveolar carcinoma. Dis Chest 1967;52:147–52.

431. Kish JK, Ro JY, Ayala AG, et al. Primary mucinous adenocarcinoma of the lung with signet-ring cells. Hum Pathol 1989;20:1097–102.

432. Hayashi H, Kitamura H, Nakatani Y, et al. Primary signet-ring cell carcinoma of the lung: Histochemical and immunohistochemical characterization. Hum Pathol 1999;30:378–83.

433. Castro CY, Moran CA, Flieder DG, et al. Primary signet ring cell adenocarcinomas of the lung: a clinicopathological study of 15 cases. Histopathology 2001;39:397–401.

434. Merchant SH, Amin MB, Tamboli P, et al. Primary signet-ring cell carcinoma of lung: immunohistochemical study and comparison with non-pulmonary

signet-ring cell carcinomas. Am J Surg Pathol 2001;25:1515–19.

435. Tsuta K, Ishii G, Yoh K, et al. Primary lung carcinoma with signet-ring cell carcinoma components: clinicopathological analysis of 39 cases. Am J Surg Pathol 2004;28:868–74.

436. Tsuta K, Ishii G, Nitadori J, et al. Comparison of the immunophenotypes of signet-ring cell carcinoma, solid adenocarcinoma with mucin production, and mucinous bronchioloalveolar carcinoma of the lung characterized by the presence of cytoplasmic mucin. J Pathol 2006;209:78–87.

437. Iwasaki T, Ohta M, Lefor AT, et al. Signet-ring cell carcinoma component in primary lung adenocarcinoma: potential prognostic factor. Histopathology 2008;52:639–40.

438. Moran CA, Hochholzer L, Fishback N, et al. Mucinous (so-called colloid) carcinomas of lung. Mod Pathol 1992;5:634–8.

439. Rossi G, Murer B, Cavazza A, et al. Primary mucinous (So-called colloid) carcinomas of the lung – A clinicopathologic and immunohistochemical study with special reference to CDX-2 homeobox gene and MUC2 expression. Am J Surg Pathol 2004;28:442–52.

440. Graeme-Cook F, Mark EJ. Pulmonary mucinous cystic tumors of borderline malignancy. Hum Pathol 1991;22:185–90.

441. Davison AM, Lowe JW, DaCosta P. Adenocarcinoma arising in a mucinous cystadenoma of the lung. Thorax 1992;47:129–30.

442. Dixon AY, Moran JF, Wesselius LJ, et al. Pulmonary mucinous cystic tumor – case report with review of the literature. Am J Surg Pathol 1993;17:722–8.

443. Kragel PJ, Devaney KO, Meth BM, et al. Mucinous cystadenoma of the lung. A report of two cases with immunohistochemical and ultrastructural analysis. Arch Pathol Lab Med 1990;114:1053–6.

444. Roux FJ, Lantuejoul S, Brambilla E, et al. Mucinous cystadenoma of the lung. Cancer 1995;76:1540–4.

445. Gowar FJS. An unusual mucous cyst of the lung. Thorax 1978;33:796–9.

446. Tan DF, Li Q, Deeb G, et al. Thyroid transcription factor-1 expression prevalence and its clinical implications in non-small cell lung cancer: A high-throughput tissue microarray and immunohistochemistry study. Hum Pathol 2003;34:597–604.

447. Kimula Y. A histochemical and ultrastructural study of adenocarcinoma of the lung. Am J Surg Pathol 1978;2:253–64.

448. Marcus PB, Martin JH, Green RH, et al. Glycocalyceal bodies and microvillous core rootlets, their value in tumour typing. Arch Pathol Lab Med 1979;103:89–92.

449. Weidner N. Intriguing case – pulmonary adenocarcinoma with intestinal- type differentiation. Ultrastruct Pathol 1992;16:7–10.

450. Tsutahara S, Shijubo N, Hirasawa M, et al. Lung adenocarcinoma with type-II pneumocyte characteristics. Eur Respir J 1993;6:135–7.

451. Dekmezian R, Ordonez NG, Mackay B. Bronchioloalveolar adenocarcinoma with myoepithelial cells. Cancer 1991;57:2356–60.

452. Hiroshima K, Toyozaki T, Iyoda A, et al. Ultrastructural study of intranuclear inclusion bodies of pulmonary adenocarcinoma. Ultrastruct Pathol 1999;23:383–9.

453. Tsumuraya M, Kodama T, Kameya T, et al. Light and electron microscopic analysis of intranuclear inclusions in papillary adenocarcinoma of the lung. Acta Cytol 1981;25:523–32.

454. Ladanyi M, Pao W. Lung adenocarcinoma: guiding EGFR-targeted therapy and beyond. Mod Pathol 2008;21:S16–22.

455. Shigematsu H, Gazdar AF. Somatic mutations of epidermal growth factor receptor signaling pathway in lung cancers. Int J Cancer 2006;118:257–62.

Small cell carcinoma

456. Souhami RL, Law K. Longevity in small cell lung cancer – A report to the Lung Cancer Subcommittee of the United Kingdom Coordinating Committee for Cancer Research. Br J Cancer 1990;61:584–9.

457. Shore DF, Paneth M. Survival after resection of small cell carcinoma of the bronchus. Thorax 1980;35:819–22.

458. Prasad US, Naylor AR, Walker WS, et al. Long term survival after pulmonary resection for small cell carcinoma of the lung. Thorax 1989;44:784–7.

459. Quoix E, Fraser R, Wolkove N, et al. Small cell lung cancer presenting as a solitary pulmonary nodule. Cancer 1990;66:577–82.

460. Smit EF, Groen HJM, Timens W, et al. Surgical resection for small cell carcinoma of the lung – a retrospective study. Thorax 1994;49:20–2.

461. Shepherd FA, Crowley J, Van HP, et al. The International Association for the Study of Lung Cancer lung cancer staging project: proposals regarding the clinical staging of small cell lung cancer in the forthcoming (seventh) edition of the tumor, node, metastasis classification for lung cancer. J Thorac Oncol 2007;2:1067–77.

462. International Union Against Cancer (UICC) TNM Classification of Malignant Tumours. New York: Wiley-Liss; 2009.

463. World Health Organization. Histological Typing of Lung Tumours. 2nd ed. Geneva: World Health Organization.; 1981.

464. Hirsch FR, Osterlind K, Hansen HH. The prognostic significance of histopathologic subtyping of small cell carcinoma of the lung according to the classification of the World Health Organization. A study of 375 consecutive patients. Cancer 1983;52:2144–50.

465. Choi H, Byhardt RW, Clowry LJ, et al. The prognostic significance of histologic subtyping in small cell carcinoma of the lung. Am J Clin Oncol 1984;7:389–97.

466. Bepler G, Neumann K, Holle R, et al. Clinical relevance of histologic subtyping in small cell lung cancer. Cancer 1989;64:74–9.

467. Hirsch FR, Matthews MJ, Aisner S, et al. Histopathologic classification of small cell lung cancer. Changing concepts and terminology. Cancer 1988;62:973–7.

468. Ewing SL, Sumner HW, Ophoven JJ, et al. Small cell anaplastic carcinoma with differentiation: a report of 14 cases. Lab Invest 1980;42:115.

469. Nicholson SA, Beasley MB, Brambilla E, et al. Small cell lung carcinoma (SCLC) – A clinicopathologic study of 100 cases with surgical specimens. Am J Surg Pathol 2002;26:1184–97.

470. Azzopardi JG. Oat-cell carcinoma of the bronchus. J Pathol Bacteriol 1959;78:513–19.

471. Carter D. Small-cell carcinoma of the lung. Am J Surg Pathol 1983;7:787–95.

472. Sturgis CD, Nassar DL, DAntonio JA, et al. Cytologic features useful for distinguishing small cell from non- small cell carcinoma in bronchial brush and wash specimens. Am J Clin Pathol 2000;114:197–202.

473. Vollmer RT. The effect of cell size on the pathologic diagnosis of small and large cell carcinoma of the lung. Cancer 1982;50:1380–3.

474. Marchevsky AM, Gal AA, Shah S, et al. Morphometry confirms the presence of considerable nuclear size overlap between "small cells" and "large cells" in high-grade pulmonary neuroendocrine neoplasms. Amer J Clin Pathol 2001;116:466–72.

475. Brambilla E, Moro D, Gazzeri S, et al. Cytotoxic chemotherapy induces cell differentiation in small-cell lung carcinoma. J Clin Oncol 1991;9:50–61.

476. Yesner R. Small cell tumors of the lung. Am J Surg Pathol 1983;8:775–85.

477. Vollmer RT, Ogden L, Crissman JD. Separation of small-cell from non-small-cell lung cancer. Arch Pathol Lab Med 1984;108:792–4.

478. Maloney DJL, Morritt GN, Walbaum PR, et al. Histological features of small-cell carcinomas and survival after surgical resection. Thorax 1983;38:715.

478a. den Bakker MA, Willemsen S, Grunberg K, et al. Small cell carcinoma of the lung and large cell neuroendocrine carcinoma interobserver variability. Histopathology 2010;56:356–63.

479. Mooi WJ, Dingemans KP, van Zandwijk N. Prevalence of neuroendocrine granules in small cell lung carcinomas: usefulness of electron microscopy in lung cancer classification. J Pathol 1986;149:41–7.

480. Thunnissen FBJM, Diegenbach PC, Vanhattum AH, et al. Further evaluation of quantitative nuclear image features for classification of lung carcinomas. Pathol Res Pract 1992;188:531–5.

481. Bensch KG, Corrin B, Pariente R, et al. Oat cell carcinoma of the lung: its origin and relationship to bronchial carcinoid. Cancer 1968;22:1163–72.

482. Hattori S, Matsuda M, Tateishi R, et al. Oat-cell carcinoma of the lung containing serotonin granules. Gann 1968;59:123–9.

483. McDowell EM, Trump BF. Pulmonary small cell carcinoma showing tripartite differentiation in individual cells. Hum Pathol 1981;12:286–94.

484. Leong AS-Y, Canny AR. Small cell anaplastic carcinoma of the lung with glandular and squamous differentiation. Am J Surg Pathol 1981;5:307–9.

485. Saba SR, Azar HA, Richman AV, et al. Dual differentiation in small cell carcinoma (oat cell carcinoma) of the lung. Ultrastruct Pathol 1981;2:131–8.

486. Bolen JW, Thorning D. Histogenetic classification of lung carcinomas. Small cell carcinomas studied by light and electron microscopy. J Submicrosc Cytol Pathol 1982;149:499–514.

487. Jiminez C, Dardick I, McCaughey WTE, et al. Practical value of electron microscopy diagnoses in biopsies of lung carcinoma patients. Lab Invest 1982;46:41A–2A.

488. Neal MH, Kosinski R, Cohen P, et al. Atypical endocrine tumours of the lung. A clinicopathologic study of 19 cases. Hum Pathol 1986;17:1264–77.

489. Broers JLV, Ramaekers FCS, Klein Rot M, et al. Cytokeratin in different types of human lung cancer as monitored by chain-specific monoclonal antibodies. Cancer Res 1988;48:3221–9.

490. Moss F, Bobrow LG, Sheppard MN, et al. Expression of epithelial and neural antigens in small cell and non small cell lung carcinoma. J Pathol 1986;149:103–11.

491. DiLoreto C, DiLauro V, Puglisi F, et al. Immunocytochemical expression of tissue specific transcription factor-1 in lung carcinoma. J Clin Pathol 1997;50:30–2.

492. Gosney JR, Gosney MA, Lye M, et al. Reliability of commercially available immunocytochemical markers for identification of neuroendocrine differentiation in bronchoscopic biopsies of bronchial carcinoma. Thorax 1995;50:116–20.

493. Lyda MH, Weiss LM. Immunoreactivity for epithelial and neuroendocrine antibodies are useful in the differential diagnosis of lung carcinomas. Hum Pathol 2000;31:980–7.

494. Lantuejoul S, Laverriere MH, Sturm N, et al. NCAM (neural cell adhesion molecules) expression in malignant mesotheliomas. Hum Pathol 2001;31:415–21.

495. Kontogianni K, Nicholson AG, Butcher D, et al. CD56: a useful tool for the diagnosis of small cell lung carcinomas on biopsies with extensive crush artefact. J Clin Pathol 2005;58:978–80.

496. Zynger DL, Dimov ND, Ho LC, et al. Differential expression of neural-cadherin in pulmonary epithelial tumours. Histopathology 2008;52:348–54.

497. Hamid Q, Corrin B, Sheppard MN, et al. Expression of chromogranin A mRNA in small cell carcinoma of the lung. J Pathol 1991;163:293–7.

498. Patriarca C, Pruneri G, Alfano RM, et al. Polysialylated N-CAM, chromogranin A and B, and secretogranin II in neuroendocrine tumours of the lung. Virchows Archiv 1997;430:455–60.

499. Lantuejoul S, Moro D, Michalides RJAM, et al. Neural cell adhesion molecules (NCAM) and NCAM-PSA expression in neuroendocrine lung tumors. Am J Surg Pathol 1998;22:1267–76.

500. Lauweryns JM, Van Ranst L. Leu-7 immunoreactivity in human, monkey, and pig bronchopulmonary neuroepithelial bodies and neuroendocrine cells. J Histochem Cytochem 1987;35:687–91.

501. Ariza A, Mate JL, Isamat M, et al. Standard and variant CD44 isoforms are commonly expressed in lung cancer of the non-small cell type but not of the small cell type. J Pathol 1995;177:363–8.

502. Wagner PL, Kitabayashi N, Chen YT, et al. Combined small cell lung carcinomas: genotypic and immunophenotypic analysis of the separate morphologic components. Am J Clin Pathol 2009;131:376–82.

503. Onuki N, Wistuba II, Travis WD, et al. Genetic changes in the spectrum of neuroendocrine lung tumors. Cancer 1999;85:600–7.

Large cell carcinoma

504. Downey RS, Sewell CW, Mansour KA. Large cell carcinoma of the lung: a highly aggressive tumor with dismal prognosis. Ann Thorac Surg 1989;47:806–8.

505. Churg A. The fine structure of large cell undifferentiated carcinoma of the lung. Evidence for its relation to squamous cell carcinomas and adenocarcinomas. Hum Pathol 1978;9:143–56.

507. Nicholson AG, Gonzalez D, Shah P, et al. Refining the diagnosis and EGFR status of non-small cell carcinoma in biopsy and cytologic material, using a panel of mucin staining, TTF-1, cytokeratin 5/6, and P63, and EGFR mutation analysis. J Thorac Oncol 2010;5:436–41.

507a. Scagliotti GV, Parikh P, von Pawel J, et al. Phase III study comparing cisplatin plus gemcitabine with cisplatin plus pemetrexed in chemotherapy-naive

patients with advanced stage non-small-cell lung cancer. J Clin Oncol 2008;26:3543–51.

508. Edwards C, Carlile A. Clear cell carcinoma of the lung. J Clin Pathol 1985;38:880–5.

509. Morgan A, MacKenzie D. Clear cell carcinoma of the lung. J Pathol Bacteriol 1964;87:25–9.

510. McNamee CJ, Simpson RHW, Pagliero KM, et al. Primary clear-cell carcinoma of the lung. Respir Med 1993;87:471–3.

511. Sun L, Sakurai S, Sano T, et al. High-grade neuroendocrine carcinoma of the lung: comparative clinicopathological study of large cell neuroendocrine carcinoma and small cell lung carcinoma. Pathol Int 2009;59:522–9.

512. Travis WD, Linnoila RI, Tsokos MG, et al. Neuroendocrine tumors of the lung with proposed criteria for large-cell neuroendocrine carcinoma – an ultrastructural, immunohistochemical, and flow cytometric study of 35 cases. Am J Surg Pathol 1991;15:529–53.

513. Brambilla E, Veale D, Moro D, et al. Neuroendocrine phenotype in lung cancers – comparison of immunohistochemistry with biochemical determination of enolase isoenzymes. Am J Clin Pathol 1992;98:88–97.

514. Jiang SX, Kameya T, Shoji M, et al. Large cell neuroendocrine carcinoma of the lung: A histologic and immunohistochemical study of 22 cases. Am J Surg Pathol 1998;22:526–37.

515. Peng WX, Shibata T, Katoh H, et al. Array-based comparative genomic hybridization analysis of high-grade neuroendocrine tumors of the lung. Cancer Sci 2005;96:661–7.

516. Hiroshima K, Iyoda A, Shida T, et al. Distinction of pulmonary large cell neuroendocrine carcinoma from small cell lung carcinoma: a morphological, immunohistochemical, and molecular analysis. Mod Pathol 2006;19:1358–68.

517. Mooi WJ, Dewar A, Springall DR, et al. Non-small cell lung carcinomas with neuroendocrine features. A light microscopic, immunohistochemical and ultrastructural study of 11 cases. Histopathology 1988;13:329–37.

518. Hammond ME, Sause WT. Large cell neuroendocrine tumors of the lung. Cancer 1985;56:1624–9.

519. Linnoila RI, Mulshine JL, Steinberg SM, et al. Neuroendocrine differentiation in endocrine and nonendocrine lung carcinomas. Am J Clin Pathol 1988;90:641–52.

520. Wick MR, Berg LC, Hertz MI. Large cell carcinoma of the lung with neuroendocrine differentiation – a comparison with large cell undifferentiated pulmonary tumors. Am J Clin Pathol 1992;97:796–805.

521. Graziano SL, Mazid R, Newman N, et al. The use of neuroendocrine

immunoperoxidase markers to predict chemotherapy response in patients with non-small-cell lung cancer. J Clin Oncol 1989;7:1398–406.

522. Moertel CG, Kvols LK, O'Connell MJ, et al. Treatment of neuroendocrine carcinomas with combined etoposide and cisplatin – evidence of major therapeutic activity in the anaplastic variants of these neoplasms. Cancer 1991;68:227–32.

523. Souquet PJ, Chauvin F, Boissel JP, et al. Polychemotherapy in advanced non-small-cell lung cancer – a meta- analysis. Lancet 1993;342:19–21.

524. Ruckdeschel J, Linnoila RI, Mulshine JL, et al. The impact of neuroendocrine and epithelial differentiation on recurrence and survival in patients with lung cancer. Lung Cancer 1991;7:56.

525. Skov BG, Sorensen JB, Hirsch FR. et al. Prognostic impact of histologic demonstration of chromogranin A and neuron specific enolase in pulmonary adenocarcinoma. Ann Oncol 1991;2:355–60.

526. Schleusener JT, Tazelaar HD, Jung SH, et al. Neuroendocrine differentiation is an independent prognostic factor in chemotherapy-treated nonsmall cell lung carcinoma. Cancer 1996;77:1284–91.

527. Rossi G, Cavazza A, Marchioni A, et al. Role of chemotherapy and the receptor tyrosine kinases KIT, PDGFRalpha, PDGFRbeta, and Met in large-cell neuroendocrine carcinoma of the lung. J Clin Oncol 2005;23:8774–85.

528. Warren WH, Faber LP, Gould VE. Neuroendocrine neoplasms of the lung. A clinicopathologic update. J Thorac Cardiovasc Surg 1989;98:321–32.

529. Berendsen HH, De Leij L, Poppema S, et al. Clinical characterization of non-small-cell lung cancer tumors showing neuroendocrine differentiation features. J Clin Oncol 1989;7:1614–20.

530. Kibbelaar RE, Moolenaar KEC, Michalides RJAM, et al. Neural cell adhesion molecule expression, neuroendocrine differentiation and prognosis in lung carcinoma. Eur J Cancer 1991;27:431–5.

531. Pujol JL, Simony J, Demoly P, et al. Neural cell adhesion molecule and prognosis of surgically resected lung cancer. Am Rev Respir Dis 1993;148:1071–5.

532. Sunday ME, Choi N, Spindel ER, et al. Gastrin-releasing peptide gene expression in small cell and large cell undifferentiated lung carcinomas. Hum Pathol 1991;22:1030–9.

533. Sundaresan V, Reeve JG, Stenning S, et al. Neuroendocrine differentiation and clinical behaviour in non-small cell lung tumours. Br J Cancer 1991;64:333–8.

534. Graziano SL, Tatum AT, Newman NB, et al. The prognostic significance of neuroendocrine markers and carcinoembryonic antigen in patients with resected stage I and II non-small cell lung cancer. Cancer Res 1994;54:2908–13.

535. Abbona G, Papotti M, Viberti L, et al. Chromogranin A gene expression in non-small cell lung carcinomas. J Pathol 1998;186:151–6.

536. Howe MC, Chapman A, Kerr K, et al. Neuroendocrine differentiation in non-small cell lung cancer and its relation to prognosis and therapy. Histopathology 2005;46:195–201.

537. Sterlacci W, Fiegl M, Hilbe W, et al. Clinical relevance of neuroendocrine differentiation in non-small cell lung cancer assessed by immunohistochemistry: a retrospective study on 405 surgically resected cases. Virchows Archiv 2009;455:125–32.

538. Carles J, Rosell R, Ariza A, et al. Neuroendocrine differentiation as a prognostic factor in non-small cell lung cancer. Lung Cancer 1993;10:209–19.

539. Ionescu DN, Treaba D, Gilks CB, et al. Nonsmall cell lung carcinoma with neuroendocrine differentiation – an entity of no clinical or prognostic significance. Am J Surg Pathol 2007;31:26–32.

540. Brambilla E. Basaloid carcinoma of the lung. In: Corrin B, editor. Pathology of Lung Tumors. London: Churchill Livingstore; 1997. p. 71–82.

541. Sturm N, Lantuejoul S, Laverriere MH, et al. Thyroid transcription factor 1 and cytokeratins 1, 5, 10, 14 (34 beta E12) expression in basaloid and large-cell neuroendocrine carcinomas of the lung. Hum Pathol 2001;32:918–25.

542. Passalidou E, Trivella M, Singh N, et al. Vascular phenotype in angiogenic and non-angiogenic lung non-small cell carcinomas. Br J Cancer 2002;86:244–9.

543. Foroulis CN, Iliadis KH, Mauroudis PM, et al. Basaloid carcinoma, a rare primary lung neoplasm: report of a case and review of the literature. Lung Cancer 2002;35:335–8.

544. Begin LR, Eskandari J, Joncas J, et al. Epstein–Barr virus related lymphoepithelioma-like carcinoma of lung. J Surg Oncol 1987;36:280–3.

545. Wong MP, Chung LP, Yuen ST, et al. In situ detection of Epstein–Barr virus in non-small cell lung carcinomas. J Pathol 1995;177:233–40.

546. Chen FF, Yan JJ, Lai WW, Jin YT, et al. Epstein–Barr virus-associated nonsmall cell lung carcinoma: Undifferentiated 'lymphoepithelioma-like' carcinoma as a distinct entity with better prognosis. Cancer 1998;82:2334–42.

547. Han AJ, Xiong M, Gu YY, et al. Lymphoepithelioma-like carcinoma of the lung with a better prognosis. A clinicopathologic study of 32 cases. Am J Clin Pathol 2001;115:841–50.

548. Chang YL, Wu CT, Shih JY, et al. New aspects in clinicopathologic and oncogene studies of 23 pulmonary lymphoepithelioma-like carcinomas. Am J Surg Pathol 2002;26:715–23.

549. Wockel W, Hofler G, Popper HH, et al. Lymphoepithelioma-like carcinoma of the lung. Pathol Res Pract 1995;191:1170–4.

550. Morbini P, Riboni R, Tomaselli S, et al. EBER- and LMP-1-expressing pulmonary lymphoepithelioma- like carcinoma in a Caucasian patient. Hum Pathol 2003;34:623–5.

551. Chan ATC, Teo PML, Lam KC, et al. Multimodality treatment of primary lymphoepithelioma-like carcinoma of the lung. Cancer 1998;83:925–9.

552. Cavazza A, Colby TV, Tsokos M, et al. Lung tumors with a rhabdoid phenotype. Am J Clin Pathol 1996;105:182–8.

553. Rubenchik I, Dardick I, Auger M. Cytopathology and ultrastructure of primary rhabdoid tumor of lung. Ultrastruct Pathol 1996;20:355–60.

554. Itakura E, Tamiya S, Morita K, et al. Subcellular distribution of cytokeratin and vimentin in malignant rhabdoid tumor: Three-dimensional imaging with confocal laser scanning microscopy and double immunofluorescence. Mod Pathol 2001;14:854–61.

555. Chetty R. Combined large cell neuroendocrine, small cell and squamous carcinomas of the lung with rhabdoid cells. Pathology 2000;32:209–12.

556. Miyagi J, Tsuhako K, Kinjo T, et al. Rhabdoid tumour of the lung is a dedifferentiated phenotype of pulmonary adenocarcinoma. Histopathology 2000;37:37–44.

557. Tamboli P, Toprani TH, Amin MB, et al. Carcinoma of lung with rhabdoid features. Hum Pathol 2004;35:8–13.

558. Shimazaki H, Aida S, Sato M, et al. Lung carcinoma with rhabdoid cells: a clinicopathological study and survival analysis of 14 cases. Histopathology 2001;38:425–34.

Adenosquamous carcinoma

559. Fitzgibbons PL, Kern WH. Adenosquamous carcinoma of the lung: a clinical and pathological study of seven cases. Hum Pathol 1985;16:463–6.

560. Naunheim KS, Taylor JR, Skosey C, et al. Adenosquamous lung carcinoma: clinical characteristics, treatment, and prognosis. Ann Thorac Surg 1987;44:462–6.

561. Takamori S, Noguchi M, Morinaga S, et al. Clinicopathologic characteristics of adenosquamous carcinoma of the lung. Cancer 1991;67:649–54.

562. Shimizu J, Oda M, Hayashi Y, et al. A clinicopathological study of resected cases of adenosquamous carcinoma of the lung. Chest 1996;109:989–94.

563. Sridhar KS, Bounassi MJ, Raub W, et al. Clinical features of adenosquamous lung carcinoma in 127 patients. Am Rev Respir Dis 1990;142:19–23.

Sarcomatoid carcinoma

564. Battifora H. Spindle cell carcinoma. Ultrastructural evidence of squamous origin and collagen production by tumor cells. Cancer 1976;37:2275–82.

565. Addis BJ, Corrin B. Pulmonary blastoma, carcinosarcoma and spindle cell carcinoma: an immunohistochemical study of keratin intermediate filaments. J Pathol 1985;147:291–301.

566. Humphrey PA, Scroggs MW, Roggli VL, et al. Pulmonary carcinomas with a sarcomatoid element: an immunocytochemical and ultrastructural analysis. Hum Pathol 1988;19:155–65.

567. Holst VA, Finkelstein S, Colby TV, et al. p53 and K-ras mutational genotyping in pulmonary carcinosarcoma, spindle cell carcinoma, and pulmonary blastoma: Implications for histogenesis. Am J Surg Pathol 1997;21:801–11.

568. Dacic S, Finkelstein SD, Sasatomi E, et al. Molecular pathogenesis of pulmonary carcinosarcoma as determined by microdissection-based allelotyping. Am J Surg Pathol 2002;26:510–16.

569. Kojc N, Zidar N, Gale N, et al. Transcription factors Snail, Slug, Twist, and SIP1 in spindle cell carcinoma of the head and neck. Virchows Arch 2009;454:549–55.

570. Fishback NF, Travis WD, Moran CA, et al. Pleomorphic (spindle/giant cell) carcinoma of the lung – a clinicopathologic correlation of 78 cases. Cancer 1994;73:2936–45.

571. Rossi G, Cavazza A, Sturm N, et al. Pulmonary carcinomas with pleomorphic, sarcomatoid, or sarcomatous elements – A clinicopathologic and immunohistochemical study of 75 cases. Am J Surg Pathol 2003;27:311–24.

572. Nappi O, Glasner SD, Swanson PE, et al. Biphasic and monophasic sarcomatoid carcinomas of the lung – a reappraisal of 'carcinosarcomas' and 'spindle-cell carcinomas'. Am J Clin Pathol 1994;102:331–40.

573. Wick MR, Ritter JH, Humphrey PA. Sarcomatoid carcinomas of the lung: A clinicopathologic review. Am J Clin Pathol 1997;108:40–53.

574. Pelosi G, Fraggetta F, Nappi O, et al. Pleomorphic carcinomas of the lung show a selective distribution of gene products involved in cell differentiation, cell cycle control, tumor growth, and tumor cell motility – A clinicopathologic and immunohistochemical study of 31 cases. Am J Surg Pathol 2003;27:1203–15.

575. Ro JY, Chen JL, Lee JS, et al. Sarcomatoid carcinoma of the lung – immunohistochemical and ultrastructural studies of 14 cases. Cancer 1992;69:376–86.

576. Lucas DR, Pass HI, Madan SK, et al. Sarcomatoid mesothelioma and its histological mimics: a comparative immunohistochemical study. Histopathology 2003;42:270–9.

577. Ginsberg SS, Buzaid AC, Stern H, et al. Giant cell carcinoma of the lung. Cancer 1992;70:606–10.

578. Attanoos RL, Papagiannis A, Suttinont P, et al. Pulmonary giant cell carcinoma: pathological entity or morphological phenotype? Histopathology 1998;32:225–31.

579. Nash AD, Stout AP. Giant cell carcinoma of the lung. Report of 5 cases. Cancer 1958;11:369–76.

580. Wang N-S, Seemayer TA, Ahmed MN, et al. Giant cell carcinoma of the lung. A light and electron microscopic study. Hum Pathol 1976;7:3–16.

581. Addis BJ, Dewar A, Thurlow NP. Giant cell carcinoma of the lung – immunohistochemical and ultrastructural evidence of dedifferentiation. J Pathol 1988;155:231–40.

582. Mochizuki T, Ishii G, Nagai K, et al. Pleomorphic carcinoma of the lung: clinicopathologic characteristics of 70 cases. Am J Surg Pathol 2008;32:1727–35.

583. Kenmotsu H, Ishii G, Nagai K, et al. Pleomorphic carcinoma of the lung expressing podoplanin and calretinin. Pathol Int 2008;58:771–4.

584. Kika 1908 cited by Herxheimer G, Reinke G. Carcinoma sarcomatodes (Pathologie des Krebses). Ergeb Allg Path Pathol Anatom 1912;16:280–2.

585. Thompson L, Chang B, Barsky SH. Monoclonal origins of malignant mixed tumors (carcinosarcomas): evidence for a divergent histogenesis. Am J Surg Pathol 1996;20:277–85.

586. Stewart HL, Grady HG, Andervont HB. Development of sarcoma at site of serial transplantation of pulmonary tumours in inbred mice. J Natl Cancer Inst 1947;7:207–25.

587. Davis MP, Eagen RT, Weiland LH, et al. Carcinosarcoma of the lung: Mayo Clinic experience and response to chemotherapy. Mayo Clin Proc 1984;59:598–603.

588. Cabarcos A, Dorrojnsoro MG, Beristain JLL. Pulmonary carcinosarcoma: a case study and review of the literature. Br J Dis Chest 1985;79:83–94.

589. Koss MN, Hochholzer L, Frommelt RA. Carcinosarcomas of the lung – A clinicopathologic study of 66 patients. Am J Surg Pathol 1999;23:1514–26.

590. Haussinger K, Kohlhauffl M, Bolliger CT. Diagnostic bronchoscopy. In: Gibson GJ, Geddes DM, Costabel U, et al, editors. Respiratory Medicine. 3rd ed. London: Saunders; 2003. p. 415–30.

591. Cohen-Salmon D, Michel RP, Wang N-S, et al. Pulmonary carcinosarcoma and carcinoma: report of a case studied by electron microscopy, with critical review of the literature. Ann Pathol 1985;5:115–24.

592. Rainosek DE, Ro JY, Ordonez NG, et al. Sarcomatoid carcinoma of the lung: a case with atypical carcinoid and rhabdomyosarcomatous components. Am J Clin Pathol 1994;102:360–4.

593. Mayall FG, Gibbs AR. Pleural and pulmonary carcinosarcomas. J Pathol 1992;167:305–11.

594. Kitazawa R, Kitazawa S, Nishimura Y, et al. Lung carcinosarcoma with liposarcoma element: Autopsy case. Pathol International 2006;56:449–52.

595. Huszar M, Herczog E, Lieberman Y, et al. Distinctive immunofluorescent labeling of epithelial and mesenchymal elements of carcinosarcoma with antibodies specific for different intermediate filaments. Hum Pathol 1984;15:532–8.

596. Gatter KC, Dunnill MS, van Muijan GNP, et al. Human lung tumours may coexpress different classes of intermediate filaments. J Clin Pathol 1986;39:950–4.

597. Cupples J, Wright J. An immunohistological comparison of primary lung carcinosarcoma and sarcoma. Pathol Res Pract 1990;186:326–9.

598. Stackhouse EM, Harrison EG, Ellis FH. Primary mixed malignancies of lung: carcinosarcoma and blastoma. J Thorac Cardiovasc Surg 1969;57:385–99.

599. Spencer H. Pulmonary blastomas. J Pathol Bacteriol 1961;82:161–5.

600. Barrett NK, Barnard WG. Some unusual thoracic tumours. Br J Surg 1945;32:447–57.

601. Barnard WG. Embryoma of lung. Thorax 1952;7:299–301.

602. Roth JA, Elguezabal A. Pulmonary blastoma evolving into carcinosarcoma. Am J Surg Pathol 1978;2:407–13.

603. Edwards CW, Saunders AM, Collins F. Mixed malignant tumour of the lung. Thorax 1979;34:629–39.

604. Olenick SJ, Fan CC, Ryoo JW. Mixed pulmonary blastoma and carcinosarcoma. Histopathology 1994;25:171–4.

605. Francis D, Jacobsen M. Pulmonary blastoma. In: Muller K-M, editor. Pulmonary Diseases – Clinicopathological Correlations. Current Topics in Pathology No. 73. Berlin: Springer-Verlag; 1983. p. 265–94.

606. Koss MN, Hochholzer L, O'Leary T. Pulmonary blastomas. Cancer 1991;67:2368–81.

607. Yousem SA, Wick MR, Randhawa P, et al. Pulmonary blastoma. An immunohistochemical analysis with comparison with fetal lung in its pseudoglandular stage. Am J Clin Pathol 1990;93:167–75.

608. Inoue H, Kasai K, Shinada J, et al. Pulmonary blastoma – comparison between its epithelial components and fetal bronchial epithelium. Acta Pathol Jpn 1992;42:884–92.

609. Heckman CJ, Truang LD, Cagle PT, et al. Pulmonary blastoma with

rhabdomyosarcomatous differentiation: an electron microscopic and immunohistochemical study. Am J Surg Pathol 1988;12:35–40.

610. Cohen RE, Weaver MG, Monteregro HD, et al. Pulmonary blastoma with malignant melanoma component. Arch Pathol Lab Med 1990;114:1076–8.

611. Scully RE, Mark EJ, McNeely BU. Case records of the Massachusetts General Hospital: case 3–1984, pulmonary blastoma with major component of small cell carcinoma. N Engl J Med 1984;310:178–87.

612. Siegel RJ, Bueso-Ramos C, Cohen C, et al. Pulmonary blastoma with germ cell (yolk sac) differentiation: report of two cases. Mod Pathol 1992;4:566–70.

613. Jackson MD, Albrecht R, Roggli VL, et al. Pulmonary blastoma: an ultrastructural and histochemical study. Ultrastruct Pathol 1984;7:259–68.

614. Tamai S, Kameya T, Shimosato Y, et al. Pulmonary blastoma: an ultrastructural study of a case and its transplanted tumour in athymic nude mice. Cancer 1980;46:1389–96.

615. Berean K, Truong LD, Dudley AW, et al. Immunohistochemical characteristics of pulmonary blastoma. Am J Clin Pathol 1988;89:773–7.

616. Garcia-Escudero A, Gonzalez-Campora R, Villar-Rodriguez JL, et al. Thyroid transcription factor-1 expression in pulmonary blastoma. Histopathology 2004;44:507–8.

Prognostic factors

617. Greenberg SD, Fraire AE, Kinner BM, et al. Tumor cell type versus staging in the prognosis of carcinoma of the lung. Pathol Annu 1987;2:387–405.

618. Wetzels RH, van der Velden LA, Schaafsma HE, et al. Immunohistochemical localization of basement membrane type VII collagen and laminin in neoplasms of the head and neck. Histopathology 1992;21:459–64.

619. Holty J-EC, Kuschner WG, Gould MK. Accuracy of transbronchial needle aspiration for mediastinal staging of non-small cell lung cancer: a meta-analysis. Thorax 2005;60:949–55.

620. Kerr KM, Lamb D, Wathen CG, et al. Pathological assessment of mediastinal lymph nodes in lung cancer – implications for non-invasive mediastinal staging. Thorax 1992;47:337–41.

621. Prenzel KL, Monig SP, Sinning JM, et al. Lymph node size and metastatic infiltration in non-small cell lung cancer. Chest 2003;123:463–7.

622. Passlick B, Izbicki JR, Kubuschak B, et al. Immunohistochemical assessment of individual tumour cells in lymph nodes of patients with non-small-cell lung cancer. J Clin Oncol 1994;12:1827–32.

623. Passlick B, Izbicki JR, Kubuschok B, et al. Detection of disseminated lung cancer cells in lymph nodes: impact on staging and prognosis. Ann Thorac Surg 1996;61:177–83.

624. Salerno CT, Frizelle S, Niehans GA, et al. Detection of occult micrometastases in non-small cell lung carcinoma by reverse transcriptase-polymerase chain reaction. Chest 1998;113:1526–32.

625. Nicholson AG, Graham ANJ, Pezzella F, et al. Does the use of immunohistochemistry to identify micrometastases provide useful information in the staging of node-negative non-small cell lung carcinomas? Lung Cancer 1997;18:231–40.

626. Goldstein NS, Mani A, Chmielewski G, et al. Immunohistochemically detected micrometastases in peribronchial and mediastinal lymph nodes from patients with T1, N0, M0 pulmonary adenocarcinomas. Am J Surg Pathol 2000;24:274–9.

627. Fernando HC, Goldstraw P. The accuracy of clinical evaluative intrathoracic staging in lung cancer as assessed by postsurgical pathologic staging. Cancer 1990;65:2503–6.

628. Naruke T, Suemasu K, Ishikawa S. Lymph node mapping and curability at various levels of metastasis in resected lung cancer. J Thorac Cardiovasc Surg 1978;76:832–9.

629. International Union Against Cancer (UICC). TNM Atlas. Illustrated guide to the TNM classification of malignant tumours. 5th ed. Hoboken, New Jersey: Wiley-Liss; 2005.

630. Goldstraw P, Crowley J, Chansky K, et al. The IASLC Lung Cancer Staging Project: proposals for the revision of the TNM stage groupings in the forthcoming (seventh) edition of the TNM Classification of malignant tumours. J Thorac Oncol 2007;2:706–14.

631. Detterbeck FC, Boffa DJ, Tanoue LT. The New Lung Cancer Staging System. Chest 2009;136:260–71.

632. International Union Against Cancer (UICC). TNM classification of malignant tumours. 7th ed. New York: Wiley-Liss; 2009.

633. Pasic A, Grunberg K, Mooi WJ, et al. The natural history of carcinoma in situ involving bronchial resection margins. Chest 2005;128:1736–41.

634. Bunker ML, Raab SS, Landreneau RJ, et al. The diagnosis and significance of visceral pleural invasion in lung carcinoma – histologic predictors and the role of elastic stains. Am J Clin Pathol 1999;112:777–83.

635. Taube JM, Askin FB, Brock MV, et al. Impact of elastic staining on the staging of peripheral lung cancers. Am J Surg Pathol 2007;31:953–6.

636. Butnor KJ, Vollmer RT, Blaszyk H, et al. Interobserver agreement on what constitutes visceral pleural invasion by non-small cell lung carcinoma: an internet-based assessment of international current practices. Am J Clin Pathol 2007;128:638–47.

637. Travis WD. Reporting lung cancer pathology specimens. Impact of the anticipated 7th Edition TNM classification based on recommendations of the IASLC Staging Committee. Histopathology 2009;54:3–11.

638. Flieder DB. Commonly encountered difficulties in pathologic staging of lung cancer. Arch Pathol Lab Med 2007;131:1016–26.

639. Dacic S, Ionescu DN, Finkelstein S, et al. Patterns of allelic loss of synchronous adenocarcinomas of the lung. Am J Surg Pathol 2005;29:897–902.

640. Girard N, Ostrovnaya I, Lau C, et al. Genomic and mutational profiling to assess clonal relationships between multiple non-small cell lung cancers. Clin Cancer Res 2009;15:5184–90.

641. Girard N, Deshpande C, Azzoli CG, et al. Use of epidermal growth factor receptor/kirsten rat sarcoma 2 viral oncogene homolog mutation testing to define clonal relationships among multiple lung adenocarcinomas. Chest 2010;137:46–52.

642. Pastorino U. Benefits of neoadjuvant chemotherapy in NSCLC. Chest 1996;109:S96–101.

643. Liu-Jarin X, Stoopler MB, Raftopoulos H, et al. Histologic assessment of non-small cell lung carcinoma after neoadjuvant therapy. Mod Pathol 2003;16:1102–8.

644. van Velzen E, Snijder RJ, Brutel dlR, et al. Type of lymph node involvement influences survival rates in T1N1M0 non-small cell lung carcinoma. Lymph node involvement by direct extension compared with lobar and hilar node metastases. Chest 1996;110:1469–73.

645. Riquet M, Manac'h D, Pimpec-Barthes F, et al. Prognostic significance of surgical-pathologic N1 disease in non-small cell carcinoma of the lung. Ann Thorac Surg 1999;67:1572–6.

646. Shields TW, Yee J, Conn JH. Relationship of cell type and lymph node metastasis to survival after resection of bronchial carcinoma. Am J Thorac Surg 1975;20:501–10.

647. Mayer JE, Ewing SL, Ophoren TJ, et al. Influence of histological type on survival after curative resection for undifferentiated lung cancer. J Thorac Cardiovasc Surg 1982;84:641–8.

648. Lipford EH, Eggleston JC, Lillemore KD, et al. Prognostic factors in surgically resected limited-state, nonsmall cell carcinoma of the lung. Am J Surg Pathol 1984;8:357–65.

649. Fraire AE, Johnson EH, Yesner R, et al. Prognostic significance of histopathologic subtype and stage in small cell lung cancer. Hum Pathol 1992;23:520–8.

650. Carriaga MT, Henson DE. The histologic grading of cancer. Cancer 1995;75:406–21.

651. Ladekarl M, Boekhansen T, Henriknielsen R, et al. Objective malignancy grading of squamous cell carcinoma of the lung: stereologic estimates of mean nuclear size are of prognostic value, independent of clinical stage of disease. Cancer 1995;76:797–802.

652. Ries LA. Influence of extent of disease, histology, and demographic factors on lung cancer survival in the SEER population-based data. Semin Surg Oncol 1994;10:21–30.

653. Kimura T, Sato T, Onodera K. Clinical significance of DNA measurements in small cell lung cancer. Cancer 1993;72:3216–22.

654. Tanaka I, Masuda R, Furuhata Y, et al. Flow cytometric analysis of the DNA content of adenocarcinoma of the lung, especially for patients with stage 1 disease with long term follow-up. Cancer 1995;75:2461–5.

655. Asamura H, Ando M, Matsuno Y, et al. Histopathologic prognostic factors in resected adenocarcinomas – Is nuclear DNA content prognostic? Chest 1999;115:1018–24.

656. Zimmerman PV, Hawson GAT, Bint MH, et al. Ploidy as a prognostic determinant in surgically treated lung cancer. Lancet 1987;2:530–3.

657. Yasushira K. Flow cytometric analysis of DNA ploidy level in paraffin-embedded tissue of non-small-cell lung cancer. Eur J Cancer Clin Oncol 1988;24:455–60.

658. Ogawa J, Tsurumi T, Inoue H, et al. Relationship between tumor DNA ploidy and regional lymph node changes in lung cancer. Cancer 1992;69:1688–95.

659. Battlehner CN, Saldiva PHN, Carvalho CRR, et al. Nuclear/cytoplasmic ratio correlates strongly with survival in non-disseminated neuroendocrine carcinoma of the lung. Histopathology 1993;22:31–4.

660. Tungekar MF, Gatter KC, Dunnill MS, et al. Ki-67 immunostaining and survival in operable lung cancer. Histopathology 1991;19:545–50.

661. Theunissen PHMH, Leers MPG, Bollen ECM. Proliferating cell nuclear antigen (PCNA) expression in formalin-fixed tissue of non-small-cell lung carcinoma. Histopathology 1992;20:251–5.

662. Shiba M, Kohno H, Kakizawa K, et al. Ki-67 immunostaining and other prognostic factors including tobacco smoking in patients with resected nonsmall cell lung carcinoma. Cancer 2000;89:1457–65.

663. Poleri C, Morero JL, Nieva B, et al. Risk of recurrence in patients with surgically resected stage I non-small cell lung carcinoma – Histopathologic and immunohistochemical analysis. Chest 2003;123:1858–67.

664. Boldy DAR, Ayres JG, Crocker J, et al. Interphase nucleolar organiser regions and survival in squamous cell carcinoma of the bronchus – a ten year follow up study of 138 cases. Thorax 1991;46:871–7.

665. Ogura S, Abe S, Sukoh N, et al. Correlation between nucleolar organizer regions visualized by silver staining and the growth rate in lung adenocarcinoma. Cancer 1992;70:63–8.

666. Antonangelo L, Bernardi FD, Capelozzi VL, et al. Morphometric evaluation of argyrophilic nucleolar organizer region is useful in predicting long-term survival in squamous cell carcinoma of the lung. Chest 1997;111:110–4.

667. Fujiwara M, Okayasu I, Takemura T, et al. Telomerase activity significantly correlates with chromosome alterations, cell differentiation, and proliferation in lung adenocarcinomas. Modern Pathol 2000;13:723–9.

668. Ghosh M, Crocker J, Morris A. Apoptosis in squamous cell carcinoma of the lung: correlation with survival and clinicopathological features. J Clin Pathol 2001;54:111–5.

669. Usuda K, Saito Y, Sagawa M, et al. Tumor doubling time and prognostic assessment of patients with primary lung cancer. Cancer 1994;74:2239–44.

670. Battifora H, Sorensen HR, Mehta P, et al. Tumor-associated antigen 43–9f is of prognostic value in squamous cell carcinoma of the lung – a retrospective immunohistochemical study. Cancer 1992;70:1867–72.

671. Clarke MR, Landreneau RJ, Resnick NM, et al. Prognostic significance of CD44 expression in adenocarcinoma of the lung. J Clin Pathol Clin Mol Pathol 1995;48:M200–4.

672. Vargas SO, Leslie KO, Vacek PM, et al. Estrogen-receptor-related protein p29 in primary nonsmall cell lung carcinoma: Pathologic and prognostic correlations. Cancer 1998;82:1495–500.

673. Furukawa T, Watanabe S, Kodama T, et al. T-zone histiocytes in adenocarcinoma of the lung in relation to postoperative prognosis. Cancer 1985;56:2651–6.

674. Dammrich J, Buchwald J, Papadopoulos T, et al. Special subtypes of pulmonary adenocarcinomas indicated by different tumor cell HLA-expression and stromal infiltrates – a light, electron microscopic and immunohistologic study. Virchows Arch B Cell Pathol 1991;61:9–18.

675. Takise A, Kodama T, Shimosato Y, et al. Histopathologic prognostic factors in adenocarcinomas of the peripheral lung less than 2 cm in diameter. Cancer 1992;61:2083–8.

676. Zeid NA, Muller HK. S100 positive dendritic cells in human lung tumours associated with cell differentiation and enhanced survival. Pathology 1993;25:338–43.

677. Al-Shibli K, Al-Saad S, Donnem T, et al. The prognostic value of intraepithelial and stromal innate immune system cells in non-small cell lung carcinoma. Histopathology 2009;55:301–12.

678. Yuan A, Yang PC, Yu CJ, et al. Tumor angiogenesis correlates with histologic type and metastasis in non-small-cell lung cancer. Am J Respir Crit Care Med 1995;152:2157–62.

679. Harpole DH Jr, Richards WG, Herndon JE, et al. Angiogenesis and molecular biologic substaging in patients with stage I non-small cell lung cancer. Ann Thorac Surg 1996;61:1470–6.

680. Giatromanolaki A, Koukourakis M, Obyrne K, et al. Prognostic value of angiogenesis in operable non-small cell lung cancer. J Pathol 1996;179:80–8.

681. Fontanini G, Lucchi M, Vignati S, et al. Angiogenesis as a prognostic indicator of survival in non-small-cell lung carcinoma: A prospective study. J Nat Cancer Inst 1997;89:881–6.

682. Kayser G, Baumhakel JD, Szoke T, et al. Vascular diffusion density and survival of patients with primary lung carcinoma. Virchows Archiv 2003;442:462–7.

683. Fujisawa T, Yamaguchi Y, Saitoh Y, et al. Blood and lymphatic vessel invasion as prognostic factors for patients with primary resected nonsmall cell carcinoma of the lung with intrapulmonary metastases. Cancer 1995;76:2464–70.

684. Brechot JM, Chevret S, Charpentier MC, et al. Blood vessel and lymphatic vessel invasion in resected nonsmall cell lung carcinoma: correlation with TNM stage and disease free and overall survival. Cancer 1996;78:2111–18.

685. Sulzer MA, Leers MPG, Vannoord JA, et al. Reduced E-cadherin expression is associated with increased lymph node metastasis and unfavorable prognosis in non-small cell lung cancer. Amer J Respir Crit Care Med 1998;157:1319–23.

686. Salon C, Moro D, Lantuejoul S, et al. E-cadherin-[beta]-catenin adhesion complex in neuroendocrine tumors of the lung: a suggested role upon local invasion and metastasis. Human Pathology 2004;35:1148–55.

687. Awaya H, Takeshima Y, Amatya VJ, et al. Loss of expression of E-cadherin and beta-catenin is associated with progression of pulmonary adenocarcinoma. Pathology International 2005;55:14–18.

688. Fukuoka J, Dracheva T, Shih JH, et al. Desmoglein 3 as a prognostic factor in lung cancer. Human Pathology 2007;38:276–83.

689. Smith DR, Kunkel SL, Burdick MD, et al. Production of interleukin-10 by human bronchogenic carcinoma. Am J Pathol 1994;145:18–25.

690. Watanabe N, Nakajima I, Abe S, et al. Staining pattern of type IV collagen and prognosis in early stage adenocarcinoma of the lung. J Clin Pathol 1994;47:613–15.

691. Matsui K, Kitagawa M, Sugiyama S, et al. Distribution pattern of the basement membrane components is one of the significant prognostic correlates in peripheral lung adenocarcinomas. Hum Pathol 1995;26:186–94.

692. Kodate M, Kasai T, Hashimoto H, et al. Expression of matrix metalloproteinase (gelatinase) in T1 adenocarcinoma of the lung. Pathol Int 1997;47:461–9.

693. Karameris A, Panagou P, Tsilalis T, et al. Association of expression of metalloproteinases and their inhibitors with the metastatic potential of squamous-cell lung carcinomas – A molecular and immunohistochemical study. Amer J Respir Crit Care Med 1997;156:1930–6.

694. Thomas P, Khokha R, Shepherd FA, et al. Differential expression of matrix metalloproteinases and their inhibitors in non-small cell lung cancer. J Pathol 2000;190:150–6.

695. Carey FA, Fabbroni G, Lamb D. Expression of proliferating cell nuclear antigen in lung cancer – a systematic study and correlation with DNA ploidy. Histopathology 1992;20:499–503.

696. Brown DC, Gatter KC. Comparison of proliferation rates assessed using multiblock and conventional tissue blocks of lung carcinoma. J Clin Pathol 1992;45:579–82.

697. Maniwa Y, Yoshimura M, Obayashi C, et al. Association of p53 gene mutation and telomerase activity in resectable non-small cell lung cancer. Chest 2001;120:589–94.

698. Han H, Landreneau RJ, Santucci TS, et al. Prognostic value of immunohistochemical expressions of p53, HER-2/neu, and bcl-2 in stage I non-small-cell lung cancer. Hum Pathol 2002;33:105–10.

699. Gessner C, Liebers U, Kuhn H, et al. BAX and p16INK4A are independent positive prognostic markers for advance tumour stage of nonsmall cell lung cancer. Eur Resp J 2002;19:134–40.

700. Greatens TM, Niehans GA, Rubins JB, et al. Do molecular markers predict survival in non-small-cell lung cancer? Amer J Respir Crit Care Med 1998;157:1093–7.

701. Silvestrini R, Costa A, Lequaglie C, et al. Bcl-2 protein and prognosis in patients with potentially curable nonsmall-cell lung cancer. Virchows Archiv 1998;432:441–4.

702. Meert AP, Martin B, Delmotte P, et al. The role of EGF-R expression on patient survival in lung cancer: a systematic review with meta-analysis. Eur Resp J 2002;20:975–81.

703. Harada M, Dosakaakita H, Miyamoto H, et al. Prognostic significance of the expression of ras oncogene product in non-small-cell lung cancer. Cancer 1992;69:72–7.

704. Silini EM, Bosi F, Pellegata NS, et al. K-ras gene mutations: an unfavorable prognostic marker in stage I lung adenocarcinoma. Virchows Arch 1994;424:367–73.

705. Fujino M, Dosakaakita H, Harada M, et al. Prognostic significance of p53 and ras p21 expression in nonsmall cell lung cancer. Cancer 1995;76:2457–63.

706. Fukuyama Y, Mitsudomi T, Sugio K, et al. K-ras and p53 mutations are an independent unfavourable prognostic indicator in patients with non-small-cell lung cancer. Br J Cancer 1997;75:1125–30.

707. Selvaggi G, Scagliotti GV, Torri V, et al. HER-2/neu overexpression in patients with radically resected nonsmall cell lung carcinoma. Impact on long-term survival. Cancer 2002;94:2669–74.

708. Korkolopoulou P, Oates J, Crocker J, et al. p53 expression in oat and non-oat small cell lung carcinomas – correlations with proliferating cell nuclear antigen. J Clin Pathol 1993;46:1093–6.

709. Marchetti I, Buttitta F, Merlo G, et al. p53 alterations in non-small cell lung cancers correlate with metastatic involvement of hilar and mediastinal lymph nodes. Cancer Res 1993;53:2846–51.

710. Jiang SX, Sato YC, Kuwao S, et al. Expression of bcl-2 oncogene protein is prevalent in small cell lung carcinomas. J Pathol 1995;177:135–8.

711. Dalquen P, Sauter G, Torhorst J, et al. Nuclear p53 overexpression is an independent prognostic parameter in node-negative non-small cell lung carcinoma. J Pathol 1996;178:53–8.

712. Laudanski J, Niklinska W, Burzykowski T, et al. Prognostic significance of p53 and bcl-2 abnormalities in operable nonsmall cell lung cancer. Eur Resp J 2001;17:660–6.

713. Groeger AM, Esposito V, DeLuca A, et al. Prognostic value of immunohistochemical expression of p53, bax, Bcl-2 and Bcl-x(L) in resected non-small-cell lung cancers. Histopathology 2004;44:54–63.

714. Johnson BE, Inde DC, Makuch RW, et al. Myc family oncogene amplification in tumor cell lines established from small cell lung cancer patients and its relationship to clinical status and course. J Clin Invest 1987;79:1629–34.

715. Biedler JL. Genetic aspects of multidrug resistance. Cancer 1992;70:1799–809.

716. Wright SR, Boag AH, Valdimarsson G, et al. Immunohistochemical detection of multidrug resistance protein in human lung cancer and normal lung. Clin Cancer Res 1998;4:2279–89.

717. Scheffer GL, Pijnenborg ACLM, Smit EF, et al. Multidrug resistance related molecules in human and murine lung. J Clin Pathol 2002;55:332–9.

718. Takanami I, Imamura T, Hashizume T, et al. Transforming growth factor beta(1) as a prognostic factor in pulmonary adenocarcinoma. J Clin Pathol 1994;47:1098–100.

719. Woll PJ. New perspectives in lung cancer .2. Growth factors and lung cancer. Thorax 1991;46:924–9.

720. Weber S, Zuckerman JE, Bostwick DG, et al. Gastrin-releasing peptide is a selective mitogen for small cell carcinoma in vitro. J Clin Invest 1985;75:306–9.

721. Cuttita F, Carney DN, Mulshine J, et al. Bombesin-like peptides can function as autocrine growth factors in human small cell lung cancer. Nature 1985;316:823–6.

722. Berger MS, Gullick WJ, Greenfield C, et al. Epidermal growth factor receptors in lung tumours. J Pathol 1987;152:297–307.

723. Petty RD, Nicolson MC, Kerr KM, et al. Gene expression profiling in non-small cell lung cancer: from molecular mechanisms to clinical application. Clin Cancer Res 2004;10:3237–48.

724. Meyerson M, Franklin WA, Kelley MJ. Molecular classification and molecular genetics of human lung cancers. Seminars in Oncology 2004;31:4–19.

Developments in treatment

725. Douillard JY, Tribodet H, Aubert D, et al. Adjuvant cisplatin and vinorelbine for completely resected non-small cell lung cancer: subgroup analysis of the Lung Adjuvant Cisplatin Evaluation. J Thorac Oncol 2010;5:220–8.

726. Cullen M. Lung cancer – 4: Chemotherapy for non-small cell lung cancer: the end of the beginning. Thorax 2003;58:352–6.

727. Le Chevalier T, Scagliotti G, Natale R, et al. Efficacy of gemcitabine plus platinum chemotherapy compared with other platinum containing regimens in advanced non-small-cell lung cancer: a meta-analysis of survival outcomes. Lung Cancer 2005;47:69–80.

728. Blackhall F, Papakotoulas PI, Danson S, et al. Perspectives on novel therapies for bronchial carcinoma. Expert Opin Pharmacother 2005;6:1157–67.

729. Karp JE, Kaufmann SH, Adjei AA, et al. Current status of clinical trials of farnesyltransferase inhibitors. Curr Opin Oncol 2001;13:470–6.

730. Cross SS. The molecular pathology of new anti-cancer agents. Current Diagnostic Pathology 2005;11:329–39.

731. Taller A, Chilevers ER, Dransfield I, et al. Inhibition of neuropeptide stimulated tyrosine phosphorylation and tyrosine kinase activity stimulates apoptosis in small cell lung cancer cells. Cancer Res 1996;56:4255–63.

732. Agus DB, Bunn PA Jr, Franklin W, et al. HER-2/neu as a therapeutic target in non-small cell lung cancer, prostate cancer, and ovarian cancer. Semin Oncol 2000;27:53–63.

733. Paez JG, Janne PA, Lee JC, et al. EGFR mutations in lung cancer: correlation with clinical response to gefitinib therapy. Science 2004;304:1497–500.

734. Rosell R, Ichinose Y, Taron M, et al. Mutations in the tyrosine kinase domain of the EGFR gene associated with gefitinib response in non-small-cell lung cancer. Lung Cancer 2005;50:25–33.

735. Sequist LV, Bell DW, Lynch TJ, et al. Molecular predictors of response to epidermal growth factor receptor antagonists in non-small-cell lung cancer. J Clin Oncol 2007;25: 587–95.

736. Sequist LV. Second-generation epidermal growth factor receptor tyrosine kinase inhibitors in non-small cell lung cancer. Oncologist 2007;12:325–30.

737. Pao W. Defining clinically relevant molecular subsets of lung cancer. Cancer Chemother Pharmacol 2006;58: s11–5.

738. Olaussen KA, Mountzios G, Soria JC. ERCC1 as a risk stratifier in platinum-based chemotherapy for nonsmall-cell lung cancer. Curr Opin Pulm Med 2007;13:284–9.

739. Olaussen KA, Dunant A, Fouret P, et al. DNA repair by ERCC1 in non-small-cell lung cancer and cisplatin-based adjuvant chemotherapy. N Eng J Med 2006;355:983–91.

740. Bepler G, Kusmartseva J, Sharma S, et al. RRM1 modulated in vitro and in vivo efficacy of gemcitabine and platinum in non-small-cell lung cancer. J Clin Oncol 2006;24:4731–7.

12.2 Other epithelial tumours

CARCINOID TUMOURS, TUMOURLETS AND NEUROENDOCRINE CELL HYPERPLASIA

Carcinoid tumours

The term 'carcinoid' was introduced in 1907 to distinguish certain previously described low-grade intestinal neoplasms from adenocarcinomas.[1,2] Bronchial carcinoids were subsequently described, together with 'cylindromas' (adenoid cystic carcinomas of tracheobronchial gland origin, see p. 601), as well-differentiated bronchial tumours.[3] These two tumours came to be known as the carcinoid and cylindromatous types of bronchial adenoma, but this nomenclature was abandoned when it was realised that their histogenesis differed and that both were of at least low-grade malignancy.

It is now appreciated that carcinoid tumours are neuroendocrine neoplasms of low-grade malignancy, related to a variety of more malignant bronchopulmonary tumours that also show evidence of such differentiation.[4–6] These include small cell carcinoma, atypical carcinoid and large cell neuroendocrine carcinoma. Evidence of neuroendocrine differentiation can also be found in occasional squamous cell and adenocarcinomas but its presence there does not appear to be of any clinical significance.[7,8] Neuroendocrine tumours can all generally be distinguished with ease but together they form a spectrum and occasional examples are difficult to classify precisely. Carcinoids, the microscopic tumour-like hyperplasias of the bronchopulmonary neuroendocrine cells known as tumourlets and neuroendocrine cell hyperplasia are considered in this chapter while carcinomas showing neuroendocrine differentiation are dealt with in Chapter 12.1.

Epidemiology and aetiology

About 12% of all carcinoids arise in the lung but less than 1% of lung tumours are carcinoids.[9] The sex incidence is equal and they occur over a wide age range.[10,11] The mean age is about 50 years, significantly lower than that for carcinoma of the lung. About 8% develop in the second decade, making them the commonest primary pulmonary tumour of childhood.[12,13] Carcinoid tumours are not related to smoking or environmental pollution: it is not known what promotes their formation but they are sometimes associated with multiple foci of neuroendocrine cell hyperplasia and tumourlets, which are dealt with next.[14,15] They do not appear to de-differentiate into small cell or large cell neuroendocrine carcinomas, although focal carcinoid differentiation is sometimes observed within otherwise classic small cell carcinoma.

Clinical features

Most patients with bronchopulmonary carcinoid tumours present with cough, haemoptysis or symptoms referable to the consequences of collapse or pneumonia distal to airway obstruction.[10,11] Sometimes there is wheezing, or even stridor, and these features have occasionally been mistaken for asthma. Small central tumours and those in the periphery of the lung may be asymptomatic and only discovered by chance. Occasionally a polypoid carcinoid may be coughed up spontaneously and no trace of its origin found on bronchoscopy.

Very occasionally, bronchial carcinoids present with metastatic deposits or with a variety of paraneoplastic endocrine syndromes, including Cushing's syndrome, acromegaly or the carcinoid syndrome.[16-20] In contrast to their gastrointestinal counterparts, bronchopulmonary carcinoids may cause the carcinoid syndrome in the absence of metastases, although these are usually present. This is because they release their secretions directly into the systemic circulation rather than into portal vessels. For the same reason, the endocarditis that forms part of the carcinoid syndrome affects valves on the left side of the heart rather than the right. Bronchopulmonary carcinoids may also be associated with pituitary, parathyroid and pancreatic islet cell tumours as part of a multiple endocrine neoplasia syndrome known as MEN1.[21]

Gross appearances

Most bronchopulmonary carcinoids arise in the walls of central airways where they are seen on bronchoscopy as smooth cherry-red nodules that protrude into the airway. The bulk of the tumour often extends between the bronchial cartilages to invade the adjacent lung but sometimes the tumour grows entirely into the lumen of the airway, forming an endobronchial polyp. A combination of endobronchial and intrapulmonary growth may also be found, giving the tumour a dumb-bell or cottage-loaf appearance (Fig. 12.2.1A). Those that extend into the lung usually have a well-defined, rounded border. Bronchopulmonary carcinoids are notorious for bleeding profusely if biopsied, although this is not the experience of all groups.[10] The cut surface of the tumour has a soft pinkish-tan or yellow appearance, or is haemorrhagic. A minority of bronchopulmonary carcinoids arise in the periphery of the lung (Fig. 12.2.1B).[22] Occasionally there are multiple tumours.[23-25] These are particularly likely to be associated with multiple tumourlets, hyperplasia of bronchiolar neuroendocrine cells, a peripheral location and, rarely, obliterative bronchiolitis.[14,15,26,27] However a minority of isolated carcinoids also present in a peripheral location. These tend to be circumscribed lesions and may have no obvious association with an airway.

Histological appearances

Microscopy shows that carcinoid tumours have a thin fibrous capsule that is often incomplete. They may also exhibit infiltrative activity (Fig. 12.2.2). Several histological patterns, which may be present in combination, are recognised (Box 12.2.1).[28] The commonest patterns are the trabecular and the mosaic.[29,30] In the former the tumour cells are arranged in interlocking cords or ribbons while in the latter they form nests or islands separated by a delicate fibrovascular stroma (Fig. 12.2.3). The tumour cells are uniform and generally polygonal, with a moderate amount of eosinophilic cytoplasm and round nuclei having finely granular chromatin and inconspicuous nucleoli. Necrosis is not seen and mitoses are not readily evident, numbering less than 2/2 mm². If either necrosis or a higher mitotic rate is identified, the tumour is classified as an atypical carcinoid (see below) or, if 11 or more mitoses per 2 mm² are evident, a large cell neuroendocrine carcinoma (see p. 563).

About 40% of bronchial carcinoids are biphasic, being made up of groups of neuroendocrine cells surrounded by S-100-positive sustentacular cells, a feature that is also found in paragangliomas and which has caused these carcinoids to be termed 'paraganglioid'.[31,32] An

Figure 12.2.1 Bronchial carcinoid tumours. (A) A central carcinoid tumour that is partly endobronchial but has mainly grown into the surrounding lung. Note its well-circumscribed edge. (B) A well-circumscribed 15 mm diameter carcinoid tumour located in the periphery of the lung.

Figure 12.2.2 Bronchial carcinoid tumours showing infiltrative activity. (A) Typical carcinoid tumours have a thin fibrous capsule that is often incomplete. (B) Infiltration of cartilage may be seen in typical carcinoids.

Box 12.2.1 **Histological patterns of bronchopulmonary carcinoid tumours**

Classic patterns
Mosaic (insular)
Trabecular

Variants
Paraganglioid
Adenopapillary
Clear cell
Oncocytic
Melaninogenic
Spindle cell
Atypical

The pattern may vary within a tumour but to a limited degree histological pattern correlates with site; central tumours tend to be trabecular and peripheral growths mosaic or spindle cell.[22]

Figure 12.2.3 Bronchial carcinoid tumours. (A) Trabecular pattern, in which the tumour cells form anastomosing cords. (B) Mosaic pattern, in which the tumour cells are arranged in nests. In both patterns the groups of tumour cells are separated by a delicate vascular stroma, nuclei are regular and there are no atypical features.

alternative view is that these tumours are not carcinoids at all but paragangliomas. Support for this view comes from the identification of scanty ganglion cells in a few examples, leading to the introduction of the term 'pulmonary gangliocytic paraganglioma' (see also p. 638).[33–35] Sustentacular cells are less common in the more malignant neuroendocrine tumours.[32]

Some carcinoid tumours have an adenopapillary pattern, with small amounts of mucin contained within either tumour cells or gland lumina (Fig. 12.2.4).[28,30,36] Peripheral tumours tend to show a spindle cell pattern in which groups of fusiform cells are separated by a rich network of blood vessels (Fig. 12.2.5).[22,29,37] Other carcinoid tumours have abundant clear[38] (Fig. 12.2.6) or eosinophilic cytoplasm (Fig. 12.2.7),[39–41] the latter representing oncocytic change, something that may also be seen in occasional tracheobronchial gland tumours and in glomangiomas. Clear cell carcinoids may be confused with benign clear cell tumours (see p. 625), but the immunohistochemical and ultrastructural features, which are outlined below, are very different. Melanin is occasionally evident within the tumour cells[42–48] (Fig. 12.2.8) and rare examples contain rod-shaped crystalloid cytoplasmic inclusions.[49] Argentaffin stains are seldom positive but argyrophilia can often be demonstrated.

Figure 12.2.4 Bronchial carcinoid tumour of adenopapillary pattern.

Figure 12.2.7 An oncocytic bronchial carcinoid tumour. The tumour cells have abundant deeply eosinophilic cytoplasm.

Figure 12.2.5 A peripheral pulmonary carcinoid tumour of spindle cell pattern.

Figure 12.2.8 A bronchial carcinoid tumour in which many of the tumour cells contain melanin.

Figure 12.2.6 A bronchial carcinoid tumour of clear cell pattern.

Cartilage and bone may form in the stroma of bronchial carcinoid tumours (Fig. 12.2.9).[50] This has been variously ascribed to the tumour infiltrating the perichondrium of the bronchial cartilage or to release of various growth factors by the tumour. Apudamyloid is also occasionally found in the stroma of carcinoid tumours.[51,52] Stromal vascularity may be very marked, with dilated sinusoidal vessels separating groups of tumour cells to give an appearance resembling that of a paraganglioma, the distinction from which is based on the immunocytochemical demonstration of cytokeratin (see below). Alternatively, the hypervascularity may suggest a glomus tumour, which is distinguished by immunocytochemistry and electron microscopy.[53]

Ultrastructure

Electron microscopy shows that the cytoplasm contains abundant dense-core neurosecretory granules, which range from 100 to 250 nm in diameter and vary in shape and electron density (Fig. 12.2.10).[4–6,54–57] Epithelial features include desmosomes and

Figure 12.2.9 A bronchial carcinoid tumour in which there is stromal bone formation.

Figure 12.2.10 Bronchopulmonary carcinoid tumour. Electron microscopy shows a wealth of dense-core neuroendocrine granules.

occasional bundles of tonofilaments. Oncocytic tumours are characterised by closely packed mitochondria in addition to neurosecretory granules, but it may not be possible to demonstrate both in the same cells.[39–41]

Immunohistochemistry

Immunohistochemistry may be used to identify markers of neuroendocrine differentiation.[54,56,58,59] None of the antibodies currently available is totally specific,[60] the best probably being CD56, synaptophysin, chromogranin and N-cadherin.[61–67] Other specific components of the neurosecretory granules include biologically active amines and peptides such as serotonin, calcitonin, gastrin-releasing peptide (human bombesin), adrenocorticotrophic hormone (ACTH), vasoactive intestinal polypeptide and leu-enkephalin. Differences between central and peripheral carcinoids are described, the latter more frequently expressing immunoreactivity for gastrin-releasing peptide, calcitonin and ACTH.[59,68] One bronchial carcinoid contained eight different hormones.[69] The ability to produce more than one hormone may account for variations in granule size seen in a single cell.[57] However, neuroendocrine tumours may even store multiple peptides within a single granule.[70] Occasional tumours show evidence of dual exocrine and endocrine (so-called amphicrine differentiation[71]), for example, neuroendocrine granules have been identified in the same tumour cells as type II pneumocyte lamellar bodies, Clara cell granules and mucous vacuoles.[72,73] The intermediate filaments in the neuroendocrine cells consist of cytokeratin.[74] Although the lung marker thyroid transcription factor-1 (TTF-1) is expressed by small cell carcinoma and large cell neuroendocrine carcinoma, reports of its expression by carcinoid tumours, tumourlets and neuroendocrine cell hyperplasia vary.[75–77] However, positive staining of a carcinoid for TTF-1 makes an origin in the gastrointestinal tract or thymus unlikely.[76,77]

Behaviour

Typical carcinoids are of low-grade malignancy and infiltration of adjacent lung or bronchus is often seen. However, it is important to distinguish typical and atypical carcinoids as the latter carry a worse prognosis (see below). Nuclear pleomorphism is sometimes apparent in typical carcinoids but, as with other endocrine tumours, this is a poor indicator of metastatic potential. It is likely that most early series failed to exclude tumours that would now be regarded as atypical carcinoids, and therefore overestimated the tendency for them to metastasise. In a series of 101 bronchial carcinoids, 10 of the 12 that metastasised were histologically atypical.[11] Typical carcinoid tumours metastasise to hilar nodes in only 6–10% of cases,[59,78,79] and distant metastases, which may involve liver, lung, brain, adrenal or bone, are even less common. Deposits in bone may be osteosclerotic. Treatment usually requires lobectomy or, if the tumour involves the main bronchus, pneumonectomy. However, more limited procedures are sometimes feasible and a correct biopsy diagnosis is therefore important.

Atypical carcinoid tumours

Atypical carcinoids make up about 11% of bronchopulmonary carcinoid tumours.[22] An early report suggested that peripheral carcinoids were more likely to be atypical[80] but more recent larger studies have failed to confirm this.[81] Up to 70% of atypical carcinoids eventually metastasise.[22,59,78,79,82,83] There is little effective treatment for metastatic disease as carcinoid tumours lack the chemosensitivity of small cell carcinomas[84] and the somatostatin analogues that are successfully employed in controlling the advance of metastatic islet cell tumours are only occasionally effective.[85] The 5-year survival rate is about 60%,

Figure 12.2.11 Atypical carcinoid. Increased malignant potential is suggested by (A) mitoses numbering more than 2/mm² and (B) foci of punctate necrosis (right of centre).

which is closer to that of typical carcinoids (95%) than that of large cell neuroendocrine carcinomas and small cell carcinomas (2%). The peak age incidence (56 years, range 19–75 years) is also intermediate between that of typical carcinoid tumours (50 years, range 19–75 years) and small cell carcinoma (62 years, range 30–79 years) and they are more often seen in smokers than are their more benign counterparts. Ectopic endocrine activity is commoner with atypical than typical carcinoids.

Macroscopically, atypical carcinoids tend to be related to airways like their typical counterparts, but are more infiltrative. Microscopically, they are recognised by increased mitotic activity and necrosis being seen in a tumour with the characteristic cellular make-up and trabecular or mosaic architecture of a carcinoid (Fig. 12.2.11). The necrosis is usually punctate and confined to the centres of cell groups, and it may lead to focal dystrophic calcification. The atypical features may not be apparent in small biopsies as they are often focal. Atypical tumours were originally defined as carcinoids that showed any one or a combination of features that included pleomorphism, prominent

nucleoli, hyperchromasia, hypercellularity and disorganisation, as well as the afore-mentioned necrosis and increased mitotic activity,[78] but some of these additional features are of little prognostic importance. Nuclear pleomorphism, for example, may be found in otherwise unexceptional carcinoids that behave in an indolent manner. Necrosis and increased mitotic activity are the most reliable pointers to atypical behaviour. Mitoses number 3–10 per 2 mm² (about 10 high-power fields); more than 10 indicates small cell or large cell neuroendocrine carcinoma (see Table 12.1.12, p. 563).[86] Within a group of atypical carcinoids, those with 6–10 mitoses per 2 mm² were more aggressive than those with 2–5, and patients with tumours measuring over 3.5 cm also fared badly.[81]

Electron microscopy shows that atypical carcinoids contain fewer dense-core granules than typical carcinoids, but more than small cell carcinomas. The immunohistochemical features are generally similar to those of typical carcinoids, but with increasing malignancy there is a progressive loss of chromogranin and N-cadherin positivity, loss of heterozygosity and increased incidence of gene abnormalities.[67,87,88] Also, the C-terminal peptide of human pre-bombesin is detectable in the majority of atypical tumours whereas it can only be shown in a small number of typical carcinoids.[89] Increasing atypicality is also associated with loss of the S-100-positive sustentacular cells that characterise many typical carcinoid tumours.[31,90] Aneuploidy occurs in both typical and atypical carcinoids but is commoner in the latter.[91–94] Proliferative activity assessed by expression of the Ki-67 antigen is higher in atypical than in typical carcinoids.[95] All these features correlate with the observed behaviour of atypical carcinoids, which is intermediate between that of typical carcinoids and small cell carcinoma. Thus, in the spectrum of neuroendocrine tumours of the lung, atypical carcinoids come between typical carcinoid and the neuroendocrine carcinomas in terms of their pathological features, natural history and prognosis (Table 12.2.1).

Molecular biology and genetics of carcinoids

Comparative genomic hybridisation has shown frequent chromosomal abnormalities at 11q13 (the site of the MEN1 gene) in both typical and atypical carcinoids, a point of distinction from small cell carcinoma and neuroendocrine large cell carcinoma.[96,97] Further differences between carcinoids and the higher-grade neuroendocrine carcinomas include low Rb and p53 inactivation and a low incidence of 3p and 17p deletions in the carcinoids and differences in the ratio of bcl2:bax proteins.[88,98,99] These differences support the opinion that typical and atypical carcinoids are more closely related to each other than to large cell neuroendocrine carcinoma and small cell carcinoma.[88,100–105] Differences between typical and atypical carcinoids are relatively rare but, in general, atypical carcinoids show more extensive genetic alterations than typical carcinoids. For example, atypical carcinoids have more often shown DNA underrepresentation at 10q and 13q.[101]

Tumourlets and neuroendocrine cell hyperplasia

While neuroendocrine cells are abundant in fetal lung, few are found in adult lungs where they are normally scattered singly and sparsely along the bronchial basement membrane. Occasionally however aggregates of neuroendocrine cells are encountered in adult lungs, occurring either as clusters of cells or as linear arrays along the basement membrane. If such aggregates are confined by the basement membrane the process is termed neuroendocrine cell hyperplasia whereas if they penetrate the basement membrane the term tumourlet is used (for lesions up to a size of 5 mm; beyond 5 mm they are

Table 12.2.1 A comparison of typical carcinoid, atypical carcinoid, large cell neuroendocrine carcinoma and small cell carcinoma

	Typical carcinoid	Atypical carcinoid	Large cell neuroendocrine carcinoma	Small cell carcinoma
Behaviour				
Local invasion	Present	Present	Present	Present
Lymphatic metastases	Occasional	Not infrequent	Frequent	Usual
Distant metastases	Rare	45–70%	>50%	90–100%
5-year survival	95%	60%	27–35%	2%
Histology				
Architecture	Well-organised	Focal loss	Moderate loss	Poor
Necrosis	None	Focal	Abundant	Abundant
DNA deposition on vessels	None	None	None	Frequent
Cytology				
Mitoses	Not seen (<2/10 HPF)	Common (2–10/10 HPF)	Numerous (>10/10 HPF)	Numerous (>10/10 HPF)
Pleomorphism	Usually absent	Moderate	Marked	Small cell
Argyrophilia	Common	Variable	–	Rare
Neuroendocrine markers	Common, diffuse	Common, diffuse	Common, often patchy	Common, often patchy
Aetiology				
Role of smoking	None	Weak	Strong	Strong
Male:female ratio	0.8:1	2:1	2.5:1	Declining[a]
Mean age (years)	50	56	63	62
Ultrastructure				
Granule numbers	Many	Moderate numbers	–	Scanty
Granule size (nm)	150–250	80–140	–	80–140

[a]The male:female ratio of small cell carcinoma was formerly high but has been constantly dropping as more women smoke.

HPF, high-powered field.

regarded as carcinoid tumours) (Figs 12.2.12 and 12.2.13).[106] Neuroendocrine cell hyperplasia is more commonly found in association with neuroendocrine tumours of the lung than with non-neuroendocrine tumours and within the spectrum of neuroendocrine tumours it is especially associated with peripheral carcinoids.[26,107]

The term 'tumourlet' was coined by Whitwell[108] but Liebow had earlier noted their histological resemblance to carcinoid tumours and referred to them, perhaps more accurately, as atypical carcinoid proliferations.[109] However, Whitwell's term 'tumourlet' is in more general use. Opinion is divided on the nature of tumourlets but the secondary cases probably represent hyperplasia whereas a preneoplastic state is envisaged for those patients with diffuse idiopathic pulmonary neuroendocrine cell hyperplasia (see below). Tumourlets seldom, if ever, metastasise and if similar deposits are found in the hilar lymph nodes[110–112] or the pulmonary lesions are larger than 5 mm, they are classified as carcinoid tumours.

Clinical features

Tumourlets are most frequently associated with bronchiectasis and are often multiple.[113] Other conditions associated with neuroendocrine cell hyperplasia and tumourlets include pulmonary hypertension,[114] bronchopulmonary dysplasia,[115] chondroid 'hamartomas'[116] and various causes of focal pulmonary scarring.[117,118] However, they are not particularly associated with diffuse interstitial fibrosis.

It has generally been assumed that neuroendocrine cell hyperplasia and tumourlets are pathological curiosities devoid of any clinical import but this view has had to be revised following reports of their association with clinically significant obstructive airway disease.[14,26,119,120] Histological examination in such cases has shown fibrous obliteration of bronchioles associated with diffuse idiopathic neuroendocrine cell hyperplasia and multiple tumourlets (Fig. 12.2.14). This syndrome has been termed diffuse idiopathic pulmonary neuroendocrine cell hyperplasia.[27,106,119] It is suggested that in these cases the tumourlets are the cause rather than an effect of the fibrosis, the fibrosis being mediated by the secretion of fibrogenic cytokines such as gastrin-releasing peptide (human bombesin) by the tumourlets.[119] Similar postulates were advanced in a report of interstitial pulmonary fibrosis associated with diffuse neuroendocrine hyperplasia that extended out from the bronchioles to fill many alveoli.[121] It is now considered that diffuse neuroendocrine cell hyperplasia represents a preneoplastic lesion leading to carcinoid tumours, mainly typical but occasionally

Figure 12.2.12 Neuroendocrine cell hyperplasia. (A) A focus of neuroendocrine cell hyperplasia is present in the basal layer of the respiratory epithelium, limited by the basement membrane. (B) The hyperplastic cells are more easiliy visualised by immunohistochemistry and are demonstrated here with an immunoperoxidase stain for chromogranin.

Figure 12.2.13 Tumourlet. A neuroendocrine cell aggregate composed of small oval cells has infiltrated the peribronchiolar lung parenchyma.

atypical,[27] but not to other neuroendocrine tumours. No genetic markers have been identified that might distinguish diffuse idiopathic neuroendocrine cell hyperplasia from neuroendocrine cell hyperplasia secondary to lung damage, although diffuse idiopathic neuroendocrine cell hyperplasia is seen in occasional patients at the

extreme end of type MEN1 syndrome,[122] with mutation at the associate gene being seen frequently in carcinoid tumours (see above).

Until recently tumourlets and foci of neuroendocrine hyperplasia have been too small to be detected radiologically but with improved imaging technology this is no longer the case and increasing numbers are being identified, often leading to them being biopsied to exclude metastatic disease.[27,123]

Microscopy

Tumourlets are minute, tumour-like proliferations that are generally discovered incidentally. They arise in close proximity to bronchioles as multiple nests of cells separated by narrow connective tissue septa (see Fig. 12.2.13). Their cells are uniform and have regular, round, oval or spindle-shaped nuclei with finely dispersed chromatin. Electron microscopy shows that the cytoplasm contains granules of typical dense-core type, averaging 100 nm in diameter.[124] The immunohistochemical features are identical to those of normal bronchopulmonary neuroendocrine cells and of carcinoid tumours (see above).[58,59,125]

The relationship between tumourlets and bronchioles can often be clearly seen and it is likely that tumourlets arise from bronchiolar neuroendocrine cells.[126,127] Bronchiolar epithelium may directly overlie the cell clusters, or the bronchiole may be distended by the tumourlet. In lungs in which tumourlets have been identified, markers such as synaptophysin or chromogranin usually reveal many more but smaller clusters of cells within the basal layer of the bronchiolar epithelium. Examination of lungs resected for carcinoid tumours or carcinoma may also show a significant increase in the number of neuroendocrine cells, including clusters large enough to disturb and narrow small airways.[15,119] Occasionally, otherwise typical carcinoid tumours may be accompanied by multiple fully formed tumourlets.[14]

Differential diagnosis

Tumourlets differ from carcinoid tumours only in their size. An arbitrary upper size limit of 5 mm has been adopted.[106] Tumourlets may be confused with meningothelioid nodules (see p. 700). Unlike

Figure 12.2.14 Diffuse idiopathic neuroendocrine cell hyperplasia. (A) A dilated bronchiole shows chronic obstructive changes. (B) At the lower border of (A) there is a small focus of neuroendocrine cell hyperplasia and fibrosis. (C) An elastin stain shows that this represents fibrous obliteration of a branching bronchiole. This was just one of many such foci identified throughout the explanted lung of a patient undergoing lung transplantation for obstructive lung disease.

tumourlets, the latter are not related to air spaces but are situated within the interstitium, generally near septal veins: they lack neuroendocrine features. Localised regenerative proliferations of bronchiolar epithelium have sometimes been termed tumourlets, but they usually consist of stratified squamous epithelium and lack the pattern of a true tumourlet; they also are devoid of any neuroendocrine features.

Prognosis

Diffuse idiopathic neuroendocrine cell hyperplasia generally pursues a benign course but the condition is slowly progressive and the subsequent obliterative bronchiolitis has occasionally necessitated transplantation.[120]

TRACHEOBRONCHIAL GLAND (SALIVARY GLAND-TYPE) TUMOURS

The mixed seromucous glands of the trachea and bronchi are similar to the minor salivary glands and give rise to the same range of tumours.[128] Many are of low-grade malignancy and the term 'bronchial adenoma', previously used to cover both tracheobronchial gland tumours and bronchial carcinoid tumours,[3] has therefore been abandoned despite them very rarely occurring in combination.[129] Tracheobronchial gland tumours are less common than bronchial carcinoids, in a ratio of 1:10, and most are either adenoid cystic carcinomas or mucoepidermoid tumours. Pleomorphic adenoma, the commonest tumour of the major salivary glands, is rare in the lower respiratory tract. It is probable that some central adenocarcinomas arise in tracheobronchial glands, although the site of origin of these aggressive tumours can rarely be identified with confidence and claims that they have a distinctive morphological pattern[130,131] are not entirely convincing.

Tracheobronchial gland tumours are usually central lesions that tend to protrude into the airway lumen, causing such symptoms as cough and haemoptysis, possibly of long duration. Alternatively, there may be a history of repeated episodes of pneumonia. Occasionally a tracheobronchial gland tumour is coughed up spontaneously.[132] Clinical evaluation to exclude metastasis from a salivary gland primary is always prudent, particularly if the lung tumour is peripheral or one of many.

Adenoid cystic carcinoma

Adenoid cystic carcinoma, formerly known as cylindroma, has an equal sex incidence and is a tumour of middle age (mean about 50 years), being extremely rare under the age of 30.[128,133,134] Clinical features are as outlined above.

Pathological features

Adenoid cystic carcinomas most often involve the lower trachea or large bronchi but some are peripheral, presumably derived from glands in small bronchi.[135,136] They are slowly growing infiltrative tumours that thicken and narrow the airway wall. They form poorly defined, sessile, nodular growths that may ulcerate centrally but more usually infiltrate extensively beneath an intact mucosa, ultimately involving adjacent lung tissue and hilar lymph nodes by direct invasion.[136] Perineural infiltration is a characteristic feature.

Pulmonary adenoid cystic carcinomas are identical in their microscopical appearances to those encountered in other sites, which include salivary gland, breast, skin, oesophagus, cervix uteri and prostate. The tumour cells form well-demarcated groups within which small cysts give a cribriform or tubular appearance (Fig. 12.2.15). The cysts may contain alcianophilic connective tissue mucin, secreted by their lining myoepithelial cells. Serial sections show that these spaces are continuous with the stroma of the tumour. Whilst most of this secretion is mucoid and haematoxyphil, in places it becomes eosinophilic and hyaline, forming connective tissue cylinders that gave the tumour its former name of cylindroma. Closely packed, small, dark myoepithelial cells form the dominant cell population, but there are also true ducts lined by slightly larger cells that secrete periodic acid–Schiff (PAS)-positive epithelial mucin.[137] As in the salivary glands, these tumours may occasionally be more solid and of higher grade. The immunocytochemical profile of adenoid cystic carcinoma reflects its myoepithelial nature. the tumour cells staining for cytokeratin, vimentin and actin; S-100 staining may also be positive (Table 12.2.2). The cysts contain components of basement membrane which may stain for laminin, fibronectin and type IV collagen.[134,138,139] Molecular studies have shown polysomy of chromosome 7 in one-third of cases but neither amplification nor mutation of the epidermal growth factor receptor (EGFR) gene.[140] KIT protein expression is frequently found but KIT-activating mutations are not seen.[141]

Differential diagnosis

The histological features are usually sufficiently distinctive to allow a confident diagnosis but in small biopsies it may be difficult to distinguish adenoid cystic carcinoma from adenocarcinoma, basaloid carcinoma, small cell carcinoma and lymphoma. Identification of a myoepithelial phenotype is then helpful.

Treatment and prognosis

The central location of adenoid cystic carcinomas and their predilection for submucosal and perineural spread make it difficult to treat these tumours effectively. Despite this, resection is the treatment of choice, with stenting, local ablation and radiotherapy forming alternative options for tumours that cannot be completely resected. Because of their growth pattern it is particularly important that the resection margins are checked by frozen section before closure. Nevertheless, local recurrence is frequent, often after a period of years, and may eventually lead to fatal pulmonary infection. Metastases are uncommon but may develop in lymph nodes, bone, kidney, liver, brain and lung.[135]

Figure 12.2.15 Adenoid cystic carcinoma of bronchial gland origin. (A) The tumour is almost wholly endobronchial. (B) Histologically, these tumours are identical to those that arise in the salivary glands. Microcysts give the tumour a cribriform pattern.

Table 12.2.2 Immunohistochemistry of tracheobronchial gland tumours				
	Adenoid cystic carcinoma	**Mucoepidermoid tumour**	**Pleomorphic adenoma**	**Acinic cell tumour**
Cytokeratin	+++	+++	+++	+++
S-100 protein	+	−	++	−
Actin	+++	−	++	−
Vimentin	++	−	++	−
Glial fibrillary protein	−	−	++	−
Chromogranin	−	−	−	−

Figure 12.2.16 Low-grade mucoepidermoid carcinoma. (A) Endobronchial tumour occludes the airway. (B) At low power, this endobronchial tumour shows a mixed solid and glandular pattern. Many of the tumour acini are distended by mucus, in which there is focal dystrophic calcification. (C) An island of tumour beneath the surface epithelium consists of intermediate and goblet cells.

Mucoepidermoid carcinoma

Mucoepidermoid carcinomas comprise 0.1–0.2% of primary lung tumours.[142] All ages are affected, although approximately 50% of cases present before 30 years of age and 20% before 20 years. There is a female sex predominance.[143] The tumours show a spectrum of malignancy.[128,133,142–150] Low- and high-grade variants are recognised, the former comprising about 80% of these neoplasms. Younger patients generally have low-grade tumours, most of which are cured by surgical resection. The high-grade tumours are generally found in patients over the age of 30 years and prove fatal in 23% of cases.[143] Although typically presenting with symptoms of obstruction, occasional patients may be misdiagnosed as having asthma.[151] Imaging classically reflects airway obstruction and an endobronchial mass, sometimes with punctate calcification.[152]

Gross features

Mucoepidermoid carcinoma most commonly arises in the main, lobar or segmental bronchi but occasional examples are peripheral.[149] The gross appearances vary according to the degree of malignancy. Low-grade tumours form smooth, partly cystic, polypoid masses that project into the lumen of the bronchus (Fig. 12.2.16A) and may have a papillary stucture.[150] They grow by expansion and compress surrounding tissue. The overlying bronchial mucosa, which may show squamous metaplasia, is generally intact. More aggressive tumours tend to be less clearly defined, irregular and solid: they infiltrate surrounding lung and more closely resemble the commoner carcinomas of the lung.

Microscopy

The essential microscopic feature of mucoepidermoid carcinomas is that they contain both glands and squamous elements (Fig. 12.2.16B, C). The glands are lined by a mixture of mucous and non-secretory columnar cells, and contain epithelial mucus that may calcify or even ossify.[143] The mucous cells are also found mixed with the squamous cells in a sheet-like arrangement. The squamous cells are linked by intercellular bridges but keratinisation is not seen.[144] Sheets of regular, polygonal cells with abundant eosinophilic cytoplasm and known as transitional or intermediate cells merge with the mucous and squamous cells and may be the dominant component. In some tumours the cells have abundant clear cytoplasm or, rarely, show oncocytic change.[153] Occasional examples display a prominent lymphoplasmacytic infiltrate.[154] Low-grade tumours lack cellular atypia and mitoses, features that are seen particularly in the squamous component of the more malignant tumours. Genetic analysis has shown a variety of translocations including t(11;19)(p22;q13), t(11;19)(q14–21;p12) and t(11;19)(q21;p13) that lead to the development of a novel fusion oncogene, *MECT1-MAML2*.[152,155–157] The last of these gene rearrangements was found in 10/10 well-differentiated bronchopulmonary mucoepidermoid carcinomas, 3 of 7 poorly differentiated such tumours and in none of the several adenosquamous, squamous or adenocarcinomas examined, thus proving to be of use in both diagnosis and prognosis.[157]

Differential diagnosis

The histological features are usually sufficiently distinctive to permit a confident diagnosis but separation from mucous gland adenoma and carcinoid may be difficult in small biopsies or on frozen section. Immunohistochemistry may help exclude carcinoid tumours but, in practice, as long as the surgeons are aware that they are dealing with a low-grade malignancy or benign tumour and that bronchoplastic resection is an option, definitive classification may wait until examination of the resection specimen.

High-grade tumours show a more infiltrative growth pattern (Fig. 12.2.17) and it is difficult to draw absolute distinctions between high-grade mucoepidermoid carcinoma and adenosquamous carcinoma, both of which have a dual cell population. However, adenosquamous carcinomas tend to arise in the periphery of the lung whereas mucoepidermoid carcinomas arise in major airways. Frank keratinisation with the formation of keratin pearls suggests adenosquamous carcinoma rather than mucoepidermoid carcinoma whereas the presence of abundant cells that are transitional in appearance between squamous and mucous cells, foci of the more characteristic low-grade pattern and a lack of in situ carcinoma in the overlying epithelium all favour mucoepidermoid carcinoma. The differential diagnosis also includes necrotising sialometaplasia, a reactive, non-invasive process that generally follows prolonged tracheal intubation (see p. 51).[158]

Treatment and prognosis

Surgical resection is the treatment of choice for both low-grade and high-grade tumours, with bronchoplastic surgery an option in low-grade cases. The prognosis of low-grade tumours is generally excellent, although nodal involvement and metastases have occasionally been reported.[143,147,159] The prognosis in children appears to be slightly better than in adults, probably reflecting a higher incidence of low-grade tumours in younger patients.[12,145] The prognosis for high-grade tumours is variably reported[142,143,160] but about 25% of patients with these tumours develop metastases, typically in lymph nodes, bone or skin. Some patients with unresectable disease have responded favourably to EGFR-targeted therapy.[161]

Mucous gland adenoma

Mucous gland adenoma, or cystadenoma, is one of the rarest tumours of tracheobronchial glands and one that has no direct counterpart in the salivary glands.[128,132,162–164] Reported examples cover a wide age range, including childhood. They arise in main, lobar or segmental

Figure 12.2.17 High-grade mucoepidermoid carcinoma. (A) An endobronchial tumour occludes a segmental bronchus and an adjacent lymph node is greatly enlarged by metastastatic tumour. (B) The intermediate cells are of acinar pattern, pleomorphic and mitotically active and there is some resemblance to an adenocarcinoma.

bronchi as smooth, rounded, polypoid tumours (Fig. 12.2.18A). The overlying bronchial mucosa is usually intact and the cut surface may show irregular microcystic spaces filled with mucus. Invasion of bronchial wall or lung parenchyma is not seen and these tumours tend to remain superficial to the bronchial cartilage. Surgical resection, ideally by bronchoplastic resection, is curative.

Microscopically, glands, which sometimes form small cysts, are lined by columnar or cuboidal mucous cells and contain mucin (Fig. 12.2.18B). More solid areas consist of tubular or acinar structures or aggregates of mucus-filled cells. The intermediate and squamous cells of a mucoepidermoid carcinoma are not seen but the identification by electron microscopy of occasional squamous, myoepithelial and oncocytic elements indicates a possible overlap with low-grade mucoepidermoid carcinoma.[163,164]

normal bronchial glands, oncocytic change affects small groups of cells in ducts and acini and is seen more frequently with increasing age.[166] Bronchial carcinoids (see Fig. 12.2.7), glomus tumours, mucoepidermoid carcinomas and acinic cell carcinomas are all occasionally oncocytic, and recognition of their true nature may depend upon the use of mucous stains, immunocytochemistry or electron microscopy.[167]

Pure oncocytomas are exceedingly rare in the airways.[128,167-169] Some reported cases have been very small incidental lesions in which the oncocytes formed acinar or tubulopapillary patterns.[125,168] Grossly, oncocytomas usually form well-demarcated, solid nodules ranging in size from 1 to 3.5 cm. They are generally solitary but multiple pulmonary oncocytomas have been described.[170] Histologically, the oncocytic tumour cells are arranged in sheets or nests. They show little mitotic activity and no necrosis. Focal infiltrative growth may be noted at the periphery of lesions but this is not regarded as indicating malignancy.[169] The tumour cells stain focally for cytokeratin and vimentin, but not for actin, S-100 or neuroendocrine markers.[169] The absence of neuroendocrine markers helps exclude oncocytic carcinoid. Granular cell tumours resemble oncocytomas but are S-100-positive and cytokeratin-negative.

Oncocytoma carries an excellent prognosis. Lymph node metastasis is recorded in one case but 2 years after lobectomy the patient was free of disease.[171]

Pleomorphic adenoma

Pleomorphic adenoma, which is the commonest tumour of major salivary glands, is rare in the lower respiratory tract.[172-176] The histological features are similar to those seen in the salivary gland tumour except that ducts are relatively sparse: microscopy shows epithelial and myoepithelial cells in a myxoid or chondroid stroma (Fig. 12.2.19). The tumour cells react strongly with antibodies to cytokeratin and variably for vimentin, actin, S-100 protein and glial fibrillary acidic protein (see Table 12.2.2).[173] Occasional tumours show cytological atypia or local infiltrative activity and these tumours are prone to metastasise.[128,173,177] Frankly carcinomatous elements may also be seen arising from a pleomorphic adenoma (carcinoma ex pleomorphic adenoma). Some rare malignant endobronchial myxoid tumours resemble extraskeletal myxoid chondrosarcomas but probably represent a variant of pleomorphic adenoma.[178]

Epithelial–myoepithelial carcinoma

Terms such as adenomyoepithelioma and myoepithelioma have been previously applied to this tumour but it is of low malignant potential and the name epithelial–myoepithelial carcinoma is therefore recommended.[106] It is particularly rare in the lower respiratory tract: no more than 30 cases have been recorded.[179-191] Age at presentation ranges from 33 to 71 years, with no sex predominance.

Pathological features

Grossly, the tumour either protrudes into the bronchus or forms a large intrapulmonary mass. The cut surface may be solid or gelatinous. Microscopically, both epithelial and myoepithelial elements are usually present (Fig. 12.2.20), although purely myoepithelial tumours also occur and some also show pneumocytic differentiation.[192] The typical tubule is lined by two cell types, an inner layer of cytokeratin-positive epithelial cells surrounded by an outer mantle of myoepithelial cells, the latter expressing smooth-muscle actin and S-100 antigen. The outer cells may in turn be surrounded by a rim of PAS-positive basement membrane material. In purely myoepithelial

Figure 12.2.18 Mucous gland adenoma. (A) Endoscopic view. *(Courtesy of Dr Gaafar, Alexandria, Egypt.)* (B) The tumour consists solely of glands lined by cytologically bland mucus-secreting columnar cells.

Oncocytoma

Oncocytes, or oxyphil cells, have abundant, finely granular, eosinophilic cytoplasm due to the presence of numerous closely packed mitochondria. These organelles are very striking when examined by electron microscopy but may also be demonstrated by their affinity for phosphotungstic acid haematoxylin, with which they stain dark blue. Oncocytes are also distinguished by their strong expression of cytokeratin 14.[165] Oncocytes occur in the thyroid, parathyroid and salivary glands and give rise to oncocytic tumours in all these sites. In

Figure 12.2.19 Pleomorphic adenoma of the bronchus. Glandular structures are set in an abundant myxoid stroma showing chondroid differentiation.

areas, the tumour cells vary from polygonal to spindle-shaped and generally form solid nodules separated by a hyaline stroma.

Differential diagnosis

The differential diagnosis includes several other types of tracheobronchial gland neoplasm. Pleomorphic adenomas often contain myoepithelial cells and ducts, but chondroid or myxochondroid elements usually predominate.[173] Adenoid cystic carcinomas may resemble epithelial–myoepithelial carcinomas with a predominantly ductal pattern, but are more infiltrative and cribriform areas are usually also present. Epithelial–myoepithelial carcinoma may also enter the differential diagnosis of pulmonary clear cell tumours (see Table 12.3.1, p. 626).[187]

Treatment and prognosis

Surgical resection is the treatment of choice. Epithelial–myoepithelial carcinomas are generally indolent growths but recurrence or metastasis has been recorded in purely myoepitheliomatous cases that showed brisk mitotic activity, necrosis and atypia.[186,187]

Acinic cell carcinoma

The histological appearances of this rare tumour are identical to those of its salivary gland counterpart. It is an indolent growth and the prognosis is good.[193] The pattern is generally solid but reticulin surrounds groups of tumour cells and outlines an acinar or glandular pattern. The tumour cells are regular and have a poorly staining slightly basophilic, vacuolated or granular cytoplasm.[194,195] Diastase PAS reactions are generally weak. Electron microscopy shows dense cytoplasmic granules of about 500 nm diameter, as seen in the serous acini of the tracheobronchial glands.[194,195] The differential diagnosis includes carcinoid tumour, paraganglioma and benign clear cell tumour.

PAPILLOMAS

Several types of tumour show a tendency to endobronchial growth, which means that they grow predominantly into the lumen of the airways (Fig. 12.2.21).[196] They include squamous cell carcinomas,[196] basaloid carcinomas, carcinoids,[36] some tracheobronchial gland neoplasms,[150] carcinosarcomas, occasional metastases, inflammatory polyps and the papillomas that are dealt with here.

Solitary papilloma

Solitary papillomas are generally squamous cell in type but glandular papillomas and mixed squamous and glandular papillomas are also recognised.[197] Sometimes a bronchial papilloma of mixed squamous and mucous cell type is continuous with a mucous cell adenoma of an underlying bronchial gland.[198]

Aetiological factors concerned in the development of solitary squamous cell papillomas include human papillomavirus, which is found in over 50% of cases,[197,199–202] and cigarette smoking, perhaps acting in combination. The patients are generally middle-aged or elderly men. Types 16 and 18 papillomavirus are involved in these solitary tumours, rather than the types 6 and 11 found in papillomatosis.[200,201] About one-third show cytologic atypia and there is a spectrum of microscopic appearances, ranging from a simple benign, cytologically bland papilloma with or without an inflamed hyaline stroma to the invasive papillary squamous cell carcinoma discussed in Chapter 12.1.[198] In solitary squamous papillomas, the epithelial covering may show the whole range of changes described in the development of squamous cell carcinoma in flat bronchial epithelium: squamous metaplasia, dysplasia, carcinoma-in-situ and invasive tumour. In general, older patients are more likely to have lesions that are malignant. Most are cured by excision, but about 20% recur.[197]

Papillomas clothed entirely by mucous, simple columnar or ciliated cells are termed glandular (or columnar cell) papillomas (Fig. 12.2.22).[106,203,204] They generally develop in the larger conductive airways but peripheral examples are recorded.[204a] The age range is wide – 26–74 years.[205] Most are cured by excision but occasional cases recur[197] and some show foci of adenocarcinomatous change.[204a] Unusual glandular papillomas containing multiple cysts have been described in association with von Hippel–Lindau syndrome.[206]

Mixed squamous and columnar cell papillomas are rare. They are commoner in male smokers, as with squamous papillomas, and may show cytologic atypia. No such cases have recurred.[197]

Some bronchial tumours resemble papillary urothelial tumours and have been called transitional cell papillomas.[198,207] Tumours of this name are well known in the nose, where they are also known as schneiderian, Ringertz or inverted papilloma. Earlier editions of the

Figure 12.2.20 Epithelial–myoepithelial carcinoma. (A) The tumour shows a mixture of tubules (right) and a more solid spindle cell proliferation (left). (B) The tubules are lined by an inner layer of epithelial cells surrounded by an outer layer of myoepithelial cells which have a clear cytoplasm. The myoepithelial cells stain for both S-100 (C) and smooth-muscle actin (D).

World Health Organization's histological classification of lung tumours referred to transitional cell papillomas[208] whereas the current edition uses the term 'inverted papilloma'.[106] However, specialists in nasal pathology do not accept that the bronchial tumours are the same as those seen in the nose, where they are regarded as polyps showing squamous metaplasia[209]: those in the bronchi are a subtype of squamous cell papilloma and comparing them to tumours of the nose or urinary tract is best avoided.

Recurrent respiratory papillomatosis

Recurrent respiratory papillomatosis most commonly affects the larynx. Only 5% of patients have involvement of the trachea or large bronchi, and fewer than 1% have more distal lung involvement.[210,211]

The human papillomavirus is an aetiological factor, types 6 and 11 having been identified in the lesions.[212–217] Infection is believed to be acquired at birth during vaginal delivery. However, since papillomavirus infection is common and recurrent respiratory papillomatosis is rare, other factors probably contribute to pathogenesis. For example, an association with HLA DRB1*0301 has been reported.[213–215,217,218]

The onset is generally before the age of 11 years and most examples regress before puberty. However, repeated laser therapy may first be required because the lesions are prone to recur. If left untreated, the lesions may enlarge, spread and endanger the airway (Fig. 12.2.23).[219] Multiple laryngeal, tracheal and bronchial papillomas cause hoarseness, stridor and respiratory obstruction, whilst the rare pulmonary lesions appear on chest radiographs as solid or cystic rounded nodules.[217]

The papillomas have a narrow connective tissue stalk covered by non-keratinising stratified squamous epithelium. There is no atypia but certain cytological changes typical of a genital condyloma caused by the human papillomavirus may be found, namely koilocytosis, which is characterised by irregular nuclear shrinkage, binucleation

Figure 12.2.21 Endoscopic view of a tracheobronchial papilloma. *(Courtesy of Dr Gaafar, Alexandria, Egypt.)*

Figure 12.2.23 Papillomatosis spreading along the wall of the trachea: bronchoscopic appearances. *(Reproduced from Haussinger et al. (2003)[219] by permission of Elsevier.)*

Figure 12.2.22 A bronchial papilloma of glandular type in which the epithelium consists of columnar mucous cells.

and perinuclear clearing (Fig. 12.2.24).[220] The papillomatous proliferation may extend into the soft tissues surrounding the airways, even though there are no cytological features of malignancy. Such extension has been termed invasive papillomatosis.[221] In the lung clusters of squamous cells fill several adjacent alveoli without destroying their walls. Continued growth leads to expansion of the alveoli and compression of the surrounding lung. In larger invasive lesions, central cavitation occurs, with the danger of secondary infection.

Frank malignant change to squamous cell carcinoma, characterised by atypia, keratinisation and infiltrative growth, supervenes in about 2% of cases. Smoking and irradiation, the latter used in the past to treat the papillomatosis, appear to promote this complication, which has been recorded in patients whose ages have ranged from 6 to 35 years.[220,222–227] Malignant change has been associated with type 11 papillomavirus infection followed by increased expression of p53 and Rb proteins.[228]

ADENOMAS

Papillary adenoma

Papillary adenomas are rare well-circumscribed parenchymal lesions. Affected patients are usually asymptomatic, the lesions being found incidentally on imaging. The tumours may be encapsulated and are typically soft solid masses that range from 1 to 4 cm in size. Multiple type II cell papillary adenomas are recorded in a child with neurofibromatosis.[229]

The lining cells are cuboidal or columnar (Fig. 12.2.25). They stain for cytokeratins, TTF-1, surfactant apoproteins, carcinoembryonic antigen and epithelial membrane antigen (EMA) and have the ultrastructural features of either Clara cells or type II alveolar epithelial cells or both these cell types.[198,230–235]

Papillary adenomas are distinguished from sclerosing pneumocytoma by lacking the varied architecture of the latter and by the TTF-1 and EMA staining being limited to the surface epithelium. They are distinguished from alveolar adenoma by their papillary growth pattern and focal ciliated or Clara cell morphology. Metastases also need to be excluded, especially those from the thyroid. Occasionally, papillary adenomas show infiltrative growth, in which case their distinction from papillary adenocarcinoma is uncertain and they are probably best classified as low-grade adenocarcinomas.

Alveolar adenoma

This tumour often resembles a lymphangioma microscopically and some examples have probably been reported as such.[236,237] Its epithelial nature was established in 1986 by a combination of electron microscopy and immunocytochemistry.[238] Only a few have been reported since.[239–244] One group compared the lesion to the sclerosing

Figure 12.2.24 Bronchial papillomatosis. (A) The papillae are covered by well-differentiated non-keratinising squamous epithelium. (B) High magnification shows nuclear shrinkage with perinuclear vacuolation indicative of papilloma virus infection.

Figure 12.2.25 Papillary adenoma. The tumour consists of papillae lined by cytologically bland pneumocyte-like cells. It differs from sclerosing pneumocytoma by its lack of stromal cells.

Figure 12.2.26 Alveolar adenoma forming a well-circumscribed 13-mm peripheral nodule. *(Courtesy of Dr M Jagusch, formerly of Auckland, New Zealand.)*

Figure 12.2.27 Alveolar adenoma. Irregular spaces, deceptively resembling lymphatics, are separated by fibrous septa of varying thickness with flattened lining cells. *(Courtesy of Dr M Jagusch, formerly of Auckland, New Zealand.)*

pneumocytoma described below and suggested that it was a variant of the latter.[245]

The mean age of the patients reported to date is about 60 years. They have all had solitary peripheral lung lesions, measuring up to 2 cm in diameter, most of which were discovered incidentally as a radiographic 'coin lesion'.[238,239] None has recurred after local excision or lobectomy.[243]

Alveolar adenomas are well-circumscribed tumours with a solid grey or haemorrhagic appearance on the cut surface (Fig. 12.2.26). Microscopy typically shows irregular spaces, empty or filled with PAS-positive eosinophilic material (Fig. 12.2.27). Occasional lesions may be solid and mimic a sclerosing pneumocytoma.[245–247] The spaces are lined by flattened or cuboidal cytokeratin-positive cells that have the ultrastructural features of type I and II alveolar epithelial cells (Fig. 12.2.28). They also stain for surfactant apoprotein and TTF-1. However they are negative for the Clara cell marker, CC10[243] and they do not express endothelial markers. This latter finding helps exclude

Figure 12.2.28 Alveolar adenoma. The cells lining the spaces stain for cytokeratin, showing that the tumour is an adenoma rather than a lymphangioma. Immunoperoxidase stain.

Figure 12.2.29 Sclerosing pneumocytoma forming a well-circumscribed peripheral tumour. It shows microcystic change and is yellow because of its high lipid content. *(Courtesy of Dr M Jagusch, formerly of Auckland, New Zealand.)*

lymphangioma which the tumour may mimic morphologically. The spaces are separated by fibrous septa that are generally thin but may show exuberant connective tissue proliferation so that a mesenchymal neoplasm with cystic change enters the differential diagnosis. There may also be focal lymphoid infiltration or central stellate scarring.

SCLEROSING PNEUMOCYTOMA (SCLEROSING 'HAEMANGIOMA')

This unusual lung tumour was first described in 1956[248] under the name sclerosing haemangioma, a term that reflects two common histological features, sclerosis and vascular proliferation, that are both now thought to represent secondary changes in an essentially epithelial neoplasm. This view is based on immunohistochemical and ultrastructural evidence that the tumour cells are type II pneumocytes: they stain for epithelial rather than endothelial markers and have ultrastructural features characteristic of type II cells.[249–264]

The term 'sclerosing pneumocytoma' is therefore more appropriate than sclerosing haemangioma,[251] although the latter is still preferred by the World Health Organization for historic reasons.[106] It is suggested that these tumours are related to the peripheral papillary adenoma and the alveolar adenoma described above.[239] Several authors have proposed that they are hamartomatous[246,249,265] but rare reports of them metastasising to hilar lymph nodes[245–247,266] and evidence of clonality support them being neoplastic.[267]

Clinical features

Patients with sclerosing pneumocytoma range from 13 to 83 years of age, with a peak incidence in the fifth decade and the ratio of females to males being about 5:1.[246,250,251,255,268] The preponderance of females is reflected in the demonstration of oestrogen and progesterone receptors on the tumour.[269,270] Most of the patients with these receptors have been Asian.[258] Most patients are asymptomatic, but some complain of cough or haemoptysis. Imaging typically shows a solitary circumscribed mass that may rarely be calcified or cystic, while haemorrhagic variants are sometimes identifiable by nuclear magnetic resonance. Alternatively, multiple small nodules may be found.[271,272] The tumours are generally benign but, as noted above, hilar lymph node

Figure 12.2.30 Sclerosing pneumocytoma showing a typically mixed solid, papillary, haemorrhagic and sclerotic architecture.

metastasis is recorded.[245–247] One example was observed over a period of 47 years, at which stage it occupied the whole of the left thoracic cavity but had not metastasised.[273]

Pathological features

Sclerosing pneumocytomas are well-circumscribed but not encapsulated tumours: they show expansile growth and compress rather than infiltrate the adjacent lung. The cut surface is variegated, with red well-vascularised areas and yellow foci amid firmer grey tissue (Fig. 12.2.29). Most tumours are peripheral and solitary, but multiple lesions have been reported and occasionally there is prominent endobronchial growth.[250,271,274,275] Rare cystic examples are also recorded.[276]

Histologically, the tumours may be papillary, solid, sclerotic or angiomatoid. One of these patterns may predominate but they more commonly seen in combination (Fig. 12.2.30).[261] In the papillary

Figure 12.2.31 Sclerosing pneumocytoma. The tumour comprises cuboidal lining cells, which have eosinophilic cytoplasm, and more rounded stromal cells that have either eosinophilic or clear cytoplasm.

Figure 12.2.32 Sclerosing pneumocytoma. Only the surface tumour cells stain for cytokeratins (A) but both surface and stromal cells stain for epithelial membrane antigen (B) and thyroid transcription factor-1 (C).

areas the covering cells have moderate amounts of lightly eosinophilic cytoplasm and oval, slightly irregular nuclei with a single nucleolus (Fig. 12.2.31). Mitoses are rare and atypia is unusual. These cells may be continuous with normal bronchiolar epithelium. They stain for cytokeratin, EMA, TTF-1 and surfactant (Fig. 12.2.32).[260,261] A second cell type forms the stroma of the papillae and often fills the interpapillary spaces. These cells are rounded and uniform with distinct cell borders. Significant pleomorphism is exceptionally rare. They contain centrally located cytologically bland nuclei with fine chromatin. Their cytoplasm is either eosinophilic or clear (see Fig. 12.2.31). These cells, like those covering the surface of the papillae, express EMA and TTF-1 but not surfactant or cytokeratin (see Fig. 12.2.32).[245,260–263] The two cell types show an identical pattern of monoclonality.[267] By electron microscopy the surface cells contain lamellar bodies similar to those of type II pneumocytes whereas the round cells contain electron-dense structures that possibly represent lamellar body precursors.[261] Molecular studies suggest that the Wnt/β-catenin pathway is involved in the pathogenesis of these tumours.[277]

Secondary changes include haemorrhage, haemosiderosis, foamy macrophage accumulation, sclerosis, focal dystrophic calcification, cystic degeneration and even a granulomatous reaction (Fig. 12.2.33).[278] The formation of 'giant lamellar bodies' is a further secondary change. These structures represent extracellular accumulations of surfactant material arranged in lamellar fashion and forming roughly spherical bodies that measure up to 25 μm in diameter.[279] They are not specific to sclerosing pneumocytomas but are encountered most frequently in these tumours.

Occasional patients have multiple small sclerosing pneumocytomas intimately related to multiple tumourlets.[271]

Differential diagnosis

The most important distinction is from adenocarcinoma of the lung. A dual cell population, variegated patterns, a characteristic immunophenotype and a lack of cytological atypia all favour sclerosing pneumocytoma. One study suggests that the diagnosis can be confidently made at frozen section.[280]

Figure 12.2.33 Sclerosing pneumocytoma. Secondary features include (A) sclerosis, (B) foamy macrophage accumulation, (C) angiomatoid change and (D) dystrophic calcification.

Epithelioid haemangioendothelioma is another tumour characterised by sclerosis and a papillary structure, but it is generally multifocal and differs in its radiographic appearances and natural history as well as microscopically: furthermore its stromal cells express endothelial rather than epithelial markers (see p. 636).

Sclerosing pneumocytomas characterised by sheets of clear cells may be mistaken for the benign clear cell tumour of the lung described on page 625 and also for metastatic renal cell carcinoma but are distinguished from both these tumours by their TTF-1 and EMA positivity and from the benign clear cell tumour by failing to express HMB45. Clear cell carcinoma of the lung is distinguished by showing malignant features and lacking the two cell types seen in sclerosing pneumocytoma. Papillary adenoma and alveolar adenoma similarly lack these two cell types.

PULMONARY THYMOMA

It is rare to encounter primary thymomas outside the mediastinum but examples have been described in the neck, trachea, thyroid, lung and pleura, sometimes associated with thymic rests in these tissues.[281–289] The diagnosis of thymoma in such sites requires careful review of the clinical and radiological findings to exclude metastasis or direct spread from a primary mediastinal lesion (see Fig. 12.6.15, p. 688).

Patients with pulmonary or pleural thymomas may be asymptomatic or complain of chest pain, weight loss or breathlessness. One patient with an intrapulmonary thymoma had myasthenia gravis.[281] Radiology shows a circumscribed central or peripheral pulmonary nodule, a pleural nodule, pleural thickening or pleural effusion. Occasionally there are multiple intrapulmonary tumours, or a thymoma may involve the pleura diffusely in the manner of a mesothelioma.[288]

Pulmonary thymomas are identical to those that arise in the thymus but are not so clearly encapsulated. Infiltrative growth is therefore more difficult to assess. Some invasive tumours prove to be inoperable and others have metastasised.[287] However, most pulmonary thymomas are slowly growing tumours that can be cured by surgical resection.

Predominantly epithelial thymomas arising in the lung are likely to be mistaken for carcinoma, those of mixed cellularity for lymphoepithelial carcinoma, those predominantly lymphocytic for lymphoma or small cell carcinoma, and those of spindle cell pattern for localised fibrous tumour. Thymoma carries a better prognosis than many of these and a correct histological diagnosis is therefore important. Except in the case of lymphoepithelial carcinoma, the mixed cellularity of a thymoma is helpful in suggesting the correct diagnosis.[284] The lymphocytes within a thymoma express CD1a whereas those within a lymphoepithelial carcinoma or those reacting to a carcinoma do not. TTF-1 staining would indicate carcinoma of the lung, being found in about 30% of pulmonary large cell undifferentiated carcinomas but not in thymomas, while CD5 is more commonly expressed in thymomas.[290,291] Positive immunostaining for cytokeratin generally distinguishes spindle cell thymomas from both localised fibrous tumour and lymphoma.

REFERENCES

Carcinoid tumours, tumourlets and neuroendocrine cell hyperplasia

1. Lubarsch O. Ueber den primaren Krebs des Ileum nebst Bemerkungen uber das gleichzeitige Vorkommen von Krebs und Tuberculose. Virchows Arch A Pathol Anat Histopathol 1888;111:280–317.
2. Oberndorfer S. Karzinoide Tumoren des Dunndarmes. Frankf Z Pathol 1907;1:426–32.
3. Hamperl H. Uber gutartige Bronchialtumoren (Cylindrome und Carcinoide). Virchows Arch A Pathol Anat Histopathol 1937;300:46–88.
4. Bensch KG, Gordon GB, Miller LR. Electron microscopic and biochemical studies on the bronchial carcinoid tumor. Cancer 1965;18:592–602.
5. Gmelich JT, Bensch KG, Liebow AA. Cells of Kultchitzky type in bronchioles and their relation to the origin of peripheral carcinoid tumor. Lab Invest 1967;17:88–98.
6. Bensch KG, Corrin B, Pariente R, et al. Oat cell carcinoma of the lung: its origin and relationship to bronchial carcinoid. Cancer 1968;22:1163–72.
7. Ionescu DN, Treaba D, Gilks CB, et al. Nonsmall cell lung carcinoma with neuroendocrine differentiation – an entity of no clinical or prognostic significance. Am J Surg Pathol 2007;31:26–32.
8. Sterlacci W, Fiegl M, Hilbe W, et al. Clinical relevance of neuroendocrine differentiation in non-small cell lung cancer assessed by immunohistochemistry: a retrospective study on 405 surgically resected cases. Virchows Archiv 2009;455:125–32.
9. Godwin JD. Carcinoid tumors. Cancer 1975;36:560–9.
10. Hurt R, Bates M. Carcinoid tumours of the bronchus: a 33 year experience. Thorax 1984;39:617–23.
11. McCaughan BC, Martini N, Bains MS. Bronchial carcinoids. Review of 124 cases. J Thorac Cardiovasc Surg 1985;89:8–17.
12. Hartman GE, Shochat SJ. Primary pulmonary neoplasms of childhood: a review. Ann Thorac Surg 1983;36:108–19.
13. Wang LT, Wilkins EW, Bode HH. Bronchial carcinoid tumors in pediatric patients. Chest 1993;103:1426–8.
14. Miller MA, Mark GJ, Kanarek D. Multiple peripheral pulmonary carcinoids and tumorlets of carcinoid type, with restrictive and obstructive lung disease. Am J Med 1978;65:373–8.
15. Gould VE, Linnoila I, Memoli VA, et al. Neuroendocrine components of the bronchopulmonary tract in hyperplasias, dysplasias and neoplasms. Lab Invest 1983;15:519–37.
16. Melmon KL, Sjoerdsma A, Mason DT. Distinctive clinical and therapeutic aspects of the syndrome associated with bronchial carcinoid tumors. Am J Med 1965;39:568–81.
17. Ricci C, Patrassi N, Massa R, et al. Carcinoid syndrome in bronchial adenoma. Am J Surg 1973;126:671–7.
18. Sonksen PH, Ayres AB, Braimbridge M, et al. Acromegaly caused by pulmonary carcinoid tumours. Clin Endocrinol 1976;5:503–13.
19. Okike N, Bernatz PE, Woolner LB. Carcinoid tumors of the lung. Ann Thorac Surg 1976;22:270–7.
20. Huber RM, Schopohl J, Losa M, et al. Growth-hormone releasing hormone in a bronchial carcinoid. Cancer 1991;67:2538–42.
21. Marx SJ, Agarwal SK, Kester MB, et al. Multiple endocrine neoplasia type 1: clinical and genetic features of the hereditary endocrine neoplasias. Recent Prog Horm Res 1999;54:397–438.
22. Bonikos DS, Bensch KG, Jamplis RW. Peripheral pulmonary carcinoid tumours. Cancer 1976;37:1977–98.
23. Felton WL, Liebow AA, Lindskog GE. Peripheral and multiple bronchial adenomas. Cancer 1953;6:555–66.
24. Skinner C, Ewen SWB. Carcinoid lung: diffuse pulmonary infiltration by a multifocal bronchial carcinoid. Thorax 1976;31:212–19.
25. Aubry MC, Thomas CF Jr, Jett JR, et al. Significance of multiple carcinoid tumors and tumorlets in surgical lung specimens: analysis of 28 patients. Chest 2007;131:1635–43.
26. Miller RR, Muller NL. Neuroendocrine cell hyperplasia and obliterative bronchiolitis in patients with peripheral carcinoid tumors. Am J Surg Pathol 1995;19:653–8.
27. Davies SJ, Gosney JR, Hansell DM, et al. Diffuse idiopathic pulmonary neuroendocrine cell hyperplasia: an under-recognised spectrum of disease. Thorax 2007;62:248–52.
28. Wise WS, Bonder D, Aikawa M, et al. Carcinoid tumour of lung with varied histology. Am J Surg Pathol 1982;6:261–7.
29. Salyer DC, Salyer WR, Eggleston JC. Bronchial carcinoid tumours. Cancer 1975;36:1522–37.
30. Jones RA, Dawson IMP. Morphology and staining patterns of endocrine tumours in the gut, pancreas and bronchus and their possible significance. Histopathology 1977;1:137–50.
31. Barbareschi M, Frigo B, Mosca L, et al. Bronchial carcinoids with S-100 positive sustentacular cells. A comparative study with gastrointestinal carcinoids, pheochromocytomas and paragangliomas. Pathol Res Pract 1990;186:212–22.
32. Gosney JR, Denley H, Resi M. Sustentacular cells in pulmonary neuroendocrine tumours. Histopathology 1999;34:211–15.
33. Hironaka M, Fukayama M, Takayashiki N, et al. Pulmonary gangliocytic paraganglioma – case report and comparative immunohistochemical study of related neuroendocrine neoplasms. Am J Surg Pathol 2001;25:688–93.
34. Min KW. Spindle cell carcinoids of the lung with paraganglioid features: a

reappraisal of their histogenetic origin from paraganglia using immunohistochemical and electronmicroscopic techniques. Ultrastruct Pathol 2001;25:207–17.

35. Palau MA, Merino MJ, Quezado M. Corticotropin-producing pulmonary gangliocytic paraganglioma associated with Cushing's syndrome. Human Pathology 2006;37:623–6.

36. Mark EJ, Quay SC, Dickerson GR. Papillary carcinoid tumor of lung. Cancer 1981;48:316–24.

37. Ranchod M, Levine GD. Spindle-cell carcinoid tumours of the lung. Am J Surg Pathol 1980;4:315–31.

38. Gaffey MJ, Mills SE, Frierson HF, et al. Pulmonary clear cell carcinoid tumor: Another entity in the differential diagnosis of pulmonary clear cell neoplasia. Am J Surg Pathol 1998;22:1020–5.

39. Sklar JL, Churg A, Bensch KG. Oncocytic carcinoid tumor of the lung. Am J Surg Pathol 1980;4:287–92.

40. Scharifker D, Marchevsky A. Oncocytic carcinoid of lung: an ultrastructural analysis. Cancer 1981;47:530–2.

41. Alvarez-Fernandez E, Folque-Gomez E. Atypical bronchial carcinoid with oncocytoid features. Arch Pathol Lab Med 1981;105:428–31.

42. Cebelin MS. Melanocytic bronchial carcinoid tumor. Cancer 1980;46:1843–8.

43. Gould VE, Memoli VE, Dardi LE, et al. Neuroendocrine carcinomas with multiple immunoreactive peptides and melanin production. Ultrastruct Pathol 1981;2:199–217.

44. Grazer R, Cohen SM, Jacobs JB, et al. Melanin-containing peripheral carcinoid of the lung. Am J Surg Pathol 1982;6:73–8.

45. Carlson JA, Dickersin GR. Melanotic paraganglioid carcinoid tumor – a case report and review of the literature. Ultrastruct Pathol 1993;17:353–72.

46. Fukuda T, Kobayashi H, Kamishima T, et al. Peripheral carcinoid tumor of the lung with focal melanin production. Pathol Int 1994;44:309–16.

47. Iihara K, Yamaguchi K, Fujioka Y, et al. Pigmented neuroendocrine tumor of the lung, showing neuromelanin. Pathol Int 2002;52:734–9.

48. Goel A, Addis BJ. Pigmented atypical carcinoid of the lung. Histopathology 2007;51:263–5.

49. Grogg KL, Padmalatha C, Leslie KO. Bronchial carcinoid tumor with crystalloid cytoplasmic inclusions. Arch Pathol Lab Med 2002;126:93–6.

50. Hasleton PS, al Saffar N. The histological spectrum of bronchial carcinoid tumours. Appl Pathol 1989;7:205–18.

51. Gordon HW, Miller R, Mittman C. Medullary carcinoma of the lung with amyloid stroma: a counterpart of medullary carcinoma of the thyroid. Hum Pathol 1973;4:431–6.

52. Abe Y, Utsunomiya H, Tsutsumi Y. Atypical carcinoid tumor of the lung with amyloid stroma. Acta Pathol Jpn 1992;42:286–92.

53. Heard BE, Dewar A, Firmin RK, et al. One very rare and one new tracheal tumour found by electron microscopy: glomus tumour and acinic cell tumour resembling carcinoid tumours by light microscopy. Thorax 1982;37:97–103.

54. Hage E. Histochemistry and fine structure of bronchial carcinoid tumours. Virchows Arch A Pathol Anat Histopathol 1973;361:121–8.

55. Capella C, Gabrielli M, Polak JM, et al. Ultrastructural and histological study of 11 bronchial carcinoids. Virchows Arch A Pathol Anat Histopathol 1979;381:313–29.

56. Fisher ER, Palekar A, Paulson JD. Comparative histopathologic histochemical, electron microscopic and tissue culture studies of bronchial carcinoids and oat cell carcinomas of lung. Am J Clin Pathol 1978;69:165–72.

57. Warren WH, Memoli VA, Gould VE. Immunohistochemical and ultrastructural analysis of bronchopulmonary neuroendocrine neoplasms. I Carcinoids. Ultrastruct Pathol 1984;6:15–27.

58. Cutz E, Chan W, Kay JM, et al. Immunoperoxidase staining for serotonin, bombesin, calcitonin and leu-enkephalin in pulmonary tumourlets, bronchial carcinoids and oat cell carcinomas. Lab Invest 1982;46:16A.

59. Bonato M, Cerati M, Pagani A, et al. Differential diagnostic patterns of lung neuroendocrine tumours – a clinico-pathological and immunohistochemical study of 122 cases. Virchows Arch A Pathol Anat Histopathol 1992;420:201–11.

60. Loy TS, Darkow GVD, Quesenberry JT. Immunostaining in the diagnosis of pulmonary neuroendocrine carcinomas: an immunohistochemical study with ultrastructural correlations. Am J Surg Pathol 1995;19:173–82.

61. Totsch M, Muller LC, Hittmair A, et al. Immunohistochemical demonstration of chromogranin-A and chromogranin-B in neuroendocrine tumors of the lung. Hum Pathol 1992;23:312–16.

62. Gould VE, Wiedenmann B, Lee I, et al. Synaptophysin expression in neuroendocrine neoplasms as determined by immunocytochemistry. Am J Pathol 1987;126:243–57.

63. Gosney JR, Gosney MA, Lye M, et al. Reliability of commercially available immunocytochemical markers for identification of neuroendocrine differentiation in bronchoscopic biopsies of bronchial carcinoma. Thorax 1995;50:116–20.

64. Boers JE, Denbrok JLM, Koudstaal J, et al. Number and proliferation of neuroendocrine cells in normal human airway epithelium. Amer J Respir Crit Care Med 1996;154:758–63.

65. Lantuejoul S, Moro D, Michalides RJAM, et al. Neural cell adhesion molecules (NCAM) and NCAM-PSA expression in neuroendocrine lung tumors. Am J Surg Pathol 1998;22:1267–76.

66. Lyda MH, Weiss LM. Immunoreactivity for epithelial and neuroendocrine antibodies are useful in the differential diagnosis of lung carcinomas. Hum Pathol 2000;31:980–7.

67. Zynger DL, Dimov ND, Ho LC, et al. Differential expression of neural-cadherin in pulmonary epithelial tumours. Histopathology 2008;52:348–54.

68. Roth KA, Ritter J, Mazoujian G. Central and peripheral bronchial carcinoids possess distinct peptide immunostaining patterns. In: Fenoglio-Preiser CM, Wolff M, Rilke F, editors. Progress in Surgical Pathology. Philadelphia: Field and Wood; 1992. p. 241–50.

69. Rees LH, Bloomfield GA, Rees GM, et al. Multiple hormones in a bronchial tumor. J Clin Endocrinol Metab 1974;38:1090–7.

70. Erlandson RA, Nesland JM. Tumors of the endocrine/neuroendocrine system – an overview. Ultrastruct Pathol 1994;18:149–70.

71. Chejfec G, Capella C, Solcia E, et al. Amphicrine cells, dysplasias and neoplasias. Cancer 1985;56:2683–90.

72. Geller SA, Gordon RE. Peripheral spindle-cell carcinoid tumour of the lung with type II pneumocyte features. Am J Surg Pathol 1984;8:145–50.

73. Sheppard MN, Thurlow NP, Dewar A. Amphicrine differentiation in bronchioloalveolar cell carcinoma. Ultrastruct Pathol 1994;18:437–41.

74. Blobel GA, Gould VE, Moll R, et al. Coexpression of neuroendocrine markers and epithelial cytoskeletal proteins in bronchopulmonary neuroendocrine neoplasms. Lab Invest 1985;52:39–51.

75. Sturm N, Rossi G, Lantuejoul S, et al. Expression of thyroid transcription factor-1 in the spectrum of neuroendocrine cell lung proliferations with special interest in carcinoids. Hum Pathol 2002;33:175–82.

76. Saqi A, Alexis D, Remotti F, et al. Usefulness of CDX2 and TTF-1 in differentiating gastrointestinal from pulmonary carcinoids. Am J Clin Pathol 2005;123:394–404.

77. Du EZ, Goldstraw P, Zacharias J, et al. TTF-1 expression is specific for lung primary in typical and atypical carcinoids: TTF-1-positive carcinoids are predominantly in peripheral location. Hum Pathol 2004;35:825–31.

78. Arrigoni MG, Woolner LB, Bernatz PE. Atypical carcinoid tumours of the lung. J Thorac Cardiovasc Surg 1972;64:413–21.

79. Fink G, Krelbaum T, Yellin A, et al. Pulmonary carcinoid – presentation, diagnosis, and outcome in 142 cases in

Israel and review of 640 cases from the literature. Chest 2001;119:1647–51.

80. Mark EJ, Ramirez JF. Peripheral small-cell carcinoma of the lung resembling carcinoid tumour. Arch Pathol Lab Med 1985;109:263–9.

81. Beasley MB, Thunnissen FFJ, Brambilla E, et al. Pulmonary atypical carcinoid: Predictors of survival in 105 cases. Hum Pathol 2000;31:1255–65.

82. Mills SE, Cooper PH, Walker AN, et al. Atypical carcinoid tumor of the lung. Am J Surg Pathol 1982;6:643–54.

83. Lequaglie C, Patriarca C, Cataldo I, et al. Prognosis of resected well-differentiated neuroendocrine carcinoma of the lung. Chest 1991;100:1053–6.

84. Struyf NJA, Vanmeerbeeck JPA, Ramael MRL, et al. Atypical bronchial carcinoid tumours. Respir Med 1995;89: 133–8.

85. Christinmaitre S, Chabbertbuffet N, Mure A, et al. Use of somatostatin analog for localization and treatment of ACTH secreting bronchial carcinoid tumor. Chest 1996;109:845–6.

86. Travis WD, Rush W, Flieder DB, et al. Survival analysis of 200 pulmonary neuroendocrine tumors with clarification of criteria for atypical carcinoid and its separation from typical carcinoid. Am J Surg Pathol 1998;22:934–44.

87. Przygodzki RM, Finkelstein SD, Langer JC, et al. Analysis of p53, K-ras-2, and C-raf-1 in pulmonary neuroendocrine tumors: correlation with histological subtype and clinical outcome. Am J Pathol 1996;148:1531–41.

88. Onuki N, Wistuba II, Travis WD, et al. Genetic changes in the spectrum of neuroendocrine lung tumors. Cancer 1999;85:600–7.

89. Addis BJ, Hamid Q, Ibrahim NBN, et al. Immunohistochemical markers of small cell carcinoma and related neuroendocrine tumours of the lung. J Pathol 1987;153:137–50.

90. Barbareschi M, Detassis C, Palma PD, et al. Atypical bronchial carcinoids lack S-100 positive sustentacular cells. Pathol Res Pract 1991;187:856.

91. Jackson-York GL, Davis BH, Warren WH, et al. Flow cytometric DNA content analysis in neuroendocrine carcinoma of the lung – correlation with survival and histologic subtype. Cancer 1991;68: 374–9.

92. Travis WD, Linnoila RI, Tsokos MG, et al. Neuroendocrine tumors of the lung with proposed criteria for large-cell neuroendocrine carcinoma – an ultrastructural, immunohistochemical, and flow cytometric study of 35 cases. Am J Surg Pathol 1991;15:529–53.

93. Caulet S, Capron F, Ghorra C, et al. Flow cytometric DNA analysis of 20 bronchopulmonary neuroendocrine tumours. Eur Respir J 1993;6:83–9.

94. Padberg BC, Woenchkhaus J, Hilger G, et al. DNA cytophotometry and prognosis in typical and atypical bronchopulmonary carcinoids: a clinicomorphologic study of 100 neuroendocrine lung tumors. Am J Surg Pathol 1996;20:815–22.

95. Costes V, Martyane C, Picot MC, et al. Typical and atypical bronchopulmonary carcinoid tumors: a clinicopathologic and KI-67-labeling study. Hum Pathol 1995;26:740–5.

96. Debelenko LV, Brambilla E, Agarwal SK, et al. Identification of MEN1 gene mutations in sporadic carcinoid tumors of the lung. Hum Mol Genet 1997;6:2285–90.

97. Debelenko LV, Swalwell JI, Kelley MJ, et al. MEN1 gene mutation analysis of high-grade neuroendocrine lung carcinoma. Genes Chromosomes Cancer 2000;28:58–65.

98. Brambilla E, Negoescu A, Gazzeri S, et al. Apoptosis-related factors p53, Bcl(2), and Bax in neuroendocrine lung tumors. Am J Pathol 1996;149:1941–52.

99. Beasley MB, Lantuejoul S, Abbondanzo S, et al. The P16/cyclin D1/Rb pathway in neuroendocrine tumors of the lung. Hum Pathol 2003;34:136–42.

100. Ullmann R, Schwendel A, Klemen H, et al. Unbalanced chromosomal aberrations in neuroendocrine lung tumors as detected by comparative genomic hybridization. Hum Pathol 1998;29:1145–9.

101. Walch AK, Zitzelsberger HF, Aubele MM, et al. Typical and atypical carcinoid tumors of the lung are characterized by 11q deletions as detected by comparative genomic hybridization. Am J Pathol 1998;153:1089–98.

102. Finkelstein SD, Hasegawa T, Colby T, et al. 11q13 allelic imbalance discriminates pulmonary carcinoids from tumorlets – A microdissection-based genotyping approach useful in clinical practice. Am J Pathol 1999;155:633–40.

103. Ullmann R, Petzmann S, Klemen H, et al. The position of pulmonary carcinoids within the spectrum of neuroendocrine tumors of the lung and other tissues. Genes Chromosomes Cancer 2002;34:78–85.

104. Petzmann S, Ullmann R, Klemen H, et al. Loss of heterozygosity on chromosome arm 11q in lung carcinoids. Hum Pathol 2001;32:333–8.

105. Gugger M, Burckhardt E, Kappeler A, et al. Quantitative expansion of structural genomic alterations in the spectrum of neuroendocrine lung carcinomas. J Pathol 2002;196:408–15.

106. World Health Organization. Tumours of the lung, pleura, thymus and heart. Lyons: IARC Press; 2004.

107. Rizvi SM, Goodwill J, Lim E, et al. The frequency of neuroendocrine cell hyperplasia in patients with pulmonary neuroendocrine tumours and non-neuroendocrine cell carcinomas. Histopathology 2009;55:332–7.

108. Whitwell F. Tumourlets of the lung. J Pathol Bacteriol 1955;70:529–41.

109. Liebow AA. Tumours of the lower respiratory tract. *Atlas of Tumor Pathology.* Washington: Armed Forces Institute of Pathology; 1952. p. 16.

110. Hausman DH, Weimann RB. Pulmonary tumorlet with hilar lymph node metastasis. Cancer 1967;20:1515–19.

111. D'Agati VD, Perzin KH. Carcinoid tumorlets of the lung with metastasis to a peribronchial lymph node. Cancer 1985;55:2472–6.

112. Liu SM, Wu HH, Wu CJ, et al. Adrenocorticotropin-producing pulmonary tumorlets with lymph node metastasis. Pathol Int 2003;53:883–6.

113. Canessa PA, Santini D, Zanelli M, et al. Pulmonary tumourlets and microcarcinoids in bronchiectasis. Monaldi Arch Chest Dis 1997;52:138–9.

114. Heath D, Yacoub M, Gosney JR, et al. Pulmonary endocrine cells in hypertensive pulmonary vascular disease. Histopathology 1990;16:21–8.

115. Johnson DE, Lock JE, Elde RP, et al. Pulmonary neuroendocrine cells in hyaline membrane disease and bronchopulmonary dysplasia. Pediatr Res 1982;16:446–54.

116. Cavazza A, Paci M, Rossi G. Pulmonary hamartoma with typical carcinoid/tumourlet. Virchows Arch 2006;449:392–3.

117. Churg A, Warnock ML. Pulmonary tumorlet: a form of peripheral carcinoid. Cancer 1976;37:1469–77.

118. Pelosi G, Zancanaro C, Sbabo L, et al. Development of innumerable neuroendocrine tumorlets in pulmonary lobe scarred by intralobar sequestration – immunohistochemical and ultrastructural study of an unusual case. Arch Pathol Lab Med 1992;116:1167–74.

119. Aguayo SM, Miller YE, Waldron JA, et al. Brief report – idiopathic diffuse hyperplasia of pulmonary neuroendocrine cells and airways disease. N Engl J Med 1992;327:1285–8.

120. Sheerin N, Harrison NK, Sheppard MN, et al. Obliterative bronchiolitis caused by multiple tumourlets and microcarcinoids successfully treated by single lung transplantation. Thorax 1995;50: 207–9.

121. Armas OA, White DA, Erlandson RA, et al. Diffuse idiopathic pulmonary neuroendocrine cell proliferation presenting as interstitial lung disease. Am J Surg Pathol 1995;19:963–70.

122. Fessler MB, Cool CD, Miller YE, et al. Idiopathic diffuse hyperplasia of pulmonary neuroendocrine cells in a patient with acromegaly. Respirology 2004;9:274–7.

123. Darvishian F, Ginsberg MS, Klimstra DS, et al. Carcinoid tumorlets simulate pulmonary metastases in women with breast cancer. Human Pathology 2006;37:839–44.

124. Torikata C. Tumorlets of the lung – an ultrastructural study. Ultrastruct Pathol 1991;15:189–95.

125. Gosney J, Green ART, Taylor W. Appropriate and inappropriate neuroendocrine products in pulmonary tumourlets. Thorax 1990;45:679–83.

126. Ranchod M. The histogenesis and development of pulmonary tumorlets. Cancer 1977;39:1135–45.

127. Bonikos DS, Archibald R, Bensch KE. On the origin of the so-called tumourlets of the lung. Hum Pathol 1976;7:461–9.

Tracheobronchial gland (salivary gland-type) tumours

128. Spencer H. Bronchial mucous gland tumours. Virchows Arch A Pathol Anat Histopathology 1979;383:101–15.

129. Rodriguez J, Diment J, Lombardi L, et al. Combined typical carcinoid and acinic cell tumor of the lung: A heretofore unreported occurrence. Hum Pathol 2003;34:1061–5.

130. Kimula Y. A histochemical and ultrastructural study of adenocarcinoma of the lung. Am J Surg Pathol 1978;2: 253–64.

131. Edwards CW. Pulmonary adenocarcinoma: review of 106 cases and proposed new classification. J Clin Pathol 1987;40:125–35.

132. Terashima M, Nishimura Y, Nakata H, et al. Spontaneous coughing up of a polyp. Respiration 2000;67:101–3.

133. Conlan AA, Payne WS, Woolner LB, et al. Adenoid cystic carcinoma (cylindroma) and mucoepidermoid carcinoma of the bronchus. J Thorac Cardiovasc Surg 1978;76:370–7.

134. Moran CA, Suster S, Koss MN. Primary adenoid cystic carcinoma of the lung – a clinicopathologic and immunohistochemical study of 16 cases. Cancer 1994;73:1390–7.

135. Gallagher CG, Stark R, Teskey J, et al. Atypical manifestations of pulmonary adenoid cystic carcinoma. Br J Dis Chest 1986;80:396–9.

136. Inoue H, Iwashita A, Kanegae H, et al. Peripheral pulmonary adenoid cystic carcinoma with substantial submucosal extension to the proximal bronchus. Thorax 1991;46:147–8.

137. Azumi N, Battifora H. The cellular composition of adenoid cystic carcinoma. Cancer 1987;60:1589–98.

138. Nomori H, Kaseda S, Kobayashi K, et al. Adenoid cystic carcinoma of the trachea and main-stem bronchus. A clinical, histopathologic, and immunohistochemical study. J Thorac Cardiovasc Surg 1988;96:271–7.

139. Tsubochi H, Suzuki T, Suzuki S, et al. Immunohistochemical study of basaloid squamous cell carcinoma, adenoid cystic and mucoepidermoid carcinoma in the upper aerodigestive tract. Anticancer Res 2000;20:1205–11.

140. Macarenco RS, Uphoff TS, Gilmer HF, et al. Salivary gland-type lung carcinomas: an EGFR immunohistochemical, molecular genetic, and mutational analysis study. Mod Pathol 2008;21:1168–75.

141. Aubry MC, Heinrich MC, Molina J, et al. Primary adenoid cystic carcinoma of the lung: absence of KIT mutations. Cancer 2007;110:2507–10.

142. Heitmiller RF, Mathisen DJ, Ferry JA, et al. Mucoepidermoid lung tumours. Ann Thorac Surg 1989;47:394–9.

143. Yousem SA, Hochholzer L. Mucoepidermoid tumours of the lung. Cancer 1987;60:1346–52.

144. Klacsmann PG, Olson JL, Eggleston JC. Mucoepidermoid carcinoma of the bronchus: an electron microscopic study of the low grade and high grade variants. Cancer 1979;43:1720–33.

145. Mullins JD, Barnes RP. Childhood bronchial mucoepidermoid tumours: a case report and review of the literature. Cancer 1979;44:315–22.

146. Lack EE, Harris GBC, Eraklis AJ, et al. Primary bronchial tumours in childhood. Cancer 1983;51:492–7.

147. Metcalf JS, Maize JC, Shaw EB. Bronchial mucoepidermoid carcinoma metastatic to skin. Report of a case and review of the literature. Cancer 1986;58:2556–9.

148. Wolf KM, Mehta D, Claypool WD. Mucoepidermoid carcinoma of the lung with intracranial metastases. Chest 1988;94:435–8.

149. Green LK, Gallion TL, Gyorkey F. Peripheral mucoepidermoid tumour of the lung. Thorax 1991;46:65–6.

150. Guillou L, Deluze P, Zysset F, et al. Papillary variant of low-grade mucoepidermoid carcinoma – an unusual bronchial neoplasm – a light microscopic, ultrastructural and immunohistochemical study. Am J Clin Pathol 1994;101:269–74.

151. Cicutto LC, Chapman KR, Chamberlain D, et al. Difficult asthma: consider all of the possibilities. Can Respir J 2000;7:415–18.

152. Johansson M, Mandahl N, Johansson L, et al. Translocation 11;19 in a mucoepidermoid tumor of the lung. Cancer Genet Cytogenet 1995;80:85–6.

153. LopezTerrada D, Bloom MGK, Cagle PT, et al. Oncocytic mucoepidermoid carcinoma of the trachea. Arch Pathol Lab Med 1999;123:635–7.

154. Shilo K, Foss RD, Franks TJ, et al. Pulmonary mucoepidermoid carcinoma with prominent tumor-associated lymphoid proliferation. Am J Surg Pathol 2005;29:407–11.

155. Stenman G, Petursdottir V, Mellgren G, et al. A child with a t(11;19)(Q14–21;p12) in a pulmonary mucoepidermoid carcinoma. Virchows Archiv 1998;433:579–81.

156. Liu X, Adams AL. Mucoepidermoid carcinoma of the bronchus: a review. Arch Pathol Lab Med 2007;131:1400–4.

157. Achcar RDOD, Nikiforova MN, Dacic S, et al. Mammalian mastermind like 2 11q21 gene rearrangement in bronchopulmonary mucoepidermoid carcinoma. Human Pathol 2009;40:854–60.

158. Romagosa V, Bella MR, Truchero C, et al. Necrotizing sialometaplasia (adenometaplasia) of the trachea. Histopathology 1992;21:280–2.

159. Barsky SH, Martin SE, Matthews M, et al. 'Low grade' mucoepidermoid carcinoma of the bronchus with 'high grade' biological behavior. Cancer 1983;51:1505–9.

160. Vadasz P, Egervary M. Mucoepidermoid bronchial tumors: a review of 34 operated cases. Eur J Cardiothorac Surg 2000;17:566–9.

161. O'Neill ID. Gefitinib as targeted therapy for mucoepidermoid carcinoma of the lung: possible significance of CRTC1-MAML2 oncogene. Lung Cancer 2009;64:129–30.

162. Edwards CW, Matthews HR. Mucous gland adenoma of the bronchus. Thorax 1981;36:147–8.

163. Heard BE, Corrin B, Dewar A. Pathology of seven mucous cell adenomas of the bronchial glands with particular reference to ultrastructure. Histopathology 1985;9:687–701.

164. England DM, Hochholzer L. Truly benign 'bronchial adenoma' – report of 10 cases of mucous gland adenoma with immunohistochemical and ultrastructural findings. Am J Surg Pathol 1995;19:887–99.

165. Chu PG, Weiss LM. Cytokeratin 14 immunoreactivity distinguishes oncocytic tumour from its renal mimics: an immunohistochemical study of 63 cases. Histopathology 2001;39:455–62.

166. Matsuba K, Takizawa T, Thurlbeck W. Oncocytes in human bronchial mucous glands. Thorax 1972;27:181–4.

167. Fechner RE, Bentinck BR. Ultrastructure of bronchial oncocytoma. Cancer 1973;31:1451–7.

168. Warter A, Walter P, Sabountchi M, et al. Oncocytic bronchial adenoma. Virchows Arch A Pathol Anat Histopathol 1981;392:231–9.

169. Tashiro Y, Iwata Y, Nabae T, et al. Pulmonary oncocytoma: report of a case in conjunction with an immunohistochemical and ultrastructural study. Pathol Int 1995;45:448–51.

170. Laforga JB, Aranda FI. Multicentric oncocytoma of the lung diagnosed by fine-needle aspiration. Diagn Cytopathol 1999;21:51–4.

171. Nielsen AL. Malignant bronchial oncocytoma: case report and review of

the literature. Hum Pathol 1985;16: 852–4.

172. Sakamoto H, Uda H, Tanaka T, et al. Pleomorphic adenoma in the periphery of the lung – report of a case and review of the literature. Arch Pathol Lab Med 1991;115:393–6.

173. Moran CA, Suster S, Askin FB, et al. Benign and malignant salivary gland-type mixed tumors of the lung – clinicopathologic and immunohistochemical study of eight cases. Cancer 1994;73:2481–90.

174. Sweeney EC, McDermott M. Pleomorphic adenoma of the bronchus. J Clin Pathol 1996;49:87–9.

175. Pomp J, Pannekoek BJM, Overdiep SH. Pleomorphic adenoma and severe tracheal obstruction. Resp Med 1998;92: 889–91.

176. Ang KL, Dhannapuneni VR, Morgan WE, et al. Primary pulmonary pleomorphic adenoma – An immunohistochemical study and review of the literature. Arch Pathol Lab Med 2003;127:621–2.

177. Payne WS, Schier J, Woolner JB. Mixed tumors of the bronchus (salivary gland type). J Thorac Cardiovasc Surg 1965;49:663–8.

178. Nicholson AG, Baandrup U, Florio R, et al. Malignant myxoid endobronchial tumour: a report of two cases with a unique histological pattern. Histopathology 1999;35:313–18.

179. Strickler JG, Hegstrom J, Thomas MJ, et al. Myoepithelioma of the lung. Hum Pathol 1987;111:1082–5.

180. Strickler JG, Hegstrom J, Thomas MJ, et al. Myoepithelioma of the lung. Arch Pathol Lab Med 1991;111:1082–5.

181. Nistal M, Garciaviera M, Martinezgarcia C, et al. Epithelial myoepithelial tumor of the bronchus. Am J Surg Pathol 1994;18:421–5.

182. Tsuji N, Tateishi R, Ishiguro S, et al. Adenomyoepithelioma of the lung. Am J Surg Pathol 1995;19:956–62.

183. Wilson RW, Moran CA. Epithelial–myoepithelial carcinoma of the lung: Immunohistochemical and ultrastructural observations and review of the literature. Hum Pathol 1997;28:631–5.

184. Shanks JH, Hasleton PS, Curry A, et al. Bronchial epithelial–myoepithelial carcinoma. Histopathology 1998;33:90–1.

185. Ryska A, Kerekes Z, Hovorkova E, et al. Epithelial–myoepithelial carcinoma of the bronchus. Pathol Res Pract 1998;194:431–5.

186. Higashiyama M, Kodama K, Yokouchi H, et al. Myoepithelioma of the lung: report of two cases and review of the literature. Lung Cancer 1998;20:47–56.

187. Miura K, Harada H, Aiba S, et al. Myoepithelial carcinoma of the lung arising from bronchial submucosa. Amer J Surg Pathol 2000;24:1300–4.

188. Veeramachaneni R, Gulick J, Halldorsson AO, et al. Benign myoepithelioma of the lung – A case report and review of the literature. Arch Pathol Lab Med 2001;125:1494–6.

189. Pelosi G, Fraggetta F, Maffini F, et al. Pulmonary epithelial–myoepithelial tumor of unproven malignant potential: Report of a case and review of the literature. Modern Pathol 2001;14:521–6.

190. Fulford LG, Kamata Y, Okudera K, et al. Epithelial–myoepithelial carcinomas of the bronchus. Am J Surg Pathol 2001;25:1508–14.

191. Nguyen CV, Suster S, Moran CA. Pulmonary epithelial–myoepithelial carcinoma: a clinicopathologic and immunohistochemical study of 5 cases. Hum Pathol 2009;40:366–73.

192. Chang T, Husain AN, Colby T, et al. Pneumocytic adenomyoepithelioma: a distinctive lung tumor with epithelial, myoepithelial, and pneumocytic differentiation. Am J Surg Pathol 2007;31:562–8.

193. Ukoha OO, Quartararo P, Carter D, et al. Acinic cell carcinoma of the lung with metastasis to lymph nodes. Chest 1999;115:591–5.

194. Fechner RE, Bentinck BR, Askew JB. Acinic cell tumor of the lung. Cancer 1972;29:501–8.

195. Moran CA, Suster S, Koss MN. Acinic cell carcinoma of the lung (Fechner tumor) – a clinicopathologic, immunohistochemical, and ultrastructural study of five cases. Am J Surg Pathol 1992;16:1039–50.

Papillomas

196. Dulmet-Brender E, Jaubert F, Huchon G. Exophytic endobronchial epidermoid carcinoma. Cancer 1986;57:1358–64.

197. Flieder DB, Koss MN, Nicholson A, et al. Solitary pulmonary papillomas in adults: A clinicopathologic and in situ hybridization study of 14 cases combined with 27 cases in the literature. Am J Surg Pathol 1998;22:1328–42.

198. Spencer H, Dail DH, Areaud AJ. Non-invasive bronchial epithelial papillary tumors. Cancer 1980;45:1486–97.

199. Trillo A, Guha A. Solitary condylomatous papilloma of the bronchus. Arch Pathol Lab Med 1988;112:731–3.

200. Popper HH, Wirnsberger G, Juttner-Smolle FM, et al. The predictive value of human papilloma virus (HPV) typing in the prognosis of bronchial squamous cell papillomas. Histopathology 1992;21:323–30.

201. Popper HH, Elshabrawi Y, Wockel W, et al. Prognostic importance of human papilloma virus typing in squamous cell papilloma of the bronchus: comparison of in situ hybridization and the polymerase chain reaction. Hum Pathol 1994;25:1191–7.

202. Syrjanen KJ. HPV infections and lung cancer. J Clin Pathol 2002;55: 885–91.

203. Henry M, Landers R, Kealy WF, et al. Solitary columnar bronchial papilloma: a rare endoscopic finding. Resp Med 1998;92:878–9.

204. Aida S, Ohara I, Shimazaki H, et al. Solitary peripheral ciliated glandular papillomas of the lung: a report of 3 cases. Am J Surg Pathol 2008;32:1489–94.

204a. Arai Y, Shimizu S, Eimoto T, et al. Peripheral pulmonary papillary/glandular neoplasms with ciliated cells and a component of well-differentiated adenocarcinoma: report of three tumours. Histopathology 2010;56:265–9.

205. Basheda S, Gephardt GN, Stoller JK. Columnar papilloma of the bronchus – case report and literature review. Am Rev Respir Dis 1991;144:1400–2.

206. Klein J, Zhuang Z, Lubensky I, et al. Multifocal microcysts and papillary cystadenoma of the lung in von Hippel–Lindau disease. Am J Surg Pathol 2007;31:1292–6.

207. Assor D. A papillary transitional cell tumor of the bronchus. Am J Clin Pathol 1971;55:761–4.

208. World Health Organization. Histological typing of lung tumours. 2nd ed. Geneva: World Health Organization; 1981.

209. Michaels L, Young M. Histogenesis of papillomas of the nose and paranasal sinuses. Arch Pathol Lab Med 1995;119:821–6.

210. Singer DB, Greenberg SD, Harrison GM. Papillomatosis of the lung. Am Rev Respir Dis 1966;94:777–83.

211. Kramer SS, Wehunt WD, Kashima H. Pulmonary manifestations of juvenile laryngotracheal papillomatosis. Am J Roentgenol 1985;144:687–94.

212. Mounts P, Kashima H. Association of human papilloma virus subtype and clinical course in respiratory papillomatosis. Laryngoscope 1984;94:28–33.

213. Terry RM, Lewis FA, Griffiths S, et al. Demonstration of human papillomavirus types 6 and 11 in juvenile laryngeal papillomatosis by in-situ hybridization. J Pathol 1987;153:245–8.

214. Carey FA, Salter DM, Kerr KM, et al. An investigation into the role of human papillomavirus in endobronchial papillary squamous tumours. Respir Med 1990;84:445–7.

215. Yousem SA, Ohori NP, Sonmezalpan E. Occurrence of human papillomavirus DNA in primary lung neoplasms. Cancer 1992;69:693–7.

216. Franzmann MB, Buchwald C, Larsen P, et al. Tracheobronchial involvement of laryngeal papillomatosis at onset. J Laryngol Otol 1994;108:164–5.

217. Harada H, Miura K, Tsutsui Y, et al. Solitary squamous cell papilloma of the lung in a 40-year-old woman with recurrent laryngeal papillomatosis. Pathol Int 2000;50:431–9.

218. Gelder CM, Williams OM, Hart KW, et al. HLA class II polymorphisms and susceptibility to recurrent respiratory papillomatosis. J Virol 2003;77: 1927–39.

219. Haussinger K, Kohlhauffl M, Bolliger CT. Diagnostic bronchoscopy. In: Gibson GJ, Geddes DM, Costabel U, et al, editors. Respiratory Medicine. 3rd ed. London: Saunders; 2003. p. 415–30.

220. Helmuth RA, Strate RW. Squamous carcinoma of the lung in a nonirradiated, nonsmoking patient with juvenile laryngotracheal papillomatosis. Am J Surg Pathol 1987;11:643–50.

221. Fechner RE, Goepfert H, Alford BR. Invasive laryngeal papillomatosis. Arch Otolaryngol 1974;99:147–51.

222. Runckel D, Kessler S. Bronchogenic squamous carcinoma in nonirradiated juvenile laryngotracheal papillomatosis. Am J Surg Pathol 1980;4:293–6.

223. Dallimore NS. Squamous bronchial carcinoma arising in a case of multiple juvenile papillomatosis. Thorax 1985;40:797–8.

224. Guillou L, Sahli R, Chaubert P, et al. Squamous cell carcinoma of the lung in a nonsmoking, nonirradiated patient with juvenile laryngotracheal papillomatosis – evidence of human papillomavirus-11 DNA in both carcinoma and papillomas. Am J Surg Pathol 1991;15:891–8.

225. Wilde E, Duggan MA, Field SK. Bronchogenic squamous cell carcinoma complicating localized recurrent respiratory papillomatosis. Chest 1994;105:1887–8.

226. Orphanidou D, Dimakou K, Latsi P, et al. Recurrent respiratory papillomatosis with malignant transformation in a young adult. Respir Med 1996;90:53–5.

227. Cook JR, Hill DA, Humphrey PA, et al. Squamous cell carcinoma arising in recurrent respiratory papillomatosis with pulmonary involvement: Emerging common pattern of clinical features and human papillomavirus serotype association. Modern Pathol 2000;13:914–8.

228. Lele SM, Pou AM, Ventura K, et al. Molecular events in the progression of recurrent respiratory papillomatosis to carcinoma. Arch Pathol Lab Med 2002;126:1184–8.

Adenomas

229. Kurotaki H, Kamata Y, Kimura M, et al. Multiple papillary adenomas of type-II pneumocytes found in a 13-year-old boy with von Recklinghausen's disease. Virchows Arch A Pathol Anat Histopathol 1993;423:319–22.

230. Fantone JC, Geisinger KR, Appelman HD. Papillary adenoma of the lung with lamellar and electron dense granules. Cancer 1982;50:2839–44.

231. Noguchi M, Kodama T, Shimosato Y, et al. Papillary adenoma of type 2 pneumocytes. Am J Surg Pathol 1986;10:134–9.

232. Fine G, Chang CH. Adenoma of type-2 pneumocytes with oncocytic features. Arch Pathol Lab Med 1991;115:797–801.

233. Fukuda T, Ohnishi Y, Kanai I, et al. Papillary adenoma of the lung – histological and ultrastructural findings in 2 cases. Acta Pathol Jpn 1992;42: 56–61.

234. Hegg CA, Flint A, Singh G. Papillary adenoma of the lung. Am J Clin Pathol 1992;97:393–7.

235. Dessy E, Braidotti P, DelCurto B, et al. Peripheral papillary tumor of type-II pneumocytes: a rare neoplasm of undetermined malignant potential. Virchows Archiv 2000;436:289–95.

236. Wada A, Tateishi R, Terazawa T, et al. Lymphangioma of the lung. Arch Pathol Lab Med 1974;98:211–13.

237. Al-Hilli F. Lymphangioma (or alveolar adenoma?) of the lung. Histopathology 1987;11:979–80.

238. Yousem SA, Hochholzer L. Alveolar adenoma. Hum Pathol 1986;17:1066–71.

239. Semeraro D, Gibbs AR. Pulmonary adenoma: a variant of sclerosing haemangioma of lung? J Clin Pathol 1989;42:1222–3.

240. Siebenmann RE, Odermatt B, Hegglin J, et al. Das Alveolarzelladenom. Ein neu erkannter gutartiger Lungentumor. Pathologe 1990;11:48–54.

241. Oliveira P, Nunes JFM, Clode AL, et al. Alveolar adenoma of the lung: further characterization of this uncommon tumour. Virchows Arch 1996;429:101–8.

242. Bohm J, Fellbaum C, Bautz W, et al. Pulmonary nodule caused by an alveolar adenoma of the lung. Virchows Arch 1997;430:181–4.

243. Burke LM, Rush WI, Khoor A, et al. Alveolar adenoma: A histochemical, immunohistochemical, and ultrastructural analysis of 17 cases. Hum Pathol 1999;30:158–67.

244. Halldorsson A, Dissanaike S, Kaye KS. Alveolar adenoma of the lung: a clinicopathological description of a case of this very unusual tumour. J Clin Pathol 2005;58:1211–14.

245. Nicholson AG, Magkou C, Snead D, et al. Unusual sclerosing haemangiomas and sclerosing haemangioma-like lesions, and the value of TTF-1 in making the diagnosis. Histopathology 2002;41:404–13.

246. Spencer H, Nambu S. Sclerosing haemangiomas of the lung. Histopathology 1986;10:477–87.

247. Tanaka I, Inoue M, Matsui Y, et al. A case of pneumocytoma (so-called sclerosing hemangioma) with lymph node metastasis. Jpn J Clin Oncol 1986;16:77–86.

Sclerosing pneumocytoma (sclerosing 'haemangioma')

248. Liebow AA, Hubbell DS. Sclerosing haemangioma (histiocytoma, xanthoma) of the lung. Cancer 1956;9:53–75.

249. Hill GS, Eggleston JC. Electron microscopic study of so-called pulmonary sclerosing haemangioma. Report of a case suggesting epithelial origin. Cancer 1972;30:1092–106.

250. Katzenstein A-LA, Gmelich JT, Carrington CB. Sclerosing hemangioma of the lung. A clinicopathologic study of 51 cases. Am J Surg Pathol 1980;4:343–56.

251. Chan K-W, Gibbs AR, Lo WS, et al. Benign sclerosing pneumocytoma of lung (sclerosing haemangioma). Thorax 1982;37:404–12.

252. Nagata N, Dairaku M, Sueishi K, et al. Sclerosing hemangioma of the lung. An epithelial tumor composed of immunohistochemically heterogenous cells. Am J Clin Pathol 1987;88:552–9.

253. Aiba M, Hirayama A, Sakurada M, et al. So-called sclerosing hemangioma of the lung. An immunohistochemical, histochemical and ultrastructural study. Acta Pathol Jpn 1988;38:873–81.

254. Fukayama M, Koike M. So-called sclerosing hemangioma of the lung. An immunohistochemical, histochemical and ultrastructural study. Acta Pathol Jpn 1988;38:627–42.

255. Yousem SA, Wick MR, Singh G, et al. So-called sclerosing hemangiomas of the lung. Am J Surg Pathol 1988;12:582–90.

256. Parkinson C. So-called sclerosing hemangiomas of lung. Am J Surg Pathol 1988;12:582–90.

257. Satoh Y, Tsuchiya E, Weng S-Y, et al. Pulmonary sclerosing hemangioma of the lung. A type II pneumocytoma by immunohistochemical and immunoelectron microscopic studies. Cancer 1989;64:1310–7.

258. Leong ASY, Chan KW, Seneviratne HSK. A morphological and immunohistochemical study of 25 cases of so-called sclerosing haemangioma of the lung. Histopathology 1995;27:121–8.

259. Leong AS-Y, Chan K-W, Leong FJW-M. Sclerosing hemangioma. In: Corrin B, editor. Pathology of Lung Tumors. London: Churchill Livingstone; 1997. p. 175–88.

260. RodriguezSoto J, Colby TV, Rouse RV. A critical examination of the immunophenotype of pulmonary sclerosing hemangioma. Amer J Surg Pathol 2000;24:442–50.

261. Devouassoux-Shisheboran M, Hayashi T, Linnoila RI, et al. A clinicopathologic study of 100 cases of pulmonary sclerosing hemangioma with immunohistochemical studies – TTF-1 is expressed in both round and surface cells, suggesting an origin from primitive respiratory epithelium. Amer J Surg Pathol 2000;24:906–16.

262. Chan ACL, Chan JKC. Pulmonary sclerosing hemangioma consistently expresses thyroid transcription factor-1 (TTF-1) – A new clue to its histogenesis. Amer J Surg Pathol 2000;24:1531–6.

263. Illei PB, Rosai J, Klimstra DS. Expression of thyroid transcription factor-1 and other markers in sclerosing hemangioma of the lung. Arch Pathol Lab Med 2001;125:1335–9.

264. Keylock JB, Galvin JR, Franks TJ. Sclerosing hemangioma of the lung. Arch Pathol Lab Med 2009;133:820–5.

265. Kennedy A. Sclerosing haemangioma of the lung: an alternative view of its development. J Clin Pathol 1973;26:792–9.

266. MiyagawaHayashino A, Tazelaar HD, Langel DI, et al. Pulmonary sclerosing hemangioma with lymph node metastases – report of 4 cases. Arch Pathol Lab Med 2003;127:321–5.

267. Niho S, Suzuki K, Yokose T, et al. Monoclonality of both pale cells and cuboidal cells of sclerosing hemangioma of the lung. Am J Pathol 1998;152:1065–9.

268. Nagata N, Dairaku M, Ishida T, et al. Sclerosing haemangioma of the lung. Cancer 1985;55:116–23.

269. Ohori NP, Yousem SA, Sonmezalpan E, et al. Estrogen and progesterone receptors in lymphangioleiomyomatosis, epithelioid hemangioendothelioma, and sclerosing hemangioma of the lung. Am J Clin Pathol 1991;96:529–35.

270. Aihara T, Nakajima T. Sclerosing hemangioma of the lung – pathological study and enzyme immunoassay for estrogen and progesterone receptors. Acta Pathol Jpn 1993;43:507–15.

271. Saluja R, Pomplun S, Eisen T, et al. Multiple combined sclerosing haemangiomas and tumourlets. A report of two patients with bilateral disease. Histopathology 2008;53:614–7.

272. Choi KH, Baek HA, Park HS, et al. Sclerosing hemangioma, presenting as a pneumonic pattern with mucinous adenomatous hyperplasia of the lung. Pathol Int 2008;58:735–40.

273. Shibata R, Mukai M, Okada Y, et al. A case of sclerosing hemangioma of the lung presenting as a gigantic tumor occupying the left thoracic cavity. Virchows Archiv 2003;442:409–11.

274. Noguchi M, Kodama T, Morinaga S, et al. Multiple sclerosing haemangiomas of the lung. Am J Surg Pathol 1986;10:429–35.

275. Lee ST, Lee YC, Hsu CY, et al. Bilateral multiple sclerosing hemangiomas of the lung. Chest 1992;101:572–3.

276. Khoury JD, Shephard MN, Moran CA. Cystic sclerosing haemangioma of the lung. Histopathology 2003;43:239–43.

277. Chiang PM, Yuan RH, Hsu HC, et al. Frequent nuclear expression of (β-catenin protein but rare (β-catenin mutation in pulmonary sclerosing haemangioma. J Clin Pathol 2008;61:268–71.

278. Moran CA, Zeren H, Koss MN. Sclerosing hemangioma of the lung – granulomatous variant. Arch Pathol Lab Med 1994;118:1028–30.

279. Perry LJ, Florio R, Dewar A, et al. Giant lamellar bodies as a feature of pulmonary low-grade MALT lymphomas. Histopathology 2000;36:240–4.

280. Chan AC, Chan JK. Can pulmonary sclerosing haemangioma be accurately diagnosed by intra-operative frozen section? Histopathology 2002;41:392–403.

Pulmonary thymoma

281. McBurney R, Clagget O, McDonald JR. Primary intrapulmonary neoplasms (thymoma?) associated with myasthenia gravis. Mayo Clin Proc 1951;26:354–6.

282. Yeoh CB, Ford JM, Lattes R, et al. Intrapulmonary thymoma. J Thorac Cardiovasc Surg 1966;51:131–6.

283. Kung ITM, Loke SL, So SY, et al. Intrapulmonary thymoma: report of two cases. Thorax 1985;40:471–4.

284. Green WR, Pressoir R, Gumbs RV, et al. Intrapulmonary thymoma. Arch Pathol Lab Med 1987;111:1074–6.

285. James CL, Iyer PV, Leong AS-Y. Intrapulmonary thymoma. Histopathology 1992;21:175–7.

286. Marchevsky AM. Lung tumors derived from ectopic tissues. Semin Diagn Pathol 1995;12:172–84.

287. Moran CA, Suster S, Fishback NF, et al. Primary intrapulmonary thymoma: a clinicopathologic and immunohistochemical study of eight cases. Am J Surg Pathol 1995;19:304–12.

288. Payne CB, Morningstar WA, Chester EH. Thymoma of the pleura masquerading as diffuse mesothelioma. Am Rev Respir Dis 1960;94:441–6.

289. Shih DF, Wang JS, Tseng HH, et al. Primary pleural thymoma. Arch Pathol Lab Med 1997;121:79–82.

290. Pomplun S, Wotherspoon AC, Shah G, et al. Immunohistochemical markers in the differentiation of thymic and pulmonary neoplasms. Histopathology 2002;40:152–8.

291. Fukayama M, Maeda Y, Funata N, et al. Pulmonary and pleural thymoma. Diagnostic application of lymphocyte markers to the thymoma of unusual site. Am J Clin Pathol 1988;89:617–21.

12.3 Soft-tissue tumours

INFLAMMATORY MYOFIBROBLASTIC TUMOUR ('PLASMA CELL GRANULOMA', 'INFLAMMATORY PSEUDOTUMOUR')

Many different names have been applied to this tumour, reflecting its varied cellular composition on the one hand and the confusion that has existed over its nature on the other. It has been variously termed plasma cell granuloma, postinflammatory pseudotumour, xanthoma, xanthomatous pseudotumour, fibrous histiocytoma or histiocytoma, mast cell tumour or mast cellgranuloma and the current term, inflammatory myofibroblastic tumour.[1-14a] The lungs are a common site of origin but, these tumours have also been reported in many other sites, including the mesentery, mediastinum, soft tissue, larynx, stomach, oesophagus, intestine, liver, genitourinary tract, central nervous system, nerve, heart, skin and breast.

Aetiology[15]

Inflammatory myofibroblastic tumours form a neoplastic subgroup of the rather nebulous and broad category of 'inflammatory pseudo-tumours', which also includes several non-neoplastic fibroinflammatory mass lesions. Previous reports that they can be induced experimentally by irritants[16,17] and that in humans they represent organising pneumonia[18] or are the result of antecedent infection[12,29] probably relate to the non-neoplastic varieties of inflammatory pseudotumour rather than inflammatory myofibroblastic tumour. The possibility that some infective agents, particularly Epstein–Barr virus and human herpesvirus-8, may play a role in the development of inflammatory myofibroblastic tumours is not incompatible with them being neoplastic.[22-25]

In an early review of 118 cases no instances of malignant change were identified[26] but reports of vascular invasion,[27] sarcomatous change with distant metastasis,[12,28,29] chromosomal translocations, aneuploidy and monoclonality have steadily accumulated.[30-37] Particularly notable is the identification of the 2p23 chromosomal aberrations associated with expression of anaplastic lymphoma kinase

(ALK) in 33% of pulmonary 'pseudotumours' and of identical clonality in separate lesions, features that support a neoplastic process capable of distant metastasis.[34,38] The predominant view today is that these tumours are either myofibroblastic or fibroblastic reticulum cell neoplasms of low malignant potential.[13,39]

The term 'inflammatory pseudotumour' remains in use but is only properly applied as a generic term to lesions such as localised foci of organising pneumonia, malakoplakia (p. 216), mycobacterial spindle cell tumour (p. 212), atypical mycoses of tumour-like configuration and the lesions of hyper-IgG$_4$ disease (p. 485). The following account of inflammatory myofibroblastic tumour is necessarily based on the existing literature and may need to be modified as more soundly based series are described.

Clinical features

The age range stretches from the first year of life to the eighth decade but most patients are less than 40 years old and many are children.[7,12,40] This lesion is one of the commonest primary lung tumours seen in young people.[41] Females outnumber males but there are no significant racial or geographical differences.

About half the patients are asymptomatic, the lesion being discovered as a chance radiological finding. Other patients complain of cough, haemoptysis, chest pain or dyspnoea, sometimes accompanied by systemic features that are possibly related to interleukin production by the lesion, namely low-grade pyrexia, weight loss, microcytic hypochromic anaemia, polyclonal hyperglobulinaemia and a raised erythrocyte sedimentation rate.[42] Hypercalcaemia has also been recorded, apparently caused by the tumour secreting calcitriol.[43] High-resolution computed tomography typically shows a solitary mass with sharp regular borders, or if the tumour is endobronchial, obstructive pneumonia or atelectasis.[44]

Gross appearances

The lesions occur with equal frequency on the two sides and are slightly more common in the lower lobes. There are instances of bilateral tumours, multiple lesions in the same lung, satellite nodules about the main mass and the simultaneous occurrence of pulmonary and extrapulmonary lesions.[7,27,40,45–47a] There may be endobronchial extension with disruption of bronchial cartilage and polypoid protrusion into the lumen.[2,7,9,10] Peripheral lesions often invade the chest wall or mediastinum.

The lesions form rounded masses that can measure less than 1 cm or occupy the whole hemithorax.[7,12,48] They are sharply circumscribed and generally of firm consistency with a yellow, tan or grey cut surface (Fig. 12.3.1). Other examples may be softer and more fleshy, or even mucoid. Focal calcification, haemorrhage or necrosis may be apparent in the larger examples.[14]

Histopathology

There are two major histological patterns, fibrohistiocytic and inflammatory, but these are the ends of a spectrum and both are often seen in the same tumour. Generally, the tumours are composed of cellular fibrous tissue heavily infiltrated by plasma cells, histiocytes, lymphocytes and foam cells in varying proportion (Fig. 12.3.2).[7,9,11,12,17] Mast cells occasionally predominate.[4,5] Eosinophils and neutrophils are infrequent. Most lesions have a prominent spindle cell component with a variable degree of collagenisation. There is often hyalinisation, occasionally calcification and rarely ossification.[7,49] Central necrosis with the formation of a small cavity is occasionally seen. In more cellular areas, there may be a woven or 'storiform' pattern, mitoses may be seen and rare examples show frank sarcomatous transformation. Plasma cells and lymphocytes tend to be most conspicuous at

Figure 12.3.1 Inflammatory myofibroblastic tumour occupying the major part of the lower lobe with a satellite nodule at the hilum.

the periphery of the lesion where they often extend into adjacent lung as an interstitial infiltrate, sometimes forming lymphoid follicles. Russell bodies are often found in areas rich in plasma cells. There is no capsule and incorporation of lung tissue into the expanding mass may result in the presence of epithelial inclusions. The pulmonary architecture is generally effaced and vascular, perineural and bronchiolar invasion may be evident (Fig. 12.3.3). Histiocytes and foam cells, together with Touton giant cells, may either be interspersed with spindle cells or form discrete clusters. Some inflammatory myofibroblastic tumours consist largely of plump histiocytes set in a loose myxoid stroma in which there are few inflammatory cells.[9] Some such examples have been incorrectly termed histiocytomas or xanthomas[3,6,8,9,11] but it is important that such examples are diagnosed correctly so that clinicians are aware of their more malignant growth potential.

Immunocytochemistry demonstrates the presence of vimentin and actin in most cases, and cytokeratin in about one-third, consistent with the spindle cells being myofibroblasts.[13] Immunocytochemistry also demonstrates the polytypic nature of the plasma cells,[50–52]

Figure 12.3.2 Inflammatory myofibroblastic tumour – variations in morphology. (A) Many plasma cells and lymphocytes are mixed with the myofibroblastic cells. (B) Inflammatory areas merge with areas of dense hyaline fibrosis. (C) Focal collections of foam cells are seen. (D) Hyaline fibrosis with osseous metaplasia.

substantial numbers of CD68-positive cells and in about half the cases cytoplasmic ALK, which correlates well with the presence of ALK gene rearrangements detected by in situ hybridisation.[25,34,36,37]

Ultrastructural studies[6,9,11,16,17,48,50,53,54] confirm that the spindle cells have the features of myofibroblasts, uncommitted mesenchymal cells or fibroblasts, and that the histiocytes may contain numerous myelin figures resulting from phagosomal activity.

Differential diagnosis

The differential diagnosis of inflammatory myofibroblastic tumour includes mycobacterial spindle cell tumour, sclerosing pneumocytoma, lymphoma, plasmacytoma, localised organising pneumonia, amyloid tumour, hyalinising granuloma, intrapulmonary localised fibrous tumour, malignant fibrous histiocytoma, follicular dendritic cell tumour, lymphoepithelial carcinoma, spindle cell carcinoma, localised fibromuscular scar and invasive fibrous tumour of the trachea.

Mycobacterial spindle cell tumours, as seen in acquired immuno-deficiency syndrome (AIDS) patients (see p. 212), resemble the lesion now being considered but the spindle cells contain numerous mycobacteria and have the phenotype of macrophages rather than myofibroblasts.

In a sclerosing pneumocytoma (see p. 610), large numbers of foam cells and fibrosis may produce an appearance similar to the xanthomatous variety of inflammatory myofibroblastic tumour but there are also papillary formations and angiomatoid areas that are not seen in the latter and the stromal cells stain for epithelial membrane antigen (EMA) and thyroid transcription factor-1 (TTF-1).

Lymphomas (see p. 659) are not so well circumscribed as inflammatory myofibroblastic tumours and like plasmacytomas (see p. 666) comprise a dense and often monotonous infiltrate of atypical monoclonal cells, although they may show marked central sclerosis. In the commonest primary lymphoma of the lung, marginal zone lymphoma of mucosa-associated lymphoid tissue origin, lymphoepithelial lesions are often prominent and the dense infiltrate mainly comprises CD20-positive B lymphocytes.

Organising pneumonia may produce a chronic inflammatory mass but this is generally irregular in outline, and a connective tissue stain will reveal the underlying lung architecture to be intact.

Although hyaline areas resemble amyloid, stains for this substance are negative.[7] Hyalinising granuloma (see p. 699) differs from in-

Figure 12.3.3 Inflammatory myofibroblastic tumour. (A) Invasion of the chest wall with widespread perineural infiltration. (B) Vascular invasion may also be seen, in this instance within the lung parenchyma.

flammatory myofibroblastic tumour in being less cellular and showing less intense inflammation with what inflammation is present being more pronounced peripherally; affected patients are older and the geographical distribution of the two diseases is different.

Inflammatory myofibroblastic tumour lacks the focal calcification of a calcifying fibrous pseudotumour but rare cases showing a combination of patterns suggest that the two lesions are related, a possibility that is discussed further on page 733.[55–58]

When fibrohistiocytic elements predominate, inflammatory myofibroblastic tumour needs to be distinguished from fibrosarcoma and on addressing this problem one group found necrosis, bizarre giant cells, numerous mitoses, high cellularity and poor circumscription to be more significant histological features of malignancy than nuclear pleomorphism and atypical mitoses.[59] Others rely on inflammatory myofibroblastic tumours lacking cytological atypia, pleomorphism and abnormal mitoses, or recommend *p53* oncogene identification as an indicator of malignancy.[51,60] Occasional cases may however undergo sarcomatous transformation.

Follicular dendritic cell tumours, which may extend into the lungs from the mediastinum or more rarely arise in the lungs (see p. 653), closely resemble the fibrohistiocytic variant of inflammatory myofibroblastic tumour and may only be distinguished by the use of dendritic cell markers such as CD21 and CD35; confusion between these two entities may have led to some reports of malignant change in extrapulmonary inflammatory myofibroblastic tumours.

Intrapulmonary localised fibrous tumours are identical to those that occur in the pleura (see p. 730) and are usually subpleural. They also lack the inflammatory component of myofibroblastic tumours and their CD34 positivity is a further distinguishing feature.

Invasive fibrous tumour of the trachea[61] is not a well-defined entity and some examples may have represented inflammatory myofibroblastic tumours.

Lymphoepithelial carcinoma and inflammatory spindle cell carcinoma (see pp. 564 and 567) are both distinguished by their cytological atypia. Markers have to be interpreted with caution in this context: cytokeratin immunoreactivity is frequently patchy in spindle cell carcinoma and often positive in inflammatory myofibroblastic tumour while although ALK1 confirms the latter when positive it is often negative.

Course of the disease

In most cases growth is slow and occasional instances of arrested growth[62] or spontaneous resolution are recorded.[40] Indeed, some cases of calcified fibrous pseudotumour of the lung may represent involuted inflammatory myofibroblastic tumours.[57] The majority of lesions are resected before the diagnosis has been established and this is usually curative. Attempts at enucleation may be followed by recurrence,[26] possibly with mediastinal extension mimicking sclerosing mediastinitis.[7] If the pleural surface is involved and the tumour is adherent to chest wall or mediastinum, excision may be difficult and the usual good prognosis adversely affected. Infiltration of vessels at a distance from the main tumour mass has been reported and occasionally death is due to extension into pulmonary veins or oesophagus.[19,27,50,54] Exceptional instances of sarcomatous change have been referred to above.[12,29,63]

The histological features provide a poor prediction of behaviour. Aneuploidy appears to correlate better with a more aggressive course[64] while in one series of extrapulmonary inflammatory myofibroblastic tumours a combination of aneuploidy, atypia, ganglion-like cells and p53 expression was identified as providing the best predictor of aggressive behaviour.[65] Another group reports that ALK reactivity is associated with local recurrence but not metastasis.[66]

PLEUROPULMONARY BLASTOMA

Unlike other tumours that have been termed pulmonary blastoma (see p. 569) pleuropulmonary blastoma lacks an epithelial component and consists entirely of primitive blastema showing varying lines of sarcomatous differentiation. These tumours may be pulmonary, pleural or mediastinal and are largely confined to childhood.[67–71] In the past they have been reported under a variety of terms, including cystic blastoma and sarcomas or malignant mesenchymoma arising in congenital cysts.[72–79]

Pleuropulmonary blastoma appears to be the true embryonic tumour or blastoma of the lung. This is supported by cytogenetic analysis, which has revealed a variety of chromosomal alterations, including partial trisomy of chromosome 2q, trisomy of chromosome 8 and loss of heterozygosity on chromosome 11 involving the Wilms tumour gene WT2. These abnormalities show some overlap with those of hepatoblastoma, embryonal rhabdomyosarcoma and Wilms tumour.[80,81] It is also noteworthy that pleuropulmonary blastoma has been reported in association with familial cystic nephroma and a variety of other tumours or tumour precursors in approximately 25% of cases.[82–84] Pleuropulmonary blastoma evidently heralds a constitutional and heritable predisposition to dysplastic or neoplastic disease, indicating that family members need to be counselled and monitored accordingly.[83] Several families have shown heterozygous germline mutations in *DICER1*, a gene that encodes an endoribonuclease critical to the generation of regulatory RNAs. The DICER-1 protein is found in the blastematous component of tumours.[85]

Clinical features

Patients are usually less than 12 years old and of either sex but rare cases have been reported in adults.[86] The patient may be asymptomatic but there is usually chest pain, breathlessness and fever. Imaging shows a cystic or solid peripheral mass or masses, possibly accompanied by pneumothorax.[67–69,71,87,88] The cystic tumours are generally found in the youngest patients.[71]

Pathological features

Pleuropulmonary blastomas from large multilobed masses that may be difficult to resect. Cystic (type 1), partly cystic (type 2) and solid (type 3) varieties are described.[71] The cysts may be unilocular or multilocular. In the type 2 lesions the solid component may be limited to a nodule of tumour protruding into the cyst. The solid areas sometimes show necrosis and haemorrhage.

Microscopically, small round or spindle-shaped blastematous cells comprise the malignant component and in the cystic varieties these cells are typically concentrated immediately beneath a non-neoplastic lining of entrapped respiratory epithelium in a so-called cambium layer (Fig. 12.3.4). Solid areas consist of sheets of a similar blastema, but often with a greater degree of pleomorphism, mitotic activity and divergent sarcomatous differentiation resulting in foci of rhabdomyosarcoma or chondrosarcoma (Fig. 12.3.5). Very cellular areas alternating with others composed of looser myxoid tissue may result in an appearance resembling that of a Wilms tumour.

Differential diagnosis

Low-grade cystic examples resemble both mesenchymal cystic hamartoma and type 4 congenital cystic adenomatoid malformation, so much so that it is questionable whether these represent separate entities (see pp. 74 and 61). In the few published cases of type 4 congenital cystic adenomatoid malformation small areas of cellular blastematous proliferation may be seen[89] and these cases are certainly better classified as type 1 pleuropulmonary blastomas.[71] Staining with desmin may be helpful as it highlights foci of rhabdomyomatous differentiation, although care is needed to distinguish these from normal muscle.[71,89,90] The distinction is vital so that the child can benefit from adequate surgery and follow-up care.[91]

The differential diagnosis of high-grade pleuropulmonary blastomas depends upon the proportion of blastema and sarcoma, and includes undifferentiated sarcoma, synovial sarcoma, rhabdomyosarcoma, chondrosarcoma, malignant teratoma and metastatic Wilms tumour. Pleuropulmonary blastoma is distinguished from malignant small cell tumour of the thoracopulmonary region (Askin tumour or primitive neuroectodermal tumour (PNET), see p. 737) by its location in the periphery of the lung rather than the chest wall, cystic nature and focal sarcomatous differentiation, while in doubtful cases CD99 staining and chromosomal analysis may be helpful. Well-differentiated fetal adenocarcinoma and pulmonary blastoma are excluded by the absence of malignant epithelial elements.

Figure 12.3.4 Pleuropulmonary blastoma. Cystic (type 1) variant. (A) The tumour forms a multiloculated cyst. Even at low power, foci of stromal cellularity are identifiable. (B) Stromal hypercellularity sometimes forms a subepithelial 'cambium' layer (top).

Treatment and prognosis

The long-term survival is 25–50%,[67] with the solid variety and those involving the pleura or mediastinum having a particularly poor prognosis.[71] Five-year survival for type 1 pleuropulmonary blastoma is 83% compared to 42% for types 2 and 3.[71] Younger patients are more likely to have surgically resectable lower-grade tumours. Complete surgical resection is important because, although progression of type 1 tumours to types 2 and 3 is not inevitable, these tumours tend to recur in a more malignant form.[91–93] The requirement for family

Figure 12.3.5 Pleuropulmonary blastoma. Solid (type 3) variant. (A) Recurrence of a cystic type 1 pleuropulmonary blastoma in solid form. (B) Microscopy shows undifferentiated sarcoma with marked pleomorphism.

members to be counselled and investigated appropriately is outlined above, especially in relation to the *DICER*-1 mutation, which conveys a risk of tumours at other sites and in other family members.[85]

BENIGN CLEAR CELL TUMOUR ('SUGAR TUMOUR')

This is a particularly rare tumour that is now thought to be one of several that derive from a putative perivascular epithelioid cell (PEC, and hence PEComa).[94,95] The tumour is sometimes encountered in patients with tuberous sclerosis, which links it to other neoplasms and proliferations such as lymphangioleiomyomatosis that also show evidence of PEComatous differentiation.[96–101]

Benign clear cell tumours span a wide age range (8–73 years, mean 49 years) and have an equal sex incidence.[97,102–116] Most patients are asymptomatic and the tumour is often an incidental finding in chest radiographs, where it is seen as a solitary 'coin lesion' in the periphery

Figure 12.3.6 Benign clear cell tumour. Trabeculae of cells with clear cytoplasm are separated by thin-walled sinusoidal vessels. (A) Low power; (B) high power.

of the lung. Upper and lower lobes are equally affected. Although initially believed to be unique to the lung, examples of clear cell tumour have now been reported in the trachea, pancreas, ligamentum teres hepatis, rectum, uterus, vulva, breast and heart, a few of which have exhibited aggressive behaviour, sometimes metastasising to the lungs.[99,117–123] Certain abdominopelvic sarcomas of perivascular epithelioid cells appear to represent further malignant examples of extrapulmonary clear cell tumours.[101,124] In the lungs, lobectomy, wedge resection or even simple enucleation is generally curative, but in one case widespread metastases resulted in death 17 years after resection.[110,125]

Pathology

On gross inspection the tumour has a sharp outline and lacks any obvious connection with major airways, blood vessels or pleura. The cut surface is often haemorrhagic: otherwise it is a translucent pinkish-grey, and not yellow, as are many renal carcinomas. Necrosis is rare; it was present in the only case that metastasised and may therefore auger malignancy.[110,125–127]

The microscopic appearances are rather uniform, consisting of sheets and cords of large polygonal or spindle cells with distinct outlines and abundant clear cytoplasm that is generally rich in glycogen (Fig. 12.3.6), a feature that has given rise to the colloquial term 'sugar tumour'. A few reticulin fibres representing type IV collagen surround individual tumour cells.[116] Nuclei are hyperchromatic and often have

Table 12.3.1 Features of benign clear cell tumour and other pulmonary clear cell tumours

Tumour	Glycogen	Fat	Mucin	Vessels	NE	HMB45	S-100	CK	CK7	EMA	TTF1
Benign clear cell tumour	+	−	−	Sinusoidal	−	+	+	−	−	−	−
Metastatic renal cell carcinoma	+	+	−	−	−	−	−	+	-	+	−
Clear cell carcinoma and clear cell adenocarcinoma of the lung	−	−	−	−	−	−	−	+	+	+	+
Clear cell carcinoid	−	−	−	Sinusoidal	+	−	+[a]	+	+	+	−/+
Sclerosing pneumocytoma	−	+	−	−	−	−	−	+	+	+	+

+, present; −, absent; NE, neuroendocrine: HMB45, human melanin black 45; CK, cytokeratin, EMA, epithelial membrane antigen, TTF1, thyroid transcription factor-1.
[a]Positive in sustentacular cells.

irregular outlines. Binucleate, or even multinucleate, cells may be present. Mitoses are generally absent. Although the cytoplasm is characteristically clear it may contain fine eosinophil granules which sometimes appear to radiate from the nucleus. Lipochrome is found in some tumour cells. A rich blood supply is evident in many parts of the tumour, taking the form of large thin-walled sinusoidal vessels that lack a muscle coat (see Fig. 12.3.6). Hyaline connective tissue may form around or within vessel walls and occasionally this progresses to more extensive fibrosis with calcification. Inclusions lined by bronchiolar or alveolar epithelium probably represent entrapment of adjacent lung tissue.

Electron microscopy generally confirms the presence of glycogen but reports are otherwise inconsistent.[105,108,111,116] However, ultrastructural evidence of melanogenesis[113] is in line with human melanin black-45 (HMB45) being consistently and diffusely expressed, a feature that benign clear cell tumours share with lymphangioleiomyomatosis (see p. 293) and angiomyolipoma (see p. 630).[94,116,128,129] CD1a is a further marker found in all these lesions.[130]

Differential diagnosis

The importance of this lesion lies in its distinction from clear cell carcinoma of the lung, either primary (see p. 562) or metastatic from the kidney or elsewhere.[131] The major differences are outlined in Table 12.3.1. The characteristic vascular pattern is helpful, the wide thin-walled sinusoids of the benign tumour contrasting with the thick-walled narrow arterioles of a carcinoma. Renal carcinomas owe their seemingly empty cytoplasm to the presence of both glycogen and fat and it is useful to be able to demonstrate the latter if reserve tissue is available. A diastase-controlled periodic acid–Schiff stain is also useful in distinguishing mucus-secreting adenocarcinomas of solid pattern from the glycogen-rich benign tumour. Chemodectoma, carcinoid and haemangiopericytoma all contain sinusoidal vessels on occasion but lack significant quantities of glycogen and only haemangiopericytoma has reticulin surrounding individual cells.

'HAMARTOMA' (CHONDROID HAMARTOMA, ADENOCHONDROMA, MIXED MESENCHYMOMA)

Despite their popular name – chondroid hamartoma – it is likely that these lesions are benign connective tissue neoplasms rather than tumour-like malformations.[132–135] They are widely regarded as being hamartomatous because of their disorganised mix of the various connective and epithelial tissues normally found in the lung but their rarity in childhood and continued growth in adult life favour them being neoplasms, albeit benign. The identification of chromosomal rearrangements (6p21 and 12q14–15) similar to those found in lipomas and leiomyomas also favours neoplasia rather than malformation.[136–139] Terms such as adenochondroma, adenofibroma[140] and fibroadenoma[141] imply a benign mixed neoplasm but the role played by the epithelial components may also be questioned. It is notable that the chromosomal rearrangements referred to above are confined to the mesenchymal component. Also, it is now appreciated that epithelial structures are commonly entrapped in many lung tumours, both primary and metastatic,[142,143] and it is likely that this is how the epithelial clefts of the so-called adenochondroma or chondroid hamartoma should be regarded. A name that reflects a purely mesenchymal nature appears appropriate and, since these tumours display a variety of connective tissues, the term 'mesenchymoma' has been recommended.[134] However, the term 'hamartoma' is well entrenched and continues to be used.

Clinical features

These tumours are fairly common, constituting about 8% of all 'coin' lesions in chest radiographs.[143a] In an unselected postmortem series, an incidence of 1 in 400 was found.[144] The age range is wide but they are rare in children; the peak age incidence is the sixth decade and they are commoner in men.[134] Sequential radiographs show that most first develop in adult life and slowly increase in size thereafter (at a rate of up to 5 mm/year).[145] Most are parenchymal and asymptomatic but about 8% are endobronchial[134] and cause coughing, dyspnoea, haemoptysis, obstructive pneumonia or collapse.[146,147] Multiple lesions are uncommon, as is involvement of the trachea[134,148–151]; multiplicity raises the possibility of Carney's triad (see below).[152] An accompanying carcinoma of the lung is encountered more frequently than expected[134,153] but this may be fortuitous, the carcinoma causing the chest to be investigated so that an asymptomatic 'hamartoma' is revealed. Sarcomatous change is recorded but is exceptionally rare.[154] One study identified a high incidence of associated congenital anomalies and benign tumours, prompting the authors to envisage a 'pulmonary hamartoma syndrome'.[155] In another study, the lung adjacent to six of 38 resected chondroid hamartomas showed areas resembling the so-called placental transmogrification described on page 703.[156] Others have described 'tumourlets' in association with chondroid hamartomas.[157]

Pathological features[133–135]

There are no significant pathological differences between parenchymal and endobronchial growths, although the proportions in which the

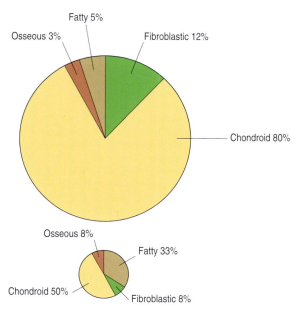

Figure 12.3.7 The predominant tissue in a series of 154 'hamartomas' comprising 142 parenchymal (top) and 12 endobronchial (bottom) tumours.[134]

Figure 12.3.8 A 'hamartoma' of the lung forming a 4.5-cm tumour that 'shelled out' at operation. Note the clefts intersecting the pale cartilaginous tissue.

various connective tissues are represented differ (Fig. 12.3.7) and epithelial clefts are less prominent in endobronchial than parenchymal tumours.[133,158,159] Most measure 1–3 cm in diameter but they range up to 9 cm. They lack a capsule but are sharply circumscribed and shell out easily at operation (Fig. 12.3.8), after which there is little risk of recurrence. Most are lobulated and the predominant tissue is cartilage (Fig. 12.3.9), which may calcify or undergo osseous change. Other connective tissues commonly found include fat, fibrous tissue and loose mesenchyme with a myxoid appearance (Fig. 12.3.10). These various components are usually present in combination, together with cells of transitional form.[135] The lesions may come close to the bronchial cartilage but there is no continuity with this tissue, as there is in tracheobronchopathia osteochondroplastica; fibromyxoid spindle cells probably represent the progenitor mesenchymal element.[135] The connective tissue components are quite regular cytologically and show no evidence of malignancy. Intersecting the connective tissue lobules are clefts lined by ciliated pseudostratified columnar epithelium, which is quite normal cytologically. The retention of cilia is notable as these are usually lost when respiratory epithelium becomes neoplastic.

Differential diagnosis

There is a close genetic relationship between 'hamartoma' and other benign mesenchymal tumours such as lipoma, chondroma and fibroma (which are discussed below) but these entities can be excluded histologically because they consist of just one mesenchymal tissue. More difficulty may be encountered if metastatic teratoma is removed from the lung following successful chemotherapy and submitted for pathological examination with inadequate clinical information (see pp. 686 and 690).

Treatment and prognosis

The parenchymal tumours are often enucleated or removed by wedge resection but lobectomy may be undertaken if there is chronic parenchymal damage. Endobronchial lesions are generally treated by

Figure 12.3.9 A 'hamartoma' composed of mature cartilage intersected by clefts lined by respiratory epithelium.

bronchoplastic resection. Recurrence is rare[134] and sarcomatous transformation even rarer.[154]

LIPOMA, CHONDROMA AND FIBROMA

If the proposed nature of the 'hamartomas' (mixed mesenchymomas) outlined above is accepted, they are obviously closely related to benign connective tissue neoplasms composed of a single tissue – lipoma,[160–163] chondroma,[164,165] fibroma,[166] fibromyxoma[167] and osteoma,[168] for example – none of which is common in the lungs.[133] Like the mixed mesenchymomas, all these neoplasms may either lie entirely within the lung substance or protrude into major bronchi

Figure 12.3.10 A 'hamartoma' formed of myxoid fibrous tissue and fat as well as cartilage.

(Fig. 12.3.11), but the proportion of lipomas and chondromas that are endobronchial is higher than the 8% found with the so-called hamartomas. Epithelial clefts are not found in single-tissue benign mesenchymal tumours, which resemble in every way their counterparts that occur more commonly in other parts of the body. Like chondroid hamartomas, they appear to have no malignant potential: the rare primary pulmonary fibrosarcomas, liposarcomas, chondrosarcomas and osteosarcomas (dealt with below) are believed to be sarcomatous from their outset.

Carney's triad

This is a rare combination of three unusual neoplasms that affects young women.[164,165,169–172] The patients are generally in the second or third decade, the youngest recorded being a girl aged 9 years. The three tumours are pulmonary chondroma, extra-adrenal paraganglioma (chemodectoma) and gastric stromal tumour (epithelioid leiomyosarcoma). Carney's triad is therefore quite different from Carney's syndrome, which lacks a pulmonary component and comprises

myxomas of various organs, blue naevi and tumours of the pituitary, adrenal cortex and Sertoli cells.

In a review of 79 patients with Carney's triad, 85% were female, 22% presented with three tumours and 78% with two tumours. The commonest combination was one that included gastric and pulmonary tumours. Intervals up to 26 years between detection of the first and second components were noted but the mean was 8 years. In half the patients there were multiple chondromas, involving either one or both lungs. A total of 13% of patients died of the disorder (but none of pulmonary chondroma) and some cases were familial.[173] Similar findings are reported in other large series.[172] Early recognition of the syndrome is important in view of the malignant potential of the gastric lesions and paragangliomas. Pulmonary metastases from one or other of these may be difficult to distinguish from chondromas clinically but calcification in pulmonary opacities is a useful radiographic pointer to the opacities being chondromas.

The chondromas have no malignant potential. They differ from chondroid 'hamartomas' in lacking both epithelial clefts and other connective tissue components (Fig. 12.3.12 and Table 12.3.2) and in being encapsulated. However, the presence of a little respiratory epithelium at the edge of the chondromas persuaded Carney that they derive from bronchial cartilage,[173] a further difference from 'chondroid hamartomas', which are believed to derive from precursor fibromyxoid cells.[135]

Concurrent duodenal stromal tumour, pulmonary chondromatous 'hamartoma' and pancreatic islet cell tumour in a 63-year-old man have been reported as a possible variant of Carney's triad.[174] Adrenocortical adenomas may also be associated with Carney's triad[173] but the significance of this observation is uncertain as these tumours are very common in the general population.

HISTIOCYTOMA

Pulmonary lesions that have all the features of benign fibrous histiocytomas, as described in other sites, have been widely regarded as forming part of a plasma cell granuloma–histiocytoma complex, but most would now be regarded as inflammatory myofibroblastic tumours (see p. 620) and every effort should be made to confirm this diagnosis. Nevertheless, true fibrous histiocytomas very rarely occur in the lungs. Most 'cystic fibrohistiocytic tumours' of the lungs are metastases from low-grade cellular fibrous histiocytomas (see p. 686).[175]

LEIOMYOMA AND FIBROLEIOMYOMA

A diagnosis of primary pulmonary leiomyoma or fibroleiomyoma should be advanced only with caution. Pulmonary tumours corresponding to these terms often prove to be multiple and confined to middle-aged women with uterine fibroids, representing examples of so-called benign metastasising leiomyomas of the uterus (see p. 686). In the rare instances in which the patient is male, a history of previous surgery for a 'soft-tissue tumour' can often be elicited. True primary leiomyomas developing in the lungs are distinctly rare.[176–181]

Patients with a pulmonary leiomyoma may be of any age, from infancy onwards. The sex incidence is equal. The tumours may involve the airways or be peripheral, the former usually giving rise to symptoms resulting from obstruction while the latter are often discovered

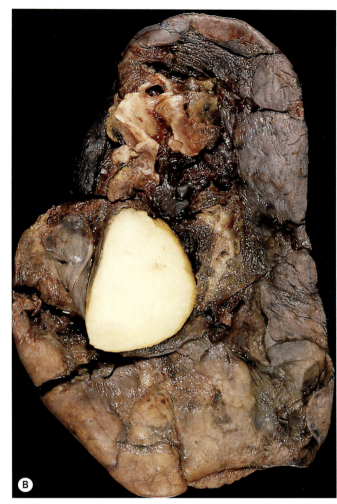

Figure 12.3.11 (A) Endobronchial and (B) parenchymal lipomas. *(B courtesy of Dr JT Gmelich, formerly of Pasadena, USA.)*

by chance in an asymptomatic person. Pulmonary leiomyomas and leiomyosarcomas developing in AIDS are referred to below under miscellaneous sarcomas.

Pulmonary leiomyomas resemble those encountered in other sites in every way (Fig. 12.3.13). They show a well-developed fascicular pattern and lack features suggesting malignancy, such as atypia, haemorrhage and necrosis. Immunostaining for smooth-muscle actin supports the diagnosis.

Leiomyomas of the lung are well-circumscribed tumours, in contrast to the more frequently seen fibromuscular scars that are stellate in outline and lack a definite edge. These may be rich in smooth muscle and are often considered to be smooth-muscle hamartomas, but if there is any appreciable degree of fibrosis a more likely explanation is that they represent old scars in which there is prominent reactive smooth-muscle hyperplasia. Diffuse changes of this nature are often seen in end-stage diffuse pulmonary fibrosis and the term 'muscular cirrhosis of the lung' has been used for this (see p. 269). A case reported as 'diffuse fibroleiomyomatous hamartomatosis'[182] is possibly just a further example of 'muscular cirrhosis'. Pulmonary lymphangioleiomyomatosis is another diffuse infiltrative process rather than a circumscribed tumour (see p. 293). Other conditions to be distinguished from leiomyoma include the CD34-positive intra-

Figure 12.3.12 Pulmonary chondroma as a component of Carney's triad. The tumour is composed solely of benign chondroid elements. *(Courtesy of Dr TV Colby, Scottsdale, USA.)*

Table 12.3.2 The chondromas of Carney's triad compared to chondroid 'hamartomas'[172]

	Carney's triad chondromas	Chondroid 'hamartomas'
Mean age	25 years	59 years
Sex	88% female	60% male
Multiple lesions	52%	2%
Central : peripheral	15 : 85	8 : 92
Fibrous pseudocapsule	93%	0
Invaginated epithelium	2%	99%
Fat and fibromyxoid tissue	Not found	Commonly present

Figure 12.3.13 Pulmonary leiomyoma involving airway wall. The tumour, which was resected from the lung of a male patient, consists of cytologically bland spindle cells with abundant eosinophilic cytoplasm, as seen in leiomyomas arising in other sites.

pulmonary localised fibrous tumour (see p. 730), nerve sheath tumours, which are S-100-positive, inflammatory myofibroblastic tumour, which generally shows a lymphoplasmacytic infiltrate, and epithelial–myoepithelial carcinoma (see p. 605), which expresses epithelial as well as muscle markers.

ANGIOMYOLIPOMA

Angiomyolipomas are rare benign tumours composed of a mixture of small to medium-sized blood vessels, smooth muscle and fat, all of which appear quite mature. They are most commonly found in the kidney, but have been reported in a variety of other sites, including the lung.[183–185] One pulmonary angiomyolipoma developed in a patient suffering from tuberous sclerosis but not lymphangioleiomyo-

matosis, two conditions that are sometimes associated with extra-pulmonary angiomyolipomas.[186] Angiomyolipomas express the melanocyte marker HMB45 and CD1a, which are also found in the 'perivascular epithelioid cells' of lymphangioleiomyomatosis (see p. 293) and the benign clear cell tumour of the lung that is dealt with above.[130,187] A histogenetic relationship is envisaged, which also encompasses a variety of clear cell neoplasms of the soft tissues. They are collectively known colloquially as PEComas.[94,101,188] Angiomyolipomas have been regarded as hamartomas rather than neoplasms but the demonstration of clonality casts doubt upon this.[189,190]

MYELOLIPOMA

Myelolipoma is best known as a tumour of the adrenal glands and examples arising in the lungs are distinctly unusual.[191] They are usually small and asymptomatic, being discovered by chance at necropsy or when radiography is undertaken for unrelated reasons. They consist of mature fat and haemopoietic tissue, occasionally with a thin rim of trabecular bone. Some have been contiguous with a bronchial cartilage but the cartilage has shown no evidence of calcification or ossification. Unlike foci of extramedullary haemopoiesis they are solitary, well circumscribed and unassociated with a blood disorder. They are quite benign. It is suggested that they may represent metaplasia rather than neoplasia.

MISCELLANEOUS SARCOMAS

Primary bronchopulmonary sarcomas are rare, outnumbered by carcinomas 700 to 1.[192,193] However, they are quite diverse and represent a diagnostically challenging group of neoplasms that need to be distinguished from sarcomatoid carcinoma of the lung and secondary sarcoma invading the lungs from adjacent structures or metastasising from distant sites.[194] Immunohistochemistry is helpful here. Cytokeratin positivity permits the recognition of sarcomatoid carcinomas and mesotheliomas while CD34 immunohistochemistry facilitates the identification of solitary (localised) fibrous tumours. Immunocytochemical markers also allow a more confident characterisation of certain sarcomas as being of muscular, vascular or neural origin. This has led to the re-categorisation of tumours that on purely morphological grounds were formerly described as malignant fibrous histiocytoma, haemangiopericytoma and fibrosarcoma. Molecular techniques are also useful in the study of soft-tissue tumours, permitting the recognition of characteristic translocations in tumours such as synovial sarcoma.

Except for a few notable exceptions that have arisen in children,[74,195,196] sarcomas of the lung generally affect the middle-aged and elderly. They usually appear to arise without antecedent lesions but occasional examples have developed in bronchial cysts[74,197] and arteriovenous fistulas,[198] or after radiation therapy.[199] However, most, if not all, of those 'arising' in bronchial cysts would now be recognised to be pleuropulmonary blastomas. More recently, leiomyosarcomas have been encountered in many organs, including the lung, in association with Epstein–Barr virus in AIDS[196,200] and following transplantation.[201]

Most pulmonary sarcomas show smooth muscle or fibrous differentiation or are anaplastic.[194,202–205] The commonest histological subtype is storiform pleomorphic but the inflammatory and giant cell

Figure 12.3.14 Synovial sarcoma of the lung. (A) A circumscribed, soft and focally haemorrhagic mass fills half a lobe. (B) Microscopy shows a monophasic synovial sarcoma surrounding residual entrapped air spaces. (C) Staining for thyroid transcription factor-1 confirms that gland-like structures are indeed entrapped lung elements and not part of a biphasic synovial sarcoma.

subtypes may also be encountered in the lung.[206] They contain foam cells, giant cells and myofibroblasts as well as fibroblasts and have to be distinguished from inflammatory myofibroblastic tumour (see above) by the usual cytological criteria of malignancy.

Synovial sarcomas of both monophasic spindle cell and biphasic pattern have been described as arising in the lung[205,207–214]: they express cytokeratins and the *bcl*-2 oncogene and show the t(X;18)(p11.2;q11.2) translocation seen in synovial sarcomas of soft tissues (Fig. 12.3.14).

Solitary fibrous tumours may be wholly intrapulmonary (see Fig. 13.28, p. 731).[215–217] They characteristically express CD34, although less so in the more malignant examples.

Malignant nerve sheath tumours arising in the lung as opposed to other intrathoracic sites are particularly rare[218,219] and, in the absence of von Recklinghausen's disease, may be mistaken for fibrosarcoma. They are dealt with more fully on page 640.

Other rare varieties include liposarcoma,[220] rhabdomyosarcoma,[221,222] chondrosarcoma,[223] osteosarcoma,[224,225] giant cell tumour,[226] alveolar soft-part sarcoma[227] and angiosarcoma.[228,229] Myxoid change may be prominent in several of these sarcomas.[230,231] Sarcomas arising in the major pulmonary blood vessels are described on page 638. Occasionally a pulmonary sarcoma may elaborate multiple mesenchymal elements such as bone, cartilage and striped muscle and is best described as a malignant mesenchymoma.[232]

A distinction is generally made between endobronchial and intrapulmonary sarcomas, the endobronchial tumours presenting earlier and consequently having a better prognosis.[233,234] Small intrapulmonary sarcomas may metastasise early but large intrapulmonary growths are equally lethal due to direct invasion of the chest wall and mediastinum. Tumour grade and mitotic activity give a good indication of the degree of malignancy.[203,235]

VASCULAR TUMOURS AND PROLIFERATIONS

Haemangioma and lymphangioma

Haemangiomas and lymphangiomas of the lung are very rare.[236–249a] Most reports comprise single cases but one German group was able to retrieve 13 haemangiomas (five capillary and eight cavernous) and two lymphangiomas from their archives.[250] Some of the cases reported before immunocytochemistry was available were possibly examples of alveolar adenoma (see p. 608) or sclerosing pneumocytoma (see p. 610),[241] the distinction from which can now be made by immunohistochemical staining for endothelial markers (see below), cytokeratins, EMA and TTF-1. Pulmonary haemangiomas and lymphangiomas resemble the commoner tumours found elsewhere: they form circumscribed lesions consisting of dilated, closely apposed, endothelium-lined vascular spaces which share adventitial connective tissue but lack a media (Fig. 12.3.15). Histologically, they differ only in their content – blood or lymph – but it is notoriously difficult to tell whether the presence of blood is genuine or artefactual, justifying the use of the non-committal term 'angioma' unless specific markers for haemangioendothelium, such as factor VIII, CD31 or CD34, and for lymphangioendothelium, such as Fli-4 or D2-40, are employed. Using CD34 and D2-40, the German group referred to above found that two of their capillary haemangiomas expressed both these markers in a mutually exclusive manner, leading the authors to recategorize these lesions as combined haemangiolymphangiomas.[250] Sometimes a haemangioma forms a pedunculated endobronchial tumour. More often it is an asymptomatic parenchymal mass (Fig. 12.3.16) but there is always the danger of life-threatening haemorrhage. Pulmonary lymphangiomas cause non-specific symptoms such as cough or dyspnoea or are discovered by chance radiographically.[249a]

Haemangiomatosis and lymphangiomatosis

Pulmonary haemangiomatosis is a rare condition in which the lungs may be affected diffusely or by multifocal nodules. The diffuse form is most frequently encountered in very young children as part of a generalised vascular malformation affecting many viscera and soft tissues.[251,252] The multifocal form is more often confined to the lungs and, although often congenital, it may present in later life.[253,254] Pulmonary lesions manifest themselves by causing haemoptysis, shortness of breath, haemorrhagic pleural effusions and pneumonia. Vascular fragility and thrombocytopenia due to platelet trapping both contribute to the haemorrhage. The lungs are infiltrated diffusely or in a multifocal manner by a network of vascular spaces of varying size. The infiltration is particularly prominent where there is abundant connective tissue – beneath the pleura, in interlobular septa and

Figure 12.3.15 Lymphangioma of the lung. A localized mass composed of interweaving vascular channels devoid of blood.

Figure 12.3.16 Haemangioma of the lung. A well-circumscribed tumour composed of many blood-filled channels is seen at the hilum of the lung. *(Courtesy of Dr T Jelihovsky, Sydney, Australia.)*

Figure 12.3.17 Haemangiomatosis. (A) High-resolution computed tomography shows a lobulated mass in the lung. (B and C) The bronchial wall and alveolar parenchyma are diffusely infiltrated by anastomosing vascular channels. (D) CD31 stain demonstrates that the channels have an endothelial lining.

around airways. Arteriovenous communication is not a feature and the disease is not hereditary. It thus differs from arteriovenous fistula and hereditary haemorrhagic telangectasia (see below). It should also be distinguished from pulmonary peliosis (see below), and from pulmonary capillary haemangiomatosis (see p. 429). Tracheobronchial haemangiomatosis (Fig. 12.3.17) is recorded in blue rubber bleb disease (see p. 482) accompanying the more usual cavernous haemangiomas of the skin and gastrointestinal tract.[255]

A similar condition involving lymphatic channels is known as lymphangiomatosis (Fig. 12.3.18).[243,256–258] Although generally a disorder of children, lymphangiomatosis may first present in adult life.[259] It causes shortness of breath, tiredness and chylous effusions. Chest radiographs show bilateral reticular infiltrates, often more marked in the lower lobes. The lung markings represent a proliferation of anastomosing endothelium-lined channels along pulmonary lymphatic routes, especially the pleura and interlobular septa, accompanied by spindle cells which stain for smooth-muscle actin. The histological appearances resemble those of congenital lymphangiectasia (see p. 77) but differ in the greater number of lymphatics while the prominent vascular lumina distinguish the condition from lymphangioleiomyomatosis (see p. 293). Haemangiomatosis is distinguished by the use of the immunomarkers described above. There may be associated abnormalities of the thoracic and retroperitoneal lymphatics.[259,260] In one example the lungs were compressed by a mass of dense connective tissue containing numerous dilated lymphatic pathways which invaded the chest wall and diaphragm.[261] Pulmonary

Figure 12.3.18 Lymphangiomatosis. (A) The pleura is markedly thickened and the interlobular septa are unduly prominent. (B) Lymphangiomatosis. An interlobular septum is thickened by the presence of numerous lymphatics.

lymphangiomatosis may also form part of the Klippel–Trenaunay syndrome, the more common manifestations of which are soft-tissue hypertrophy, angiomas and varicosities (see pp. 77 and 482). Gorham's syndrome represents a destructive non-neoplastic vascular proliferation of bone that may invade the lung if it involves the thoracic skeleton, as described on page 737.

Pulmonary telangiectasia

Telangiectasias are localised dilatations of small precapillary blood vessels, which in the lungs may be so small that they are not evident on chest radiographs. Multiple pulmonary telangiectasias occur in two unrelated conditions, hereditary haemorrhagic telangiectasia (Rendu–Osler–Weber disease, see p. 481) and cirrhosis of the liver. Patients with liver failure due to cirrhosis occasionally present with hypoxia due to pulmonary shunts through vascular lesions analogous to cutaneous spider naevi, casts of which show them to consist of both dilated existing vessels and newly formed channels.[262–265]

Pulmonary peliosis

Peliosis is well known in the liver as a rare vascular anomaly of uncertain aetiology. Extrahepatic peliosis is exceptional but, very rarely, pulmonary involvement has been reported in association with similar lesions in the liver and spleen.[266,267] One such patient was receiving anabolic steroids, which is often the case with peliosis hepatis. The pulmonary lesion was an unexpected postmortem finding in one case but another patient died of haemoptysis from rupture of a peliotic lesion in the lungs. Pulmonary peliosis consists of multiple, irregularly distributed, thin-walled blood spaces of variable size.

Haemangiopericytoma

The histological boundaries between haemangiopericytoma and localised fibrous tumour have become increasingly blurred and it is likely that most of the tumours reported as pulmonary haemangiopericytomas[235,268–274] were intrapulmonary localized fibrous tumours or synovial sarcomas. These are described on pages 730 and 631 respectively and no further attention will be paid to haemangiopericytoma.

Glomus tumour

Rare instances of glomus tumour (glomangioma) have been reported in the trachea,[275–281] bronchi[282] and lung,[283–290] suggesting that the specialised arteriovenous anastomoses familiar in the nailbeds also exist in the lower respiratory tract. The histological appearances are identical to those of glomus tumours elsewhere and for the most part they are similarly benign in their behaviour. The affected patients were adults who were asymptomatic or presented with cough or non-specific symptoms and were found to have well-demarcated nodules in their major airways or lungs.

Pathology

Glomus tumours consist of a network of vessels of capillary size surrounded by small, uniform, rounded cells with moderate amounts of eosinophilic or clear cytoplasm, set in a hyaline or myxoid stroma. Occasionally they undergo oncocytic transformation.[278] The nuclei are round with finely dispersed chromatin and indistinct nucleoli (Fig. 12.3.19). A reticulin or periodic acid–Schiff stain reveals a fine basement membrane network surrounding individual tumour cells. Immunohistochemical stains are positive for vimentin and actin, weakly so for desmin and negative for cytokeratins, melanocytic markers (HMB45, S-100 protein) and CD31. Markers of endothelium (factor VIII-related antigen, CD34) stain the vasculature but not the tumour cells. On electron microscopy there is abundant basement membrane and the cells contain prominent cytoplasmic filaments with dense bodies and rows of pinocytotic vesicles,[275,276,283] features very similar to those of smooth muscle, although there is little resemblance on light microscopy.

Differential diagnosis

Many of the immunohistochemical and ultrastructural features of glomus cells are also seen in pericytes but these cells are more elongated, and have long processes and far fewer myofilaments and dense bodies. Glomus cells, pericytes and smooth-muscle cells are closely related[291] but the differential diagnosis is unlikely to include haemangiopericytoma and leiomyoma. However, the distinction from carcinoid tumour (see p. 593) may be difficult by light microscopy, particularly in a small biopsy.[288] Helpful histological features are the distinctive reticulin pattern of a glomus tumour and the absence of immunohistochemical staining for cytokeratins and neuroendocrine differentiation.

Figure 12.3.19 An endobronchial glomus tumour. (A) The tumour surrounds entrapped gland ducts. (B) The tumour cells have clear cytoplasm, are cytologically bland and are in close apposition to capillaries.

Prognosis

Most pulmonary glomus tumours are benign. Only a few glomangiosarcomas are recorded in the lung, some disseminating widely to extrapulmonary sites.[282,286,289] Their malignant nature is evidenced histologically by brisk mitotic activity, cytological atypia and necrosis.

Kaposi's sarcoma

Epidemiology and aetiology

Kaposi's sarcoma was initially known as a rare sporadic disease of elderly European men, usually of Italian or Jewish ancestry, and as a more frequent disease affecting younger men, and occasionally women and children in central and east Africa. More recently the disease has become more widespread and immunodeficiency has

been recognised as a risk factor. Groups at particular risk now include transplant recipients, patients being treated for leukaemia or lymphoma, and those suffering from AIDS.[292–298] These patients suffer from a particularly aggressive disseminated form of the disease. Up to 70% of AIDS patients in the USA formerly developed Kaposi's sarcoma,[299–301] but the proportion is now less. A notable feature is that these cases are almost all men who acquired their human immunodeficiency virus (HIV) by homosexual contact, whereas the tumour is rare in AIDS patients infected with HIV by intravenous injection.[292 302–305] This suggests sexual transmission of a causative agent, presumably a virus distinct from, but often transmitted with, HIV.[306] This is supported by a reduction in the incidence of the tumour as homosexual promiscuity lessens and by the identification of human herpesvirus-8 in lesional tissue from patients Kaposi's sarcoma.[307–314] DNA sequences unique to this virus appear to be preferentially associated with Kaposi's sarcoma, serosal lymphoma, some inflammatory myofibroblastic tumours and multicentric Castleman's disease.[315] Their identification in bronchoalveolar lavage fluid appears to be highly sensitive and specific for pulmonary involvement by Kaposi's sarcoma.[316]

Following the identification of human herpesvirus 8-associated Kaposi sarcoma in the Uygurs of Xinjiang, northwest China, a serological survey of the region identified the virus in a high proportion of the population, leading to speculation that it had been carried thither (or thence) by travellers on the ancient silk road connecting Europe and China.[317]

Clinical features

The sporadic European form of the disease is characterised by purple macules on the skin of the legs and feet. It generally runs an indolent course. Visceral lesions are present in 10–20% of patients, with lymph nodes, gastrointestinal tract, liver, lungs, heart, bone and spleen involved in descending order of frequency.[318] Very rarely, predominantly pulmonary involvement is seen without skin lesions.[294,319–321] In Africa, Kaposi's sarcoma accounts for up to 15% of all tumours and is more aggressive: lymphoadenopathy and pulmonary involvement are common.[322,323]

Pulmonary involvement by Kaposi's sarcoma is often overlooked, partly because coexisting opportunistic infections blur the clinical and radiographic appearances and partly because open-lung biopsy is often thought necessary to make the diagnosis. In most cases, visceral lesions are preceded by cutaneous disease but this is not always true.[297,298,319,321,322] About 16% of one group of HIV-positive patients had bronchial lesions but no mucocutaneous disease.[324]

The commonest symptom of pulmonary Kaposi's sarcoma is breathlessness, which may be accompanied by cough, wheezing or haemoptysis. Pleural effusion is frequently present. Chest radiographs show diffuse pulmonary infiltrates, fine nodularity or a combination of the two. The changes are often bilateral.[325] Mucosal lesions may be seen at bronchoscopy as bright red raised areas. The prognosis in AIDS is adversely affected by the development of pulmonary Kaposi's sarcoma as this introduces the added risks of pulmonary haemorrhage, pulmonary oedema due to lymphatic obstruction and airway narrowing.

Pathology[320,322,326,327]

At autopsy, multiple small haemorrhagic nodules are found scattered throughout the lungs and visible in the tracheobronchial mucosa or on the visceral pleura. The nodules may aggregate to form larger masses.

Histologically, there is often interstitial infiltration in addition to the nodules visible macroscopically. Low-power microscopy reveals a

Figure 12.3.20 (A) Kaposi's sarcoma surrounds and infiltrates a pulmonary artery and its accompanying bronchiole in a patient with acquired immunodeficiency syndrome (AIDS). (B) Higher magnification shows the tumour to consist of spindle cells separated by slit-like vascular spaces.

characteristic distribution of the infiltrative disease along lymphatic pathways: the interlobular septa and visceral pleura are thickened and a cuff of neoplastic tissue forms around arteries and their accompanying airways (Fig. 12.3.20). The infiltrate consists of spindle cells and variable numbers of inflammatory cells, particularly plasma cells. The spindle cells closely resemble fibroblasts or endothelial cells and may form a network of irregular vascular channels. Red blood cells are often scattered between the spindle cells or may be present in the vascular spaces. Obvious features of malignancy are often lacking but scanty mitoses are usually evident. The histogenesis of Kaposi's sarcoma is still debated but it is likely that the malignant cells are endothelial, originating either in lymphatics or in blood vessels.[328–331] The tumour cells express the haemangioendothelial markers CD31, CD34 and factor VIII and the lymphangioendothelial marker D2–40. The infiltrate extends into the walls of airways but the bronchial epithelium usually remains intact. Arteries and veins appear to offer more resistance, although some separation of muscle fibres may occur. The intervening lung shows non-specific features such as alveolar oedema, haemosiderosis and the development of lymphoid aggregates. A variant of Kaposi's sarcoma, described as 'inflammatory'[301] or 'polymorphous',[326] is characterised by a predominant infiltrate of lymphocytes and plasma cells with inconspicuous spindle cells: in contrast to other forms of the disease it forms a diffuse infiltrate and seldom produces a mass lesion. The inflammatory form is particularly common in AIDS patients.

Diagnosis by bronchial or transbronchial biopsies requires a high index of suspicion.[326,327] The inflammatory form of Kaposi's sarcoma is particularly likely to be mistaken for inflammatory granulation tissue, but with a knowledge of the different variants of the disease and of its distribution, the diagnosis should be evident. Mycobacterial spindle cell pseudotumour also enters the differential diagnosis and, as both conditions are predisposed to by severe immunodeficiency, they may coexist. The mycobacterial lesion consists of shorter spindle-shaped or even polygonal cells with voluminous eosinophilic cytoplasm. It lacks the blood-filled slit-like spaces seen in Kaposi's sarcoma and mitoses are not observed. The component cells are histiocytic, staining for CD68 and strongly with the Ziehl–Nielsen method, but not for the vascular markers such as CD31 and CD34, which are evinced by Kaposi's sarcoma.

Epithelioid haemangioendothelioma

Dail and Liebow provided the first comprehensive description of this tumour but mistakenly believed it to be epithelial in type and named it 'intravascular bronchioloalveolar tumour'.[332,333] Earlier reports had suggested a possible decidual origin[334] and other examples had been mistaken for chondrosarcoma. The endothelial nature of the neoplastic cells was established by the identification of Weibel–Palade bodies in the cytoplasm by electron microscopy[335,336] and the later demonstration of immunoreactivity for factor VIII-related antigen.[333,337,338] This led to the introduction of terms such as sclerosing angiogenic tumour,[336] sclerosing interstitial vascular sarcoma,[339] sclerosing epithelial angiosarcoma[340] and low-grade sclerosing angiosarcoma.[338] The neoplasm was also included among the so-called histiocytoid haemangiomas.[341] Soft-tissue[342,343] and hepatic[338,344,345] counterparts were then recognised, and nomenclature was standardised by the adoption of the term 'epithelioid haemangioendothelioma'. It is now included in the spectrum of angiosarcomas as one of the less malignant members. A non-random chromosomal translocation t(1;3)(p36.3;q25) has been identified.[346]

Clinical features

Although pulmonary epithelioid haemangioendothelioma occurs over a wide age range (12–71 years) and in both sexes, about 50% of patients are less than 40 years of age and 80% are female.[333,347] Oestrogen receptors have been detected in a minority of tumours.[348] Symptoms are slight at first but shortness of breath slowly increases. Occasionally the tumour presents as a solitary pulmonary nodule[349] but initial chest radiographs usually show numerous small nodular opacities, mostly less than 1 cm in diameter, scattered throughout both lungs. Calcification is not usually evident radiographically and hilar lymphadenopathy is uncommon. The nodules enlarge only slowly and patients may survive for as long as 15 years after diagnosis before dying of restrictive pulmonary failure. One patient presented with hypertrophic pulmonary osteoarthropathy and following treatment with azathioprine remained well with no apparent progression for 16 years.[350]

Unusual intrathoracic forms of the disease include an anterior mediastinal mass, diffuse pleural thickening resembling malignant mesothelioma,[351–353] a solitary peripheral calcified nodule,[351] widespread vascular occlusion resulting in pulmonary hypertension,[354] alveolar haemorrhage and pleural effusion.[355] Diffuse pleural thickening and widespread vascular occlusion are seen more often in men. They indicate more aggressive growth and a correspondingly worse prognosis.[356,357]

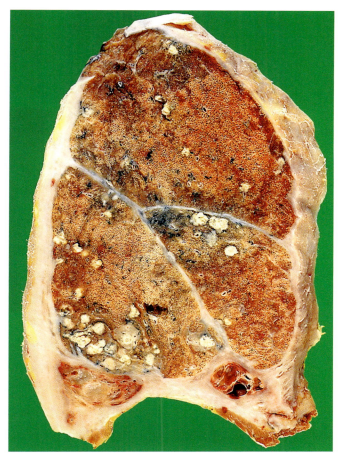

Figure 12.3.21 Epithelioid haemangioendothelioma forming multiple pulmonary nodules and thickening the pleura diffusely in the manner of a mesothelioma. *(Courtesy of Dr CGB Simpson, Aberystwyth, UK.[352])*

Figure 12.3.22 Epithelioid haemangioendothelioma. (A) The tumour nodules are more cellular at the periphery, where they protrude into neighbouring air spaces, giving them a micropolypoid structure. (B) The centres of the nodules show hyaline sclerosis, and sometimes calcification.

Pathology

At autopsy, the lungs are studded by multiple hard nodules and the pleura may be diffusely thickened (Fig. 12.3.21). Microscopically, the nodules have a central core of myxoid or hyaline connective tissue, which may show central calcification, chondrification or ossification (Fig. 12.3.22). Elastin stains reveal compressed alveolar walls and obliterated vessels. Congo red staining may be positive but the characteristic birefringence and dichroism of amyloid are absent. The nodules are more cellular at the periphery where the stroma contains single, or small clusters of tumour cells. Tumour cell nuclei are oval with dispersed granular chromatin and a small nucleolus; they lack atypia and mitoses are infrequent. The cytoplasm is abundant, eosinophilic and often contains vacuoles, which may coalesce to form an intracellular lumen (Fig. 12.3.23). These minature lumina sometimes contain a few red blood cells but if not they are apt to be confused with the mucin vacuoles of an adenocarcinoma.[358]

At the periphery, the nodules extend into adjacent bronchioles and alveoli as papillary processes that are often clothed by cuboidal cells (see Fig. 12.3.23). In paraffin sections these are not clearly distinguishable from stromal cells but marked differences are evident on electron microscopy.[335,336] The surface cells are type II alveolar epithelial cells and are presumably reactive. The tumour cells have ultrastructural features more suggestive of vasoformative cells in that they contain Weibel–Palade bodies, and immunoreactive factor VIII-related antigen is demonstrable both in the cytoplasm and within vacuoles (Fig. 12.3.24).[335–338] Positive reactions are usually obtained with other endothelial markers, including Fli-1, CD 31 and CD34.[359]

Extension within the lung may occur by lymphatic spread, producing appearances similar to those seen in cases of lymphatic permeation by carcinoma (so-called carcinomatous lymphangitis – see p. 682),[351] and the pleura may be involved diffusely, resulting in a gross appearance that resembles that of a mesothelioma (see Fig. 12.3.21).[351–353] Extrathoracic spread is rare but extrapulmonary deposits are recorded in sites such as the liver, bone and skin.[333,338,344,348,349,360] The characteristic micropolypoid structure is not seen outside the lung and is evidently a product of the alveolar architecture.

With such a slow-growing multifocal tumour, the identification of a solitary deposit in the liver raises the question whether the pulmonary lesions are metastases from an occult hepatic primary.[361,362] Based on a study of basement membrane composition it has been claimed that the pulmonary tumours represent multicentric primary growths rather than metastases,[363] but this issue is unsettled.[348] There are cases in which the multiple pulmonary lesions have developed long after epithelioid haemangioendothelioma has been diagnosed in an extrapulmonary site.[352,364]

Figure 12.3.23 Epithelioid haemangioendothelioma. (A) The tumour nodules have a micropolypoid structure at their periphery. (B) Vacuolation of tumour cells is sometimes evident, probably representing primitive angiogenesis.

Figure 12.3.24 Epithelioid haemangioendothelioma. The tumour cells stain for the endothelial marker CD31.

Differential diagnosis

The differential diagnosis includes lesions containing cartilage or myxoid connective tissue, such as chondroid 'hamartoma', metastatic chondrosarcoma and sclerosing pneumocytoma. Sclerosing pneumocytoma is typically a solitary lesion and contains sclerotic areas and papillary processes that may resemble those of epithelioid haemangioendothelioma, but the presence of prominent vascular spaces in the sclerosing pneumocytoma usually enables the distinction to be made.

Non-chromaffin paraganglioma (chemodectoma)

Paraganglia of the head, neck and thorax are closely aligned with the parasympathetic nervous system and blood vessels such as the carotid arteries, aorta and the main pulmonary arteries, locations that fit well with their proposed chemoreceptor function. They are not well described in the lungs. The existence of chemoreceptors on intrapulmonary blood vessels is based on functional observations[365] backed up by a single morphological description of 'glomera' (paraganglia, chemoreceptors) in the outer coats of pulmonary arteries at their branching points closely related to adjacent nerves (see p. 23).[366] Primary pulmonary paragangliomas could develop from such structures. However, most intrathoracic paragangliomas arise outside the lung[367–370] or, if intrapulmonary, eventually prove to be metastases from an occult growth in the neck. Apart from the so-called multiple minute chemodectomas of the lung described separately (see meningothelioid nodules, p. 700), few cases of primary pulmonary paraganglioma have been reported, and it is debatable whether these represent paragangliomas or carcinoids.[371–377] Carcinoids and paragangliomas both contain dense-core granules, which are indistinguishable in size and structure. The nature of the dense-core granules is obscure but one reputed pulmonary paraganglioma was shown to contain noradrenaline (norepinephrine),[378] whilst a few others have secreted catecholamines.[379,380] Cytokeratin immunocytochemistry was formerly thought to provide a clear means of distinguishing carcinoids from paragangliomas but it is now recognised that positive reactions may be obtained with both.[381–384] Paragangliomas are characterised by S-100-positive sustentacular cells surrounding cells with neuroendocrine characteristics but this feature is also described in a substantial number of bronchopulmonary carcinoids. However, some workers prefer to regard tumours of this description as paragangliomas and have substantiated this claim by demonstrating scanty ganglion cells in occasional examples, terming these tumours gangliocytic paragangliomas.[385–387] These few examples have included both a central peribronchial tumour of *Zellballen* pattern and peripheral spindle cell growths. All have been benign. One was responsible for Cushing's syndrome.[387]

Sarcoma of the major pulmonary blood vessels

A rare form of sarcoma arises within the pulmonary trunk, the main pulmonary arteries or the right side of the heart and gives rise to multiple pulmonary tumours.[388–398] Less commonly, similar tumours arise in the pulmonary veins, the chambers on the left side of the heart or the aorta and metastasise via the systemic circulation.[178,227,395,399–402]

Clinical features

Patients with sarcoma of the pulmonary arteries cover a wide age range, from 21 to 80 years, but most tumours occur between the ages

Figure 12.3.25 Pulmonary trunk sarcoma. (A and B) A pulmonary artery is plugged and almost totally occluded by metastatic tumour, which consists of (C) undifferentiated spindle cell sarcoma. *(Courtesy of Dr W Kenyon, Liverpool, UK.)*

or 45 and 65 and there appears to be a predominance of females. Radiation induction is recorded.[403] Dyspnoea, chest pain and cough may be accompanied by episodes of haemoptysis, syncope, a systolic murmur or right ventricular dilatation and failure.[404] Plain chest radiography shows increased hilar shadowing and hypoperfusion of the lung fields, often leading to a mistaken diagnosis of pulmonary thromboembolism.[405–407] Weight loss, fever and anaemia are additional features more suggestive of malignancy.[408] Diagnosis during life has been unusual but modern imaging techniques, such as angiography and computed tomography, make this possible.[409,410] Fragmentation and tumour embolization result in multiple pulmonary metastases, which appear as peripheral rounded nodules or masses. Metastatic sites beyond the lungs include lymph nodes, brain, diaphragm, thyroid and pancreas.

Pathology

At surgery or autopsy the pulmonary trunk is distended by soft, grey, polypoid tumour, often mixed with thrombus. This frequently extends distally into one or both main pulmonary arteries and, less often, proximally to involve the pulmonary valve and right ventricular outflow tract. Sometimes the tumour appears to arise in the right ventricle or atrium. The intima and media of the pulmonary trunk are infiltrated but often quite superficially. In about half the cases tumour extends directly into smaller intrapulmonary branches (Fig.

12.3.25a, b). It may spread from the arteries to present as a diffuse pulmonary infiltrate.[229]

In biopsy material, pathologists often misinterpret the pulmonary deposits as infarcts, haemorrhagic pneumonia or haemorrhage as many are well vascularised and liable to bleed. Other deposits, however, are more solid. Some tumours consist of a fairly uniform population of polygonal or spindle cells whereas others show marked pleomorphism and giant tumour cells (Fig. 12.3.25c). They are most frequently termed undifferentiated, pleomorphic or intimal sarcomas but other terms reflect their ability to differentiate in a number of directions and include, in descending order of frequency, leiomyosarcoma, rhabdomyosarcoma, chondrosarcoma, fibromyxosarcoma, mesenchymoma (containing mixed elements), osteosarcoma, myxosarcoma, angiosarcoma and malignant fibrous histiocytoma.[411] Thus, some tumours show the formation of bone or cartilage. The few examples subjected to electron microscopy have shown striated[388] or smooth muscle[392,412] or have been undifferentiated.[413] Occasional cases are examples of epithelioid angiosarcoma,[394] and are likely to be confused with poorly differentiated carcinoma, particularly pseudovascular variants[414]: both carcinoma and epithelioid angiosarcoma express cytokeratin[415] but only the latter expresses endothelial markers.

The prognosis is usually poor but some well-differentiated myofibroblastic tumours have been associated with prolonged patient survival and rare examples reported under terms such as myxoma appear to have been benign.[416]

Figure 12.3.26 Neurofibroma. (A) As in the skin, the tumour surrounds rather than destroys glands. (B) The tumour consists of cytologically bland wavy spindle cells, and mast cells are evident in the stroma. *(Courtesy of Dr A Herbert, London, UK.)*

NEURAL TUMOURS

Nerve sheath tumours

Posterior mediastinal or paravertebral nerve sheath tumours are fairly common but in the lower respiratory tract tumours of nerve sheath origin are distinctly rare.[219,235,417–422] They develop in both sexes and may be endobronchial or parenchymal.[235] They comprise both neurofibromas and neurilemmomas (schwannomas), some of which are malignant. Neurofibromas are more frequent in men, whereas schwannomas are more common in women. The gross, microscopical, immunocytochemical and ultrastructural appearances are identical to those of nerve sheath tumours elsewhere (Fig. 12.3.26). Melanin production is occasionally encountered[423] and rhabdomyoblastic differentiation is recorded in rare malignant nerve sheath tumours (so-called triton tumours) of the lung.[424]

It is uncertain what proportion of patients with intrapulmonary nerve sheath tumours have neurofibromatosis but most have no other features of the disease. Such patients are often asymptomatic, their tumours having reached a considerable size by the time they are discovered on a routine chest radiograph. Others have chest symptoms attributable to the obstructive effect of the tumour. Some lesions are visible bronchoscopically as a polypoid mass bulging into the lumen of an airway, and this may cause bronchiectasis.[425] The airways may also be affected diffusely and require stenting[421] or there may be multiple endobronchial lesions.[426] A unique case of multiple neurofibromas has been described with severe hypoxaemia due to right-to-left shunts within the tumours.[427]

In addition to these true neoplasms, traumatic (amputation) neuromas may be observed, generally at bronchoscopy following pulmonary resection when they are liable to be mistaken for recurrence of the original tumour or a stitch granuloma.[428] They resemble similar lesions encountered elsewhere, consisting of disorganised, hypertrophic bundles of axons surrounded by Schwann cells, perineurium, fibroblasts and collagenous scar tissue.

Granular cell tumour

Granular cell tumours were first described by Abrikossof in 1926 and in the respiratory tract shortly afterwards.[429–431] They were initially considered to be of striated muscle origin but a neural derivation is now thought more likely[432–435] and the original term 'granular cell myoblastoma' has therefore been modified. The tongue is the commonest site but they occur in many other locations, including the lip, skin, breast, muscle, neurohypophysis and other viscera. A small proportion, about 8%, arise in the tracheobronchial tree or the periphery of the lung.[436–442]

Clinical features

Patients with bronchopulmonary granular cell tumour range in age from 20 to 47 years (median 45 years) and show no sex predilection.[439,442] The tumours are either incidental findings or cause obstructive symptoms or haemoptysis. A small number of patients have multiple pulmonary lesions[438] and some have associated soft-tissue granular cell tumours.[438,440] Imaging usually shows obstructive changes. At bronchoscopy, granular cell tumours usually appear as endobronchial nodules at points of bifurcation but others are plaque-like. They range in size up to 6.5 cm in diameter.

Pathology

Bronchoscopic biopsy is usually diagnostic, showing the characteristic cells lying directly beneath the epithelium, which may undergo squamous metaplasia. The tumour cells are closely packed in cords, sheets or nests. They are polygonal or spindle-shaped and have small, densely staining nuclei and abundant, coarsely granular, eosinophilic and periodic acid–Schiff-positive cytoplasm (Fig. 12.3.27A). Nerve fibres may be seen among the tumour cells. Infiltration of the adjacent lung is often seen and lymph nodes may be directly involved but metastasis is not a feature.

Ultrastructurally, the cytoplasmic granules are consistent with them being of lysosomal autophagic or cell membrane origin[432,433,443] and the presence of axons and an incomplete basement membrane around the cells is thought to point to a Schwann cell origin.[444] This is supported by the immunohistochemical demonstration of S-100 neural protein (Fig. 12.3.27B).[432,442,445] Negative reactions are obtained for cytokeratin and neuroendocrine markers.

Figure 12.3.27 A granular cell tumour that formed a bronchial polyp. (A) The tumour is composed of polygonal cells with abundant eosinophilic cytoplasm. (B) The tumour cells are strongly positive for S-100 protein.

Figure 12.3.28 Meningioma of the lung. There was no evidence of an intracranial lesion and electron microscopy supported the diagnosis. *(Courtesy of Dr TV Colby, Scottsdale, USA.)*

Differential diagnosis

Granular cell tumours may be confused with oncocytic carcinoid tumours (see p. 595) or oncocytic tumours of bronchial gland origin (see p. 605). Carcinoid tumours are typically much more vascular than granular cell tumours. Electron microscopy of oncocytic tumours shows closely packed mitochondria rather than the autophagic granules of granular cell tumours. Some carcinoid tumours may stain weakly for S-100 protein but both carcinoid tumours and bronchial gland tumours also stain for cytokeratin whereas granular cell tumours do not.

Prognosis

Granular cell tumours generally grow slowly and no malignant examples are described in the lung. Nevertheless, effective therapy usually requires formal resection.

Meningioma

Occasional meningiomas, identical to those found within the cranium but apparently primary to the lungs, have been described.[446–458] It has been suggested that they arise from ectopic arachnoid cells,[452] but it is likely that arachnoid-like cells are an inherent part of the normal lung (see p. 23) and that this is the source of the pulmonary tumours. This relates them to the meningothelioid nodules (so-called multiple minute chemodectomas, see p. 700) but pulmonary meningiomas are generally solitary and are not minute.[459]

Clinical features

The reported cases have ranged from 51 to 70 years of age. The patients have generally been asymptomatic, their tumour being discovered on routine chest examination. The tumours have generally been solitary but in one case there were multiple pulmonary meningiomas and the patient also had neurofibromatosis.[448]

Pathology

The tumours are well circumscribed but are not encapsulated. They have no obvious connection with airways, blood vessels or pleura. Histologically, they consist of sheets of regular ovoid or spindle cells forming the 'menigothelial whorls' and psammoma bodies characteristic of the intracranial growths (Fig. 12.3.28). Immunohistochemistry shows that the tumour cells stain positively for vimentin and EMA but negatively for cytokeratin and S-100 protein. Electron microscopy shows complex cellular interdigitations and many desmosomes.

Differential diagnosis

An occult primary in the cranium obviously needs to be excluded before the diagnosis of primary pulmonary meningioma can be countenanced. The degree of atypia is of no significance as some metastases appear quite benign histologically, giving rise to the term 'benign metastasising meningioma'.[460]

Treatment and prognosis

Treatment is by surgical resection, following which recurrence is very rare.[456]

Ependymoma

Rare examples of ependymomas occurring outside the central nervous system have been described in the pelvis and posterior mediastinum and, in one patient only, the lung.[461] This was an elderly woman who also had a small cell carcinoma treated by chemotherapy and it is uncertain whether the ependymoma represented metaplastic change in the carcinoma, perhaps due to the chemotherapy, or whether it arose in ectopic ependyma. The tumour had the usual morphology of a malignant ependymoma and showed strong immunoreactivity for glial fibrillary protein with less intense staining for vimentin, EMA and S-100 protein.

REFERENCES

Inflammatory myofibroblastic tumour

1. Umiker WO, Iverson L. Postinflammatory 'tumors' of the lung. Report of four cases simulating xanthoma, fibroma or plasma cell tumor. J Thorac Surg 1954;28:55–63.

2. Bates T, Hull OH. Histiocytoma of the bronchus. A report of a case in a six-year-old child. Am J Dis Child 1958;95:53–6.

3. Fisher ER, Beyer FD. Post-inflammatory tumour (xanthoma) of lung. Dis Chest 1959;36:43–8.

4. Sherwin RP, Kern WH, Jones JC. Solitary mast cell granuloma (histiocytoma) of the lung. Cancer 1965;18:634–41.

5. Charette EE, Mariano AV, LaForet EG. Solitary mast cell 'tumour' of the lung. Arch Intern Med 1966;118:358–62.

6. Dentworth P, Lynch MJ, Fallis JC. Xanthomatous pseudotumor of lung: a case report with electron microscope and lipid studies. Cancer 1968;22:345–55.

7. Bahadori M, Liebow AA. Plasma cell granulomas of the lung. Cancer 1973;31:191–208.

8. Narodick BG. Fibrous histiocytoma or xanthoma of the lung with bronchial involvement. J Thorac Cardiovasc Surg 1973;65:653–7.

9. Buell R, Wang N-S, Seemayer TA, et al. Endobronchial plasma cell granuloma (xanthomatous pseudotumor). A light and electron microscopic study. Hum Pathol 1976;7:411–26.

10. Bates HR, Buis LJ, Johns TNP. Endobronchial histiocytoma. Chest 1976;69:705–6.

11. Katzenstein A-LA, Maurer JJ. Benign histiocytic tumor of the lung. A light and electron-microscopic study. Am J Surg Pathol 1979;3:61–8.

12. Spencer H. The pulmonary plasma cell/histiocytoma complex. Histopathology 1984;8:903–16.

13. Coffin CM, Watterson J, Priest JR, et al. Extrapulmonary inflammatory myofibroblastic tumor (inflammatory pseudotumor) – a clinicopathologic and immunohistochemical study of 84 cases. Am J Surg Pathol 1995;19:859–72.

14. Gleason BC, Hornick JL. Inflammatory myofibroblastic tumours: where are we now? J Clin Pathol 2008;61:428–37.

14a. Yi E, Aubry MC. Pulmonary pseudoneoplasms. Arch Pathol Lab Med 2010;134:417–26.

15. Dehner LP. The enigmatic inflammatory pseudotumours: the current state of our understanding, or misunderstanding. J Pathol 2000;192:277–9.

16. Alvarez-Fernandez E, Escalona-Zapata J. Pulmonary plasma cell granuloma – an electron microscopic and tissue culture study. Histopathology 1983;7:279–86.

17. Chen HP, Lee SS, Berardi RS. Inflammatory pseudotumor of the lung. Ultrastructural and light microscopic study of a myxomatous variant. Cancer 1984;54:861–5.

18. Matsubara O, Tan-Liu NS, Kenney RM, et al. Inflammatory pseudotumors of the lung: progression from organizing pneumonia to fibrous histiocytoma or to plasma cell granuloma in 32 cases. Hum Pathol 1988;19:807–14.

19. Kubicz ST, Paradowska W, Czarnowska-Nastula B, et al. Pseudo-tumor of the lung in children. Ann Radiol (Paris) 1975;18:447–52.

20. Janigan DJ, Marrie TJ. An inflammatory pseudotumor of the lung in Q fever pneumonia. N Engl J Med 1983;308:86–7.

21. Lipton JH, Fong TC, Gill MJ, et al. Q fever inflammatory pseudotumor of the lung. Chest 1987;92:756–7.

22. Arber DA, Kamel OW, Vanderijn M, et al. Frequent presence of the Epstein–Barr virus in inflammatory pseudotumor. Hum Pathol 1995;26:1093–8.

23. Gomez-Roman JJ, Ocejo-Vinyals G, Sanchez-Velasco P, et al. Presence of human herpesvirus-8 DNA sequences and overexpression of human IL-6 and cyclin D1 in inflammatory myofibroblastic tumor (inflammatory pseudotumor). Lab Invest 2000;80:1121–6.

24. Gomez-Roman JJ, Sanchez-Velasco P, Ocejo-Vinyals G, et al. Human herpesvirus-8 genes are expressed in pulmonary inflammatory myofibroblastic tumor (inflammatory pseudotumor). Am J Surg Pathol 2001;25:624–9.

25. Farris AB III, Mark EJ, Kradin RL. Pulmonary 'inflammatory myofibroblastic' tumors: a critical examination of the diagnostic category based on quantitative immunohistochemical analysis. Virchows Arch 2007;450:585–90.

26. Berardi RS, Lee SS, Chen HP, et al. Inflammatory pseudotumors of the lung. Surg Gynecol Obstet 1988;156:89–96.

27. Warter A, Satge D, Roeslin N. Angioinvasive plasma cell granulomas of the lung. Cancer 1987;59:435–43.

29. Donner LR, Trompler RA, White RR. Progression of inflammatory myofibroblastic tumor (inflammatory pseudotumor) or soft tissue into sarcoma after several recurrences. Hum Pathol 1996;27:1095–8.

30. Treissman SP, Gillis DA, Lee CLY, et al. Omental-mesenteric inflammatory pseudotumor. Cytogenetic demonstration of genetic changes and monoclonality in one tumor. Cancer 1994;73:1433–7.

31. Snyder CS, Dellaquila M, Haghighi P, et al. Clonal changes in inflammatory pseudotumor of the lung: a case report. Cancer 1995;76:1545–9.

32. Biselli R, Ferlini C, Fattorossi A, et al. Inflammatory myofibroblastic tumor

(inflammatory pseudotumor): DNA flow cytometric analysis of nine pediatric cases. Cancer 1996;77:778–84.

33. Su LD, Atayde-Perez A, Sheldon S, et al. Inflammatory myofibroblastic tumor: cytogenetic evidence supporting clonal origin. Mod Pathol 1998;11:364–8.

34. Yousem SA, Shaw H, Cieply K. Involvement of 2p23 in pulmonary inflammatory pseudotumors. Hum Pathol 2001;32:428–33.

35. Bridge JA, Kanamori M, Ma ZG, et al. Fusion of the ALK gene to the clathrin heavy chain gene, CLTC, in inflammatory myofibroblastic tumor. Am J Pathol 2001;159:411–15.

36. Cook JR, Dehner LP, Collins MH, et al. Anaplastic lymphoma kinase (ALK) expression in the inflammatory myofibroblastic tumor – A comparative immunohistochemical study. Am J Surg Pathol 2001;25:1364–71.

37. Cessna MH, Zhou H, Sanger WG, et al. Expression of ALK1 and p80 in inflammatory myofibroblastic tumor and its mesenchymal mimics: A study of 135 cases. Modern Pathol 2002;15:931–8.

38. Debelenko LV, Arthur DC, Pack SD, et al. Identification of CARS-ALK fusion in primary and metastatic lesions of an inflammatory myofibroblastic tumor. Lab Invest 2003;83:1255–65.

39. Nonaka D, Birbe R, Rosai J. So-called inflammatory myofibroblastic tumour: a proliferative lesion of fibroblastic reticulum cells? Histopathology 2005;46:604–13.

40. Mandalbaum I, Brashear RE, Hull MT. Surgical treatment and course of pulmonary pseudotumour (plasma cell granuloma). J Thorac Cardiovasc Surg 1981;82:77–82.

41. Hartman GE, Shochat SJ. Primary pulmonary neoplasms of childhood: a review. Ann Thorac Surg 1983;36:108–19.

42. Rohrlich P, Peuchmaur M, Cocci SD, et al. Interleukin-6 and interleukin-1 beta production in a pediatric plasma cell granuloma of the lung. Am J Surg Pathol 1995;19:590–5.

43. Helikson MA, Havey AD, Zerwekh JE, et al. Plasma cell granuloma producing calcitriol and hypercalcemia. Ann Intern Med 1986;105:379–81.

44. Agrons GA, Rosado-de-Christenson ML, Kirejczyk WM, et al. Pulmonary inflammatory pseudotumor: radiologic features. Radiology 1998;206:511–18.

45. Titus JL, Harrison EG, Clagett OT, et al. Xanthomatous and inflammatory pseudotumors of the lung. Cancer 1962;15:522–38.

46. Strutynsky N, Balthazar EJ, Klein RM. Inflammatory pseudotumours of the lung. Br J Radiol 1974;47:94–6.

47. Lemarchadour F, Lavielle JP, Guilcher C, et al. Coexistence of plasma cell granulomas of lung and central nervous system – a case report. Pathol Res Pract 1995;191:1038–45.

47a. Athanassiadi K, Laenger F, Dickgreber N, et al. Multiple inflammatory myofibroblastic tumors involving lung and mediastinum: a rare clinical entity. Thorac Cardovasc Surg 2009;57:343–6.

48. Shirakusa T, Miyazaki N, Kitagawa T, et al. Ultrastructural study of pulmonary plasma cell granuloma – report of a case. Br J Dis Chest 1979;73:289–96.

49. Tomita T, Dixon A, Watanabe I, et al. Sclerosing vascular variant of plasma cell granuloma. Hum Pathol 1980;11:197–202.

50. Muraoka S, Sato T, Takahashi T, et al. Plasma cell granuloma of the lung with extrapulmonal extension. Immunohistochemical and electron microscopic studies. Acta Pathol Jpn 1985;35:933–44.

51. Ramachandra S, Hollowood K, Bisceglia M, et al. Inflammatory pseudotumour of soft tissues: a clinicopathological and immunohistochemical analysis of 18 cases. Histopathology 1995;27:313–23.

52. Rose AG, McCormick S, Cooper K, et al. Inflammatory pseudotumor (plasma cell granuloma) of the heart: report of two cases and literature review. Arch Pathol Lab Med 1996;120:549–54.

53. Kuzela DC. Ultrastructural study of postinflammatory 'tumor' of the lung. Cancer 1975;36:149–56.

54. Pettinato G, Manivel JC, De Rosa N, et al. Inflammatory myofibroblastic tumor (plasma cell granuloma) – clinicopathologic study of 20 cases with immunohistochemical and ultrastructural observations. Am J Clin Pathol 1990;94:538–46.

55. Van Dorpe J, Ectors N, Geboes K, et al. Is calcifying fibrous pseudotumor a late sclerosing stage of inflammatory myofibroblastic tumor? Am J Surg Pathol 1999;23:329–35.

56. Weynand B, Draguet AP, Bernard P, et al. Calcifying fibrous pseudotumour: first case report in the peritoneum with immunostaining for CD34. Histopathology 1999;34:86–7.

57. Pomplun S, Goldstraw P, Davies SE, et al. Calcifying fibrous pseudotumour arising within an inflammatory pseudotumour: evidence of progression from one lesion to the other? Histopathology 2000;37:380–2.

58. Hill KA, GonzalezCrussi F, Chou PM. Calcifying fibrous pseudotumor versus inflammatory myofibroblastic tumor: A histological and immunohistochemical comparison. Modern Pathol 2001;14:784–90.

59. Gal AA, Koss MN, McCarthy WF, et al. Prognostic factors in pulmonary fibrohistiocytic lesions. Cancer 1994;73:1817–24.

60. Ledet SC, Brown RW, Cagle PT. p53 immunostaining in the differentiation of inflammatory pseudotumor from sarcoma involving the lung. Mod Pathol 1995;8:282–6.

61. Tan-Liu NS, Matsubara O, Grillo HC, et al. Invasive fibrous tumor of the tracheobronchial tree: clinical and pathologic study of seven cases. Hum Pathol 1989;20:180–4.

62. Bush A, Sheppard MN, Wahn U, et al. Spontaneous arrest of growth of a plasma cell granuloma. Respir Med 1992;86:161–4.

63. Maier HC, Sommers SC. Recurrent and metastatic pulmonary fibrous histiocytoma/plasma cell granuloma in a child. Cancer 1987;60:1073–6.

64. Biselli R, Boldrini R, Ferlini C, et al. Myofibroblastic tumours: neoplasias with divergent behaviour. Ultrastructural and flow cytometric analysis. Pathol Res Pract 1999;195:619–32.

65. Hussong JW, Brown M, Perkins SL, et al. Comparison of DNA ploidy, histologic, and immunohistochemical findings with clinical outcome in inflammatory myofibroblastic tumors. Mod Pathol 1999;12:279–86.

66. Coffin CM, Hornick JL, Fletcher CD. Inflammatory myofibroblastic tumor: comparison of clinicopathologic, histologic, and immunohistochemical features including ALK expression in atypical and aggressive cases. Am J Surg Pathol 2007;31:509–20.

Pleuropulmonary blastoma

67. Manivel JC, Priest JR, Watterson J, et al. Pleuropulmonary blastoma. The so-called pulmonary blastoma of childhood. Cancer 1988;62:1516–26.

68. Cohen M, Emms M, Kaschula R. Childhood pulmonary blastoma: a pleuropulmonary variant of the adult-type pulmonary blastoma. Pediatr Pathol 1991;11:737–49.

69. Hachitanda Y, Aoyama C, Sato JK, et al. Pleuropulmonary blastoma in childhood – a tumor of divergent differentiation. Am J Surg Pathol 1993;17:382–91.

70. Pacinda SJ, Ledet SC, Gondo MM, et al. p53 and MDM2 immunostaining in pulmonary blastomas and bronchogenic carcinomas. Hum Pathol 1996;27:542–6.

71. Priest JR, McDermott MB, Bhatia S, et al. Pleuropulmonary blastoma: a clinicopathologic study of 50 cases. Cancer 1997;80:147–61.

72. Weinblatt ME, Siegel SE, Isaacs H. Pulmonary blastoma associated with cystic lung disease. Cancer 1982;49:669–71.

73. Ueda K, Gruppo R, Unger F, et al. Rhabdomyosarcoma of lung arising in congenital cystic adenomatoid malformation. Cancer 1977;40:383–8.

74. Hedlund GL, Bisset GSI, Bove KE. Malignant neoplasms arising in cystic hamartomas of the lung in childhood. Radiology 1989;173:77–9.

75. d'Agostino S, Bonoldi E, Dante S, et al. Embryonal rhabdomyosarcoma of the lung arising in cystic adenomatoid malformation: case report and review of the literature. J Pediatr Surg 1997;32:1381–3.

76. Ozcan C, Celik A, Ural Z, et al. Primary pulmonary rhabdomyosarcoma arising within cystic adenomatoid malformation: a case report and review of the literature. J Pediatr Surg 2001;36:1062–5.

77. Domizio P, Liesner RJ, Dicks-Mireaux C et al. Malignant mesenchymoma associated with a congenital lung cyst in a child: case report and review of the literature. Pediatr Pathol 1990;10:785–97.

78. Krous HF, Sexauer CL. Embryonal rhabdomyosarcoma arising within a congenital bronchogenic cyst in a child. J Pediatr Surg 1981;16:506–8.

79. Weinberg AG, Currarino G, Moore GC, et al. Mesenchymal neoplasia and congenital pulmonary cysts. Pediatr Radiol 1980;9:179–82.

80. Sciot R, Cin PD, Brock P, et al. Pleuropulmonary blastoma (pulmonary blastoma of childhood): genetic link with other embryonal malignancies? Histopathology 1994;24:559–63.

81. Yang P, Hasegawa T, Hirose T, et al. Pleuropulmonary blastoma: Fluorescence in situ hybridization analysis indicating trisomy 2. Am J Surg Pathol 1997;21:854–9.

82. Delahunt B, Thomson KJ, Ferguson AF, et al. Familial cystic nephroma and pleuropulmonary blastoma. Cancer 1993;71:1338–42.

83. Priest JR, Watterson J, Strong L, et al. Pleuropulmonary blastoma: a marker for familial disease. J Pediatr 1996;128:220–4.

84. Boman F, Hill DA, Williams GM, et al. Familial association of pleuropulmonary blastoma with cystic nephroma and other renal tumors: a report from the International Pleuropulmonary Blastoma Registry. J Pediatr 2006;149:850–4.

85. Hill DA, Ivanovich J, Priest JR, et al. DICER1 mutations in familial pleuropulmonary blastoma. Science 2009;325:965.

86. Hill DA, Sadeghi S, Schultz MZ, et al. Pleuropulmonary blastoma in an adult: an initial case report. Cancer 1999;85:2368–74.

87. Indolfi P, Casale F, Carli M, et al. Pleuropulmonary blastoma: management and prognosis of 11 cases. Cancer 2000;89:1396–401.

88. Dehner LP. Pleuropulmonary blastoma is THE pulmonary blastoma of childhood. Semin Diagn Pathol 1994;11:144–51.

89. MacSweeney F, Papagiannopoulos K, Goldstraw P, et al. An assessment of the expanded classification of congenital cystic adenomatoid malformations and their relationship to malignant transformation. Am J Surg Pathol 2003;27:1139–46.

90. Hill DA, Dehner LP. A cautionary note about congenital cystic adenomatoid malformation (CCAM) type 4. Am J Surg Pathol 2004;28:554–5.

91. Hill DA, Jarzembowski JA, Priest JR, et al. Type I pleuropulmonary blastoma: pathology and biology study of 51 cases from the international pleuropulmonary blastoma registry. Am J Surg Pathol 2008;32:282–95.

92. Wright JR Jr. Pleuropulmonary blastoma: a case report documenting transition from type I (cystic) to type III (solid). Cancer 2000;88:2853–8.

93. Papagiannopoulos KA, Sheppard M, Bush A, et al. Pleuropulmonary blastoma: is prophylactic resection of congenital lung cysts effective? Ann Thorac Surg 2001;72:604–5.

Benign clear cell tumour

94. Bonetti F, Pea M, Martignoni G, et al. Clear cell ('sugar') tumor of the lung is a lesion strictly related to angiomyolipoma – the concept of a family of lesions characterized by the presence of the perivascular epithelioid cells (PEC). Pathology 1995;26:230–6.

95. Pea M, Martignoni G, Zamboni G, et al. Perivascular epithelioid cell. Am J Surg Pathol 1996;20:1149–53.

96. Hironaka M, Fukayama M. Regional proliferation of HMB-45-positive clear cells of the lung with lymphangioleiomyomatosislike distribution, replacing the lobes with multiple cysts and a nodule. Am J Surg Pathol 1999;23:1288–93.

97. Flieder DB, Travis WD. Clear cell 'Sugar' tumor of the lung: Association with lymphangioleiomyomatosis and multifocal micronodular pneumocyte hyperplasia in a patient with tuberous sclerosis. Am J Surg Pathol 1997;21:1242–7.

98. Chuah KL, Tan PH. Multifocal micronodular pneumocyte hyperplasia, lymphangiomyomatosis and clear cell micronodules of the lung in a Chinese female patient with tuberous sclerosis. Pathology 1998;30:242–6.

99. Vang R, Kempson RL. Perivascular epithelioid cell tumor ('PEComa') of the uterus – a subset of HMB-45-positive epithelioid mesenchymal neoplasms with an uncertain relationship to pure smooth muscle tumors. Am J Surg Pathol 2002;26:1–13.

100. Pileri SA, Cavazza A, Schiavina M, et al. Clear-cell proliferation of the lung with lymphangioleiomyomatosis-like change. Histopathology 2004;44:156–63.

101. Folpe AL, Kwiatkowski DJ. Perivascular epithelioid cell neoplasms: pathology and pathogenesis. Human Pathology 2010;41:1–15.

102. Liebow AA, Castleman B. Benign 'clear cell tumors' of the lung. Am J Pathol 1963;43:13a–4a.

103. Liebow AA, Castleman B. Benign clear cell ('sugar') tumors of the lung. Yale J Biol Med 1971;43:213–22.

104. Becker NH, Soifer I. Benign clear cell tumour ('sugar tumor') of the lung. Cancer 1971;27:712–19.

105. Hoch WS, Patchefsky AS, Takeda M, et al. Benign clear cell tumor of the lung. Cancer 1974;33:1328–36.

106. Harbin WP, Mark GJ, Greene RE. Benign clear cell tumor ('sugar tumor') of the lung: case report and review of the literature. Radiology 1978;129:595–6.

107. Zolliker A, Jacques J, Goldstein AS. Benign clear cell tumor of the lung. Arch Pathol Lab Med 1979;103:526–30.

108. Andrion A, Mazzucco G, Gugliotta P, et al. Benign clear cell ('sugar') tumor of the lung. A light microscopic, histochemical and ultrastructural study with a review of the literature. Cancer 1985;56:2657–63.

109. Fukuda T, Machinami R, Jashita T, et al. Benign clear cell tumor of the lung in an 8-year-old girl. Arch Pathol Lab Med 1986;110:664–6.

110. Sale GE, Kulander BG. 'Benign' clear-cell tumor (sugar tumor) of the lung with hepatic metastases ten years after resection of pulmonary primary tumor. Arch Pathol Lab Med 1988;112:1177–8.

111. Nguyen G-K. Aspiration biopsy cytology of benign clear cell ('sugar') tumor of the lung. Acta Cytol 1989;33:511–15.

112. Gaffey MJ, Mills SE, Askin FB, et al. Clear cell tumor of the lung. A clinicopathologic, immunohistochemical and ultrastructural study of eight cases. Am J Surg Pathol 1990;14:248–59.

113. Gaffey MJ, Mills SE, Zarbo RJ, et al. Clear cell tumor of the lung – immunohistochemical and ultrastructural evidence of melanogenesis. Am J Surg Pathol 1991;15:644–53.

114. Gal AA, Koss MN, Hochholzer L, et al. An immunohistochemical study of benign clear cell (sugar) tumor of the lung. Arch Pathol Lab Med 1991;115:1034–8.

115. Lantuejoul S, Isaac S, Pinel N, et al. Clear cell tumor of the lung: An immunohistochemical and ultrastructural study supporting a pericytic differentiation. Modern Pathol 1997;10:1001–8.

116. Hashimoto T, Oka K, Hakozaki H, et al. Benign clear cell tumor of the lung. Ultrastruct Pathol 2001;25:479–83.

117. Kung M, Landa JF, Lubin J. Benign clear cell tumor (sugar tumor) of the trachea. Cancer 1984;54:517–19.

118. Zamboni G, Pea M, Martignoni G, et al. Clear cell "sugar" tumor of the pancreas: a novel member of the family of lesions characterized by the presence of perivascular epithelioid cells. Am J Surg Pathol 1996;20:722–30.

119. Folpe AL, Goodman ZD, Ishak KG, et al. Clear cell myomelanocytic tumor of the falciform ligament/ligamentum teres: a

novel member of the perivascular epithelioid clear cell family of tumors with a predilection for children and young adults. Am J Surg Pathol 2000;24:1239–46.

120. Tanaka Y, Ijiri R, Kato K, et al. HMB-45/melan-A and smooth muscle actin-positive clear-cell epithelioid tumor arising in the ligamentum teres hepatis: additional example of clear cell 'sugar' tumors. Am J Surg Pathol 2000;24:1295–9.

121. Tazelaar HD, Batts KP, Srigley JR. Primary extrapulmonary sugar tumor (PEST): A report of four cases. Modern Pathol 2001;14:615–22.

122. Govender D, Sabaratnam RM, Essa AS. Clear cell 'sugar' tumor of the breast – Another extrapulmonary site and review of the literature. Amer J Surg Pathol 2002;26:670–5.

123. Dimmler A, Seitz G, Hohenberger W, et al. Late pulmonary metastasis in uterine PEComa. J Clin Pathol 2003;56:627–8.

124. Bonetti F, Martignoni G, Colato C, et al. Abdominopelvic sarcoma of perivascular epithelioid cells. Report of four cases in young women, one with tuberous sclerosis. Modern Pathol 2001;14:563–8.

125. Sale GE, Kulander BG. Benign clear cell tumor of lung with necrosis. Cancer 1976;37:2355–8.

126. Ozdemir A, Zaman NU, Rullis I, et al. Benign clear cell tumor of the lung. J Thorac Cardiovasc Surg 1974;68:131–3.

127. Dahms BB. Benign clear cell tumor of lung with necrosis. Cancer 1976;37:2355–8.

128. Pea M, Bonetti F, Zamboni G, et al. Clear cell tumour and angiomyolipoma. Am J Surg Pathol 1991;15:199–202.

129. Kaiserling E, Krober S, Xiao JC, et al. Angiomyolipoma of the kidney. immunoreactivity with HMB-45. light- and electron-microscopic findings. Histopathology 1994;25:41–8.

130. Adachi Y, Horie Y, Kitamura Y, et al. CD1a expression in PEComas. Pathology International 2008;58:169–73.

131. Leong AS-Y, Meredith DJ. Clear cell tumors of the lung. In: Corrin B, editor. Pathology of Lung Tumors. London: Churchill Livingstone; 1997. p. 159–74.

Chondroid 'hamartoma'

132. Bateson EM. So-called hamartoma of the lung – a true neoplasm of fibrous connective tissue of the bronchi. Cancer 1973;31:1458–67.

133. Tomashefski JF. Benign endobronchial mesenchymal tumors. Their relationship to parenchymal pulmonary hamartomas. Am J Surg Pathol 1982;6:531–40.

134. van den Bosch JMM, Wagenaar SjSc, Corrin B, et al. Mesenchymoma of the lung (so called hamartoma): a review of 154 parenchymal and endobronchial cases. Thorax 1987;42:790–3.

135. Takemura T, Kusafuka K, Fujiwara M, et al. An immunohistochemical study of the mesenchymal and epithelial components of pulmonary chondromatous hamartomas. Pathol Int 1999;49:938–46.

136. Xiao S, Lux ML, Reeves R, et al. HMGI(Y) activation by chromosome 6p21 rearrangements in multilineage mesenchymal cells from pulmonary hamartoma. Am J Pathol 1997;150:901–10.

137. Kazmierczak B, Meyer-Bolte K, Tran KH, et al. A high frequency of tumors with rearrangements of genes of the HMGI(Y) family in a series of 191 pulmonary chondroid hamartomas. Genes Chromosomes Cancer 1999;26:125–33.

138. Tallini G, Vanni R, Manfioletti G, et al. HMGI-C and HMGI(Y) immunoreactivity correlates with cytogenetic abnormalities in lipomas, pulmonary chondroid hamartomas, endometrial polyps, and uterine leiomyomas and is compatible with rearrangement of the HMGI-C and HMGI(Y) genes. Lab Invest 2000;80:359–69.

139. Kayser K, Dunnwald D, Kazmierczak B, et al. Chromosomal aberrations, profiles of expression of growth-related markers including galectins and environmental hazards in relation to the incidence of chondroid pulmonary hamartomas. Pathol Res Pract 2003;199:589–98.

140. Suster S, Moran CA. Pulmonary adenofibroma – report of two cases of an unusual type of hamartomatous lesion of the lung. Histopathology 1993;23:547–51.

141. Scarff RW, Gowar FJS. Fibroadenoma of the lung. J Pathol Bacteriol 1944;56:257–9.

142. Wolff M, Kaye G, Silva F. Pulmonary metastases (with admixed epithelial elements) from smooth muscle neoplasms. Report of nine cases, including three males. Am J Surg Pathol 1979;3:325–42.

143. Alvarez-Fernandez E. Alveolar trapping in pulmonary carcinomas. Diag Histopathol 1982;5:59–64.

143a. Toomes H, Delphendahl A, Manke H-G, Vogt-Moykopf I. The coin lesion of the lung. A review of 955 resected coin lesions. Cancer 1983;51:534–7.

144. McDonald JR, Harrington SW, Clagett OT. Hamartoma (often called chondroma) of the lung. J Thorac Surg 1945;14:128–43.

145. Jensen KG, Schiodt T. Growth conditions of hamartoma of the lung: a study based on 22 cases operated on after radiographic observation for from one to 18 years. Thorax 1958;13:233–7.

146. Sharkey RA, Mulloy EMT, O'Neil S. Endobronchial hamartoma presenting as massive haemoptysis. Eur Respir J 1996;9:2179–80.

147. Cosio BG, Villena V, EchaveSustaeta J, et al. Endobronchial hamartoma. Chest 2002;122:202–5.

148. King TE, Christopher KL, Schwarz MI. Multiple pulmonary chondromatous hamartomas. Hum Pathol 1982;13:496–7.

149. Laroche CM, Stewart S, Wells F, et al. Multiple recurrent intrapulmonary and endobronchial mesenchymomas (hamartomas). Thorax 1993;48:572–3.

150. Suzuki N, Ohno S, Ishii Y, et al. Peripheral intrapulmonary hamartoma accompanied by a similar endotracheal lesion. Chest 1994;106:1291–3.

151. Dominguez H, Hariri J, Pless S. Multiple pulmonary chondrohamartomas in trachea, bronchi and lung parenchyma. Review of the literature. Respir Med 1996;90:111–14.

152. Kiryu T, Kawaguchi S, Matsui E, et al. Multiple chondromatous hamartomas of the lung – A case report and review of the literature with special reference to Carney syndrome. Cancer 1999;85:2557–61.

153. Karasik A, Modan M, Jacob CO, et al. Increased risk of lung cancer in patients with chondromatous hamartoma. J Thorac Cardiovasc Surg 1980;80:217–20.

154. Basile A, Gregoris A, Antoci B, et al. Malignant change in a benign pulmonary hamartoma. Thorax 1989;44:232–3.

155. Gabrail NY, Zara BY. Pulmonary hamartoma syndrome. Chest 1990;97:962–5.

156. Xu R, Murray M, Jagirdar J, et al. Placental transmogrification of the lung is a histologic pattern frequently associated with pulmonary fibrochondromatous hamartoma. Arch Pathol Lab Med 2002;126:562–6.

157. Cavazza A, Paci M, Rossi G. Pulmonary hamartoma with typical carcinoid/tumourlet. Virchows Arch 2006;449:392–3.

158. Bateson EM. Cartilage-containing tumours of the lung. Relationship between the purely cartilaginous type (chondroma) and the mixed type (so-called hamartoma): an unusual case of multiple tumours. Thorax 1967;22:256–9.

159. Bateson EM. Histogenesis of intrapulmonary and endobronchial hamartomas and chondromas (cartilage-containing tumours): a hypothesis. J Pathol 1970;101:77–83.

Lipoma, chondroma, fibroma, histiocytoma, leiomyoma, fibroleiomyoma, angiomyolipoma, myelolipoma and miscellaneous sarcomas

160. Moran CA, Suster S, Koss MN. Endobronchial lipomas – a clinicopathologic study of four cases. Mod Pathol 1994;7:212–4.

161. Huisman C, vanKralingen KW, Postmus PE, et al. Endobronchial lipoma: A series of three cases and the role of electrocautery. Respiration 2000;67:689–92.

162. Muraoka M, Oka T, Akamine S, et al. Endobronchial lipoma – Review of 64

cases reported Japan. Chest 2003;123:293–6.

163. Kim NR, Kim HJ, Kim JK, et al. Intrapulmonary lipomas: report of four cases. Histopathology 2003;42:305–6.

164. Carney JA, Sheps SG, Go VLW, et al. The triad of gastric leiomyosarcoma, functioning extra-adrenal paraganglioma and pulmonary chondroma. N Engl J Med 1977;296:1517–18.

165. Carney JA. The triad of gastric epithelioid leiomyosarcoma, functioning extra-adrenal paraganglioma, and pulmonary chondroma. Cancer 1979;43:374–82.

166. Engelman RM. Pulmonary fibroma: a rare benign tumor. Am Rev Respir Dis 1967;96:1242–5.

167. Shilo K, Miettinen M, Travis WD, et al. Pulmonary microcystic fibromyxoma: Report of 3 cases. Am J Surg Pathol 2006;30:1432–5.

168. Markert E, Gruber-Moesenbacher U, Porubsky C, et al. Lung osteoma – a new benign lung lesion. Virchows Archiv 2006;449:117–20.

169. Margulies KB, Sheps SG. Carney's triad: guidelines for management. Mayo Clin Proc 1988;63:496–502.

170. Raafat F, Salman WD, Roberts K, et al. Carney's triad: gastric leiomyosarcoma, pulmonary chondroma and extra-adrenal paraganglioma in young females. Histopathology 1986;10:1325–33.

171. Carney JA. The triad of gastric epithelioid leiomyosarcoma, pulmonary chondroma, and functioning extra-adrenal paraganglioma: a five-year review. Medicine (Baltimore) 1983;62:159–69.

172. Rodriguez FJ, Aubry MC, Tazelaar HD, et al. Pulmonary chondroma: a tumor associated with Carney triad and different from pulmonary hamartoma. Am J Surg Pathol 2007;31:1844–53.

173. Carney JA. Gastric stromal sarcoma, pulmonary chondroma, and extra-adrenal paraganglioma (Carney Triad): natural history, adrenocortical component, and possible familial occurrence. Mayo Clin Proc 1999;74:543–52.

174. Ngadiman S, Horenstein MG, Campbell WG. The concurrence of duodenal epithelioid stromal sarcoma, pulmonary chondromatous hamartoma, and nonfunctioning pancreatic islet cell tumor – a possible analogue of Carney's triad? Arch Pathol Lab Med 1994;118:840–3.

175. Osborn M, Mandys V, Beddow E, et al. Cystic fibrohistiocytic tumours presenting in the lung: primary or metastatic disease? Histo Pathology 2003;43:556–62.

176. Williams RB, Daniel RA. Leiomyoma of the lung. J Thorac Surg 1950;19:806–10.

177. Vera-Roman JM, Sobonya RE, Gomez-Garcia JL, et al. Leiomyoma of the lung. Cancer 1983;52:936–41.

178. Peters P, Trotter SE, Sheppard MN, et al. Primary leiomyoma of the pulmonary vein. Thorax 1992;47:393–4.

179. Naresh KN, Pai SA, Vyas JJ, et al. Leiomyoma of the bronchus – a case report. Histopathology 1993;22:288–9.

180. Ozcelik U, Kotiloglu E, Gocmen A, et al. Endobronchial leiomyoma: a case report. Thorax 1995;50:101–2.

181. Olgun N, Ozaksoy D, Ucan ES, et al. Paediatric endobronchial leiomyoma mimicking asthma. Respir Med 1995;89:581–2.

182. Cruickshank DB, Harrison GK. Diffuse fibro-leiomyomatous hamartomatosis of the lung. Thorax 1953;8:316–18.

183. Guinee DG, Thornberry DS, Azumi N, et al. Unique pulmonary presentation of an angiomyolipoma: analysis of clinical, radiographic, and histopathologic features. Am J Surg Pathol 1995;19:476–80.

184. Ito M, Sugamura Y, Ikari H, et al. Angiomyolipoma of the lung. Arch Pathol Lab Med 1998;122:1023–5.

185. Garcia TR, deJuan MJM. Angiomyolipoma of the liver and lung: A case explained by the presence of perivascular epithelioid cells. Pathol Res Pract 2002;198:363–7.

186. Wu K, Tazelaar HD. Pulmonary angiomyolipoma and multifocal micronodular pneumocyte hyperplasia associated with tuberous sclerosis. Hum Pathol 1999;30:1266–8.

187. Stone CH, Lee MW,, Amin MB, et al. Renal angiomyolipoma – further immunophenotypic characterization of an expanding morphologic spectrum. Arch Pathol Lab Med 2001;125:751–8.

188. Hornick JL, Fletcher CD. PEComa: what do we know so far? Histopathology 2006;48:75–82.

189. Paradis V, Laurendeau I, Vieillefond A, et al. Clonal analysis of renal sporadic angiomyolipomas. Hum Pathol 1998;29:1063–7.

190. Kenerson H, Folpe AL, Takayama TK, et al. Activation of the mTOR pathway in sporadic angiomyolipomas and other perivascular epithelioid cell neoplasms. Human Pathology 2007;38:1361–71.

191. Sato K, Ueda Y, Katsuda S, et al. Myelolipoma of the lung: a case report and brief review. J Clin Pathol 2007;60:728–30.

192. Cameron EWJ. Primary sarcoma of the lung. Thorax 1975;30:516–20.

193. Miller DL, Allen MS. Rare pulmonary neoplasms. Mayo Clin Proc 1993;68:492–8.

194. Litzky LA. Pulmonary sarcomatous tumors. Arch Pathol Lab Med 2008;132:1104–17.

195. Pettinato G, Manivel JC, Saldana MJ, et al. Primary bronchopulmonary fibrosarcoma of childhood and adolescence: reassessment of a low-grade malignancy. Clinicopathologic study of five cases and review of the literature. Hum Pathol 1989;20:463–71.

196. McClain KL, Leach CT, Jenson HB, et al. Association of Epstein–Barr virus with leiomyosarcomas in young people with AIDS. N Engl J Med 1995;332:12–18.

197. Bernheim J, Griffel B, Versano S, et al. Mediastinal leiomyosarcoma in the wall of a bronchial cyst. Arch Pathol Lab Med 1980;104:221.

198. Wang N-S, Seemayer TA, Ahmed MN, et al. Pulmonary leiomyosarcoma associated with an arteriovenous fistula. Arch Pathol 1974;98:100–5.

199. Chowdhury LN, Swerdlow MA, Jao W, et al. Postirradiation malignant fibrous histiocytoma of the lung. Am J Clin Pathol 1980;74:820–6.

200. Bluhm JM, Yi ES, Diaz G, et al. Multicentric endobronchial smooth muscle tumors associated with the Epstein–Barr virus in an adult patient with the acquired immunodeficiency syndrome: A case report. Cancer 1997;80:1910–3.

201. Somers CR, Tesoriero AA, Hartland E, et al. Multiple leiomyosarcomas of both donor and recipient origin arising in a heart–lung transplant patient. Am J Surg Pathol 1998;22:1423–8.

202. Yousem SA, Hochholzer L. Malignant fibrous histiocytoma of the lung. Cancer 1987;60:2532–41.

203. Moran CA, Suster S, Abbondanzo SL, et al. Primary leiomyosarcomas of the lung: a clinicopathologic and immunohistochemical study of 18 cases. Mod Pathol 1997;10:121–8.

204. Shimizu J, Sasaki M, Nakamura Y, et al. Simultaneous lung and liver resection for primary pulmonary leiomyosarcoma. Respiration 1997;64:179–81.

205. Keel SB, Bacha E, Mark EJ, et al. Primary pulmonary sarcoma: A clinicopathologic study of 26 cases. Modern Pathol 1999;12:1124–31.

206. Kimizuka G, Okuzawa K, Yarita T. Primary giant cell malignant fibrous histiocytoma of the lung: A case report. Pathol Int 1999;49:342–6.

207. Zeren H, Moran CA, Suster S, et al. Primary pulmonary sarcomas with features of monophasic synovial sarcoma: a clinicopathological, immunohistochemical, and ultrastructural study of 25 cases. Hum Pathol 1995;26:474–80.

208. Kaplan MA, Goodman MD, Satish J, et al. Primary pulmonary sarcoma with morphologic features of monophasic synovial sarcoma and chromosome translocation t(x;18). Am J Clin Pathol 1996;105:195–9.

209. Hisaoka M, Hashimoto H, Iwamasa T, et al. Primary synovial sarcoma of the lung: report of two cases confirmed by molecular detection of SYT-SSX fusion gene transcripts. Histopathology 1999;34:205–10.

210. Mikami Y, Nakajima M, Hashimoto H, et al. Primary poorly differentiated monophasic synovial sarcoma of the lung. A case report with immunohistochemical

and genetic studies. Pathol Res Pract 2003;199:827–33.

211. Okamoto S, Hisaoka M, Daa T, et al. Primary pulmonary synovial sarcoma: a clinicopathologic, immunohistochemical, and molecular study of 11 cases. Hum Pathol 2004;35:850–6

212. Niwa H, Masuda S, Kobayashi C, et al. Pulmonary synovial sarcoma with polypoid endobronchial growth: A case report, immunohistochemical and cytogenetic study. Pathology International 2004;54:611–15.

213. Begueret H, Galateau-Salle F, Guillou L, et al. Primary intrathoracic synovial sarcoma: a clinicopathologic study of 40 t(X;18)-positive cases from the French Sarcoma Group and the Mesopath Group. Am J Surg Pathol 2005;29:339–46.

214. Hartel PH, Fanburg-Smith JC, Frazier AA, et al. Primary pulmonary and mediastinal synovial sarcoma: a clinicopathologic study of 60 cases and comparison with five prior series. Mod Pathol 2007;20:760–9.

215. Abrahamson JR, Friedman NB. Intrapulmonary stromal mesothelioma. J Thorac Cardiovasc Surg 1966;51:300–6.

216. Alvarez-Fernandez E, Escalona-Zapata J. Intrapulmonary mesotheliomas: their identification by tissue culture. Virchows Arch A Pathol Anat Histopathol 1982;395:331–43.

217. Yousem SA, Flynn SD. Intrapulmonary localized fibrous tumor. Intraparenchymal so-called localized fibrous mesothelioma. Am J Clin Pathol 1988;89:365–9.

218. Bartley TD, Arean VM. Intrapulmonary neurogenic tumours. J Thorac Cardiovasc Surg 1965;50:114–23.

219. Oosterwijk WM, Swierenga J. Neurogenic tumours with an intrathoracic localization. Thorax 1968;23:374–84.

220. Krygier G, Amado A, Salisbury S, et al. Primary lung liposarcoma. Lung Cancer 1997;17:271–5.

221. Comin CE, Santucci M, Novelli L, et al. Primary pulmonary rhabdomyosarcoma: Report of a case in an adult and review of the literature. Ultrastruct Pathol 2001;25:269–73.

222. Gupta A, Sharma MC, Kochupillai V, et al. Primary pulmonary rhabdomyosarcoma in adults: case report and review of literature. Clin Lung Cancer 2007;8:389–91.

223. Steurer S, Huber M, Lintner F. Dedifferentiated chondrosarcoma of the lung: case report and review of the literature. Clin Lung Cancer 2007;8:439–42.

224. Chapman AD, Pritchard SC, Yap WW, et al. Primary pulmonary osteosarcoma: case report and molecular analysis. Cancer 2001;91:779–84.

225. Shenjere P, Travis WD, Franks TJ, et al. Primary pulmonary osteosarcoma: a report of four cases and a review of the literature. Int J Surg Pathol 2009 (in press).

226. Kuroda M, Oka T, Horiuchi H, et al. Giant cell tumor of the lung – an autopsy case

report with immunohistochemical observations. Pathol Int 1994;44:158–63.

227. Tsutsumi Y, Deng YL. Alveolar soft part sarcoma of the pulmonary vein. Acta Pathol Jpn 1991;41:771–7.

228. Tralka GA, Katz S. Hemangioendothelioma of the lung. Am Rev Respir Dis 1963;87:107–15.

229. Yousem SA. Angiosarcoma presenting in the lung. Arch Pathol Lab Med 1986;110:112–15.

230. Koizumi N, Fukuda T, Ohnishi Y, et al. Pulmonary myxoid leiomyosarcoma. Pathol Int 1995;45:879–84.

231. Inayama Y, Hayashi H, Ogawa N, et al. Low-grade pulmonary myxoid sarcoma of uncertain histogenesis. Pathol Int 2001;51:204–10.

232. Kalus M, Rahman F, Jenkins DE, et al. Malignant mesenchymoma of the lung. Arch Pathol 1973;95:199–202.

233. Guccion JG, Rosen SH. Bronchopulmonary leiomyosarcoma and fibrosarcoma. A study of 32 cases and review of the literature. Cancer 1972;30:836–47.

234. Hayashi T, Tsuda N, Iseki M, et al. Primary chondrosarcoma of the lung – a clinicopathologic study. Cancer 1993;72:69–74.

235. Attanoos RL, Appleton MAC, Gibbs AR. Primary sarcomas of the lung: a clinicopathological and immunohistochemical study of 14 cases. Histopathology 1996;29:29–36.

Vascular tumours and proliferations

236. Harding JR, Williams J, Seal RME. Pedunculated capillary haemangioma of the bronchus. Br J Dis Chest 1978;72:336–42.

237. Paul KP, Borner C, Muller KM, et al. Capillary hemangioma of the right main bronchus treated by sleeve resection in infancy. Am Rev Respir Dis 1991;143:876–9.

238. Bowyer JJ, Sheppard M. Capillary haemangioma presenting as a lung pseudocyst. Arch Dis Child 1990;65:1162–4.

239. Hamada K, Ishii Y, Nakaya M, et al. Solitary lymphangioma of the lung. Histopathology 1995;27:482–3.

240. Wada A, Tateishi R, Terazawa T, et al. Lymphangioma of the lung. Arch Pathol Lab Med 1974;98:211–13.

241. Al-Hilli F. Lymphangioma (or alveolar adenoma?) of the lung. Histopathology 1987;11:979–80.

242. Holden WE, Morris JF, Antonovic R, et al. Adult intrapulmonary and mediastinal lymphangioma causing haemoptysis. Thorax 1987;42:635–6.

243. Faul JL, Berry GJ, Colby TV, et al. Thoracic lymphangiomas, lymphangiectasis, lymphangiomatosis, and lymphatic dysplasia syndrome. Amer J Respir Crit Care Med 2000;161:1037–46.

244. Wilson C, Askin FB, Heitmiller RF. Solitary pulmonary lymphangioma. Ann Thorac Surg 2001;71:1337–8.

245. Nagayasu T, Hayashi T, Ashizawa K, et al. A case of solitary pulmonary lymphangioma. J Clin Pathol 2003;56:396–8.

246. Irani S, Brack T, Pfaltz M, et al. Tracheal lobular capillary hemangioma – A rare cause of recurrent hemoptysis. Chest 2003;123:2148–9.

247. Kobayashi A, Ohno S, Bando M, et al. Cavernous hemangiomas of lungs and liver in an asymptomatic girl. Respiration 2003;70:647–50.

248. Fugo K, Matsuno Y, Okamoto K, et al. Solitary capillary hemangioma of the lung: report of 2 resected cases detected by high-resolution CT. Am J Surg Pathol 2006;30:750–3.

249. Rose AS, Mathur PN. Endobronchial capillary hemangioma: case report and review of the literature. Respiration 2008;76:221–4.

249a. Ehara R, Koga T, Higaki K, et al. Complex cystic lung lesion presenting in a 41-year-old woman. Chest 2010;138:208–12.

250. Copeland J, Muller KM, Muller AM. Pulmonary haemangiolymphangioma – a new entity of pulmonary vascular tumours? Histopathology 2008;52:527–9.

251. Holden KR, Alexander F. Diffuse neonatal hemangiomatosis. Pediatrics 1970;46:411–21.

252. Rowen M, Thompson JR, Williamson RA, et al. Diffuse pulmonary hemangiomatosis. Radiology 1978;127:445–51.

253. Fine SW, Whitney KD. Multiple cavernous hemangiomas of the lung: a case report and review of the literature. Arch Pathol Lab Med 2004;128:1439–41.

254. Quijano G, Drut R. Multiple congenital infantile hemangiomas of the lung in partial trisomy D. J Clin Pathol 2007;60:943–5.

255. Gilbey LK, Girod CE. Blue rubber bleb nevus syndrome – Endobronchial involvement presenting as chronic cough. Chest 2003;124:760–3.

256. Swank DW, Hepper NGG, Folkert KE, et al. Intrathoracic lymphangiomatosis mimicking lymphangioleiomyomatosis in a young woman. Mayo Clin Proc 1989;64:1264–8.

257. Ramani P, Shah A. Lymphangiomatosis – histologic and immunohistochemical analysis of four cases. Am J Surg Pathol 1993;17:329–35.

258. Tazelaar HD, Kerr D, Yousem SA, et al. Diffuse pulmonary lymphangiomatosis. Hum Pathol 1993;24:1313–22.

259. Takahashi K, Takahashi H, Maeda K, et al. An adult case of lymphangiomatosis of the mediastinum, pulmonary interstitium and retroperitoneum complicated by chronic disseminated intravascular coagulation. Eur Respir J 1995;8:1799–802.

260. Joshi M, Cole S, Knibbs D, et al. Pulmonary abnormalities in Klippel–

Trenaunay syndrome – a histologic, ultrastructural, and immunocytochemical study. Chest 1992;102:1274–7.

261. Carlson KC, Parnassus WN, Klatt CC. Thoracic lymphangiomatosis. Arch Pathol Lab Med 1987;111:475–7.

262. Rydell R, Hoffbauer FW. Multiple pulmonary arteriovenous fistulas in juvenile cirrhosis. Am J Med 1956;21:450–60.

263. Berthelot P, Walker JG, Sherlock S, et al. Arterial changes in the lungs in cirrhosis of the liver – lung spider nevi. N Engl J Med 1966;274:291–8.

264. Stanley NN, Williams AJ, Dewar CA, et al. Hypoxia and hydrothoraces in a case of liver cirrhosis: correlation of physiological, radiographic, scintigraphic, and pathological findings. Thorax 1977;32:457–71.

265. Macnee W, Buist TAS, Finlayson NDC, et al. Multiple microscopic pulmonary arteriovenous connections in the lungs presenting as cyanosis. Thorax 1985;40:316–18.

266. Ichijima K, Kobashi Y, Yamabe H, et al. Peliosis hepatis: an unusual case involving multiple organs. Acta Pathol Jpn 1980;30:109–20.

267. Lie JT. Pulmonary peliosis. Arch Pathol Lab Med 1985;109:878–9.

268. Davis Z, Berliner WP, Weiland LH, et al. Primary pulmonary hemangiopericytoma. J Thorac Cardiovasc Surg 1972;64:882–25.

269. Meade JB, Whitwell F, Bickford BJ, et al. Primary haemangiopericytoma of lung. Thorax 1974;29:1–15.

270. Razzuk MA, Nassur A, Gardner MA, et al. Primary pulmonary hemangiopericytoma. J Thorac Cardiovasc Surg 1977;74:227–9.

271. Shin MS, Ho K-J. Primary hemangiopericytoma of the lung: radiography and pathology. Am J Roentgenol 1979;133:1077–83.

272. Yousem SA, Hochholzer L. Primary pulmonary hemangiopericytoma. Cancer 1987;59:549–55.

273. Rusch VW, Shuman WP, Schmidt R, et al. Massive pulmonary hemangiopericytoma. An innovative approach to evaluation and treatment. Cancer 1989;64:1928–36.

274. Rothe TB, Karrer W, Gebbers JO. Recurrent haemoptysis in a young woman – a case of a malignant haemangiopericytoma of the lung. Thorax 1994;49:188–9.

275. Fabich DR, Hafez G-R. Glomangioma of the trachea. Cancer 1980;45:2337–41.

276. Heard BE, Dewar A, Firmin RK, et al. One very rare and one new tracheal tumour found by electron microscopy: glomus tumour and acinic cell tumour resembling carcinoid tumours by light microscopy. Thorax 1982;37:97–103.

277. Sheffield EA, Dewar A, Corrin B, et al. Glomus tumour of the trachea. Histopathology 1988;13:234–6.

278. Shin DH, Park SS, Lee JH, et al. Oncocytic glomus tumor of the trachea. Chest 1990;98:1021–3.

279. Garcia-Prats MD, Sotelo-Rodriguez MT, Ballestin C, et al. Glomus tumour of the trachea – report of a case with microscopic, ultrastructural and immunohistochemical examination and review of the literature. Histopathology 1991;19:459–64.

280. Arapantoni-Dadioti P, Panayiotides J, Fatsis M, et al. Tracheal glomus tumour. Respiration 1995;62:160–2.

281. Menaissy YM, Gal AA, Mansour KA. Glomus tumor of the trachea. Ann Thorac Surg 2000;70:295–7.

282. Katabami M, Okamoto K, Ito K, et al. Bronchogenic glomangiomyoma with local intravenous infiltration. Eur Respir J 2006;28:1060–4.

283. Tang C, Toker CK, Foris NP, et al. Glomangioma of the lung. Am J Surg Pathol 1978;2:103–9.

284. Brooks JJ, Miettinen M, Virtanen I. Desmin immunoreactivity in glomus tumors. Am J Clin Pathol 1987;87:292–4.

285. Koss MN, Hochholzer L, Moran CA. Primary pulmonary glomus tumor: a clinicopathologic and immunohistochemical study of two cases. Modern Pathol 1998;11:253–8.

286. Gaertner EM, Steinberg DM, Huber M, et al. Pulmonary and mediastinal glomus tumors – report of five cases including a pulmonary glomangiosarcoma: a clinicopathologic study with literature review. Amer J Surg Pathol 2000;24:1105–14.

287. Oizumi S, Kon Y, Ishida T, et al. A rare case of bronchial glomus tumor. Respiration 2001;68:95–8.

288. Yilmaz A, Bayramgurler B, Aksoy F, et al. Pulmonary glomus tumour: a case initially diagnosed as carcinoid tumour. Respirology 2002;7: 369–71.

289. Hishida T, Hasegawa T, Asamura H, et al. Malignant glomus tumor of the lung. Pathol Int 2003;53:632–6.

290. Rossle M, Bayerle W, Lohrs U. Glomangioma of the lungs: a rare differential diagnosis of a pulmonary tumour. J Clin Pathol 2006;59:1000.

291. Granter SR, Badizadegan K, Fletcher CDM. Myofibromatosis in adults, glomangiopericytoma, and myopericytoma: a spectrum of tumors showing perivascular myoid differentiation. Am J Surg Pathol 1998;22:513–25.

292. Gottlieb GJ, Ackerman AB. Kaposi's sarcoma: an extensively disseminated form in young homosexual men. Hum Pathol 1982;13:882–42.

293. Gunawardena KA, Al-Hasani MK, Haleem A, et al. Pulmonary Kaposi's sarcoma in two recipients of renal transplants. Thorax 1988;43:653–6.

294. Khan GA, Klapper P. Pulmonary haemorrhage following renal transplantation. Thorax 1995;50:98–9.

295. Yousem SA. Lung tumors in the immunocompromised host. In: Corrin B, editor. Pathology of Lung Tumors. London: Churchill Livingstone; 1997. p. 189–212.

296. Aboulafia DM. The epidemiologic, pathologic, and clinical features of AIDS-associated pulmonary Kaposi's sarcoma. Chest 2000;117:1128–45.

297. Miller RF, Tomlinson MC, Cottrill CP, et al. Bronchopulmonary Kaposi's sarcoma in patients with AIDS. Thorax 1992;47:721–5.

298. Mitchell DM, McCarty M, Fleming J, et al. Bronchopulmonary Kaposi's sarcoma in patients with AIDS. Thorax 1992;47:726–9.

299. Reichert CM, O'Leary TJ, Levens DL, et al. Autopsy pathology in the acquired immune deficiency syndrome. Am J Pathol 1983;112:357–82.

300. Guarda LA, Luna MA, Smith JL, et al. Acquired immune deficiency syndrome and postmortem findings. Am J Clin Pathol 1984;81:549–57.

301. Moskowitz LB, Hensley GT, Gould EW, et al. Frequency and anatomic distribution of lymphadenopathic Kaposi's sarcoma in the acquired immunodeficiency syndrome. Hum Pathol 1985;16:447–56.

302. Farber HW, Mark EJ, Moore EH, et al. A 29-year-old man with a positive test for HIV and a reticulonodular pulmonary infiltrate – pulmonary Kaposi's sarcoma – acquired immunodeficiency syndrome (AIDS). N Engl J Med 1990;322: 43–51.

303. Beral V, Peterman TA, Berkelman R, et al. Kaposi's sarcoma among persons with AIDS: a sexually transmitted infection? Lancet 1990;335:123–8.

304. Nash G, Said JW, Nash SV, et al. The pathology of AIDS – Kaposi's sarcoma. Mod Pathol 1995;8:208–9.

305. Cadranel J, Mayaud C. Intrathoracic Kaposi's sarcoma in patients with AIDS. Thorax 1995;50:407–14.

306. Siegal B, Levinton-Kriss S, Schiffer A, et al. Kaposi's sarcoma in immunosuppression. Possibly the result of a dual viral infection. Cancer 1990;65:492–8.

307. Chang Y, Cesarman E, Pessin MS, et al. Identification of herpesvirus-like DNA sequences in AIDS-associated Kaposi's sarcoma. Science 1994;266:1865–9.

308. Moore PS, Chang YA. Detection of herpesvirus-like DNA sequences in Kaposi's sarcoma in patients with and those without HIV infection. N Engl J Med 1995;332:1181–5.

309. Cesarman E, Chang YA, Moore PS, et al. Kaposi's sarcoma-associated herpesvirus-like DNA sequences in AIDS-related body-cavity-based lymphomas. N Engl J Med 1995;332:1186–91.

310. Roizman B. New viral footprints in Kaposi's sarcoma. N Engl J Med 1995;332:1227–8.

311. Jin YT, Tsai ST, Yan JJ, et al. Detection of Kaposi's sarcoma-associated herpesvirus-like DNA sequence in vascular lesions: a reliable diagnostic marker for Kaposi's sarcoma. Am J Clin Pathol 1996;105:360–3.

312. Li JJ, Huang YQ, Cockerell CJ, et al. Localization of human herpes-like virus type 8 in vascular endothelial cells and perivascular spindle-shaped cells of Kaposi's sarcoma lesions by in situ hybridization. Am J Pathol 1996;148:1741–8.

313. Dictor M, Rambech E, Way D, et al. Human herpesvirus 8 (Kaposi's sarcoma-associated herpesvirus) DNA in Kaposi's sarcoma lesions, AIDS Kaposi's sarcoma cell lines, endothelial Kaposi's sarcoma simulators, and the skin of immunosuppressed patients. Am J Pathol 1996;148:2009–16.

314. Kennedy MM, Cooper K, Howells DD, et al. Identification of HHV8 in early Kaposi's sarcoma: implications for Kaposi's sarcoma pathogenesis. J Clin Pathol Mol Pathol 1998;51:14–20.

315. Chadburn A, Cesarman E, Nador RG, et al. Kaposi's sarcoma-associated herpesvirus sequences in benign lymphoid proliferations not associated with human immunodeficiency virus. Cancer 1997;80:788–97.

316. Tamm M, Reichenberger F, McGandy CE, et al. Diagnosis of pulmonary Kaposi's sarcoma by detection of human herpes virus 8 in bronchoalveolar lavage. Amer J Respir Crit Care Med 1998;157:458–63.

317. Dilnur P, Katano H, Wang ZH, et al. Classic type of Kaposi's sarcoma and human herpesvirus 8 infection in Xinjiang, China. Pathol Int 2001;51:845–52.

318. Dantzig PI, Richardson D, Rayhanzadeh S, et al. Thoracic involvement of non-African Kaposi's sarcoma. Chest 1974;66:522–5.

319. Loring WE, Wolman SR. Idiopathic multiple hemorrhagic sarcoma of lung (Kaposi's sarcoma). N Y State J Med 1965;65:668–75.

320. Misra DP, Sunderrajan EV, Hurst DJ, et al. Kaposi's sarcoma of the lung: radiography and pathology. Thorax 1982;37:155–6.

321. Chin R, Jones DF, Pegram PS, et al. Complete endobronchial occlusion by Kaposi's sarcoma in the absence of cutaneous involvement. Chest 1994;105:1581–2.

322. Templeton AC. Studies in Kaposi's sarcoma: post mortem findings and disease patterns in women. Cancer 1972;30:854–67.

323. Pozniak AL, Latif AS, Neill P, et al. Pulmonary Kaposi's sarcoma in Africa. Thorax 1992;47:730–3.

324. Schnapp LM, Gruden JF, Hopewell PC, et al. Presentation of AIDS-related pulmonary Kaposi's sarcoma diagnosed by bronchoscopy. Am J Respir Crit Care Med 1996;153:1385–90.

325. Maduri GU, Stover DE, Lee M, et al. Pulmonary Kaposi's sarcoma in the acquired immune deficiency syndrome. Am J Med 1986;81:11–18.

326. Purdy LJ, Colby TV, Yousem SA, et al. Pulmonary Kaposi's sarcoma: premortem histologic diagnosis. Am J Surg Pathol 1986;10:301–11.

327. Hamm PG, Judson MA, Aranda CP. Diagnosis of pulmonary Kaposi's sarcoma with fiberoptic bronchoscopy and endobronchial biopsy: a report of five cases. Cancer 1987;59:807–10.

328. Russell Jones R, Paull JS, Spry C, et al. Histogenesis of Kaposi's sarcoma in patients with and without acquired immune deficiency syndrome (AIDS). J Clin Pathol 1986;39:742–9.

329. Marguart KH. Weibel–Palade bodies in Kaposi's sarcoma. J Clin Pathol 1987;40:933.

330. Kostianovsky M, Lamy Y, Greco MA. Immunohistochemical and electron microscopic profiles of cutaneous Kaposi's sarcoma and bacillary angiomatosis. Ultrastruct Pathol 1992;16:629–40.

331. Kahn HJ, Bailey D, Marks A. Monoclonal antibody D2-40, a new marker of lymphatic endothelium, reacts with Kaposi's sarcoma and a subset of angiosarcomas. Mod Pathol 2002;15:434–40.

332. Dail DH, Liebow AA. Intravascular bronchioloalveolar tumour. Am J Pathol 1975;78:6a–7a.

333. Dail DH, Liebow AA, Gmelich JT, et al. Intravascular, bronchiolar and alveolar tumour of the lung (IVBAT). Cancer 1983;51:452–64.

334. Farinacci CJ, Blauw MD, Jennings EM. Multifocal pulmonary lesions of possible decidual origin (so-called pulmonary deciduosis): report of a case. Am J Clin Pathol 1973;59:508–14.

335. Corrin B, Manners B, Millard M, et al. Histogenesis of the so-called 'intravascular bronchioloalveolar tumour'. J Pathol 1979;128:163–7.

336. Weldon-Linne CM, Victor TA, Christ ML, et al. Angiogenic nature of the 'intravascular tumor' of the lung: an electron microscopic study. Arch Pathol Lab Med 1981;105:174–9.

337. Weldon-Linne CM, Victor TA, Christ ML. Immunohistochemical identification of factor VIII-related antigen in the intravascular bronchioloalveolar tumor of the lung. Arch Pathol Lab Med 1981;105:628–9.

338. Corrin B, Harrison WJ, Wright DH. The so-called intravascular bronchioloalveolar tumour of the lung (low-grade sclerosing angiosarcoma): presentation with extrapulmonary deposits. Diag Histopathol 1983;6:229–37.

339. Azumi N, Churg A. Intravascular and sclerosing bronchioloalveolar tumour: a pulmonary sarcoma of probable vascular origin. Am J Surg Pathol 1981;5:587–96.

340. Bhagavan BS, Dorfman HD, Murthy MSN. Intravascular bronchioloalveolar tumor (IVBAT). Am J Surg Pathol 1982;6:41–52.

341. Rosai J, Gold J, Landy R. The histiocytoid hemangiomas. A unifying concept embracing several previously described entities of skin, soft tissues, large vessels, bone and heart. Hum Pathol 1979;10:707–30.

342. Weidner N. Intriguing case – atypical tumor of the mediastinum – epithelioid hemangioendothelioma containing metaplastic bone and osteoclastlike giant cells. Ultrastruct Pathol 1991;15:481–8.

343. Weiss SW, Enzinger FM. Epithelioid hemangioendothelioma. A vascular tumor often mistaken for carcinoma. Cancer 1982;50:970–81.

344. Gledhill A, Kay JM. Hepatic metastases in a case of intravascular bronchioloalveolar tumour. J Clin Pathol 1984;37:279–82.

345. Ishak KG, Sesterhenn IA, Goodman ZD, et al. Epithelioid hemangioendothelioma of the liver. Hum Pathol 1984;15:839–52.

346. Mendlick MR, Nelson M, Pickering D, et al. Translocation t(1;3)(P36.3;q25) is a nonrandom aberration in epithelioid hemangioendothelioma. Am J Surg Pathol 2001;25:684–7.

347. Kitaichi M, Nagai S, Nishimura K, et al. Pulmonary epithelioid haemangioendothelioma in 21 patients, including three with partial spontaneous regression. Eur Resp J 1998;12:89–96.

348. Bollinger BK, Laskin WB, Knight CB. Epithelioid hemangioendothelioma with multiple site involvement – literature review and observations. Cancer 1994;73:610–15.

349. Nagata N, Takatsu H, Sato Y, et al. Metastatic pulmonary epithelioid hemangioendothelioma with peculiar radiographic features. Respiration 1999;66:78–80.

350. Ledson MJ, Convery R, Carty A, et al. Epithelioid haemangioendothelioma. Thorax 1999;54:560–1.

351. Yousem SA, Hochholzer L. Unusual thoracic manifestations of epithelioid hemangioendothelioma. Arch Pathol Lab Med 1981;111:459–63.

352. Corrin B, Dewar A, Simpson CGB. Epithelioid hemangioendothelioma of the lung. Ultrastruct Pathol 1996;20:345–7.

353. Lin BTY, Colby T, Gown AM, et al. Malignant vascular tumors of the serous membranes mimicking mesothelioma: a report of 14 cases. Am J Surg Pathol 1996;20:1431–9.

354. Yi ES, Auger WR, Friedman PJ, et al. Intravascular bronchioloalveolar tumor of the lung presenting as pulmonary thromboembolic disease and pulmonary hypertension. Arch Pathol Lab Med 1995;119:255–60.

355. Kradin RL, Aquino S, Christiani DC, et al. Hemoptysis in a 20-year-old man with multiple pulmonary nodules. Epithelioid

450. Flynn SD, Yousem SA. Pulmonary meningiomas: a report of two cases. Hum Pathol 1991;22:469–74.

451. Drlicek M, Grisold W, Lorber J, et al. Pulmonary meningioma – immunohistochemical and ultrastructural features. Am J Surg Pathol 1991;15:455–9.

452. Robinson PG. Pulmonary meningioma – report of a case with electron microscopic and immunohistochemical findings. Am J Clin Pathol 1992;97:814–97.

453. Moran CA, Hochholzer L, Rush W, et al. Primary intrapulmonary meningiomas: a clinicopathologic and immunohistochemical study of ten cases. Cancer 1996;78:2328–33.

454. Lockett L, Chiang V, Scully N. Primary pulmonary meningioma: Report of a case and review of the literature. Am J Surg Pathol 1997;21:453–60.

455. Kaleem Z, Fitzpatrick MM, Ritter JH. Primary pulmonary meningioma: Report of a case and review of the literature. Arch Pathol Lab Med 1997;121:631–6.

456. Prayson RA, Farver CF. Primary pulmonary malignant meningioma. Amer J Surg Pathol 1999;23:722–6.

457. Falleni M, Roz E, Dessy E, et al. Primary intrathoracic meningioma: histopathological, immunohistochemical and ultrastructural study of two cases. Virchows Archiv 2001;439:196–200.

458. Rowsell C, Sirbovan J, Rosenblum MK, et al. Primary chordoid meningioma of lung. Virchows Arch 2005;446:333–7.

459. Ionescu DN, Sasatomi E, Aldeeb D, et al. Pulmonary meningothelial-like nodules – A genotypic comparison with meningiomas. Am J Surg Pathol 2004;28:207–14.

460. Cerda-Nicolas M, Lopez-Gines C, Perez-Bacete M, et al. Histologically benign metastatic meningioma: morphological and cytogenetic study. Case report. J Neurosurg 2003;98:194–8.

461. Crotty TB, Hooker RP, Swensen SJ, et al. Primary malignant ependymoma of the lung. Mayo Clin Proc 1992;67:373–8.

12.4 Lymphoproliferative disease

CHAPTER CONTENTS

Lymphoproliferative disease is a useful term as it covers lymphoid infiltrates of the lung of questionable status as well as those that are evidently reactive or neoplastic. Until recently those of questionable status included lymphoid interstitial pneumonia and so-called pseudolymphoma but the application of modern laboratory techniques has clarified the nature of both these conditions. However, the emergence of seemingly malignant posttransplantation and acquired immunodeficiency syndrome (AIDS)-related lymphoid lesions that regress when immunity is restored has again blurred the distinction between lymphoid hyperplasia and neoplasia.

In this chapter we follow the World Health Organization (WHO) classification of extranodal lymphomas, considering reactive lesions and lymphoproliferative disease complicating severe immune impair-
ment before the various lymphomas that affect the lungs.[1] Whereas the lungs are often involved in disseminated nodal lymphomas of all types, primary pulmonary lymphoma is relatively rare, accounting for less than 0.5% of all primary lung neoplasms. There are several varieties but marginal-zone non-Hodgkin lymphoma of mucosa-associated lymphoid tissue (MALT) origin makes up approximately 80% of the total and diffuse large B-cell non-Hodgkin lymphoma approximately 15%.[2–6] The other 5% comprises lymphomatoid granulomatosis, plasmacytoma, Hodgkin lymphoma, anaplastic large cell lymphoma, CD56-positive (natural killer cell) lymphoma,[7,8] the CD21- and CD35-positive follicular dendritic cell tumour,[9,10,11] solitary mast cell tumours of the lung,[12,13] Langerhans cell sarcoma[14] and exceptional cases that appear to be of follicle centre cell origin and are therefore directly comparable to nodal lymphomas.[15]

INTRAPULMONARY LYMPH NODES

The lymphoid elements of the lung consist of intrapulmonary lymph nodes and airway-associated lymphoid tissue, details of which are provided on p. 26. The two are best considered separately. Intrapulmonary lymph nodes have a normal follicular and sinusoidal architecture, and may undergo all those changes encountered in lymph nodes elsewhere. In the lungs they are also often heavily pigmented with carbon. Most are situated at the hilum but they may be found anywhere in the lung, occasionally as far out as the pleura (Fig. 12.4.1). In one necropsy study intrapulmonary lymph nodes were identified in 18% of patients.[16] They are generally asymptomatic and discovered incidentally on chest radiographs, following which they may be excised to exclude cancer, increasingly so since the advent of high-resolution computed tomography (HRCT).[17,18] Otherwise they are of no clinical significance.

LYMPHOID HYPERPLASIA

Hyperplasia of the airway-associated lymphoid tissue may be seen in a variety of diseases and is often no more than an epiphenomenon.

Figure 12.4.1 An intrapulmonary lymph node lies just beneath the pleura.

Thus, lung tumours and many focal pulmonary infections are often attended by a chronic inflammatory infiltrate comprising a mixture of lymphocytes, plasma cells and histiocytes, sometimes with lymphoid follicles. Such an infiltrate is also a general feature of viral, rickettsial and *Mycoplasma* pneumonia. Similarly, extrinsic allergic alveolitis is characterised by an interstitial lymphoid infiltrate that histologically may closely resemble lymphoid interstitial pneumonia. Chronic interstitial inflammation is particularly marked in obstructive pneumonia. It is also a component of all patterns of chronic idiopathic interstitial pneumonia, although the intensity of the infiltrate varies considerably, being light in desquamative interstitial pneumonia, moderate in cellular non-specific interstitial pneumonia and heavy in lymphoid interstitial pneumonia. Expansion of the bronchus-associated lymphoid tissue is particularly conspicuous in follicular bronchiectasis. However, all these conditions have their own specific features that facilitate their recognition.

Hyperplasia of the pulmonary lymphoid tissue also occurs in the absence of any accompanying morphological pointers to its aetiology, although the conditions with which it is associated often provide a clue to its causation. Three forms are recognised: follicular bronchiolitis, lymphoid interstitial pneumonia and nodular lymphoid hyperplasia.[19,20] The first of these is centriacinar, the second diffuse and the last forms a localised tumour-like nodule. Castleman's disease may also present as primary pulmonary disease, but more commonly involves the lung as part of a multiorgan disorder and is discussed below under secondary involvement.

Although follicular bronchiolitis and lymphoid interstitial pneumonia are traditionally regarded as distinct, they frequently coexist and have overlapping clinical and histological features. Both are encompassed by the term 'diffuse pulmonary lymphoid hyperplasia'.

Follicular bronchiolitis

Follicular bronchitis/bronchiolitis consists of a predominantly centriacinar lymphocytic infiltrate with abundant germinal centres. It represents an expansion of the normally sparse peribronchiolar lymphoid

tissue.[19,21,22] There may be extension of the process into the bronchiolar epithelium and into the walls of neighbouring alveoli but the air spaces are spared. In extreme cases the lymphoid follicles are evenly distributed throughout the lung, perhaps even involving the pleura, when the term 'diffuse lymphoid hyperplasia' has sometimes been applied,[23] but this process does not otherwise differ materially from follicular bronchiolitis.[19,24]

Clinical features

Patients commonly present in middle age. They complain of breathlessness and cough and suffer from recurrent episodes of fever or pneumonia.[21] There are several clinical association, which are listed in Box 12.4.1.[21,25-38] The sexes are affected equally, apart from the patients in whom follicular bronchiolitis is associated with connective tissue disorders, in which females predominate.[21,25,39] Chest X-ray findings are similar to those seen in lymphoid interstitial pneumonia, but HRCT typically shows bilateral centrilobular and peribronchial nodules rather than ground-glass opacification.[25,33,39,40]

Aetiology

Follicular bronchiolitis is associated with a range of conditions similar to that found with lymphoid interstitial pneumonia. Their aetiology is probably similar and is therefore dealt with together (see p. 655).

Pathological features

Follicular bronchiolitis is characterised by prominent peribronchial and peribronchiolar lymphoid follicles with only minor interstitial inflammatory component (Fig. 12.4.2). Hyperplastic follicles may also be seen in the interlobular septa and the visceral pleura. Compression of the airways may lead to an obstructive endogenous lipoid pneumonia or secondary infection with pus in the bronchioles and the alveoli showing focal organising pneumonia.

Differential diagnosis

The differential diagnosis of follicular bronchiolitis is from the other forms of bronchiolitis described in Chapter 3. It also has to be distinguished from follicular bronchiectasis, a term used when prominent follicular hyperplasia accompanies airway dilatation. Lymphoid follicles may also be prominent in the middle-lobe syndrome (see p. 92), but this is a localised disease. Extrinsic allergic alveolitis may also

Figure 12.4.2 Follicular bronchiolitis. (A) A lymphoid follicle is closely related to a small bronchiole, compressing the lumen. (B) The bronchiolar lumen contains retained proteinaceous debris and cholesterol because of narrowing by hyperplastic lymphoid follicles.

show prominent peribronchial lymphoid follicles, but there are usually granulomas and a significant interstitial inflammatory component.

Treatment and prognosis

Most patients respond well to corticosteroid therapy, although non-resolving alveolar collapse, fibrosis and even bulla formation may occur. Occasional cases show obliterative bronchiolitis but this probably represents an independent manifestation of an associated connective tissue disorder rather than progression of the follicular bronchiolitis.

Lymphoid interstitial pneumonia

Lymphoid (or lymphocytic or lymphoplasmacytic) interstitial pneumonia is characterised by a prominent, diffuse, alveolar infiltrate of lymphocytes and plasma cells.[41] Occasional cases are idiopathic but it is generally associated with a variety of clinical conditions that reflect impaired immunity (Box 12.4.1).[21,25–27,28–31,32–36,21,37,38]

Clinical features

The age and sex distribution tend to reflect the associated diseases listed in Box 12.4.1 so the age range is broad. Cases have been described in both infants and the elderly but most cases occur in middle age. There is a slight female preponderance[21] and occasionally there is a familial pattern of inheritance.[42,43] Most patients have cough and dyspnoea accompanied by systemic symptoms such as weight loss and low-grade pyrexia.[28] Many also have hypergammaglobulinaemia but some show low levels of gammaglobulins.[26,32,44–47] Pulmonary function tests show a restrictive defect.[28] Chest radiographs show ground-glass opacities or reticular, coarse reticulonodular or fine reticulonodular opacities[19,26,32,45] while HRCT may also show cystically dilated air spaces, which occasionally dominate the image.[28,47–50]

Aetiology

The aetiology of lymphoid interstitial pneumonia is probably multifactorial as there is evidence that both viruses and immune processes contribute. The viruses include Epstein–Barr virus (EBV)[51–53] and in children particularly human immunodeficiency virus (HIV).[51,54–57] The identification of monoclonal gammopathy in some patients[44] and of clones of lymphoid cells with high sequence homology to autoreactive lymphocytes suggests autoimmunity[58] while the association with congenital immunodeficiency suggests further pathways of lymphocyte dysregulation.[46,59] In the acquired immunodeficiency of HIV infection, high levels of chemokines such as interleukin-18 may be in part responsible for recruitment of inflammatory cells into the interstitium.[60]

Pathological features

The involved lung tissue may appear consolidated on gross inspection but microscopy shows that it is the alveolar walls that are affected rather than the air spaces, being expanded by an interstitial infiltrate. The infiltrate is predominantly composed of small lymphocytes but these are mixed with plasma cells, a few larger mononuclear cells and histiocytes (Fig. 12.4.3). The distribution is typically diffuse but may be similar to that encountered in the more diffuse forms of pulmonary lymphoma, being particularly prominent in relation to lymphatics and thus most marked around bronchovascular bundles, bordering interlobular septa and beneath the pleura. It also forms rounded nodular aggregates about small intralobular vessels but the alveolar walls are nevertheless considerably thickened (see Fig. 12.4.3). Lymphoid follicles are frequent and there may be poorly formed granulomas.[23,26] The follicles largely consist of B cells (see Fig. 12.4.3) but the interstitial infiltrate predominantly comprises T cells. Occasionally there is local deposition of amyloid (Fig. 12.4.4).[23,61] Molecular studies show no immunoglobulin heavy-chain restriction or gene rearrangement.[19,22,23,32,62,63] Lymphoid interstitial pneumonia may occasionally overlap with follicular bronchiolitis (see above); these two conditions represent different patterns of lymphoid hyperplasia and are seen together particularly in patients with connective tissue disorders (Fig. 12.4.5).[19,22,24]

Differential diagnosis

The differential diagnosis includes both reactive conditions and interstitial patterns of low-grade B-cell lymphoma. The former include HIV and EBV infection. In comparison with the other idiopathic interstitial pneumonias the infiltrate of lymphoid interstitial pneumonia is much denser and is generally not accompanied by any significant degree of fibrosis. It most closely resembles cellular non-specific interstitial pneumonia, from which it is only distinguished by a subjective

Figure 12.4.3 Lymphoid interstitial pneumonia. (A) A heavy infiltrate of small lymphocytes cuffs the intralobular blood vessels and thickens the alveolar walls. (B) Although the alveolar walls are markedly expanded, there is little involvement infiltration of the air space. (C) At high power, the interstitial infiltrate comprises small round lymphocytes, plasma cells and histiocytes. (D) CD20 staining shows tight aggregates of B cells, mainly within follicles (compare with the lymphomatous infiltration in Fig. 12.4.15a).

assessment of the intensity of the infiltrate, which is less marked in non-specific interstitial pneumonia. Extrinsic allergic alveolitis is also characterised by a predominantly T-cell infiltrate with occasional granulomas, but a peribronchiolar concentration of the infiltrate and the presence of organising pneumonia distinguish it from lymphoid interstitial pneumonia.[64] Extrinsic allergic alveolitis, sarcoidosis and lymphoid interstitial pneumonia are compared in Table 6.1.6 (p. 281). Distinguishing these conditions is greatly facilitated by correlation with clinical data, especially the HRCT findings (Table 12.4.1).[65] The distinction of lymphoid interstitial pneumonia from marginal-zone lymphomas of MALT origin is considered on p. 660.

Treatment and prognosis

Older reports probably included cases that were lymphomatous from the outset, which would explain why the condition has been regarded as having a propensity to evolve into frank lymphoma. More recent studies, taking advantage of molecular techniques, suggest that apart from the cases complicating AIDS,[51,52,66] lymphomatous change is unusual.[28] The prognosis is therefore better than was formerly believed, although it remains unpredictable.[45] Some patients recover completely, others remain stable[46] or slowly progress to end-stage fibrosis[50] and some die within months.[19,32,45] One group reported that 7 of 15 patients died with a median survival of 11.5 years.[28] Causes of death include progression to interstitial fibrosis and infection.[47] Treatment is usually with corticosteroids, with or without cytotoxic therapy. Patients with symptomatic HIV-related lymphoid interstitial pneumonia have improved following highly active antiretroviral therapy.[67]

Nodular lymphoid hyperplasia[23,68,68a]

Over the last two decades, it has become apparent that most localised lymphoid lesions arising in the lung are marginal-zone non-Hodgkin

Figure 12.4.4 Lymphoid interstitial pneumonia. Rare cases may be associated with the deposition of either amyloid or, as in this case, light chains.

Figure 12.4.6 Nodular lymphoid hyperplasia. A pulmonary nodule is composed of hyperplastic germinal centres interspersed by a mixed infiltrate of plasma cells and small lymphocytes. The features are similar to those of marginal-zone lymphomas of mucosa-associated lymphoid tissue (MALT) origin, but no evidence of clonality was found on immunohistochemistry or molecular analysis.

Figure 12.4.5 Histological overlap in lymphoid hyperplasia. On the left, the inflammatory infiltrate is mainly interstitial, whereas on the right there is follicular bronchiolitis.

lymphomas.[4,15,69] However, a few prove to be polyclonal and reactive in nature and the term 'nodular lymphoid hyperplasia' is now applied to these, having superseded pseudolymphoma.

Clinical features

Patients have a mean age of 65 years (range 19–80) and show a slight female preponderance.[68] The lesions are generally chance radiographic finding. Symptoms include cough, shortness of breath and pleuritic pain. Most lesions are solitary and, if multiple, unilateral. Surgical resection is curative.

Pathological features

Nodular lymphoid hyperplasia forms a well circumscribed nodule measuring up to 6 cm, which is of fleshy or rubbery consistence and usually subpleural. Histologically, lymphoid follicles are well developed and plasma cells are prominent between the follicles (Fig. 12.4.6). There may be extensive central scarring. Any infiltrative acti-

vity at the periphery is quite limited. Atypical cells are not seen. Immunochemistry shows that the reactive follicles are populated by B cells expressing both κ and λ light chains while the interfollicular lymphocytes are largely T cells. Staining for bcl-2 protein is negative and no immunoglobulin heavy-chain gene rearrangement is detectable.

Differential diagnosis

Nodular lymphoid hyperplasia differs from lymphoid interstitial pneumonia in being focal rather than diffuse. The principal alternatives are inflammatory myofibroblastic tumour (see p. 620) and marginal-zone non-Hodgkin lymphoma of MALT type (see below). It differs from inflammatory myofibroblastic tumour in lacking spindle cells. The distinction from marginal-zone non-Hodgkin lymphoma of MALT type is particularly difficult and often uncertain without molecular studies but any significant degree of infiltrative activity along side adjacent lymphatics would favour lymphoma.

LYMPHOPROLIFERATIVE DISEASE COMPLICATING SEVERE IMMUNE IMPAIRMENT

The spread of AIDS and the development of organ transplantation have both seen the appearance of a remarkable spectrum of lymphoproliferative disease from which the lungs have not been spared. The chief pulmonary manifestations have been lymphoid hyperplasia, including lymphoid interstitial pneumonia (see above), and a variety of lesions that have many of the features of lymphoma.[70–73] In the case of posttransplantation lymphoproliferative disease, which is touched upon again in Chapter 11 (see p. 521), some of these lesions regress when immunosuppressive therapy is withdrawn or even reduced, while in the case of AIDS-related lymphomas tumour grade appears

Table 12.4.1 Clinical and pathological characteristics of lymphoid interstitial pneumonia, cellular non-specific interstitial pneumonia and extrinsic allergic alveolitis[65]

	Lymphoid interstitial pneumonia	Cellular non-specific interstitial pneumonia	Extrinsic allergic alveolitis
Age	Wide age range	26–50 years	Wide age range
Sex	Female preponderance in adults	Male preponderance	Dependent on causative agent
Associated diseases			
Autoimmunity	Common	Fairly common	No
Immunodeficiency	Common (especially in HIV+ve children)	May be seen in HIV+ve patients	No
Idiopathic disease	Rare	Fairly common	No
Amyloidosis	Rare	No	No
Environmental allergens	No	No	Yes
Hypogammaglobulinaemia	Common	No	No
Lavage lymphocytosis	Common	Common	Common
Imaging			
Chest radiograph	Ground-glass or reticulonodular shadowing Occasionally normal	Non-specific, variable shadowing May be normal	Variable (dependent on stage of disease) May wax and wane on serial radiographs
HRCT	Spectrum of randomly distributed nodules (1–4 mm) through to ground-glass opacification with the latter sometimes accompanied by thin-walled cystic air spaces	Ground-glass opacification without architectural disturbance or honeycombing	Subacute disease characterised by ground-glass opacification and poorly defined centrilobular nodularity. Expiratory scans show air-trapping reflecting bronchiolitis Chronic disease shows fibrosis of non-specific pattern and distribution
Histopathology			
Distribution	Diffuse	Diffuse	Often centrilobular
Inflammation	Severe interstitial infiltrate	Mild interstitial infiltrate	Variable interstitial infiltrate
Architecture	Little architectural destruction	No architectural destruction	May be lost in chronic disease
Interstitial fibrosis	Rare	None	May be present in chronic disease
Interstitial cell types	Small round lymphocytes, plasma cells, histiocytes	Small round lymphocytes, plasma cells, histiocytes, some fibroblasts	Small round lymphocytes, plasma cells, histiocytes, some fibroblasts
Granulomas	Rare	No	Common
Organising pneumonia	Rare	Rare (less than 10% of cases)	Common (70% of cases)

HIV, human immunodeficiency virus; HRCT, high-resolution computed tomography.

to vary with the patient's immune status, the more severely immunodepleted developing more aggressive neoplasms.[74]

Lymphoproliferative disease complicating profound immunosuppression generally involves B cells: T cells are poorly represented. The B-cell proliferation is probably attributable to T-lymphocyte deficiency for in normal individuals T cells control the division of B cells. T-cell deficiency also permits the proliferation of latent EBV infection. This virus is a further stimulus to B-cell proliferation and its constituents have been identified in most of the resultant tumours.[75–79] It would appear that after a period of unchecked poly-

clonal B-lymphocyte proliferation, a clone of malignant cells may emerge. The resultant B-cell tumours are often high-grade and notable for affecting extranodal tissues, including the lungs on occasion.[75,80,81] There is a particularly high risk of pulmonary involvement, around 60%, after heart–lung transplantation. Transplantation of lungs alone carries less of a risk.

Lung involvement by these high-grade tumours generally takes the form of multiple nodules that are relatively well circumscribed and show extensive necrosis. Histologically, the lesions may be monomorphic or polymorphic: the former consist of immuno-

Figure 12.4.7 Marginal-zone lymphoma of mucosa-associated lymphoid tissue (MALT) origin. High-resolution computed tomography shows an area of consolidation with ground-glass changes at its periphery. Air bronchograms are present within the consolidation.

Figure 12.4.8 Marginal-zone lymphoma of mucosa-associated lymphoid tissue (MALT) origin. Bronchial washings show a moderately dense infiltrate of small lymphocytes, which proved to be of B-cell phenotype.

blasts or large or small non-cleaved lymphoid cells, whilst the latter consist of a variety of cell types, including immunoblasts, centroblast-like and centrocyte-like cells, plasmacytoid cells and histiocytes. The infiltrate tends to involve blood vessels, so that the features may resemble those of lymphomatoid granulomatosis (see below).[81] AIDS-related lymphoma of the pleura is considered separately on page 734.

MARGINAL-ZONE B-CELL LYMPHOMA OF MALT TYPE

Clinical features

More than 80% of patients with these tumours are over 40 years of age. The mean age is about 55 years; children are rarely affected.[15] There is a slight male preponderance. The majority of patients are asymptomatic at presentation, the disease being first detected on routine radiographs. Other patients suffer from cough, dyspnoea, chest pain and haemoptysis, sometimes accompanied by malaise, weight loss or pyrexia.[2] Paraproteinaemia is present in up to 20% of cases and this is usually of IgM type (macroglobulinaemia).[82] Evidence of Sjögren's syndrome or, less often, another connective tissue disorder such as lupus erythematosus, may be present,[27] and there may be a history of lymphoma in other extranodal sites, such as the gastrointestinal tract, salivary glands, orbit or skin. Some patients have systemic ('type B') symptoms such as fever, weight loss and night sweats. Imaging shows variable patterns, with unilateral or bilateral disease, isolated or multiple opacities, diffuse infiltration, reticulonodular shadowing and pleural effusions. HRCT scans typically show multiple or solitary areas of consolidation, with associated air bronchograms and haloes of ground-glass shadowing at lesion margins (Fig. 12.4.7).[83] Mediastinal lymphadenopathy is unusual.[5] Diagnosis is possible with cytological specimens (Fig. 12.4.8) or small biopsies,[4,84–86] but more often a surgical lung biopsy and correlation with HRCT data are needed. Immunohistochemistry, flow cytometry and molecular analysis may be required.[87,88]

Aetiology

Whereas gastric marginal-zone lymphomas of MALT origin show a strong relation to *Helicobacter pylori* infection, less is known of the aetiology of the comparable tumours arising in the lungs. However, there is evidence that smoking,[89] autoimmune disorders,[76,90] immunosuppressive therapy,[91,92] AIDS, tuberculosis[93] and hepatitis C[94] may all play a role. Neoplastic change in the bronchus-associated lymphoid tissue is therefore likely to be multifactorial. These associations are all characterised by an expansion of the bronchus-associated lymphoid tissue and this is probably a common factor in the pathogenesis of these tumours.

Molecular studies have shown various translocations, trisomy of chromosome 3 and mutation of the *bcl*-10 gene.[95–99] The commonest translocations are t(11;18)(q21;q21), t(14;18)(q32;q21) and t(1;14)(p22;q32), being seen in 40%, 5–25% and 8% of pulmonary marginal-zone lymphomas respectively.[99] They result in fusion, and hence inactivation, of genes concerned in apoptosis, or overexpression of oncogenes such as *bcl*-10 and MALT-1.[99]

Pathological features

The macroscopic appearances vary from a localised tan or grey tumour to areas of apparent pulmonary consolidation (Fig. 12.4.9). Preserved bronchovascular bundles can sometimes be seen on the cut surface.

Microscopically, the tumours consist of small lymphocytes, which may be centrocyte-like, lymphocyte-like or monocytoid, although all are thought to be variations of the same neoplastic cell (Fig. 12.4.10A). They first proliferate around the bronchovascular bundles and then spread out in the connective tissue planes alongside blood vessels and their accompanying lymphatics. At this stage there is prominent involvement of the interlobular septa (Fig. 12.4.10B) and there may be pleural infiltration. As the disease progresses there is invasion of the alveolar walls, which are first expanded and then destroyed leading to filling of the air spaces and obliteration of the alveolar architecture (Fig. 12.4.10C, D).[100] This ultimately results in a tumour mass in which only the larger airways and blood vessels are spared. The latter may be infiltrated[101] but not on the scale seen with the angiocentric

Figure 12.4.9 Marginal-zone lymphoma of mucosa-associated lymphoid tissue (MALT) origin. The tumour forms a cream-coloured mass which is less dense peripherally, in keeping with the ground-glass changes at the edges of the mass noted on high-resolution computed tomography in Figure 12.4.7.

lymphoproliferative disorders. Ultimately, the tumour cells also infiltrate the pleura and bronchial cartilage. Hyaline sclerosis is common and lymphoid follicles are often evident, particularly when stains for the CD21 marker of follicular dendritic cells are employed (Fig. 12.4.11). Epithelioid and giant cell granulomas may rarely be observed (Fig. 12.4.12) and lymphoepithelial lesions are often present, recognition of which is facilitated by cytokeratin staining (Fig. 12.4.13). Giant lamellar bodies derived from type II pneumocytes may be seen within the tumour, possibly related to airway obstruction (Fig. 12.4.14).[102] Amyloid is present in up to 10% of cases.[5,6,103,104] Necrosis is rarely observed.

Immunohistochemistry

The more numerous B lymphocytes can be identified with stains for CD20 or CD79a and the background reactive T cells with CD3 (Fig. 12.4.15A, B). Immunostains for κ and λ light chains may provide evidence of clonality but are successful in only a minority of cases, less so than at any other site where lymphomas of this type arise.[100] However, amplification of the immunoglobulin heavy-chain gene by the polymerase chain reaction may provide firmer evidence of mono-

clonality.[4] The *bcl-2* oncogene is not expressed in the follicle centre cells but is positive in the colonising neoplastic lymphocytes. The neoplastic cells are also CD5- and CD10-negative. If there is nodal involvement the features there are those of nodal marginal-zone B-cell non-Hodgkin lymphomas.[105,106]

Differential diagnosis

The principal histological difficulty lies in distinguishing this type of lymphoma from lymphoid interstitial pneumonia. These conditions share many histological features but involvement of alveolar spaces, destruction of alveolar walls, the presence of giant lamellar bodies and infiltration of the pleura and bronchial cartilage all favour lymphoma. Immunohistochemical characterisation of the infiltrate is of considerable help for whereas the small lymphocytes in lymphoid interstitial pneumonia are predominantly T cells, the interstitial infiltrate in marginal-zone lymphoma has a predominantly B-cell phenotype (compare Figs 12.4.3D and 12.4.11D).[4,6,19] Finally, molecular studies may provide firm supportive evidence; amplification of the immunoglobulin heavy chain gene favours lymphoma and identification of the chromosomal translocations described above points to marginal-zone B-cell lymphoma of MALT type.

Distinguishing lymphoma from nodular lymphoid hyperplasia is described above (p. 657). Distinguishing primary from secondary lymphoma depends upon clinical data. Lymphocyte-rich variants of thymoma (WHO type B1) involving the lung may resemble lymphoma but are easily recognised by their cytokeratins CD3 and CD1a positivity.[107]

In cases of lymphoma with extensive amyloid deposition, the intensity of the lymphocytic infiltration, lymphatic tracking and pleural invasion are all clues to the lymphomatous nature of the disease.

Clinically, the differential diagnosis often includes local or multifocal mucinous adenocarcinoma and organising pneumonia, in which case a cytological specimen or endoscopic biopsy showing a dense lymphocytic infiltrate with the appropriate immunophenotype may be sufficient to identify marginal-zone lymphoma.

Treatment and prognosis

These tumours are either stage Ie (confined to the lungs) or IIe (Ie plus hilar/mediastinal involvement) and resection has often resulted in prolonged remission.[108] In some elderly patients with asymptomatic disease, a 'wait and watch' policy is often appropriate for these indolent tumours. The 5-year survival exceeds 90%.[3,4,15,109] Metastases involve other mucosal sites rather than lymph nodes.[2,4] Recurrence is associated with a tendency towards transition to diffuse large B-cell lymphoma.[15] Extensive pulmonary involvement that is not amenable to resection is associated with a worse prognosis. Chlorambucil is the medical treatment of choice.[109]

DIFFUSE LARGE B-CELL NON-HODGKIN LYMPHOMA

Clinical features

Diffuse large B-cell non-Hodgkin lymphoma forms about 20% of pulmonary lymphomas. The age range is similar to that of marginal-zone non-Hodgkin lymphoma of MALT origin but the patients are usually symptomatic at presentation, complaining of cough, haemoptysis, dyspnoea and systemic ('B') symptoms such as fever,

Figure 12.4.10 Marginal-zone lymphoma of mucosa-associated lymphoid tissue (MALT) origin. (A) The tumour is composed of a monotonous sheet of small mature lymphocytes. (B) At its periphery, the tumour has spread primarily along the pulmonary lymphatics. (C) As the lymphoma expands, so the interstitium becomes increasingly widened and alveoli are filled by tumour cells. (D) Centrally, alveolar walls are destroyed, but as yet bronchovascular bundles are preserved.

weight loss and night sweats. Imaging shows solid masses, which are often multiple.

Aetiology

It is likely that these tumours represent blastic transformation of marginal-zone non-Hodgkin lymphomas of MALT origin, probably through further mutation. There is a rare association with fibrosing alveolitis and connective tissue diseases. Diffuse large B-cell lymphomas are also found in immunodeficient individuals, notably those undergoing immunosuppression following organ transplantation or suffering from AIDS.[4,73,76,90,110]

Pathological features

Macroscopically, areas of pulmonary involvement typically form solid or necrotising cream-coloured masses. Microscopically, the lung architecture is destroyed by sheets of tumour cells that have large irregular vesicular nuclei and moderate amounts of cytoplasm. The cells are pleomorphic and there are many mitoses (Fig. 12.4.16). Lymphoid follicles, lymphoepithelial lesions and granulomas are seldom evident but bronchial MALT may be found in the distant non-involved lung. Foci of marginal-zone non-Hodgkin lymphomas of MALT origin may be seen.[4] The neoplastic cells are of B-cell phenotype, mixed with reactive T cells. Evidence of monoclonality is occasionally obtained by demonstrating heavy-chain gene amplification with the polymerase chain reaction.[4]

Table 12.4.2 Clinical and pathological characteristics of lymphoid interstitial pneumonia, mucosa-associated lymphoid tissue (MALT) lymphoma, nodular lymphoid hyperplasia and lymphomatoid granulomatosis[65]

	Lymphoid interstitial pneumonia	MALT lymphoma	Nodular lymphoid hyperplasia	Lymphomatoid granulomatosis
Age	Wide age range	Usually between 50 and 70 years	19–80 years	4–80 years
Sex	In adults, female preponderance	Slight male preponderance	Slight male preponderance	Male preponderance
Associated diseases				
Autoimmunity	Common	Rare	None	None
Immunodeficiency	Common (especially HIV+ve children)	Rare	None	Occasional
Amyloidosis	Rare	Rare	None	None
Imaging				
Chest radiograph	Ground-glass or reticulonodular shadowing. Occasionally normal	Consolidation (single or multifocal) Air bronchograms	Variably sized nodules (occasionally multiple)	Multiple bilateral nodules (may be cavitating)
HRCT	Spectrum of randomly distributed nodules (1–4 mm) through to ground-glass opacification with the latter sometimes accompanied by thin-walled cystic air spaces	Consolidation (single or multifocal) with ground glass at periphery of lesions. Air bronchograms	Not known	Cavitating nodules, sometimes with peripheral ground-glass attenuation
Histopathology				
Architecture	Heavy diffuse interstitial infiltrate with little architectural destruction	Consolidated mass (alveolar + interstitial) May be multifocal, or rarely diffuse	Single or multiple nodules	Multiple nodules, usually with focal necrosis Infiltrate usually angiocentric
Cell type	Mainly T lymphocytes with lesser numbers of plasma cells and histiocytes	Mainly B lymphocytes (lymphocyte-like, plasmacytoid and/or monocytoid)	Mainly T lymphocytes with some plasma cells and histiocytes	Mainly T lymphocytes with some plasma cells and histiocytes, and a variable population of atypical B cells
Germinal centres	Yes	Yes	Yes	Occasional (secondary reactive phenomenon)
Dutcher bodies	No	Yes	No	No
Monoclonality	No	Yes	No	Yes

HIV, human immunodeficiency virus; HRCT, high-resolution computed tomography.

Differential diagnosis

There are few difficulties in identifying the confluent sheets of blast cells of a high-grade lymphoma, other than distinguishing the condition from other undifferentiated neoplasms, which may be accomplished by applying stains for lymphocyte markers (CD45), cytokeratins, alpha-fetoprotein, and epithelial membrane antigen. A surgical lung biopsy may be required to identify the angiocentric lesions of lymphomatoid granulomatosis but, although both are B-cell proliferations, B cells are comparatively scarce in lymphomatoid granulomatosis and they are usually positive for EBV, while those in immunocompetent patients with diffuse large B-cell non-Hodgkin lymphoma are negative.[111] Sclerosing mediastinal B-cell lymphoma may invade the lung but the anatomical position of the main mass and the younger age of these mediastinal tumours enable them to be distinguished from the pulmonary growths.

Treatment and prognosis

Extensive involvement of the lung usually precludes resection and most patients require combination chemotherapy. Five-year survival figures range from 0 to 60%.[3,4,15]

Figure 12.4.11 (A) Marginal-zone lymphoma of mucosa-associated lymphoid tissue (MALT) origin in which there are prominent reactive lymphoid follicles. (B) The follicles are particularly well demonstrated with the CD21 marker of follicular dendritic cells (immunoperoxidase stain for CD21).

Figure 12.4.13 Lymphoepithelial lesions in a marginal-zone lymphoma of mucosa-associated lymphoid tissue (MALT) origin. These lesions may be difficult to recognise in haematoxylin and eosin stains (A) but are readily apparent in sections immunostained for cytokeratin (B).

Figure 12.4.12 Tuberculoid granulomas in a marginal-zone lymphoma of mucosa-associated lymphoid tissue (MALT) origin.

Figure 12.4.14 Giant lamellar bodies in a marginal-zone lymphoma of mucosa-associated lymphoid tissue (MALT) origin. A low-grade lymphoma of MALT origin contains abundant giant lamellar bodies within the alveolar spaces.

Figure 12.4.15 Marginal-zone lymphoma of mucosa-associated lymphoid tissue (MALT) origin. (A) The cells within the interstitium are predominantly CD20-positive, (B) with variable numbers of admixed CD3-positive T lymphocytes. (Compare with lymphoid interstitial pneumonia in Fig. 12.4.3D).

LYMPHOMATOID GRANULOMATOSIS

Aetiology and nomenclature

Lymphomatoid granulomatosis is a rare disease characterised by a necrotising, angiocentric, polymorphous and usually atypical lymphoid infiltrate that typically forms tumour-like masses in the lungs, brain, skin and other tissues. It was first described by Liebow in 1972, the rather ambiguous term chosen reflecting initial uncertainty concerning the nature of the condition.[112–114]

Early attempts to characterise the lymphoid cells established that the majority were T cells and the condition was therefore included, together with polymorphic reticulosis (lethal midline granuloma of the nose), in a spectrum of so-called postthymic T-cell proliferations.[115,116] However, although further studies substantiated the pre-

Figure 12.4.16 Diffuse large B-cell lymphoma. (A) The tumour is very cellular and shows focal necrosis. (B) At high power, the neoplastic B cells show considerable cellular pleomorphism and mitotic activity.

dominant T-cell phenotype, rearrangement of the T-cell receptor genes could be identified in only a minority of cases[116–120] and it was subsequently shown that the scanty atypical cells were of B-cell phenotype, often with rearrangement of the immunoglobulin heavy-chain gene.[121–124] EBV was localised to the atypical B cells[81,120–123,125–127] and lymphomatoid granulomatosis is now regarded as representing a T-cell-rich, EBV-driven, angiocentric B-cell proliferation, distinct from polymorphic reticulosis.[121]

Note has to be taken however of occasional cases that are histologically identical to lymphomatoid granulomatosis yet consist entirely of T cells. These are generally not associated with EBV and may represent peripheral T-cell lymphomas.[122] Other lymphomas may also show an angiocentric pattern resembling that seen in lymphomatoid granulomatosis.[7] Thus, what appears to be a distinct morphological entity may be mimicked by various lymphoproliferative diseases showing angiocentricity and secondarily involving the lung, the identification of which will probably become important as treatment evolves.[22]

Conversely, what were initially described as separate conditions are now widely regarded as different grades of lymphomatoid granulomatosis. Thus, based on the degree of atypia and necrosis, benign lymphocytic angiitis and granulomatosis[128–130] is now considered to be the lowest grade of lymphomatoid granulomatosis while the highest grade conforms to what has been termed angiocentric lymphoma.[101,116,131]

Clinical features

Patients with lymphomatoid granulomatosis cover a wide age range but most are middle-aged with the median age at diagnosis being in the sixth decade: men are affected twice as frequently as women.[132–135] Most patients present with pyrexia, weight loss and general malaise in addition to chest symptoms such as cough, chest pain and dyspnoea. About a quarter have neurological symptoms at presentation and half develop an erythematous, macular rash or subcutaneous nodules some time during their illness.[136] An appreciable degree of lymphadenopathy is unusual. CD4 lymphocyte counts may be low.[133] Chest radiographs and HRCT scans typically reveal bilateral, multiple, rounded masses, located in the middle and lower zones.[137] These vary in size and may coalesce or cavitate; they are frequently mistaken for metastases. Unilateral lesions or a diffuse infiltrative process are less often seen. Hilar node enlargement is not a feature in the early stages of the disease, although lymph node involvement is present in 22% of cases at autopsy[114] and can be more readily recognised as malignant than the lesions in the lungs.

Lymphomatoid granulomatosis may also present in other organs. Neurological symptoms may result either from similar involvement of small vessels in the central nervous system or peripheral nerves or from the formation of tumour-like masses in the brain. In the kidney there may be a diffuse interstitial infiltrate or distinct tumours[138] but, in contrast to Wegener's granulomatosis, there is no glomerulonephritis. Other affected sites include skin, liver, spleen, adrenals, heart, pancreas, gastrointestinal tract and pancreas.[114] Extrapulmonary lesions generally resemble those in the lungs but in the skin it is unusual to find cells bearing the EBV genome. This has led to suggestions that the skin lesions may be caused by cytokines released by lesions elsewhere rather than direct involvement.[139] Extrapulmonary involvement is unusual in benign lymphocytic angiitis and granulomatosis.

Aetiology

Apart from its close association with EBV, the aetiology of lymphomatoid granulomatosis is obscure, although the patients sometimes have obvious underlying defects in their cell-mediated immunity. These may be congenital, as in the Wiskott–Aldrich syndrome,[140] or acquired, as in AIDS,[141] angiogenic myeloid metaplasia[142] and the treatment of other forms of lymphoma.[143,144] There is also some similarity between lymphomatoid granulomatosis and posttransplantation lymphoproliferative disorders (see p. 521): both are essentially angiocentric B-cell proliferations, both bear the EBV genome and both vary in their clonality, but they differ in the proportion of reactive T cells.[145,146] It appears likely that impaired immunity underlies the development of both these diseases.

Pathological features

Macroscopically, the lungs contain nodules of pinkish-grey tissue, the largest of which show central necrosis and cavitation (Fig. 12.4.17). Alternatively, areas of confluent consolidation may be seen. The pleura is frequently thickened but effusions are unusual.

Microscopically, most cases show broad tracts of necrosis separated by a mixed angiocentric infiltrate that includes usually scanty pleomorphic atypical lymphoid cells (Fig. 12.4.18). While most of the lymphocytes stain for T-cell markers,[147] the atypical lymphoid cells stain as B cells, analogous to the findings in T-cell-rich B-cell lymphomas. The B cells may also be positive for CD30 but are negative for CD15. Eosinophils and giant cells are not usually

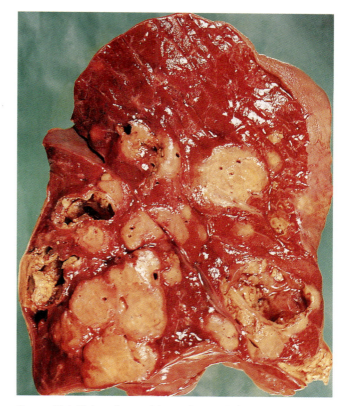

Figure 12.4.17 Lymphomatoid granulomatosis forming large fleshy masses within the lung. *(Courtesy of Dr P King, Johannesburg, South Africa.)*

present in significant numbers and sarcoid-like granulomas are not a feature.

The degree of cellular atypia varies considerably, from lymphocytes with irregular, folded nuclei in lymphomatoid granulomatosis to larger blast-like cells with prominent nucleoli and condensed marginal chromatin in angiocentric lymphoma. The lesions are graded 1–3 on the degree of lymphocytic atypia, the presence of necrosis and the polymorphic/monomorphic nature of the infiltrate, grade 3 lesions being synonymous with angiocentric lymphomas.[116] The B-cell proliferation index correlates well with histological grade.[148]

Differential diagnosis

In contrast to true vasculitis, in which the vessel wall is destroyed by a necrotising inflammatory process, vascular involvement is characterised by separation of the components of the wall by the infiltrating cells. This is usually best seen in the intima, which becomes greatly thickened as the infiltrate lifts the endothelium and obliterates the lumen. Similar cells infiltrate the alveolar and bronchiolar walls, giving rise to additional non-specific reactive changes, such as organising intra-alveolar fibrinous exudates, proliferation of alveolar epithelial cells and bronchiolitis obliterans. However, the cardinal feature that distinguishes lymphomatoid granulomatosis from other granulomatous vasculitides is the presence of the atypical B lymphocytes. These are poorly represented in the lower grades. Gene rearrangement studies may be of value in doubtful cases.[123] Distinction from diffuse large B-cell non-Hodgkin lymphomas is discussed above. IgG4-related systemic sclerosing disease (see p. 485) is a further condition that may be confused with lymphomatoid granulomatosis. It is characterised by a sclerosing vasculitis and a heavy infiltrate of IgG4-bearing plasma cells, the recognition of which is key to the diagnosis.

Figure 12.4.18 Lymphomatoid granulomatosis. (A) The wall of a small pulmonary blood vessel is heavily infiltrated. (B) Atypical lymphoid cells infiltrate the intima of a pulmonary artery but do not destroy the vessel wall. Immunostaining shows that, although many T cells are present, the atypical cells are B cells.

Treatment and prognosis

Survival varies from a few months to many years, according to grade, but is generally short.[114,122,123] High-dose corticosteroids, cyclophosphamide and combination chemotherapy have been used, and good responses to interferon-alpha 2b,[127] bone marrow transplantation and, in line with the B-cell nature of the lesion, response to anti-CD20 (rituxiab) have been achieved.[149,150]

HODGKIN DISEASE

Primary pulmonary Hodgkin disease is very uncommon, much rarer than secondary involvement.[151] The diagnosis is only justified if hilar lymph nodes are uninvolved and disease elsewhere has been excluded.

Clinical features, treatment and prognosis

Reported cases cover a wide age range (18–82 years, mean 43 years) and, as with nodal Hodgkin disease, the age incidence is bimodal, with peaks at 21–30 and 60–80 years of age.[152] There is a slight female predominance.[152-157] Most patients complain of breathlessness and cough and about half also have systemic symptoms such as weight loss and fever. Chest radiographs may show multiple nodules or solitary tumours with cavitation in some of the larger lesions. Following treatment, relapse occurs in the majority of cases, either in the lungs or elsewhere. Solitary tumours are less frequently associated with systemic symptoms and have a better prognosis than bilateral growths.[155]

Pathological features

The microscopic appearances are typical of Hodgkin disease, usually of either nodular sclerosing or mixed cellularity type. Bronchi are frequently involved, with resultant obstructive changes distally, but presentation as an endobronchial lesion is rare.[158] Larger lesions usually undergo extensive central necrosis. Away from the nodules, a lymphatic or vascular distribution of spread is discernible, the pleura may be infiltrated and atypical cells may be found in air spaces.[154] As in other organs, the lesions of Hodgkin disease may be accompanied by sarcoid-like epithelioid and giant cell granulomas.[159]

Differential diagnosis

The differential diagnosis of pulmonary Hodgkin disease includes necrotising granulomatous inflammation, particularly Wegener's granulomatosis, sarcoidosis and infection, Langerhans cell histiocytosis, undifferentiated carcinoma and other forms of malignant lymphoma. Wegener's granulomatosis can be excluded if clearly atypical lymphoid cells are present. Large numbers of eosinophils may cause Langerhans cell histiocytosis to be considered, but the extensive necrosis is not a feature of this disorder and the Langerhans cells lack the malignant characteristics of mononuclear Hodgkin cells and Reed–Sternberg cells. Undifferentiated carcinomas occasionally appear extremely pleomorphic, sometimes with the multilobed nuclei and large nucleoli of Reed–Sternberg cells. Neutrophils are frequently present in undifferentiated carcinomas but eosinophils are seldom a feature. In debatable cases, immunostaining for keratin intermediate filaments and leukocyte common antigen can be decisive.

Exclusion of other forms of malignant lymphoma may be impossible when only standard histological preparations are available: immunocytochemistry, which has often been lacking in reported cases, may be required. Some forms of T-cell lymphoma may simulate Hodgkin disease by showing extreme degrees of cellular pleomorphism and a background of reactive inflammatory cells.

PLASMACYTOMA

Extramedullary plasmacytomas are rare tumours. The majority occur in the upper respiratory tract and only 6% arise in the bronchi or lungs.[160-165] Some earlier cases may have represented inflammatory myofibroblastic tumours,[166,167] whilst others were probably marginal-zone lymphomas of MALT origin showing predominantly plasmacytoid differentiation.

Only about 7% of patients with multiple myeloma have intrathoracic disease[168] and this is rarely confined to the lung. However, pulmonary plasmacytoma occasionally precedes or accompanies other manifestations of disseminated disease.[169,170] The presence of a paraprotein is not necessarily indicative of multifocal disease: resection of a solitary intrapulmonary plasmacytoma may be followed by disappearance of a circulating paraprotein,[171] or of urinary Bence Jones protein.[172] However, as in myelomatosis, the gammopathy may lead to renal failure.[165]

Pathological features

Microscopically, plasmacytomas consist of sheets of plasma cells: many may appear normal but others have multiple nuclei and some show nuclear pleomorphism. The spindle-shaped and inflammatory cells seen in inflammatory myofibroblastic tumours are lacking. Immunohistochemical investigation confirms the diagnosis by demonstrating light-chain restriction. Occasionally, amyloid is found in the stroma,[160] or there is material that resembles amyloid but fails to stain as such and consists of monotypic immunoglobulin.[163,173] Sometimes the plasma cells are overshadowed by numerous macrophages distended by large amounts of ingested immunoglobulin (crystal-storing histiocytosis), which renders the cytoplasm eosinophilic and can be shown to be monoclonal (see Fig. 12.7.5, p. 700).[174,175] Monoclonality needs to be verified as similar appearances can be produced by reactive conditions that result in excessive immunoglobulin production.[176]

Prognosis

The overall 2- and 5-year survival rates of pulmonary plasmacytomas are 66% and 40%, respectively.[177]

LARGE CELL ANAPLASTIC LYMPHOMA

Large cell anaplastic lymphoma characteristically involves the lymph nodes or skin, but rare cases are limited to the lungs.[178–181] The tumour is considered to be a T-cell lymphoma, although many cases fail to express the typical T-cell phenotype, being CD3- and CD45-negative. However, on molecular analysis most show clonal rearrangement of the T-cell receptor genes. The large, pleomorphic tumour cells are also CD15-negative and sometimes epithelial membrane antigen-positive. CD30 expression is a characteristic feature and many cases also stain for large cell lymphoma kinase (ALK). A t(2:5)(p23:35) translocation involving the ALK gene may be demonstrated. EBV is not detected. Negative reactions for cytokeratins distinguish large cell anaplastic lymphoma from primary or secondary carcinoma, conditions for which it is most easily mistaken. Patient ages range from childhood to the seventh decade with the sexes affected equally. Radiographic features include nodules, masses, air space consolidation, pleural effusion, cavitations and cystic change. Response to treatment is variable.

INTRAVASCULAR LYMPHOMA (ANGIOTROPIC LYMPHOMA)

Intravascular (or angiotropic) lymphoma is to be distinguished from the angiocentric lymphoma described above. It was originally considered to represent a form of malignant 'angioendotheliomatosis' but is now recognised to be a lymphoma of unusual distribution, the malignant cells being almost exclusively confined to the lumen of capillaries and small arteries and veins throughout the body.[182,183] The lung is generally involved at a late stage of the disease but rare cases are reported in which the process is apparently confined to the lungs.[184–187]

Clinical features

Intravascular lymphoma usually presents with fever and features referable to the skin or central nervous system.[182] However, involvement of the pulmonary vasculature is sometimes so extensive that pulmonary hypertension is the presenting feature.[188] Alternatively, the

Figure 12.4.19 Intravascular lymphoma. (A) Atypical lymphoid cells are evident within the small blood vessels of the lung. (B) With CD 20 staining the tumour is categorised as an intravascular large B-cell lymphoma. *(Courtesy of Dr AC Wotherspoon, London, UK.)*

process may present as interstitial lung disease[185,189] or even obstructive airway disease with air trapping.[190] Affected patients are usually in the fifth to seventh decades of life. Chest radiographs may be normal or show non-specific infiltrates. Laboratory findings are also often unhelpful. Despite the presence of numerous malignant cells within small blood vessels, only rarely are they identified in blood films. Most cases are diagnosed postmortem but the disease is relatively sensitive to combination chemotherapy if treated early.[187]

Pathological features

Microscopic examination shows a proliferation of neoplastic round or spindle-shaped cells confined to capillaries and small arteries and veins throughout the body. Affected vessels may show intimal fibrosis. The neoplastic cells have large, vesicular, indented nuclei, eosinophilic nucleoli and moderate amounts of cytoplasm. They are usually B cells and stain for the appropriate lymphoid markers (Fig. 12.4.19) but occasional cases have been reported to have a T-cell phenotype. Monoclonality may be demonstrated with immunohistochemical stains for κ and λ chains and by gene rearrangement studies.[186,191] The neoplastic cells lack CD29 (beta1-integrin), a molecule integral to lymphocyte trafficking, which presumably underlies the peculiar intravascular localisation of this neoplasm.[192] Gene mutations on chromosome 1 and trisomy 18 have also been reported.[193]

Differential diagnosis

The differential diagnosis of angiotropic lymphoma includes metastatic carcinoma and melanoma, leukaemia and lymphoid interstitial pneumonia. The first of these are distinguished by immunohistochemical identification of lymphoma, epithelial cell and melanocyte markers (CD45, cytokeratin, S-100 and HMB45). Leukaemia may be distinguished by reference to blood counts and bone marrow examination and lymphoid interstitial pneumonia by the intravascular rather than interstitial location of the cells.

SECONDARY PULMONARY INVOLVEMENT BY LYMPHOPROLIFERATIVE DISORDERS

Secondary involvement of the lung in patients with nodal lymphoma is common and may be due to direct invasion from involved mediastinal lymph nodes or metastasis via the blood stream or lymphatics.[151] At presentation only about 12% of patients with Hodgkin disease and 4% of patients with non-Hodgkin lymphoma have radiographic evidence of lung involvement[194] but the figure is much higher in patients dying with disseminated disease.[195] Whereas non-Hodgkin lymphomas tend to involve the lungs in a diffuse fashion, following the perivascular and pleural lymphatics, the pulmonary lesions of Hodgkin disease are often nodular, and polypoid endobronchial masses are occasionally seen.[158,195]

Less commonly, *angioimmunoblastic lymphadenopathy* may also involve the lungs, when the microscopic features are similar to those in the lymph nodes, showing a mixed infiltrate of plasma cells and immunoblasts and hyperplasia of the capillary endothelium.[196–198] *Multiple myelomatosis* is another condition that may involve the lungs and be associated there with the deposition of material similar to that better known in the renal tubules.[199] Lymphocytic infiltrates of the lung, pleura and hilar lymph nodes are also described in *Waldenstrom's macroglobulinaemia*.[200,201] *Systemic mast cell disease* has also presented as diffuse parenchymal lung disease.[202] *Cutaneous T-cell lymphoma* (mycosis fungoides or Sézary syndrome) involves the lungs in about two-thirds of cases at autopsy. The interstitial infiltrate of convoluted or cerebriform cells follows the bronchovascular bundles in a lymphatic distribution and may form nodular aggregates[203] or simulate pneumonia.[204] A similar lymphatic distribution is described in *malignant histiocytosis*[205–207] and *leukaemia*.[208,209]

PULMONARY PROBLEMS IN LEUKAEMIA

Respiratory distress often develops in advanced leukaemia and in these circumstances it can be difficult clinically to distinguish leukaemic infiltration of the lungs from opportunistic infection and from the cytotoxic effects of antileukaemic chemotherapy.[210] Furthermore, the chemotherapy may well have been augmented with bone marrow transplantation.[210–213] Posttransplantation lymphoproliferative disease is rare with bone marrow transplantation and, although usually extranodal, seldom affects the lungs.[214] However, bone marrow trans-

Box 12.4.2 **Causes of breathlessness in leukaemia**

Leukaemic infiltration
Infection
Cytotoxic drug damage
Irradiation injury
Graft-versus-host disease
Alveolar haemorrhage

Box 12.4.3 **Pulmonary complications found at autopsy in 71 adult bone marrow transplant recipients[215]**

Infectious complications	
Bacterial bronchopneumonia	13
Aspergillosis	11
Cytomegalovirus pneumonia	2
Candida infection	1
Non-infectious complications	
Diffuse alveolar damage	35
Diffuse alveolar haemorrhage	10
Amyloidosis	9
Pulmonary embolism	5
Lymphoma/leukaemia	4
Bronchiolitis obliterans	2
Organising pneumonia	2
Aspiration	1
Alveolar proteinosis	1

plantation is preceded by whole-body irradiation and introduces the possibility of both radiation injury and graft-versus-host disease. Haemostasis may also be impaired and these patients are liable to suffer diffuse alveolar haemorrhage. There are therefore six possible conditions to consider when such patients complain of breathlessness (Box 12.4.2). In one autopsy study of adult patients treated by bone marrow transplantation, pulmonary complications were the commonest cause of death: the detailed findings are listed in Box 12.4.3.[215] Another group reported that the important late-onset non-infectious pulmonary complications of haemopoietic stem cell transplantation were bronchiolitis obliterans, organising pneumonia and interstitial pneumonia and that, whereas the organising pneumonia responded to corticosteroids, fewer than 15% of the patients with interstitial pneumonia survived 1 year while the bronchiolitis obliterans carried a 61% mortality.[216]

The chest radiograph is generally non-specific and seldom of help in distinguishing these conditions and even after full haematological and microbiological investigations the diagnosis may remain uncertain. However, bronchoalveolar lavage is generally of value in distinguishing leukaemic infiltration, opportunistic infections and haemorrhage, the last of these being characterised by haemosiderin-laden macrophages as well as fresh blood. If bronchoalveolar lavage is not diagnostic, the histopathological appearances of leukaemic infiltration, infection and cytotoxic damage are sufficiently distinctive to make biopsy a worthwhile procedure,[217–221] particularly as these three categories of disease fit well with the therapeutic regimens available to the clinician, namely, further antileukaemic drugs, antimicrobials and corticosteroids respectively. It matters little to patient management that the pathological changes induced by radiotherapy and antileukaemic drugs are virtually identical, or that they are difficult to distinguish from some of the features of graft-versus-host disease.

Leukaemic infiltration of the lungs initially involves the bronchioloalveolar bundles, interlobular septa and pleura, wherein run the lymphatics, but it later spills out into the air spaces. Micronodular aggregates of leukaemic cells may form, as in secondary involvement of the lung by lymphoma,[209] and rarely myeloid leukaemia may present as a granulocytic sarcoma of the lungs.[222–224] In some cases of myeloid leukaemia coming to autopsy with very high white blood cell counts, diffuse accumulations of leukaemic cells are found filling minor blood vessels, especially those of the lungs, a process known as leukostasis.[225] Lysis of these many leukaemic cells may develop within 48 hours of the initiation of chemotherapy, releasing toxic metabolites that may ultimately lead to diffuse alveolar damage.[226] Chronic lymphocytic leukemia may also occasionally extend into the lung parenchyma in a bronchiolocentric fashion, mimicking bronchiolitis.[227] High-grade transformation (Richter syndrome) causing bronchial obstruction due to massive peribronchial lymphadenopathy and bronchial infiltration is also described.[228]

The spectrum of opportunistic infection is wide but, as well as the common bacterial pneumonias, invasive aspergillosis, cytomegalovirus infection and *Pneumocystis* pneumonia are particularly common.[220,229–231] Herpes, parainfluenza and respiratory syncytial virus pneumonias are also recorded.[231–234] Infection is a likely cause of the bronchiolitis obliterans organising pneumonia that has been reported in bone marrow recipients.[235–237]

The pathology in the cytotoxic group consists of interstitial pneumonitis, diffuse alveolar damage and vascular disease.[38,217–220] It carries a high mortality.[238] Biopsy shows lymphocytic infiltration and fibrosis of the alveolar walls, oedema, fibrinous exudates, haemorrhage and hyaline membranes. Regenerating alveolar epithelium may show atypia, regardless of whether cytomegalovirus is present.[239] Small blood vessels show organising thrombus and intimal thickening, sometimes resulting in pulmonary veno-occlusive disease.[240,241] It is probable that such changes reflect the toxicity of antileukaemic drugs or whole-body irradiation rather than graft-versus-host disease for they occur in the absence of the better-known extrapulmonary manifestations of this condition and occur with syngeneic as well as allogeneic grafts.[242,243] However, some patients develop obstructive airway disease a year or more after the marrow transplant, and this may be a manifestation of graft-versus-host disease[211,244–249] mediated by tumour necrosis factor.[250] Biopsy shows lymphocytic bronchiolitis and bronchitis with bronchiolitis obliterans of constrictive pattern.[237,244,246,248,251] Lymphoid interstitial pneumonia is also recorded and it is suggested that this is also a manifestation of graft-versus-host disease.[38,252]

Late manifestations of bone marrow transplantation include the development of solid tumours but the risk of lung cancer does not appear to be increased.[253] However, impaired lung function of uncertain nature can be detected in many long-term survivors who are free of respiratory symptoms.[254]

ANGIOFOLLICULAR LYMPH NODE HYPERPLASIA (GIANT LYMPH NODE HYPERPLASIA, CASTLEMAN'S DISEASE)

Clinical features and prognosis

Angiofollicular lymph node hyperplasia typically affects mediastinal lymph nodes but the condition has also been reported in the trachea,[255] the lung,[256–258] the pleura[259] and the chest wall,[260] in addition to many

extrathoracic sites. Some patients have multicentric disease. Two histological patterns are described, hyaline-vascular and plasma cell. The hyaline-vascular pattern is much the commoner. It is seen more often in the localised form of the disease and generally forms a mass lesion that is either asymptomatic or causes pressure effects. The plasma cell pattern is more often seen in multicentric disease. This is a systemic disease that is characterised by fever, sweating, fatigue, anaemia, lymphadenopathy, hepatosplenomegaly, skin rashes, an elevated erythrocyte sedimentation rate, polyclonal hypergammaglobulinaemia and bone marrow plasmacytosis. Pulmonary involvement results in diffuse reticulonodular infiltrates involving the bronchovascular bundles and interlobular septa, often accompanied by thin-walled cysts and occasionally by subpleural nodules or bronchiectasis.[258,261] In contrast to the solitary form of the disease, which is quite benign and usually cured by surgery, the multicentric variety has an aggressive course with a mean survival of 5 years: some patients with multicentric disease develop lymphoma.[262–265] Others are AIDS patients who are also suffering from Kaposi's sarcoma and in these patients DNA sequences of the Kaposi sarcoma virus (human herpesvirus-8) have been identified within the Castleman's disease, raising the possibility of this virus playing a causative role in both diseases.[266] The same virus is incriminated in body cavity-based lymphoma (see p. 734), which is also recorded in association with multicentric Castleman's disease.[267]

Pathological features

In the hyaline-vascular variant, which is the type most likely to be seen in the lungs, there are prominent lymphoid follicles of abnormal pattern. The germinal centres are reduced in size and contain increased numbers of follicular dendritic cells and reduced numbers of follicular centre cells. The reduced germinal centres are surrounded by an expanded layer of mantle cells arranged in concentric layers, resulting in an onion-skin appearance. Blood vessels enter the germinal centres while between the follicles there are increased numbers of high-endothelial venules and clusters of plasmacytoid monocytes (Fig. 12.4.20).

The plasma cell variant is characterised by a dense interstitial infiltrate of plasma cells and lymphocytes (Fig. 12.4.21).[258] It overlaps

Figure 12.4.20 Hyaline vascular variant of Castleman's disease. Germinal centres within the bronchial mucosa-associated lymphoid tissue (MALT) contain prominent hyalinised capillaries.

Figure 12.4.21 Plasma cell variant of Castleman's disease. (A) Lymphoid cells infiltrate the parenchymal interstitium and an interlobular septum. (B) The infiltrate is markedly plasma cell-rich and proved to be polyclonal in nature.

histologically with both lymphoid interstitial pneumonia and marginal-zone lymphoma of MALT origin. Ancillary investigations are required to exclude the latter, along the line of those undertaken for nodular lymphoid hyperplasia, as the lesions may form solid masses that are rich in plasma cells and therefore mimic plasmacytoid vari-

ants of lymphoma. Such nodularity argues against lymphoid interstitial pneumonia, which does not usually have aggregations of plasma cells. Ultimately the diagnosis may be easier to make on any lymph nodes that may be involved.

REFERENCES

1. World Health Organization. Tumours of the lung, pleura, thymus and heart. Lyons: IARC Press; 2004.

2. Cordier JF, Chailleux E, Lauque D, et al. Primary pulmonary lymphomas – a clinical study of 70 cases in nonimmunocompromised patients. Chest 1993;103:201–8.

3. Fiche M, Capron F, Berger F, et al. Primary pulmonary non-Hodgkin's lymphomas. Histopathology 1995;26:529–37.

4. Nicholson AG, Wotherspoon AC, Diss TC, et al. Pulmonary B-cell non-Hodgkin's lymphomas. The value of immunohistochemistry and gene analysis in diagnosis. Histopathology 1995;26:395–403.

5. Kurtin PJ, Myers JL, Adlakha H, et al. Pathologic and clinical features of primary pulmonary extranodal marginal zone B-cell lymphoma of MALT type. Amer J Surg Pathol 2001;25:997–1008.

6. Begueret H, Vergier B, Parrens M, et al. Primary lung small B-cell lymphoma versus lymphoid hyperplasia – Evaluation of diagnostic criteria in 26 cases. Amer J Surg Pathol 2002;26:76–81.

7. Wong KF, Chan JK, Ng CS, et al. CD56 (NKH1)-positive hematolymphoid

malignancies: an aggressive neoplasm featuring frequent cutaneous/mucosal involvement, cytoplasmic azurophilic granules, and angiocentricity. Hum Pathol 1992;23:798–804.

8. Laohaburanakit P, Hardin KA. NK/T cell lymphoma of the lung: a case report and review of literature. Thorax 2006;61:267–70.

9. Shah RN, Ozden O, Yeldandi A, et al. Follicular dendritic cell tumor presenting in the lung: A case report. Hum Pathol 2001;32:745–9.

10. Kovacs RB, Sattar HA, Krausz T, et al. Primary follicular dendritic cell sarcoma of the lung. Histopathology 2006;49:431–3.

11. Denning KL, Olson PR, Maley RH Jr, et al. Primary pulmonary follicular dendritic cell neoplasm: a case report and review of the literature. Arch Pathol Lab Med 2009;133:643–7.

12. Kudo H, Morinaga S, Shimosato Y, et al. Solitary mast cell tumor of the lung. Cancer 1988;61:2089–94.

13. Li XH. Case for the panel. Microvillous structure in a mast cell tumor of lung. Ultrastruct Pathol 1990;14:95–100.

14. Julg B, Weidner S, Mayr D. Pulmonary manifestation of a Langerhans cell sarcoma: case report and review of the literature. Virchows Archiv 2006;448:369–74.

15. Li G, Hansmann M-L, Zwingers T, et al. Primary lymphomas of the lung: morphological, immunohistochemical and clinical features. Histopathology 1990;16:519–31.

Intrapulmonary lymph nodes and lymphoid hyperplasia

16. Trapnell DH. Recognition and incidence of intrapulmonary lymph nodes. Thorax 1964;19:44–50.

17. Kradin RL, Spirn PW, Mark EJ. Intrapulmonary lymph nodes. Clinical, radiologic and pathologic features. Chest 1985;87:662–7.

18. Yokomise H, Mizuno H, Ike O, et al. Importance of intrapulmonary lymph nodes in the differential diagnosis of small pulmonary nodular shadows. Chest 1998;113:703–6.

19. Nicholson AG, Wotherspoon AC, Diss TC, et al. Reactive pulmonary lymphoid disorders. Histopathology 1995;26:405–12.

20. Travis WD, Galvin JR. Non-neoplastic pulmonary lymphoid lesions. Thorax 2001;56:964–71.

21. Yousem SA, Colby TV, Carrington CB. Follicular bronchitis/bronchiolitis. Hum Pathol 1985;16:700–6.

22. Nicholson AG. Lymphoproliferative lung disease. In: Corrin B, editor. Pathology of Lung Tumors. London: Churchill Livingstone; 1997. p. 213–24.

23. Kradin RL, Mark EJ. Benign lymphoid disorders of the lung with a theory regarding their development. Hum Pathol 1983;14:857–67.

24. Scully RE, McNeely WF, McNeely BU, et al. A 30-year-old man with a dry cough, dyspnea, and nodular pulmonary lesions – diffuse lymphoid hyperplasia of lungs, peribronchiolar (follicular bronchiolitis) and interstitial (lymphocytic interstitial pneumonitis). N Engl J Med 1993;328:1696–705.

25. Fortoul TI, Cano Valle F, Oliva E, et al. Follicular bronchiolitis in association with connective tissue diseases. Lung 1985;163:305–14.

26. Liebow AA, Carrington CB. Diffuse pulmonary lymphoreticular infiltrations associated with dysproteinaemia. Med Clin North Am 1973;57:809–43.

27. Strimlan CV, Rosenov EC, Divertie MB, et al. Pulmonary manifestations of Sjögren's syndrome. Chest 1976;70:354–61.

28. Cha SI, Fessler MB, Cool CD, et al. Lymphoid interstitial pneumonia: clinical features, associations and prognosis. Eur Respir J 2006;28:364–9.

29. Levison AI, Hopewell PC, Stites DP, et al. Coexistent lymphoid interstitial pneumonia, pernicious anaemia and agammaglobulinaemia; comment on autoimmune pathogenesis. Arch Intern Med 1976;136:213–16.

30. DeCouteau WE, Tourville D, Ambrus JL, et al. Lymphoid interstitial pneumonia and autoerythrocyte sensitisation syndrome. Arch Intern Med 1974;134:519–22.

31. Helman CA, Keeton GR, Benatar SR. Lymphoid interstitial pneumonia with associated chronic active hepatitis and renal tubular acidosis. Am Rev Respir Dis 1977;115:161–4.

32. Koss MN, Hochholzer L, Langloss JM, et al. Lymphoid interstitial pneumonia: clinicopathological and immunopathological findings in 18 cases. Pathology 1987;19:178–85.

33. Chatte G, Streichenberger N, Boillot O, et al. Lymphocytic bronchitis/bronchiolitis in a patient with primary biliary cirrhosis. Eur Respir J 1995;8:176–9.

34. Solal-Celigny P, Couderc LJ, Herman P, et al. Lymphoid interstitial pneumonitis in acquired immunodeficiency syndrome-related complex. Am Rev Respir Dis 1985;131:956–60.

35. Grieco MH, Chinoy-Achara P. Lymphocytic interstitial pneumonia associated with the acquired immune deficiency syndrome. Am Rev Respir Dis 1985;131:952–5.

36. Morris JC, Rosen MJ, Marchevsky A, et al. Lymphocytic interstitial pneumonia in patients at risk from the acquired immune deficiency syndrome. Chest 1987;91:63–7.

37. Joshi VV. Pathology of AIDS in children. Pathol Annu 1989;24:355–81.

38. Perreault C, Cousineau S, D'Angelo G, et al. Lymphoid interstitial pneumonia after allogeneic bone marrow transplantation: a possible manifestation of chronic graft-versus-host disease. Cancer 1985;55:1–9.

39. Howling SJ, Hansell DM, Wells AU, et al. Follicular bronchiolitis: thin-section CT and histologic findings. Radiology 1999;212:637–42.

40. Romero S, Barroso E, Gil J, et al. Follicular bronchiolitis: clinical and pathologic findings in six patients. Lung 2003;181:309–19.

41. Liebow AA, Carrington CB. The interstitial pneumonias. In: Simon M, editor. Frontiers of Pulmonary Radiology. New York: Grune & Stratton; 1969. p. 102–41.

42. O'Brodovich HM, Moser MM, Lu L. Familial lymphoid interstitial pneumonia: a long-term follow up. Pediatrics 1980;65:523–8.

43. Thomas H, Risma KA, Graham TB, et al. A kindred of children with interstitial lung disease. Chest 2007;132:221–30.

44. Montes T, Tomasi TB, Noebreu TH, et al. Lymphoid interstitial pneumonia with monoclonal gammopathy. Am Rev Respir Dis 1968;98:277–80.

45. Strimlan CV, Rosenow EC, Weiland LH, et al. Lymphocytic interstitial pneumonitis. Ann Intern Med 1978;88:616–21.

46. Church JA, Isaacs H, Saxon A, et al. Lymphoid interstitial pneumonitis and hypogammaglobulinemia. Am Rev Respir Dis 1981;124:491–8.

47. Swigris JJ, Berry GJ, Raffin TA, et al. Lymphoid interstitial pneumonia – A narrative review. Chest 2002;122: 2150–64.

48. Desai SR, Nicholson AG, Stewart S, et al. Benign pulmonary lymphocytic infiltration and amyloidosis: computed tomographic and pathologic features in three cases. J Thorac Imaging 1997;12:215–20.

49. Johkoh T, Muller NL, Pickford HA, et al. Lymphocytic interstitial pneumonia: thin-section CT findings in 22 patients. Radiology 1999;212:567–72.

50. Johkoh T, Ichikado K, Akira M, et al. Lymphocytic interstitial pneumonia: follow-up CT findings in 14 patients. J Thorac Imaging 2000;15:162–7.

51. Kramer MR, Saldana MJ, Ramos M, et al. High titers of Epstein–Barr virus antibodies in adult patients with lymphocytic interstitial pneumonitis associated with AIDS. Respir Med 1992;86:49–52.

52. Barbera JA, Hayashi S, Hegele RG, et al. Detection of Epstein–Barr virus in lymphocytic interstitial pneumonia by in situ hybridization. Am Rev Respir Dis 1992;145:940–6.

53. Kaan PM, Hegele RG, Hayashi S, et al. Expression of bcl-2 and Epstein–Barr virus LMP1 in lymphocytic interstitial pneumonia. Thorax 1997;52:12–16.

54. Itescu S, Brancato LJ, Winchester R. A sicca syndrome in HIV infection: association with HLA-DR5 and CD8 lymphocytosis. Lancet 1989;ii:466–8.

55. Travis WD, Fox CH, Devaney KO, et al. Lymphoid pneumonitis in 50 adult patients infected with the human immunodeficiency virus – lymphocytic interstitial pneumonitis versus nonspecific interstitial pneumonitis. Hum Pathol 1992;23:529–41.

56. Koga M, Umemoto Y, Nishikawa M, et al. A case of lymphoid interstitial pneumonia in a 3-month-old boy not associated with HIV infection: Immunohistochemistry of lung biopsy specimens and serum transforming growth factor-beta 1 assay. Pathol Int 1997;47:698–702.

57. Kurosu K, Yumoto N, Rom WN, et al. Aberrant expression of immunoglobulin heavy chain genes in Epstein–Barr virus-negative, human immunodeficiency virus-related lymphoid interstitial pneumonia. Lab Invest 2000;80: 1891–903.

58. Kurosu K, Yumoto N, Furukawa M, et al. Third complementarity-determining-region sequence analysis of lymphocytic interstitial pneumonia: most cases demonstrate a minor monoclonal population hidden among normal lymphocyte clones. Am J Respir Crit Care Med 1997;155:1453–60.

59. Nicholson AG, Kim H, Corrin B, et al. The value of classifying interstitial pneumonitis in childhood according to defined histological patterns. Histopathology 1998;33:203–11.

60. TeruyaFeldstein J, Kingma DW, Weiss A, et al. Chemokine gene expression and clonal analysis of B cells in tissues involved by lymphoid interstitial pneumonitis from HIV-infected pediatric patients. Modern Pathol 2001;14:929–36.

61. Kradin RL, Young RH, Kradin LA, et al. Immunoblastic lymphoma arising in chronic lymphoid hyperplasia of the pulmonary interstitium. Cancer 1982;50:1339–43.

62. Julsrud PR, Brown LR, Li C-Y, et al. Pulmonary processes of mature-appearing lymphocytes: pseudolymphoma, well-differentiated lymphocytic lymphoma and lymphocytic interstitial pneumonitis. Diag Radiology 1978;127:289–96.

63. Kawabuchi B, Tsuchiya S, Nakagawa K, et al. Immunophenotypic and molecular analysis of a case of lymphocytic interstitial pneumonia. Acta Pathol Jpn 1993;43:260–4.

64. Colby TV, Coleman A. The histologic diagnosis of extrinsic allergic alveolitis and

its differential diagnosis. Prog Surg Pathol 1989;10:11–25.

65. Nicholson AG. Lymphocytic interstitial pneumonia and other lymphoproliferative disorders in the lung. Seminars in Respiratory and Critical Care Medicine 2001;22:409–22.

66. Teruya-Feldstein J, Temeck BK, Sloas MM, et al. Pulmonary malignant lymphoma of mucosa-associated lymphoid tissue (MALT) arising in a pediatric HIV-positive patient. Am J Surg Pathol 1995;19:357–63.

67. Dufour V, Wislez M, Bergot E, et al. Improvement of symptomatic human immunodeficiency virus-related lymphoid interstitial pneumonia in patients receiving highly active antiretroviral therapy. Clin Infect Dis 2003;36:e127–30.

68. Abbondanzo SL, Rush W, Bijwaard KE, et al. Nodular lymphoid hyperplasia of the lung – a clinicopathologic study of 14 cases. Amer J Surg Pathol 2000;24:587–97.

68a. Yi E, Aubry MC. Pulmonary pseudoneoplasms. Arch Pathol Lab Med 2010;13:417–26.

69. Addis BJ, Hyjek E, Isaacson PG. Primary pulmonary lymphoma: a re-appraisal of its histogenesis and its relationship to pseudolymphoma and lymphoid interstitial pneumonia. Histopathology 1988;13:1–17.

Lymphoproliferative disease complicating severe immune impairment

70. Di Carlo EF, Amberson JB, Metroka CE, et al. Malignant lymphomas and the acquired immunodeficiency syndrome. Evaluation of 30 cases using a working formulation. Arch Pathol Lab Med 1986;110:1012–16.

71. Nalesnik MA, Jaffe R, Starzl TE, et al. The pathology of posttransplant lymphoproliferative disorders occurring in the setting of cyclosporine A-prednisone immunosuppression. Am J Pathol 1988;133:173–92.

72. Yousem SA, Randhawa P, Locker J, et al. Posttransplant lymphoproliferative disorders in heart–lung transplant recipients: primary presentation in the allograft. Hum Pathol 1989;20:361–9.

73. Ray P, Antoine M, MaryKrause M, et al. AIDS-related primary pulmonary lymphoma. Am J Respir Crit Care Med 1998;158:1221–9.

74. Gaidano G, Carbone A, DallaFavera R. Pathogenesis of AIDS-related lymphomas: Molecular and histogenetic heterogeneity. Am J Pathol 1998;152:623–30.

75. Hamilton-Dutoit SJ, Pallesen G, Franzmann MB, et al. AIDS-related lymphoma – histopathology, immunophenotype, and association with Epstein–Barr virus as demonstrated by in situ nucleic acid hybridization. Am J Pathol 1991;138:149–63.

76. Kamel OW, van de Rijn M, Lebrun DP, et al. Lymphoid neoplasms in patients with rheumatoid arthritis and dermatomyositis: frequency of Epstein–Barr virus and other features associated with immunosuppression. Hum Pathol 1994;25:638–43.

77. Thomas JA, Crawford DH, Burke M. Clinicopathologic implications of Epstein–Barr virus related B cell lymphoma in immunocompromised patients. J Clin Pathol 1995;48:287–90.

78. Baumforth KRN, Young LS, Flavell KJ, et al. Demystified … The Epstein–Barr virus and its association with human cancers. J Clin Pathol Mol Pathol 1999;52:307–22.

79. Rezk SA, Weiss LM. Epstein–Barr virus-associated lymphoproliferative disorders. Human Pathology 2007;38:1293–304.

80. Ioachim HL, Dorsett B, Cronin W, et al. Acquired immunodeficiency syndrome-associated lymphomas – clinical, pathologic, immunologic, and viral characteristics of 111 cases. Hum Pathol 1991;22:659–73.

81. Haque AK, Myers JL, Hudnall SD, et al. Pulmonary lymphomatoid granulomatosis in acquired immunodeficiency syndrome: lesions with Epstein–Barr virus infection. Mod Pathol 1998;11:347–56.

Marginal zone B-cell lymphoma of MALT type and diffuse large B-cell non-Hodgkin lymphoma

82. Valdez R, Finn WG, Ross CW, et al. Waldenström macroglobulinemia caused by extranodal marginal zone B-cell lymphoma – A report of six cases. Am J Clin Pathol 2001;116:683–90.

83. King LJ, Padley SP, Wotherspoon AC, et al. Pulmonary MALT lymphoma: imaging findings in 24 cases. Eur Radiol 2000;10:1932–8.

84. Davis WB, Gadek JE. Detection of pulmonary lymphoma by bronchoalveolar lavage. Chest 1987;91:787–90.

85. Sprague RI, deBlois GG. Small lymphocytic pulmonary lymphoma. Diagnosis by transthoracic fine needle aspiration. Chest 1989;96:929–30.

86. Betsuyaku T, Munakata M, Yamaguchi E, et al. Establishing diagnosis of pulmonary malignant lymphoma by gene rearrangement analysis of lymphocytes in bronchoalveolar lavage fluid. Am J Respir Crit Care Med 1994;149:526–9.

87. Meda BA, Buss DH, Woodruff RD, et al. Diagnosis and subclassification of primary and recurrent lymphoma. The usefulness and limitations of combined fine-needle aspiration cytomorphology and flow cytometry. Am J Clin Pathol 2000;113:688–99.

88. Murphy BA, Meda BA, Buss DH, et al. Marginal zone and mantle cell lymphomas: assessment of cytomorphology in subtyping small B-cell lymphomas. Diagn Cytopathol 2003;28:126–30.

89. Richmond I, Pritchard GE, Ashcroft T, et al. Bronchus associated lymphoid tissue (BALT) in human lung – its distribution in smokers and non-smokers. Thorax 1993;48:1130–4.

90. Nicholson AG, Wotherspoon AC, Jones AL, et al. Pulmonary B-cell non-Hodgkin's lymphoma associated with autoimmune disorders: a clinicopathological review of six cases. Eur Respir J 1996;9:2022–5.

91. Symmons DP. Neoplasms of the immune system in rheumatoid arthritis. Am J Med 1985;78:22–8.

92. Frizzera G. Immunosuppression, autoimmunity, and lymphoproliferative disorders. Hum Pathol 1994;25:627–9.

93. Inadome Y, Ikezawa T, Oyasu R, et al. Malignant lymphoma of bronchus-associated lymphoid tissue (BALT) coexistent with pulmonary tuberculosis. Pathol Int 2001;51:807–11.

94. Luppi M, Longo G, Ferrari MG, et al. Additional neoplasms and HCV infection in low-grade lymphoma of MALT type. Br J Haematol 1996;94:373–5.

95. Wotherspoon AC, Finn TM, Isaacson PG. Trisomy 3 in low-grade B-cell lymphomas of mucosa-associated lymphoid tissue. Blood 1995;85:2000–4.

96. Kubonishi I, Sugito S, Kobayashi M, et al. A unique chromosome translocation, t(11;12;18)(q21;q13;q21) [correction of t(11;12;18)(q13;q13;q12)], in primary lung lymphoma. Cancer Genet Cytogenet 1995;82:54–6.

97. Ye H, Liu H, Attygalle A, et al. Variable frequencies of t(11;18)(q21;q21) in MALT lymphomas of different sites: significant association with CagA strains of H pylori in gastric MALT lymphoma. Blood 2003;102:1012–18.

98. Ohshima K, Muta H, Kawasaki C, et al. Bcl10 expression, rearrangement and mutation in MALT lymphoma: correlation with expression of nuclear factor-kappaB. Int J Oncol 2001;19:283–9.

99. Bacon CM, Du MQ, Dogan A. Mucosa-associated lymphoid tissue (MALT) lymphoma: a practical guide for pathologists. J Clin Pathol 2007;60:361–72.

100. Rawal A, Finn WG, Schnitzer B, et al. Site-specific morphologic differences in extranodal marginal zone B-cell lymphomas. Arch Pathol Lab Med 2007;131:1673–8.

101. Colby TV, Carrington CB. Pulmonary lymphomas simulating lymphomatoid granulomatosis. Am J Surg Pathol 1982;6:19–32.

102. Perry LJ, Florio R, Dewar A, et al. Giant lamellar bodies as a feature of pulmonary low-grade MALT lymphomas. Histopathology 2000;36:240–4.

103. Dacic S, Colby TV, Yousem SA. Nodular amyloidoma and primary pulmonary lymphoma with amyloid production: A

differential diagnostic problem. Modern Pathol 2000;13:934–40.

104. Lim JK, Lacy MQ, Kurtin PJ, et al. Pulmonary marginal zone lymphoma of MALT type as a cause of localised pulmonary amyloidosis. J Clin Pathol 2001;54:642–6.

105. Ortiz-Hidalgo C, Wright DH. The morphological spectrum of monocytoid B-cell lymphoma and its relationship to lymphomas of mucosa-associated lymphoid tissue. Histopathology 1992;21:555–61.

106. Ngan BY, Warnke RA, Wilson M, et al. Monocytoid B-cell lymphoma: a study of 36 cases. Hum Pathol 1991;22:409–21.

107. Moran CA, Suster S, Fishback NF, et al. Primary intrapulmonary thymoma: a clinicopathologic and immunohistochemical study of eight cases. Am J Surg Pathol 1995;19:304–12.

108. Uppal R, Goldstraw P. Primary pulmonary lymphoma. Lung Cancer 1992;8:95–100.

109. Borie R, Wislez M, Thabut G, et al. Clinical characteristics and prognostic factors of pulmonary MALT lymphoma. Eur Respir J 2009;34:1408–16.

110. Orchard TR, Eraut CD, Davison AG. Non-Hodgkin's lymphoma arising in cryptogenic fibrosing alveolitis. Thorax 1998;53:228–9.

111. Sabourin JC, Kanavaros P, Briere J, et al. Epstein–Barr virus (EBV) genomes and EBV-encoded latent membrane protein (LMP) in pulmonary lymphomas occurring in nonimmunocompromised patients. Am J Surg Pathol 1993;17:995–1002.

Lymphomatoid granulomatosis

112. Liebow AA, Carrington CRB, Friedman PJ. Lymphomatoid granulomatosis. Hum Pathol 1972;3:457–558.

113. Liebow AA. Pulmonary angiitis and granulomatosis. Am Rev Respir Dis 1973;108:1–18.

114. Katzenstein ALA, Carrington CB, Liebow AA. Lymphomatoid granulomatosis. A clinicopathologic study of 152 cases. Cancer 1979;43:360–73.

115. Jaffe ES. Post-thymic lymphoid neoplasia. Surgical Pathology of the Lymph Nodes and Related Organs. Major Problems in Pathology No. 16. Philadelphia: Saunders; 1985.

116. Lipford EH, Margolick JB, Longo DL, et al. Angiocentric immunoproliferative lesions: a clinicopathologic spectrum of post-thymic T-cell proliferations. Blood 1988;72:1674–81.

117. Harris TJ, Bhan AK, Murphy GF, et al. Lymphomatoid papulosis and lymphomatoid granulomatosis: T cell subset populations. Am J Invest Dermatol 1981;76:326.

118. Gaulard P, Henni T, Marolleau J-P, et al. Lethal midline granuloma (polymorphic reticulosis) and lymphomatoid granulomatosis – evidence for a

monoclonal T-cell lymphoproliferative disorder. Cancer 1988;62:705–10.

119. Nichols PW, Koss M, Levine AM, et al. Lymphomatoid granulomatosis: a T-cell disorder. Am J Med 1982;72:467–71.

120. Tanaka Y, Sasaki Y, Kurozumi H, et al. Angiocentric immunoproliferative lesion associated with chronic active Epstein–Barr virus infection in an 11-year-old boy. Clonotopic proliferation of Epstein–Barr virus-bearing CD4+ T lymphocytes. Am J Surg Pathol 1994;18:623–31.

121. Guinee D, Jaffe E, Kingma D, et al. Pulmonary lymphomatoid granulomatosis – evidence for a proliferation of Epstein–Barr virus infected B-lymphocytes with a prominent T-cell component and vasculitis. Am J Surg Pathol 1994;18:753–64.

122. Myers JL, Kurtin PJ, Katzenstein ALA, et al. Lymphomatoid granulomatosis: evidence of immunophenotypic diversity and relationship to Epstein–Barr virus infection. Am J Surg Pathol 1995;19:1300–12.

123. Nicholson AG, Wotherspoon AC, Diss TC, et al. Lymphomatoid granulomatosis: evidence that some cases represent Epstein–Barr virus-associated B-cell lymphoma. Histopathology 1996;29:317–24.

124. Taniere P, ThivoletBejui F, Vitrey D, et al. Lymphomatoid granulomatosis – a report on four cases: evidence for B phenotype of the tumoral cells. Eur Resp J 1998;12:102–6.

125. Katzenstein AA, Peiper SC. Detection of Epstein–Barr virus genomes in lymphomatoid granulomatosis: analysis of 29 cases by the polymerase chain reaction. Mod Pathol 1990;3:435–41.

126. Peiper SC. Angiocentric lymphoproliferative disorders of the respiratory system: incrimination of Epstein–Barr virus in pathogenesis. Blood 1993;82:687–90.

127. Wilson WH, Kingma DW, Raffeld M, et al. Association of lymphomatoid granulomatosis with Epstein–Barr viral infection of B lymphocytes and response to interferon-alpha 2b. Blood 1996;87:4531–7.

128. Saldana MJ, Patchefsky AS, Israel HI, et al. Pulmonary angiitis and granulomatosis: the relationship between histological features, organ involvement and response to treatment. Hum Pathol 1977;8:391–409.

129. Israel HL, Patchefsky AJ, Saldana MJ. Wegener's granulomatosis, lymphomatoid granulomatosis and benign lymphocytic angiitis and granulomatosis. Ann Intern Med 1977;87:691–9.

130. Gracey DR, DeRemee RA, Colby TV, et al. Benign lymphocytic angiitis and granulomatosis: experience with three cases. Mayo Clin Proc 1988;63:323–31.

131. Norton AJ. Angiocentric lymphoma. Current Diagnostic Pathology 1994;1:158–66.

132. Bone RC, Vernon M, Sobonya RE, et al. Lymphomatoid granulomatosis: report of a case and review of the literature. Am J Med 1978;65:709–16.

133. Sordillo PP, Epremian B, Koziner B, et al. Lymphomatoid granulomatosis. An analysis of clinical and immunologic characteristics. Cancer 1982;49:2070–6.

134. Fauci AS, Haynes BF, Costa J, et al. Lymphomatoid granulomatosis. Prospective clinical and therapeutic experience over 10 years. N Engl J Med 1982;306:68–74.

135. Koss MN, Hochholzer L, Langloss JM, et al. Lymphomatoid granulomatosis: a clinicopathologic and immunopathologic study of 42 patients. Pathology 1986;18:283–8.

136. Key S, Fu Y-S, Minars N, et al. Lymphomatoid granulomatosis of the skin: light microscopic and ultrastructural studies. Cancer 1974;34:1675–82.

137. Frazier AA, Rosado-de-Christenson ML, Galvin JR, et al. Pulmonary angiitis and granulomatosis: radiologic–pathologic correlation. Radiographics 1998;18:687–710.

138. Klein FA. Lymphomatoid granulomatosis masquerading as hypernephroma with lung masses. J Urol 1984;131:942–4.

139. Teruya Feldstein J, Jaffe ES, Burd PR, et al. The role of Mig, the monokine induced by interferon-gamma, and IP-10, the interferon-gamma-inducible protein-10, in tissue necrosis and vascular damage associated with Epstein–Barr virus-positive lymphoproliferative disease. Blood 1997;90:4099–105.

140. Ilowite NT, Fligner CL, Ochs HD, et al. Pulmonary angiitis with atypical lymphoreticular infiltrates in Wiskott–Aldrich syndrome: possible relationship to lymphomatoid granulomatosis and EBV infection. Clin Immunol Immunopathol 1986;41:479–84.

141. Colby TV. Central nervous system lymphomatoid granulomatosis in AIDS? Hum Pathol 1989;20:301–2.

142. Naschitz JE, Yeshurun D, Grishkan A, et al. Lymphomatoid granulomatosis of the lung in a patient with agnogenic myeloid metaplasia. Respiration 1984;45:316–20.

143. Bekassy AN, Cameron R, Garwicz S, et al. Lymphomatoid granulomatosis during treatment of acute lymphoblastic lymphoma in a 6 year old girl. Am J Paed Hematol -Oncol 1985;7:377–80.

144. Imai Y, Yamamoto K, Suzuki K, et al. Lymphomatoid granulomatosis (LYG) occurring in a patient with follicular lymphoma during remission. Jpn J Clin Hematol 1992;33:507–13.

145. Swerdlow SH. Post-transplant lymphoproliferative disorders: a morphologic, phenotypic and genotypic

146. Burke MM. Complications of heart and lung transplantation and of cardiac surgery. In: Anthony PP, MacSween RNM, editors. Recent Advances in Histopathology. vol. 16. New York: Churchill Livingstone; 1994. p. 95–122.

147. Morice WG, Kurtin PJ, Myers JL. Expression of cytolytic lymphocyte-associated antigens in pulmonary lymphomatoid granulomatosis. Am J Clin Pathol 2002;118:391–8.

148. Guinee DG Jr, Perkins SL, Travis WD, et al. Proliferation and cellular phenotype in lymphomatoid granulomatosis: implications of a higher proliferation index in B cells. Am J Surg Pathol 1998;22:1093–100.

149. Bernstein ML, Reece ER, de Chadarevian JP, et al. Bone marrow transplantation in lymphomatoid granulomatosis. Report of a case. Cancer 1986;58:969–72.

150. Jordan K, Grothey A, Grothe W, et al. Successful treatment of mediastinal lymphomatoid granulomatosis with rituximab monotherapy. Eur J Haematol 2005;74:263–6.

Hodgkin disease

151. Berkman N, Breuer R. Pulmonary involvement in lymphoma. Respir Med 1993;87:85–92.

152. Radin AI. Primary pulmonary Hodgkin's disease. Cancer 1990;65:550–63.

153. Kern WGH, Crepeau AG, Jones JC. Primary Hodgkin's disease of the lung. Cancer 1961;14:1151–65.

154. Yousem SA, Weiss LM, Colby TV. Primary pulmonary Hodgkin's disease. Cancer 1986;57:1217–24.

155. Schee ACvd, Dinkla BA, Knapen Av. Primary pulmonary manifestation of Hodgkin's disease. Respiration 1990;57:127–8.

156. Pinson P, Joos G, Praet M, et al. Primary pulmonary Hodgkin's disease. Respiration 1992;59:314–6.

157. Boshnakova T, Michailova V, Koss M, et al. Primary pulmonary Hodgkin's disease – report of two cases. Resp Med 2000;94:830–1.

158. Harper PG, Fisher C, McLennan K, et al. Presentation of Hodgkin's disease as an endobronchial lesion. Cancer 1984;53:147–50.

159. Daly PA, O'Brian DS, Robinson I et al. Hodgkin's disease with a granulomatous pulmonary presentation mimicking sarcoidosis. Thorax 1988;43:407–9.

Plasmacytoma

160. Okada S, Ohtsuki H, Midorikawa O, et al. Bronchial plasmacytoma identified by immunoperoxidase technique on paraffin embedded section. Acta Pathol Jpn 1982;32:149–55.

161. Dux S, Pitlik S, Rosenfeld JB, et al. Localised visceral immunocytoma associated with serological findings suggesting systemic lupus erythematosus. BMJ 1984;288:898–9.

162. Roikjaer O, Thomsen JK. Plasmacytoma of the lung. A case report describing two tumors of different immunologic type in a single patient. Cancer 1986;58:2671–4.

163. Morinaga S, Watanabe H, Gemma A, et al. Plasmacytoma of the lung associated with nodular deposits of immunoglobulin. Am J Surg Pathol 1987;11:989–95.

164. Brackett LE, Myers JR, Sherman CB. Laser treatment of endobronchial extramedullary plasmacytoma. Chest 1994;106:1276–7.

165. Wise JN, Schaefer RF, Read RC. Primary pulmonary plasmacytoma – a case report. Chest 2001;120:1405.

166. Childness WG, Adie GC. Plasma cell tumors of the mediastinum and lung. J Thorac Surg 1950;19:794–9.

167. Cotton BM, Pinedo JR. Plasma cell tumours of the lung: report of a case. Dis Chest 1952;21:218–21.

168. Herskovic T, Anderson HA, Bayrd ED. Intrathoracic plasmacytomas. Dis Chest 1952;47:1–6.

169. Kernan JA, Meyer BW. Malignant plasmacytoma of the lung with metastases. J Thorac Cardiovasc Surg 1966;51:739–44.

170. Amin R. Extramedullary plasmacytoma of the lung. Cancer 1985;56:152–6.

171. Baroni CD, Mineo TC, Ricci C, et al. Solitary secretory plasmacytoma of the lung in a 14 year old boy. Cancer 1977;40:2329–32.

172. Wile A, Olinger G, Peter JB, et al. Solitary intraparenchymal pulmonary plasmacytoma associated with production of an M-protein. Cancer 1976;37:2338–42.

173. Piard F, Yaziji N, Jarry D, et al. Solitary plasmacytoma of the lung with light chain extracellular deposits: a case report and review of the literature. Histopathology 1998;32:356–61.

174. Kazzaz B, Dewar A, Corrin B. An unusual pulmonary plasmacytoma. Histopathology 1992;21:285–7.

175. Prasad ML, Charney DA, Sarlin J, et al. Pulmonary immunocytoma with massive crystal storing histiocytosis : a case report with review of literature. Am J Surg Pathol 1998;22:1148–53.

176. Jones D, Renshaw AA. Recurrent crystal-storing histiocytosis of the lung in a patient without a clonal lymphoproliferative disorder. Arch Pathol Lab Med 1996;120:978–80.

177. Koss MN, Hochholzer L, Moran CA, et al. Pulmonary plasmacytomas: a clinicopathologic and immunohistochemical study of five cases. Ann Diagn Pathol 1998;2:1–11.

Large cell anaplastic lymphoma

178. Rush WL, Andriko JAW, Taubenberger JK, et al. Primary anaplastic large cell lymphoma of the lung: A clinicopathologic study of five patients. Modern Pathol 2000;13:1285–92.

179. Beltran S, Tomas Labat ME, Ferreras FP. Primary Ki-1 positive anaplastic large cell non-Hodgkin's lymphoma of the lung. A case study and review of the literature. An Med Interna 2001;18:587–90.

180. Guerra J, Echevarria-Escudero M, Barrio N, et al. Primary endobronchial anaplastic large cell lymphoma in a pediatric patient. P R Health Sci J 2006;25:159–61.

181. Yang HB, Li J, Shen T. Primary anaplastic large cell lymphoma of the lung. Report of two cases and literature review. Acta Haematol 2007;118:188–91.

Intravascular lymphoma (angiotropic lymphoma)

182. Wick MR, Mills SE, Scheithauer BW, et al. Reassessment of malignant angioendotheliomatosis. Am J Surg Pathol 1986;10:112–13.

183. Theaker JM, Gatter KC, Esiri MM, et al. Neoplastic angioendotheliomatosis – further evidence supporting a lymphoid origin. Histopathology 1986;10:1261–70.

184. Remberger K, Nawrath-Koll I, Gokel JM, et al. Systemic angioendotheliomatosis of the lung. Pathol Res Pract 1987;182:265–70.

185. Tan TB, Spaander PJ, Blaisse M, et al. Angiotropic large cell lymphoma presenting as interstitial lung disease. Thorax 1988;43:578–9.

186. Yousem SA, Colby TV. Intravascular lymphomatosis presenting in the lung. Cancer 1990;65:349–53.

187. Takamura K, Nasuhara Y, Mishina T, et al. Intravascular lymphomatosis diagnosed by transbronchial lung biopsy. Eur Respir J 1997;10:955–7.

188. Snyder LS, Harmon KR, Estensen RD. Intravascular lymphomatosis (malignant angioendotheliomatosis) presenting as pulmonary hypertension. Chest 1989;96:1199–200.

189. Ko YH, Han JH, Go JH, et al. Intravascular lymphomatosis: a clinicopathological study of two cases presenting as an interstitial lung disease. Histopathology 1997;31:555–62.

190. Walls JG, Hong G, Cox JE, et al. Pulmonary intravascular – lymphomatosis presentation with dyspnea and air trapping. Chest 1999;115:1207–10.

191. Demirer T, Dail DH, Aboulafia DM. Four varied cases of intravascular lymphomatosis and a literature review. Cancer 1994;73:1738–45.

192. Owa M, Koyama J, Asakawa K, et al. Intravascular lymphomatosis presenting as reversible severe pulmonary hypertension. Int J Cardiol 2000;75:283–4.

193. Tsukadaira A, Okubo Y, Ogasawara H, et al. Chromosomal aberrations in intravascular lymphomatosis. Am J Clin Oncol 2002;25:178–81.

Secondary pulmonary involvement by lymphoproliferative disorders

194. Filly R, Blauk N, Castellino RA. Radiographic distribution of intrathoracic disease in previously untreated patients with Hodgkin's disease and non-Hodgkin's lymphoma. Radiology 1976;120: 277–81.

195. Costa MB, Siqueira SA, Saldiva PH, et al. Histologic patterns of lung infiltration of B-cell, T-cell, and Hodgkin lymphomas. Am J Clin Pathol 2004;121:718–26.

196. Zylak CJ, Banerjee R, Galbraith PA, et al. Lung involvement in angioimmunoblastic lymphadenopathy (AIL). Radiology 1976;121:513–9.

197. Iseman MD, Schwarz MI, Stanford RE. Interstitial pneumonia in angio-immunoblastic lymphadenopathy with dysproteinaemia: a case report with special histologic studies. Ann Intern Med 1976;85:752–5.

198. Myers TJ, Cole SR, Pastuszak WT. Angioimmunoblastic lymphadenopathy: pleural-pulmonary disease. Cancer 1978;40:266–71.

199. Chejfec G, Natarelli J, Gould VE. 'Myeloma lung' – A previously unreported complication of multiple myeloma. Hum Pathol 1983;14:558–61.

200. Rausch PG, Herion JC. Pulmonary manifestations of Waldenström's macroglobulinaemia. Am J Hematol 1980;9:201–9.

201. Lin P, Bueso-Ramos C, Wilson CS, et al. Waldenström macroglobulinemia involving extramedullary sites: morphologic and immunophenotypic findings in 44 patients. Am J Surg Pathol 2003;27:1104–13.

202. Schmidt M, Dercken C, Loke O, et al. Pulmonary manifestation of systemic mast cell disease. Eur Resp J 2000;15: 623–5.

203. Rappaport H, Thomas LB. Mycosis fungoides: the pathology of extracutaneous involvement. Cancer 1974;34: 1198–229.

204. Rubin DL, Blank N. Rapid pulmonary dissemination in mycosis fungoides simulating pneumonia. A case report and review of the literature. Cancer 1985;56:649–51.

205. Colby TV, Carrington CB, Mark GJ. Pulmonary involvement in malignant histiocytosis. A clinicopathologic spectrum. Am J Surg Pathol 1981;5:61–73.

206. Wongchaowart B, Kennealy JA, Crissman J, et al. Respiratory failure in malignant histiocytosis. Am Rev Respir Dis 1981;124:640–2.

207. Stempel DA, Volberg FM, Parker BR, et al. Malignant histiocytosis presenting as interstitial pulmonary disease. Am Rev Respir Dis 1982;126:726–8.

208. Colby TV, Carrington CB. Lymphoreticular tumours and infiltrates of the lung. Pathol Annu 1983;18:27–70.

209. Rollins SD, Colby TV. Lung biopsy in chronic lymphocytic leukemia. Arch Pathol Lab Med 1988;112:607–11.

Pulmonary problems in leukaemia

210. Breuer R, Lossos IS, Berkman N, et al. Pulmonary complications of bone marrow transplantation. Respir Med 1993;87:571–9.

211. Sloane JP, Norton J. Invited review – the pathology of bone marrow transplantation. Histopathology 1993;22:201–9.

212. Soubani AO, Miller KB, Hassoun PM. Pulmonary complications of bone marrow transplantation. Chest 1996;109: 1066–77.

213. Roychowdhury M, Pambuccian SE, Aslan DL, et al. Pulmonary complications after bone marrow transplantation: an autopsy study from a large transplantation center. Arch Pathol Lab Med 2005;129:366–71.

214. Orazi A, Hromas RA, Neiman RS, et al. Posttransplantation lymphoproliferative disorders in bone marrow transplant recipients are aggressive diseases with a high incidence of adverse histologic and immunobiologic features. Am J Clin Pathol 1997;107:419–29.

215. Sharma S, Nadrous HF, Peters SG, et al. Pulmonary complications in adult blood and marrow transplant recipients: autopsy findings. Chest 2005;128:1385–92.

216. Afessa B, Litzow MR, Tefferi A. Bronchiolitis obliterans and other late onset non-infectious pulmonary complications in hematopoietic stem cell transplantation. Bone Marrow Transplant 2001;28:425–34.

217. Moir DH, Turner JJ, Ma DDF, et al. Autopsy findings in bone marrow transplantation. Pathology 1982;14:197–204.

218. Sloane JP, Depledge MH, Powles RL, et al. Histopathology of the lung after bone marrow transplantation. J Clin Pathol 1983;36:546–54.

219. Bombi JA, Cardesa A, Llebaria C, et al. Main autopsy findings in bone marrow transplant patients. Arch Pathol Lab Med 1987;111:125–9.

220. Doran HM, Sheppard MN, Collins PW, et al. Pathology of the lung in leukaemia and lymphoma – a study of 87 autopsies. Histopathology 1991;18:211–19.

221. White DA, Wong PW, Downey R. The utility of open lung biopsy in patients with hematologic malignancies. Am J Respir Crit Care Med 2000;161:723–9.

222. Callahan M, Wall S, Askin F, et al. Granulocytic sarcoma presenting as pulmonary nodules and lymphadenopathy. Cancer 1987;60:1902–4.

223. Hicklin GA, Drevyanko TF. Primary granulocytic sarcoma presenting with pleural and pulmonary involvement. Chest 1988;94:655–6.

224. Stafford CM, Herndier B, Yi ES, et al. Granulocytic sarcoma of the tracheobronchial tree: bronchoscopic and pathologic correlation. Respiration 2004;71:529–32.

225. van Buchem MA, Wondergem JH, Kool LJ, et al. Pulmonary leukostasis: radiologic-pathologic study. Radiology 1987;165:739–41.

226. Tryka AF, Godleski JJ, Fanta CH. Leukemic cell lysis pneumonopathy. A complication of treated myeloblastic leukemia. Cancer 1982;50:2763–70.

227. Trisolini R, Lazzari AL, Poletti V. Bronchiolocentric pulmonary involvement due to chronic lymphocytic leukemia. Haematologica 2000;85:1097.

228. Snyder LS, Cherwitz DL, Dykoski RK, et al. Endobronchial Richter's syndrome. A rare manifestation of chronic lymphocytic leukemia. Am Rev Respir Dis 1988;138:980–3.

229. Beschorner WE, Hutchins GM, Burns WH, et al. Cytomegalovirus pneumonia in bone marrow transplant recipients: miliary and diffuse patterns. Am Rev Respir Dis 1980;122:107–14.

230. Stals FS, Steinhoff G, Wagenaar SS, et al. Cytomegalovirus induces interstitial lung disease in allogeneic bone marrow transplant recipient rats independent of acute graft-versus-host response. Lab Invest 1996;74:343–52.

231. Harrington SW, Hooton TM, Hackman RC, et al. An outbreak of respiratory syncytial virus in a bone marrow transplant center. J Infect Dis 1989;158:987–93.

232. Carrigan DR, Drobyski WR, Russler SK, et al. Interstitial pneumonitis associated with human herpesvirus-6 infection after marrow transplantation. Lancet 1991;338:147–9.

233. Wendt CH, Weisdorf DJ, Jordan MC, et al. Parainfluenza virus respiratory infection after bone marrow transplantation. N Engl J Med 1992;326:921–6.

234. Cone RW, Hackman RC, Huang MLW, et al. Human herpesvirus-6 in lung tissue from patients with pneumonitis after bone marrow transplantation. N Engl J Med 1993;329:156–61.

235. Thirman MJ, Devine SM, O'Toole K, et al. Bronchiolitis obliterans organizing pneumonia as a complication of allogeneic bone marrow transplantation. Bone Marrow Transplantation 1992;10:307–11.

236. Thirman MJ, Devine SM, O'Toole K, et al. Bronchiolitis obliterans organizing pneumonia as a complication of allogeneic bone marrow transplantation. Bone Marrow Transplantation 1992;10:307–11.

237. Yousem SA. The histological spectrum of pulmonary graft versus host disease in bone marrow transplant recipients. Hum Pathol 1995;26:668–75.

238. Crawford SW, Hackman RC. Clinical course of idiopathic pneumonia after bone

marrow transplantation. Am Rev Respir Dis 1993;147:1393–400.

239. Elias AD, Mark EJ, Trotman-Dickenson B. A 60-year-old man with pulmonary infiltrates after a bone marrow transplantation – Busulfan pneumonitis. N Engl J Med 1997;337:480–9.

240. Williams LM, Fussell S, Veith RW, et al. Pulmonary veno-occlusive disease in an adult following bone marrow transplantation: case report and review of the literature. Chest 1996;109:1388–91.

241. Hackman RC, Madtes DK, Petersen FB, et al. Pulmonary veno-occlusive disease following bone marrow transplantation. Transplantation 1989;47:989–92.

242. Appelbaum FR, Meyers JD, Fefer A, et al. Nonbacterial nonfungal pneumonia following marrow transplantation in 100 identical twins. Transplantation 1982;33:265–8.

243. Clark JG, Hansen JA, Hertz MI, et al. Idiopathic pneumonia syndrome after bone marrow transplantation. Am Rev Respir Dis 1993;147:1601–6.

244. Roca J, Granena A, Rodriguez-Roisin R, Alvarez P, et al. Fatal airway disease in an adult with chronic graft-versus-host disease. Thorax 1982;37:77–8.

245. Ralph DD, Springmeyer SC, Sullivan KM, et al. Rapidly progressive air-flow obstruction in marrow transplant recipients. Possible association between obliterative bronchiolitis and chronic graft-versus-host disease. Am Rev Respir Dis 1984;129:641–4.

246. Urbanski SJ, Kossakowska AE, Curtis J, et al. Idiopathic small airways pathology in patients with graft-versus-host disease following allogeneic bone marrow transplantation. Am J Surg Pathol 1987;11:965–71.

247. Epler GR. Bronchiolitis obliterans and airway obstruction associated with graft-versus-host disease. Clin Chest Med 1988;9:551–6.

248. Ralph DD, Springmeyer SC, Sullivan KM, et al. Rapidly progressive air-flow obstruction in marrow transplant recipients. Possible association between

obliterative bronchiolitis and chronic graft-versus-host disease. Am Rev Respir Dis 1994;129:641–4.

249. Paz HL, Crilley P, Topolsky DL, et al. Bronchiolitis obliterans after bone marrow transplantation – the effect of preconditioning. Respiration 1993;60:109–14.

250. Piguet PF, Grau GE, Collart MA, et al. Pneumopathies of the graft-versus-host reaction. Alveolitis associated with an increased level of tumor necrosis factor mRNA and chronic interstitial pneumonitis. Lab Invest 1989;61:37.

251. Yokoi T, Hirabayashi N, Ito M, et al. Broncho-bronchiolitis obliterans as a complication of bone marrow transplantation: a clinicopathological study of eight autopsy cases. Virchows Archiv 1997;431:275–82.

252. Perreault C, Coosineau S, D'Angelo G, et al. Lymphoid interstitial pneumonia after allogeneic bone marrow transplantation. Cancer 1985;55:1–9.

253. Curtis RE, Rowlings PA, Deeg HJ, et al. Solid cancers after bone marrow transplantation. N Engl J Med 1997;336:897–904.

254. Cerveri I, Zoia MC, Fulgoni P, et al. Late pulmonary sequelae after childhood bone marrow transplantation. Thorax 1999;54:131–5.

Angiofollicular lymph node hyperplasia (giant lymph node hyperplasia, Castleman's disease)

255. Pham TT, Harrell JH, Harrell JH, et al. Endotracheal Castleman disease: A case report. Chest 2007;131:590–2.

256. Awotedu AA, Otulana BA, Ukoli CO. Giant lymph node hyperplasia of the lung (Castleman's disease) associated with recurrent pleural effusion. Thorax 1990;45:775–6.

257. Barrie JR, English JC, Muller N. Castleman's disease of the lung: radiographic, high-resolution CT, and pathologic findings. Am J Roentgenol 1996;166:1055–6.

258. Iyonaga K, Ichikado K, Muranaka H, et al. Multicentric Castleman's disease manifesting in the lung: clinical, radiographic, and pathologic findings and successful treatment with corticosteroid and cyclophosphamide. Intern Med 2003;42:182–6.

259. Mohamedani AA, Bennett MK. Angiofollicular lymphoid hyperplasia in a pulmonary fissure. Thorax 1985;40:686–7.

260. Matsuda H, Mori M, Yasumoto K, et al. Angiofollicular lymph node hyperplasia arising from the intercostal space. Thorax 1988;43:337–8.

261. Johkoh T, Muller NL, Ichikado K, et al. Intrathoracic multicentric Castleman disease: CT findings in 12 patients. Radiology 1998;209:477–81.

262. Weisenburger DD, Nathwani BN, Winberg CD, et al. Multicentric angiofollicular lymph node hyperplasia: A clinicopathologic study of 16 cases. Hum Pathol 1985;16:162–72.

263. Baruch Y, Ben-Arie Y, Kerner H, et al. Giant lymph node hyperplasia (Castleman's disease): a clinical study of eight patients. Postgrad Med J 1991;67:366–70.

264. Abdelreheim FA, Koss W, Rappaport ES, et al. Coexistence of Hodgkin's disease and giant lymph node hyperplasia of the plasma-cell type (Castleman's disease). Arch Pathol Lab Med 1996;120:91–6.

265. Guihot A, Couderc LJ, Agbalika F, et al. Pulmonary manifestations of multicentric Castleman's disease in HIV infection: a clinical, biological and radiological study. Eur Respir J 2005;26:118–25.

266. Dupin N, Gorin I, Deleuze J, et al. Herpes-like DNA sequences, AIDS-related tumors, and Castleman's disease. New Engl J Med 1995;333:798–9.

267. TeruyaFeldstein J, Zauber P, Setsuda JE, et al. Expression of human herpesvirus-8 oncogene and cytokine homologues in an HIV-seronegative patient with multicentric Castleman's disease and primary effusion lymphoma. Lab Invest 1998;78:1637–42.

12.5   Miscellaneous tumours

Six tumours were listed as miscellaneous in the 2004 World Health Organization/International Association for the Study of Lung Cancer Histological Classification of Lung Tumours, of which we have dealt with two (sclerosing 'haemangioma' and thymoma) in Chapter 12.2 (Other epithelial tumours) and two ('hamartoma' and benign clear cell tumour) in Chapter 12.3 (Soft-tissue tumours), as we believe this reflects their histogenesis more accurately. This leaves only melanoma and germ cell tumours to be considered in this chapter.

MELANOMA

Whereas melanoma commonly metastasises to the lungs, primary bronchopulmonary melanoma is extremely rare. Embryologically, melanocytes derive from the neural crest. They are not a normal feature of the lower respiratory tract and descriptions of a blue naevus[1] and primary melanomas of the bronchi are therefore surprising, particularly one arising in an albino patient.[2–13] Whether these tumours can be presumed to arise from ectopic melanocytes is not entirely clear since melanin production is documented in bronchopulmonary carcinoid tumours,[14–18] which are thought to be of endodermal rather than neural crest origin. Melanin pigmentation has also been recorded in a bronchial schwannoma,[19] a pulmonary blastoma[20] and 'pecomas' such as the benign clear cell tumour of the lung (see p. 625).[21]

Clinical features, treatment and prognosis

Age at presentation ranges from 29 to 80 years (median 51 years) and there is no sex predilection.[7,11] The tumours nearly always involve large bronchi or the trachea and the patients complain of persistent cough and haemoptysis or symptoms attributable to obstructive pneumonia. Treatment is surgical but the prognosis is poor.[10]

Pathological features

Tracheobronchial melanomas are generally polypoid but occasional 'flat' examples are reported.[3] Microscopically, they are identical to those that occur elsewhere, being predominantly pigmented, probably because amelanotic melanomas in the lung are likely to be interpreted as anaplastic carcinomas (Fig. 12.5.1). If there is no pigmentation, or if pigmented carcinoid tumour is suspected, the presence of S-100 protein and HMB-45 antigen, the absence of cytokeratin expression and neuroendocrine markers, and the identification of melanosomes by electron microscopy are helpful diagnostic features.

Differential diagnosis

Strict criteria must be applied before a diagnosis of primary malignant melanoma of the lower respiratory tract can be accepted.[8] Very few reported cases withstand close scrutiny. There should be no evidence of a current or previous primary melanoma elsewhere and any previously resected lesions of the skin, adjacent mucosal surfaces or the eye should be reviewed. The phenomenon of spontaneous regression of an extrapulmonary melanoma after metastasis has occurred bedevils the exclusion of a bronchial melanoma having such an origin. Junctional change in bronchial epithelium is regarded as the best histological evidence of a primary bronchial origin, particularly if it is well away from the tumour because neoplastic melanocytes may directly infiltrate the overlying epithelium and mimic junctional activity. True junctional change has been well described in only a few melanomas of the lower respiratory tract.[2,3,6,9] In a review of 18 previously published cases, only two were considered to be proven, eight were thought to be near proven, four probable and four improbable.[6]

GERM CELL TUMOURS

Primary germ cell tumours of the lung are extremely rare[22–40a] and the possibility of metastasis should always be excluded. Germ cell tumours of the anterior mediastinum arise in the thymus and the presence of thymic tissue in several reported cases of intrapulmonary teratoma

Figure 12.5.1 Melanoma. A primary endobronchial lesion shows malignant polygonal cells, within which only a little melanin pigment can be seen. (*Courtesy of Dr TV Colby, Scottsdale, USA.*)

suggests that these may have originated in heterotopic thymic tissue.[24,26]

Clinical features, treatment and prognosis

Pulmonary germ cell tumours show a wide age range (3 months to 68 years) and a slight female preponderance.[26] They are also more prevalent in the upper lobes and on the left side.[34,38] The presenting symptoms are usually not specific, apart from the expectoration of hair, a dramatic but rare manifestation of a cystic pulmonary teratoma.[28,41] Choriocarcinomas are often haemorrhagic and one that arose in the lungs caused diffuse pulmonary haemorrhage.[40]

Pancreatic enzymes released from a teratoma may erode adjacent tissue and this has been a frequent cause of haemoptysis.[40a] Surgical treatment is the treatment of choice. Prognosis depends on tumour type.

Pathological features and differential diagnosis

Pulmonary teratomas tend to be large and cystic, and may be partly or entirely endobronchial, resulting in bronchiectasis.[34] The cysts are often in continuity with the bronchi. About two-thirds are benign and consist solely of mature tissues such as skin (with its usual appendages, including hair), bronchus, pancreas (which is also a frequent feature of mediastinal teratomas), cartilage and neural tissue. Malignant primary teratomas of the lung show the usual variety of differentiated and anaplastic tissues.

Some of the reported malignant germ cell tumours have been choriocarcinomas associated with elevated levels of serum human chorionic gonadotrophin,[29–31,37,40] and a few of these have arisen in infants[22] or men.[25,31,39] They have displayed the usual mixture of cytotrophoblastic and syncytiotrophoblastic elements.

Other pulmonary germ cell tumours have contained yolk sac elements and secreted α-fetoprotein.[32,36] Mixed yolk sac and blastematous differentiation is also described.[33,35] The immunohistochemical demonstration of β-human chorionic gonadotrophin and α-fetoprotein is of little value as these trophoblastic markers may be seen in carcinoma of the lung.[42] It is notable that some of the few primary choriocarcinomas of the lung reported in men have been combined with carcinoma of more conventional pattern,[39] suggesting that they represent carcinomas showing unusual differentiation rather than primary germ cell tumours.

The differential diagnosis also includes metastatic teratoma, either by direct spread from a mediastinal tumour (see Fig.12.6.14, p. 687) or blood-borne. In the latter context, it is important to remember that chemotherapy may ablate all the malignant elements of the tumour so that the pulmonary metastases may only contain totally mature elements and appear quite benign (see Fig.12.6.13, p. 687).[43,44] Pleuropulmonary blastoma, pulmonary blastoma and carcinosarcoma do not form the organoid structures seen in a teratoma.

REFERENCES

Melanoma

1. Ferrara G, Boscaino A, Derosa G. Bronchial blue naevus. A previously unreported entity. Histopathology 1995;26:581–3.
2. Reid JD, Mehta VT. Melanoma of the lower respiratory tract. Cancer 1966;19:627–31.
3. Mori K, Cho H, Som M. Primary 'flat' melanoma of the trachea. J Pathol Bacteriol 1977;121:101–5.
4. Gephardt GN. Malignant melanoma of the bronchus. Hum Pathol 1981;12:671–3.
5. Santos F, Entrenas LM, Sebastian F, et al. Primary bronchopulmonary malignant melanoma. Case report. Scand J Thorac Cardiovasc Surg 1987;21:187–9.
6. Herbert A. Primary malignant melanoma of the lung. In: Williams CJ, Krikorian JG, Green MR, et al, editors. Textbook of Uncommon Cancer. Chichester: John Wiley; 1988. p. 383–97.
7. Jennings TA, Axiotis CA, Kress Y, et al. Primary malignant melanoma of the lower

respiratory tract – report of a case and literature review. Am J Clin Pathol 1990;94:649–55.
8. Littman CD. Metastatic melanoma mimicking primary bronchial melanoma. Histopathology 1991;18:561–3.
9. Farrell DJ, Kashyap AP, Ashcroft T, et al. Primary malignant melanoma of the bronchus. Thorax 1996;51:223–4.
10. Wilson RW, Moran CA. Primary melanoma of the lung: A clinicopathologic and immunohistochemical study of eight cases. Am J Surg Pathol 1997;21:1196–202.
11. Ost D, Joseph C, Sogoloff H, et al. Primary pulmonary melanoma: case report and literature review. Mayo Clin Proc 1999;74:62–6.
12. Ozdemir N, Cangir AK, Kutlay H, et al. Primary malignant melanoma of the lung in oculocutaneous albino patient. Eur J Cardiothorac Surg 2001;20:864–7.

13. Filosso PL, Donati G, Ruffini E, et al. Primary malignant melanoma of the bronchus intermedius. J Thorac Cardiovasc Surg 2003;126:1215–17.
14. Cebelin MS. Melanocytic bronchial carcinoid tumor. Cancer 1980;46:1843–8.
15. Gould VE, Memoli VE, Dardi LE, et al. Neuroendocrine carcinomas with multiple immunoreactive peptides and melanin production. Ultrastruct Pathol 1981;2:199–217.
16. Grazer R, Cohen SM, Jacobs JB, et al. Melanin-containing peripheral carcinoid of the lung. Am J Surg Pathol 1982;6:73–8.
17. Carlson JA, Dickersin GR. Melanotic paraganglioid carcinoid tumor – a case report and review of the literature. Ultrastruct Pathol 1993;17:353–72.
18. Fukuda T, Kobayashi H, Kamishima T, et al. Peripheral carcinoid tumor of the lung with focal melanin production. Pathol Int 1994;44:309–16.

19. Rowlands D, Edwards C, Collins F. Malignant melanotic schwannoma of the bronchus. J Clin Pathol 1987;40:1449–55.
20. Cohen RE, Weaver MG, Montenegro HD, et al. Pulmonary blastoma with malignant melanoma component. Arch Pathol Lab Med 1990;114:1076–8.
21. Gaffey MJ, Mills SE, Zarbo RJ, et al. Clear cell tumor of the lung – immunohistochemical and ultrastructural evidence of melanogenesis. Am J Surg Pathol 1991;15:644–53.

Germ cell tumours

22. Kay S, Reed WG. Chorioepithelioma of the lung in a female infant seven months old. Am J Pathol 1955;29:555–60.
23. Pound AW, Willis RA. A malignant teratoma of the lung in an infant. J Pathol 1969;98:111–14.
24. Day DW, Taylor SA. An intrapulmonary teratoma associated with thymic tissue. Thorax 1975;30:582–6.
25. Hayakawa K, Takahashi M, Sasaki K, et al. Primary choriocarcinoma of the lung. Acta Pathol Jpn 1977;27:123–35.
26. Holt S, Deverall PB, Boddy JE. A teratoma of the lung containing thymic tissue. J Pathol 1978;126:85–9.
27. Jamieson MPG, McGowan AR. Endobronchial teratoma. Thorax 1982;37:157–9.
28. Filho JCC, Coehlo JCMR. Benign lung teratomas. Report of two cases. J. Pneumologia 1985;11:82–8.

29. Tanimura A, Natsuyama H, Kawano M, et al. Primary choriocarcinoma of the lung. Hum Pathol 1985;16:1281–4.
30. Pushchak MJ, Farhi DC. Primary choriocarcinoma of the lung. Arch Pathol Lab Med 1987;111:477–9.
31. Sullivan LG. Primary choriocarcinoma of the lung in a man. Arch Pathol Lab Med 1989;113:82–3.
32. Hunter S, Hewan-Lowe K, Costa MJ. Primary pulmonary alpha-fetoprotein-producing malignant germ cell tumor. Hum Pathol 1990;21:1074–6.
33. Siegel RJ, Bueso-Ramos C, Cohen C, et al. Pulmonary blastoma with germ cell (yolk sac) differentiation: report of two cases. Mod Pathol 1992;4:566–70.
34. Morgan DE, Sanders C, McElvein RB, et al. Intrapulmonary teratoma: a case report and review of the literature. J Thorac Imaging 1992;7:70–7.
35. Miller RR, Champagne K, Murray RCN. Primary pulmonary germ cell tumor with blastomatous differentiation. Chest 1994;106:1595–6.
36. Kakkar N, Vasishta RK, Banerjee AK, et al. Primary pulmonary malignant teratoma with yolk sac element associated with hematologic neoplasia. Respiration 1996;63:52–4.
37. Aparicio J, Oltra A, Martinez-Moragon E, et al. Extragonadal nongestational choriocarcinoma involving the lung: a report of three cases. Respiration 1996;63:251–3.

38. Asano S, Hoshikawa Y, Yamane Y, et al. An intrapulmonary teratoma associated with bronchiectasia containing various kinds of primordium: a case report and review of the literature. Virchows Archiv 2000. APR;436(4):384–388 2000;436:384–8.
39. Chen FS, Tatsumi A, Numoto S. Combined choriocarcinoma and adenocarcinoma of the lung occurring in a man – Case report and review of the literature. Chest 2001;91:123–9.
40. Shintaku M, Hwang MH, Amitani R. Primary choriocarcinoma of the lung manifesting as diffuse alveolar hemorrhage. Arch Pathol Lab Med 2006;130:540–3.
40a. Macht M, Mitchell JD, Cool C, et al. A 31-year-old woman with hemoptysis and an intrathoracic mass. Chest 2010;138:213–19.
41. Ustun MO, Demircan A, Paksoy N, et al. A case of intrapulmonary teratoma presenting with hair expectoration. Thorac Cardiovasc Surg 1996;44:271–3.
42. Boucher LD, Yoneda K. The expression of trophoblastic cell markers by lung carcinomas. Hum Pathol 1995;26:1201–6.
43. Madden M, Goldstraw P, Corrin B. Effect of chemotherapy on the histological appearances of testicular teratoma metastatic to the lung: correlation with patient survival. J Clin Pathol 1984;37:1212–14.
44. Cagini L, Nicholson AG, Horwich A, et al. Thoracic metastasectomy for germ cell tumours: long term survival and prognostic factors. Ann Oncol 1998;9:1185–91.

Chapter |12|

12.6 Secondary tumours of the lungs

ROUTES OF TUMOUR SPREAD TO THE LUNGS

Extrapulmonary neoplasms may involve the lungs by direct extension or by metastasis. Direct extension may be through the pleura or along lymphatic or blood vessels. Metastasis is by way of the pulmonary or bronchial arteries and possibly within the lungs via the airways (aerial metastasis).

Direct extension

Direct invasion of the lungs through the pleura complicates primary or metastatic growths in the pleura, mediastinal lymph nodes, thymus, oesophagus, chest wall, breast, thyroid or abdomen. No particular route is followed, other than penetration of the fused pleurae. Alternatively, there may be retrograde spread through pulmonary lymphatics once the lymphatic pathway is obstructed by tumour emboli in the mediastinal lymph nodes. Further dissemination within pulmonary lymphatics may be widespread and this is one route (but not the commonest) by which secondary tumours produce the characteristic appearances of so-called lymphangitis carcinomatosa (see below).

Direct invasion of the lungs along veins is rare as this entails invasion of pulmonary veins between the lungs and the left atrium and retrograde venous extension into the lungs. Direct extension along the pulmonary arteries is also rare but is occasionally seen with sarcomas originating in the pulmonary trunk or the right side of the heart (see p. 638).

Metastasis

With their vast capillary network and unique position in the circulation it is not surprising that the lungs are frequently the site of metastatic tumours. The incidence of lung involvement in metastatic disease is second only to that of the liver; pulmonary metastases are found at necropsy in 30–50% of patients dying of cancer.[1] The commoner extrathoracic tumours may be ranked in the following descending order in regard to the frequency with which they metastasise to the lungs: kidney, skin, breast, thyroid, pancreas, prostate, stomach, uterus and colon (Box 12.6.1). Tumours of the lung itself and certain rare tumours, notably choriocarcinoma and osteosarcoma, also commonly metastasise to the lungs. Some tumours with a high tendency to metastasise to the lungs are not themselves common. Therefore they are not the first to be considered when trying to identify the origin of pulmonary metastases. Thus, an order of frequency different from the above applies when considering possible sites of origin following the identification of pulmonary metastases (see Box 12.6.1). If these organs are grouped regionally it is found that the genitourinary tract accounts for 28% of pulmonary metastases, the gastrointestinal tract for 28%, the breasts for 17% and sarcomas for 11%.[2] In a patient with sarcoma or melanoma elsewhere, even a solitary pulmonary lesion is most often a metastasis. Conversely, if the patient has a nodal lymphoma, a solitary parenchymal lesion in the lung is more likely to be an independent primary carcinoma.[3]

PATTERNS OF TUMOUR SPREAD WITHIN THE LUNGS

Secondary growth in the lung may take the form of discrete nodules, diffuse lymphatic permeation, diffuse consolidation, endobronchial growth or massive tumour embolism (Box 12.6.2).[11–13] Metastases in the pleura are usually multinodular but occasionally form a continuous sheet and mimic the appearances of a mesothelioma. They are dealt with in Chapter 13 (see p. 736).

Blood-borne metastases

Discrete tumour nodules

Metastases in the lung commonly take the form of discrete nodules or well-circumscribed masses, which are generally multiple and bilateral (Fig. 12.6.1). They affect the lower lobes more often than the upper, and are commonest in the outer parts of the lungs, in accordance with the distribution of blood within the lungs and with the sites of embolic lodgement.[1,5,14,15] Metastatic deposits may be of any size, and whereas they are sometimes all the same size, in other cases growths of many different sizes are seen. Although metastatic tumours are generally multiple, solitary deposits forming 'coin lesions' may be encountered.[15a] Pulmonary metastases generally have well-circumscribed margins, in contrast to the ill-defined infiltrating edge usually seen with primary malignant lung tumours. On its cut surface a metastasis is generally white and opaque but may show necrosis and haemorrhage. Cavitation and calcification are occasionally seen.[16] Appearances indicative of the site of origin are considered below.

Massive tumour embolism

Tumour emboli occluding the main pulmonary arteries are rare[12] but tumours such as renal cell carcinomas and hepatocellular carcinomas have a propensity to invade the systemic veins and may present with massive tumour embolism. This may also occur with tumours arising in the right side of the heart and pulmonary trunk (See p. 638).

Metastases in the lung almost all arise from tumour emboli arrested in small pulmonary arteries.[4] Bronchial arterial dissemination is far less common but may account for some endobronchial metastases. Groups of tumour cells enter the circulation by invasion of small peripheral veins or through the thoracic duct, and generally come to rest in pulmonary arteries between 400 and 800 μm in diameter.[5] Occasionally there is widespread occlusion of medium-sized pulmonary arteries by tumour or tumour-associated thrombus (see below).

Pulmonary arteries are less resistant to invasion by malignant tumour than their counterparts in the systemic circulation.[6] Nevertheless, although microscopic emboli are very common in the lungs, most fail to establish themselves. In many cases of abdominal carcinoma, malignant cells in the lungs are only to be found in thrombus within the pulmonary arteries, and many of these intraluminal malignant cells are degenerate.[1] Although viable cells within tumour emboli are in the minority, it is of course these which invade the walls of the pulmonary arteries to form secondary lung tumours, and then promote further tumour dissemination via the pulmonary veins and systemic arteries. It is very unusual to encounter widespread systemic metastases in the total absence of tumour deposits in the lungs. Systemic dissemination is dependent as much on pulmonary metastases invading pulmonary venules as single cancer cells traversing the lung capillaries.

Although the high incidence of lung involvement in metastatic disease owes much to the special position of the lungs in the circulation, other factors are also involved. Many cancers display characteristic organ colonisation patterns that do not conform to simple mechanical trapping. Organ preferences of metastatic spread appear to be influenced by selective attachment of tumour cells to endothelium, based on particular cell surface components.[7] This appears to be under genetic control. For example, in breast cancer certain genes selectively facilitate the establishment of metastases in the lung whereas others mediate skeletal metastasis.[8] On the other hand hyperoxic injury to the pulmonary endothelium increases the number of pulmonary metastases.[9] An intriguing correlation between cigarette smoking and a high risk of breast cancer metastasising to the lungs has been noted.[10]

Figure 12.6.1 Pulmonary metastases forming well-circumscribed masses.

Figure 12.6.2 Embolic choriocarcinoma occludes the pulmonary arteries.

Figure 12.6.3 Carcinomatous microangiopathy. Tumour has filled the lumen of a small pulmonary artery in a man with occult gastric carcinoma who died of rapidly progressive pulmonary hypertension.

Microscopic tumour angiopathy

Microscopic tumour emboli are found in up to 26% of cancer patients coming to autopsy,[12,17–19] typically occluding small muscular pulmonary arteries and arterioles (Fig. 12.6.2). Symptoms are generally similar to those seen with lymphangitic spread (see below)[11] but rarely the emboli may be sufficiently extensive to cause pulmonary hypertension and right ventricular failure.[20–23] This is alternatively termed carcinomatous thrombotic microarteriopathy or carcinomatous pulmonary endarteritis (Fig. 12.6.3).[19] Carcinomas of the stomach and breast are the commonest tumours to have this effect but it may also be seen with tumours of the liver and placenta. The emboli may consist purely of tumour cells, a mixture of cells and fibrin, or show severe fibrointimal hyperplasia with scanty tumour cells. The last of these patterns is particularly characteristic of metastatic gastric adenocarcinoma.[13] It has been attributed to the expression of osteopontin (a multifunctional cytokine and adhesive protein), platelet-derived growth factor and vascular endothelial growth factor, by the tumour.[24,24a] Such arteriopathy is generally first diagnosed postmortem but is sometimes detected by lung biopsy or from examining material obtained at pulmonary artery catheterisation.[25] Survival in such patients has seldom exceeded 12 weeks.[19–23]

Lymphatic spread within the lung

'Lymphangitis carcinomatosa'

The major route of spread within the lung of both metastatic and primary tumours is along lymphatics. When very marked this results in so-called lymphangitis carcinomatosa, a condition in which the entire lymphatic system of the lungs is brought into sharp relief by pale threads of tumour tissue filling these vessels (Fig. 12.6.4).[26] A network of occluded lymph channels is clearly visible on the visceral pleural surface whilst on the cut surface the bronchoarterial bundles in the centres of the acini and the veins in the interlobular septa are cuffed by tumour spreading along their accompanying lymphatics. The bronchus is richly supplied with lymphatics and fibreoptic bronchial biopsy may detect lymphatic permeation even when bronchoscopy is normal.[27]

Although lymphangitis carcinomatosa may be produced by direct extension from tumour deposits in hilar lymph nodes, a more common source of involvement is multiple minute tumour emboli reaching the lungs via the pulmonary arteries and subsequently invading the lymphatics.[1,5,28] The main evidence for this is the high incidence of tumour emboli within small pulmonary arteries and the frequent absence of marked hilar lymph node enlargement in lymphangitis carcinomatosa. There is also a high incidence of minute blood-borne tumour emboli in organs other than the lung in this condition, notably in the bone marrow. In one case, previous thoraco-

Figure 12.6.4 'Lymphangitis carcinomatosa'. (A) Tumour fills lymphatics throughout the lung, thickening the interlobular septa and periarterial sheaths. (B) Pleural lymphatics permeated by tumour. *(Courtesy of Dr GA Russell, Tunbridge Wells, UK.)* (C) Microscopy shows tumour filling the periarterial lymphatics.

plasty, which reduces pulmonary perfusion as well as ventilation, appeared to have caused the lung on that side to be spared the widespread lymphatic permeation present in the other.[29] Tumours most likely to give rise to lymphangitis carcinomatosa are those arising in the stomach, pancreas, breast and colon, and in the lung itself.

Endobronchial metastases

In following lymphatics to the hilum of the lung, neoplastic cells may occlude mucosal lymph channels and thereby develop into secondary tumours in the main air passages, so simulating primary growths of the bronchus. Sometimes these metastases protrude into the lumen of the bronchus (Fig. 12.6.5).[30,31] Such endobronchial metastases are encountered with a wide variety of tumours but most commonly originate from growths in the intestine, cervix uteri and breast.[30] Primary tumours of the bronchus with a propensity to grow in this way include carcinosarcomas, carcinoids and bronchial gland tumours.

Intra-alveolar spread

Microscopical examination of the growing edge may show tumour extending into the lumen of neighbouring alveoli, by which means it

Figure 12.6.5 Metastatic osteosarcoma showing endobronchial growth.

Figure 12.6.6 Metastatic carcinoma growing from one alveolus to the next without disturbing the alveolar architecture.

Figure 12.6.8 Metastatic adenocarcinoma of the pancreas growing along the alveolar walls and simulating adenocarcinoma-in-situ (formerly in bronchioloalveolar cell carcinoma).

Figure 12.6.7 Poorly cohesive cells of metastatic carcinoma fill the alveolar spaces, mimicking desquamative interstitial pneumonia.

spreads from one air space to the next (Fig 12.6.6). When this occurs the alveolar septa are generally compressed. Only older parts eventually are obliterated. Elastin stains often demonstrate the skeletal remains of alveolar septa in what appears to be solid tumour tissue.

Alternatively, non-cohesive tumour cells may fill many alveoli without affecting the alveolar walls, resulting in appearances that simulate desquamative interstitial pneumonia (Fig. 12.6.7).[32,33] This is distinguished by careful attention to the cytological features of the free cells, aided by the immunocytochemical demonstration of cytokeratin, which is present in carcinoma and mesothelioma cells but not in the macrophages of desquamative interstitial pneumonia.[32] This pattern has been shown to be non-angiogenic, the tumour cells depending on the pre-existent alveolar capillaries rather than inducing neoangiogenesis.[34] Some metastatic breast and renal carcinomas showing such non-angiogenic alveolar spread have apparently been confined to the lungs, with obvious implications regarding prognosis and treatment.[35,36] Such non-angiogenic spread is also seen with some primary pulmonary tumours. It indicates a relatively favourable prognosis whatever the tumour.[34,37–39]

Lepidic spread

A further route of tumour spread within the alveolar tissues of the lung is one in which the tumour cells grow along the surface of alveolar walls. The tumour replaces the alveolar epithelium, usually in a layer no more than one cell thick. Neither the alveolar walls nor the air spaces are obliterated; the tumour uses the alveolar walls as a supporting scaffold (Fig. 12.6.8). This is termed a lepidic growth pattern. It is the pattern of growth found with adenocarcinoma-in-situ (formerly bronchioloalveolar cell carcinoma, see p. 536), but is one that may be adopted by any adenocarcinoma, either primary or metastatic.[40,41] Pancreatic, gastric and colorectal growths are the commonest metastatic tumours to grow in this way. Because it does not destroy the lung tissue, this growth is likely to mimic an area of pneumonic consolidation both radiographically and on macroscopical examination of the cut surface of the lung. There may be a single area of diffuse involvement or multiple foci may develop in both lungs. A mucoid appearance may be evident, depending on the secretory status of the tumour. Considerable controversy attends the possibility of aerial metastases accounting for the frequent multifocal distribution of primary lung tumours which evince this pattern of growth but in cases of metastatic tumour vascular dissemination provides an adequate explanation.

Interstitial spread

Another extralymphatic route of tumour spread in the alveolar tissues of the lung is within the alveolar interstitium, which is correspondingly thickened (Fig. 12.6.9). The air spaces are eventually obliterated by this encroachment. Total destruction of the alveolar architecture may take place in the older parts of the tumour as with intra-alveolar growth.

PRIMARY OR METASTATIC TUMOUR?

The development of metastatic disease long after the primary growth has been eradicated is well recognised[42] but mention of previous operations is often neglected when a new specimen is submitted to the laboratory.

Figure 12.6.9 Metastatic mesothelioma growing within the alveolar walls.

Figure 12.6.10 Metastatic melanoma. The heavy pigmentation of this tumour provides a strong clue to its nature.

A multiplicity of growths in the lungs always suggests metastatic disease but solitary metastases are not uncommon and the question whether a given tumour is primary or metastatic arises particularly in patients with a solitary lung nodule. Up to 9% of solitary lung nodules prove to be metastases.

Whether the lung is the site of single or multiple growths, recognition of the site of origin assumes particular clinical importance where there is site-specific therapy. Testicular teratoma and carcinoma of the breast, ovary, prostate and thyroid fall into this category. Familiarity with the histological appearances of tumours is of limited help in the hunt for the primary site for there can be no certainty in distinguishing, for example, one adenocarcinoma from another by this means.

Gross appearances

The gross appearances are seldom informative with regard to the tissue of origin but obvious mucin secretion, melanin production (Fig. 12.6.10) or bone or cartilage formation may be helpful on occasion. Similarly, the metastases of choriocarcinomas and angiosarcomas are often grossly haemorrhagic and smooth-muscle tumours may display a recognisable fascicular pattern.[42a,b]

Histological appearances

Sometimes the microscopic pattern gives a clear indication of an extrapulmonary derivation, but often the tumour is anaplastic or the pattern of differentiation is one seen in both pulmonary and extrapulmonary primary growths. All the common carcinomas of the lung may be mimicked microscopically by metastases. Adenocarcinomas are broadly similar whether they arise in lung, alimentary tract or the female genital tract. Adenosquamous carcinomas of lung and uterus are similar histologically while squamous cell carcinomas are identical regardless of origin. Similarly, recognising the source of anaplastic large cell carcinomas is a common histopathological problem wherever they are encountered, and even small cell carcinomas may arise outside the lungs.[42c] However, there are some purely morphological characteristics that may point to particular types of tumour arising in the lungs themselves rather than in some other parts of the body and these will now be described.

Squamous cell carcinoma of the bronchus arises in foci of dysplasia and develops through an in-situ phase. Such lesions are multifocal and recognition of these premalignant changes in the surface epithelium of neighbouring airways may help in deciding that a squamous cell carcinoma is primary rather than metastatic. Continuity between invasive and apparently in-situ carcinoma is less helpful because metastases can erode a bronchus and replace the surface epithelium to mimic pre-existent in situ carcinoma.

Adenocarcinoma presents particular difficulties in distinguishing primary from secondary growths.[3,43] Scarring may suggest the possibility of a primary scar cancer but it is notoriously difficult to prove that such fibrosis antedates the tumour (see p. 534). Central fibrosis may be a consequence of tissue destruction in either primary or metastatic pulmonary tumours, rather than the cause of the tumour, whilst metastases sometimes develop in lung scars. However, premalignant epithelial atypia suggests that a tumour is a primary scar cancer rather than a metastasis.

Some metastases appear quite benign and are therefore likely to be mistaken for primary growths. So-called ' benign metastasising leiomyoma of the uterus is a notable example of this.[44–49] Obviously, a tumour that metastasises to the lung cannot be truly benign but in this entity neither the primary growth nor its metastases shows any microscopic evidence of malignancy whatsoever (Fig. 12.6.11). Primary leiomyoma of the lung is rare and, before such a diagnosis is contemplated, metastatic tumour must be excluded, particularly in a middle-aged woman with multiple lung tumours. Some may evolve from benign tumour emboli released at myomectomy, some from intravenous leiomyomatosis of the myometrium[50] and some may represent metastases of a very well-differentiated leiomyosarcoma. Very rarely, the patient is male, and the primary tumour then arises in sites such as the skin.[51] The metastases may be discovered by chance radiographically, appearing as multiple rounded opacities in an individual with no respiratory complaints. They grow quite slowly in the lungs, leading to gradually increasing breathlessness and eventually fatal respiratory failure. The median survival is quoted as 94 months after excision of the pulmonary metastases, compared with 22 months with metastatic leiomyosarcoma.[48] During pregnancy or after oophorectomy or the menopause, growth is even slower or may stop completely.[52,53] Antioestrogen drugs may be beneficial; in this, and the almost exclusively female predilection, the condition resembles pulmonary lymphangioleiomyomatosis (see p. 293) but the latter is characterised radiographically by an interstitial infiltrate rather than multiple discrete opacities.

Other tumours that have metastasised despite entirely benign histological appearances include thymoma,[54] giant cell tumours of bone,[55] dermatofibroma,[56] adenomyoepithelioma of the breast[57] and meningioma.[58]

Secondary changes within metastases may also confuse the unwary pathologist. For example, metastases in the lung often engulf pre-existent structures and the survival of entrapped air spaces in a metastatic sarcoma must not be mistaken for the epithelial component of a primary mixed tumour such as pulmonary blastoma or carcinosarcoma.[51,59] Obstruction of engulfed air spaces may lead to marked cystic change,[60–65] occasionally resulting in pneumothorax, haemopneumothorax or pneumomediastinum.[66] This change appears to be particularly common in the condition of 'benign metastasising leiomyoma' described above (see Fig. 12.6.11) and metastatic endometrial stromal sarcoma.[65] It may also have led to some low-grade metastatic sarcomas being described as primary pulmonary tumours under terms such as multiple cystic fibrohistiocytic tumour or mesenchymal cystic hamartoma[62,63,67]: most cases classified as such have been shown to represent metastatic cellular fibrous histiocytomas (Fig. 12.6.12). They show a male predominance and long-term survival despite extensive disease.[68]

A further trap for the pathologist arises from the surgeon withholding information that the patient has had a testicular teratoma treated by chemotherapy. Subsequent metastases are thought to be worth excising and the pathologist can give useful prognostic information, or, if ignorant of the clinical circumstances, make a totally wrong diagnosis. For example, complete chemotherapeutic ablation may result in totally necrotic tissue encompassed by granulation tissue, the whole resembling a granuloma. Alternatively, fibrous scars may be the only remnants of successfully treated metastases. In other cases metastases consist only of well-differentiated tissues with limited growth potential. All these findings indicate that chemotherapy has been successful, whereas viable malignant tumour indicates that it has failed.[69,70]

On occasion, chemotherapy results in metastatic teratoma being reduced to such well-differentiated cartilage that the residual tumour

Figure 12.6.11 'Benign metastasising leiomyoma' of the uterus. (A, B) This was one of many pulmonary nodules in a woman with uterine fibroids. No cytological evidence of malignancy was apparent in any of the uterine or pulmonary tumours. (C) The pulmonary metastases of these tumours may be cystic.

Figure 12.6.13 Pulmonary metastasis of testicular teratoma excised after chemotherapy. Histologically, the tumour appears entirely benign, indicating that the chemotherapy has been successful and that the prognosis is favourable. In this example, the predominant component of the tumour is cartilage and it is easy to see how the lesion could be erroneously diagnosed as a chondroid hamartoma if the necessary clinical information was lacking.

Figure 12.6.14 Secondary teratoma. This differentiated teratoma infiltrated the lung directly from the mediastinum.

Figure 12.6.12 Metastatic cellular fibrous histiocytoma. (A) Multiple thin-walled cystic masses are present within the lung in a case originally diagnosed as mesenchymal cystic hamartoma.[67] It was later found that the patient had a cellular fibrous histiocytoma resected over a decade earlier. (B, C) The walls of the cysts consist of a cytologically bland fibrohistiocytic proliferation and the diagnosis was revised to metastatic cellular fibrous histiocytoma.

closely mimics a 'hamartoma' (Fig. 12.6.13).[69,71] At other times successful chemotherapy causes cystic change and, if there is also chemo-resistant cartilage, a bronchogenic cyst may be simulated.[72] In these circumstances immunocytochemical study of the epithelial elements along the lines described below is helpful because, whereas a teratoma may express both intestinal and respiratory markers, the former are not found in these primary lesions.

Teratomas spreading directly from the mediastinum need also to be considered (Fig. 12.6.14), as does direct spread from a thymoma into the lung (Fig. 12.6.15).

Other secondary tumours that may mimic primary lung growths include low-grade endometrial stromal sarcoma[60,65,73,74] and clear cell odontogenic carcinoma.[75]

Figure 12.6.15 Secondary thymoma. Tumour has infiltrated the lung directly from the thymus.

Figure 12.6.16 A positive immunoperoxidase reaction for surfactant apoprotein enables this pleural deposit of adenocarcinoma to be recognised as having originated in the lung.

Ultrastructural features

Electron microscopy might be thought to reveal cytological features indicative of a particular cell type or tissue but, apart from the Birbeck granules of Langerhans cells and the Weibel–Palade bodies of endothelial cells, there are few such marker organelles. However, in trying to identify the origin of an adenocarcinoma the identification of Clara cell granules or lamellar (surfactant) bodies is indicative of a primary origin in the lung: conversely, terminal webs are diagnostic of intestinal carcinomas.[76] Glycocalyceal bodies and microvillous core rootlets are characteristic of adenocarcinomas of the gastrointestinal tract but are also found on occasion in primary lung carcinomas.[77–79]

Cytochemistry

Cytochemical characterisation of mucin has been utilised to distinguish primary and secondary mucus-secreting adenocarcinomas[80,81] but the specificity is low. However, a diastase-controlled periodic acid–Schiff stain identifying both mucin and glycogen can be useful in distinguishing primary and secondary clear cell carcinomas. Clear cell carcinoma of the kidney contains glycogen but no mucin whereas some pulmonary clear cell carcinomas are mucin-rich. If a clear cell tumour evinces no features of malignancy such as excessive mitotic activity and necrosis, the possibility of benign clear cell tumour of the lung (see p. 625) arises: like a renal metastasis, this stains for glycogen rather than mucin. In this case any available reserve tissue should be utilised for a fat stain, with a positive reaction favouring a renal origin. There are also vascular differences between these tumours, the metastases of a renal carcinoma lacking the thin-walled wide sinusoids that characterise the benign clear cell tumour of lung (see Table 12.3.1, p. 626). Immunocytochemistry is also helpful.

Immunocytochemistry

Immunocytochemistry is very helpful in distinguishing primary and metastatic tumours in the lung, particularly carcinomas and especially adenocarcinomas.[82,83] Identification of the various cytokerains is important in this and it is worth noting how these are classified. Their enumeration is not random but is based firstly upon their acid–base profile and secondly upon their molecular weights. Thus 1–8 represent basic cytokeratins of progressively increasing molecular weight while 9–20 are similarly ranked among the acidic cytokeratins.

Some particular problems that lend themselves to immunocytochemical elucidation will now be considered.

Pulmonary versus extrapulmonary adenocarcinoma

Primary adenocarcinoma may be recognised by the immunocytochemical demonstration of thyroid transcription factor-1 (TTF-1), napsin A, surfactant apoprotein or Clara cell antigens (Fig. 12.6.16).[84–93b] Conversely, these markers enable the lungs to be recognised as the origin of tumours in other organs (Fig. 12.6.17).[94] TTF-1 is the more sensitive lung marker and its antibody is the method of choice for establishing origin in the lung, although being both a lung and thyroid marker, it may need to be supplemented by thyroglobulin and surfactant apoprotein on occasion.[86,91] It is applicable to frozen as well as paraffin sections.[95] Attention should be confined to the nuclei as cytoplasmic TTF-1 immunoreactivity is occasionally encountered as a non-specific feature in various neoplasms.[96] TTF-1 is relatively specific for lung and thyroid.[89,90,92,97–103] It is positive in the nuclei of up to 76% of primary adenocarcinomas of the lung (but seldom in mucinous varieties) and 40% of large cell carcinomas.[92,93b]

Immunocytochemical markers specific for other organs occasionally help in identifying an extrapulmonary origin, e.g. thyroglobulin, prostate-specific antigen, hepatocyte paraffin-1, renal cell carcinoma marker and kidney-specific cadherin,[104,105] while a mammary origin is likely if a lung tumour expresses oestrogen receptors and cystic disease fluid protein-15.[93b,106–109] Similarly, the immunocytochemical demonstration of CDX-2 strongly favours an adenocarcinoma as having originated in the large bowel[110,111] (except in the case of primary colloid carcinoma of the lung, which also expresses CDX-2).[112] A panel of immunocytochemical markers that proved useful in distinguishing adenocarcinomas of various origin is shown in Table 12.6.1.[82] Other proposed discriminants are of less value. For example, villin is expressed in a substantial proportion of pulmonary as well as gastrointestinal adenocarcinomas,[113,114] while the Wilms tumour suppressor gene WT-1 is expressed in pulmonary adenocarcinomas as well as renal, ovarian and mesothelial neoplasms.[115] A useful website for assessing the specificities and sensitivities of antibodies in relation to primary sites is available at http://e-immunohistochemistry.info.

Figure 12.6.17 (A) Non-small cell carcinoma in a hilar node in a patient with a pulmonary mass and a history of previous breast carcinoma. (B) The tumour cells seen in (A) stain for thyroid transcription factor-1, indicating metastasis from the lung.

Individual cytokeratins can be helpful in narrowing the list of potential primary sites in a TTF-1-negative adenocarcinoma, particularly if a combination of cytokeratins 7 and 20 is used.[116,117] Thus, while adenocarcinomas arising in the lung, endometrium, thyroid and breast are generally cytokeratin 7-positive and cytokeratin 20-negative, the converse is seen with colonic carcinomas. However, mucinous adenocarcinoma of lepidoic pattern (formerly bronchiolo-alveolar carcinoma) differs from other adenocarcinomas of the lung in that it is generally cytokeratin 20-positive. It is also TTF-1 negative and may therefore be confused with metastatic bowel cancer growing in this fashion but it lacks the CDX-2 reactivity found with bowel cancer.[118] Pulmonary adenocarcinomas showing enteric differentiation may fail to stain for TTF-1 and surfactant apoprotein but usually retain cytokeratin-7 expression; they also fail to stain for the enteric marker CDX-2.[119,120] The combination of cytokeratins 7 and 20 does not distinguish pulmonary adenocarcinoma from pleural mesothelioma of epithelioid pattern, techniques for which are consid-

ered on page 722. The expression of cytokeratin 7 and 20 applied in combination is shown in Box 12.6.3.

Pulmonary versus extrapulmonary clear cell tumours

In distinguishing primary and secondary clear cell tumours, immuno-histochemistry augments the mucin, fat and glycogen stains referred to above. Renal cell carcinoma reacts for the broad-spectrum cyto-keratins detected by Cam 5.2 but is distinguished from primary clear cell carcinoma of the lung by failing to stain for TTF-1 or cytokeratin-7, and from the benign cell tumour of the lung by failing to stain for HMB45 (see Table 12.3.1, p. 626). Renal cell carcinoma antigen and kidney-specific cadherin may also be helpful.[104,105,121]

Pulmonary versus extrapulmonary neuroendocrine neoplasms

Small cell carcinomas have been described in many organs other than the lungs and may of course metastasise to the lungs. TTF-1 and the neuroendocrine markers CD56, chromogranin and synaptophysin are of limited value as they are expressed by small cell carcinomas wherever they arise.

However, the distinction between primary and metastatic small cell carcinomas is of limited importance if it is assumed that the patient has extensive disease and is to be treated systemically irrespective of where the tumour arose. Similarly with large cell neuroendocrine carcinomas: if staging identifies deposits in extrapulmonary organs as well as the lungs the patient will be referred for appropriate chemotherapy irrespective of the site of origin.

With the less malignant carcinoid tumours, CD56 and TTF-1 are again of debatable utility, the former being universally expressed and the latter variably so, positivity being reported in 0–69% of cases, with more peripheral than central carcinoids being positive.[122–124] Cytokeratin-20 and CDX2 are of more value as these markers are frequently positive in gastrointestinal carcinoids and islet cell tumours but not in bronchopulmonary carcinoids.[122] Metastatic islet cell tumours also react for neurosecretory protein-55.[125] Medullary carcinoma of the thyroid may be distinguished from carcinoids by its expression of calcitonin[104] and the identification of stromal amyloid in some cases.

Paraganglioma is distinctly rare in the lung (see p. 638) and when a patient appears to have a primary paraganglioma of the lung cyto-keratin positivity usually indicates that it is a carcinoid or subsequent events suggest that it has metastasised from sites such as the glomus jugulare. When considering the possibility of carcinoid tumour or any neuroendocrine tumour of cribriform pattern, metastatic adeno-carcinoma of the prostate needs to be kept in mind and prostate-specific markers sought.[126]

Pulmonary versus extrapulmonary squamous cell carcinoma

While the high specificity and relatively good sensitivity of TTF-1 make it a valuable antibody in distinguishing primary and metastatic adenocarcinomas, it is of limited value with squamous cell carcino-mas because these tumours generally fail to stain for this epitope, irrespective of site of origin. However, cytokeratin-5/6 is a sensitive and specific marker for primary pulmonary growths of this phenotype (Table 12.6.2).[127] Also, there is a high chance that a squamous cell carcinoma positive for cytokeratin-7 has originated in the uterine cervix because most other squamous cell carcinomas (but not several tumours of other phenotype) fail to express this epitope.[116] Similarly, p16 is almost always strongly expressed in squamous cell carcinomas of the cervix but less frequently in such growths arising in the lungs.[128]

Table 12.6.1 A panel of immunostains that correctly predicted the site of origin of 75% of 314 test samples of metastatic adenocarcinoma of known primary site[82]

	TTF-1	CDX2	CK7	CK20	CEA	MUC2	MUC5AC	ER	GCDFP15
Lung (n = 50)	+	−	+	−	−		−	−	−
Colorectal (n = 50)	−	+	−	+					
or	−	+	−	−	+	+			
Ovary (n = 14)	−	−	+	−			+		−
Breast (n = 50)	−	−	+	−					+
or	−	−		−			−	+	
Pancreas (n = 50)	−	−	+		+		+		
Bile duct (n = 50)	−	−	+		+		+		
Stomach (n = 50)	−	+	+	−					

TTF-1, thyroid transcription factor-1; CK, cytokeratin; CEA, carcinoembryonic antigen; MUC, mucin; ER, oestrogen receptor; GCDFP, gross cystic disease fluid protein.

Box 12.6.3 CK7/CK20 combinations

CK7+/CK20−

Adenocarcinoma of lung
Small cell carcinoma of lung
Squamous cell carcinoma of cervix
Adenocarcinoma of endometrium
Non-mucinous carcinoma of ovary
Epithelioid mesothelioma

CK7−/CK20+

Adenocarcinoma of large bowel

CK7−/CK20−

Squamous cell carcinoma of lung
Adenocarcinoma of prostate
Thymoma
Renal carcinoma
Hepatocellular carcinoma

CK7+/CK20+

Mucinous carcinoma of ovary
Transitional cell carcinoma
Adenocarcinoma of pancreas

Table 12.6.2 Expression of cytokeratins (CK) 5, 6 and 7 in squamous cell carcinomas

Primary site	CK 5/6	CK 7
Lung	Positive	Negative
Cervix uteri	Negative	Positive
Other	Negative	Negative

Table 12.6.3 Antibodies for undifferentiated malignancies

	EMA	HMB-45	LCA	PLAP
Carcinoma	+	−	−	−
Melanoma	−	+	−	−
Lymphoma	−	−	+	−
Germ cell neoplasm	−	−	−	+

EMA, epithelial membrane antigen; HMB-45, human melanin black-45; LCA, leukocyte common antigen (CD45); PLAP, placental-like alkaline phosphatase.

Undifferentiated malignancy of uncertain origin

Undifferentiated large cell carcinoma is a common pattern of primary lung tumour that may be mimicked by certain undifferentiated non-epithelial malignancies metastasising to the lung. Important examples include melanoma, lymphoma and germ cell tumours. Key screening antibodies that distinguish these undifferentiated growths are shown in Table 12.6.3. Others include the germ cell-specific transcription factors OCT3/4, NANOG and SOX2.[129]

Metastatic teratoma simulating primary chondroid lesions

It has been mentioned above that successful chemotherapy may result in the metastases of a teratoma being composed wholly of well-differentiated tissues of benign appearance and that if cartilage is the predominant element a diagnosis of bronchogenic cyst or 'hamartoma' may be considered in the differential diagnosis. Attention to the epithelial elements can be helpful here for whereas a teratoma may include respiratory epithelium (complete with cilia and expressing respiratory markers such as TTF-1) there may also be gastrointestinal epithelium expressing markers such as CDX2 foreign to the lung.

Molecular techniques

In the future, immunocytochemistry will be augmented by molecular techniques: organ-specific gene profiles that enable adenocarcinomas of the lung, colon and ovary to be distinguished have already been identified[130] and the recognition of cytogenetic aberrations has enabled a endometrial synovial sarcoma metastasising to the lung to be correctly categorised.[131] Similarly, molecular techniques have been used to distinguish specific human papillomavirus genotypes in patients with squamous cell carcinoma in both the lung and other organs in which these tumours originate, identical genotypes favouring pulmonary metastasis and dissimilar genotypes favouring independent tumours.[132] One group found that this allowed almost certain discrimination in 57% of cases.[133] Others have successfully distinguished pulmonary from head and neck squamous cell carcinomas by applying molecular techniques to routine specimens.[133a]

EFFECTS OF SECONDARY LUNG TUMOURS AND THEIR CLINICAL FEATURES

The capillary bed of the lungs is an effective filter of tumour emboli and secondary tumours in the lungs are therefore the usual immediate source of metastases in other organs, except of course those that reach the liver via the portal circulation. Pulmonary metastases, like primary tumours in the lung, may also result in non-neoplastic systemic disturbances, such as hypertrophic pulmonary osteoarthropathy and blood eosinophilia.[134]

Local effects on the lung are inevitable if there is extensive replacement of lung tissue, but it is remarkable how few symptoms pulmonary metastases generally cause. The commonest effects are compression of the lung and mediastinal shift by an effusion caused by pleural rather than pulmonary metastases, and terminal bronchopneumonia. The latter is largely attributable to general debility but pneumonia and abscess formation may also follow airway obstruction by secondary lung tumours. Haemoptysis is seldom severe except with metastatic choriocarcinoma or angiosarcoma. Massive pulmonary metastases result in a significant reduction in lung volume, whilst lymphangitis carcinomatosa renders the lung stiff and impairs gas transfer, but is only occasionally severe enough to cause respiratory failure.[135] Widespread pulmonary artery occlusion may cause pulmonary hypertension (see patterns of spread above)[5,136-141] while repeated episodes of tumour embolism may result in recurrent infarction.[142] Massive tumour embolism has proved fatal[143,144] or necessitated emergency embolectomy.[145] Even successful chemotherapy is not without its complications; an arteriovenous fistula has been reported in an ablated pulmonary metastasis.[146]

PROLONGED SURVIVAL DESPITE METASTATIC DISEASE

The prognosis in patients with secondary lung tumours is of course very poor but instances of prolonged survival[147] and even spontaneous regression are well known. Spontaneous regression of metastatic tumours is commonest with renal carcinomas[148,149]: it sometimes follows resection of the primary tumour,[150] whilst in other cases hormonal influences are possibly responsible.[53,148]

Although chemotherapy and radiotherapy are the mainstays of treatment of metastatic disease there is increasing interest in the resection of solitary and even multiple pulmonary metastases.[70,151-154] An International Registry for Lung Metastases has shown an actuarial survival after complete metastasectomy of 36% at 5 years, 26% at 10 years, and 22% at 15 years.[155] Favourable prognostic indicators are solitary metastases, prolonged interval between primary tumour and metastasis, completeness of resection and certain tumour types such as metastatic teratoma, breast carcinoma and melanoma.[70,156-158] Incomplete resection does not usually offer any survival advantage but the 'debulking' of certain tumours, for example metastatic thyroid tumours resistant to chemotherapy, helps control symptoms and may also prolong survival.[159] Opinions currently differ on the value of metastatectomy for metastatic bowel cancer.[160,161]

REFERENCES

Routes of tumour spread to the lungs

1. Willis RA. The spread of Tumours in the Human Body. 3rd ed. London: Butterworths; 1973. p. 170.
2. Shepherd MP. Thoracic metastases. Thorax 1982;37:366-70.
3. Cahan WG, Castro EB, Hajdu SI. The significance of a solitary lung shadow in patients with colon carcinoma. Cancer 1974;33:414-21.
4. Wong CW, Song C, Grimes MM, et al. Intravascular location of breast cancer cells after spontaneous metastasis to the lung. Amer J Pathol 2002;161:749-53.
5. Morgan AD. The pathology of subacute cor pulmonale in diffuse carcinomatosis of the lungs. J Pathol Bacteriol 1949;61:75-84.
6. Kolin A, Koutoulakis T. Invasion of pulmonary arteries by bronchial carcinomas. Hum Pathol 1987;18:1165-71.
7. Pauli BU, Lee C-C. Organ preference of metastasis. The role of organ-specifically modulated endothelial cells. Lab Invest 1988;58:379-87.

8. Minn AJ, Gupta GP, Siegel PM, et al. Genes that mediate breast cancer metastasis to lung. Nature 2005;436:518-24.
9. Adamson IYR, Young L, Orr FW. Tumor metastasis after hyperoxic injury and repair of the pulmonary endothelium. Lab Invest 1987;57:71-7.
10. Murin S, Inciardi J. Cigarette smoking and the risk of pulmonary metastasis from breast cancer. Chest 2001;19:1635-40.

Patterns of tumour spread within the lungs

11. Soares FA, Pinto AP, Landell GA, et al. Pulmonary tumor embolism to arterial vessels and carcinomatous lymphangitis. A comparative clinicopathological study. Arch Pathol Lab Med 1993;117:827-31.
12. Winterbauer RH, Elfenbein IB, Ball WC Jr. Incidence and clinical significance of tumor embolization to the lungs. Am J Med 1968;45:271-90.
13. Shields DJ, Edwards WD. Pulmonary hypertension attributable to neoplastic emboli: an autopsy study of 20 cases and a

review of the literature. Cardiovasc Pathol 1992;1:279-87.
14. Pryce DM, Heard BE. The distribution of experimental pulmonary emboli in the rabbit. J Pathol Bacteriol 1956;71:15-25.
15. Crow J, Slavin G, Kreel L. Pulmonary metastasis: a pathologic and radiologic study. Cancer 1981;47:2595-602.
15a. Toomes H, Delphendahl A, Manke H-G, et al. The coin lesion of the lung. A review of 955 resected coin lesions. Cancer 1983;51:534-7.
16. Semple J, West LR. Calcified pulmonary metastases from testicular and ovarian tumours. Thorax 1955;10:287-92.
17. Filderman AE, Coppage L, Shaw C, et al. Pulmonary and pleural manifestations of extrathoracic malignancies. Clin Chest Med 1989;10:747-807.
18. Le Cam Y, Tuel N, Zimbacca F, et al. Neoplastic pulmonary embolism. An uncommon cause of acute respiratory distress with normal pulmonary radiography. Rev Pneumol Clin 1997;53:355-9.

100. Comperat E, Zhang F, Perrotin C, et al. Variable sensitivity and specificity of TTF-1 antibodies in lung metastatic adenocarcinoma of colorectal origin. Mod Pathol 2005;18:1371–6.

101. Lim TK-H, Teo C, Giron DM, et al. Thyroid transcription factor-1 may be expressed in ductal adenocarcinoma of the prostate:a potential pitfall. J Clin Pathol 2007;60:941–3.

102. Jones TD, Kernek KM, Yang XJ, et al. Thyroid transcription factor 1 expression in small cell carcinoma of the urinary bladder: an immunohistochemical profile of 44 cases. Human Pathology 2005;36:718–23.

103. Siami K, McCluggage WG, Ordonez NG, et al. Thyroid transcription factor-1 expression in endometrial and endocervical adenocarcinomas. Am J Surg Pathol 2007;31:1759–63.

104. Ordonez NG. The diagnostic utility of immunohistochemistry in distinguishing between mesothelioma and renal cell carcinoma: a comparative study. Hum Pathol 2004;35:697–710.

105. Shen SS, Krishna B, Chirala R, et al. Kidney-specific cadherin, a specific marker for the distal portion of the nephron and related renal neoplasms. Mod Pathol 2005;18:933–40.

106. Chaubert P, Hurlimann J. Mammary origin of metastases – immunohistochemical determination. Arch Pathol Lab Med 1992;116:1181–8.

107. Raab SS, Berg LC, Swanson PE, et al. Adenocarcinoma in the lung in patients with breast cancer – a prospective analysis of the discriminatory value of immunohistology. Am J Clin Pathol 1993;100:27–35.

108. Canver CC, Memoli VA, Vanderveer PL, et al. Sex hormone receptors in non-small cell lung cancer in human beings. J Thorac Cardiovasc Surg 1994;108:153–7.

109. Ollayos CW, Riordan P, Rushin JM. Estrogen receptor detection in paraffin sections of adenocarcinoma of the colon, pancreas and lung. Arch Pathol Lab Med 1994;118:630–2.

110. Barbareschi M, Murer B, Colby TV, et al. CDX-2 homeobox gene expression is a reliable marker of colorectal adenocarcinoma metastases to the lungs. Am J Surg Pathol 2003;27:141–9.

111. Saad RS, Cho P, Silverman JF, et al. Usefulness of Cdx2 in separating mucinous bronchioloalveolar adenocarcinoma of the lung from metastatic mucinous colorectal adenocarcinoma. Am J Clin Pathol 2004;122:421–7.

112. Rossi G, Murer B, Cavazza A, et al. Primary mucinous (So-called colloid) carcinomas of the lung – A clinicopathologic and immunohistochemical study with special reference to CDX-2 homeobox gene and MUC2 expression. Am J Surg Pathol 2004;28:442–52.

113. Tan JY, Sidhu G, Greco MA, et al. Villin, cytokeratin 7, and cytokeratin 20 expression in pulmonary adenocarcinoma with ultrastructural evidence of microvilli with rootlets. Hum Pathol 1998;29:390–6.

114. Sharma S, Tan JY, Sidhu G, et al. Lung adenocarcinomas metastatic to the brain with and without ultrastructural evidence of rootlets: An electron microscopic and immunohistochemical study using cytokeratins 7 and 20 and villin. Ultrastruct Pathol 1998;22:385–91.

115. Oates J, Edwards C. HBME-1, MOC-31, WT1 and calretinin: an assessment of recently described markers for mesothelioma and adenocarcinoma. Histopathology 2000;36:341–7.

116. Chu P, Wu E, Weiss LM. Cytokeratin 7 and cytokeratin 20 expression in epithelial neoplasms: A survey of 435 cases. Modern Pathol 2000;13:962–72.

117. Chu PG, Weiss LM. Keratin expression in human tissues and neoplasms. Histopathology 2002;40:403–39.

118. Goldstein NS, Thomas M. Mucinous and nonmucinous bronchioloalveolar adenocarcinomas have distinct staining patterns with thyroid transcription factor and cytokeratin 20 antibodies. Amer J Clin Pathol 2001;116:319–25.

119. Inamura K, Satoh Y, Okumura S, et al. Pulmonary adenocarcinomas with enteric differentiation: histologic and immunohistochemical characteristics compared with metastatic colorectal cancers and usual pulmonary adenocarcinomas. Am J Surg Pathol 2005;29:660–5.

120. Yousem SA. Pulmonary intestinal-type adenocarcinoma does not show enteric differentiation by immunohistochemical study. Mod Pathol 2005;18:816–21.

121. Bakshi N, Kunju LP, Giordano T, et al. Expression of renal cell carcinoma antigen (RCC) in renal epithelial and nonrenal tumors: diagnostic Implications. Appl Immunohistochem Mol Morphol 2007;15:310–5.

122. Cai YC, Banner B, Glickman J, et al. Cytokeratin 7 and 20 and thyroid transcription factor 1 can help distinguish pulmonary from gastrointestinal carcinoid and pancreatic endocrine tumors. Hum Pathol 2001;32:1087–93.

123. Sturm N, Rossi G, Lantuejoul S, et al. Expression of thyroid transcription factor-1 in the spectrum of neuroendocrine cell lung proliferations with special interest in carcinoids. Hum Pathol 2002;33:175–82.

124. Du EZ, Goldstraw P, Zacharias J, et al. TTF-1 expression is specific for lung primary in typical and atypical carcinoids: TTF-1-positive carcinoids are predominantly in peripheral location. Hum Pathol 2004;35:825–31.

125. Srivastava A, Padilla O, Fischer-Colbrie R, et al. Neuroendocrine secretory protein-55 (NESP-55) expression discriminates

pancreatic endocrine tumors and pheochromocytomas from gastrointestinal and pulmonary carcinoids. Am J Surg Pathol 2004;28:1371–8.

126. Anton RC, Schwartz MR, Kessler ML, et al. Metastatic carcinoma of the prostate mimicking primary carcinoid tumor of the lung and mediastinum. Pathol Res Pract 1998;194:753–8.

127. Jerome Marson V, Mazieres J, Groussard O, et al. Expression of TTF-1 and cytokeratins in primary and secondary epithelial lung tumours: correlation with histological type and grade. Histopathology 2004;45:125–34.

128. Wang CW, Wu TI, Yu CT, et al. Usefulness of p16 for differentiating primary pulmonary squamous cell carcinoma from cervical squamous cell carcinoma metastatic to the lung. Am J Clin Pathol 2009;131:715–22.

129. Santagata S, Ligon KL, Hornick JL. Embryonic stem cell transcription factor signatures in the diagnosis of primary and metastatic germ cell tumors. Am J Surg Pathol 2007;31:836–45.

130. Giordano TJ, Shedden KA, Schwartz DR, et al. Organ-specific molecular classification of primary lung, colon, and ovarian adenocarcinomas using gene expression profiles. Am J Pathol 2001;159:1231–8.

131. Shukunami K, Hirabuki S, Kaneshima M, et al. Well-differentiated papillary mesothelioma involving the peritoneal and pleural cavities: successful treatment by local and systemic administration of carboplatin. Tumori 2000;86:419–21.

132. Zannoni GF, Sioletic S, Fadda G, et al. The role of HPV detection and typing in diagnosis of pulmonary metastatic squamous cell carcinoma of the uterine cervix. Histopathology 2008;53:604–6.

133. Weichert W, Schewe C, Denkert C, et al. Molecular HPV typing as a diagnostic tool to discriminate primary from metastatic squamous cell carcinoma of the lung. Am J Surg Pathol 2009;33:513–20.

133a. Mercer RR, Lucas NC, Simmons AN, et al. Molecular discrimination of multiple primary cersus metastatic squamous cell cancers of the head/neck and lung. Exp Mol Pathol 2009;86:1–9.

Effects of secondary lung tumours and their clinical features

134. Lowe D, Fletcher CDM. Eosinophilia in squamous cell carcinoma of the oral cavity, external genitalia and anus – clinical correlations. Histopathology 1984;8:627–32.

135. Fujita J, Yamagishi Y, Kubo A, et al. Respiratory failure due to pulmonary lymphangitis carcinomatosis. Chest 1993;103:967–8.

136. Bagshawe KD, Brooks WDW. Subacute pulmonary hypertension due to chorionepithelioma. Lancet 1959;1:653–8.

137. He XW, Tang YH, Luo ZQ, et al. Subacute cor pulmonale due to tumor embolization to the lungs. Angiology 1989;40:11–7.

138. Seckl MJ, Rustin GJS, Newlands ES, et al. Pulmonary embolism, pulmonary hypertension, and choriocarcinoma. Lancet 1991;338:1313–15.

139. Veinot JP, Ford SE, Price RG. Subacute cor pulmonale due to tumor embolization. Arch Pathol Lab Med 1992;116:131–4.

140. Soares FA, Landell GAM, Deoliveira JAM. Pulmonary tumor embolism to alveolar septal capillaries – an unusual cause of sudden cor pulmonale. Arch Pathol Lab Med 1992;116:187–8.

141. Hibbert M, Braude S. Tumour microembolism presenting as 'primary pulmonary hypertension'. Thorax 1997;52:1016–17.

142. Edmondstone WM. Flitting radiographic shadows: an unusual presentation of cancer in the lungs. Thorax 1998;53:906–8.

143. Storey PD, Goldstein W. Pulmonary embolization from primary hepatic carcinoma. Arch Intern Med 1962;110:262–9.

144. Wakasa K, Sakurai M, Uchida A, et al. Massive pulmonary tumor emboli in osteosarcoma: occult and fatal complication. Cancer 1990;66:583–6.

145. Watanabe S, Shimokawa S, Sakasegawa K, et al. Choriocarcinoma in the pulmonary artery treated with emergency pulmonary embolectomy. Chest 2002;121:654–6.

146. Casson AG, McCormack D, Craig I, et al. A persistent pulmonary lesion following chemotherapy for metastatic choriocarcinoma. Chest 1993;103:269–70.

Prolonged survival despite metastatic disease

147. Casciato DA, Nagurka C, Tabbarah HJ. Prolonged survival with unresected pulmonary metastases. Ann Thorac Surg 1983;36:202–8.

148. Bloom HJG, Wallace DM. Hormones and the kidney: possible therapeutic role of testosterone in a patient with regression of metastases from renal adenocarcinoma. BMJ 1964;2:476–80.

149. Palmer MA, Viswanath S, Desmond AD. Spontaneous regression of metastatic renal cell carcinoma. J R Soc Med 1993;86:113–14.

150. Everson TC. Spontaneous regression of cancer. Ann N Y Acad Sci 1964;14:721–35.

151. Casson AG, Putnam JB, Natarajan G, et al. Five-year survival after pulmonary metastatectomy for adult soft tissue sarcoma. Cancer 1992;69:662–8.

152. Matthay RA, Arroliga AC. Resection of pulmonary metastases. Am Rev Respir Dis 1993;148:1691–6.

153. Sakamoto T, Tsubota N, Iwanaga K, et al. Pulmonary resection for metastases from colorectal cancer. Chest 2001;119:1069–72.

154. Davidson RS, Nwogu CE, Brentjens MJ, et al. The surgical management of pulmonary metastasis: current concepts. Surg Oncol 2001;10:35–42.

155. Long-term results of lung metastasectomy: prognostic analyses based on 5206 cases. The International Registry of Lung Metastases. J Thorac Cardiovasc Surg 1997;113:37–49.

156. Kaltreider HB. Alveolar macrophages. Enhancers or suppressors of pulmonary immune reactivity? Chest 1982;82:261–2.

157. Leo F, Cagini L, Rocmans P, et al. Lung metastases from melanoma: when is surgical treatment warranted? Br J Cancer 2000;83:569–72.

158. Friedel G, Pastorino U, Ginsberg RJ, et al. Results of lung metastasectomy from breast cancer: prognostic criteria on the basis of 467 cases of the International Registry of Lung Metastases. Eur J Cardiothorac Surg 2002;22:335–44.

159. Protopapas AD, Nicholson AG, Vini L, et al. Thoracic metastasectomy in thyroid malignancies. Ann Thorac Surg 2001;72:1906–8.

160. Negri F, Musolino A, Cunningham D, et al. Retrospective study of resection of pulmonary metastases in patients with advanced colorectal cancer: the development of a preoperative chemotherapy strategy. Clin Colorectal Cancer 2004;4:101–6.

161. Treasure T. Pulmonary metastasectomy for colorectal cancer: weak evidence and no randomised trials. Eur J Cardiothorac Surg 2008;33:300–2.

Chapter | 12 |

12.7   Tumour-like conditions

This chapter deals with certain tumour-like lesions of the lower respiratory tract, these being non-neoplastic processes that present as masses or nodules within the lung and thereby simulate true neoplasms. However, several such lesions are considered in other chapters, for example endometriosis under systemic disorders and localised areas of organising pneumonia, Langerhans cell histiocytosis and lymphangioleiomyomatosis under diffuse parenchymal diseases. Similarly, inflammatory pseudotumour is dealt with in the chapter on soft-tissue neoplasms (Chapter 12.3) under the title inflammatory myofibroblastic tumour, following recognition that at least some of these lesions are neoplastic rather than reactive. Tumourlets are not considered to be neoplastic but are nevertheless considered with the related carcinoid tumours, as in the context of diffuse neuroendocrine cell hyperplasia they are probably preneoplastic (see p. 598). The term 'pseudolymphoma' has simply become obsolete.

REGENERATIVE CONDITIONS MIMICKING NEOPLASIA

Throughout the lower respiratory tract regenerative processes may be so atypical that carcinomatous transformation has to be considered in the differential diagnosis. This impression is often augmented by excessive mitotic activity and metaplasia. Thus, at the alveolar level necrotising lesions such as infarcts and the granulomatoses may be bordered by foci of atypical squamous hyperplasia that are easily mistaken for squamous cell carcinoma. Similarly, damage to the bronchial epithelium is often followed by atypical regeneration that is easily mistaken for carcinoma, particularly when exfoliated cells are being examined. Bronchoscopy inevitably involves bronchial injury and cytopathologists have to be aware of the atypicalities that follow this procedure. Necrotising lesions of the larynx are sometimes accompanied by atypical regeneration that involves both the surface epithelium and the submucosal glands: the term 'necrotising sialometaplasia' has been applied to this and to a similar process involving the trachea in patients with herpetic tracheitis undergoing repeated intubation (see p. 97).

AMYLOID TUMOUR

Amyloidosis of the lower respiratory tract may develop as part of generalised amyloidosis or in isolation (Table 12.7.1).[1-5] Pulmonary involvement in generalised amyloidosis is dealt with on page 489 and this section deals only with amyloidosis confined to the lower respiratory tract. The disease is usually confined to either the lung parenchyma or the major airways but occasionally affects both.[6] It generally takes the form of tumour-like nodules. In the airways the tumours may be solitary or multifocal, whereas parenchymal tumours are usually solitary. Rarely, however, there may be extensive pulmonary

Figure 12.7.7 Pulmonary hyalinising granuloma. A mass of densely fibrotic tissue with a peripheral rim of chronic inflammation. The fibrotic tissue consists of thick interweaving collagen bundles.

Figure 12.7.6 Inflammatory polyp. (A) A mixed polyp protrudes into a segmental bronchus. (B) The polyp is lined by respiratory epithelium and there is moderate chronic inflammation of the stroma.

There is a marked ultrastructural and immunohistochemical resemblance to meningeal arachnoid granulations and meningiomas,[68–72] in which context it is of interest that a few primary pulmonary meningiomas have been reported (see p. 641). The term 'meningothelioid (or arachnoid) nodules' is therefore preferred to minute pulmonary chemodectomas. Some authors suggest that they have a similar function to the meningeal arachnoid granulations that absorb cerebrospinal fluid and return it to the dural veins: it is suggested that in the lung they may return interstitial fluid to the pulmonary veins and so minimise the danger of pulmonary oedema.[73] Clonality and loss of heterozygosity have been reported but not so frequently as in meningiomas.[72] Reported increases in their number and size probably represent hyperplasia induced by local changes in perfusion, rather than neoplasia. They are confined to the lung and have no malignant potential.

These lesions are generally found fortuitously at autopsy or in surgical samples. Dyspnoea with diffuse radiographic opacification is unusual.[74] An incidence of 1 in every 200–300 autopsies is reported, but this can be increased to around 1 in 25 if a specific search is made.[66,68,75–77] They are more common in patients with thromboembolic disease, other forms of chronic pulmonary disease in which scarring occurs and cardiac failure.[75,76,78] They also appear to be commoner in people who reside at high altitude.[73] A tendency to pulmonary oedema may be the linking factor. The age range is wide but most patients are in their fifth or sixth decade.[78] There is a female preponderance of about 5 to 1, in connection with which it is notable that the lesions bear a progesterone receptor.[78,79]

Pathology

Meningothelioid nodules measure up to 3 mm in diameter. They are occasionally visible beneath the pleura or on the cut surface of the lung but most are discovered only when randomly selected tissue is examined microscopically. They are situated in the pulmonary interstitium close to the walls of veins, causing distension of adjacent alveoli. They consist of aggregated small nests of closely packed cells separated by collagen and elastic tissue (Fig. 12.7.8). The cells have moderate amounts of lightly eosinophilic cytoplasm and often appear elongated. Nuclei are oval or reniform, and vesicular, with a small nucleolus, so differing from the finely dispersed chromatin pattern of tumourlets.

Unlike chemodectomas, sustentacular cells are not present and, unlike tumourlets, argyrophilia and immunohistochemical stains for neuroendocrine markers are negative. Meningothelioid nodules stain for epithelial membrane antigen, progesterone receptor[79] and vimentin but not for cytokeratin, S-100 or actin. The location of tumourlets adjacent to small airways rather than veins is another helpful point of distinction.

MULTIFOCAL MICRONODULAR TYPE II PNEUMOCYTE HYPERPLASIA

Micronodular type II pneumocyte hyperplasia is largely, though not exclusively, confined to patients with tuberous sclerosis, of which it is a particularly rare manifestation.[80–88] It may be seen in otherwise normal lungs or in association with pulmonary

Figure 12.7.8 Meningothelioid nodule (so-called minute pulmonary chemodectoma). (A) Islands of round to oval cells lie within a fibrous stroma. (B) The cells have oval nuclei and eosinophilic cytoplasm without clear cell boundaries.

Figure 12.7.9 (A) Low- and (B) high-power views of micronodular type II cell hyperplasia in tuberous sclerosis.

Figure 12.7.10 Bullous placentoid lesion, (A) Multiple papillary processes as seen leaving a spurious resemblance to chorionic villi few clotted by an attenuated cytokeratin-positives and TTF-1-positives epithelium. The core of the papillae contain a mix of connective tissues, including fat, which is will seen in (B). *(Courtesy of Professor D.W. Henderson, Adelaide, Australia.)*

lymphangioleiomyomatosis. Unlike lymphangioleiomyomatosis, it affects tuberous sclerosis patients of either sex and the hyperplastic type II cells fail to stain for HMB-45.[87] The condition is multifocal and microscopic and usually of no clinical significance. However, in rare cases the lesions are of an appreciable size and so numerous that pulmonary function is severely compromised.[89] The hyperplastic cells stain for cytokeratin, surfactant apoprotein and epithelial membrane antigen. They show no atypia and appear to be devoid of any malignant potential (Fig. 12.7.9).

BULLOUS PLACENTOID LESION (PLACENTAL TRANSMOGRIFICATION)

The nature of this rare lesion is poorly understood but the name by which it is best known, placental transmogrification,[90] is inaccurate: the term 'placentoid'[91] is to be preferred to 'placental' for the condition represents a localised accumulation of papillary processes that bear only a superficial histological resemblance to chorionic villi, being clothed by an attenuated layer of epithelium rather than trophoblast, as shown by cytokeratin immunocytochemistry.

Patients are typically young to middle-aged adults[90,92,93] who often present with pneumothorax related to an associated bullous component.[91,92] The lesion is widely regarded as being reactive to the bullous change but this is disputed as the lung seldom shows bullous change elsewhere, suggesting that the converse may be more correct, namely that the bullous change is the result of the placentoid lesion.[93,94] Attention has therefore switched to the interstitial cores of the papillary processes. These contain a variety of connective tissues, including fibroblasts, fat, smooth muscle, clear cells, blood vessels and lymphatics (Fig. 12.7.10), giving rise to suggestions that the lesion is a benign connective tissue tumour or tumour-like process sharing some features with the common 'chondroid hamartoma' described on page 626.[92,95,96] This suggestion derives support from the lesion being identified adjacent to six of 38 resected 'chondroid hamartomas'.[95]

REFERENCES

Amyloid tumour

1. Thompson PJ, Citron KM. Amyloid and the lower respiratory tract. Thorax 1983;38:84–7.
2. Hui AN, Koss MN, Hochholzer L, et al. Amyloidosis presenting in the lower respiratory tract. Arch Pathol Lab Med 1986;110:212–18.
3. Cordier JF, Loire R, Brune J. Amyloidosis of the lower respiratory tract. Chest 1986;90:827–31.
4. Utz JP, Swensen SJ, Gertz MA. Pulmonary amyloidosis. The Mayo Clinic experience from 1980 to 1993. Ann Intern Med 1996;124:407–13.
5. Gillmore JD, Hawkins PN. Amyloidosis and the respiratory tract. Thorax 1999;54:444–51.
6. Schulz C, Hauck RW, Nathrath WBJ, et al. Combined amyloidosis of the upper and lower respiratory tract. Respiration 1995;62:163–6.
7. Thompson PJ, Jewkes J, Corrin B, et al. Primary bronchopulmonary amyloid tumour with massive hilar lymphadenopathy. Thorax 1983;38:153–4.
8. Laden SA, Cohen ML, Harley RA. Nodular pulmonary amyloidosis with extrapulmonary involvement. Hum Pathol 1984;15:594–7.
9. Knapp MJ, Roggli VL, Kim J, et al. Pleural amyloidosis. Arch Pathol Lab Med 1988;112:57–60.
10. Adams AL, Castro CY, Singh SP, et al. Pleural amyloidosis mimicking mesothelioma: a clinicopathologic study of two cases. Ann Diagn Pathol 2001;5:229–32.
11. Shah PL, Gillmore JD, Copley SJ, et al. The importance of complete screening for amyloid fibril type and systemic disease in patients with amyloidosis in the respiratory tract. Sarcoidosis Vasc Diffuse Lung Dis 2002;19:134–42.
12. Gordon HW, Miller R, Mittman C. Medullary carcinoma of the lung with amyloid stroma: a counterpart of medullary carcinoma of the thyroid. Hum Pathol 1973;4:431–6.
13. Al-Kaisi N, Abdul-Karim FW, Mendelsohn G, et al. Bronchial carcinoid tumour with amyloid stroma. Arch Pathol Lab Med 1988;112:211–14.
14. Abe Y, Utsunomiya H, Tsutsumi Y. Atypical carcinoid tumor of the lung with amyloid stroma. Acta Pathol Jpn 1992;42:286–92.
15. Davis CJ, Butchart EG, Gibbs AR. Nodular pulmonary amyloidosis occurring in association with pulmonary lymphoma. Thorax 1991;46:217–18.
16. Michaels L, Hyams VJ. Amyloid in localised deposits and plasmacytomas of the respiratory tract. J Pathol 1979;128:29–38.
17. Jenkins MCF, Potter M. Calcified pseudotumoural mediastinal amyloidosis. Thorax 1991;46:686–7.
18. Ihling C, Weirich G, Gaa A, et al. Amyloid tumours of the lung – an immunocytoma? Pathol Res Pract 1996;192:446–52.
19. Dacic S, Colby TV, Yousem SA. Nodular amyloidoma and primary pulmonary lymphoma with amyloid production: A differential diagnostic problem. Modern Pathol 2000;13:934–40.
20. Lim JK, Lacy MQ, Kurtin PJ, et al. Pulmonary marginal zone lymphoma of MALT type as a cause of localised pulmonary amyloidosis. J Clin Pathol 2001;54:642–6.
21. Lantuejoul S, Moulai N, Quetant S, et al. Unusual cystic presentation of pulmonary nodular amyloidosis associated with MALT-type lymphoma. Eur Respir J 2007;30:589–92.
22. Bonner H, Ennis RS, Geelhoed GW, et al. Lymphoid infiltration and amyloidosis of lung in Sjögren's syndrome. Arch Pathol Lab Med 1973;95:42–4.
23. Kobayashi H, Matsuoka R, Kitamura S, et al. Sjögren's syndrome with multiple bullae and pulmonary nodular amyloidosis. Chest 1988;94:438–40.
24. Zatloukal P, Bezdicek P, Schimonova M, et al. Waldenström's macroglobulinemia with pulmonary amyloidosis. Respiration 1998;65:414–6.
25. Smith RRL, Hutchins GM, Moore GW, et al. Type and distribution of pulmonary parenchymal and vascular amyloid: correlation with cardiac amyloidosis. Am J Med 1979;66:96–104.
26. DaCosta P, Corrin B. Amyloidosis localized to the lower respiratory tract: probable immunoamyloid nature of the tracheobronchial and nodular pulmonary forms. Histopathology 1985;9:703–10.
27. Miura K, Shirasawa H. Lambda III subgroup immunoglobulin light chains are precursor proteins of nodular pulmonary amyloidosis. Am J Clin Pathol 1993;100:561–6.
28. Toyoda M, Ebihara Y, Kato H, et al. Tracheobronchial AL amyloidosis – histologic, immunohistochemical, ultrastructural, and immunoelectron microscopic observations. Hum Pathol 1993;24:970–6.
29. Page DL, Isersky C, Harada M, et al. Immunoglobulin origin of localized nodular pulmonary amyloidosis. Res Exp Med 1972;159:75–86.
30. Stokes MB, Jagirdar J, Burchstin O, et al. Nodular pulmonary immunoglobulin light chain deposits with coexistent amyloid and nonamyloid features in an HIV-infected patient. Modern Pathol 1997;10:1059–65.

31. Sakula A. Tracheobronchopathia osteoplastica. Its relationship to primary tracheobronchial amyloidosis. Thorax 1968;23:105–10.

32. Alroy GG, Lichtig C, Kaftori JK. Tracheobronchopathia osteoplastica: end stage of primary lung amyloidosis? Chest 1972;61:465–8.

33. Jones AW, Chatterji AN. Primary tracheobronchial amyloidosis with tracheobronchopathia osteoplastica. Br J Dis Chest 1977;71:268–72.

34. Khoor A, Myers JL, Tazelaar HD, et al. Amyloid-like pulmonary nodules, including localized light-chain deposition. Am J Clin Pathol 2004;121:200–4.

35. Dyke PC, Demaray MJ, Delavan JW, et al. Pulmonary amyloidoma. Am J Clin Pathol 1974;61:301–5.

Light-chain deposition disease

36. Kijner CH, Yousem SA. Systemic light chain deposition disease presenting as multiple pulmonary nodules. A case report and review of the literature. Am J Surg Pathol 1988;12:405–13.

37. Morinaga S, Watanabe H, Gemma A, et al. Plasmacytoma of the lung associated with nodular deposits of immunoglobulin. Am J Surg Pathol 1987;11:989–95.

38. Piard F, Yaziji N, Jarry O, et al. Solitary plasmacytoma of the lung with light chain extracellular deposits: a case report and review of the literature. Histopathology 1998;32:356–61.

39. Rostagno A, Frizzera G, Ylagan L, et al. Tumoral non-amyloidotic monoclonal immunoglobulin light chain deposits ('aggregoma'): presenting feature of B-cell dyscrasia in three cases with immunohistochemical and biochemical analyses. Br J Haematol 2002;119:62–9.

40. Colombat M, Stern M, Groussard O, et al. Pulmonary cystic disorder related to light chain deposition disease. Am J Respir Crit Care Med 2006;173:777–80.

41. Bhargava P, Rushin JM, Rusnock EJ, et al. Pulmonary light chain deposition disease: report of five cases and review of the literature. Am J Surg Pathol 2007;31:267–76.

42. Colombat M, Caudroy S, Lagonotte E, et al. Pathomechanisms of cyst formation in pulmonary light chain deposition disease. Eur Respir J 2008;32:1399–403.

Crystal-storing histiocytosis

43. Kazzaz B, Dewar A, Corrin B. An unusual pulmonary plasmacytoma. Histopathology 1992;21:285–7.

44. Jones D, Renshaw AA. Recurrent crystal-storing histiocytosis of the lung in a patient without a clonal lymphoproliferative disorder. Arch Pathol Lab Med 1996;120:978–80.

45. Renshaw AA, Dean BR, Antman KH, et al. The role of cytologic evaluation of pleural fluid in the diagnosis of malignant mesothelioma. Chest 1997;111:106–9.

46. Prasad ML, Charney DA, Sarlin J, et al. Pulmonary immunocytoma with massive crystal storing histiocytosis: A case report with review of literature. Am J Surg Pathol 1998;22:1148–53.

47. Ionescu DN, Pierson DM, Qing G, et al. Pulmonary crystal-storing histiocytoma. Arch Pathol Lab Med 2005;129:1159–63.

48. Fairweather PM, Williamson R, Tsikleas G. Pulmonary extranodal marginal zone lymphoma with massive crystal storing histiocytosis. Am J Surg Pathol 2006;30:262–7.

49. Lewis JT, Candelora JN, Hogan RB, et al. Crystal-storing histiocytosis due to massive accumulation of Charcot–Leyden crystals: a unique association producing colonic polyposis in a 78-year-old woman with eosinophilic colitis. Am J Surg Pathol 2007;31:481–5.

Bronchial inflammatory polyp

50. McShane D, Nicholson AG, Goldstraw P, et al. Inflammatory endobronchial polyps in childhood: clinical spectrum and possible link to mechanical ventilation. Pediatr Pulmonol 2002;34:79–84.

51. Roberts C, Devenny AM, Brooker R, et al. Inflammatory endobronchial polyposis with bronchiectasis in cystic fibrosis. Eur Resp J 2001;18:612–15.

52. Yamagishi M, Harada H, Kurihara M, et al. Inflammatory endotracheal polyp resolved after antibiotic treatment. Respiration 1993;60:193–6.

Hyalinizing granuloma

53. Engleman P, Liebow AA, Gmelich J, et al. Pulmonary hyalinizing granuloma. Am Rev Respir Dis 1977;115:997–1008.

54. Schlosnagle DC, Check IJ, Sewell CW, et al. Immunologic abnormalities in two patients with pulmonary hyalinizing granuloma. Am J Clin Pathol 1982;78:231–5.

55. Guccion JG, Rohatgi PK, Saini N. Pulmonary hyalinizing granuloma. Electron microscopic and immunologic studies. Chest 1984;85:571–3.

56. Yousem SA, Hochholzer L. Pulmonary hyalinizing granuloma. Am J Clin Pathol 1987;87:1–6.

57. Patel Y, Ishikawa S, Macdonnell KF. Pulmonary hyalinizing granuloma presenting as multiple cavitary calcified nodules. Chest 1991;100:1720–1.

58. Russell AFR, Suggit RIC, Kazzi JC. Pulmonary hyalinising granuloma: A case report and literature review. Pathology 2000;32:290–3.

59. Dent RG, Godden DJ, Stovin PGI, et al. Pulmonary hyalinising granuloma in association with retroperitoneal fibrosis. Thorax 1983;38:955–6.

60. Kuramochi S, Kawai T, Yakumaru K, et al. Multiple pulmonary hyalinizing granulomas associated with systemic idiopathic fibrosis. Acta Pathol Jpn 1991;41:375–82.

61. Basoglu A, Findik S, Celik B, et al. Pulmonary hyalinizing granuloma mimicking lung carcinoma. Thorac Cardiovasc Surg 2006;54:282–3.

62. Drasin H, Blume MR, Rosenbaum EH, et al. Pulmonary hyalinizing granulomas in a patient with malignant lymphoma, with development nine years later of multiple myeloma and systemic amyloidosis. Cancer 1979;44:215–20.

63. Ren YF, Raitz EN, Lee KR, et al. Pulmonary small lymphocytic lymphoma (mucosa-associated lymphoid tissue type) associated with pulmonary hyalinizing granuloma. Chest 2001;120:1027–30.

64. Atagi S, Sakatani M, Akira M, et al. Pulmonary hyalinizing granuloma with Castleman's disease. Intern Med 1994;33:689–91.

65. John PG, Rahman J, Payne CB. Pulmonary hyalinizing granuloma: an unusual association with multiple sclerosis. South Med J 1995;88:1076–7.

Multiple minute meningothelioid nodules

66. Korn D, Bensch K, Liebow AA, et al. Multiple minute pulmonary tumours resembling chemodectomas. Am J Pathol 1960;37:641–72.

67. Zak FG, Chabes A. Pulmonary chemodectomatosis. JAMA 1963;183:887–9.

68. Churg AM, Warnock ML. So-called 'minute pulmonary chemodectoma'. A tumour not related to paragangliomas. Cancer 1976;37:1759–69.

69. Kuhn C, Askin FB. The fine structure of so-called minute pulmonary chemodectomas. Hum Pathol 1975;6:681–91.

70. Gaffey MJ, Mills SE, Askin FB. Minute pulmonary meningothelial-like nodules. A clinicopathologic study of so-called minute pulmonary chemodectoma. Am J Surg Pathol 1988;12:167–75.

71. Torikata C, Mukai M. So-called minute chemodectoma of the lung. An electron microscopic and immunohistochemical study. Virchows Arch A Pathol Anat Histopathol 1990;417:113–18.

72. Niho S, Yokose T, Nishiwaki Y, et al. Immunohistochemical and clonal analysis of minute pulmonary meningothelial-like nodules. Hum Pathol 1999;30:425–9.

73. Heath D, Williams D. Arachnoid nodules in the lungs of high altitude Indians. Thorax 1993;48:743–5.

74. Suster S, Moran CA. Diffuse pulmonary meningotheliomatosis. Am J Surg Pathol 2007;31:624–31.

75. Spain DM. Intrapulmonary chemodectomas in subjects with organising pulmonary thromboemboli. Am Rev Respir Dis 1967;96:1158–64.

76. Ichinose H, Hewitt RL, Drapanas T. Minute pulmonary chemodectoma. Cancer 1971;28:692–700.

77. Mizutani E, Tsuta K, Maeshima AM, et al. Minute pulmonary meningothelial-like nodules: clinicopathologic analysis of 121 patients. Human Pathology 2009;40:678–82.

78. Mukhopadhyay S, El-Zammar OA, Katzenstein ALA. Pulmonary meningothelial-like nodules: new insights into a common but poorly understood entity. Am J Surg Pathol 2009;33:487–95.

79. Pelosi G, Maffini F, Decarli N, et al. Progesterone receptor immunoreactivity in minute meningothelioid nodules of the lung. Virchows Archiv 2002;440: 543–6.

Multifocal micronodular type II pneumocyte hyperplasia

80. Corrin B, Liebow AA, Friedman PJ. Pulmonary lymphangiomyomatosis. Am J Pathol 1975;79:347–82.

81. Lie JT, Miller RD, Williams DE. Cystic disease of the lungs in tuberous sclerosis. Clinicopathologic correlation, including body plethysmographic lung function tests. Mayo Clin Proc 1980;55:547–53.

82. Popper HH, Juettner-Smolle FM, Pongratz MG. Micronodular hyperplasia of type-II pneumocytes – a new lung lesion associated with tuberous sclerosis. Histopathology 1991;18:347–54.

83. Popper HH. Micronodular hyperplasia of type-II pneumocytes. Histopathology 1992;20:281.

84. Guinee D, Singh R, Azumi N, et al. Multifocal micronodular pneumocyte hyperplasia: a distinctive pulmonary manifestation of tuberous sclerosis. Mod Pathol 1995;8:902–6.

85. Bonetti F, Chiodera P. The lung in tuberous sclerosis. In: Corrin B, editor. Pathology of Lung Tumors. London: Churchill Livingstone; 1997. p. 225–40.

86. Lantuejoul S, Ferretti G, Negoescu A, et al. Multifocal alveolar hyperplasia associated with lymphangioleiomyomatosis in tuberous sclerosis. Histopathology 1997;30:570–5.

87. Muir TE, Leslie KO, Popper H, et al. Micronodular pneumocyte hyperplasia. Am J Surg Pathol 1998;22:465–72.

88. Yamanaka A, Kitaichi M, Fujimoto T, et al. Multifocal micronodular pneumocyte hyperplasia in a postmenopausal woman with tuberous sclerosis. Virchows Archiv 2000. APR;436(4):389–92 2000;436:389–92.

89. Cancellieri A, Poletti V, Corrin B. Respiratory failure due to micronodular type II pneumocyte hyperplasia. Histopathology 2002;41:263–5.

Bullous placentoid lesion (placental transmogrification)

90. Fidler ME, Koomen M, Sebek B, et al. Placental transmogrification of the lung, a histologic variant of giant bullous emphysema: clinicopathological study of three further cases. Am J Surg Pathol 1995;19:563–70.

91. Mark EJ, Muller KM, McChesney T, et al. Placentoid bullous lesion of the lung. Hum Pathol 1995;26:74–9.

92. Hochholzer L, Moran CA, Koss MN. Pulmonary lipomatosis: A variant of placental transmogrification. Modern Pathol 1997;10:846–9.

93. Marchevsky AM, Guintu R, Koss M, et al. Swyer–James (MacLeod) syndrome with placental transmogrification of the lung: a case report and review of the literature. Arch Pathol Lab Med 2005;129:686–9.

94. Cavazza A, Lantuejoul S, Sartori G, et al. Placental transmogrification of the lung: clinicopathologic, immunohistochemical and molecular study of two cases, with particular emphasis on the interstitial clear cells. Hum Pathol 2004;35:517–21.

95. Xu R, Murray M, Jagirdar J, et al. Placental transmogrification of the lung is a histologic pattern frequently associated with pulmonary fibrochondromatous hamartoma. Arch Pathol Lab Med 2002;126:562–6.

96. Santana AN, Canzian M, Stelmach R, et al. Placental transmogrification of the lung presenting as giant bullae with soft-fatty components. Eur J Cardiothorac Surg 2008;33:124–6.

Chapter |13|

Pleura and chest wall

NORMAL STRUCTURE AND FUNCTION OF THE PLEURA

The lung is surrounded by a smooth glistening membrane, the visceral pleura, which is reflected at the hilum over the mediastinum and the inside of the chest wall as the parietal pleura. The potential space thus created extends from the root of the neck, 3 cm above the midpoint of the clavicle, down behind the abdominal cavity and the kidney as

©2010 Elsevier Ltd
DOI: 10.1016/B978-0-7020-3369-8.00013-6

the costodiaphragmatic recess as far as the 12th rib. The two layers of the pleura are in close contact and slide easily over each other because of a thin mucinous film between them. Although this facilitates respiratory movements, there is little respiratory embarrassment if the pleural space is obliterated. Indeed, elephants and other large animals that generate large negative intrathoracic pressures lose their pleural cavities early in development without suffering any evident respiratory disability. The pleural cavities have therefore been called 'an anatomical luxury and a pathological hazard'.[1]

Each pleural surface consists of connective tissue covered by a single layer of flattened mesothelial cells which secrete fluid rich in hyaluronic acid. However, most of the pleural fluid (which normally amounts to no more than a few millilitres) is a transudate of blood plasma with a protein concentration of less than 2 g/dl, mainly albumin. Although the parietal and visceral layers of the pleura both receive blood from systemic arteries – distal branches of the intercostal and bronchial arteries respectively – the visceral layer is largely supplied by pulmonary vessels and, because of the different pressures in the systemic and pulmonary circulations, most of the pleural fluid enters through the parietal pleura. Initial views that it was absorbed by the visceral pleura were based on the false assumption that the two pleurae were morphologically similar and that Starling principles would apply. In fact the parietal and visceral pleurae differ considerably in structure.[2,3] Whereas the connective tissue of the parietal pleura is thin and capillaries and lymphatics within this tissue are no more than a few microns from the pleural space, the connective tissue of the visceral pleura is relatively thick. The pulmonary blood vessels lie deep to the pleura and are separated from the pleural space by as much as 60–70 μm. Furthermore, the parietal pleura is equipped with specialised stomata, described below, which provide a direct exit from the pleural space.[4] Under normal circumstances most of the fluid therefore both enters and leaves the pleural space through the parietal pleura (Fig. 13.1).

The uptake of macromolecules and particles less than 4 nm in diameter probably takes place by passive diffusion through the gap junctions that connect many mesothelial cells[5] and by active vesicular transport across the mesothelial cytoplasm.[6,7] Larger particles are mainly cleared in the caudal portions of the parietal pleura. The systemic lymphatic network is particularly rich here, and mesothelial and lymphatic endothelial cells are in direct apposition, without an intervening basement membrane. Here too, stomata in the parietal pleura provide a direct connection between the pleural cavity and the underlying lymphatics.[8] Over the lower mediastinum the stomata are associated with collections of macrophages and lymphoid cells, visible macroscopically as pale spots known as Kampmeier's foci. Particles up to about 10 μm are absorbed by the stomata-membrana-cribriformis complex, a process that is monitored by the lymphoreticular cells of Kampmeier's foci. Many particles are rapidly cleared by this route[9] but some are retained in Kampmeier's foci to form what are termed black spots.[10–12]

Mesothelial cells express epithelial markers such as cytokeratin and are joined by desmosomes which contribute to the formation of either tight or gap junctions. However, many mesothelial cells merely overlap one another, like lymphatic endothelial cells. Pinocytotic vesicles are plentiful in the cytoplasm which also contains rough endoplasmic reticulum and bundles of fine filaments. The mesothelial cell surface is not smooth but bears long, slender microvilli measuring up to 3 μm in length and 0.3 μm in width, suggesting an absorptive function. The numbers of microvilli vary from cell to cell. They are sparse over the ribs but increase towards the base of the lung and are more numerous on the visceral than the parietal pleura.[13] With their surface mucopolysacharide coat, microvilli may also counter frictional forces.[14]

Except at the stomata in the parietal pleura described above, both layers of mesothelium rest upon a continuous basement membrane,

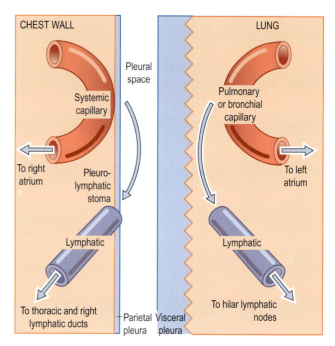

Figure 13.1 The normal formation and drainage of pleural fluid. Pleural fluid is normally derived from the high-pressure systemic blood vessels in the parietal pleura and most of it leaves the pleural space through stomata in the parietal pleura. This changes when the pulmonary venous pressure rises (as in left heart failure) and when the pulmonary vasculature is unduly leaky (as in pneumonia), in which circumstances fluid enters the pleural space through the visceral pleura (the inner elastin layer of which is represented here by the thin red zigzag line).

beneath which there is a connective tissue network, which, as noted above, is thicker in the visceral pleura than in the parietal pleura. In the parietal pleura the amount and distribution of elastin are irregular whereas in the visceral pleura a thin inner and a thick outer elastic lamina can generally be discerned. Thus, the visceral pleura comprises five layers (Fig. 13.2):

1. The flattened mesothelium and its basement membrane
2. A thin submesothelial layer of loose connective tissue
3. A thin outer layer of elastin, which is continuous around the lobe and does not dip into the interlobular septa
4. A thicker layer of loose connective tissue in which are found the pleural veins, the pleural arteries (which are branches of the systemic bronchial arteries) and the pleural lymphatics. The lymphatics are valved whereas the veins are not, the opposite to what appertains elsewhere in the body
5. A relatively thick layer of elastin, which dips into the interlobular septa and is continuous with the elastic tissue of the peripheral alveoli.

Mesothelial cells are readily damaged and desquamate in large numbers in many pathological conditions. Unlike epithelium, mesothelial repair does not solely involve centripetal migration of adjacent cells, as evidenced by the fact that large and small pleural lesions heal in exactly the same time. Mesothelial repair depends upon the differentiation of submesothelial connective tissue cells[15–19] and exfoliated mesothelial cells resettling on the denuded areas[20,21] as well as the centripetal migration of adjacent mesothelial cells.[21,22] Macrophages also settle out from the pleural fluid[23,24] but do not appear to differentiate into mesothelial cells.[15,25] Differentiation of proliferating submesothelial cells involves the acquisition of cytok-

Figure 13.2 The normal visceral pleura at its intersection with an interlobular septum. The visceral pleura comprises five layers, the presence and thickness of which vary regionally: (1) the surface mesothelium and its basement membrane; (2) a thin layer of connective tissue; (3) a prominent outer elastin layer; (4) a band of collagen; and (5) an inner elastin layer (which is continuous with the alveolar elastin). Whereas the outer layer of elastin forms a continuous band around each lobe, the inner elastin layer turns inwards wherever interlobular septa join the pleura. In decortication it is the collagen layer that forms the plane of cleavage but it is the outer elastin layer that needs to be addressed when assessing tumour spread (see tumour staging, p. 571).

eratin antigens, markers of mesothelial cells not normally found in connective tissue; this complicates the interpretation of immunocytochemical stains used to distinguish granulation tissue from mesothelioma of sarcomatous pattern (see p. 728).[17]

PLEURAL EFFUSIONS

Pleural effusions may be serous (hydrothorax), bloody (haemothorax) or chylous (chylothorax), or consist of frank pus (pyothorax or empyema thoracis). Most are caused by malignancy or infection.[26] Their rapid therapeutic removal occasionally alters pulmonary haemodynamics to such an extent that pulmonary oedema or even pulmonary haemorrhage results.[27,28]

Hydrothorax

Serous effusions may be clear or cloudy, the former usually denoting a transudate low in protein content and the latter a protein-rich exudate. The traditional demarcation point between transudates and exudates is 3 g protein/dl but pleural fluid-to-serum ratios of protein, lactic dehydrogenase and cholesterol are now widely used.[29–31]

Transudates develop in cardiac failure, overhydration, constrictive pericarditis and fibrosing mediastinitis, the fluid accumulation resulting from an imbalance between hydrostatic and osmotic forces in each case. In cardiac failure the effusion is commonly unilateral. It is often stated that the right side is more frequently involved than the left but several studies have failed to confirm this. Pleural effusion is more likely to develop when cardiac failure is accompanied by pulmonary venous hypertension than when there is systemic venous hypertension. Thus pleural effusion is common with left ventricular failure but rare with cor pulmonale.

Exudates are of varying aetiology, being the result of pleural or pulmonary irritation from any cause. The irritation is often due to acute infection, which is usually pneumonic but may be a pulmonary or subdiaphragmatic abscess. Other causes include acute pancreatitis,[32] rheumatoid disease, lupus erythematosus, tuberculosis, pulmonary infarction, a drug reaction (notably to practolol, methysergide and bromocriptine), non-malignant asbestos pleurisy, cancer and lymphatic obstruction or deficiency, and even pleural amyloidosis.[33] Acute irritation typically leads to an accumulation of neutrophils in the fluid and chronic disease to increased numbers of lymphocytes. Pleural exudates due to defective lymphatic drainage are also rich in lymphocytes. A predominance of eosinophils is occasionally found, even in the absence of blood eosinophilia. The most common associations of an eosinophil-rich pleural effusion are malignancy, infection and trauma but often no cause can be identified.[34] Exudates caused by cancer and pulmonary infarction are commonly bloodstained.[26] The presence of tumour markers in the exudate may contribute to the diagnosis.[35]

Ascites may also result in pleural effusion due to ascitic fluid crossing the diaphragm, in which case the nature of the pleural effusion is similar to that of the ascitic fluid from which it derives. The passage is through mesothelium-lined channels, which are generally microscopic but may measure up to 5 mm.[36] The sudden development of a pleural effusion in association with ascites secondary to a pelvic tumour is known as Meig's syndrome (see p. 495). Hydrothorax is also recorded in patients with ascites secondary to cirrhosis[36] and in those undergoing peritoneal dialysis.[37] Ovarian stimulation undertaken for in vitro fertilisation is a more recently recognised cause of pleural effusion accompanying ascites.[38]

Chylothorax

The accumulation of chyle in the pleural space is due to obstruction or rupture of the thoracic duct.[39] Rupture is usually traumatic whilst obstruction may be developmental, neoplastic or surgical, or due to rare conditions such as lymphangioleiomyomatosis (see p. 293), angiofollicular lymphoid hyperplasia (Castleman's disease, see p. 669) or the yellow-nail syndrome.[40] Chyle is rich in dietary fat and a chylous effusion appears milky (Fig. 13.3A). Diagnosis involves cholesterol and triglyceride measurement in the pleural fluid. Pseudochylothorax may develop in a long-standing serous exudate: this also looks milky and has a high content of cholesterol but it lacks the triglycerides and chylomicrons found in chyle.[41] Complications include malnutrition, immunosuppression and respiratory distress.

Yellow-nail syndrome

This syndrome, first described in 1964, consists of chylous effusions, lymphoedema of varied distribution and yellow discoloration and distortion of the nails, all of which are attributed to defective lymphatic drainage (Fig. 13.3B).[42] It is often associated with repeated pulmonary infections, bronchiectasis and an immunological disorder such as lymphopenia, hypogammaglobulinaemia or macroglobulinaemia.[42–47] Although widely regarded as representing a hereditary disorder, the family history is generally negative and the clinical features are seldom evident before adult life: the median age at diagnosis is 61 years (range 18–82 years).[48,49] The yellow nails may return to normal if the pulmonary problems are treated successfully.[49]

Figure 13.3 Yellow-nail syndrome. (A) A chylous pleural exudate aspirated from a patient with the yellow-nail syndrome. (B) Dilated pleural lymphatics in another patient with the syndrome. *(B courtesy of Dr Fiona Roberts, Glasgow, UK)*

Haemothorax

Haemorrhage into a pleural sac may follow trauma to the chest, pulmonary embolism or spontaneous rupture of an aneurysm of the thoracic aorta.[50] Occasionally, rupture of an emphysematous bulla is followed by haemopneumothorax, with blood and air escaping simultaneously from the damaged lung into the sac.[51] Thoracic endometriosis may also cause haemopneumothorax (see p. 495). Carcinomatous involvement of the pleura typically causes a blood-stained pleural effusion but seldom gives rise to frank haemorrhage.

Biliothorax (thoracobilia)

The removal of gallstones from the pleural cavity is one of the more unusual thoracic operations.[52] Such calculi enter the thorax by producing a cholecystopleural fistula. The accompanying bile is liable to cause a chemical pleuritis resulting in severe respiratory insufficiency.

Silicone thorax

Pleural nodules representing a foreign-body reaction to silicone is described in a woman whose breast implant had burst and who had subsequently undergone cardiac surgery, which admitted the silicone into the pleural cavity.[53]

PNEUMOTHORAX

Air may enter the pleural sac through either the chest wall or the visceral pleura. In the former case the condition is almost always due to trauma, a fractured clavicle or rib lacerating the parietal pleura and allowing the ingress of air through an associated wound of the skin. Sometimes, the local blood vessels may also be damaged and the condition becomes one of haemopneumothorax. In surgical operations on the thorax the pleural sac is often opened and allowed to fill with air. Formerly, air was deliberately introduced into the pleural sac in the treatment of chronic respiratory tuberculosis, to collapse and thus rest the lung (artificial pneumothorax). Further consideration will be limited to air entering the pleural sac through the visceral pleura. Such pneumothoraces may be open or closed: in the former, the aperture remains patent, so that air can pass freely into and out of the sac; in the latter, the opening soon becomes sealed, and thus traps the air that has entered. Once the air leak has been sealed, the air in the pleural sac is gradually absorbed over the ensuing weeks – oxygen first and nitrogen later. Occasionally, and particularly in older people, the tissues near the orifice act as a valve, allowing air to enter but not to escape. In these cases pressure builds up in the sac, displacing the structures of the mediastinum to the opposite side, with consequent grave embarrassment of respiration. This is known as pressure or tension pneumothorax and constitute a medical emergency.

Clinical features

Pneumothorax is usually sudden in onset, and often occurs during physical exertion. It is generally unilateral. Bilateral pneumothorax is more serious since there is interference with the inflation of both lungs. The onset is painful, and quickly followed by shortness of breath, especially in patients with emphysema or other extensive chronic pulmonary disease that already impairs their respiratory capacity. In the cases in which the tissues create a valve at the site of perforation, the pneumothorax may build up slowly without any

Air entry through the chest wall

Trauma

Air entry through the visceral pleura

Emphysema
Langerhans cell histiocytosis
Lymphangioleiomyomatosis
Cystic fibrosis
Thoracic endometriosis
Lymphoid interstitial pneumonia
Light-chain deposition disease
Marfan's syndrome
Ehlers–Danlos syndrome
Birt–Hogg–Dubé syndrome
Necrotising pneumonia, as with *Pneumocystis*

Figure 13.4 A bulla, rupture of which had caused pneumothorax, associated with a focus of fibrosis, the so-called apical cap. The overlying visceral pleura is oedematous and contains pockets of air. These represent interstitial emphysema and are termed blebs, in contrast to bullae, such as that seen to the left, which represent enlarged alveolar spaces.

sudden symptoms; in these instances the displacement of the mediastinum is apt to be greater.

Epidemiology

Epidemiological studies show that men are affected more than women (in a ratio of 2.4 : 1), that there is a biphasic age distribution and that most deaths occur in older patients.[54] Cigarette smoking increases the risk in a dose-dependent manner[55] and cannabis use further increases this risk.[56,57]

Pathogenesis and pathological features

Escape of air into the pleural space from the lungs may be due to trauma or some pathological change in the lungs, usually emphysema. It causes the lung to collapse and if bilateral may prove fatal (see Fig. 7.2.7, p. 377). Other conditions in which pneumothorax occur particularly frequently are listed in Box 13.1. A sudden drop in atmospheric pressure may be the precipitating factor and occasionally loud music has also had this effect, pressure changes presumably being again responsible.[58,59]

Pneumothorax also occurs in healthy young individuals who appear to have normal lungs. This is known as idiopathic spontaneous pneumothorax. When treatment in such cases has necessitated thoracotomy it has usually been found that at the apex of the lung there is an area of fibrosis, 2–3 cm in its greatest dimension, surmounted by one or more bullae up to 1 cm or so in diameter.[60,61] A hole may be found in the pleural surface adjoining the bullae, or one of the bullae may have a tear in its wall. Microscopy shows subpleural alveolar collapse and fibrosis, and an accumulation of chronic inflammatory cells (Fig. 13.4), but no evidence of tuberculosis or other specific disease. Such lesions are not uncommon. They were identified in 15 (6%) of 250 young, healthy adults undergoing bilateral thoracoscopic sympathectomy for hyperhidrosis.[62] It has been suggested that, since most of these patients are tall, thin men, the changes in the apical region of the lungs – demonstrably affected bilaterally in some cases – may be developmental in origin and possibly related to rapid somatic growth. Their tall build will result in the apices of these individuals' lungs being particularly poorly perfused when they stand erect. This ischaemia may damage the apices directly or contribute to the fibrosis by impairing the resolution of any inflammatory process.[63] Because the apical changes are frequently bilateral, there is often recurrence on the opposite side.

Pneumothorax causes a reactive mesothelial hyperplasia associated with an inflammatory infiltrate that is frequently rich in eosinophils and is sometimes called 'reactive eosinophilic pleuritis'.[64,65] The infiltrate is superficial, penetrating only a short distance into the substance of the lung beneath the pleura: this distinguishes the process from eosinophilic granuloma of the lung and eosinophilic pneumonia. Small blood vessels may be involved but limitation of the process to the subpleural region of the lung distinguishes it from a true vasculitis. Reactive type II pneumocyte hyperplasia may also develop and be atypical enough to arouse suspicion of adenocarcinoma.[66]

If air is maintained in the pleural cavity for many months, as was once customary in the treatment of pulmonary tuberculosis, the mesothelium may undergo extensive squamous change. It is uncertain whether this represents metaplasia of the mesothelium, extension of metaplastic bronchial epithelium through a bronchopleural fistula or implantation of skin, but progression to malignancy has been noted.[67] In cystic fibrosis, focal replacement of the visceral pleural mesothelium by ciliated columnar or squamous epithelium has been described, possibly due to rupture of bronchiectatic abscesses[68] and perhaps contributing to the pathogenesis of pneumothorax in this condition.[69] Unexplained columnar or mucous cell metaplasia of the pleura has also been reported.[70]

Pleurodesis

If a patient suffers from repeated pneumothoraces, it may be necessary to obliterate the pleural cavity, a procedure termed 'pleurodesis'. This may be effected surgically, by stripping the pleura, or by the instillation of sclerosing substances such as talc or tetracycline. Intractable pleural effusions may also require such treatment, especially in the palliation of malignant effusions. However, before performing pleurodesis consideration should be given to the possibility of the underlying condition requiring lung transplantation at some future date as pleurodesis would make this technically difficult. The histological observation of numerous birefringent crystals in a fibrotic pleura indicates that pleurodesis has been undertaken in the past (Fig. 13.5). Neoplasia involving the chest wall 2 years after talc pleurodesis is recorded but the tumour was an adenocarcinoma of the peripheral lung rather than a pleural mesothelioma[71] and is therefore likely to have been coincidental, particularly as no mesotheliomas developed in any of 80 patients who had undergone talc pleurodesis 22–35 years previously.[72] Although commercial talc is often contaminated by tremolite asbestos and talc miners have developed mesothelioma, cosmetic talc and that used in medicine are rigorously screened to ensure their purity; they appear to be entirely non-carcinogenic but there are reports of acute lung enjury following pleural talc insufflation.[73,73a]

INFLAMMATION AND FIBROSIS OF THE PLEURA (PLEURITIS, PLEURISY)

Inflammation of the pleural sac can develop in many conditions (Box 13.2). Usually, it is secondary to inflammation of one of the adjoining thoracic or subdiaphragmatic structures, particularly the lungs. Sometimes, it is a manifestation of systemic lupus erythematosus or another connective tissue disorder (see below). Asbestos and certain drugs may also cause pleural inflammation and fibrosis (see pp. 715 and 391). Silicotic nodules developing along the pleural lymphatics have been likened to pearls or drops of candle wax[74] while eosinophilic pleuritis as a reaction to air in the pleural cavity has been mentioned above. Occasionally, no cause is evident.[75]

Acute inflammation of the pleura commences with hyperaemia, which is followed by exudation of fluid and leukocytes into the sac. Initially, before the exudate has fully formed, the pleurisy is dry (fibrinous pleurisy). This is accompanied by considerable pain on breathing and a rub that is audible on auscultation. With the development of an exudate (serofibrinous pleurisy) the visceral and parietal pleural surfaces separate and the pain and rub diminish. If the cause is bacterial, the serofibrinous exudate may be replaced by suppuration, the cavity becoming filled by pus – the condition known as empyema thoracis or pyothorax (see below).

In many cases of serofibrinous pleurisy the inflammation regresses as time or treatment brings about recovery from the underlying disease. In such cases, the exudate is absorbed, and unless the pleura has been extensively denuded of its mesothelium the sac recovers its smooth lining. Where mesothelium has been lost, adhesions may form between the lung and the chest wall: at first the adhesions are fibrinous, but later, through organisation, they become fibrous. In this way, part or all of the cavity may be obliterated. This generally occasions no great functional disadvantage. However, an appreciable degree of diffuse fibrous thickening of the pleura of any cause impairs movement of the chest. Accordingly, bilateral diffuse pleural fibrosis has important clinical consequences. The causes are as numerous as those of pleuritis (see Box 13.2) but asbestos is particularly important and the condition is therefore dealt with below under the heading of non-malignant asbestos-induced pleural disease.

The organisation of surface fibrin often involves the development of abundant granulation tissue and this may mimic sarcomatoid mesothelioma. The expression of keratin by such spindle cells is generally taken as evidence that they are mesothelial rather than fibroblastic, but it is not necessarily indicative of mesothelioma because reactive submesothelial spindle cells stain similarly.[17] However, cytokeratin staining is a useful marker of malignancy if it is positive in irregular cells in the deeper parts of the process for, as granulation tissue matures away from the surface, the intensity of the cytokeratin staining lessens.

Figure 13.5 Talc pleurodesis. (A) A linear inflammatory infiltrate is seen within densely fibrotic pleura. (B) The inflammation is of foreign-body granulomatous type. (C) Polarisation readily identifies birefringent talc crystals amongst the macrophages and giant cells.

Box 13.2 **Causes of pleural inflammation and fibrosis**

Infection, particularly of the lungs
Other pulmonary lesions, e.g. infarction
Connective tissue disease
Drug reaction
Asbestos
Pneumothorax
Sarcoidosis
Pancreatitis
Post cardiac injury (Dressler's syndrome)
Radiation
Renal failure
Trauma
Malignancy

Figure 13.6 Empyema thoracis. There is shaggy fibrinopurulent thickening of both pleural surfaces over the lower lobe.

Empyema thoracis (pyothorax)

Empyema thoracis represents a collection of pus in the pleural space (Fig. 13.6). It is usually a complication of pneumonia and, with the advent of antibiotics, is now rare. When it does occur there is usually some underlying debilitating condition such as diabetes or alcoholism, chronic lung disease such as bronchiectasis or carcinoma, or the patient is on long-term immunosuppressive therapy. In about a third of cases the condition is associated with a necrotising pneumonia or 'primary' lung abscess, due to aspirated anaerobes (see pp. 189–191). Often there is a mixture of bacteria, the predominant ones being the anaerobic or microaerophilic *Streptococcus milleri*, peptostreptococci, peptococci, *Fusobacterium nucleatum*, *Bacteroides melaninogenicus*, *B. fragilis*, clostridia, *Escherichia coli* and *Pseudomonas aeruginosa*.[76–79] *Klebsiella pneumoniae* is common in patients with diabetes mellitus[80] whereas in children *Staphylococcus aureus* is common, the empyema generally complicating underlying staphylococcal pneumonia or pneumatocele (see p. 182). If it complicates a staphylococcal pneumatocele the empyema may be associated with pneumothorax. This combination is known as pyopneumothorax and may also develop when a cavitating rheumatoid nodule establishes a bronchopleural fistula.[81,82] Empyema may also follow thoracotomy, or less commonly thoracocentesis, penetrating injuries or rupture of the oesophagus during instrumentation or by a sharp foreign body. Blood-borne and transdiaphragmatic infection are rare causes of empyema.

In empyema thoracis the whole of the sac or merely a part, usually the lower part, may be filled with thick viscous pus (see Fig. 13.6). Sometimes the pus is confined to an interlobar fissure. Organisation of parts of the exudate leads to the formation of firm adhesions that restrict spread of the infection and localise the pus. Alternatively, the pus may extend into the lung and rupture into a bronchus, leading to the sudden dissemination of infected material throughout the bronchial tree. If the patient survives this, there remains a chronic bronchopleural fistula. Occasionally, the pleural infection erodes the chest wall, leading to discharge of pus through the skin (empyema necessitans).

Empyema thoracis is a serious condition which, if inadequately treated, has a high mortality. Sometimes infection is overcome without intervention, and the pus is eventually replaced by granulation tissue and fibrous tissue. Even in favourable cases the damage to the serosa is severe: when the suppuration subsides, fibrous adhesions develop and eventually obliterate the cavity. The lining of the cavity may undergo calcification during the succeeding years. Malignant change is a further complication (see pleural sarcoma and pleural lymphoma, p. 734).

Tuberculosis of the pleura

Pleural involvement is common in tuberculosis, usually taking the form of an effusion in an apparently healthy young person soon after the primary infection. Pleural involvement may also complicate obvious active pulmonary tuberculosis or even apparently healed disease. The effusion is usually clear but occasionally blood-tinged. It contains numerous lymphocytes. Tubercle bacilli may be demonstrable, for the condition is truly infective rather than an allergic reaction as was once thought. Occasionally there is a dry painful pleurisy.

The pleura may be infected directly or by blood-borne spread from either the Ghon focus or caseous hilar lymph nodes. Bilateral effusion suggests blood spread but one pleural cavity may be infected directly from the other, as may the pericardium.

In the early stages of a tuberculous pleurisy the appearance of the visceral and parietal serosal surfaces does not differ greatly from that seen in the usual serofibrinous form of pleurisy. Discrete miliary granulomas may stud the pleura but more often there is diffuse surface involvement. However, typical tubercles can be seen histologically. Pleural biopsy with both histological and bacteriological examination has a sensitivity of greater than 90%,[83] confirming that the condition is infective rather than allergic. Ultimately, there is caseation and, in time, this may undergo calcification.

Even before effective antituberculosis drugs were available, such an effusion usually disappeared within 3–4 months, leaving at most a minor degree of obliteration of the costophrenic angle in the radiographs. However, some patients developed extensive thick rigid adhesions with consequent restriction of pulmonary ventilation.

A more severe form of tuberculous infection of the pleura may develop in the course of postprimary tuberculosis if a tuberculous cavity erodes into the pleural sac. The result is the condition conventionally described as a tuberculous empyema (see Fig. 5.3.8, p. 202), although the semifluid matter that collects is caseous and not true pus, except when there is a simultaneous or subsequent infection by pyogenic bacteria. The exudate in the pleural sac becomes encased in a thick, fibrosing layer of tuberculous granulation tissue. The same condition may result from rupture of a juxtavertebral abscess in cases of tuberculosis of the thoracic spine. Similarly, tuberculosis of a rib may be complicated by pleural effusion or 'empyema'. Bronchopleural fistula may be present in association with tuberculous 'empyema'. This increases the liability to secondary infection, which in some cases is caused by fungi.[84]

The formerly common establishment of an artificial pneumothorax to rest a tuberculous lung has been mentioned above. Other manipulations favoured in the past for the same purpose included the resection of several ribs (thoracoplasty) or the introduction of some inert material into the pleural sac, a procedure known as plombage: decades later, patients may find worm-like threads of wax in their sputum,[85] or pathologists unfamiliar with this outdated procedure may be surprised to find at autopsy one side of a deceased elderly patient's chest largely filled with what look remarkably like white billiard balls. More often, complications such as infection led to the removal of the plombe within a few years of its insertion.[86] Various forms of plombage material were favoured: plastic in the form of sponge or lucite spheres, packets of shredded plastic and injections of paraffin wax or vegetable oil (oleothorax).[87] The development of carcinoma of the lung underlying lucite spheres is mentioned on page 735.

Connective tissue disorders

Pleural involvement is common in rheumatoid disease and systemic lupus erythematosus, but rare in systemic sclerosis, polymyositis and dermatomyositis.[88]

Rheumatoid disease

Pleurisy and pleural effusions are the most common of the several respiratory manifestations of rheumatoid disease (see Box 10.1, p. 473). The pleural inflammation may be non-specific or represented by classic rheumatoid nodules.[89] Sometimes a subpleural rheumatoid nodule discharges into the pleural space and the characteristic palisade of cells forms a linear pattern over the surface of the pleura (Fig. 13.7).[90] An effusion, unilateral or bilateral, generally forms. This is an exudate, rich in immunoglobulins and other proteins, and sometimes cloudy or opalescent due to a high cholesterol content. Glucose levels in the fluid are low, apparently due to impaired glucose transport.[91] Lymphocytes are the predominant leukocytes, but sometimes there is a unique microscopical pattern – a combination of large elongated multinucleate cells, cholesterol crystals, clumps of eosinophilic granular material and a dearth of mesothelial cells.[92-94] The elongated cells are believed to come from the palisade layer of the granuloma. Their bizarre shape makes them liable to be mistaken for carcinoma cells. Rheumatoid pleural effusions are liable to become infected, sometimes resulting in empyema. At other times a cavitating intrapulmonary rheumatoid nodule leads to the development of a bronchopleural fistula and pyopneumothorax.[81,82]

Systemic lupus erythematosus

Pleurisy, with or without effusion, is among the most common visceral manifestations of systemic lupus erythematosus, far exceeding

Figure 13.7 (A) A rheumatoid nodule is seen discharging into the pleural space, following which (B) the palisade of histiocytes fronts the pleural space rather than the centre of a granuloma.

pulmonary involvement in frequency. The pleural effusions are usually bilateral and the fluid is an exudate rich in proteins. Glucose concentrations are normal. The cells are usually unremarkable but occasionally lupus erythematosus cells may form. These are phagocytes that have taken up effete nuclear material so that their own nuclei are stretched around a large haemotoxyphil inclusion. Biopsy shows non-specific chronic inflammation or fibrosis.

Nodular histiocytic/mesothelial hyperplasia

Nodular histiocytic/mesothelial hyperplasia is found on serosal surfaces as small discrete aggregates of histiocytes intermingled with occasional mesothelial cells. The condition is well known on the pericardium where the aggregates are often termed mesothelial/monocytic incidental cardiac excrescences (cardiac MICE), and upon the peritoneum in hernial sacs. The aggregates are also found on the pleura, probably developing in response to non-specific pleural irritation.[95] They are symptomless and of no clinical importance unless an unwary pathologist mistakes them for something more sinister, such as carcinoma or mesothelioma. Recognising the numerous histiocytes as such is the key to the correct diagnosis; these cells stain strongly for CD68 and greatly outnumber the calretinin- and cytokeratin5/6-positive mesothelial cells and any reactive thyroid transforming factor-1 (TTF-1)-positive pulmonary epithelial cells present at the deeper aspect of a lesion on the visceral pleura.[96]

NON-MALIGNANT ASBESTOS-INDUCED PLEURAL DISEASE

Besides asbestosis, carcinoma of the lung and pleural mesothelioma, respiratory disease attributable to the inhalation of asbestos includes pleurisy, which is generally accompanied by an effusion, and pleural fibrosis.[97] The latter takes several forms: distinctive plaques and less distinct pleural fibrosis that may be focal or diffuse, and either of no clinical consequence or responsible for particular clinical syndromes.

In contrast to asbestosis and asbestos-induced lung cancer, both of which generally require relatively high exposure levels, all pleural diseases attributable to asbestos are associated with relatively low asbestos burdens in the lung.[98] Furthermore, it is very difficult to identify asbestos in the pleural lesions themselves, although they are attributable to asbestos inhalation.

Benign asbestos pleurisy and pleural effusion

An exudative pleurisy may develop within 10 years of first contact with asbestos and therefore be found in persons currently at work in the industry. The effusion may be asymptomatic[97] or the patient may complain of pleuritic pain, sometimes accompanied by fever, leukocytosis and an elevated blood sedimentation rate.[99] The effusion is usually small and blood-stained, giving rise to suspicion of malignancy. It often resolves spontaneously, only to recur, perhaps on the other side. It may progress to diffuse pleural fibrosis that requires decortication.[99] Asbestos-induced pleurisy is thought to play no part in the development of pleural mesothelioma.

Asbestos-induced pleural fibrosis

Bilateral obliteration of the costophrenic angles is a common radiographic finding in healthy asbestos workers. It presumably reflects the organisation of previous asymptomatic effusions. Pleural fibrosis of non-specific character is common in such workers, and in those suffering from asbestosis a diffuse but thin fibrous thickening of the visceral pleura is almost invariably present. Indeed, apart from the presence of asbestos in the lungs, this is one of the few pathological features that distinguish asbestosis from idiopathic pulmonary fibrosis.

This thin fibrous thickening of the visceral pleura is of no clinical consequence but occasionally asbestos-exposed individuals develop extensive, thick fibrosis of the pleura in the absence of asbestosis (Fig. 13.8) and this may severely compromise expansion of the chest.[24,100–104] It may be bilateral or limited to one side.[105] The resultant restrictive defect in lung function is responsible for incapacitating breathlessness and this form of pleural fibrosis is one of the industrial diseases recognised by several governments for compensation purposes. Medicolegal definitions vary from country to country and with time. In the UK the current definition is unilateral or bilateral diffuse pleural thickening with obliteration of the costophrenic angle.[106] Mesothelioma may develop in patients with such restrictive pleural fibrosis but the tumour is thought to arise independently. Although generally limited to the pleura, the fibrosis occasionally extends into the chest wall[107] and mediastinum.[108] The lung parenchyma immediately beneath the thickened pleura may show diffuse

Figure 13.8 Diffuse thick fibrous thickening of the pleura in an asbestos worker. At the base of the lower lobe there is also a localised area of pleural thickening (Blesovsky's disease).

interstitial fibrosis but this should not be interpreted as asbestosis unless there is also evidence of substantial asbestos exposure.

Asbestos-induced pleural fibrosis has to be distinguished from pleural plaque, which is described below, and from a cryptogenic form of bilateral fibrosing pleuritis that has been reported in a few patients in whom asbestos, systemic connective tissue disorders, tuberculosis and all other recognised causes of pleural fibrosis have been excluded.[109] Such cryptogenic diffuse pleural fibrosis has been reported in three sisters.[110] In other patients it has been associated with a thin rim of subpleural fibrosis and been termed idiopathic pleuroparenchymal fibroelastosis.[111,112]

Blesovsky's disease (folded lung, rounded atelectasis)

Localised patches of pleural fibrosis may be important clinically, not for their functional effects, but because they may mimic a peripheral lung tumour radiographically. The contracture of the pleural scar draws the adjacent lung tissue to it, causing a localised area of collapse. The bases of the lungs are particularly affected (Figs 13.8 and 13.9 and Table 13.1). The collapsed lung often appears to be folded upon itself and the resultant radiographic opacity has a comet's tail appearance. The condition is variously known as Blesovsky's disease, folded lung or rounded atelectasis.[24,113–117a] In 25% of cases the lesion is bilateral.[105] There is often a history of asbestos exposure, but like the other forms of asbestos-induced pleural fibrosis, the condition is thought to play no part in the pathogenesis of mesothelioma.

Figure 13.9 Folded lung (Blesovsky's disease). A white Y-shaped band of scarred pleura is surrounded by collapsed lung. *(Courtesy of Dr T Jelihovsky, Sydney, Australia.)*

Table 13.1 Lobar distribution of Blesovsky's disease in 100 reported cases[113]

	Right	Left
Upper lobe	2	3
Middle lobe/lingual	11	10
Lower lobe	47	27

Pleural plaques

Pleural plaques are a further form of asbestos-induced pleural fibrosis, described separately because of their distinctive pathological appearance.[24] Although they are occasionally found in persons with no history of asbestos exposure, the association with asbestos is a firm one, based on both epidemiological evidence[118,119] and the identification of asbestos in the underlying lung.[120] Pleural plaques therefore provide strong evidence of asbestos exposure, which may be occupational or environmental. They occur after exposure to all types of asbestos but anthophyllite is particularly potent. Plaques are common in areas where the soil is contaminated with asbestiform minerals, for example parts of Finland and Greece.[121,122] The longer and heavier the exposure, the more extensive the plaques, but even slight exposure can be sufficient. Very few develop within 15 years of first exposure and most appear after 30 years. Postmortem studies show that plaques are more common than can be appreciated from radiological

Figure 13.10 Pleural plaques. (A) The eviscerated thoracic cavity showing pearly white and irregular plaques on the inner side of the chest wall. (B) Microscopically, the plaques are practically acellular, consisting of hyaline collagen that has a 'basket-weave' pattern. They provide strong evidence of asbestos exposure.

examination in life.[118] Pleural plaques are harmless and have no relationship to mesothelioma, or lung cancer, other than their association with asbestos.[123]

Pathology

Plaques are localised raised areas that are generally multifocal and bilateral. They may occur on the visceral pleura or even the peritoneum[124] but usually affect the parietal pleura, particularly in relation to the ribs and the central tendon of the diaphragm. They have an irregular outline, a smooth shiny pearly-grey surface and a low profile, typically about 5 mm in height: their other dimensions are very variable (Fig. 13.10A). Microscopically, plaques are hyaline, avascular and almost acellular (Fig. 13.10B). In a pleural biopsy, even a small number of spindle cells in a hyaline lesion should suggest the possibility of paucicellular hyaline mesothelioma (see p. 722) rather than plaque. The hyaline collagen bundles have a characteristic pattern that is often likened to basket weave. Calcification is common. Inflammation is not found, except at the periphery and there it is mild.

Pathogenesis

Although the connection between asbestos and plaques is firmly established, the pathogenetic mechanism is obscure. Organisation of exudates probably underlies the other less distinctive forms of pleural fibrosis found in asbestos workers but it is difficult to envisage a special type of exudate that may give rise to plaques. Furthermore, the plaques are covered by an intact mesothelium and are not usually attended by adhesions. It has been suggested that the parietal pleura is particularly affected because it is abraded by asbestos fibres projecting through the visceral pleura, but no such projections have been identified. A further possibility derives from consideration of the lymphatic drainage of the pleural cavity, which is largely through the parietal pleura. Short asbestos fibres have been identified in the visceral pleura[125] and it is likely that some reach the pleural cavity, whence their disposal would be by the stomata and lymphatics of the parietal pleura (see p. 708). Any fibres arrested by the ribs or the tendinous portion of the diaphragm would elicit submesothelial fibrosis at these sites.[24] Ferruginous bodies are not usually seen in the plaques but they have been recorded there.[126]

PLEURAL TUMOURS

Pleuropulmonary blastoma is dealt with on page 623 and this section will consider only those tumours that are initially confined to the pleura, of which mesothelioma is by far the most important.

Mesothelioma

Mesotheliomas arise most commonly in the pleura but also develop in the peritoneum and occasionally in the pericardium or tunica vaginalis of the testis.[127,128] They are malignant neoplasms: the terms 'benign fibrous mesothelioma' and 'multicystic mesothelioma' are misnomers in that the former is not of mesothelial origin and the latter is not neoplastic (see solitary fibrous tumour on page 730 and multicystic mesothelioma on page 729). A benign mesothelial neoplasm is encountered in the peritoneum and rarely in the pleura but is termed adenomatoid tumour rather than benign mesothelioma (see p. 729). Well-differentiated papillary mesothelioma is a low-grade mesothelioma that warrants separate consideration (see p. 729).

Incidence

Mesothelioma was very rare in the nineteenth and early twentieth centuries. Indeed, as late as the 1950s, some eminent authorities denied its existence. However, it is now recognised to be one of the most important occupational diseases. Its incidence has been steadily rising and in industrialised countries mesothelioma now accounts for about 1% of all cancer deaths. The highest annual crude incidence rates (about 30 cases per million) are observed in Australia, Belgium and the UK.[129,130]

Measures to curtail exposure to its principal cause, asbestos, were introduced and progressively strengthened in many countries in the latter half of the twentieth century but such is the long latent interval between exposure and disease that these do not have an effect for several decades. The durability of asbestos is another factor hampering efforts to reduce the incidence of mesothelioma. It is calculated that the numbers mesotheliomas in the UK will triple between 1991 and 2020 and only then decline.[131] In contrast, there is already a decline in the incidence of mesothelioma in the USA where the use of amphibole asbestos was restricted as early as the 1960s.[132]

Aetiology

In the mid twentieth century it was increasingly suspected that mesothelioma was related to asbestos exposure and substance was given to this in 1960, when Wagner and colleagues showed a high incidence of the tumour in the area near Kimberley, northern Cape province, South Africa, where blue asbestos is mined.[133,134] The relationship between asbestos exposure and mesothelioma was subsequently confirmed in other countries where asbestos is mined and in those that import and process the ore.[135-139] Asbestos and similar fibrous substances are virtually the only recognised causes of mesothelioma. Smoking does not increase the risk of mesothelioma. Cases that can be attributed to causes such as radiation, chronic inflammation and scarring are exceptionally rare.[140-146] Despite the predominant role of asbestosis, there is evidence that simian virus 40 (SV40) may also play a role in the development of mesothelioma, acting either independently or synergistically with asbestos. This virus contaminated monkey kidney cells used in the manufacture of early batches of poliomyelitis vaccine and may have reached humans in this way. SV40 sequences are selectively expressed in many mesotheliomas, the development of which has been attributed to the ability of the sequences to inactivate the *p53* and *Rb* tumour suppressor genes and promote the secretion of various growth factors.[147-150] However, subsequent investigations have resulted in both supportive and contrary findings[151-156] and the relationship of SV40 infection to development of mesotheliomas remains uncertain.

The risk of mesothelioma is substantial in the mining, transportation and processing of asbestos but is dose-related and can be minimised by precautionary measures based on good industrial hygiene.[157] The principal manufacturing industries using asbestos are those producing items such as specialised cement products, insulating materials and brake linings. All industries applying and refitting asbestos insulation carry a potential risk and many cases have been seen in construction and demolition work, ship-fitting and other dockyard work, and railway carriage maintenance. Many joiners, heating engineers, boilermen, railwaymen and former naval servicemen have been exposed unknowingly[158] whilst some exposure is para-occupational, incurred by men such as shipyard welders who work alongside those applying or stripping asbestos. The families of asbestos workers are also at increased risk through being exposed to asbestos dust carried home on work clothes. Such exposure may occur very early in life.[159] Others appear to have developed mesothelioma because they live in the vicinity of asbestos mines or factories, but it is always difficult to exclude occupational, para-occupational or domestic exposure in such cases.[160,161] However, environmental exposure undoubtedly occurs in parts of the world such as Turkey and the Metsovo region of Greece where the soil contains asbestos,[121,122,162,163] and town dwellers are subjected to continuous low levels of asbestos exposure from sources such as brake linings. Thus, exposure to asbestos may be:

- direct, from the handling of asbestos ore or its products
- para-occupational, from working alongside asbestos workers, as in shipyards
- household, for example from the clothes of an asbestos worker
- neighbourhood, from living near an asbestos mine or factory
- ambient.

The carcinogenicity of asbestos depends on its physical properties and it is notable that not all forms of asbestos carry the same risk of mesothelioma.[164] The various types of asbestos have been described on page 342, where a broad division was drawn between the serpentine chrysotile (white asbestos) and the straight-fibred amphiboles, crocidolite (blue asbestos), amosite (brown asbestos), anthophyllite, tremolite and actinolite. Chrysotile accounts for more than 90% of all asbestos used and of the others only crocidolite and amosite are now produced commercially. The principal cause of mesothelioma in the UK is crocidolite whilst in North America it is amosite. Chrysotile is thought not to cause mesothelioma[165,166] and the few mesotheliomas associated with this form of asbestos are probably due to contamination of the chrysotile by tremolite.[167-169] Contamination with tremolite is also the probable explanation of the occasional mesotheliomas observed in talc and vermiculate miners[167] and of mesotheliomas reported in southeast Turkey amongst inhabitants of houses whitewashed with a non-asbestiform ore.[170]

The particular physical properties of asbestos that determine its carcinogenicity are fibre diameter, length and biodegradability. Its dimensions determine whether a fibre reaches the lung and all three factors determine whether it is retained there or cleared. Fibres thinner than 0.25 μm and longer than 5 μm carry the greatest risk of mesothelioma.[171] The curly chrysotile fibres tend to settle in large airways and to be eliminated by ciliary action, whilst those that reach the lung break up more readily than the amphiboles and are cleared more rapidly. Because of this a former chrysotile miner may ultimately have more tremolite than chrysotile in his lungs, although the tremolite is only a contaminant of the mined ore.

The physical properties of asbestos not only govern whether it reaches, and is cleared from the lung, but are also responsible for its carcinogenicity. Thus, whereas the injection of fibrous tremolite into the pleural cavity of rats produced mesotheliomas, an equal dose of non-asbestiform tremolite did not.[172]

Fibrous minerals other than asbestos may have fibres of the same shape and size as the dangerous amphibole forms of asbestos. In central Turkey a high incidence of mesothelioma is associated with environmental exposure to erionite, which is a fine fibrous form of the volcanic silicate, zeolite.[125,173] In inhalation experiments, erionite exceeds asbestos in its ability to induce mesotheliomas.[174] Much attention therefore centres on the many other naturally occurring fibrous minerals, some of which are in commercial use as oil absorbents or cat litter, and on synthetic fibres.[175] Fortunately, many of these fibres are not in the respirable range but the potential dangers are shown by the high incidence of mesothelioma in rats injected with fibreglass and other fibres particles of respirable size.[176-178] A variety of bronchopulmonary abnormalities is reported in workers exposed to fine fibreglass[179] but so far at least there have been no convincing reports of synthetic fibres causing cancer in humans.[180-182]

Susceptibility to mesothelioma is probably influenced by genetic factors. Thus, the prevalence of mesotheliomas induced experimentally with asbestos was found to vary according to the strain of mice studied.[183] Genetic factors are also suggested by the development of mesothelioma in families[184,185] but it must be remembered that one family member may inadvertently expose others to asbestos, for example by bringing home soiled work clothes.

The age incidence of mesothelioma is largely determined by the time at which an individual is first exposed to asbestos and the latent interval between exposure and presentation, which is generally over 20 years, with a mean of about 40 years, but may be as short as 15 years.[186-188] Where environmental exposure occurs from birth, mesotheliomas start to develop from about the age of 14.[189] The cause of mesotheliomas occurring in younger children is unknown.[190-194] Cases without evidence of asbestos exposure are touched upon again below.

The sex incidence of mesothelioma is also largely determined by asbestos exposure, men greatly outnumbering women, a difference that is not so marked in the rare cases where asbestos does not appear to be involved. In all other respects mesothelioma in women is identical to mesothelioma in men.[195]

The cumulative dose of asbestos is of greater importance than the duration of exposure: short periods of high exposure can be very hazardous. Some women who developed mesotheliomas after making military gas masks in Nottingham during the Second World War had only short periods of exposure, in some cases as little as 3 months, but their exposure was heavy. Nevertheless, the level of exposure necessary to cause pleural mesothelioma is far less than that required to cause asbestosis (Table 7.1.5, p. 346). Peritoneal tumours are generally associated with relatively heavy exposure and the proportion of mesotheliomas arising in the peritoneum diminishes as occupational hygiene improves: in one asbestos manufacturing company the ratio of peritoneal to pleural tumours fell from 5:1 before 1921 to 1:3 after 1950.[196] The proportion of peritoneal cases has always been low in mining. Ingested asbestos fibres do not penetrate the walls of the gastrointestinal tract, and peritoneal mesothelioma is presumed to be caused by inhaled asbestos crossing both the pleura and the diaphragm.[197]

The assessment of asbestos load is described on page 344 but a simple first step is to examine thick (20–30-μm) unstained sections of the lungs for asbestos bodies. In cases of mesothelioma the presence of as few as one asbestos body in a standard 5-μm thick section of lung is regarded as evidence of substantial exposure,[198-200] obviating the need for more sophisticated procedures. However, an inability to identify asbestos bodies in histological sections does not exclude asbestos causation.

Even after an exhaustive occupational history and the most detailed analysis, no cause can be identified for some mesotheliomas. The proportion of such cases varies considerably, probably depending upon the degree of industrialisation so that in a non-industrialised country the low background incidence becomes important. In the UK and the USA, 10–20% of mesotheliomas appear to be unrelated to asbestos exposure.[201-206] One group reported that asbestos bodies were identified in histological sections in 57% of mesothelioma cases, that the figure reached 83% when asbestos bodies were sought in lung digests by light microscopy and 89% when electron microscopy was used to identify coated and uncoated fibres in lung digests (Fig. 13.11).[205,207] Another group, which confined their attention to a careful occupational history or the presence of asbestos bodies in lung sections, identified asbestos exposure in 87% of cases.[206]

Evidence that there is a low background of mesothelioma unrelated to asbestos derives from several sources:

- Mortality trends in industrialised countries record an equal sex incidence in the early twentieth century.
- The subsequent increase is largely confined to men.
- Mesothelioma in childhood is rare, but well established.[190-194]
- Although rare, associations with possible causes such as radiotherapy and chronic infection are recorded.[140-145]

Pathogenesis

Three main hypotheses have been adduced to explain the induction of mesothelioma by asbestos: (1) an oxidative stress theory based on the fact that macrophages release large amounts of free radicals when they ingest asbestos fibres; (2) a chromosome-tangling theory that envisages asbestos fibres damaging chromosomes during cell division; and (3) an absorptive theory that postulates carcinogens being concentrated on the surface of the fibres.[207a]

It is likely that most mesotheliomas commence as localised lesions on the parietal pleura and evolve through a non-invasive phase

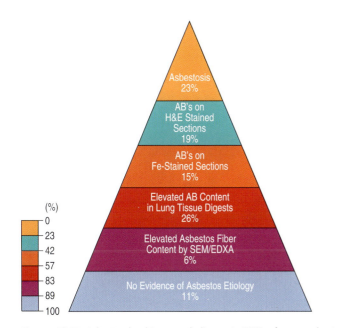

Figure 13.11 Asbestos load in mesothelioma. In 23% of cases asbestosis is evident (ABs), in another 19% there is no pulmonary fibrosis but asbestos bodies; can be identified in standard sections; in a further 15% asbestos bodies are detected when iron stains are employed; in a further 26% asbestos body counts in lung digests are elevated; in a further 6% excess asbestos fibre is found when lung digests are examined by scanning electron microscopy; leaving 11% in which a link with asbestos cannot be established.[205,207] H&E, haematoxylin and eosin; Fe, iron; SEM, scanning electron microscopy; EDXA, energy-dispersive X-ray analysis. *(Courtesy of Professor V Roggli, Durham, USA.)*

known as mesothelioma-in-situ (see below).[208,209] These morphological changes are preceded by molecular alterations that activate receptors, inactivate tumour suppression and promote cell signalling. Both asbestos exposure and SV40 transfection of human mesothelial cells cause genetic modifications such as AP-1 activation that favour cell growth and malignant change.[150] The tumour suppressor genes p 16 and p 21 are often inactivated in mesothelioma[209a] and several autocrine growth factors have been identified in mesotheliomas. The latter include platelet-derived growth factor, transforming growth factor-β, vascular endothelial growth factor, tumour necrosis factor-α and inhibitors of apotosis[210-220] while oncogenes identified within mesotheliomas include *p53*, *RAS* and *bcl-2*.[221-223] Mesotheliomas are often infiltrated by lymphoid cells that might be expected to suppress tumour growth but they include regulatory T cells that suppress an efficient immune response.[224] Chromosomal abnormalities are common but there is no single, specific defect, indicating a broad spectrum of heterogeneity, as reflected in the tumour's morphology.[225,225a]

Clinical features

Mesothelioma is more common in men, reflecting their greater exposure to asbestos. It generally presents after the age of 50 years but may arise at any age.

Patients with pleural mesothelioma complain of continuous chest pain due to infiltration of the chest wall and dyspnoea due to pleural effusion or encasement of the lung by tumour restricting chest movement. The effusion is often blood-stained. Mediastinal infiltration may result in superior vena caval compression, Horner's syndrome or recurrent laryngeal nerve palsy.[226] Invasion of the spinal canal may cause paraplegia.[227] Chest radiographs typically show diffuse pleural thickening on the affected side but at first the tumour may be localised or multifocal. Symptoms due to metastases generally develop only terminally, if at all, but rarely they are the initial manifestation of the disease.[228-230] Paraneoplastic syndromes include thrombocytosis due to the production of interleukin-6 by the tumour, which may also be responsible for in amyloidosis and pseudohyperkalaemia (high serum but normal plasma potassium levels).[213,231-233]

Pleural aspiration

As well as relieving breathlessness, aspiration of pleural fluid can be helpful diagnostically, particularly in the recognition of metastatic tumour.[234,235] Its sensitivity in the diagnosis of mesothelioma depends upon the expertise of the cytologist and a biopsy is often preferred.[236] Opinions vary as to the volume of fluid required for diagnosis of malignancy but 50–60 ml appears to be a reasonable compromise.[237,238] The International Mesothelioma Interest Group recommends that a cytological suspicion of mesothelioma be followed by tissue confirmation supported by both clinical and radiological data.[239]

Exfoliated cells may be examined in films in the conventional way or concentrated into cell blocks which may be sectioned for light or electron microscopy. Immunocytochemical procedures (see below) may be applied to either smears or sections of these cells.[240-242] Pleural fluid is particularly suitable for flow cytometry, cytogenetic and molecular studies and scanning electron microscopy.[209a-244]

The cytological diagnosis of adenocarcinoma or other types of metastatic tumour in serous effusions is often relatively straightforward for, in addition to reactive mesothelial cells, recognisable by their microvillous border and denser perinuclear staining, a separate population of malignant cells can be recognised.[245-247] Adenocarcinoma cells form clumps with a smooth border rather than a scalloped edge, which is characteristic of mesothelioma.[239] On the other hand, the distinction between benign and malignant mesothelial cells is notoriously difficult.[236] Reactive mesothelial cells can be alarmingly large and binucleate or multinucleate. The nuclear-to-cytoplasmic ratio is often not significantly increased in mesothelioma but nuclear irregularity and prominent multiple nucleoli may suggest malignancy. A feature particularly suggestive of epithelioid mesothelioma is the presence of papillary aggregates or morulae containing up to 100 or so cells and having a scalloped edge (Fig. 13.12).

Although attention is usually concentrated on the cellular component, the supernatant fluid can also be informative. Many mesotheliomas, but not carcinomas, secrete hyaluronic acid which can then reach high levels in the pleural fluid.[248,249] Some immunocytochemical tumour markers may be detected in pleural fluid. For example, the demonstration of carcinoembryonic antigen (CEA) in a pleural effusion favours metastatic carcinoma.[250-252] Conversely, raised levels of soluble mesothelin favour mesothelioma.[253,254]

Macroscopic features

Pleural mesothelioma is commoner on the right than the left, in a ratio of 3:2.[206] The reason for this is poorly understood but may depend upon differences in airway orientation, fibre burden, pleural area and chest wall movement on the two sides.

Asbestos fibres reaching the pleural cavity are concentrated in Kampmeier's foci (see p. 708)[10] and thoracoscopy has shown that mesothelioma first develops in the parietal pleura where these foci are found, appearing there as multiple small grape-like nodules; involvement of the visceral pleura follows.[208] Progression of the tumour

Figure 13.12 Mesothelioma in a pleural aspirate. (A) The exfoliated malignant cells are clumped together in so-called morulae. (B) The cells stain strongly for epithelial membrane antigen, a feature supportive, but not diagnostic, of malignancy.

Figure 13.13 Pleural mesothelioma. Dense white tumour encases the lung and spreads along a fissure.

Microscopic features

Needle biopsy of the pleura is often disappointing and a firm diagnosis of mesothelioma is sometimes not possible until thorascopic or open biopsy, or even autopsy, is undertaken.[262] Reactive mesothelial cells may form loose aggregates and it is important that in small biopsies these are not mistaken for true papillae, which are suggestive, but not pathognomonic, of mesothelioma.[246,263]

Despite their epithelioid appearance, mesothelial cells are of mesodermal origin and their malignant counterparts display a wide diversity of differentiation, which has led to the alternative name of mesodermoma being suggested.[264–266] This diversity is reflected in the traditional histological classification of mesotheliomas as epithelioid, sarcomatoid (or fibrous) and biphasic (or mixed).[267] The epithelioid type is the commonest in most series[268,269] but widespread sampling of the tumour, which is possible postmortem, increases the proportion of biphasic tumours.[270,271]

A mixed (biphasic) pattern combining the epithelioid and sarcomatoid features described below is the classic pattern of mesothelioma (Fig. 13.14). The two components often merge where they meet and the combination makes a distinctive picture that presents few diagnostic problems (which are considered below).

In well-differentiated tumours of purely epithelioid type a tubulopapillary pattern is most commonly seen (Fig. 13.15), but the pattern may be purely tubular, composed of well-formed glandular spaces, or purely papillary, in which small, irregular, cystic spaces are lined by tumour cells and filled by papillary projections with delicate cores of connective tissue and a covering of tumour cells. As in other papillary neoplasms, psammoma bodies (calcospherites) may be formed. Mesothelioma may also be strikingly glandular in morphology (Fig. 13.16). Individual tumour cells are generally cuboidal or polygonal with moderate amounts of eosinophilic cytoplasm and round nuclei containing a single nucleolus. Sometimes they are peg-shaped, with only a narrow base (Fig. 13.17). In many cases mitoses are infrequent

results in coalescence of the nodules to form plaques and, ultimately, a continuous sheet of tumour fusing the visceral and parietal pleura and obliterating the pleural space (Fig. 13.13), except for occasional residual loculi containing glairy fluid or blood. Areas of necrosis or haemorrhage and softer areas of mucoid consistency may be seen and occasionally the whole tumour appears gelatinous. In the late stage, tumour encases the lung as a layer of dense white tissue up to several centimetres thick, which extends into fissures and infiltrates the peripheral lung parenchyma so that at autopsy the lung has to be forcibly dissected from the chest wall. It is very rare for a mesothelioma to remain localised and form a solitary mass; not surprisingly, such localised mesotheliomas have a comparatively good prognosis.[255–260] A feature of mesothelioma that is often stressed is a supposed predeliction to infiltrate along biopsy tracks or surgical incisions, but this is a feature of all malignant tumours.[261] Metastasis is late but at death may be widespread (see below).

Figure 13.14 Biphasic mesothelioma comprising both epithelioid and sarcomatoid elements.

Figure 13.16 Epithelioid mesothelioma in which the glands closely resemble those of an adenocarcinoma. In (A) the stroma is fibrous while in (B) it is myxoid.

Figure 13.15 Epithelioid mesothelioma of tubulopapillary pattern. (A) A papillary pattern is seen on the surface while (B) a tubular pattern is seen invading the stroma.

Figure 13.17 Epitheliod mesothelioma in which some of the tumour cells are peg-shaped.

Figure 13.18 Mesothelioma-in-situ. This term should only be used when there is unequivocal invasion adjacent to the surface proliferation (as there is on the right).

and there may be little cellular pleomorphism. Occasionally there is atypia but no evidence of invasive activity; this appears to be a pre-malignant state.[272] The term 'mesothelioma-in-situ' has been introduced to describe such changes but it is recommended by its originators that the term should only be used when the surface changes are accompanied by invasive tumour (Fig. 13.18).[209] Vacuoles may develop within the cytoplasm of tumour cells, compressing the nuclei and simulating signet ring cell carcinoma.[273] In some tumours the glands are lined by flattened cells, giving the tumour a lace-like microcystic appearance (Fig. 13.19A). The stroma around the tumour cells is typically myxoid and may be abundant, with wide separation of the gland spaces, but may be sclerotic (see Fig. 13.16). Undifferentiated epithelioid mesotheliomas often consist of sheets of cells with abundant eosinophilic cytoplasm but few other characteristic features and little intervening stroma (Fig. 13.19B). Alternatively there may be little cytoplasm and a focal resemblance to small cell carcinoma.[274,275] The diversity of these tumours is shown by reports of focal trophoblastic differentiation and chorionic gonadotrophin secretion,[276,277] or the tumour having a deciduoid (Fig. 13.19C),[146,233,278-282] small cell,[274] rhabdoid[283,284] or clear cell (Fig. 13.19D, E)[285-287] phenotype. Their diversity is further emphasised by reports of chromogranin being demonstrated immunocytochemically in mesotheliomas of glandular pattern[288] and rare cases showing a marked lymphohistiocytoid reactive infiltrate (Fig. 13.19F) being mistakenly diagnosed as lymphomas.[289-291]

In the sarcomatoid (fibrous) type of mesothelioma the cells are spindle-shaped and set in a varying amount of collagenised stroma so that the cellularity varies greatly. Markedly pleomorphic, cellular foci showing mitotic activity are indistinguishable from other forms of undifferentiated sarcoma or the tumour may consist of bland spindle cells widely scattered in a densely collagenised stroma constituting the so-called desmoplastic variant, which may be very difficult to distinguish from scar tissue (Fig. 13.20).[291a] Cartilaginous, osseous, muscular or fatty differentiation is occasionally seen and, if no epithelioid elements are present, the tumour may resemble a primary sarcoma of one of these tissues (Fig. 13.21).[264,265,292-296] However, it is uncommon for these heterologous patterns to dominate the histological picture and the adoption of nomenclature such as osteosarcoma

of the pleura for an otherwise typical mesothelioma in an asbestos worker is inappropriate and may prejudice a justifiable claim for industrial compensation.[296] Lymphangiomatoid is another rare pattern.[297]

Mesotheliomas frequently evince distinctive features when stained for mucus or examined by immunocytochemistry or electron microscopy. These procedures are often invaluable in the differential diagnosis of a tumour involving the serous cavities of the body and will now be considered.

Differential diagnosis of mesothelioma

The classic gross appearance of a pleural mesothelioma, that of a firm pale tumour encasing the lung, may be mimicked by extensive pleural fibrosis or by a peripheral carcinoma of the lung growing along the pleura – so-called pseudomesotheliomatous carcinoma of the lung,[298-300] as well as other tumours growing in a similar manner (see Fig. 12.3.21, p. 637).[301,302] Each of the histological types of mesothelioma presents its own diagnostic problems. A distinction has to drawn between:

1. biphasic mesothelioma and other biphasic tumours
2. epithelioid mesothelioma and adenocarcinoma
3. poorly differentiated epithelioid mesothelioma and poorly differentiated squamous cell carcinoma
4. epithelioid mesothelioma and reactive mesothelial hyperplasia
5. sarcomatoid mesothelioma and other spindle cell tumours
6. sarcomatoid mesothelioma and fibrosis.

These will now be considered in turn:

Biphasic mesothelioma versus other biphasic tumours

The distinctive biphasic pattern of the mixed type of mesothelioma presents few diagnostic problems, but pleural involvement by sarcomatoid carcinoma[303,304] or biphasic synovial sarcoma[305-307] may need to be considered, although both are rare and generally form localised rather than diffuse growths. The key to distinguishing these tumours from mesotheliomas of mixed pattern lies in their epithelioid component: if this is squamous, sarcomatoid carcinoma can be assumed, but if it is glandular the problem is similar to that encountered in distinguishing metastatic adenocarcinoma from mesothelioma of purely epithelioid type, which is considered next. The special techniques considered in the next section are equally applicable to the epithelial component of a sarcomatoid carcinoma or biphasic synovial sarcoma. Synovial sarcomas also stain strongly and diffusely for bcl-2 protein,[308] which is only rarely expressed in mesothelioma, and they show an x:18 translocation, which is not seen in mesothelioma.

Epithelioid mesothelioma versus adenocarcinoma

Mucin stains afford one of the simplest and most effective means of distinguishing epithelioid mesotheliomas from carcinomas (Table 13.2). Mesotheliomas do not produce the epithelial mucins so often seen in adenocarcinomas and the periodic acid–Schiff (PAS) stain is therefore a useful first step in this differential diagnosis (Fig. 13.22). The presence of PAS-positive mucin within tumour cells or glands is generally regarded as excluding a diagnosis of mesothelioma, although rare exceptions to this are reported in which crystals of hyaluronic acid are responsible for the PAS-positivity.[128,273,309,310] PAS-positive material in mesotheliomas may also represent basement membranes rather than epithelial mucin.[311] Attention should therefore be confined to the contents of the glands or cytoplasmic vacuoles: finely granular cytoplasmic PAS-positivity should be disregarded. Diastase predigestion is essential because mesotheliomas are frequently rich in glycogen,

Figure 13.19 Rarer variants of epithelioid mesothelioma. These include (A) microcystic, (B) solid, (C) deciduoid, (D and E) clear cell and (F) lymphohistiocytoid. (E, cytokeratin stain.)

Figure 13.20 Sarcomatoid (fibrous) mesothelioma. (A) A cellular tumour showing pleomorphism and cytological atypia. (B) The desmoplastic variant showing densely hyaline fibrosis and little cellularity. Here the distinction from scar tissue depends on finding atypical cytokeratin-positive spindle cells. A lack of zonation, a storiform pattern, numerous mitoses and foci of necrosis are further features suggestive of malignancy.

Figure 13.21 Sarcomatoid mesothelioma showing (A) cartilaginous and (B) osseous differentiation.

occasionally to the extent that the tumour cells have abundant clear cytoplasm.[312]

The glycosaminoglycan hyaluronic acid is an acid mucopolysaccharide produced by both normal and neoplastic mesothelial cells. Alcian blue (pH 2.5) can be used to demonstrate its presence on the apical surface of tumour cells, and within glandular spaces and intracellular vacuoles: the staining is abolished by prior treatment with hyaluronidase, in contrast to acidic glycoproteins produced by some adenocarcinomas.[313] Attention must be confined to the epithelial component because stromal glycosaminoglycans include hyaluronic acid. Fixation in alcohol or cetyl pyridyl formalin is desirable as it preserves hyaluronic acid, which is water-soluble and may be leached out by prolonged fixation in aqueous solutions.

Mucicarmine stains both epithelial mucin and hyaluronic acid and has no place in the distinction of mesothelioma from adenocarcinoma unless hyaluronidase controls are employed.[314]

These traditional mucus stains are now widely augmented, or indeed replaced, by immunohistochemical staining (see Table 13.3). Antibodies of diagnostic utility fall into two groups, those that recognise epithelial epitopes and those that recognise mesothelial charac-

teristics. The first group includes antibodies against CEA, Leu-M1, B72.3, AUA1, BerEP4, MOC-31, claudin-4 and E-cadherin. Some of these reagents are not without their critics and it is best to employ a panel of such antibodies. Hyaluronic acid may account for some spuriously positive immunocytochemical results so these procedures may be worth repeating after predigestion with hyaluronidase.[314] The commonest adenocarcinoma mimicking mesothelioma is that arising in the underlying lung and antibodies specific to the lung such as those reacting with surfactant apoprotein and TTF-1 are therefore helpful.[315,316] The following sensitivities/specificities are quoted for pulmonary adenocarcinoma involving the pleura: TTF-1 72/100; CEA 93/95; Ber-EP4 80/90; B72.3 80/93; E-cadherin 86/82.[317]

Monoclonal antibodies that react with mesotheliomas but seldom with adenocarcinomas include those directed against cytokeratin 5/6, thrombomodulin (CD141), calretinin, Wilms tumour product-1, N-cadherin and podoplanin (D2-40).[239,317,318,318a] Initial enthusiasm for HMBE1, OV632, mesothelin and CD44 hyaluronate receptor has waned. More recently h-caldesmon and caveolin-1 have also been reported as being highly specific for mesothelioma.[319,320] With calretinin it is important to confine attention to the nuclei of the malig-

Table 13.2 Staining characteristics of mesothelioma and adenocarcinoma

Mesothelioma	Adenocarcinoma
Cytoplasm contains glycogen but no diastase-resistant PAS-positive material	Glycogen content is small. May contain diastase-resistant PAS-positive mucin
Alcianophilic hyaluronic acid in glands or on tumour cell surface	No hyaluronic acid within or on tumour cells
CEA, Leu M_1, BerEp4 and AUA1 negative	CEA, Leu M_1, BerEp4 and AUA1 positive
EMA positive at cell membrane	EMA positive in cytoplasm and at cell periphery
Cytokeratin 5/6, thrombomodulin and calretinin[a] positive	Cytokeratin 5/6, thrombomodulin and calretinin[a] negative

[a]Attention should be confined to nuclear staining as cytoplasmic staining for calretinin is non-specific.

PAS, periodic acid–Schiff; CEA, carcinoembryonic antigen; EMA, epithelial membrane antigen.

Figure 13.22 Metastatic adenocarcinoma. A diastase-controlled periodic acid–Schiff stain is strongly positive, confirming that the tumour is a metastatic adenocarcinoma rather than an epithelioid mesothelioma.

Figure 13.23 Immunohistochemistry for epithelioid mesothelioma. In contrast to metastatic adenocarcinomas, epithelioid mesotheliomas typically stain for (A) calretinin (nuclear stain), (B) cytokeratin 5/6 (cytoplasmic stain) and (C) thrombomodulin (membrane stain).

nant cells as cytoplasmic staining is far less specific for cells of mesothelial origin (Fig. 13.23). Podoplanin is specific for mesotheliomas but whereas the staining is membranous with epithelioid mesotheliomas, it is cytoplasmic with sarcomatoid mesotheliomas.[321] The International Mesothelioma Interest Group recommends that markers have either sensitivity or specificity greater than 80% for the lesion in question,[239] although how many markers are required for confident diagnosis remains a matter of debate.[322] Figures quoted for epithelioid mesothelioma are shown in Table 13.3.[317]

Whilst these mesothelial markers are relatively dependable in distinguishing mesothelioma from adenocarcinoma, they are not so dependable in relation to other carcinomas of the lung. They not infrequently stain squamous cell, small cell, large cell and giant cell carcinomas,[323,324] but most of these are distinguishable on their morphology and their expression of other epitopes such as TTF-1.

Table 13.3 Sensitivities and specificities of epithelioid mesothelioma markers versus adenocarcinoma[317]

Immunocytochemical marker	Sensitivity (%)	Specificity (%)
Cytokeratin 5/6	83	85
Calretinin	82	85
N-cadherin	78	84
Wilms tumour product-1	77	96
Thrombomodulin	61	80

Figure 13.24 Transmission electron micrograph of an epithelioid mesothelioma showing long curly microvilli intermingled with collagen.

Table 13.4 Ultrastructural distinction between mesothelioma and adenocarcinoma

Mesothelioma	Adenocarcinoma
Microvilli elongated, slender and bushy without glyocalyceal bodies. May mingle with collagen fibrils	Microvilli short and stubby with glycocalyceal bodies. Generally confined to the luminal surface and seldom mingle with collagen fibrils
Apical tight junctions	Terminal bars near lumen
Long, well-developed desmosomes	Short, less well-developed desmosomes
Perinuclear tonofilaments	Irregularly distributed intermediate filaments
No mucin granules	May contain mucin granules
Abundant glycogen	Variable amount of glycogen
Scanty fat droplets	No fat

Extrapulmonary carcinomas that may express some of these mesothelial markers include transitional cell and renal cell carcinomas, the latter exceptional in also failing to express the epithelial marker CEA. Results obtained with mesothelial markers therefore need to be viewed with some caution and assessed in conjunction with clinical, radiological and morphological features.[325,326] Separation of the rare clear cell type of mesothelioma[285–287] from metastatic clear cell carcinoma of the kidney can be problematic. One authority recommends the mesothelioma markers cytokeratin 5/6, podoplanin and mesothelin and the renal markers CD15 and RCC Ma.[239] It is advisable to correlate these laboratory results with imaging studies.

In distinguishing peritoneal mesothelioma of epithelioid pattern from serous carcinoma of the ovary a similar panel of antibodies may be employed but calretinin is more sensitive than thrombomodulin, cytokeratin 5/6 and BerEP4 than CEA.[327] It is also worth adding oestrogen receptor antibody as a specific marker of ovarian serous carcinoma.[328,329]

Electron microscopy is now used less than formerly but when the sample is small (as in cell block preparations) or the histological and immunohistochemical findings are of uncertain significance, it can be very helpful in distinguishing mesotheliomas from other tumours.[330,331] Although epithelioid mesotheliomas have several ultrastructural features in common with adenocarcinomas, sufficient differences may be present to enable a confident diagnosis to be made

(Table 13.4).[332–337] Adenocarcinomas often contain secretory granules, which are never found in mesotheliomas. Conversely, mesotheliomas generally have long, slender, curved microvilli that give a bush-like appearance to the surface of the cells (Fig. 13.24) and differ from the short stubby microvilli of an adenocarcinoma. The long microvilli are easily recognisable by scanning electron microscopy. They cover all free surfaces of the mesothelioma cells, including both intracellular and intercellular lumina, and may come into direct contact with stromal collagen through deficiencies in the basement membrane (see Fig. 13.24), a feature that is rarely encountered in carcinomas. Neither long curly microvilli nor contact between microvilli and collagen is totally specific but either of these findings is very suggestive of mesothelioma.[338] At points of contact between mesothelioma cells, well-developed and often unusually long desmosomes are found. Abundant intermediate filaments (tonofilaments) form bundles that may converge on cell junctions, or more characteristically are perinuclear. Large collections of glycogen and occasional fat droplets are often evident in the cytoplasm of mesothelioma cells. Tubular structures that possibly represent crystallised proteoglycan have been identified in the rare mesotheliomas referred to above as containing hyaluronidase-resistant PAS-positive droplets.[310]

Separation of small cell anaplastic mesothelioma[274,275] from small cell carcinoma involving the pleura[339] depends upon wide sampling to identify more characteristic areas. The neuroendocrine markers chromogranin, neuron-specific enolase, Leu-7 and neural cell adhesion molecule (CD56) are not specific, being found in a proportion of mesotheliomas.[288,340,341]

Flow cytometric ploidy studies have been conducted in the hope of discriminating better between carcinoma and mesothelioma. Differences are reported but these are not absolute and therefore of limited use in individual cases: 47–78% of mesotheliomas are diploid whereas 85–88% of carcinomas are aneuploid.[342–344] Despite the relative lack of aneuploidy in mesotheliomas, cytogenetic studies have documented abnormal karyotypes in about three-quarters of cases but no consistent abnormality has been identified.[344] However, microarray data assessing expression levels of a small number of genes as ratios have shown similar specificity to immunohistochemistry in distinguishing mesothelioma from metastatic adenocarcinoma.[345]

Many asbestos workers are also cigarette smokers and it is therefore inevitable that occasional cases of synchronous pulmonary carcinoma and mesothelioma will arise, necessitating particularly careful evaluation.[346]

Poorly differentiated epithelioid mesothelioma versus poorly differentiated squamous cell carcinoma

Specific markers of squamous cell carcinoma are as yet not as well substantiated as those for adenocarcinoma, which is unfortunate

Table 13.5 Immunohistochemical distinction of sarcomatoid mesothelioma, sarcoma and sarcomatoid carcinoma[364,378]

	Pankeratin	**CK5/6**	**Calretinin**	**Thrombomodulin**	**SMA**	**TTF-1**	**D2-40**
Sarcomatoid mesothelioma	70%	Rare	70%	70%	60%	0/10	87%
Sarcoma	17%	Rare	17%	38%	58%	Negative	
Sarcomatoid carcinoma	90%	Rare	60%	40%	10%	Pulmonary may be positive	26%

SMA, smooth-muscle actin; TTF-1, thyroid transcription factor-1.

because without obvious evidence of keratinisation it may be difficult to distinguish squamous cell carcinoma from poorly differentiated epithelioid mesothelioma. Furthermore, markers such as cytokeratin 5/6 and calretinin that distinguish mesothelioma from adenocarcinoma are expressed by some squamous cell carcinomas.[323,347] At present discrimination is best achieved with a combination of the mesothelioma marker Wilms tumour suppressor gene-1 and the squamous cell carcinoma markers p63 and MOC-31.[239,348]

Epithelioid mesothelioma versus reactive mesothelial hyperplasia

The epithelioid pattern of mesothelioma may be simulated both by papillary hyperplasia of the surface mesothelium and by the presence of groups of hyperplastic mesothelial cells trapped in granulation tissue beneath the surface. Cellular pleomorphism and mitotic activity may be lacking in mesothelioma and there are often few other pointers to malignancy. However, mesothelial inclusions entrapped by granulation tissue differ from an invasive mesothelioma in that they are often aligned parallel to the surface because they represent the line of the former pleural surface, and they do not invade the fat underlying the parietal pleura. Invasion of fat, muscle or lung is undoubtedly the best indicator of neoplasia.[349,350] Caution is needed in the interpretation of non-invasive papillary proliferation of the surface mesothelium in view of the possibility that it may represent a premalignant state (see Fig. 13.15a and mesothelioma-in-situ[209] above). In effusions, macrophages may mimic exfoliated mesothelial cells, both reactive and malignant, but may be recognised by the inclusion of the macrophage marker CD68 in the immunohistochemical panel. The spread of non-malignant mesothelial cells to regional lymph nodes is another trap for the unwary.[351–358]

Immunohistochemistry has a limited role in the recognition of pleural malignancy. Epithelial membrane antigen (EMA) and p53 are found more often in malignant mesothelioma than reactive hyperplasia, whereas the reverse is found with desmin,[308,359,360] but many find these antibodies unhelpful in the individual case.[349] The following sensitivity/specificity figures are quoted: EMA 74/89; p53 58/91; desmin 83/83.[317] The combination of EMA and p53 positivity, together with lack of desmin expression, may give additional weight to a benign or malignant diagnosis, but should not override the morphological features.[349,361] When there is doubt a report of 'atypical mesothelial proliferation' is recommended.[350] It is likely that in the near future the definition of genetic abnormalities will contribute to the distinction of malignant and reactive mesothelial proliferation.[361a]

Sarcomatoid mesothelioma versus other spindle cell tumours

Sarcomatoid mesotheliomas may mimic a wide range of connective tissue tumours and it is necessary to consider these in the differential

diagnosis, especially if the tumour is localised and there is no history of exposure to asbestos.[362] Sarcomatoid mesotheliomas frequently express broad-spectrum cytokeratins[363] and this provides strong but not infallible support for the tumour being a sarcomatoid mesothelioma rather than a sarcoma (Table 13.5),[364] and helps in the distinction of lymphohistiocytoid mesothelioma from lymphoma. However, it has to be remembered that the submesothelial spindle cells of reactive pleural fibrosis also express cytokeratin[18,365]: attention should therefore be concentrated on the deeper parts of the lesion. Conversely, between 16 and 40% of sarcomatoid mesotheliomas fail to stain for cytokeratin.[128,366] It is therefore helpful that calretinin and thrombomodulin react with some sarcomatoid as well as epithelioid mesotheliomas,[364,367] although their specificity and sensitivity in relation to primary pleural sarcomas and sarcomatoid carcinomas of lung are sufficiently low that they are of questionable diagnostic value.[322] For example, calretinin often stains synovial sarcomas.[368] However, podoplanin staining is more specific, decorating the cytoplasm of sarcomatoid mesothliomas but not staining synovial sarcomas.[321] Sarcomatoid mesothelioma also lacks the SYT-SSX fusion of synovial sarcoma.[369,370]

The diversity of differentiation seen with mesotheliomas means that the expression of markers such as vimentin and smooth-muscle actin does not exclude a diagnosis of mesothelioma, even if the tumour is cytokeratin-negative.[293,363,371,372] However, a combination of cytokeratin-negativity and CD34-positivity would favour localised fibrous tumour of the pleura. Epithelioid haemangioendothelioma and other vascular tumours may mimic mesothelioma both grossly and microscopically but can be distinguished by their positive endothelial markers (factor VIII-related antigen, von Willebrand factor, CD31, CD34 and *Ulex europaeus* agglutinin).[302,373–376]

Sarcomatoid mesotheliomas also need to be distinguished from a variety of epithelial spindle cell tumours, notably the pleural metastases of monophasic sarcomatoid carcinomas of the lung, renal carcinomas of spindle cell or eosinophilic polygonal cell type, and melanomas. The last of these differs from mesothelioma in lacking cytokeratins and staining for S-100 and HMB45 antigens. Lung markers such as surfactant apoprotein and TTF-1 may occasionally be useful in distinguishing spindle cell carcinoma of the lung (see Table 13.5)[364] and wider sampling of many apparently monophasic sarcomatoid carcinomas of the lung reveals that they are biphasic, permitting a distinction based upon the properties of the epithelioid component,[377] as described above. Of 13 other immunomarkers, one group reported that only D2-40 (antipodoplanin) stained most sarcomatoid mesotheliomas (87%) and few sarcomatoid carcinomas of the lung (26%), the specificity for mesothelioma being 75% (see Table 13.5).[378] Sarcomatoid renal carcinoma may be very difficult to distinguish from mesothelioma, as there is some overlap in their immunohistochemical profiles.[325,326] If a renal origin is suspected it is perhaps best to advise a non-invasive investigation of that area by computed tomography or ultrasound.[325,379] Thymomas involving the pleura may also mimic mesothelioma in their gross structure but generally retain their distinctive microscopic morphology.[380-383]

In mesotheliomas that appear purely sarcomatoid by light microscopy, electron microscopy may demonstrate the classic biphasic pattern by revealing cells with such epithelial features as desmosomes and microvilli.[334,384,385]

Sarcomatoid mesothelioma versus fibrosis

Desmoplastic sarcomatoid mesotheliomas may mimic scar tissue very closely (see Fig. 13.20B)[386] whilst cellular sarcomatoid mesotheliomas may be impossible to distinguish from granulation tissue if, as is sometimes the case, they lack cellular pleomorphism and invasion is not evident in the area sampled. Cytokeratin may be expressed in either reactive or neoplastic fibrous pleural lesions because as submesothelial cells mature to replace lost mesothelial cells they acquire mesothelial characteristics.[17,18,365] In the absence of invasion, features suggestive of mesothelioma include:

- an absence of the zoning usually seen in reparative processes whereby cellular granulation overlies denser scar tissue
- a storiform pattern
- necrosis
- numerous abnormal mitoses
- severe cytological atypia.

Conversely, elongated capillaries aligned at right angles to the surface favour granulation tissue rather than mesothelioma.[239,349] Often however wider sampling to identify frankly malignant foci may be the only solution. In such cases, orientation of the specimen at the time of processing may help in distinguishing the organised maturation of granulation tissue from the more disorganised growth pattern of a desmoplastic mesothelioma.

When sarcomatoid mesotheliomas invade the mediastinum the appearances may mimic those of sclerosing mediastinitis,[226] in which case cytokeratin staining may be helpful.

Desmoplastic mesothelioma is seldom so lacking in cells as the hyaline pleural plaque, which is virtually acellular.

Spread and prognosis of mesothelioma

Instances of mesothelioma being operable are exceptionable.[255,260] There is usually widespread pleural involvement at presentation. However, once the lung is surrounded, there is a period during which the tumour expands locally before metastasising and it is in cases such as these that surgery in the form of pleurectomy or extrapleural pneumonectomy is practised, sometimes preceded by neoadjuvant chemotherapy.[387] However, the place of radical surgery remains controversial,[130] as does chemotherapy,[388] although drugs such as pemetrexed show promise in selected patients.[389,390] Peritoneal mesothelioma is similar, coating the abdominal viscera for some time before disseminating more widely. It is unusual for patients to present because of distant metastases.[228,391,392] Eventually however, dissemination may be widespread and should not detract from a diagnosis of mesothelioma.[393-396]

If the tumour is pleural, there is ultimately invasion of the lung and lymphatic spread to the hilar lymph nodes.[397] Infiltration of the diaphragm results in spread to the peritoneum and upper abdominal lymph nodes, particularly the pancreaticosplenic nodes. The parietal pericardium is infiltrated and multiple deposits may develop in the opposite pleural cavity. Late in the disease, blood-borne metastases may develop in the other lung, liver, adrenals, kidneys, brain, meninges, bone, skeletal muscle and elsewhere.[393-396] Most patients succumb within 2 years of diagnosis[206,269,398-400] but exceptional cases survive for more than 10 years.[401]

To some extent the pattern of spread and prognosis are influenced by the histological type. Epithelioid mesothelioma has a slightly better prognosis than the other histological types.[208,269,400,402-406] They tend to behave like carcinomas and spread to the regional lymph nodes whilst sarcomatoid mesotheliomas tend to behave like sarcomas and metastasise to distant sites; mixed tumours have features of both,[269,407] but these differences are by no means absolute.[394,408] The expression of factors influencing epithelial mesenchymal transition is touched upon below. Evidence has been presented that mesothelioma patients without a history of asbestos exposure survive slightly longer but it is uncertain whether this is independent of histological type.[409,410] Adverse prognostic factors also include male sex, older age, advanced stage, weight loss, poor performance status[208,406,411] and the expression of proliferation markers.[412-414]

Various staging systems are in use[208,406,415] and protocols for examining mesothelioma specimens have been established.[416] The latest TNM classification of pleural mesothelioma and stage groupings are shown in Box 13.3 and Table 13.6.[417] In assessing mesothelial inclusions in

---

Box 13.3 TNM classification of pleural mesothelioma[417]

TX	Primary tumour cannot be assessed
T0	No evidence of primary tumour
T1	Tumour involves ipsilateral parietal pleura with or without involvement of the visceral pleura
T1a	Tumour involves ipsilateral parietal pleura. No involvement of visceral pleura
T1b	Tumour involves ipsilateral parietal pleura, with focal involvement of visceral pleura
T2	Tumour involves any of the ipsilateral pleura surfaces, with at least one of the following: confluent visceral pleural tumour including the fissure invasion of the diaphragmatic muscle invasion of lung parenchyma
T3[a]	Tumour involves any of the ipsilateral pleural surfaces, with at least one of the following: invasion of endothoracic fascia invasion of mediastinal fat solitary focus of tumour invading soft tissue of chest wall non-transmural involvement of pericardium
T4[b]	Tumour involves any of the ipsilateral pleural surfaces, with at least one of the following: diffuse or multifocal invasion of soft tissues of the chest wall any involvement of rib invasion through the diaphragm to the peritoneum invasion of any mediastinal organ direct extension to the contralateral pleura invasion into the spine extension to the internal surface of the pericardium pericardial effusion with positive cytology invasion of the myocardium
NX	Regional lymph nodes cannot be assessed
N0	No regional lymph node metastasis
N1	Metastasis in ipsilateral peribronchial and/or ipsilateral hilar lymph nodes
N2	Metastasis in subcarinal lymph nodes and/or ipsilateral internal mammary or mediastinal lymph nodes
N3	Metastasis in contralateral mediastinal, internal mammary or hilar nodes and/or ipsilateral or contralateral supraclavicular or scalene lymph nodes

Notes: [a]T3 describes locally advanced but potentially resectable tumour.

[b]T4 describes locally advanced, technically unresectable tumour.

Table 13.6 Stage grouping of pleural mesothelioma TNM subsets

Stage	T	N	M
IA	1a	0	0
IB	1b	0	0
II	2	0	0
III	1 or 2	1	0
	1 or 2	2	0
	3	0,1 or 2	0
IV	4	Any N	0
	Any	3	0
	Any	Any	1

Figure 13.25 Well-differentiated papillary mesothelioma. This tumour is composed of papillae in which a mainly single layer of cuboidal cells covers delicate connective tissue cores.

mediastinal lymph nodes it should be remembered that these are not always neoplastic.[351–358]

The production of autocrine growth factors by mesotheliomas would be expected to exert an adverse influence on survival, and several have been identified, including platelet-derived growth factor, transforming growth factor-β and vascular endothelial growth factor.[210–217] An immediate consequence of autocrine activity would be increased mitotic activity and the production of proliferating cell nuclear antigen, both of which correlate with the degree of malignancy and may be of prognostic[418] and future therapeutic value.[419] Microarray data assessing expression levels of a small number of genes as ratios have been used to identify patients with a better prognosis.[420] However, the expression of osteopontin, a glycoprotein involved in cell/matrix interactions and epithelial mesenchymal transition, is an adverse prognostic factor.[421,422] Oncogenes such as *p53*, *RAS* and *bcl-2* have been identified within mesotheliomas[221–223] and the effectiveness of antioncogenes such as veglin, which blocks the action of vascular endothelial growth factor, is being assessed in clinical trials. Other potential therapeutic targets overexpressed in mesothelioma include epidermal growth factor, YAP1, MUC1, p21/WAF1, nicotinic acetyl choline receptor and mesenchymal–epithelial transition factor.[423–429]

Well-differentiated papillary mesothelioma

Well-differentiated papillary mesothelioma is a rare, low-grade variant of epithelioid mesothelioma. Most examples have arisen in the peritoneum of young women but some have been pleural, predominantly affecting middle-aged or elderly patients of either sex.[430,431] Some patients give a history of asbestos exposure.[275,430,431] The tumours may be solitary but more often are multifocal. They generally grow slowly and show no histological evidence of malignancy but occasional examples pursue an aggressive course. Of 11 patients with a minimal follow-up period of 24 months, survival ranged from 36 to 180 months with an average of 74 months and a 10-year survival of 31%.[431]

Patients with pleural involvement present with dyspnoea due to recurrent pleural effusions. Thoracoscopy shows the pleura to be studded with firm nodules measuring less than 1 cm or that there is a single arborescent tumour measuring up to 5 cm. Histology shows papillae consisting of a single layer of bland cuboidal cells covering a delicate connective tissue core (Fig. 13.25). The surface cells have small, regular nuclei. They do not contain nucleoli and mitoses are rare. The cytochemical and ultrastructural features are those of an epithelioid mesothelioma, as described above.

Multicystic mesothelioma (multicystic mesothelial proliferation)

Multicystic mesothelioma is a rare but well-recognised condition of the peritoneum,[432,433] that has occasionally been described in the pleura.[434] Confusion as to its true nature has led to a plethora of names, but it is now recognised to be a reactive lesion and the term 'multicystic mesothelial proliferation' better reflects its true nature. The prognosis is good but it is often difficult to eradicate completely and the lesion is therefore prone to recur.

Patients with peritoneal lesions are generally young adult women with a history of pelvic inflammation or surgery. Typically, multicystic lesions attached to the pelvic organs rise up into the abdomen. The patient with pleural disease was a 37-year-old woman complaining of pleuritic pain. As a child she came into contact with asbestos insulation but the condition is not thought to be related to this pollutant. A large unilateral multicystic mass continuous with the parietal pleura and tightly adherent to the visceral pleura was identified at thoracotomy: there were frequent connections between the cyst lining and the normal parietal pleura.[434]

Histologically the cysts were lined by a monolayer of flattened cells showing papillary infoldings. There was no invasive or mitotic activity. The lining cells stained with antibodies to cytokeratin and EMA while staining for factor VIII-related antigen and CEA was negative. Electron microscopy confirmed the mesothelial nature of the cyst lining. Immunocytochemistry and electron microscopy are useful in distinguishing this lesion from a lymphangioma, with which it is readily confused.

Adenomatoid tumour

Adenomatoid tumours are distinctive benign mesothelial tumours that have mainly been described in the scrotum or in relation to the female generative organs. Despite the abundance of mesothelium in the pleura, adenomatoid tumours are rare in this site.[135,436] They appear as small circumscribed nodules on imaging. Histologically, the cells are often vacuolated, giving the tumours a lace-like appearance.

Immunocytochemical reactions and electron microscopical appearances are those expected of a mesothelial tumour of epithelioid pattern, as described above, and the distinction from an early localised mesothelioma therefore arises. The sharp circumscription and bland cytological features of an adenomatoid tumour are helpful in this respect.

Solitary fibrous tumour of the pleura (localised fibrous tumour)

In the past this tumour has been known as benign or localised mesothelioma because, although there is no obvious mesothelial differentiation, early tissue culture experiments were thought to show biphasic differentiation into 'epithelial' and mesenchymal elements.[437] This may have been due to the inadvertent inclusion of normal mesothelial cells in the culture medium.[438] An alternative proposal envisages origin from subpleural mesenchyme and, despite some contrary views,[439,440] immunocytochemical and ultrastructural findings generally favour this theory. The tumour cells express vimentin and actin intermediate filaments but not cytokeratin or EMA[18,365,441–446] and the ultrastructural features are those of fibroblasts or myofibroblasts.[82,443,446–448] Occasional microvilli and poorly formed junctions are described[441,442,447,449] but it is difficult to distinguish neoplastic mesothelial cells from inclusions of reactive mesothelium by electron microscopy.[439,450] Similarly, it may be difficult to decide whether cells containing keratin intermediate filaments are an inherent part of the tumour or mere inclusions of either mesothelium or alveolar epithelium. However, the bulk of the evidence points to these cells representing entrapment of non-neoplastic elements.[451] Accordingly, the term 'solitary fibrous tumour' is preferred.

Solitary fibrous tumour of the pleura differs from mesothelioma in being unrelated to asbestos exposure and in having a much better prognosis. Several hundred have now been reported.[443,447]

Clinical features

These tumours have a wide age range (8–86 years) but most are discovered in middle-aged or older adults. There is no sex predilection. Some patients are asymptomatic but the majority complain of chest pain, cough and breathlessness. Many develop finger clubbing and hypertrophic pulmonary osteoarthropathy. Some experience hypoglycaemic episodes due to the secretion of insulin-like growth factors.[443,452–455] Recurrent pleural effusion is also recorded.[456]

Pathogenesis

The insulin receptor pathway is consistently activated in these tumours, which, together with their secretion of insulin-like growth factor-2 and expression of p53, platelet-derived growth factors alpha and beta, and hepatocyte growth factor, suggests that their growth is maintained by autocrine activity.[457,458]

Pathological features

The tumours occur with equal frequency on the left and right sides, and three to four times as many arise from the visceral pleura as from the parietal pleura. Often they are attached to the surface of the lung by a pedicle and are mobile within the pleural cavity (Fig. 13.26). Tumours of the parietal pleura tend to be sessile with a broader base (Fig. 13.27). Similar tumours are wholly intrapulmonary[459–461] (Fig. 13.28) whilst others arise in the mediastinum[462] and more distant sites.[444,463–482] Solitary fibrous tumours may also have been included in a series of invasive fibrous tumours of the trachea.[483]

Figure 13.26 Solitary fibrous tumour of the pleura, 9 cm in diameter, excised with its pedicle and a small portion of lung.

Figure 13.27 Solitary fibrous tumour of the pleura. The tumour has a broad base and is mainly encapsulated.

Typically, solitary fibrous tumours of the pleura are well circumscribed and have a smooth, often bosselated, surface covered by serosa. They may attain a weight of 2–3 kg and a diameter of 30 cm or more. The cut surface is pale grey or white, often with a whorled pattern. Small areas of softening or necrosis may be present in larger tumours and some have very vascular areas which may become haemorrhagic.

Microscopically, the appearances are those of a low-grade spindle cell neoplasm of variable cellularity with the tumour cells dispersed in a variably hyaline collagenous stroma (Fig. 13.29). The oval or spindle-shaped nuclei are fairly small and regular with finely dis-

Figure 13.28 An intrapulmonary solitary fibrous tumour, 12 cm in diameter. *(Courtesy of Dr W Downey, Melbourne, Australia.)*

persed chromatin. In more cellular areas mitoses may be present, but they are rarely numerous. A storiform pattern, reminiscent of malignant fibrous histiocytoma, is sometimes seen. Very vascular areas may resemble haemangiopericytoma, but often the vessels have a narrow cuff of hyaline material. There may be focal, or even extensive, myxoid change.[484,485] Liposarcomatous differentiation is recorded as an exceptional feature.[486] At the periphery, inclusions of non-neoplastic mesothelium or bronchioloalveolar epithelium are frequently present. Another variable feature is the presence of microscopic irregular fissures or small cysts, lined by flattened cells. Occasionally these spaces are very conspicuous, giving a lace-like microcystic pattern (Fig. 13.30). Electron microscopy shows that their lining cells resemble the other tumour cells and lack mesothelial or epithelial features. Rare biphasic tumours are reported in which there are foci of malignant epithelioid differentiation.[487]

Immunohistochemistry

Immunocytochemical features distinguishing solitary fibrous tumour (positive reactions for vimentin and actin and negative reactions for cytokeratin or EMA) have been mentioned above. In addition, positive immunostaining for CD34 is obtained in about 80% of solitary fibrous tumours: this is useful in distinguishing solitary fibrous tumour from mesothelioma, malignant fibrous histiocytoma and haemangiopericytoma, in all of which CD34 reactivity is limited to blood vessels.[468,488,489] However, the higher the grade of a solitary fibrous tumour, the less likely is it to express CD34, and the more likely to express p53.[470] Solitary fibrous tumours may be distinguished from inflammatory pseudotumours by positive staining for the p53

Figure 13.29 Solitary fibrous tumour of the pleura. (A) The tumour is encapsulated and of variable cellularity. (B) The stroma may be myxoid or fibrous. (C) The cells are rounded or spindle-shaped cells show no atypia.

Figure 13.30 Solitary fibrous tumour of the pleura of varying cellularity and showing microcystic degeneration.

Figure 13.31 Malignant solitary fibrous tumour of the pleura. (A) In places the tumour shows marked pleomorphism and mitotic activity. (B) Here, the tumour cells are more rounded, but there is still considerable cellularity and mitoses are easily seen.

oncogene product,[491] and from gastrointestinal stromal tumours, to which they have been likened (both being positive for CD99), by their failure to stain for CD117.[492] Nerve sheath tumours rarely arise in the pleura but the occasional examples reported in this site have resembled solitary fibrous tumours both histologically and by showing patchy CD34 positivity. However, they are distinguished by also expressing S-100.[493]

Prognosis

The prognosis following resection is generally good but in a minority there is local recurrence and then usually a fatal outcome.[443,447,494–496] Exceptional cases present with widespread pleural dissemination.[497] Hypercellularity, pleomorphism, necrosis and excessive mitotic activity (more than 4 mitoses per 10 high-power fields) (Fig. 13.31) suggest that the lesion will behave aggressively[443] but the most important prognostic factor is the completeness of excision, fundamental to which is the presence or absence of a pedicle. A staging system has been proposed and subsequently validated (Table 13.7).[458,498] In general, pedunculated tumours, which can be removed with their attachment, do not recur.[447,499] In a review of 360 previously reported cases it was found that 88% behaved in a benign fashion after surgical resection,[447] while in another series of 223 cases, 45 patients (20%) died due to invasion, recurrence or metastasis.[443] In a third series, local recurrence occurred in 6 of 40 cases and metastasis in 5, and tumour size and cellularity correlated with malignancy.[494] In a fourth series of 88 cases, 10% of patients died of their tumour and another 18% experienced recurrence.[458]

Pleural fibromatosis (desmoid tumour)

Desmoid tumours, also known as aggressive fibromatosis or musculoaponeurotic fibromatosis, generally arise in subcutaneous tissue but origin in the pleura is also described, often following surgery or other trauma.[500,501] The pleural examples are liable to be confused with solitary fibrous tumour, both clinically and histologically. They generally form large localised growths with a broad-based attachment to either the parietal or visceral pleura (Fig. 13.32A). The surface is bosselated but infiltrative activity is evident on the deeper aspect. The tumours are firm and show a pale trabeculated pattern on their cut surface. Histologically, they consist of hypocellular fibrous tissue: sparse spindle cells are set in a collagenous stroma (Fig. 13.32B). The spindle cells are myofibroblasts and therefore stain for vimentin, desmin and smooth-muscle actin but lack the CD34-positivity of a solitary fibrous tumour and the cytokeratin positivity of a desmoplastic sarcomatous mesothelioma, the two lesions with which they are liable to be confused.[502] Nuclear staining for β-catenin is positive in most (~80%) desmoid tumours but also in a minority (~20%) of solitary fibrous tumours.[502,503] Recurrence is likely unless excision is wide but metastasis is not a problem.

Calcifying fibrous pseudotumour

Calcifying fibrous pseudotumour, as described in soft tissues, has also been reported in the pleura, peritoneum and mediastinum.[504–506] The patients with pleural tumours were young adults who were either asymptomatic or complained of chest pain. They had a plaque-like, well-circumscribed but non-encapsulated tumour of the visceral

Table 13.7 The de Perrot staging system for localised pleural solitary fibrous tumours[498]

Stage 0	Pedunculated tumour with no histological evidence of malignancy
Stage I	Sessile tumour with no histological evidence of malignancy
Stage II	Pedunculated tumour with histological evidence of malignancy
Stage III	Sessile tumour with histological evidence of malignancy
Stage IV	Multiple synchronous metastases

Figure 13.33 Calcifying fibrous pseudotumour of the pleura. The tumour consists of thick bundles of hyaline fibrous tissue in which there is focal psammomatous calcification. *(Courtesy of Dr A Gibbs, Penarth, UK.)*

Figure 13.32 Pleural fibromatosis (desmoid tumour). (A) A discrete firm fibrous mass is present deep to the chest wall. (B) Microscopy shows a paucicellular, cytologically bland spindle cell proliferation with dense background fibrosis, typical of fibromatosis. There is extension into the peripheral lung, in keeping with the infiltrative properties of this disorder. The residual visceral pleura elastin can be seen as a corrugated line across the centre of the image (arrow).

pleura. Multiple such tumours were identified in one case.[507] Microscopically, these tumours are characterised by abundant hyaline collagen containing sparse thin spindle cells and foci of psammomatous dystrophic calcification (Fig. 13.33). The nature of this lesion is uncertain but it may represent the late stage of an inflammatory myofibroblastic tumour, a possibility that derives some support from the presence of sparse areas of lymphoplasmacytic infiltration, reactivity of both lesions for CD34 and factor XIIIa, and rare reports of cases showing transitional features.[508–511] Local excision appears adequate but it is suggested that if it behaves in a similar fashion to those in the soft tissues, a low rate of local recurrence might be expected.[504]

Desmoplastic small round cell tumour

This is a rare tumour that typically presents with widespread abdominal involvement.[512–514] It is not organ-related and appears to be of mesothelial or submesothelial origin. A few examples arising in the pleura or lung have been reported.[515–517]

The tumour generally affects children and young adults, and has a male-to-female ratio of 4. The tumours that affect the pleura do so in a diffuse manner so that the clinical, radiological and gross features all mimic mesothelioma. However, there is no association with asbestos and the histological features are quite different.

Microscopy shows discrete islands of small cells set in an abundant desmoplastic stroma. The islands of tumour cells vary greatly in size and shape and are sometimes necrotic. The tumour cells are uniform but show many mitoses. They have little cytoplasm and round or oval hyperchromatic nuclei with clumped chromatin and scanty nucleoli. Pseudorosettes are present but no glands or tubules are evident, although entrapped mesothelial islands may be seen.

Although the histological features are those of an anaplastic growth, immunocytochemistry indicates diverse differentiation, with epithelial, neuronal and myogenic expression.[518] The most consistent immunocytochemical finding is strong focal dot-like positivity for vimentin, corresponding to a collection of intermediate filaments evident near the nucleus on electron microscopy. Other ultrastructural features include numerous desmosomes, dense-core granules and occasional gland lumina with microvilli.[519] Further positive reactions are obtained with antibodies to desmin and less consistently to cytokeratin, EMA, neuron-specific antigen, S-100 and glial fibrillary acidic protein. The tumour cells are negative for actin, lymphocyte markers and mesothelial markers such as cytokeratin 5/6.

The differential diagnosis is firstly from mesothelioma, which this tumour simulates in its gross form. The mixed keratin, vimentin and neuron-specific enolase expression is compatible with a mesothelioma, of which a small cell variant has been described, but the combined histological, immunocytochemical and ultrastructural features distinguish the two. There is a closer histological similarity to the malignant small cell tumour of the primitive neuroectodermal tumour series (PNETs), first described in the chest wall (see below), but the diverse differentiation towards muscle, nerve and epithelium shown by immunocytochemistry in the tumour now under discussion is wider than the purely neural differentiation of the PNETs.[520] However, both express CD99 and there is a close cytogenetic similarity, a t(11;22)(p13;q11 or q12) translocation nearly matching the t(11;12)(q24;q12) abnormality found in PNETs and Ewing's sarcoma. 11p13 is the locus of the Wilms tumour suppressor gene and it is notable that the desmoplastic small round cell tumour reacts with an antibody to the C-terminal region of the Wilms tumour protein WT1, in contrast to PNETs, which fail to react with this antibody.[521] The phenotype of the desmoplastic small round cell tumour is intermediate between the purely neural phenotype of the PNETs and the mixed but predominantly epithelial phenotype of a Wilms tumour, reflecting its Ewings/PNET and WT1 gene fusion.[522,523].

The prognosis with pleural tumours appears to be as poor as that of patients with abdominal desmoplastic small round cell tumours. Of three patients with pleural tumours, two died 15 months and 2 years respectively after presentation and the third was alive with tumour 18 months later.[516]

Pleural lymphoma

Most patients with pleural lymphoma have evidence of simultaneous systemic involvement but occasionally the lymphoma appears to be confined to this site.[524] Two unusual lymphomas arise here. One complicates pyothorax and forms a mass lesion whereas the other is seen in acquired immunodeficiency syndrome (AIDS) patients and is generally manifest as a pleural, pericardial or peritoneal effusion. They have become known as pyothorax-associated lymphoma and primary effusion (or body cavity-based) lymphoma respectively. Both are associated with Epstein–Barr virus but the primary effusion lymphoma is also associated with human herpesvirus 8 and human immunodeficiency virus (HIV), supporting the view that they are distinct entities (Table 13.8).[525] Reports of other types of lymphoma arising in the pleura are quite exceptional.[526]

Primary effusion lymphoma (body cavity-based lymphoma)

Most patients with primary effusion lymphoma are HIV-positive homosexual men with advanced AIDS who also test positively for human herpesvirus 8.[527–531] Occasional patients are human herpesvirus-8-positive but HIV-negative.[530,532] An inflammatory effusion associated with human herpesvirus-8 may represent the precursor of primary effusion lymphoma.[530,533] Human herpesvirus-8 is also found in Kaposi's sarcoma and multicentric Castleman's disease and there are reports of patients who have developed both Castleman's disease and primary effusion lymphoma.[534,535] Many patients with primary effusion lymphoma also show evidence of Epstein–Barr virus co-infection.[528,529,536]

Table 13.8 Comparison of primary effusion (body cavity-based) and pyothorax-associated pleural lymphomas

	Primary effusion (body cavity-based) pleural lymphoma	Pyothorax-associated pleural lymphoma
Gross structure	Effusion	Mass lesion
Aetiology	Immunosuppression, typically in an HIV-positive male homosexual	Chronic pleuritis, typically following repeated artificial pneumothoraces
HIV status	Positive	Negative
HHV8 status	Positive	Negative
EBV status	Positive	Positive
CD20/CD3	Negative/negative (null cell)	Positive/negative (B-cell)

HIV, human immunodeficiency virus; HHV, human herpesvirus; EBV, Epstein–Barr virus.

Smears from the pleural fluid show dyscohesive, round to ovoid malignant lymphoid cells with large round nuclei. Some cells have irregular or multiple nuclei. Many mitoses are evident. The cells express CD45 but neither B- nor T-cell antigens (i.e. they have a null cell phenotype).[527–531] Although this lymphoma takes the form of an effusion, a tumour mass may develop late in the course of the disease.[531] Radiographs show a unilateral or bilateral pleural, pericardial or peritoneal effusion, usually associated with slight serosal thickening. The prognosis is poor, with treatment affording only slightly improved survival.[537]

Pyothorax-associated lymphoma

Pyothorax-associated lymphoma is an extranodal non-Hodgkin lymphoma of B-cell phenotype, rich in reactive T cells.[538–542] In contrast to primary effusion lymphoma, pyothorax-associated lymphoma forms a tumour mass. It has largely been reported from Japan but a few cases have been reported from the west.[540,543–548] Patients give a long history of chronic pleuritis, which has generally been consequent upon repeated artificial pneumothoraces for pulmonary tuberculosis.[548] Rarer causes of the pleuritis include asbestos.[549] In many cases there is evidence of Epstein–Barr virus infection and it is suggested that immunosuppressive cytokines or growth factors produced by the inflammatory cells favour the clonal evolution of Epstein–Barr virus-infected B cells.[536,540,546,550,551]

Patients are elderly and present with chest pain, cough and haemoptysis.[548] Radiographs show a pleura-based mass. Histology shows a diffuse proliferation of large, mitotically active lymphoid cells, which are usually CD20-positive but may show aberrant CD3 expression.[548,552] Necrosis and angioinvasion may be evident. Epstein–Barr virus may be demonstrated, but not human herpesvirus 8.[546] The prognosis is poor – only 35% of patients survive 5 years.[548]

Synovial sarcoma

Synovial sarcoma is another tumour that may arise in the pleura, usually as a localised mass but occasionally involving the pleura diffusely and so mimicking mesothelioma.[305,306,369,553–555] The age range is wide (9–79 years, mean 42 years) and males are affected twice as often as females. Reported examples have generally been aggressive tumours, proving fatal within 3 years of initial diagnosis, although occasional localised examples appear to have been cured by surgical excision.

Both biphasic and monophasic examples have been reported, resembling mesothelioma of mixed and sarcomatoid pattern respectively. Localised monophasic examples need to be distinguished from solitary fibrous tumour. Subtle differences are described: monophasic synovial sarcomas are typically composed of closely packed spindle cells arranged in interweaving bundles (so-called herringbone pattern). The cells appear to overlap and numerous mitoses are evident, but pleomorphism is not prominent, as is often the case in mesotheliomas. Mesotheliomas and localised fibrous tumours are also generally less cellular than synovial sarcoma. Immunohistochemical similarities to a mesothelioma of mixed pattern include positive reactions for calretinin, EMA and cytokeratin but the epithelial component of a synovial carcinoma also stains for mucus and carcinoma markers such as BerEP4, while the spindle cell component expresses the *bcl2* oncogene.[553] Solitary fibrous tumours may also express *bcl2* but they also react for CD34. Cytogenetic analysis for the SYT-SSX transcript resulting from t(X;18)(p11;q11) chromosomal translocation is another approach to establishing the diagnosis, this being a characteristic marker of synovial sarcoma: it can be accomplished on paraffin-embedded tissues by fluorescence in situ hybridisation.[556]

Vascular tumours

Vascular tumours such as angiosarcoma, epithelioid angiosarcoma and epithelioid haemangioendothelioma have been reported in the pleura, generally mimicking the diffuse distribution of a mesothelioma (see Fig. 12.3.21, p. 637).[374,375,557–560] The sarcomas were particularly aggressive growths. All had morphological features typical of these growths elsewhere in the body, including reactivity for the endothelial markers factor VIII-related antigen, CD31 and CD34.[302,373–376] Some angiosarcomas have complicated pyothoraces.[561,562]

Nerve sheath tumours

The visceral pleura is innervated by branches of the vagus nerve and the parietal pleura by the intercostal nerves, yet primary nerve sheath tumours of the pleura are distinctly rare. Reports are limited to one of a malignant nerve sheath tumour that mimicked a mesothelioma[563] and another describing two localised neurofibromas that mimicked solitary fibrous tumours.[493] The latter showed patchy positivity for CD34 but were distinguished from solitary fibrous tumour by expressing S-100. In contrast to their rarity in the pleura, nerve sheath tumours are common in the posterior mediastinum and these may impinge upon the pleura. They may also arise in the chest wall (see below).

Other primary sarcomas of the pleura

When considering the possibility of a primary tumour of the pleura other than mesothelioma, it must be remembered that the versatility of malignant mesothelial cells enables them to mimic many other types of primary mesenchymal tumour; for example, osteogenic sarcomatous mesotheliomas may be indistinguishable histologically from primary osteogenic sarcoma.[292] Features suggesting a non-mesothelial sarcoma include the gross appearance of a localised mass, an absence of asbestos exposure and failure to stain for cytokeratin,[564,565] but none of these features is entirely reliable. Origin from the chest wall, diaphragm, mediastinum and lung needs to be excluded. All these caveats need to be considered when evaluating reports of pleural malignant fibrous histiocytoma,[557,566–568] angiosarcoma,[557] liposarcoma,[569,570] rhabdomyosarcoma,[571,572] leiomyoma

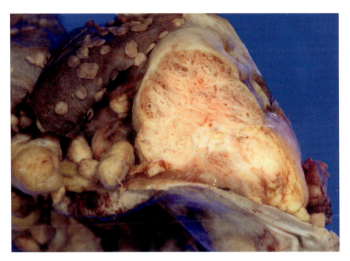

Figure 13.34 Thymoma seeding in the pleural space. A primary mediastinal thymoma adheres to the medial surface of the lung and many tumour seedlings are seen on the visceral pleura.

or leiomyosarcoma,[573–577] chondrosarcoma[578,579] and malignant nerve sheath tumour.[563] However, pleural sarcomas of various type may complicate chronic pleurisy.[557,561,562]

Thymoma

Thymoma has been reported to have arisen in the pleura on occasion, presumably arising from ectopic thymic tissue.[380–383,580] However, it is always difficult to exclude seeding of the pleura from an undetected primary in the thymus (Fig. 13.34). The reported patients have been adults complaining of chest pain, dyspnoea or loss of weight, or occasionally free of symptoms, while the tumours have generally formed localised masses or, less frequently, a diffuse mantle encasing the lung in the manner of a mesothelioma. Growth has generally been indolent but recurrence, metastasis and death from respiratory failure have all been reported. Histologically, the tumours have generally resembled those encountered in the thymus, showing lobules separated by fibrous septa and composed of epithelial cells and lymphocytes in varying proportions. Cytokeratin 5/6 and thrombomodulin (CD141) may be expressed, causing further confusion with mesothelioma, but calretinin staining is negative.[383] The lymphocytes are mainly CD3-positive T cells but CD1a, CD2 and CD99 may also be demonstrated.[383,581]

Carcinoma

Rare instances of pleural 'epidermoid' (squamous cell) carcinoma are recorded, all of which arose in pleural cavities that showed widespread squamous change following the induction of long-standing artificial pneumothoraces.[67,582] It is possible that the squamous change represented metaplasia of the mesothelium but implantation of epidermal fragments is equally likely because numerous injections of air were required to maintain these chronic pneumothoraces. Furthermore, some cases were associated with a bronchopulmonary fistula which also showed squamous change and malignancy and in these a bronchogenic origin cannot be excluded. The tumours were typically well differentiated with abundant keratinisation; although of low grade they showed undoubted infiltrative activity with destruction of adjacent tissues. Carcinoma is also reported in association with lucite ball plombage, apparently arising in the periphery of the lung but closely associated with the lucite in the pleural cavity.[383] Primary muco-

Figure 13.35 Carcinoma of the lung permeating the pleural lymphatics. *(Courtesy of W Edwards, Gordon Museum, Guy's Hospital, London, UK.)*

Figure 13.36 Schwannoma arising from an intercostal nerve.

epidermoid carcinoma of the pleura is also recorded, apparently arising spontaneously.[584]

Secondary tumours of the pleura

Pleural metastases are common in patients with malignant tumours, the commonest primary neoplasms in descending order being adeno-carcinomas of the breast, lung, ovary, stomach, large bowel, carcinoma of the kidney, lymphoma, various sarcomas and melanoma.[247] In many cases the primary site is not determined during life.[247,585,586] Breast carcinoma generally first involves the parietal pleura underlying the affected breast[587] whereas lung cancer more often involves the visceral pleura, either by direct extension (see Fig. 12.1.10, p. 543) or lymphatic permeation (Fig. 13.35 and Fig. 12.6.4B, p. 683).[588] However, at autopsy metastases generally involve both pleural surfaces.[589] Whatever the source, blood-borne metastases are generally multifocal (see Fig. 13.34) and commoner in the lower half of the thorax.[590] However, some peripheral adenocarcinomas of the lung, and, more rarely, squamous carcinomas, spread over the pleural surfaces in a manner similar to mesothelioma and it may be difficult to establish where in the lung such tumours have originated (pseudomeso-theliomatous carcinoma).[298–300] Thymomas may behave similarly.[381]

In distinguishing between secondary adenocarcinoma of the pleura and mesothelioma of epithelioid pattern, mucus stains, immuno-histochemistry and electron microscopy are all helpful (see p. 722). Thymomas spreading on to the pleura should not cause any difficulty to the histopathologist, showing as they do the lobulation and mixed cellularity that are typical of these tumours. They are distinguished from pleural lymphomas by their epithelioid component staining for cytokeratin. The metastatic nature of some pleural tumours can be recognised because they carry site-specific markers that can be detected by immunocytochemistry; for example, surfactant apoprotein as a

marker of a pulmonary origin[591] and TTF-1 as a marker of origin in the lung or thyroid.

A pleural effusion in a patient with lung cancer does not necessarily indicate that the tumour is inoperable. Other causes of a pleural effusion in these patients include secondary infection, lymphatic and venous obstruction and hypoproteinaemia. Involvement of the pleura is more likely if the effusion is blood-stained, or the lung tumour is an adenocarcinoma.[588]

Pleural splenosis

Splenosis results from the implantation of fragments of splenic tissue after traumatic rupture of this organ.[592,593] The implantation is usually on the peritoneum but if the diaphragm is also torn thoracic splenosis is a further potential complication. This may affect the left pleural cavity or pericardium. Splenosis has not been described in the right side of the chest or within the substance of either lung. The condition was first described as a chance autopsy finding in 1937[594,595] and by 1994 only 22 cases had been reported. It is generally asymptomatic and the interval between the trauma and the diagnosis of thoracic splenosis is long (9–32 years, average 20 years). In this time the implant may grow into a large mass, which is only discovered by chance when chest radiographs are taken for some other purpose. The diagnosis is generally made when the lesion is excised and submitted for histological examination. This shows all the components of normal splenic tissue, including both red and white pulp.[596]

CHEST WALL DISEASE

Chest wall tumours

The chest wall may be directly invaded by carcinoma of the breast or lung, it may be the seat of metastases from more distant organs or it may be the site of origin of a range of primary soft-tissue tumour. Attention here is confined to this latter group.[597]

Primary tumours of the chest wall include extra-abdominal desmoid tumours (aggressive fibromatosis, sometimes developing at the site of a previous thoracotomy),[598,599] elastofibroma dorsi (which particularly involves the scapular region), myositis ossificans[600] and tumours of muscle, fat, blood vessel, nerve sheath (Fig. 13.36) and bone.[601,602]

Figure 13.37 Chondrosarcoma of the rib. The tumour forms a bosselated mass on the inner aspect of the anterior chest wall, but is quite localised, a feature against it being a sarcomatoid mesothelioma showing chondroid differentiation.

The bone tumours include multiple myeloma, chondroma, chondrosarcoma (Fig. 13.37), fibrous dysplasia and Langerhans cell histiocytosis. Of the soft-tissue sarcomas, about half are fibrous (fibrosarcoma or dermatofibrosarcoma protuberans), while liposarcoma and nerve sheath malignancies each form 14%, 8% show muscle differentiation, 4% are vascular and 2% are synovial.[603] Some of these tumours follow radiation for breast carcinoma or Hodgkin disease.[604] All are well described in texts devoted to skeletal and soft-tissue tumours and attention here will be confined to two that have a particular predilection for the chest wall and a reactive condition that may be mistaken for a neoplasm.

Malignant small cell tumour of the thoracopulmonary region (Askin tumour)

This high-grade tumour occurs predominantly in the first two decades of life (average age 14 years) and 75% of patients are female.[605,606] Solitary or multiple nodules occur in the chest wall, eroding the ribs and subsequently spreading to involve the pleura, pericardium, diaphragm and periphery of the lung. The tumour tends to recur locally and does not disseminate widely, but the prognosis is dismal, with a 2-year survival of 38% and a 6-year survival of only 14%.[606] Rare examples develop entirely within the lung and are more amenable to surgery.[607–609]

The microscopic features are those of a malignant tumour composed of sheets of undifferentiated small hyperchromatic cells, with rosettes of radially arranged cells around a central tangle of fibrillary cytoplasmic processes (Fig. 13.38). Electron microscopy reveals dense-core neurosecretory granules, and neuroectodermal markers such as S-100 protein, synaptophysin and neuron-specific enolase can be shown by immunohistochemistry, evidence that the tumour is of neural or neuroendocrine derivation.[605,610–613] Further support for this stems from the experimental induction of neuronal differentiation in Askin tumour cell lines.[614] However, the dense-core granules are scanty and the tumour therefore fails to stain for chromogranin.[606]

Figure 13.38 Malignant small cell tumour of the thoracopulmonary region (Askin tumour). The tumour is composed of undifferentiated small hyperchromatic cells.

Extrathoracic examples have subsequently been described and collectively they are now known as primitive neuroectodermal tumours (and colloquially as PNETs), of which those arising in the thoracopulmonary region comprise about a third. Suggestions that PNETs are related to Ewing's sarcoma are supported by cytogenetic studies showing that they carry the Ewing's karyotype, a t(11;22)(q24;q12) translocation[615] and frequently express the Ewing-specific antigen MIC2 (CD99).[616–618] Malignant small cell tumour of the thoracopulmonary region also shows histological and cytogenetic similarities to the desmoplastic small round cell tumour described above, but differs in failing to react with antibodies against the Wilms tumour protein WT1.[521]

Separation of PNETs and Ewing's sarcoma from neuroblastoma is facilitated by their expression of MIC2, neuroblastomas being negative for this antigen. However, chromosomal confirmation is desirable because a small proportion of PNETs and Ewing's sarcoma are also MIC2-negative and positive reactions are obtained with occasional rhabdomyosarcomas and synovial sarcomas.[618] Separation of PNETs from lymphoblastic lymphoma may be effected by the application of lymphocyte markers.[619] Pleuropulmonary blastoma is distinguished by its location in the periphery of the lung rather than the chest wall, its cystic nature and focal sarcomatous differentiation, while in doubtful cases CD99 staining and chromosomal analysis are helpful.[620]

Figure 13.39 Gorham's syndrome. (A) Radiographs show osteolysis of the left second to fifth ribs. (B) Microscopy shows loose connective tissue in which there is a mild lymphocytic infiltrate and prominent vascular proliferation. *(Courtesy of Drs H Aziz and C. Lam, Gothenberg, Sweden.)*

Mesenchymal hamartoma of the chest wall

This tumour-like malformation[621–623] is a distinctive lesion that presents at birth or soon after as an extrapleural chest wall mass with involvement of one or more ribs. It was formerly thought to be neoplastic but is now recognised to be a malformation. The few deaths that have been recorded are attributable to pressure effects on the thoracic viscera by lesions that grew to fill much of the hemithorax. Metastasis has not been observed. Former terms that are now redundant include osteochondroma, osteochondrosarcoma, chondroblastoma and mesenchymoma.

Growth may be rapid but spontaneous regression has been recorded. The lesion is usually solitary but may be multifocal or even bilateral. It generally forms a lobulated, well-circumscribed mass composed of bone, cartilage and blood-filled cysts set in a myxoid matrix. Aneurysmal bone cyst is the principal differential diagnosis but, although this condition affects the young, it is infrequent in the newborn and does not show the prominent cartilage seen in mesenchymal hamartoma.

Gorham's syndrome

This rare condition of unknown aetiology represents a florid proliferation of thin-walled vascular channels that predominantly involves bone and causes marked osteolysis (Fig. 13.39).[624,625] Underlying soft tissues may be invaded, including the lung if the disease is centred on a rib or vertebra. Respiratory function may be further impaired by thoracospinal deformity or pleural effusion.[626,627] Young adults of either sex are predominantly affected. The process may arrest spontaneously and is therefore not considered to be neoplastic, yet the histological appearances are quite alarming. The vascular channels are lined by plump atypical cells and together with evident invasive activity the appearances suggest a malignant process, either angiosarcoma or angiomatoid carcinoma, the latter condition being excluded by negative epithelial and positive endothelial markers (cytokeratin and CD34 respectively). Bilateral effusions, which may be chylous because of thoracic duct involvement, and vertebral collapse carry an adverse prognosis and may warrant radiotherapy, to which the condition has sometimes responded.

REFERENCES

Normal structure and function of the pleura

1. Barrett NR. The pleura. Thorax 1970;25:515–24.
2. Albertine KH, Wiener-Kronish JP, Ross PJ, et al. Structure, blood supply, and lymphatic vessels of the sheep's visceral pleura. Anat Rec 1982;165:277.
3. Albertine KH, Wiener-Kronish JP, Staub NC. The structure of the parietal pleura and its relationship to pleural liquid dynamics in sheep. Anat Rec 1984;208:401.
4. Miserocchi G. Physiology and pathophysiology of pleural fluid turnover. Eur Respir J 1997;10:219–25.
5. Cotran RS, Karnovsky MJ. Ultrastructural studies on the permeability of the mesothelium to horseradish peroxidase. J Cell Biol 1968;37:123–37.
6. Fedorko ME, Hirsch JG. Studies on transport of macromolecules and small particles across mesothelial cells of the mouse omentum. I. Morphologic aspects. Exp Cell Res 1971;69:113–27.
7. Fedorko ME, Hirsch JG, Fried B. Studies of transport of macromolecules and small particles across mesothelial cells of the mouse omentum. II.Kinetic features and metabolic requirements. Exp Cell Res 1971;69:313–23.
8. Wang N-S. The preformed stomas connecting the pleural cavity and the lymphatics in the parietal pleura. Am Rev Respir Dis 1975;111:12–20.

9. Perira AS, Grande NR. Particle clearance from the canine pleural space into thoracic lymph nodes: an experimental study. Lymphology 1992;25:120–8.

10. Boutin C, Dumortier P, Rey F, et al. Black spots concentrate oncogenic asbestos fibers in the parietal pleura: thoracoscopic and mineralogic study. Am J Respir Crit Care Med 1996;153:444–9.

11. Mitchev K, Dumortier P, Devuyst P. 'Black spots' and hyaline pleural plaques on the parietal pleura of 150 urban necropsy cases. Amer J Surg Pathol 2002;26:1198–206.

12. Muller KM, Schmitz I, Konstantinidis K. Black spots of the parietal pleura: Morphology and formal pathogenesis. Respiration 2002;69:261–7.

13. Wang N-S. The regional difference of pleural mesothelial cells in rabbits. Am Rev Respir Dis 1974;110:623–33.

14. Andrews PM, Potter KR. The ultrastructural morphology and possible functional significance of mesothelial microvilli. Anat Rec 1973;177:409–26.

15. Raftery AT. Regeneration of parietal and visceral peritoneum. A light microscopical study. Br J Surg 1973;60:293–9.

16. Raftery AT. Regeneration of peritoneal and visceral peritoneum in the immature animal: a light and electron microscopical study. Br J Surg 1973;60:969–75.

17. Bolen JW, Hammar SP, McNutt MA. Reactive and neoplastic serosal tissue. A light-microscopic, ultrastructural, and immunocytochemical study. Am J Surg Pathol 1986;10:34–47.

18. Al-Izzi M, Thurlow NP, Corrin B. Pleural mesothelioma of connective tissue type, localized fibrous tumour of the pleura, and reactive submesothelial hyperplasia. An immunohistochemical comparison. J Pathol 1989;158:41–4.

19. Gonzalez S, Friemann J, Muller KM, et al. Ultrastructure of mesothelial regeneration after intraperitoneal injection of asbestos fibres on rat omentum. Pathol Res Pract 1991;187:931–5.

20. Ryan GB, Grobety J, Majno G. Mesothelial injury and recovery. Am J Pathol 1973;71:93–102.

21. Whitaker D, Papadimitriou J. Mesothelial healing: morphological and kinetic investigations. J Pathol 1985;145:159–75.

22. Mutsaers SE, Whitaker D, Papadimitriou JM. Mesothelial regeneration is not dependent on subserosal cells. J Pathol 2000;190:86–92.

23. Eskeland G. Regeneration of parietal peritoneum in rats. A light microscopical study. Acta Path Microbiol Scand 1966;68:355–78.

24. Herbert A. Pathogenesis of pleurisy, pleural fibrosis, and mesothelial proliferation. Thorax 1986;41:176–89.

25. Raftery AT. Regeneration of parietal and visceral peritoneum: an electron microscopical study. J Anat 1973;115:375–92.

Pleural effusions

26. Porcel JM, Vives M. Etiology and pleural fluid characteristics of large and massive effusions. Chest 2003;124:978–83.

27. Waller DA, Saunders NR. Unilateral pulmonary oedema following the removal of a giant pleural tumour. Thorax 1989;44:682–3.

28. Schwartz DR, Maroo A, Malhotra A, et al. Negative pressure pulmonary hemorrhage. Chest 1999;115:1194–7.

29. Light RW. Pleural effusion. N Engl J Med 2002 346:1971–7.

30. Gazquez I, Porcel JM, Vives M, et al. Comparative analysis of Light's criteria and other biochemical parameters for distinguishing transudates from exudates. Resp Med 1998;92:762–5.

31. RomeroCandeira S, Hernandez L, RomeroBrufao S, et al. Is it meaningful to use biochemical parameters to discriminate between transudative and exudative pleural effusions? Chest 2002;122:1524–9.

32. Cooper CB, Bardsley PA, Rao SS, et al. Pleural effusions and pancreatico-pleural fistulae associated with asymptomatic pancreatic disease. Br J Dis Chest 1988;82:315–20.

33. Berk JL, Keane J, Seldin DC, et al. Persistent pleural effusions in primary systemic amyloidosis – Etiology and prognosis. Chest 2003;124:969–77.

34. Krenke R, Nasilowski J, Korczynski P, et al. Incidence and aetiology of eosinophilic pleural effusion. Eur Respir J 2009;34:1111–7.

35. Porcel JM, Vives M, Esquerda A, et al. Use of a panel of tumor markers (carcinoembryonic antigen, cancer antigen 125, carbohydrate antigen 15–3, and cytokeratin 19 fragments) in pleural fluid for the differential diagnosis of benign and malignant effusions. Chest 2004;126:1757–63.

36. Leiberman FL, Peters RL. Cirrhotic hydrothorax. Further evidence that an acquired diaphragmatic defect is at fault. Arch Intern Med 1970;125:114–7.

37. Green A, Logan M, Medawar W, et al. The management of hydrothorax in continuous ambulatory peritoneal dialysis (CAPD). Perit Dial Int 1990;10:271–4.

38. Roden S, Juvin K, Homasson JP, et al. An uncommon etiology of isolated pleural effusion – The ovarian hyperstimulation syndrome. Chest 2000;118:256–8.

39. McGrath EE, Blades Z, Anderson PB. Chylothorax: aetiology, diagnosis and therapeutic options. Respiratory Medicine 2010;104:1–8.

40. Blankenship ME, Rowlett J, Timby JW, et al. Giant lymph node hyperplasia (Castleman's disease) presenting with chylous pleural effusion. Chest 1997;112:1132–3.

41. Hillerdal G. Chylothorax and pseudochylothorax. Eur Respir J 1997;10:1157–62.

42. Samman PD, White WF. The 'yellow nail' syndrome. Br J Dermatol 1964;76:153–7.

43. Emerson PA. Yellow nails, lymphoedema and pleural effusions. Thorax 1966;21:247–53.

44. Beer DJ, Pereira W, Snider GL. Pleural effusion associated with primary lymphedema: a perspective on the yellow nail syndrome. Am Rev Respir Dis 1978;117:595–9.

45. Solal-Celigny P, Cormier Y, Fournier M. The yellow nail syndrome. Arch Pathol Lab Med 1983;107:183–5.

46. Parry CM, Powell RJ, Johnston IDA. Yellow nails, bronchiectasis and low circulating B-cells. Respir Med 1994;88:475–6.

47. DAlessandro A, Muzi G, Monaco A, et al. Yellow nail syndrome: does protein leakage play a role? Eur Resp J 2001;17:149–52.

48. Hoque SR, Mansour S, Mortimer PS. Yellow nail syndrome: not a genetic disorder? Eleven new cases and a review of the literature. Br J Dermatol 2007;156:1230–4.

49. Maldonado F, Tazelaar HD, Wang CW, et al. Yellow nail syndrome: analysis of 41 consecutive patients. Chest 2008;134:375–81.

50. Martinez FJ, Villanueva AG, Pickering R, et al. Spontaneous hemothorax. Report of 6 cases and review of the literature. Medicine Baltimore 1992;71:354–68.

51. Tatebe S, Kanazawa H, Yamazaki Y, et al. Spontaneous hemopneumothorax. Ann Thorac Surg 1996;62:1011–5.

52. Delco F, Domenighetti G, Kauzlaric D, et al. Spontaneous biliothorax (thoracobilia) following cholecystopleural fistula presenting as an acute respiratory insufficiency – successful removal of gallstones from the pleural space. Chest 1994;106:961–3.

53. Levine RL, Allen TC, Cartwright J, Jr, et al. Silicone thorax due to a ruptured breast implant. Chest 2005;127:1854–7.

Pneumothorax

54. Gupta D, Hansell A, Nichols T, et al. Epidemiology of pneumothorax in England. Thorax 2000;55:666–71.

55. Sahn SA, Heffner JE. Spontaneous pneumothorax. N Engl J Med 2000;342:868–74.

56. Feldman AL, Sullivan JT, Passero MA, et al. Pneumothorax in polysubstance-abusing marijuana and tobacco smokers: three cases. J Subst Abuse 1993;5:183–6.

57. Gill AF. Bong lung: regular smokers of cannabis show relatively distinctive histologic changes that predispose to pneumothorax (letter). American Journal of Surgical Pathology 2005;29:980–2.

58. Alifano M, Forti Parri SN, Bonfanti B, et al. Atmospheric pressure influences the risk of pneumothorax: beware of the storm! Chest 2007;131:1877–82.

59. Noppen M, Verbanck S, Harvey J, et al. Music: a new cause of primary spontaneous pneumothorax. Thorax 2004;59:722–4.

60. Lichter I, Gwynne JF. Spontaneous pneumothorax in young subjects. A clinical and pathological study. Thorax 1971;26:409–17.

61. Renner RR, Markarian B, Pernice NJ, et al. The apical cap. Radiology 1974;110:569–73.

62. Amjadi K, Alvarez GG, Vanderhelst E, et al. The prevalence of blebs or bullae among young healthy adults: a thoracoscopic investigation. Chest 2007;132:1140–5.

63. Editorial. Spontaneous pneumothorax and apical lung disease. BMJ 1971;2:573.

64. Askin FB, McGann BG, Kuhn C. Reactive eosinophilic pleuritis. A lesion to be distinguished from pulmonary eosinophilic granuloma. Arch Pathol Lab Med 1977;101:187–91.

65. Luna E, Tomashefski JF, Brown D, et al. Reactive eosinophilic pulmonary vascular infiltration in patients with spontaneous pneumothorax. Am J Surg Pathol 1994;18:195–9.

66. McGee JK, Chen LC, Cohen MD, et al. Chemical analysis of World Trade Center fine particulate matter for use in toxicologic assessment. Environ Health Perspect 2003;111:972–80.

67. Willen R, Bruce T, Dahlstroem G, et al. Squamous epithelial carcinoma in metaplastic pleura following extrapleural pneumothorax for pulmonary tuberculosis. Virchows Arch A Pathol Anat Histopathol 1976;370:225–31.

68. Dunnill MS. Metaplastic changes in the visceral pleura in a case of fibrocystic disease of the pancreas. J Pathol Bacteriol 1959;77:299–302.

69. Tomashefski JF, Dahms B, Bruce M. Pleura in pneumothorax. Comparison of patients with cystic fibrosis and 'idiopathic' spontaneous pneumothorax. Arch Pathol Lab Med 1985;109:910–6.

70. Bashir MS, Cowen PN. Mucous metaplasia of the pleura. J Clin Pathol 1992;45:1030–1.

71. Jackson JW, Bennett MH. Chest wall tumour following iodized talc pleurodesis. Thorax 1969;28:788–93.

72. Lange P, Mortensen J, Groth S. Lung function 22–35 years after treatment of idiopathic spontaneous pneumothorax with talc poudrage or simple drainage. Thorax 1988;43:559–61.

73. Bignon J. Pour et contre la pleurodèse au talc. Rev Mal Resp 1995;12:193–5.

73a. Gonzalez AV, Bezwada V, Beamis JF, Villanueva AG. Lung injury following thoracoscopic talc insufflation. Chest 2010;137:1375–81.

Inflammation of the pleura

74. Rashid AMH, Green FHY. Pleural pearls following silicosis: a histological and electronmicroscopic study. Histopathology 1995;26:84–7.

75. Venekamp LN, Velkeniers B, Noppen M. Does 'idiopathic pleuritis' exist? Natural history of non-specific pleuritis diagnosed after thoracoscopy. Respiration 2005;72:74–8.

76. Bartlett JG, Thadepalli H, Gorbach SL, et al. Bacteriology of empyema. Lancet 1974;1:338–40.

77. Neild JE, Eykyn SJ, Phillips I. Lung abscess and empyema. Q J Med 1985;57:875–82.

78. Brook I, Frazier EH. Aerobic and anaerobic microbiology of empyema – a retrospective review in two military hospitals. Chest 1993;103:1502–7.

79. Porta G, RodriguezCarballeira M, Gomez L, et al. Thoracic infection caused by Streptococcus milleri. Eur Resp J 1998;12:357–62.

80. Chen KY, Hsueh PR, Liaw YS, et al. A 10-year experience with bacteriology of acute thoracic empyema – Emphasis on Klebsiella pneumoniae in patients with diabetes mellitus. Chest 2000;117: 1685–9.

81. Hindle W, Yates DAH. Pyopneumothorax complicating rheumatoid lung disease. Ann Rheum Dis 1965;24:57–60.

82. Davies D. Pyopneumothorax in rheumatoid lung disease. Thorax 1966;21:230–5.

83. Levine H, Metzger W, Lacera D, et al. Diagnosis of tuberculous pleurisy by culture of pleural biopsy specimen. Arch Intern Med 1970;126:269–71.

84. Krakowka P, Rowinska E, Halweg H. Infection of the pleura by Aspergillus fumigatus. Thorax 1970;25:245–53.

85. Wood JB, Watson DCT. Sputum wax-worms after plombage. Br J Dis Chest 1988;82:321–3.

86. Weissberg D, Weissberg D. Late complications of collapse therapy for pulmonary tuberculosis. Chest 2001;120:847–51.

87. Shepherd MP. Plombage in the 1980s. Thorax 1985;40:328–40.

88. Joseph J, Sahn SA. Connective tissue diseases and the pleura. Chest 1993;104:262–70.

89. Ellman P, Cudkowicz L, Elwood JS. Widespread serous membrane involvement by rheumatoid nodules. J Clin Pathol 1954;7:239–44.

90. Gruenwald P. Visceral lesions in a case of rheumatoid arthritis. Arch Pathol 1948;46:59–67.

91. Dodson WH, Hollingsworth JW. Pleural effusion in rheumatoid arthritis. Impaired transport of glucose. N Engl J Med 1966;275:1337–42.

92. Nosanchuk JS, Naylor B. A unique cytologic picture in pleural fluid from patients with rheumatoid arthritis. Am J Clin Pathol 1968;50:330–5.

93. Engel U, Aru A, Francis D. Rheumatoid pleurisy. Acta Path Microbiol Immunol 1986;94:53–6.

94. Anderson RJ, Hansen KK, Kuzo RS, et al. A 38-year-old woman with chronic rheumatoid arthritis and a new pleural effusion – rheumatoid pleuritis. N Engl J Med 1994;331:1642–7.

95. Chan JK, Loo KT, Yau BK, et al. Nodular histiocytic/mesothelial hyperplasia: a lesion potentially mistaken for a neoplasm in transbronchial biopsy. Am J Surg Pathol 1997;21:658–63.

96. Rossi G, Cavazza A, Guicciardi N, et al. Nodular histiocytic/mesothelial hyperplasia on transthoracic biopsy: another source of potential pitfall in a lesion frequently present in spontaneous pneumothorax. Histopathology 2008;52:250–2.

Non-malignant asbestos-induced pleural disease

97. Hillerdal G. Non-malignant asbestos pleural disease. Thorax 1981;36:669–75.

98. Gibbs AR, Stephens M, Griffiths DM, et al. Fibre distribution in the lungs and pleura of subjects with asbestos related diffuse pleural fibrosis. Br J Ind Med 1991;48:762–70.

99. Gaensler EA, Kaplan AI. Asbestos pleural effusion. Ann Intern Med 1971;74:178–91.

100. Herbert A, Sterling GM. Lung en cuirasse: histopathology of restrictive pleurisy with asbestos exposure. Thorax 1980;35:715.

101. Stephens M, Gibbs AR, Pooley FD, et al. Asbestos induced diffuse pleural fibrosis: pathology and mineralogy. Thorax 1987;42:583–8.

102. Kee ST, Gamsu G, Blanc P. Causes of pulmonary impairment in asbestos-exposed individuals with diffuse pleural thickening. Am J Respir Crit Care Med 1996;154:789–93.

103. Yates DH, Browne K, Stidolph PN, et al. Asbestos-related bilateral diffuse pleural thickening: natural history of radiographic and lung function abnormalities [see comments]. Am J Respir Crit Care Med 1996;153:301–6.

104. Miles SE, Sandrini A, Johnson AR, et al. Clinical consequences of asbestos-related diffuse pleural thickening: A review. J Occup Med Toxicol 2008;3:20.

105. Gevenois PA, Demaertelaer V, Madani A, et al. Asbestosis, pleural plaques and diffuse pleural thickening: three distinct benign responses to asbestos exposure. Eur Resp J 1998;11:1021–7.

106. www.official-documents.gov.uk/document/ cm70/7003.pdf; 2007.

107. Hoffbrand BI, Goldstraw P, Hetzel MR. Fibrosing pleuritis with extrathoracic extension. J R Soc Med 1985;78:953–4.

108. O'Brien CJ, Franks AJ. Paraplegia due to massive asbestos-related pleural and

mediastinal fibrosis. Histopathology 1987;11:541–8.

109. Buchanan DR, Johnston IDA, Kerr IH, et al. Cryptogenic bilateral fibrosing pleuritis. Br J Dis Chest 1988;82:186–93.

110. Azoulay E, Paugam B, Heymann MF, et al. Familial extensive idiopathic bilateral pleural fibrosis. Eur Resp J 1999;14:971–3.

111. Frankel SK, Cool CD, Lynch DA, et al. Idiopathic pleuroparenchymal fibroelastosis: description of a novel clinicopathologic entity. Chest 2004;126:2007–13.

112. Becker CD, Gil J, Padilla ML. Idiopathic pleuroparenchymal fibroelastosis: an unrecognized or misdiagnosed entity? Mod Pathol 2008;21:784–7.

113. Hillerdal G. Rounded atelectasis. Clinical experience with 74 patients. Chest 1989;95:836–41.

114. Blesovsky A. The folded lung. Br J Dis Chest 1966;60:19–22.

115. Stark P. Rounded atelectasis: another pulmonary pseudotumor. Am Rev Respir Dis 1982;125:248–50.

116. Mintzer RA, Cugell DW. The association of asbestos-induced pleural disease and rounded atelectasis. Chest 1982;81:457–60.

117. Menzies R, Fraser R. Round atelectasis. Pathologic and pathogenic features. Am J Surg Pathol 1987;11:674–81.

117a. Yi E, Aubry MC. Pulmonary pseudoneoplasms. Arch Pathol Lab Med 2010;13:417–26.

118. Hourihane DO, Lessof L, Richardson PC. Hyaline and calcified pleural plaques as an index of exposure to asbestos. A study of the radiological and pathological features of 100 cases with a consideration of epidemiology. BMJ 1966;1:1069–74.

119. Hillerdal G. Pleural plaques in a health survey material. Scand J Respir Dis 1978;59:257–63.

120. Roberts GH. The pathology of parietal pleural plaques. J Clin Pathol 1971;24:348–53.

121. Langer AM, Nolan RP, Constantopoulos SH, et al. Association of Metsovo lung and pleural mesothelioma with exposure to tremolite-containing whitewash. Lancet 1987;1:965–7.

122. Constantopoulos SH, Theodoracopoulos P, Dascalopoulos G, et al. Metsovo lung outside Metsovo – endemic pleural calcifications in the ophiolite belts of Greece. Chest 1991;99:1158–61.

123. Weiss W. Asbestos-related pleural plaques and lung cancer. Chest 1993;103:1854–9.

124. Andrion A, Pira E, Mollo F. Peritoneal plaques and asbestos exposure. Arch Pathol Lab Med 1983;107:609–10.

125. Baris YI, Sahin AA, Ozesmi M, et al. An outbreak of pleural mesothelioma and chronic fibrosing pleurisy in the village of Karain/Urgup in Anatolia. Thorax 1978;33:181–92.

126. Rosen P, Gordon P, Savino A, et al. Ferruginous bodies in benign fibrous pleural plaques. Am J Clin Pathol 1973;60:608–12.

Pleural tumours

127. Jones MA, Young RH, Scully RE. Malignant mesothelioma of the tunica vaginalis: a clinicopathologic analysis of 11 cases with review of the literature. Am J Surg Pathol 1995;19:815–25.

128. Henderson DW, Comin CE, Hammar SP, et al. Malignant mesothelioma of the pleura: current surgical pathology. In: Corrin B, editor. Pathology of lung tumors. London: Churchill Livingstone; 1997. p. 241–80.

129. Bianchi C, Bianchi T. Malignant mesothelioma: global incidence and relationship with asbestos. Ind Health 2007;45:379–87.

130. Treasure T, Waller D, Tan C, et al. The mesothelioma and radical surgery randomized controlled trial: The MARS feasibility study. J Thorac Oncol 2009;4:1254–8.

131. Peto J, Hodgson JT, Matthews FE, et al. Continuing increase in mesothelioma mortality in Britain. Lancet 1995;345:535–9.

132. Weill H, Hughes JM, Churg AM. Changing trends in US mesothelioma incidence. Occup Environ Med 2004;61:438–41.

133. Wagner JC, Sleggs CA, Marchand P. Diffuse pleural mesotheliomas and asbestos exposure in Northwestern Cape Province. Br J Ind Med 1960;17:260–71.

134. Wagner JC. The discovery of the association between blue asbestos and mesotheliomas and the aftermath. Br J Ind Med 1991;48:399–403.

135. Hourihane DO. The pathology of mesotheliomata and analysis of their association with asbestos exposure. Thorax 1964;19:268–78.

136. Newhouse ML, Thompson H. Mesothelioma of pleura and peritoneum following exposure to asbestos in the London area. Br J Ind Med 1965;2:261–9.

137. Selikoff IJ, Churg J, Hammond EC. Relation between asbestos exposure and neoplasia. N Engl J Med 1965;272:560–5.

138. Whitwell F, Rawcliffe RM. Diffuse malignant pleural mesothelioma and asbestos exposure. Thorax 1971;26:6–22.

139. Selikoff IJ, Hammond EC, Churg J. Carcinogenicity of amosite asbestos. Arch Env Health 1972;25:183–6.

140. Anderson KA, Hurley WC, Hurley BT, et al. Malignant pleural mesothelioma following radiotherapy in a 16 year old boy. Cancer 1985;56:273–6.

141. Gilks B, Hegedus C, Freeman H, et al. Malignant peritoneal mesothelioma after remote abdominal radiation. Cancer 1988;61:2019–21.

142. Hillerdal G, Berg J. Malignant mesothelioma secondary to chronic inflammation and old scars. Two new cases and review of the literature. Cancer 1985;55:1968–72.

143. Shannon VR, Nesbitt JC, Libshitz HI. Malignant pleural mesothelioma after radiation therapy for breast cancer – a report of two additional patients. Cancer 1995;76:437–41.

144. Cavazza A, Travis LB, Travis WD, et al. Post-irradiation malignant mesothelioma. Cancer 1996;77:1379–85.

145. Neugut AI, Ahsan H, Antman KH. Incidence of malignant pleural mesothelioma after thoracic radiotherapy. Cancer 1997;80:948–50.

146. Henley JD, Loehrer PJ, Ulbright TM. Deciduoid mesothelioma of the pleura after radiation therapy for Hodgkin's disease presenting as a mediastinal mass. Am J Surg Pathol 2001;25:547–8.

147. Cicala C, Pompetti F, Carbone M. SV40 induces mesotheliomas in hamsters. Am J Pathol 1993;142:1524–33.

148. Carbone M, Pass HI, Rizzo P, et al. Simian virus 40-like DNA sequences in human pleural mesothelioma. Oncogene 1994;9:1781–90.

149. Cacciotti P, Strizzi L, Vianale G, et al. The presence of simian-virus 40 sequences in mesothelioma and mesothelial cells is associated with high levels of vascular endothelial growth factor. Amer J Respir Cell Molec Biol 2002;26:189–93.

150. Mossman BT, Gruenert DC. SV40, Growth factors, and mesothelioma. Another piece of the puzzle. Am J Respir Cell Mol Biol 2002;26:167–70.

151. Galateau-Salle F, Bidet P, Iwatsubo Y, et al. SV40-like DNA sequences in pleural mesothelioma, bronchopulmonary carcinoma, and non-malignant pulmonary diseases. J Pathol 1998;184:252–7.

152. Mulatero C, Surentheran T, Breuer J, et al. Simian virus 40 and human pleural mesothelioma. Thorax 1999;54:60–1.

153. Ramael M, Nagels J, Heylen H, et al. Detection of SV40 like viral DNA and viral antigens in malignant pleural mesothelioma. Eur Resp J 1999;14:1381–6.

154. Rizzo P, Carbone M, Fisher SG, et al. Simian virus 40 is present in most United States human mesotheliomas, but it is rarely present in non-Hodgkin's lymphoma. Chest 1999;116:470S–473S.

155. Pilatte Y, Vivo C, Renier A, et al. Absence of SV40 large T-antigen expression in human mesothelioma cell lines. Amer J Respir Cell Molec Biol 2000;23:788–93.

156. Mayall F, Barratt K, Shanks J. The detection of Simian virus 40 in mesotheliomas from New Zealand and England using real time FRET probe PCR protocols. J Clin Pathol 2003;56:728–30.

157. Rake C, Gilham C, Hatch J, et al. Occupational, domestic and environmental mesothelioma risks in the

British population: a case-control study. Br J Cancer 2009;100:1175–83.

158. Huncharek M. Changing risk groups for malignant mesothelioma. Cancer 1992;69:2704–11.

159. Cazzadori A, Malesani F, Romeo L. Malignant pleural mesothelioma caused by nonoccupational childhood exposure to asbestos. Br J Ind Med 1992;49:599.

160. Rey F, Viallat JR, Boutin C, et al. Les mesotheliomes environnementaux en Corse du nord-est. Rev Mal Resp 1993;10:339–45.

161. Magnani C, Terracini B, Ivaldi C, et al. Pleural malignant mesothelioma and non-occupational exposure to asbestos in Casale Monferrato, Italy. Occup Environ Med 1995;52:362–7.

162. Constantopoulos SH, Malamou-Mitsi V, Goudevenos J, et al. High incidence of malignant pleural mesothelioma in neighbouring village of North-western Greece. Respiration 1987;51:266–71.

163. Metintas S, Metintas M, Ucgun I, et al. Malignant mesothelioma due to environmental exposure to asbestos – Follow-up of a Turkish cohort living in a rural area. Chest 2002;122:2224–9.

164. Wagner JC. Mesothelioma and mineral fibres. Cancer 1986;57:1905–11.

165. Wagner JC, Newhouse ML, Corrin B, et al. Correlation between fibre content of the lung and disease in east London asbestos factory workers. Br J Ind Med 1988;45:305–8.

166. Churg A, Vedal S. Fiber burden and patterns of asbestos-related disease in workers with heavy mixed amosite and chrysotile exposure. Am J Respir Crit Care Med 1994;150:663–9.

167. McDonald JC, Armstrong B, Case B, et al. Mesothelioma and asbestos fiber type. Evidence from lung tissue analyses. Cancer 1989;63:1544–7.

168. Churg A, Wright JL, Vedal S. Fiber burden and patterns of asbestos-related disease in chrysotile miners and millers. Am Rev Respir Dis 1993;148:25–31.

169. McDonald JC, McDonald AD. The epidemiology of mesothelioma in historical context. Eur Respir J 1996;9:1932–42.

170. Senyigit A, Babayigit C, Gokirmak M, et al. Incidence of malignant pleural mesothelioma due to environmental asbestos fiber exposure in the southeast of Turkey. Respiration 2000;67:610–14.

171. Wagner JC. Experimental production of mesothelial tumours of the pleura by implantation of dusts in laboratory animals. Nature 1962;196:180–1.

172. Wagner JC, Berry G, Timbrell V. Mesotheliomata in rats after inoculation with asbestos and other materials. Br J Cancer 1973;28:173–85.

173. Metintas M, Hillerdal G, Metintas S. Malignant mesothelioma due to environmental exposure to erionite:

174. Johnson NF, Edwards RE, Munday DE, et al. Pluripotential nature of mesotheliomata induced by inhalation of erionite in rats. Br J Exp Pathol 1984;65:377–88.

175. Doll R. Symposium on man-made mineral fibres, Copenhagen, October 1986: overview and conclusions. Ann Occup Hyg 1987;31:805–20.

176. Stanton MF, Layard M, Tegeris A, et al. Carcinogenicity of fibrous glass: pleural response in the rat in relation to fibre dimension. J Natl Cancer Inst 1977;58:587–603.

177. Fraire AE, Greenberg SD, Spjut HJ, et al. Effect of fibrous glass on rat pleural mesothelium histopathologic observations. Am J Respir Crit Care Med 1994;150:521–7.

178. Takagi A, Hirose A, Nishimura T, et al. Induction of mesothelioma in p53+/− mouse by intraperitoneal application of multi-wall carbon nanotube. J Toxicol Sci 2008;33:105–16.

179. Kilburn KH, Powers D, Warshaw RH. Pulmonary effects of exposure to fine fibreglass – irregular opacities and small airways obstruction. Br J Ind Med 1992;49:714–20.

180. Shannon HS, Jamieson E, Julian JA, et al. Mortality of glass filament (textile) workers. Br J Ind Med 1990;47:533–6.

181. Hughes JM, Jones RN, Glindmeyer HW, et al. Follow up study of workers exposed to man made mineral fibres. Br J Ind Med 1993;50:658–67.

182. Devuyst P, Dumortier P, Swaen GMH, et al. Respiratory health effects of man-made vitreous (mineral) fibres. Eur Respir J 1995;8:2149–73.

183. Craighead JE, Richards SA, Calore JD, et al. Genetic factors influence malignant mesothelioma development in mice. Eur Respir Rev 1993;3:118–20.

184. Hammar SP, Bockus D, Remington F, et al. Familial mesothelioma: a report of two families. Hum Pathol 1989;20:107–12.

185. Dawson A, Gibbs A, Browne K, et al. Familial mesothelioma – details of 17 cases with histopathologic findings and mineral analysis. Cancer 1992;70:1183–7.

186. Browne K. The epidemiology of mesothelioma. J Soc Occup Med 1983;33:190–4.

187. Lanphear BP, Buncher CR. Latent period for malignant mesothelioma of occupational origin. J Occup Med 1992;34:718–21.

188. Yates DH. Malignant mesothelioma in south east England: clinicopathological experience of 272 cases (Correction to Vol 52, pg 507, 1997). Thorax 1997;52:1018.

189. Andrion A, Bosia S, Paoletti L, et al. Malignant peritoneal mesothelioma in a 17-year-old boy with evidence of previous

exposure to chrysotile and tremolite asbestos. Hum Pathol 1994;25:617–22.

190. Brenner J, Sardillo PP, Magill CB. Malignant mesothelioma in children – report of seven cases and review of the literature. Med Pediatr Oncol 1981;9:367–73.

191. Fraire AE, Cooper S, Greenberg SD, et al. Mesothelioma of childhood. Cancer 1988;62:838–47.

192. Cooper SP, Fraire EA, Buffler PA, et al. Epidemiologic aspects of childhood mesothelioma. Pathol Immunopathol Res 1989;8:276–86.

193. Marie LC, Lee YJ, Ho MY. Malignant mesothelioma in infancy. Arch Pathol Lab Med 1989;113:409–10.

194. Moran CA, Albores-Saavedra J, Suster S. Primary peritoneal mesotheliomas in children: a clinicopathological and immunohistochemical study of eight cases. Histopathology 2008;52:824–30.

195. Dawson A, Gibbs AR, Pooley FD, et al. Malignant mesothelioma in women. Thorax 1993;48:269–74.

196. Browne K, Smither WJ. Asbestos-related mesothelioma: factors discriminating between pleural and peritoneal sites. Br J Ind Med 1983;40:145–52.

197. Gross P, Harley RA, Swinburne LM, et al. Ingested mineral fibres: do they penetrate tissues or cause cancer? Arch Env Health 1974;29:341–7.

198. Roggli VL, Pratt PC. Numbers of asbestos bodies on iron-stained tissue sections in relation to asbestos body counts in lung tissue digests. Hum Pathol 1983;14:355–61.

199. Roggli VL, Pratt PC, Brody AR. Asbestos content of lung tissue in asbestos associated diseases: a study of 110 cases. Br J Ind Med 1986;43:18–28.

200. De Vuyst P, Karjalainen A, Dumortier P, et al. Guidelines for mineral fibre analyses in biological samples: report of the ERS Working Group. Eur Resp J 1998;11:1416–26.

201. Peterson JT, Greenberg SD, Butler PA. Non-asbestos related malignant mesothelioma. Cancer 1984;54:951–60.

202. Gibbs AR, Jones JSP, Pooley FD, et al. Non-occupational malignant mesotheliomas. In: Bignon J, Peto J, Saracci R, editors. Non-occupational exposure to mineral fibres. Lyon: International Agency for Research on Cancer; 1989. p. 219–28.

203. Gibbs AR. Role of asbestos and other fibres in the development of diffuse malignant mesothelioma. Thorax 1990;45:649–54.

204. Rom WN, Travis WD, Brody AR. Cellular and molecular basis of the asbestos-related diseases. Am Rev Respir Dis 1991;143:408–22.

205. Srebro SH, Roggli VL, Samsa GP. Malignant mesothelioma associated with

low pulmonary tissue asbestos burdens: a light and scanning electron microscopic analysis of 18 cases. Mod Pathol 1995;8:614–21.

206. Yates DH, Corrin B, Stidolph PN, et al. Malignant mesothelioma in south east England: clinicopathological experience of 272 cases. Thorax 1997;52:507–12.

207. Roggli VL. Quantitative and analytical studies in the diagnosis of mesothelioma. Semin Diagn Pathol 1992;9:162–8.

207a. Toyokuni S. Mechanisms of asbestos-induced carcinogenesis. Nagoya J Med Sci 2009;71:1–10

208. Boutin C, Rey F, Gouvernet J, et al. Thoracoscopy in pleural malignant mesothelioma – a prospective study of 188 consecutive patients 2. Prognosis and staging. Cancer 1993;72:394–404.

209. Whitaker D, Henderson DW, Shilkin KB. The concept of mesothelioma in situ: implications for diagnosis and histogenesis. Semin Diagn Pathol 1992;9:151–61.

209a. Savic S, Franco N, Grilli B, et al. Fluorescence in situ hybridization in the definitive diagnosis of malignant mesothelioma in effusion cytology. Chest 2010;138:137–44.

210. Dazzi H, Thatcher N, Hasleton PS, et al. DNA analysis by flow cytometry in malignant pleural mesothelioma: relationship to histology and survival. J Pathol 1990;162:51–5.

211. Donna A, Betta PG, Ribotta M, et al. Mitogenic effects of a mesothelial cell growth factor: evidence for a potential autocrine regulation of normal and malignant mesothelial cell proliferation. Int J Exp Pathol 1992;73:193–202.

212. Ramael M, Buysse C, Vandenbossche J, et al. Immunoreactivity for the beta-chain of the platelet-derived growth factor receptor in malignant mesothelioma and non-neoplastic mesothelium. J Pathol 1992;167:1–4.

213. Motoyama T, Honma T, Watanabe H, et al. Interleukin 6-producing malignant mesothelioma. Virchows Arch B Cell Pathol 1993;64:367–72.

214. Gerwin BI. Asbestos and the mesothelial cell: a molecular trail to mitogenic stimuli and suppressor gene suspects. Am J Respir Cell Mol Biol 1994;11:507–8.

215. Fitzpatrick DR, Peroni DJ, Bielefeldt-Ohmann H. The role of growth factors and cytokines in the tumorigenesis and immunobiology of malignant mesothelioma. Am J Respir Cell Mol Biol 1995;12:455–60.

216. Langerak AW, de Laat PAJM, van der Linden-van Beurden CAJ, et al. Expression of platelet-derived growth factor (PDGF) and PDGF receptors in human malignant mesothelioma in vitro and in vivo. J Pathol 1996;178:151–60.

217. Strizzi L, Catalano A, Vianale G, et al. Vascular endothelial growth factor is an autocrine growth factor in human malignant mesothelioma. J Pathol 2001;193:468–75.

218. Gordon GJ, Mani M, Mukhopadhyay L, et al. Inhibitor of apoptosis proteins are regulated by tumour necrosis factor-alpha in malignant pleural mesothelioma. J Pathol 2007;211:439–46.

219. Gordon GJ, Mani M, Mukhopadhyay L, et al. Expression patterns of inhibitor of apoptosis proteins in malignant pleural mesothelioma. J Pathol 2007;211:447–54.

220. Kothmaier H, Quehenberger F, Halbwedl I, et al. EGFR and PDGFR differentially promote growth in malignant epithelioid mesothelioma of short and long term survivors. Thorax 2008;63:345–51.

221. Ramael M, Lemmens G, Eerdekens C, et al. Immunoreactivity for p53 protein in malignant mesothelioma and non-neoplastic mesothelium. J Pathol 1992;168:371–5.

222. Ramael M, Deblier I, Eerdekens C, et al. Immunohistochemical staining of RAS oncogene product in neoplastic and non-neoplastic mesothelial tissues – immunoreactivity for n-RAS and lack of immunohistochemical staining for ha-RAS and k-RAS. J Pathol 1993;169:421–4.

223. Segers K, Ramael M, Singh SK, et al. Immunoreactivity for bcl-2 protein in malignant mesothelioma and non-neoplastic mesothelium. Virchows Arch 1994;424:631–4.

224. Hegmans JPJJ, Hemmes A, Hammad H, et al. Mesothelioma environment comprises cytokines and T-regulatory cells that suppress immune responses. Eur Respir J 2006;27:1086–95.

225. Krismann M, Muller KM, Jaworska M, et al. Molecular cytogenetic differences between histological subtypes of malignant mesotheliomas: DNA cytometry and comparative genomic hybridization of 90 cases. J Pathol 2002;197:363–71.

225a. Musti M, Kettunen E, Dragonieri S, et al. Cytogenetic and molecular genetic changes in malignant mesothelioma. Cancer Genet Cytogenet 2006;170:9–15.

226. Crotty TB, Colby TV, Gay PC, et al. Desmoplastic malignant mesothelioma masquerading as sclerosing mediastinitis – a diagnostic dilemma. Hum Pathol 1992;23:79–82.

227. Brenner J, Sardillo PP, Magill GB, et al. Malignant mesothelioma of the pleura. Review of 123 patients. Cancer 1982;49:2431–5.

228. Sussman J, Rosai J. Lymph node metastasis as the initial manifestation of malignant mesothelioma: report of six cases. Am J Surg Pathol 1990;14:819–28.

229. Ohishi N, Oka T, Fukuhara T, et al. Extensive pulmonary metastases in malignant pleural mesothelioma: a rare clinical and radiographic presentation. Chest 1996;110:296–8.

230. Ogata S, Hiroi S, Tominaga A, et al. Malignant pleural mesothelioma initially diagnosed on cervical lymph node biopsy. Pathol Int 2009;59:592–4.

231. Higashihara M, Sunaga S, Tange T, et al. Increased secretion of interleukin-6 in malignant mesothelioma cells from a patient with marked thrombocytosis. Cancer 1992;70:2105–8.

232. Elmarimi A, Kendall A, Ellis P, et al. Mesothelioma and a high potassium. J R Soc Med 2004;97:390.

233. Kimura N, Ogasawara T, Asonuma S, et al. Granulocyte-colony stimulating factor- and interleukin 6-producing diffuse deciduoid peritoneal mesothelioma. Mod Pathol 2005;18:446–50.

234. Ghosh AK, Mason DY, Spriggs AI. Immunocytochemical staining with monoclonal antibodies in cytologically 'negative' serous effusions from patients with malignant disease. J Clin Pathol 1983;36:1150–3.

235. Ghosh AK, Spriggs AI, Taylor-Papadimitriou J, et al. Immunocytochemical staining of cells in pleural and peritoneal effusions with a panel of monoclonal antibodies. J Clin Pathol 1983;36:1154–64.

236. Scherpereel A, Astoul P, Baas P, et al. Guidelines of the European Respiratory Society and the European Society of Thoracic Surgeons for the management of malignant pleural mesothelioma. Eur Respir J 2010;35:479–95

237. Swiderek J, Morcos S, Donthireddy V, et al. Prospective study to determine the volume of pleural fluid required to diagnose malignancy. Chest 2010;137:68–73.

238. Abouzgheib W, Bartter T, Dagher H, et al. A prospective study of the volume of pleural fluid required for accurate diagnosis of malignant pleural effusion. Chest 2009;135:999–1001.

239. Husain AN, Colby TV, Ordonez NG, et al. Guidelines for pathologic diagnosis of malignant mesothelioma: a consensus statement from the International Mesothelioma Interest Group. Arch Pathol Lab Med 2009;133:1317–31.

240. Esteban JM, Yokota S, Husain S, et al. Immunocytochemical profile of benign and carcinomatous effusions – a practical approach to difficult diagnosis. Am J Clin Pathol 1990;94:698–705.

241. Singer S, Boddington MM, Hudson EA. Immunocytochemical reaction of Ca1 and HMFG2 monoclonal antibodies with cells from serous effusions. J Clin Pathol 1985;38:180–4.

242. de Angelis M, Buley ID, Heryet A, et al. Immunocytochemical staining of serous effusions with the monoclonal antibody Ber-EP4. Cytopathol 1992;3:111–7.

243. Yamashita K, Kuba T, Shinoda H, et al. Detection of K-ras point mutations in the supernatants of peritoneal and pleural

effusions for diagnosis complementary to cytologic examination. Am J Clin Pathol 1998;109:704–11.

244. Chen LM, Lazcano O, Katzmann JA, et al. The role of conventional cytology, immunocytochemistry, and flow cytometric DNA ploidy in the evaluation of body cavity fluids: A prospective study of 52 patients. Am J Clin Pathol 1998;109:712–21.

245. Tao L. The cytopathology of mesothelioma. Acta Cytol 1979;23:209–13.

246. Whitaker D, Shilkin KB. Diagnosis of pleural malignant mesothelioma in life – a practical approach. J Pathol 1984;143:147–75.

247. Sears D, Hajdu SI. The cytologic diagnosis of malignant neoplasms in pleural and peritoneal effusions. Acta Cytol 1987;31:85–97.

248. Roboz J, Greaves J, Silides D, et al. Hyaluronic acid content of effusions as a diagnostic aid for malignant mesothelioma. Cancer Res 1985;45:1850–4.

249. Welker L, Muller M, Holz O, et al. Cytological diagnosis of malignant mesothelioma – improvement by additional analysis of hyaluronic acid in pleural effusions. Virchows Arch 2007;450:455–61.

250. Faravelli B, D'Amore E, Nosenzo M, et al. Carcinoembryonic antigen in pleural effusions. Cancer 1984;53:1194–7.

251. Faravelli B, Nosenzo M, Razzetti A, et al. The role of concurrent determinations of pleural fluid and tissue carcinoembryonic antigen in the distinction of malignant mesothelioma from metastatic pleural malignancies. Eur J Cancer Clin Oncol 1985;21:1083–7.

252. Mezger J, Permanetter W, Gerbes AL, et al. Tumour associated antigens in diagnosis of serous effusions. J Clin Pathol 1988;41:633–43.

253. Creaney J, Yeoman D, Naumoff LK, et al. Soluble mesothelin in effusions: a useful tool for the diagnosis of malignant mesothelioma. Thorax 2007;62:569–76.

254. Davies HE, Sadler RS, Bielsa S, et al. Clinical impact and reliability of pleural fluid mesothelin in undiagnosed pleural effusions. Am J Respir Crit Care Med 2009;180:437–44.

255. Crotty TB, Myers JL, Katzenstein ALA, et al. Localized malignant mesothelioma – a clinicopathologic and flow cytometric study. Am J Surg Pathol 1994;18:357–63.

256. Okamura H, Kamei T, Mitsuno A, et al. Localized malignant mesothelioma of the pleura. Pathol Int 2001;51:654–60.

257. Erkilic S, Sari I, Tuncozgur B. Localized pleural malignant mesothelioma. Pathol Int 2001;51:812–5.

258. Hirano H, Takeda S, Sawabata Y, et al. Localized pleural malignant mesothelioma. Pathol Int 2003;53:616–21.

259. Asioli S, Dal Piaz G, Damiani S. Localised pleural malignant mesothelioma. Report of two cases simulating pulmonary carcinoma and review of the literature. Virchows Arch 2004;445:206–9.

260. Allen TC, Cagle PT, Churg AM, et al. Localized malignant mesothelioma. Am J Surg Pathol 2005;29:866–73.

261. Denton KJ, Cotton DWK, Nakielny RA, et al. Secondary tumour deposits in needle biopsy tracks: an underestimated risk? J Clin Pathol 1990;43:83.

262. Attanoos RL, Gibbs AR. The comparative accuracy of different pleural biopsy techniques in the diagnosis of malignant mesothelioma. Histopathology 2008;53:340–4.

263. Herbert A, Gallagher PJ. Pleural biopsy in the diagnosis of malignant mesothelioma. Thorax 1982;37:816–21.

264. Donna A, Betta PG. Mesodermomas: a new embryological approach to primary tumours of coelomic surfaces. Histopathology 1981;5:31–44.

265. Donna A, Betta PG. Differentiation towards cartilage and bone in a primary tumour of pleura. Further evidence in support of the concept of mesodermoma. Histopathology 1986;10:101–8.

266. Donna A, Betta PG, Bianchi V, et al. A new insight into the histogenesis of mesodermomas – malignant mesotheliomas. Histopathology 1991;19:239–43.

267. Attanoos RL, Gibbs AR. Pathology of malignant mesothelioma. Histopathology 1997;30:403–18.

268. Suzuki Y. Pathology of human malignant mesothelioma. Semin Oncol 1981;8:268–81.

269. Law MR, Hodson ME, Heard BE. Malignant mesothelioma of the pleura: relation between histological type and clinical behaviour. Thorax 1982;37:810–5.

270. Vangelder T, Hoogsteden HC, Vandenbroucke JP, et al. The influence of the diagnostic technique on the histopathological diagnosis in malignant mesothelioma. Virchows Arch A Pathol Anat Histopathol 1991;418:315–7.

271. Arrossi AV, Lin E, Rice D, et al. Histologic assessment and prognostic factors of malignant pleural mesothelioma treated with extrapleural pneumonectomy. Am J Clin Pathol 2008;130:754–64.

272. Klima M, Gyorkey F. Benign pleural lesions and malignant mesothelioma. Virchows Arch A Pathol Anat Histopathol 1977;376:181–93.

273. Cook DS, Attanoos RL, Jalloh SS, et al. 'Mucin-positive' epithelial mesothelioma of the peritoneum: an unusual diagnostic pitfall. Histopathology 2000;37:33–6.

274. Mayall FG, Gibbs AR. The histology and immunohistochemistry of small cell mesothelioma. Histopathology 1992;20:47–51.

275. Battifora H, McCaughey WTE. Tumors of the serosal membranes. 3rd ed. Washington: Armed Forces Institute of Pathology; 1995.

276. Okamoto H, Matsuno Y, Noguchi M, et al. Malignant pleural mesothelioma producing human chorionic gonadotropin – report of two cases. Am J Surg Pathol 1992;16:969–74.

277. Burdick CO. HCG positive mesothelioma. Am J Surg Pathol 1993;17:749–50.

278. Nascimento AG, Keeney GL, Fletcher CDM. Deciduoid peritoneal mesothelioma – an unusual phenotype affecting young females. Am J Surg Pathol 1994;18:439–45.

279. Shanks JH, Harris M, Banerjee SS, et al. Mesotheliomas with deciduoid morphology – A morphologic spectrum and a variant not confined to young females. Am J Surg Pathol 2000;24:285–94.

280. Serio G, Scattone A, Pennella A, et al. Malignant deciduoid mesothelioma of the pleura: report of two cases with long survival. Histopathology 2002;40:348–52.

281. Shia J, Erlandson RA, Klimstra DS. Deciduoid mesothelioma: A report of 5 cases and literature review. Ultrastruct Pathol 2002;26:355–63.

282. Mourra N, de Chaisemartin C, Goubin-Versini I, et al. Malignant deciduoid mesothelioma: a diagnostic challenge. Arch Pathol Lab Med 2005;129:403–6.

283. Puttagunta L, Vriend RA, Nguyen GK. Deciduoid epithelial mesothelioma of the pleura with focal rhabdoid change. Am J Surg Pathol 2000;24:1440–3.

284. Ordonez NG. Mesothelioma with rhabdoid features: an ultrastructural and immunohistochemical study of 10 cases. Mod Pathol 2006;19:373–83.

285. Ordonez NG, Myhre M, Mackay B. Clear cell mesothelioma. Ultrastruct Pathol 1996;20:331–6.

286. Dessy E, Falleni M, Braidotti P, et al. Unusual clear cell variant of epithelioid mesothelioma. Arch Pathol Lab Med 2001;125:1588–90.

287. Ordonez NG. Mesothelioma with clear cell features: an ultrastructural and immunohistochemical study of 20 cases. Human Pathology 2005;36:465–73.

288. Hurlimann J. Desmin and neural marker expression in mesothelial cells and mesotheliomas. Hum Pathol 1994;25:753–7.

289. Henderson DW, Attwood HD, Constance TJ, et al. Lymphohistiocytoid mesothelioma: a rare lymphomatoid variant of predominantly sarcomatoid mesothelioma. Ultrastruct Pathol 1988;12:367–84.

290. Khalidi HS, Medeiros LJ, Battifora H. Lymphohistiocytoid mesothelioma – an often misdiagnosed variant of sarcomatoid

malignant mesothelioma. Amer J Clin Pathol 2000;113:649–54.

291. Galateau-Salle F, Attanoos R, Gibbs AR, et al. Lymphohistiocytoid variant of malignant mesothelioma of the pleura: a series of 22 cases. Am J Surg Pathol 2007;31:711–6.

291a. Klebe S, Brownlee NA, Mahar A, et al. Sarcomatoid mesothelioma: a clinical-pathologic correlation of 326 cases. Mod Pathol 2010;23:470–9.

292. Yousem S, Hochholzer L. Malignant mesotheliomas with osseous and cartilagenous differentiation. Arch Pathol Lab Med 1987;111:62–6.

293. Mayall FG, Goddard H, Gibbs AR. Intermediate filament expression in mesotheliomas – leiomyoid mesotheliomas are not uncommon. Histopathology 1992;21:453–7.

294. Krishna J, Haqqani MT. Liposarcomatous differentiation in diffuse pleural mesothelioma. Thorax 1993;48: 409–10.

295. Chang HT, Yantiss RK, Nielsen GP, et al. Lipid-rich diffuse malignant mesothelioma: A case report. Hum Pathol 2000;31:876–9.

296. Klebe S, Mahar A, Henderson DW, et al. Malignant mesothelioma with heterologous elements: clinicopathological correlation of 27 cases and literature review. Mod Pathol 2008;21:1084–94.

297. Ruangchira-urai R, Mark E. Lymphangiomatoid pattern in diffuse malignant mesothelioma of the pleura: a report of six cases. Virchows Archiv 2009;455:143–8.

298. Harwood TR, Gracey DR, Yokoo H. Pseudomesotheliomatous carcinoma of the lung – a variant of peripheral lung cancer. Am J Clin Pathol 1976;65: 159–67.

299. Dessy E, Pietra GG. Pseudomesotheliomatous carcinoma of the lung – an immunohistochemical and ultrastructural study of three cases. Cancer 1991;68:1747–53.

300. Koss M, Travis W, Moran C, et al. Pseudomesotheliomatous adenocarcinoma: a reappraisal. Semin Diagn Pathol 1992;9:117–23.

301. Taylor DR, Page W, Hughes D, et al. Metastatic renal cell carcinoma mimicking pleural mesothelioma. Thorax 1987;42:901–2.

302. Attanoos RL, Suvarna SK, Rhead E, et al. Malignant vascular tumours of the pleura in "asbestos" workers and endothelial differentiation in malignant mesothelioma. Thorax 2000;55:860–3.

303. Zimmerman KG, Sobonya RE, Payne CM. Histochemical and ultrastructural features of an unusual pulmonary carcinosarcoma. Hum Pathol 1981;12:1046–51.

304. Mayall FG, Gibbs AR. Pleural and pulmonary carcinosarcomas. J Pathol 1992;167:305–11.

305. Gaertner E, Zeren EH, Fleming MV, et al. Biphasic synovial sarcomas arising in the pleural cavity: a clinicopathologic study of five cases. Am J Surg Pathol 1996;20:36–45.

306. Jawahar DA, Vuletin JC, Gorecki P, et al. Primary biphasic synovial sarcoma of the pleura. Resp Med 1997;91:568–70.

307. Kashima T, Matsushita H, Kuroda M, et al. Biphasic synovial sarcoma of the peritoneal cavity with t(X;18) demonstrated by reverse transcriptase polymerase chain reaction. Pathol Int 1997;47:637–41.

308. Attanoos RL, Griffin A, Gibbs AR, et al. The use of immunohistochemistry in distinguishing reactive from neoplastic mesothelium. A novel use for desmin and comparative evaluation with epithelial membrane antigen, p53, platelet-derived growth factor-receptor, P-glycoprotein and Bcl-2. Histopathology 2003;43:231–8.

309. Macdougall DB, Wang SE, Zidar BL. Mucin-positive epithelial mesothelioma. Arch Pathol Lab Med 1992;116:874–80.

310. Hammar SP, Bockus DE, Remington FL, et al. Mucin-positive epithelial mesotheliomas: a histochemical, immunohistochemical, and ultrastructural comparison with mucin-producing pulmonary adenocarcinomas. Ultrastruct Pathol 1996;20:293–325.

311. Adams SA, Sherwood AJ, Smith MEF. Malignant mesothelioma: PAS-diastase positivity and inversion of polarity in intravascular tumour. Histopathology 2002;41:260–2.

312. Ordonez NG, Mackay B. Glycogen-rich mesothelioma. Ultrastruct Pathol 1999;23:401–6.

313. Wagner JC, Munday DE, Harington JS. Histochemical demonstration of hyaluronic acid in pleural mesothelioma. J Pathol Bacteriol 1962;84:73–8.

314. Robb JA. Mesothelioma versus adenocarcinoma: false-positive CEA and Leu-M1 staining due to hyaluronic acid. Hum Pathol 1989;20:400.

315. Noguchi M, Nakajima T, Hirohashi S, et al. Immunohistochemical distinction of malignant mesothelioma from pulmonary adenocarcinoma with anti-surfactant apoprotein, anti-Lewis[a], and anti-Tn antibodies. Hum Pathol 1989;20: 53–7.

316. Khoor A, Whitsett JA, Stahlman MT, et al. Utility of surfactant protein B precursor and thyroid transcription factor 1 in differentiating adenocarcinoma of the lung from malignant mesothelioma. Hum Pathol 1999;30:695–700.

317. King JE, Thatcher N, Pickering CA, et al. Sensitivity and specificity of immunohistochemical markers used in the diagnosis of epithelioid mesothelioma: a detailed systematic analysis using published data. Histopathology 2006;48:223–32.

318. Chu AY, Litzky LA, Pasha TL, et al. Utility of D2-40, a novel mesothelial marker, in the diagnosis of malignant mesothelioma. Mod Pathol 2004;18:105–10.

318a. Ordonez NG. What are the current best immunohistochemical markers for the diagnosis of epithelial mesothelioma? A review and update. Hum Pathol 2007;38:1–16.

319. Comin CE, Dini S, Novelli L, et al. h-Caldesmon, a useful positive marker in the diagnosis of pleural malignant mesothelioma, epithelioid type. Am J Surg Pathol 2006;30:463–9.

320. Amatya VJ, Takeshima Y, Kohno H, et al. Caveolin-1 is a novel immunohistochemical marker to differentiate epithelioid mesothelioma from lung adenocarcinoma. Histopathology 2009;55:10–9.

321. Padgett DM, Cathro HP, Wick MR, et al. Podoplanin is a better immunohistochemical marker for sarcomatoid mesothelioma than calretinin. Am J Surg Pathol 2008;32:123–7.

322. Marchevsky AM. Application of immunohistochemistry to the diagnosis of malignant mesothelioma. Arch Pathol Lab Med 2008;132:397–401.

323. Miettinen M, SarlomoRikala M. Expression of calretinin, thrombomodulin, keratin 5, and mesothelin in lung carcinomas of different types – An immunohistochemical analysis of 596 tumors in comparison with epithelioid mesotheliomas of the pleura. Amer J Surg Pathol 2003;27:150–8.

324. Attanoos RL, Gibbs AR. 'Pseudomesotheliomatous' carcinomas of the pleura: a 10-year analysis of cases from the Environmental Lung Disease Research Group, Cardiff. Histopathology 2003;43:444–52.

325. Osborn M, Pelling N, Walker MM, et al. The value of 'mesothelium-associated' antibodies in distinguishing between metastatic renal cell carcinomas and mesotheliomas. Histopathology 2002;41:301–7.

326. Ordonez NG. The diagnostic utility of immunohistochemistry in distinguishing between mesothelioma and renal cell carcinoma: a comparative study. Hum Pathol 2004;35:697–710.

327. Attanoos RL, Webb R, Dojcinov SD, et al. Value of mesothelial and epithelial antibodies in distinguishing diffuse peritoneal mesothelioma in females from serous papillary carcinoma of the ovary and peritoneum. Histopathology 2002;40:237–44.

328. Ordonez NG. Value of estrogen and progesterone receptor immunostaining in distinguishing between peritoneal mesotheliomas and serous carcinomas. Human Pathology 2005;36:1163–7.

329. Comin CE, Saieva C, Messerini L. h-caldesmon, calretinin, estrogen receptor, and Ber-EP4: a useful combination of immunohistochemical markers for

with malignant pleural mesothelioma – a basis for checklists. Arch Pathol Lab Med 1999;123:39–44.

417. International Union Against Cancer (UICC). TNM Classification of Malignant Tumours. 7th ed. New York: Wiley-Liss; 2009.

418. Ramael M, Jacobs W, Weyler J, et al. Proliferation in malignant mesothelioma as determined by mitosis counts and immunoreactivity for proliferating cell nuclear antigen (PCNA). J Pathol 1994;172:247–53.

419. Upham JW, Garlepp MJ, Musk AW, et al. Malignant mesothelioma: new insights into tumour biology and immunology as a basis for new treatment approaches. Thorax 1995;50:887–93.

420. Gordon GJ, Jensen RV, Hsiao LL, et al. Using gene expression ratios to predict outcome among patients with mesothelioma. J Natl Cancer Inst 2003;95:598–605.

421. Cappia S, Righi L, Mirabelli D, et al. Prognostic role of osteopontin expression in malignant pleural mesothelioma. Am J Clin Pathol 2008;130:58–64.

422. Schramm A, Opitz I, Thies S, et al. Prognostic significance of epithelial-mesenchymal transition in malignant pleural mesothelioma. Eur J Cardiothorac Surg 2010; 37: 566–72.

423. Dobra K, Hjerpe A. Targeted therapy – possible new therapeutic option for malignant mesothelioma? Connect Tissue Res 2008;49:270–2.

424. Okuda K, Sasaki H, Kawano O, et al. Epidermal growth factor receptor gene mutation, amplification and protein expression in malignant pleural mesothelioma. J Cancer Res Clin Oncol 2008;134:1105–11.

425. Yokoyama T, Osada H, Murakami H, et al. YAP1 is involved in mesothelioma development and negatively regulated by Merlin through phosphorylation. Carcinogenesis 2008;29:2139–46.

426. Creaney J, Segal A, Sterrett G, et al. Overexpression and altered glycosylation of MUC1 in malignant mesothelioma. Br J Cancer 2008;98:1562–9.

427. Lazzarini R, Moretti S, Orecchia S, et al. Enhanced antitumor therapy by inhibition of p21waf1 in human malignant mesothelioma. Clin Cancer Res 2008;14:5099–107.

428. Catassi A, Paleari L, Servent D, et al. Targeting alpha7-nicotinic receptor for the treatment of pleural mesothelioma. Eur J Cancer 2008;44:2296–311.

429. Cipriani NA, Abidoye OO, Vokes E, et al. MET as a target for treatment of chest tumors. Lung Cancer 2009;63:169–79.

430. Butnor KJ, Sporn TA, Hammar SP, et al. Well-differentiated papillary mesothelioma. Amer J Surg Pathol 2001;25:1304–9.

431. GalateauSalle F, Vignaud JM, Burke L, et al. Well-differentiated papillary mesothelioma of the pleura – A series of 24 cases. Am J Surg Pathol 2004;28:534–40.

432. Derosa G, Donofrio V, Boscaino A, et al. Multicystic mesothelial proliferation – immunohistochemical, ultrastructural and DNA analysis of 5 cases. Virchows Arch A Pathol Anat Histopathol 1992;421:379–85.

433. Sawh RN, Malpica A, Deavers MT, et al. Benign cystic mesothelioma of the peritoneum: A clinicopathologic study of 17 cases and immunohistochemical analysis of estrogen and progesterone receptor status. Hum Pathol 2003;34:369–74.

434. Ball NJ, Urbanski SJ, Green FHY, et al. Pleural multicystic mesothelial proliferation. The so-called multicystic mesothelioma. Am J Surg Pathol 1990;14:375–8.

435. Kaplan MA, Tazelaar HD, Hayashi T, et al. Adenomatoid tumors of the pleura. Am J Surg Pathol 1996;20:1219–23.

436. Minato H, Nojima T, Kurose N, et al. Adenomatoid tumor of the pleura. Pathol Int 2009;59:567–71.

437. Stout AP, Murray MR. Localized pleural mesothelioma. Arch Pathol 1942;34:951–64.

438. Alvarez-Fernandez E, Diez-Nau MD. Malignant fibrosarcomatous mesothelioma and benign pleural fibroma (localized fibrous mesothelioma) in tissue culture. Cancer 1979;43:1658–63.

439. Dardick I, Srigley JR, McCaughey WTE, et al. Ultrastructural aspects of the histogenesis of diffuse and localized mesothelioma. Virchows Arch A Pathol Anat Histopathol 1984;402:373–88.

440. Doucet J, Dardick I, Srigley JR, et al. Localized fibrous tumour of serosal surfaces. Immunohistochemical and ultrastructural evidence for a type of mesothelioma. Virchows Arch A Pathol Anat Histopathol 1986;409:349–63.

441. Said JW, Nash G, Banks-Schlegal S, et al. Localized fibrous mesothelioma: an immunohistochemical and electron microscopic study. Hum Pathol 1984;15:440–3.

442. Kawai T, Suzuki M. Nonmalignant tumors of the pleura. In: Chretien J, Bignon J, Hirsch A, editors. The Pleura in Health and Disease. Vol 30 of Lung Biology in Health and Disease. New York: Marcel Dekkar; 1985.

443. England DM, Hochholzer L, McCarthy MJ. Localized benign and malignant fibrous tumors of the pleura. A clinicopathologic review of 223 cases. Am J Surg Pathol 1989;13:640–58.

444. Goodlad JR, Fletcher CDM. Solitary fibrous tumour arising at unusual sites – analysis of a series. Histopathology 1991;19:515–22.

445. Carter D, Otis CN. Three types of spindle cell tumors of the pleura. Fibroma, sarcoma, and sarcomatoid mesothelioma. Am J Surg Pathol 1988;12:747–53.

446. Steinetz C, Clarke R, Jacobs GH, et al. Localized fibrous tumors of the pleura. Correlation of histopathological, immunohistochemical and ultrastructural features. Pathol Res Pract 1990;186:344–57.

447. Briselli M, Mark EJ, Dickersin GR. Solitary fibrous tumors of the pleura: eight new cases and review of 360 cases in the literature. Cancer 1981;47:2678–89.

448. El-Naggar AK, Ro JY, Ayala AG, et al. Localized fibrous tumor of the serosal cavities. Immunohistochemical, electron-microscopic, and flow-cytometric DNA study. Am J Clin Pathol 1989;92:561–5.

449. Osamura RY. Ultrastructure of localized fibrous mesothelioma of the pleura. Cancer 1977;39:139–42.

450. Burrig K-F, Kastendieck H. Ultrastructural observations on the histogenesis of localized fibrous tumours of the pleura (benign mesothelioma). Virchows Arch A Pathol Anat Histopathol 1984;403: 413–24.

451. Keating S, Simon GT, Alexopoulou I, et al. Solitary fibrous tumour of the pleura: an ultrastructural and immunohistochemical study. Thorax 1987;42:976–9.

452. Masson EA, Macfarlane IA, Graham D, et al. Spontaneous hypoglycaemia due to a pleural fibroma – role of insulin like growth factors. Thorax 1991;46:930–1.

453. Moat NE, Teale JD, Lea RE, et al. Spontaneous hypoglycaemia and pleural fibroma – role of insulin like growth factors. Thorax 1991;46:932–3.

454. Sakamoto T, Kaneshige H, Takeshi A, et al. Localized pleural mesothelioma with elevation of high molecular weight insulin-like growth factor II and hypoglycemia. Chest 1994;106:965–7.

455. Fukasawa Y, Takada A, Tateno M, et al. Solitary fibrous tumor of the pleura causing recurrent hypoglycemia by secretion of insulin-like growth factor II. Pathol Int 1998;48:47–52.

456. Ulrik CS, Viskum K. Fibrous pleural tumour producing 171 litres of transudate. Eur Resp J 1998;12:1230–2.

457. Li Y, Chang Q, Rubin BP, et al. Insulin receptor activation in solitary fibrous tumours. J Pathol 2007;211:550–4.

458. Schirosi L, Lantuejoul S, Cavazza A, et al. Pleuro-pulmonary solitary fibrous tumors: a clinicopathologic, immunohistochemical, and molecular study of 88 cases confirming the prognostic value of de Perrot staging system and p53 expression, and evaluating the role of c-kit, BRAF, PDGFRs (alpha/beta), c-met, and EGFR. Am J Surg Pathol 2008;32:1627–42.

459. Abrahamson JR, Friedman NB. Intrapulmonary stromal mesothelioma. J Thorac Cardiovasc Surg 1966;51:300–6.

460. Alvarez-Fernandez E, Escalona-Zapata J. Intrapulmonary mesotheliomas: their identification by tissue culture. Virchows Arch A Pathol Anat Histopathol 1982;395:331–43.

461. Yousem SA, Flynn SD. Intrapulmonary localized fibrous tumor. Intraparenchymal so-called localized fibrous mesothelioma. Am J Clin Pathol 1988;89:365–9.

462. Weidner N. Intriguing case – solitary fibrous tumor of the mediastinum. Ultrastruct Pathol 1991;15:489–92.

463. Witkin GB, Rosai J. Solitary fibrous tumor of the upper respiratory tract – a report of six cases. Am J Surg Pathol 1991;15:842–8.

464. Kottke-Marchant K, Hart WR, Broughan T. Localized fibrous tumor (localized fibrous mesothelioma) of the liver. Cancer 1989;64:1096–102.

465. Ibrahim NBN, Briggs JC, Corrin B. Double primary localized fibrous tumours of the pleura and retroperitoneum. Histopathology 1993;22:282–4.

466. Dorfman DM, To K, Dickersin GR, et al. Solitary fibrous tumor of the orbit. Am J Surg Pathol 1994;18:281–7.

467. Cameselleteijeiro J, Vareladuran J, Fonseca E, et al. Solitary fibrous tumor of the thyroid. Am J Clin Pathol 1994;101:535–8.

468. Hanau CA, Miettinen M. Solitary fibrous tumor: histological and immunohistochemical spectrum of benign and malignant variants presenting at different sites. Hum Pathol 1995;26:440–9.

469. O'Connell JX, Logan PM, Beauchamp CP. Solitary fibrous tumor of the periosteum. Hum Pathol 1995;26:460–2.

470. Suster S, Nascimento AG, Miettinen M, et al. Solitary fibrous tumors of soft tissue: a clinicopathologic and immunohistochemical study of 12 cases. Am J Surg Pathol 1995;19:1257–66.

471. Fukunaga M, Ushigome S, Nomura K, et al. Solitary fibrous tumor of the nasal cavity and orbit. Pathol Int 1995;45:952–7.

472. Sciot R, Goffin J, Fossion E, et al. Solitary fibrous tumour of the orbit. Histopathology 1996;28:188–91.

473. Ferreiro JA, Nascimento AG. Solitary fibrous tumour of the major salivary glands. Histopathology 1996;28:261–4.

474. Barnoud R, Arvieux C, Pasquier D, et al. Solitary fibrous tumour of the liver with CD34 expression. Histopathology 1996;28:551–4.

475. Carneiro SS, Scheithauer BW, Nascimento AG, et al. Solitary fibrous tumor of the meninges: a lesion distinct from fibrous meningioma: a clinicopathologic and immunohistochemical study. Am J Clin Pathol 1996;106:217–24.

476. Mentzel T, Bainbridge TC, Katenkamp D. Solitary fibrous tumour: Clinicopathological, immunohistochemical, and ultrastructural analysis of 12 cases arising in soft tissues, nasal cavity and nasopharynx, urinary bladder and prostate. Virchows Archiv 1997;430:445–53.

477. Nielsen GP, OConnell JX, Dickersin GR, et al. Solitary fibrous tumor of soft tissue: a report of 15 cases, including 5 malignant examples with light microscopic, immunohistochemical, and ultrastructural data. Modern Pathol 1997;10:1028–37.

478. Takeshima Y, Yoneda K, Sanda N, et al. Solitary fibrous tumor of the prostate. Pathol Int 1997;47:713–7.

479. Chan JKC. Solitary fibrous tumour – everywhere, and a diagnosis in vogue. Histopathology 1997;31:568–76.

480. Brunnemann RB, Ro JY, Ordonez NG, et al. Extrapleural solitary fibrous tumor: a clinicopathologic study of 24 cases. Modern Pathol 1999;12:1034–42.

481. Hasegawa T, Matsuno Y, Shimoda T, et al. Extrathoracic solitary fibrous tumors: Their histological variability and potentially aggressive behavior. Hum Pathol 1999;30:1464–73.

482. Alawi F, Stratton D, Freedman PD. Solitary fibrous tumor of the oral soft tissues – a clinicopathologic and immunohistochemical study of 16 cases. Amer J Surg Pathol 2001;25:900–10.

483. Tan-Liu NS, Matsubara O, Grillo HC, et al. Invasive fibrous tumor of the tracheobronchial tree: clinical and pathologic study of seven cases. Hum Pathol 1989;20:180–4.

484. Somerhausen NDA, Rubin BP, Fletcher CDM. Myxoid solitary fibrous tumor: a study of seven cases with emphasis on differential diagnosis. Modern Pathol 1999;12:463–71.

485. Lau S, Weiss L, Chu P. Myxoid solitary fibrous tumor: a clinicopathologic study of three cases. Virchows Archiv 2009;454:189–94.

486. Bai HW, Aswad BI, Gaissert H, et al. Malignant solitary fibrous tumor of the pleura with liposarcomatous differentiation. Arch Pathol Lab Med 2001;125:406–9.

487. Awasthi R, O'Neill J, Keen C, et al. Biphasic solitary fibrous tumour: a report of two cases with epithelioid features. Virchows Archiv 2006;448:306–10.

488. van de Rijn M, Lombard CM, Rouse RV. Expression of CD34 by solitary fibrous tumors of the pleura, mediastinum, and lung. Am J Surg Pathol 1994;18:814–20.

489. Flint A, Weiss SW. CD-34 and keratin expression distinguishes solitary fibrous tumor (fibrous mesothelioma) of pleura from desmoplastic mesothelioma. Hum Pathol 1995;26:428–31.

490. Yokoi T, Tsuzuki T, Yatabe Y, et al. Solitary fibrous tumour: significance of p53 and CD34 immunoreactivity in its malignant transformation. Histopathology 1998;32:423–32.

491. Ledet SC, Brown RW, Cagle PT. p53 immunostaining in the differentiation of inflammatory pseudotumor from sarcoma involving the lung. Mod Pathol 1995;8:282–6.

492. Shidham VB, Chivukula M, Gupta D, et al. Immunohistochemical comparison of gastrointestinal stromal tumor and solitary fibrous tumor. Arch Pathol Lab Med 2002;126:1189–92.

493. Langman G, Rathinam S, Papadaki L. Primary localised pleural neurofibroma: expanding the spectrum of spindle cell tumours of the pleura. J Clin Pathol 2010;63:116–8.

494. Dalton WT, Zolliker AS, McCaughey WTE, et al. Localised primary tumours of the pleura. Cancer 1979;44:1465–75.

495. Kanthan R, Torkian B. Recurrent solitary fibrous tumor of the pleura with malignant transformation. Arch Pathol Lab Med 2004;128:460.

496. Bini A, Grazia M, Stella F, et al. Giant malignant fibrous histiocytoma of the pleura arising from solitary fibrous tumour. Thorax 2004;59:544.

497. Zhang HQ, Lucas DR, Pass HI, et al. Disseminated malignant solitary fibrous tumor of the pleura. Pathol Int 2004;54:111–15.

498. de Perrot M, Fischer S, Brindler MA, et al. Solitary fibrous tumors of the pleura. The Annals of Thoracic Surgery 2002;74:285–93.

499. Scharifker D, Kaneko M. Localised fibrous 'mesothelioma' of pleura (submesothelial fibroma). A clinicopathologic study of 18 cases. Cancer 1979;43:627–35.

500. Kaplan J, Davidson T. Intrathoracic desmoids: report of two cases. Thorax 1986;41:894–5.

501. Wilson RW, GallateauSalle F, Moran CA. Desmoid tumors of the pleura: A clinicopathologic mimic of localized fibrous tumor. Modern Pathol 1999;12:9–14.

502. Andino L, Cagle PT, Murer B, et al. Pleuropulmonary desmoid tumors: immunohistochemical comparison with solitary fibrous tumors and assessment of beta-catenin and cyclin D1 expression. Arch Pathol Lab Med 2006;130:1503–9.

503. Carlson JW, Fletcher CD. Immunohistochemistry for beta-catenin in the differential diagnosis of spindle cell lesions: analysis of a series and review of the literature. Histopathology 2007;51:509–14.

504. Pinkard NB, Wilson RW, Lawless N, et al. Calcifying fibrous pseudotumor of pleura: a report of three cases of a newly described entity involving the pleura. Am J Clin Pathol 1996;105:189–94.

505. Kocova L, Michal M, Sulc M, et al. Calcifying fibrous pseudotumour of visceral peritoneum. Histopathology 1997;31:182–4.

506. Dumont P, de Muret A, Skrobala D, et al. Calcifying fibrous pseudotumor of the

749

507. Mito K, Kashima K, Daa T, et al. Multiple calcifying fibrous tumors of the pleura. Virchows Arch 2005;446:78–81.

508. Van Dorpe J, Ectors N, Geboes K, et al. Is calcifying fibrous pseudotumor a late sclerosing stage of inflammatory myofibroblastic tumor? Amer J Surg Pathol 1999;23:329–35.

509. Weynand B, Draguet AP, Bernard P, et al. Calcifying fibrous pseudotumour: first case report in the peritoneum with immunostaining for CD34. Histopathology 1999;34:86–7.

510. Pomplun S, Goldstraw P, Davies SE, et al. Calcifying fibrous pseudotumour arising within an inflammatory pseudotumour: evidence of progression from one lesion to the other? Histopathology 2000;37:380–2.

511. Hill KA, GonzalezCrussi F, Chou PM. Calcifying fibrous pseudotumor versus inflammatory myofibroblastic tumor: a histological and immunohistochemical comparison. Modern Pathol 2001;14:784–90.

512. Gerald WL, Miller HK, Battifora H, et al. Intra-abdominal desmoplastic small round-cell tumor. Report of 19 cases of a distinctive type of high-grade polyphenotypic malignancy affecting young individuals. Am J Surg Pathol 1991;15:499–513.

513. Ordonez NG. Desmoplastic small round cell tumor I: A histopathologic study of 39 cases with emphasis on unusual histological patterns. Am J Surg Pathol 1998;22:1303–13.

514. Ordonez NG. Desmoplastic small round cell tumor II: An ultrastructural and immunohistochemical study with emphasis on new immunohistochemical markers. Am J Surg Pathol 1998;22:1314–27.

515. Bian YL, Jordan AG, Rupp M, et al. Effusion cytology of desmoplastic small round cell tumor of the pleura – a case report. Acta Cytol 1993;37:77–82.

516. Parkash V, Gerald WL, Parma A, et al. Desmoplastic small round cell tumor of the pleura. Am J Surg Pathol 1995;19:659–65.

517. Syed S, Haque AK, Hawkins HK, et al. Desmoplastic small round cell tumor of the lung. Arch Pathol Lab Med 2002;126:1226–8.

518. Chang F. Desmoplastic small round cell tumors: cytologic, histologic, and immunohistochemical features. Arch Pathol Lab Med 2006;130:728–32.

519. Pasquinelli G, Montanaro L, Martinelli GN. Desmoplastic small round-cell tumor: A case report on the large cell variant with immunohistochemical, ultrastructural, and molecular genetic analysis. Ultrastruct Pathol 2000;24:333–7.

520. Sebire NJ, Gibson S, Rampling D, et al. Immunohistochemical findings in embryonal small round cell tumors with molecular diagnostic confirmation. Appl Immunohistochem Mol Morphol 2005;13:1–5.

521. Hill DA, Pfeifer JD, Marley EF, et al. WT1 staining reliably differentiates desmoplastic small round cell tumor from Ewing sarcoma/primitive neuroectodermal tumor – An immunohistochemical and molecular diagnostic study. Amer J Clin Pathol 2000;114:345–53.

522. Barnoud R, Delattre O, Peoch M, et al. Desmoplastic small round cell tumor: RT-PCR analysis and immunohistochemical detection of the Wilms tumor gene WT1. Pathol Res Pract 1998;194:693–700.

523. Zhang PJ, Goldblum JR, Pawel BR, et al. Immunophenotype of desmoplastic small round cell tumors as detected in cases with EWS-WT1 gene fusion product. Modern Pathol 2003;16:229–35.

524. Mitchell A, Meunier C, Ouellette D, et al. Extranodal marginal zone lymphoma of mucosa-associated lymphoid tissue with initial presentation in the pleura. Chest 2006;129:791–4.

525. Taniere P, Manai A, Charpentier R, et al. Pyothorax-associated –lymphoma: relationship with Epstein–Barr virus, human herpes virus-8 and body cavity-based high grade lymphomas. Eur Resp J 1998;11:779–83.

526. Steiropoulos P, Kouliatsis G, Karpathiou G, et al. Rare cases of primary pleural Hodgkin and non-Hodgkin lymphomas. Respiration 2009;77:459–63.

527. Green I, Espiritu E, Ladanyi M, et al. Primary lymphomatous effusions in AIDS: a morphological, immunophenotypic, and molecular study. Mod Pathol 1995;8:39–45.

528. Cesarman E, Chang YA, Moore PS, et al. Kaposi's sarcoma-associated herpesvirus-like DNA sequences in AIDS-related body-cavity-based lymphomas. N Engl J Med 1995;332:1186–91.

529. Ansari MQ, Dawson DB, Nador R, et al. Primary body cavity-based AIDS-related lymphomas. Am J Clin Pathol 1996;105:221–9.

530. Cesarman E, Nador RG, Aozasa K, et al. Kaposi's sarcoma-associated herpesvirus in non-AIDS-related lymphomas occuring in body cavities. Am J Pathol 1996;149:53–7.

531. Hsi ED, Foreman KE, Duggan J, et al. Molecular and pathologic characterization of an AIDS-related body cavity-based lymphoma, including ultrastructural demonstration of human herpesvirus-8: A case report. Am J Surg Pathol 1998;22:493–9.

532. Ascoli V, Scalzo CC, Danese C, et al. Human herpes virus-8 associated primary effusion lymphoma of the pleural cavity in HIV-negative elderly men. Eur Resp J 1999;14:1231–4.

533. Ascoli V, Sirianni MC, LoCoco F. Heterogeneity of Kaposi's sarcoma-associated herpesvirus (HHV-8)-positive effusions. Amer J Surg Pathol 2000;24:1036.

534. TeruyaFeldstein J, Zauber P, Setsuda JE, et al. Expression of human herpesvirus-8 oncogene and cytokine homologues in an HIV-seronegative patient with multicentric Castleman's disease and primary effusion lymphoma. Lab Invest 1998;78:1637–42.

535. Ascoli V, Signoretti S, OnettiMuda A, et al. Primary effusion lymphoma in HIV-infected patients with multicentric Castleman's disease. J Pathol 2001;193:200–9.

536. Ohsawa M, Tomita Y, Kanno H, et al. Role of Epstein–Barr virus in pleural lymphomagenesis. Mod Pathol 1995;8:848–53.

537. Boulanger E, Daniel MT, Agbalika F, et al. Combined chemotherapy including high-dose methotrexate in KSHV/HHV8-associated primary effusion lymphoma. Am J Hematol 2003;73:143–8.

538. Shuman LS, Libshutz HI. Solid pleural manifestations of lymphoma. AJR Am J Roentgenol 1984;142:269–73.

539. Iuchi K, Ichimiya A, Akashi A, et al. Non-Hodgkin's lymphoma of the pleural cavity developing from long-standing pyothorax. Cancer 1987;60:1771–5.

540. Martin A, Capron F, Liguory-Brunaud MD, et al. Epstein–Barr virus-associated primary malignant lymphomas of the pleural cavity occurring in longstanding pleural chronic inflammation. Hum Pathol 1994;25:1314–8.

541. Hsu NY, Chen CY, Pan ST, et al. Pleural non-Hodgkin's lymphoma arising in a patient with a chronic pyothorax. Thorax 1996;51:103–4.

542. Mori N, Yatabe Y, Narita M, et al. Pyothorax-associated lymphoma: an unusual case with biphenotypic character of T and B cells. Am J Surg Pathol 1996;20:760–6.

543. Ibuka T, Fukayama M, Hayashi Y, et al. Pyothorax-associated pleural lymphoma – a case evolving from T-cell-rich lymphoid infiltration to overt B-cell lymphoma in association with Epstein–Barr virus. Cancer 1994;73:738–44.

544. Nakamura S, Sasajima Y, Koshikawa T, et al. Ki-1 (CD30) positive anaplastic large cell lymphoma of T-cell phenotype developing in association with longstanding tuberculous pyothorax: report of a case with detection of Epstein–Barr virus genome in the tumor cells. Hum Pathol 1995;26:1382–5.

545. Molinie V, Pouchot J, Navratil E, et al. Primary Epstein–Barr virus-related non-Hodgkin's lymphoma of the pleural cavity following long-standing tuberculous empyema. Arch Pathol Lab Med 1996;120:288–91.

546. Petitjean B, Jardin F, Joly B, et al. Pyothorax-associated lymphoma – A peculiar clinicopathologic entity derived from B cells at late stage of differentiation

mediatinum. Ann Thorac Surg 1997;63:543–4.

and with occasional aberrant dual B- and T-cell phenotype. Amer J Surg Pathol 2002;26:724–32.

547. Androulaki A, Drakos E, Hatzianastassiou D, et al. Pyothorax-associated lymphoma (PAL): a western case with marked angiocentricity and review of the literature. Histo Pathol 2004;44:69–76.

548. Narimatsu H, Ota Y, Kami M, et al. Clinicopathological features of pyothorax-associated lymphoma; a retrospective survey involving 98 patients. Ann Oncol 2007;18:122–8.

549. Parisio E, Bianchi C, Rovej R, et al. Pulmonary asbestosis associated to pleural non-Hodgkin lymphoma. Tumori 1999;85:75–7.

550. Fukayama M, Ibuka T, Hayashi Y, et al. Epstein–Barr virus in pyothorax-associated pleural lymphoma. Am J Pathol 1993;143:1044–9.

551. Yamato H, Ohshima K, Suzumiya J, et al. Evidence for local immunosuppression and demonstration of c-myc amplification in pyothorax-associated lymphoma. Histopathology 2001;39:163–71.

552. Nakatsuka S, Yao M, Hoshida Y, et al. Pyothorax-associated lymphoma: a review of 106 cases. J Clin Oncol 2002;20:4255–60.

553. Nicholson AG, Goldstraw P, Fisher C. Synovial sarcoma of the pleura and its differentiation from other primary pleural tumours: a clinicopathological and immunohistochemical review of three cases. Histopathology 1998;33:508–13.

554. Ng SB, Ahmed Q, Tien SL, et al. Primary pleural synovial sarcoma – a case report and review of the literature. Arch Pathol Lab Med 2003;127:85–90.

555. Begueret H, Galateau-Salle F, Guillou L, et al. Primary intrathoracic synovial sarcoma: a clinicopathologic study of 40 t(X;18)-positive cases from the French Sarcoma Group and the Mesopath Group. Am J Surg Pathol 2005;29:339–46.

556. Nagao K, Ito H, Yoshida H. Chromosomal translocation t(X;18) in human synovial sarcomas analyzed by fluorescence in situ hybridization using paraffin-embedded tissue. Am J Pathol 1996;148:601–9.

557. Myoui A, Aozasa K, Iuchi K, et al. Soft tissue sarcoma of the pleural cavity. Cancer 1991;68:1550–4.

558. Falconieri G, Bussani R, Mirra M, et al. Pseudomesotheliomatous angiosarcoma: a pleuropulmonary lesion simulating malignant pleural mesothelioma. Histopathology 1997;30:419–24.

559. Zhang PJ, Livolsi VA, Brooks JJ. Malignant epithelioid vascular tumors of the pleura: report of a series and literature review. Hum Pathol 2000;31:29–34.

560. Al Shraim M, Mahboub B, Neligan PC, et al. Primary pleural epithelioid haemangioendothelioma with metastases to the skin. A case report and literature review. J Clin Pathol 2005;58:107–9.

561. Hattori H. Epithelioid angiosarcoma arising in the tuberculous pyothorax – report of an autopsy case. Arch Pathol Lab Med 2001;125:1477–9.

562. Kimura M, Ito H, Furuta T, et al. Pyothorax-associated angiosarcoma of the pleura with metastasis to the brain. Pathol Int 2003;53:547–51.

563. Ordonez NG, Tornos C. Malignant peripheral nerve sheath tumor of the pleura with epithelial and rhabdomyoblastic differentiation: report of a case clinically simulating mesothelioma. Am J Surg Pathol 1997;21:1515–21.

564. Cohn L, Hall AD. Extraosseous osteogenic sarcoma of the pleura. Ann Thorac Surg 1968;5:545–9.

565. Reingold IM, Amromin GD. Extraosseous osteosarcoma of the lung. Cancer 1971;28:491–8.

566. Walters KL, Martinez AJ. Malignant fibrous mesothelioma. Metastatic to brain and liver. Acta Neuropath (Berl.) 1975;33:173–7.

567. Yang H-Y, Weaver LL, Foti PR. Primary malignant fibrous histiocytoma of the pleura. Acta Cytol 1983;27:683–7.

568. Rizkalla K, Ahmad D, Garcia B, et al. Primary malignant fibrous histiocytoma of the pleura a case report and review of the literature. Respir Med 1994;88:711–4.

569. Gupta RK, Paolini FA. Liposarcoma of the pleura, report of a case with a review of the literature and views on histogenesis. Am Rev Respir Dis 1967;95:298–304.

570. Wong WW, Pluth JR, Grado GL, et al. Liposarcoma of the pleura. Mayo Clin Proc 1994;69:882–5.

571. Duhig JT. Solitary rhabdomyosarcoma of the pleura. Report of a case with a note on the nomenclature of pleural tumours. J Thorac Surg 1969;37:236–41.

572. Saenz NC, Ghavimi F, Gerald W, et al. Chest wall rhabdomyosarcoma. Cancer 1997;80:1513–7.

573. Moran CA, Suster S, Koss MN. Smooth muscle tumours presenting as pleural neoplasms. Histopathology 1995;27:227–34.

574. Gibbs AR. Smooth muscle tumours of the pleura. Histopathology 1995;27:295–6.

575. Moran CA, Suster S, Koss MN. Smooth muscle tumours of the pleura. Histopathology 1997;30:97–8.

576. Gibbs AR. Smooth muscle tumours of the pleura. Histopathology 1997;30:98.

577. Proca DM, Ross P, Pratt J, et al. Smooth muscle tumor of the pleura – a case report and review of the literature. Arch Pathol Lab Med 2000;124:1688–92.

578. Goetz SP, Robinson RA, Landas SK. Extraskeletal myxoid chondrosarcoma of the pleura – report of a case clinically simulating mesothelioma. Am J Clin Pathol 1992;97:498–502.

579. Luppi G, Cesinaro AM, Zoboli A, et al. Mesenchymal chondrosarcoma of the pleura. Eur Respir J 1996;9:840–3.

580. Fushimi H, Tanio Y, Kotoh K. Ectopic thymoma mimicking diffuse pleural mesothelioma: A case report. Hum Pathol 1998;29:409–10.

581. Fukayama M, Maeda Y, Funata N, et al. Pulmonary and pleural thymoma. Diagnostic application of lymphocyte markers to the thymoma of unusual site. Am J Clin Pathol 1988;89:617–21.

582. Sapino A, Cavallo A, Donna A, et al. Pleural epidermoid carcinoma from displaced skin following extrapleural pneumothorax in a patient exposed to asbestos. Virchows Arch 1996;429:173–6.

583. Harland RW, Sharma M, Rosenzweig DY. Lung carcinoma in a patient with lucite sphere plombage thoracoplasty. Chest 1993;103:1295–7.

584. Moran CA, Suster S. Primary mucoepidermoid carcinoma of the pleura. Am J Clin Pathol 2003;120:381–5.

585. Chernow B, Sahn SA. Carcinomatous involvement of the pleura. An analysis of 96 patients. Am J Med 1977;63:695–702.

586. Shepherd MP. Thoracic metastases. Thorax 1982;37:366–70.

587. Canto-Armengod A. Macroscopic characteristics of pleural metastases arising from the breast and observed by diagnostic thoracoscopy. Am Rev Respir Dis 1990;142:616–8.

588. Canto A, Ferrer G, Romagosa V, et al. Lung cancer and pleural effusion. Clinical significance and study of pleural metastatic locations. Chest 1985;87:649–52.

589. Meyer PC. Metastatic carcinoma of the pleura. Thorax 1966;21:437–40.

590. Canto A, Rivas J, Saumench J, et al. Points to consider when choosing a biopsy method in cases of pleurisy of unknown origin. Chest 1983;84:176–9.

591. Nicholson AG, McCormick CJ, Shimosato Y, et al. The value of PE-10, a monoclonal antibody against pulmonary surfactant, in distinguishing primary and metastatic lung tumours. Histopathology 1995;27:57–60.

592. Gaines JJ, Crosby JH, Kamath MV. Diagnosis of thoracic splenosis by Tru-cut needle biopsy. Am Rev Respir Dis 1986;133:1199–201.

593. Cordier JF, Gamondes JP, Marx P, et al. Thoracic splenosis presenting with hemoptysis. Chest 1992;102:626–7.

594. Madjar S, Weissberg D. Thoracic splenosis. Thorax 1994;49:1020–2.

595. Shaw AFB, Shafi A. Traumatic autoplastic transplantation of splenic tissue in man with observations on the late results of splenectomy in six cases. J Pathol 1937;45:215–35.

596. Carr NJ, Turk EP. The histological features of splenosis. Histopathology 1992;21:549 53.

Chest wall disease

597. Tsukushi S, Nishida Y, Sugiura H, et al. Soft tissue sarcomas of the chest wall. J Thorac Oncol 2009;4:834–7.

598. Delaney TF, Shepard JO, Chakravarti A, et al. A 45-year-old woman with a thoracic mass and Pancoast's syndrome – intrathoracic fibromatosis (Desmoid tumor). N Engl J Med 2000;342:1814–21.

599. Kabiri EH, al Aziz S, el Maslout A, et al. Desmoid tumors of the chest wall. Eur J Cardiothorac Surg 2001;19:580–3.

600. Nisolle JF, Delaunois L, Trigaux JP. Myositis ossificans of the chest wall. Eur Respir J 1996;9:178–9.

601. Gordon MS, Hajdu SI, Bains SM, et al. Soft tissue sarcomas of the chest wall. Results of surgical resection. J Thorac Cardiovasc Surg 1991;101:843–54.

602. Gross JL, Younes RN, Haddad FJ, et al. Soft-Tissue Sarcomas of the chest wall: prognostic factors. Chest 2005;127:902–8.

603. Greager JA, Patel MK, Briele HA, et al. Soft tissue sarcomas of the adult thoracic wall. Cancer 1987;59:370–3.

604. Souba WW, McKenna RJ, Meis J, et al. Radiation-induced sarcomas of the chest wall. Cancer 1986;57:610–5.

605. Askin FB, Rosai J, Sibley RK, et al. Malignant small cell tumor of the thoracopulmonary region in childhood. Cancer 1979;43:2435–52.

606. Hicks MJ, Smith JD, Carter AB, et al. Recurrent intrapulmonary malignant small cell tumor of the thoracopulmonary region with metastasis to the oral cavity: review of literature and case report. Ultrastruct Pathol 1995;19:297–303.

607. Tsuji S, Hisaoka M, Morimitsu Y, et al. Peripheral primitive neuroectodermal tumour of the lung: report of two cases. Histopathology 1998;33:369–74.

608. Mikami Y, Nakajima M, Hashimoto H, et al. Primary pulmonary primitive neuroectodermal tumor (PNET) – A case report. Pathol Res Pract 2001;197:113–9.

609. Kahn AG, Avagnina A, Nazar J, et al. Primitive neuroectodermal tumor of the lung. Am Pathol Lab Med 2001;125:397–9.

610. Gonzalez-Crussi F, Wolfson SL, Misingi K, et al. Peripheral neuroectodermal tumors of the chest wall in childhood. Cancer 1984;54:2519–27.

611. Seemayer TA, Vekemans M, de Chadarevian JP. Histological and cytogenetic findings in a malignant tumor of the chest wall and lung (Askin tumor). Virchows Arch A Pathol Anat Histopathol 1985;408:289–96.

612. Schmidt D, Herrmann C, Jurgens H, et al. Malignant peripheral neuroectodermal tumor and its necessary distinction from Ewing's sarcoma – a report from the Kiel Pediatric Tumor Registry. Cancer 1991;68:2251–9.

613. Contesso G, Llombartbosch A, Terrier P, et al. Does malignant small round cell tumor of the thoracopulmonary region (Askin tumor) constitute a clinicopathologic entity? An analysis of 30 cases with immunohistochemical and electron-microscopic support treated at the Institute-Gustave-Roussy. Cancer 1992;69:1012–20.

614. Kim MS, Kim CJ, Jung HS, et al. Fibroblast growth factor 2 induces differentiation and apoptosis of Askin tumour cells. J Pathol 2004;202:103–12.

615. Delattre O, Zucman J, Melot T, et al. The Ewing family of tumors – a subgroup of small-round-cell tumors defined by specific chimeric transcripts. N Engl J Med 1994;331:294–9.

616. Ambros IM, Ambros PF, Strehl S, et al. MIC2 is a specific marker for Ewing's sarcoma and peripheral primitive neuroectodermal tumors. Cancer 1991;67:1886–93.

617. Nagao K, Ito H, Yoshida H, et al. Chromosomal rearrangement t(11;22) in extraskeletal Ewing's sarcoma and primitive neuroectodermal tumour analysed by fluorescence in situ hybridization using paraffin-embedded tissue. J Pathol 1997;181:62–6.

618. Folpe AL, Hill CE, Parham DM, et al. Immunohistochemical detection of FLI-1 protein expression – a study of 132 round cell tumors with emphasis on CD99-positive mimics of Ewing's sarcoma/ primitive neuroectodermal tumor. Amer J Surg Pathol 2000;24:1657–62.

619. Lucas DR, Bentley G, Dan ME, et al. Ewing sarcoma vs lymphoblastic lymphoma –

a comparative immunohistochemical study. Am J Clin Pathol 2001;115:11–17.

620. Yamaguchi U, Hasegawa T, Morimoto Y, et al. A practical approach to the clinical diagnosis of Ewing's sarcoma/primitive neuroectodermal tumour and other small round cell tumours sharing EWS rearrangement using new fluorescence in situ hybridisation probes for EWSR1 on formalin fixed, paraffin wax embedded tissue. J Clin Pathol 2005;58:1051–6.

621. Odell JM, Benjamin DR. Mesenchymal hamartoma of chest wall in infancy: natural history of two cases. Pediatr Pathol 1986;5:135–46.

622. Cohen MC, Drut R, Garcia C, et al. Mesenchymal hamartoma of the chest wall: a cooperative study with review of the literature. Pediatr Pathol 1992;12:525–34.

623. SerranoEgea A, SantosBriz A, GarciaMunoz H, et al. Chest wall hamartoma – report of two cases with secondary aneurysmal bone cysts. Pathol Res Pract 2001;197:835–9.

624. Gorham LW, Wright AW, Shultz HH, et al. Disappearing bones: a rare form of massive osteolysis; report of two cases, one with autopsy findings. Am J Med 1954;17:674–82.

625. Gorham LW, Stout AP. Massive osteolysis (acute spontaneous absorption of bone, phantom bone, disappearing bone); its relation to hemangiomatosis. J Bone Joint Surg Am 1955;37-A:985–1004.

626. McNeil KD, Fong KM, Walker QJ, et al. Gorham's syndrome: a usually fatal cause of pleural effusion treated successfully with radiotherapy. Thorax 1996;51:1275–6.

627. Riantawan P, Tansupasawasdikul S, Subhannachart P. Bilateral chylothorax complicating massive osteolysis (Gorham's syndrome). Thorax 1996;51:1277–8.

Appendix

The processing of lung specimens

Whilst the value of cytopathology is fully acknowledged,[1–3] this book is concerned with histopathology and except for a section on broncho-alveolar lavage, consideration will be largely limited to specimens submitted for histology. Lung specimens are obtained by a variety of procedures and vary greatly in size (Box A.1). It is desirable that all specimens be received in the laboratory unfixed but this is best waived in the case of small biopsies because of their greater risk of drying in transit. For these specimens the clinician should be provided with small containers of fixative; for larger specimens dry containers should be provided with instructions that they should be brought to the laboratory straight away. A refrigerator should be available for specimens brought to the laboratory out of hours. The various types of specimen will be dealt with in turn but consideration must first be given to laboratory safety.

SAFE A HANDLING OF LUNG SPECIMENS

The examination of lung tissue entails two particular risks: infection and that associated with formaldehyde vapour. To minimise these, protective clothing, masks and eye shields are either desirable or (as is the case in the UK) mandatory.

It is incumbent upon the clinician to inform the pathologist if there is any possibility of the specimen being infectious but this cannot always be relied upon and it is good practice to regard all fresh tissue as being potentially infectious. To minimise the risk of laboratory infection the tissue should be immersed in formaldehyde, ideally for 72 hours before it is examined,[4] but this is not generally practicable. Not infrequently, the clinical situation demands a frozen section. Then the selection of tissue should take place in a microbiological safety cabinet and afterwards the cryostat cabinet should be fumigated with formaldehyde vapour overnight. Other specimens also need to be first handled in a microbiological safety cabinet, either to immerse or fill them with formaldehyde. By the next day most microbes will no longer be viable but tubercle bacilli and prions can survive much longer and continued caution is necessary.

Formaldehyde is categorised as a probable carcinogen by the International Agency for Research on Cancer.[5] Several governments have therefore stipulated maximum airborne levels in the workplace. These levels are easily exceeded when copious amounts are used to distend lungs unless an adequately ventilated bench or cabinet is used.

NEEDLE ASPIRATION

Needle aspiration is appropriate for solid lesions such as tumours whereas pulmonary infiltrates seldom produce satisfactory specimens if sampled by this technique. Whatever the site of the lesion within the thorax, special sampling procedures are required, namely bron-

©2010 Elsevier Ltd
DOI: 10.1016/B978-0-7020-3369-8.00014-8

Needle aspiration
Fibreoptic bronchoscopy
    Bronchial biopsy
    Transbronchial biopsy
Rigid bronchoscopic bronchial biopsy
Mediastinoscopy or mediastinotomy lymph node biopsy
Transcutaneous drill biopsy
Pleural punch biopsy
'Medical' thoracoscopy
Pleural biopsy
Thoracotomy or 'surgical' (video-assisted) thoracoscopy
    Pleural biopsy
    Wedge lung biopsy
    Segmentectomy
    Lobectomy
    Pneumonectomy
Postmortem

Figure A1 The bronchial tree showing the extent visualised with the rigid bronchoscope (seldom further than the segmental bronchi) compared with the flexible fibroptic bronchoscope (usually down to the fifth- or sixth-order bronchi. The tan-coloured airways represent the additional area visualised with the flexible instrument.

choscopy for transbronchial aspiration, oesophagoscopy for trans-oesophageal aspiration and radiography for transcutaneous aspiration. The pathologist is therefore seldom involved in the actual sampling procedure, which is generally undertaken by a clinician or a radiologist. Ultrasound guidance has greatly improved the accuracy of transbronchial and transoesophageal needle aspiration, which are being increasingly used for the diagnosis of diseases affecting the mediastinal lymph nodes, such as stage 1 sarcoidosis, and in the assessment of mediastinal lymph node status when staging lung cancer.[6–10]

The usual fine needles (22-gauge) produce a cell suspension that is suitable for cytology but it is increasingly the case that extensive immunocytochemistry and gene mutational analysis are required in addition to a microscopical diagnosis. These can all be achieved if the aspirate is centrifuged to produce a cell pellet, which may be sectioned, or submitted intact for gene analysis (see below).[10,11] Alternatively, the slightly wider 18- or 19-gauge needles may be used. These produce a thin core of tissue that can be processed for histology in the conventional way,[12,13] especially if the transcutaneous needle is inserted with the aid of a spring-loaded firing device.[14–16] With this technique the aspirated material (which may be contained in the needle as much as the syringe) can be rinsed directly into the fixative as soon as practicable and processed in the laboratory in the same way as small biopsies. The principal complications are a relatively small pneumothorax and haemoptysis, encountered in 23% and 4% of patients respectively at one institution, with no fatalities.[17] As with any invasive technique the danger of tumour seeding in the needle track has to be kept in mind.[18,19]

BRONCHIAL AND TRANSBRONCHIAL BIOPSY

The rigid bronchoscope is nowadays largely confined to therapeutic procedures such as stemming haemorrhage, the extraction of a foreign body, the insertion of a stent and laser ablation. The flexible fibreoptic bronchoscope is generally preferred for diagnostic use. It reaches further and can enter upper-lobe airways (Fig. A.1). The specimens are smaller but several may be taken.

Bronchoscopic biopsies may contain only bronchus, only pulmonary parenchyma or both. If the specimen floats it is more likely to contain alveoli than not but no less likely to be diagnostic or abnormal than if it sinks.[20,21] A note of the number of fragments received provides a useful check on laboratory procedures but if this information is incorporated in the report it may be disputed by bronchoscopists who have made their own count. Discrepancies are often due to the clinician counting flecks of mucus as tissue fragments. Reporting the number of fragments received is therefore not conducive to good professional relationships. However, it is imperative that no fragment be lost in processing and to minimise this risk it is advisable that the fragments are handled just once, if at all. It is advantageous if the clinician wipes the specimens on to a small strip of filter paper and puts this into the specimen jar. Alternatively, if loose fragments are received they should be transferred with fine-toothed forceps into a capture vehicle such as tissue paper, a fine-mesh wire cage or molten agar, which when set can be further processed as if it were a button of tissue. The agar survives processing and can seen around the tissue when the slide is examined by the naked eye but is invisible when the section is examined microscopically.[22] Imprisoning the fragments in sponge is likely to cause tissue artefacts.[23] Free tumour cells may remain in the fixative or other transport medium after all fragments have been removed and the sensitivity of the bronchoscopy procedure is marginally improved if the residual fluid is submitted for cytology.[24]

The largest fragments of lung obtained by transbronchial biopsy each contain about 100 alveoli. If the changes are non-specific and few alveoli have been obtained, the paucity of lung tissue should be made clear in the report. At least three step sections should be prepared, keeping spares at each level for any special stains that might be required.[25] If no abnormalities are identified at any of these levels and tissue remains in the block, further step sections should be prepared. Many laboratories, particularly those dealing with specimens from lung transplant or otherwise immunocompromised patients, routinely examine step sections, or even serial sections through the block. In immunodeficient patients it is advisable to stain for fungi and mycobacteria routinely as the histopathological changes may be atypical.[26]

The main indication for endoscopic biopsy is the diagnosis of bronchogenic neoplasia but transbronchial biopsy is also useful in the investigation of suspected lung infection and graft rejection. It is also often the first procedure undertaken to obtain tissue in the investigation of diffuse parenchymal disease.

Several diagnostic pitfalls are inherent in the interpretation of fibreoptic biopsies:

- Crush artefact. This can lead to lymphocytes being mistaken for small cell carcinoma. Fortunately, markers such as CD56 (for small cell carcinoma) and CD45 (for lymphocytes) are retained in crushed tissue.
- Collapse artefact. It is not possible to reinflate these small biopsies and it may therefore be difficult to appreciate individual alveoli so that on occasion normal lung tissue may be thought to be fibrotic. Reticulin and elastin stains and immunostains for epithelial markers may circumvent this problem.
- Bubble artefact. Trapped air bubbles may simulate fat globules, suggesting exogenous lipid pneumonia, but the foreign-body giant cells that characterise this condition are not evident.
- Stripping artefact. Epithelium is liable to be stripped away from its basement membrane and misinterpreted as carcinoma but the lack of atypia or evidence of invasion should warn against this.
- Presence of pleural cells. If the biopsy forceps reach as far as the pleura the patient generally yelps but the pathologist knows nothing of this and unless alert to the possibility may mistake hyperplastic mesothelium for carcinoma.[27] The mesothelial markers calretinin and cytokeratin 5/6 are helpful in this situation.
- Haemorrhage. Blood filling the alveoli is probably the result of operative trauma and may be ignored unless there is also substantial haemosiderosis.

When a tumour is visible to the bronchoscopist the sensitivity of a forceps biopsy ranges between 70% and 100%.[28–31] When the tumour is not visible the diagnostic sensitivity is less and varies with the location and size of the lesion. The yield is increased if multiple specimens are obtained. One study found that with central tumours a single biopsy succeeded in establishing the diagnosis in 92% of cases, a figure that increased to 96% if four samples were taken, but was not further improved upon with six. For peripheral tumours, positive results increased progressively from 45% through 55% and 60% to 75% when one, four, five and six samples respectively were taken.[32] Sputum examination is probably not cost-effective except when the patient has a tumour that is evidently unresectable.[33] However, cytology is appropriate for the evaluation of fine-needle transbronchial needle aspirates of mediastinal lymph nodes, which contributes to the staging of lung cancer. In some circumstances cytology and histology augment each other (Box A.2).[32,34–36]

In many of the diffuse parenchymal lung diseases a transbronchial biopsy is often uninformative, but it may provide an unexpected tissue diagnosis, obviating the need for more invasive procedures. Thus, in a patient suspected of having idiopathic pulmonary fibrosis, a disease in which fibreoptic specimens are seldom diagnostic, a bronchoscopic biopsy may identify unsuspected sarcoidosis and so circumvent the necessity for a surgical procedure. Indeed, this condition is often recognisable histologically even if an attempted transbronchial procedure samples only the bronchus. This is because the bronchus has

Box A.2 **Yield of various sampling methods in the diagnosis of peripheral lung cancer as percentages**				
First author	Washing	Brushing	Biopsy	All methods
Kvale[34]	13	26	37	47
Cortese[35]	36	36	49	62
Popovich[32]	–	40	70	75
Mak[36]	38	29	37	56

Box A.3 **Fibreoptic biopsy: utility in various lung diseases**	
	Examples
Excellent for diffuse bronchial or lung disease	Sarcoidosis 'Lymphangitis carcinomatosa' Systemic amyloidosis
Good for mass lesions or patchy disease that can be targeted	Tumours *Pneumocystis* pneumonia Eosinophilic pneumonia Alveolar lipoproteinosis Langerhans cell histiocytosis
May help in patchy disease that cannot be targeted	
Poor in diseases with scanty specific features or those in which study of the lobular architecture is important to the diagnosis	Extrinsic allergic alveolitis Interstitial pneumonias (idiopathic pulmonary fibrosis)

a rich lymphatic supply and sarcoidosis has a lymphangitic distribution. The likelihood of transbronchial biopsy giving a diagnosis in various lung diseases is shown in Box A.3.

The diseases unlikely to be identified in these small specimens are those such as idiopathic pulmonary fibrosis and extrinsic allergic alveolitis in which diagnosis depends upon their lobular distribution.[37–39] The number of fibreoptic specimens required to give diagnostic material has been studied in regard to sarcoidosis. One group found that a single biopsy provided a tissue diagnosis of sarcoidosis in 46% of cases, increasing progressively to 90% when four biopsies were taken but not appreciably increasing further thereafter.[40] On comparing the diagnostic yield in patients with pulmonary infiltrates a diagnosis is reported to be provided by transbronchial biopsy in 59% and by open-lung biopsy in 94%.[41] In the diagnosis of cryptogenic organising pneumonia, transbronchial biopsy is reported to have a sensitivity of 64% and a specificity of 86%.[42]

OPEN AND VIDEO-ASSISTED THORACOSCOPIC LUNG BIOPSIES

From the pathologist's point of view there is little difference between a biopsy obtained at thoracotomy (open biopsy)[43,44] and one obtained at video-assisted thoracoscopy.[45–48] Both give good-sized specimens and both afford the surgeon a choice of biopsy site. The optimum biopsy site often depends upon the nature of the disease being investigated. Nodules are best excised in their entirety or if this is impracticable a wedge should be taken to include both the core of the lesion and its interface with its surroundings. Diffuse lung disease often shows a zonal difference in disease activity and it is therefore advantageous if both the upper and lower lobes are sampled. Alternatively, a site thought to show intermediate changes may be chosen. Some advise that the tip of the lingula, or indeed the tip of any lobe, should be avoided as these sites often show non-specific scarring,[49] but this is disputed.[50,51] As noted above the biopsy procedure often gives rise to alveolar haemorrhage and care is needed in the interpretation of blood in the air spaces. It is likely to be genuine if there is also haemosiderosis.

In many cases the lung sample will have collapsed on removal and, if fixed in this state, there will be close apposition of the alveolar walls. This makes it difficult to study the architecture of the lung and can lead to considerable misinterpretation. The lung can however be rein-flated by vacuum[52] or better by injection, the latter achieved by gently instilling a little fixative into the specimen with a syringe, taking care not to overexpand the tissue.[53] Airways cannot easily be identified by eye in these peripheral lung specimens and it is sufficient to inject the fixative directly into the lung parenchyma. The only disadvantage of this procedure is that free cells may be cleared from consolidated alveoli and diagnoses such as desquamative interstitial pneumonia obscured. However, the benefits of gentle inflation–fixation outweigh this single disadvantage.

Before the specimen is fixed, thought should be given to the desir-ability of ancillary procedures that require unfixed or specially fixed tissue, particularly microbiological culture. Immunofluorescence microscopy and gene or chromosomal studies may also require fresh or snap-frozen tissue. However, the primary purpose of the biopsy is histopathological evaluation and it is essential that sufficient tissue remains for this.

Electron microscopy requires very little tissue but has its own requirements, the most important of which is prompt fixation. Whereas light microscopy is often satisfactory despite delayed fixation, this is not true of electron microscopy. If the recommended fixative (glutaraldehyde or methanol-free formaldehyde) is not available, commercial formalin is an acceptable alternative so long as fixation is rapid. Archival tissue rescued from old paraffin blocks is often sat-isfactory for electron microscopy if it had been fixed without delay. Rapid fixation for electron microscopy is also possible postmortem by injecting fixative through the chest wall immediately after death; a marker dye in the fixative facilitates recognition of the injected site when autopsy is undertaken.[54] Special care should be taken against 'crush' artefact when selecting small tissue samples for electron micro-scopy; a new razor blade should be used for each specimen and cutting effected with a to-and-fro motion rather than by exerting downwards pressure.

PLEURAL BIOPSY

The pleura has traditionally been sampled blind using a reverse-bevel needle such as the Abrams or Cope. The sensitivity rises with the number of specimens obtained, four to six being the optimum.[55,56] Some report that at best blind biopsy has a sensitivity of 40–50%,[56] which may be improved by the use of image guidance by computed tomography or ultrasound to about 90%[57] but for mesothelioma others report that blind biopsy has a sensitivity of only 16% and therefore recommend sampling by open or video-assisted thora-coscopy, when the sensitivity rises to 100%.[58] If fluid is found opinions vary with regard to the volume there should be sent for assessment of malignancy, but 50–60 ml is a reasonable compromise.[59,60]

FROZEN SECTION

Most frozen sections of lung tissue are performed for the evaluation of solid lesions, the assessment of tumour margins or the detection of mediastinal lymph node metastasis.[61] It is best avoided on lung tissue that is not consolidated but if it is necessary the tissue may first be inflated with frozen section mounting medium. Intraoperative assessment of mediastinal lymph node status by frozen section has diminished with the improvement in preoperative assessment by ultrasound-guided fine-needle. If a tumour of uncertain origin is iden-tified by frozen section, immunohistochemistry is feasible for distin-guishing primary from secondary lung tumours in this setting.[62]

WHOLE LUNGS AND LUNG LOBES

Artefactual collapse is inevitable when a lung is removed from the chest and inflation fixation is highly desirable for these large speci-mens. This can be effected by having a reservoir of fixative on the top of an exhaust-ventilated cut-up cabinet and running fixative into the specimen from a height of about 25 cm via tubing that terminates in a tapering nozzle wedged into the supplying bronchus. Fixative is infused until the pleural surface is smooth. The specimen is then immersed or floated in a container of fixative overnight with a cover-ing of lint or filter paper to prevent drying. It is not necessary to clamp the bronchus. This procedure is equally applicable in autopsy and surgical pathological practice. If the specimen needs to be examined the same day even a few hours of inflation–fixation is preferable to opening an unfixed lung. However, as with biopsies, thought should be given to the desirability of first sampling the lung for procedures that are impossible after fixation, notably culture. Whatever the type of fresh specimen, culture should always be considered before the opportunity for this is lost by fixation. It is good practice to establish a protocol determining who should be responsible for this, the surgeon or the pathologist.

Other procedures that might be considered before either fixation or cut-up include injection of blood vessels or airways, taking care to remove as much clot or bronchial secretions as possible and after-wards excluding these as possible causes of any blockages or apparent stenoses. A coloured or radiopaque gelatine mixture (e.g. Micropaque barium sulphate suspension 330 ml, gelatine 33 g, water 130 ml) containing thymol as a preservative may be stored for this purpose, melting the solid mix as required by immersion in warm water, but not heating it above 56 °C as this would denature the gelatine (see Figs 1.35 and 3.14B, pp. 21 and 104).[63,64]

Radiography is also possible after fixation if the lungs are inflated with formaldehyde fume[65] or if lung slices are air-dried after being fixed with liquid formaldehyde.[66–68] Air-drying is facilitated if the fixa-tive comprises 10 parts polyethylene glycol 400, 5 parts ethanol, 2 parts formalin and 3 parts water. However, both these procedures have been rendered largely redundant by preoperative contrast-enhanced studies that generally provide far superior images.

The choice of cut-up procedure is wide and depends upon the nature of the underlying disease. Different procedures are appropriate for studying a widespread process such as emphysema than for a localised one such as a tumour. In other circumstances it may be desirable to open the airways or the blood vessels widely, or possibly both without cutting across either. This can be achieved if the airways are opened from the hilum and the arteries from the oblique fissure.[69]

Corrosion casts of pulmonary blood vessels or airways constitute another way of demonstrating abnormalities in the lung,[70] albeit at the cost of losing all intervening tissue (see Figs 1.3 and 1.10, pp. 4 and 8). However, bronchial cartilage can be studied without losing the intervening tissue by staining the cartilage with toluidine blue and clearing the specimen with an organic solvent such as cedarwood oil or xylol.[71]

Diffuse lung disease

To demonstrate emphysema, or other diffuse disease, sagittal slicing is customary, and for this a particularly good result can be obtained with an electric meat-slicer. Conditions such as emphysema and fibrosis can then be demonstrated more convincingly with the barium sulphate technique.[72] This requires the lung slice to be squeezed gently in a 7.5% solution of barium chloride and then for a 10% solution of sodium sulphate to be poured on, the resultant white precipitate of barium sulphate emphasising structural differences in the lung substance (see Figs 3.14B, 3.15B, 3.16B and 7.1.23, pp. 104–106 and 347). Similar contrast can be achieved by fixing the lung in Bouin's solution.[73] Paper-mounted whole-lung sections[74,75] provide an excellent permanent demonstration of conditions such as emphysema (see Figs 1.7, 3.14A, 3.15A, 3.16B, 7.1.9A, 7.1.10A, 7.1.15 and 7.1.16, pp. 7, 104, 105, 106, 334, 335, 340) but an easy alternative is to bag or laminate in plastic the thinnest slices obtainable with a meat-slicer.[76]

Lung tumours

It is often of interest to investigate the relationship of a tumour to the airways and for this, and its subsequent demonstration, the Liebow technique cannot be bettered. This entails a probe being passed down the airways to the tumour and then cutting along the line of the probe from the hilum to the pleura, passing through all the successive airways leading to the tumour and the centre of the tumour itself (Fig. A2). The fact that the plane of the cut is neither sagittal nor coronal is immaterial and is not evident when the cut surface is presented to the viewer.

In dealing with specimens excised in the treatment of lung cancer certain information is essential for staging and to circumvent some of these points being overlooked protocols have been produced by the Association of Directors of Anatomic and Surgical Pathology, the College of American Pathologists and the Royal College of Pathologists for both carcinoma and mesothelioma[77–80] Some institutions also collect data on biopsies. Copies of such protocols and datasets may be downloaded from these organisations' websites: www.adasp.org, www.cap.org and www.rcpath.org. Particular points to be covered include:

- The size of the tumour, paying particular attention to those around 3 cm in size: 3 cm or less is one criterion categorising a tumour as stage T1 whereas a size greater than 3 cm places it in stage T2.
- The relation of the tumour to the pleura. Many tumours abut the pleura and it often requires histology with elastin staining[81,82] to ascertain whether the pleura is invaded (see Fig. 12.1.49, p. 573).
- The relation of the tumour to the bronchial resection margin, giving the apparent distance of the tumour from the margin and sampling this for microscopic evidence of involvement.
- Lymph node involvement, sampling the hilar nodes in the lung specimen: extrapulmonary lymph nodes are usually submitted separately.
- The presence of other disease, particularly further tumours.
- Microscopic confirmation of the diagnosis.

It is also useful to sample lung tissue distant from, as well as distal to, the tumour, to investigate the possibility of asbestosis having caused the tumour: it is embarrassing to be asked this when medico-legal proceedings have been instituted long after the specimen has been discarded if appropriate areas have not been sampled. Other points that should be described include the type of specimen (segment, lobe or whole lung), the size and weight of the specimen, the location of the tumour (segment involved) and its relation to the airways, the appearance of the tumour, and its effects on the surrounding lung, but the above are the ones the clinician will be particularly looking for, mainly to refine the preoperative staging of the tumour and thus prognosticate. It is of course customary to grade the tumour but the reproducibility of this is dubious. In resection specimens, tumour typing should adhere to the World Health Organization International Association for the Study of Lung Cancer classification of lung and pleural tumours, as outlined in Ch. 12.1.[83]

Image display

Pictures are more informative than a description and both gross and histological images, generated with either a digital camera or a flatbed scanner can now be easily incorporated in a computer-generated report.[84–87] Flatbed scanners are useful for making very low magnification images of histological sections as well as depicting large specimens.

SPECIAL MICROSCOPICAL PROCEDURES

The most useful special stains and immunohistochemical markers in pulmonary pathology are listed in Tables A.1 and A.2, with more detail being provided in the relevant chapters. Molecular techniques can also be applied to tissue sections and are being increasingly used in the diagnosis of infection,[88] lymphoproliferative disease[89] and the better categorisation of tumours.[90] Mineral analysis is dealt with in Chapter 7.1 .

GENE MUTATIONAL ANALYSIS

Gene mutational analysis is being increasingly required to assess the likelihood of a tumour responding to drugs such as gefitinib, which have been designed to counter particular gene mutations driving tumour growth (epidermal growth factor receptor in the case of gefitinib).[10,11] Further tissue sections may be utilised but meticulous attention is required to avoid DNA contamination. Few sections are required and they do not need to be mounted but it is advantageous if they are cut close to the section used for diagnosis to ensure that they largely consist of viable tumour rather than necrotic tissue, stroma or tumour capsule. Cell pellets of needle aspirates may also be used. Patients who may benefit from the new anticancer drugs generally have advanced disease and some procedural planning is required in consultation with the clinical team so that a very small specimen can provide both histological diagnosis and mutational analysis as quickly as possible.

BRONCHOALVEOLAR LAVAGE

This section concerns the relatively small-volume lavages (up to 300 ml) that are performed with a flexible fibreoptic bronchoscope rather than the massive washouts (up to 30 litres) used in the treatment of alveolar lipoproteinosis. Small-volume lavage is used in the diagnosis of several types of lung disease, infectious, neoplastic and interstitial.

The diagnosis of infection by bronchoalveolar lavage is usually the province of the microbiology department[91,92] and the histo(cyto)

Figure A2 Demonstration of the airways related to a lung tumour. (A) A probe is passed through the successive airways to the centre of the tumour and the lung sliced by cutting down on to the probe. (B) Cut surface of the lung showing the probe in place. (C) The same with the probe removed.

pathology department is more concerned with the identification of malignant cells and the enumeration of inflammatory cells.

Malignant cells may be searched for in smears or sections of the centrifuged deposit or in Cytospin preparations in the usual way.[93] Inflammatory cell counts are informative in interstitial lung disease

both in regard to pathogenesis and diagnostically, although their diagnostic specificity is probably low.[94,95] They can also be used to monitor the activity of the disease.[96] In the normal person the lavaged cells are mainly macrophages, whereas various leukocytes appear in a variety of infiltrative lung diseases.[97] It follows therefore that the pro-

Table A.1 Special stains of particular use in pulmonary pathology

Stain	Material stained	Indications
Ziehl–Neelsen	Acid-fast bacilli	Detection of mycobacteria
Grocott–Gomori methenamine silver	Fungi	Identification of fungi
Elastin van Gieson	Elastin, collagen	Assessment of vascular disease
Perl's Prussian blue	Ferric iron	Identification of haemosiderin
Periodic acid–Schiff (PAS)	Glycogen and other carbohydrates	Categorisation of clear cell tumours Alveolar lipoproteinosis
PAS after diastase digestion	Neutral mucin	Subclassification of non-small cell carcinomas Adenocarcinoma vs mesothelioma
Alcian blue	Acidic mucins	Mesothelioma vs adenocarcinoma Subclassification of non-small carcinomas
Congo red	Amyloid	Amyloidosis

Table A.2 Immunohistochemical markers of particular use in pulmonary pathology

Marker	Diagnostic uses
Cytokeratins	Carcinoma vs lymphoma and melanoma Sarcomatous mesothelioma vs sarcoma
Cytokeratin 5/6, calretinin, thrombomodulin	Epithelioid mesothelioma vs adenocarcinoma
Carcinoembryonic antigen	Adenocarcinoma vs epithelioid mesothelioma
CD56, chromogranin, synaptophysin	Neuroendocrine differentiation
TTF-1	Primary vs metastatic adenocarcinoma
S100	Carcinoma vs melanoma Langerhans cell histiocytosis
CD1	Langerhans cell histiocytosis
CD34	Localised fibrous tumour vs sarcomatoid mesothelioma and sarcoma
Smooth muscle actin and HMB45	Lymphangioleiomyomatosis
Leukocyte common antigen	Lymphoma vs carcinoma
T (CD3) and B (CD20 and CD79a) cell markers[a]	Lymphoproliferative disorders
Pneumocystis sp.	*Pneumocystis* pneumonia
Cytomegalovirus	Cytomegalovirus pneumonia
Legionella sp.	*Legionella* pneumonia

[a]Basic markers for analysis of lymphoid infiltrates. Consultation with a regional lymphoma pathology specialist is recommended for complex cases.

portion of macrophages will diminish whenever leukocytes are also present, but total cell counts show that macrophage numbers are always increased in these circumstances. Macrophages are also more numerous in healthy smokers than in non-smokers. It is as well to bear total cell numbers in mind when considering pathogenetic mechanisms, but for diagnostic purposes attention may be concentrated on the differential cell count, performed on Geimsa-stained smears or Cytospin preparations, augmented if required by immunocytochemical identification of lymphocyte type (B and T) and subset (T helper and suppressor), and of Langerhans cells.

The changes in cell proportions in various lung diseases are shown in Table A.3.[42,94,95,97–106] The proportions seen in lavage fluid do not necessarily represent those seen histologically, within either the air spaces or the lung as a whole.[101,107] In idiopathic pulmonary fibrosis, for example, the low numbers of lymphocytes recovered by lavage do not reflect the large numbers evident histologically, perhaps because these cells are located in the interstitium rather than the air spaces. Also in idiopathic pulmonary fibrosis, lavage recovers a higher proportion of polymorphonuclear leukocytes than is evident histologically, presumably reflecting the presence of honeycombing, the spaces of which often contain entrapped neutrophils. Macrophages may also be harder to dislodge as whenever numbers are increased electron microscopy shows that they have unusually long pseudopodia and the pseudopodia of adjacent cells intertwine. Lavage findings do not discriminate between usual interstitial pneumonia and non-specific interstitial pneumonia.[106] For these reasons bronchoalveolar lavage fluid analysis now has little clinical application in determining prognosis and response to treatment in idiopathic pulmonary fibrosis.[107a]

Further information of diagnostic value may be obtained by studying macrophage inclusions. For example, although in many diseases the macrophages recovered by lavage contain a few Perls-positive granules, in pulmonary haemosiderosis almost all these cells are heavily laden with such granules.[108] Similarly, in lipid pneumonia the macrophages have a foamy cytoplasm.[109]

The nature of any mineral particles present may also be identified by analytical electron microscopy (see p. 330),[110–112] but it should be noted that their presence indicates exposure rather than disease. The number of asbestos bodies in lung lavage fluid correlates with their number in lung sections,[113] but again their mere presence does not indicate that there is asbestosis.

Lavage fluid may also be examined for the characteristic proteinaceous aggregates of pulmonary alveolar lipoproteinosis (see Fig. 6.2.16, p. 318)[114,115] and the microliths of alveolar microlithiasis (see p. 320).[116,117] Bronchoalveolar lavage is also used in the evaluation of lung transplants,[118,119] but as in many conditions the findings are best considered in conjunction with biopsy findings.[118]

Lastly, bronchoalveolar lavage is capable of providing valuable information relevant to pathogenesis, for example in identifying various inflammatory cells, cytokines and enzymes in a variety of conditions.[120–123]

Appendix

REFERENCES

1. Suprun H, Pedio G, Ruttner GR. The diagnostic reliability of cytologic typing in primary lung cancer with a review of the literature. Acta Cytol 1980;24:494–500.
2. Popp W, Rauscher H, Ritschka L, et al. Diagnostic sensitivity of different techniques in the diagnosis of lung tumors with the flexible fiberoptic bronchoscope – comparison of brush biopsy, imprint cytology of forceps biopsy, and histology of forceps biopsy. Cancer 1991;67:72–5.
3. Bocking A, Klose KC, Kyll HJ, et al. Cytologic versus histologic evaluation of needle biopsy of the lung, hilum and mediastinum – sensitivity, specificity and typing accuracy. Acta Cytol 1995;39:463–71.

Safe a handling of lung specimens
4. Gibbs AR, Attanoos RL. Examination of lung specimens. J Clin Pathol 2000;53:507–12.
5. International Agency for Research on Cancer. An evaluation of carcinogenic risk to humans. Overall evaluation of carcinogenicity: an updating of IARC monographs vols 1–42. Supplement 7. Lyons: IARC; 1987.

Needle aspiration
6. Nakajima T, Yasufuku K, Kurosu K, et al. The role of EBUS-TBNA for the diagnosis of sarcoidosis – comparisons with other bronchoscopic diagnostic modalities. Respiratory Medicine 2009;103:1796–800.
6a. Natu S, Hoffman J, Siddiqui M, et al. The role of endobronchial ultrasound guided transbronchial needle aspiration cytology in the investigation of mediastinal lymphadenopathy and masses, the North Tees experience. J Clin Pathol 2010;63:445–51.

7. Shah PL, Singh S, Bower M, et al. The role of transbronchial fine needle aspiration in an integrated care pathway for the assessment of patients with suspected lung cancer. J Thorac Oncol 2006;1:324–7.
7a. Wallace NAH, Monaghan HM, Salter DM, et al. Endobrachial ultra-sound guided find-needle aspiration and liquid-based thin-layer cytology. J Clin Pathol 2007;60:388–91.
8. Garwood S, Judson MA, Silvestri G, et al. Endobronchial ultrasound for the diagnosis of pulmonary sarcoidosis. Chest 2007;132:1298–304.
9. Tremblay A, Stather DR, Maceachern P, et al. A randomized controlled trial of standard vs endobronchial ultrasonography-guided transbronchial needle aspiration in patients with suspected sarcoidosis. Chest 2009;136:340–6.
10. Garcia-Olive I, Monso E, Andreo F, et al. Endobronchial ultrasound-guided transbronchial needle aspiration for identifying EGFR mutations. Eur Respir J 2010;35:391–5.
11. Nicholson AG, Gonzalez D, Shah P, et al. Refining the diagnosis and EGFR status of non-small cell carcinoma in biopsy and cytologic material, using a panel of mucin staining, TTF-1, cytokeratin 5/6, and P63, and EGFR mutation analysis. Journal of Thoracic Oncology 2010 (in press).
12. Yang PC, Lee YC, Yu CJ, et al. Ultrasonographically guided biopsy of thoracic tumors – a comparison of large-bore cutting biopsy with fine-needle aspiration. Cancer 1992;69:2553–60.
13. Stratakos G, Porfyridis I, Papas V, et al. Exclusive diagnostic contribution of the histology specimens obtained by 19-gauge transbronchial aspiration needle in

suspected malignant intrathoracic lymphadenopathy. Chest 2008;133: 131–6.
14. Milman N. Percutaneous lung biopsy with a semi-automatic, spring-driven fine needle – preliminary results in 13 patients. Respiration 1993;60:289–91.
15. Smyth RL, Carty H, Thomas H, et al. Diagnosis of interstitial lung disease by a percutaneous lung biopsy sample. Arch Dis Child 1994;70:143–4.
16. Lohela P, Tikkakoski T, Ammala K, et al. Diagnosis of diffuse lung disease by cutting needle biopsy. Acta Radiol 1994;35:251–4.
17. Yeow KM, Su IH, Pan KT, et al. Risk factors of pneumothorax and bleeding: multivariate analysis of 660 CT-guided coaxial cutting needle lung biopsies. Chest 2004;126:748–54.
18. Denton KJ, Cotton DWK, Nakielny RA, et al. Secondary tumour deposits in needle biopsy tracks: an underestimated risk? J Clin Pathol 1990;43:83.
19. Sawabata N, Ohta M, Maeda H. Fine-needle aspiration cytologic technique for lung cancer has a high potential of malignant cell spread through the tract. Chest 2000;118:936–9.

Bronchial and transbronchial biopsy
20. Anders GT, Linville KC, Johnson JE, et al. Evaluation of the float sign for determining adequacy of specimens obtained with transbronchial biopsy. Am Rev Respir Dis 1991;144:1406–7.
21. Curley FJ, Johal JS, Burke ME, et al. Transbronchial lung biopsy: Can specimen quality be predicted at the time of biopsy? Chest 1998;113:1037–41.
22. Cook RW, Hotchkiss GR. A method for handling small tissue fragments in

histopathology. Med Lab Sci 1977;34:93–4.

23. Kepes JJ, Oswald O. Tissue artefacts caused by sponge in embedding cassettes. Am J Surg Pathol 1991;15:810–12.

24. Rosell A, Monso E, Lores L, et al. Cytology of bronchial biopsy rinse fluid to improve the diagnostic yield for lung cancer. Eur Resp J 1998;12:1415–18.

25. Nagata N, Hirano H, Takayama K, et al. Step section preparation of transbronchial lung biopsy. Significance in the diagnosis of diffuse lung disease. Chest 1991;100:959–62.

26. Askin FB, Katzenstein ALA. *Pneumocystis* infection masquerading as diffuse alveolar damage. A potential source of diagnostic error. Chest 1981;79:420–2.

27. Bejarano PA, Garcia MT, Ganjei-Azar P. Mesothelial cells in transbronchial biopsies: a rare complication with a potential for a diagnostic pitfall. Am J Surg Pathol 2007;31:914–18.

28. Arroliga AC, Matthay RA. The role of bronchoscopy in lung cancer. Clin Chest Med 1993;14:87–98.

29. Govert JA, Kopita JM, Matchar D, et al. Cost-effectiveness of collecting routine cytologic specimens during fiberoptic bronchoscopy for endoscopically visible lung tumor. Chest 1996;109:451–6.

30. Gasparini S. Bronchoscopic biopsy techniques in the diagnosis and staging of lung cancer. Monaldi Arch Chest Dis 1997;52:392–8.

31. Mazzone P, Jain P, Arroliga AC, et al. Bronchoscopy and needle biopsy techniques for diagnosis and staging of lung cancer. Clin Chest Med 2002;23:137–58, ix.

32. Popovich J, Kvale PA, Eichenhorn MS, et al. Diagnostic accuracy of multiple biopsies from flexible fiberoptic bronchoscopy. A comparison of central versus peripheral carcinoma. Am Rev Respir Dis 1982;125:521–3.

33. Goldberg-Kahn B, Healy JC, Bishop JW. The cost of diagnosis: A comparison of four different strategies in the workup of solitary radiographic lung lesions. Chest 1997;111:870–6.

34. Kvale PA, Bode FR, Kini S. Diagnostic accuracy in lung cancer; comparison of techniques used in association with flexible fiberoptic bronchoscopy. Chest 1976;69:752–7.

35. Cortese DA, McDougall JC. Bronchoscopic biopsy and brushing with fluoroscopic guidance in nodular metastatic lung cancer. Chest 1981;79:610–11.

36. Mak VH, Johnston ID, Hetzel MR, et al. Value of washings and brushings at fibreoptic bronchoscopy in the diagnosis of lung cancer. Thorax 1990;45:373–6.

37. Wall CP, Gaensler EA, Carrington CB, et al. Comparison of transbronchial and open lung biopsies in chronic infiltrative lung diseases. Am Rev Respir Dis 1981;123:280–5.

38. Johnston IDA, Gomm SA, Kalra S, et al. The management of cryptogenic fibrosing alveolitis in three regions of the United Kingdom. Eur Respir J 1993;6:891–3.

39. Lacasse Y, Fraser RS, Fournier M, et al. Diagnostic accuracy of transbronchial biopsy in acute farmer's lung disease. Chest 1997;112:1459–65.

40. Gilman MJ, Wang K. Transbronchial lung biopsy in sarcoidosis: an approach to determine the optimal number of biopsies. Am Rev Respir Dis 1980;122:721–4.

41. Burt ME, Flye W, Webber BL, et al. Prospective evaluation of aspiration needle, cutting needle, transbronchial and open lung biopsy in patients with pulmonary infiltrates. Ann Thorac Surg 1981;32:146–53.

42. Poletti V, Cazzato S, Minicuci N, et al. The diagnostic value of bronchoalveolar lavage and transbronchial lung biopsy in cryptogenic organizing pneumonia. Eur Respir J 1996;9:2513–16.

Open and video-assisted thoracoscopic lung biopsies

43. Venn GE, Kay PH, Midwood CJ, et al. Open lung biopsy in patients with diffuse pulmonary shadowing. Thorax 1985;40:931–5.

44. Shah SS, Tsang V, Goldstraw P. Open lung biopsy – a safe, reliable and accurate method for diagnosis in diffuse lung disease. Respiration 1992;59:243–6.

45. Bensard DD, McIntyre RC, Waring BJ, et al. Comparison of video thoracoscopic lung biopsy to open lung biopsy in the diagnosis of interstitial lung disease. Chest 1993;103:765–70.

46. Carnochan FM, Walker WS, Cameron EW. Efficacy of video assisted thoracoscopic lung biopsy: an historical comparison with open lung biopsy. Thorax 1994;49:361–3.

47. Kadokura M, Colby TV, Myers JL, et al. Pathologic comparison of video-assisted thoracic surgical lung biopsy with traditional open lung biopsy. J Thorac Cardiovasc Surg 1995;109:494–8.

48. Ravini M, Ferraro G, Barbieri B, et al. Changing strategies of lung biopsies in diffuse lung diseases: the impact of video-assisted thoracoscopy. Eur Resp J 1998;11:99–103.

49. Newman SL, Michel RP, Wang NS. Lingula lung biopsy: is it representative? Am Rev Respir Dis 1985;132:1084–6.

50. Wetstein L. Sensitivity and specificity of lingular segmental biopsies of the lung. Chest 1986;90:383–6.

51. Miller RR, Nelems B, Muller NL, et al. Lingular and right middle lobe biopsy in the assessment of diffuse lung disease. Ann Thorac Surg 1987;44:269–73.

52. vanKuppevelt TH, Robbesom AA, Versteeg EMM, et al. Restoration by vacuum inflation of original alveolar dimensions in small human lung specimens. Eur Resp J 2000;15:771–7.

53. Churg AC. An inflation procedure for open-lung biopsies. Am J Surg Pathol 1983;7:69–71.

54. Bachofen M, Weibel ER, Roos B. Postmortem fixation of human lungs for electron microscopy. Am Rev Respir Dis 1975;111:247–56.

Pleural biopsy

55. Jimenez D, PerezRodriguez E, Diaz G, et al. Determining the optimal number of specimens to obtain with needle biopsy of the pleura. Resp Med 2002;96:14–7.

56. Chakrabarti B, Ryland I, Sheard J, et al. The role of Abrams percutaneous pleural biopsy in the investigation of exudative pleural effusions. Chest 2006;129:1549–55.

57. Adams RF, Gleeson FV. Percutaneous image-guided cutting-needle biopsy of the pleura in the presence of a suspected malignant effusion. Radiology 2001;219:510–14.

58. Attanoos RL, Gibbs AR. The comparative accuracy of different pleural biopsy techniques in the diagnosis of malignant mesothelioma. Histopathology 2008;53:340–4.

59. Abouzgheib W, Bartter T, Dagher H, et al. A prospective study of the volume of pleural fluid required for accurate diagnosis of malignant pleural effusion. Chest 2009;135:999–1001.

60. Swiderek J, Morcos S, Donthireddy V, et al. Prospective study to determine the volume of pleural fluid required to diagnose malignancy. Chest 2010;137:68–73.

Frozen section

61. Sienko A, Allen TC, Zander DS, et al. Frozen section of lung specimens. Arch Pathol Lab Med 2005;129:1602–9.

62. Butcher DN, Goldstraw P, Ladas G, et al. Thyroid transcription factor 1 immunohistochemistry as an intraoperative diagnostic tool at frozen section for distinction between primary and secondary lung tumors. Arch Pathol Lab Med 2007;131:582–7.

Whole lungs and lung lobes

63. Reid LM. Selection of tissue for microscopic study from lungs injected with radio-opaque material. Thorax 1955;10:197–8.

64. Hales MR, Carrington CB. A pigmented gelatin mass for vascular injection. Yale J Biol Med 1971;43:257–70.

65. Wright BM, Slavin G, Kreel L, et al. Postmortem inflation and fixation of human lungs. A technique for pathological and radiological correlations. Thorax 1974;29:189–94.

66. Itoh M, Tokunaga S, Asamoto H, et al. Radiologic-pathologic correlations of small

lung nodules with special reference to peribronchiolar nodules. Am J Roentgenol 1978;130:223–31.

67. Sutinen S, Paakko P, Lahti R. Post-mortem inflammation, radiography and fixation of human lungs. A method for radiological and pathological correlations and morphometric studies. Scand J Respir Dis 1979;60:29–35.

68. Langlois SLP, Henderson DW. Radiological-pathological correlations in pulmonary disease: a simplified method for the study of post-mortem lungs. Australas Radiol 1980;24:262–9.

69. McCulloch TA, Rutty GN. Postmortem examination of the lungs: a preservation technique for opening the bronchi and pulmonary arteries individually without transection problems. J Clin Pathol 1998;51:163–4.

70. Liebow AA, Hales MR, Lindskog GE, et al. Plastic demonstration of pulmonary pathology. Bull Internat Assoc Med museums 1947;27:116–29.

71. MonforteMunoz H, Walls RL. Intrapulmonary airways visualized by staining and clearing of whole- lung sections: the transparent human lung. Modern Pathol 2004;17:22–7.

72. Heard BE. A pathological study of emphysema of the lungs with chronic bronchitis. Thorax 1958;13:136–49.

73. Miller RR. Bronchioloalveolar cell adenomas. Am J Surg Pathol 1990;14:904–12.

74. Gough J, Wentworth JE. Thin sections of entire organs mounted on paper. In: Harrison CV, editor. Recent Advances in Pathology. 7th ed. London: Churchill; 1960. p. 80–6.

75. Whimster WF. Rapid giant paper sections of lungs. Thorax 1969;24:737–41.

76. Cote RA, Korthy AL, Kory RC. Laminated lung macrosections: a new dimension in the study and teaching of pulmonary pathology. Dis Chest 1963;43:1–7.

77. Nash G, Hutter RVP, Henson DE. Practice protocol for the examination of specimens from patients with lung cancer. Arch Pathol Lab Med 1995;119:695–700.

78. Gal AA, Marchevsky AM, Travis WD. Updated protocol for the examination of specimens from patients with carcinoma of the lung. Arch Pathol Lab Med 2003;127:1304–13.

79. Gibbs AR, Nicholson AG. Dataset for lung cancer histopathology reports. 2nd ed. London: Royal College of Pathologists; 2007.

80. Butnor KJ, Sporn TA, Ordonez NG. Recommendations for the reporting of pleural mesothelioma: Association of Directors of Anatomic and Surgical Pathology. Am J Clin Pathol 2007;127:15–19.

81. Bunker ML, Raab SS, Landreneau RJ, et al. The diagnosis and significance of visceral pleural invasion in lung carcinoma – histologic predictors and the role of elastic stains. Am J Clin Pathol 1999;112:777–83.

82. Butnor KJ, Vollmer RT, Blaszyk H, et al. Interobserver agreement on what constitutes visceral pleural invasion by non-small cell lung carcinoma: an internet-based assessment of international current practices. Am J Clin Pathol 2007;128:638–47.

83. World Health Organization. Tumours of the Lung, Pleura, Thymus and Heart. Lyons: IARC Press; 2004.

84. Olson DR. Specimen photocopying for surgical pathology reports. Am J Clin Pathol 1978;70:94–5.

85. Beer TW. Scanning of gross specimens. Am J Surg Pathol 2000;24:1170–1.

86. Mai KT, Stinson WA, Swift J, et al. Creating digital images of pathology specimens by using a flatbed scanner. Histopathology 2001;39:323–5.

87. Ventura L. Creating digital images of pathology specimens by using a flatbed scanner. Histopathology 2002;40:294.

Special microscopical procedures

88. Unger ER, Budgeon LR, Myerson D, et al. Viral diagnosis by in situ hybridization. Description of a rapid simplified colorimetric method. Am J Surg Pathol 1986;10:1–8.

89. Nicholson AG, Wotherspoon AC, Diss TC, et al. Pulmonary B-cell non-Hodgkin's lymphomas. The value of immunohistochemistry and gene analysis in diagnosis. Histopathology 1995;26:395–403.

90. Coate LE, John T, Tsao MS, et al. Molecular predictive and prognostic markers in non-small-cell lung cancer. Lancet Oncol 2009;10:1001–10.

Bronchoalveolar lavage

91. Griffiths MH, Kocjan G, Miller RF, et al. Diagnosis of pulmonary disease in human immunodeficiency virus infection: role of transbronchial biopsy and bronchoalveolar lavage. Thorax 1989;44:554–8.

92. Baughman RP. Use of bronchoscopy in the diagnosis of infection in the immunocompromised host [editorial]. Thorax 1994;49:3–7.

93. Poletti V, Romagna M, Allen KA, et al. Bronchoalveolar lavage in the diagnosis of disseminated lung tumors. Acta Cytol 1995;39:472–7.

94. Winterbauer RH, Lammert J, Selland M, et al. Bronchoalveolar lavage cell populations in the diagnosis of sarcoidosis. Chest 1993;104:352–61.

95. Kantrow SP, Meyer KC, Kidd P, et al. The CD4/CD8 ratio in BAL fluid is highly variable in sarcoidosis. Eur Resp J 1997;10:2716–21.

96. Turner-Warwick M, Haslam PL. The value of serial bronchoalveolar lavages in assessing the clinical progress of patients with cryptogenic fibrosing alveolitis. Am Rev Respir Dis 1987;135:26–34.

97. The BAL Cooperative Steering Committee. Bronchoalveolar lavage constituents in healthy individuals, idiopathic pulmonary fibrosis, and selected comparison groups. Am Rev Respir Dis 1990;141:S169–202.

98. Reynolds HY, Fulmer JD, Kazmierowski JA, et al. Analysis of cellular and protein content of broncho-alveolar lavage fluid from patients with idiopathic pulmonary fibrosis and chronic hypersensitivity pneumonitis. J Clin Invest 1977;59:165–75.

99. Weinberger SE, Kelman JA, Elson NA, et al. Bronchoalveolar lavage in interstitial lung disease. Ann Intern Med 1978;89:459–66.

100. Casolaro MA, Bernaudin J-F, Saltini C, et al. Accumulation of Langerhans' cells on the epithelial surface of the lower respiratory tract in normal subjects in association with cigarette smoking. Am Rev Respir Dis 1988;137:406–11.

101. Haslam PL, Turton CWG, Heard B, et al. Bronchoalveolar lavage in pulmonary fibrosis: comparison of cells obtained with lung biopsy and clinical features. Thorax 1980;35:9–18.

102. Haslam PL, Turton CW, Lukoszek A, et al. Bronchoalveolar lavage fluid cell counts in cryptogenic fibrosing alveolitis and their relation to therapy. Thorax 1980;35:328–39.

103. Chollet S, Soler P, Dournovo P, et al. Diagnosis of pulmonary histiocytosis X by immunodetection of Langerhans cells in bronchoalveolar lavage fluid. Am J Pathol 1984;115:225–32.

104. Auerswald U, Barth J, Magnussen H. Value of CD-1-positive cells in bronchoalveolar lavage fluid for the diagnosis of pulmonary histiocytosis-X. Lung 1991;169:305–9.

105. Merchant RK, Schwartz DA, Helmers RA, et al. Bronchoalveolar lavage cellularity – the distribution in normal volunteers. Am Rev Respir Dis 1992;146:448–53.

106. Veeraraghavan S, Latsi PI, Wells AU, et al. BAL findings in idiopathic nonspecific interstitial pneumonia and usual interstitial pneumonia. Eur Resp J 2003;22:239–44.

107. Nagata N, Takayama K, Nikaido Y, et al. Comparison of alveolar septal inflammation to bronchoalveolar lavage in interstitial lung diseases. Respiration 1996;63:94–9.

107a. Pesci A, Ricchiuti E, Ruggiero R, et al. Bronchoalveolar lavage in idiopathic pulmonary fibrosis: what does it tell us? Res Med 2010;104(Supplement 1):570–3.

108. Perezarellano JL, Garcia JEL, Macias MCG, et al. Hemosiderin-laden macrophages in bronchoalveolar lavage fluid. Acta Cytol 1992;36:26–30.

109. Midulla F, Strappini PM, Ascoli V, et al. Bronchoalveolar lavage cell analysis in a child with chronic lipid pneumonia. Eur Resp J 1998;11:239–42.

110. Davison AG, Haslam PL, Corrin B, et al. Interstitial lung disease and asthma in hard-metal workers: bronchoalveolar lavage, ultrastructural, and analytical findings and results of bronchial provocation tests. Thorax 1983;38:119–28.

111. Johnson NF, Haslam PL, Dewar A, et al. Identification of inorganic dust particles in bronchoalveolar lavage macrophages by energy dispersive X-ray microanalysis. Arch Environ Health 1986;41:133–44.

112. Lusuardi M, Capelli A, Donner CF, et al. Semi-quantitative X-ray microanalysis of bronchoalveolar lavage samples from silica-exposed and nonexposed subjects. Eur Respir J 1992;5:798–803.

113. Karjalainen A, Piipari R, Mantyla T, et al. Asbestos bodies in bronchoalveolar lavage in relation to asbestos bodies and asbestos fibres in lung parenchyma. Eur Respir J 1996;9:1000–5.

114. Costello JF, Moriarty DC, Branthwaite MA, et al. Diagnosis and management of alveolar proteinosis: the role of electron microscopy. Thorax 1975;30:121–32.

115. Martin RJ, Coalson JJ, Rogers RM, et al. Pulmonary alveolar proteinosis: the diagnosis by segmental lavage. Am Rev Respir Dis 1980;121:819–25.

116. Palombini B, Da Silva Porto N, Wallau CU, et al. Bronchopulmonary lavage in alveolar microlithiasis. Chest 1981;80:242–3.

117. Pracyk JB, Simonson SG, Young SL, et al. Composition of lung lavage in pulmonary alveolar microlithiasis. Respiration 1996;63:254–60.

118. Clelland C, Higenbottam T, Stewart S, et al. Bronchoalveolar lavage and transbronchial lung biopsy during acute rejection and infection in heart–lung transplant patients – studies of cell counts, lymphocyte phenotypes, and expression of HLA-DR and interleukin-2 receptor. Am Rev Respir Dis 1993; 147:1386–92.

119. Guilinger RA, Paradis IL, Dauber JH, et al. The importance of bronchoscopy with transbronchial biopsy and bronchoalveolar lavage in the management of lung transplant recipients. Am J Respir Crit Care Med 1995;152:2037–43.

120. Redington AE, Madden J, Frew AJ, et al. Transforming growth factor-beta 1 in asthma: measurement in bronchoalveolar lavage fluid. Am J Respir Crit Care Med 1997;156:642–7.

121. Ashitani J, Mukae H, Nakazato M, et al. Elevated concentrations of defensins in bronchoalveolar lavage fluid in diffuse panbronchiolitis. Eur Resp J 1998;11:104–11.

122. Yamanouchi H, Fujita J, Hojo S, et al. Neutrophil elastase: alpha-1-proteinase inhibitor complex in serum and bronchoalveolar lavage fluid in patients with pulmonary fibrosis. Eur Resp J 1998;11:120–5.

123. Bouros D, Wells AU, Nicholson AG, et al. Histopathologic subsets of fibrosing alveolitis in patients with systemic sclerosis and their relationship to outcome. Am J Respir Crit Care Med 2002;165:1581–6.

Index

Index

Index

Index

Tracheobronchopathia osteochondroplastica 94–95, 94f
  pathology 94–95
Tracheo-oesophageal fistula 53, 53f
Trachiectasis (Mounier-Kuhn's syndrome) 52, 63
Transplantation
  bone marrow 668, 668b
  see also Lung transplantation
Traumatic wet lung 142–143
Trematodes 254–255
Treponema pallidum 48
Trichinella spiralis 460b
Trichomonas hominis 254
Trichomonas tenax 254, 460b
Trichomonas vaginalis 254
Trichomoniasis 254
Trichosporon cutaneum 244
Tropheryma whippelii 487
Trophoblastic embolism 410, 411f
L-tryptophan 389, 389f, 460b
Tubercle bacilli 200f
Tuberculin skin test 205, 206t
Tuberculoma 208–209, 210f
Tuberculosis 197–211
  bacteriology 197–199
  complicating silicosis 335–336
  epidemiology 198–199, 198f
  HIV/AIDS and 199, 199t
  hypersensitivity and 205–207, 206t, 207f
  immunity and 205–207, 206t, 207f
  infection patterns 200b
  non-reactive 210–212
  of pleura 713–714
  postmortem recognition 211
  postprimary *see* Postprimary tuberculosis
  primary *see* Primary tuberculosis
  route of infection 198
  silicosis and 335–336
  treatment 211
  types 199, 200b, 200f
  see also Mycobacterium tuberculosis
Tuberculous empyema 202, 202f
Tuberculous granuloma 200, 200f–201f
Tuberous sclerosis 293, 294t, 488
  children and 297
  non-malignant lung disease and 494
Tularaemia 156, 187
Tularaemic pneumonia 187
Tumour
  embolism 411
  necrosis factor 143
  suppressor genes 540–541
  see also specific tumours
Tumourlets and neuroendocrine cell hyperplasia 598–601, 600f
  clinical features 599–600, 601f
  differential diagnosis 600–601
  microscopy 600, 600f–601f
  prognosis 601
Tumour-like conditions 696–705
  amyloid tumour 696–698, 697t
  bronchial inflammatory polyp 699, 701f
  bullous placentoid lesion (placental transmogrification) 702f, 703
  crystal-storing histiocytosis 698–699, 700f
  hyalinising granuloma 699–700
  light-chain deposition disease (LCDD) 698

meningothelioid nodules 700–701
multifocal micronodular type II pneumocyte hyperplasia 701–703, 702f
regenerative, mimicking neoplasia 696

U

Ulcerative colitis 486, 487f
Undifferentiated malignancy 690, 690t
Upper-lobe fibrosis 519
Usual interstitial pneumonia (UIP) 263–264, 472
Usual interstitial pneumonia (UIP)/idiopathic pulmonary fibrosis (IFP) 263–264, 266–276
  aetiology/pathogenesis 272–275, 275f–276f
  clinical features 266–267, 267f
  course of disease 267, 268f
  differential diagnosis 272, 273t, 274f
  electron microscopy and 272
  epidemiology 266–275
  histological changes 269, 270f–271f, 272t, 273f
  morbid anatomy 267, 268f–269f
  scar cancer in 275–276

V

Varicella virus 43, 167, 168f
Varicella-zoster (chickenpox) 43, 165, 167, 520–521, 521f
  pathological features 167, 168f
Variola major (smallpox) 156, 167–168
Vascular anastomosis 512–514, 513f
Vascular development 41
Vascular disease, pulmonary 477, 480–482, 481f, 487
  polymyositis and 477–478
  systemic lupus erythematosus and 477
Vascular endothelium growth factor 541, 541t
Vascular rings 481, 482f
Vascular tumours 632–639, 735
Vasculitides 494
Vasculitis, pulmonary 475
  in connective tissue disease 445, 446f
  differential diagnosis with granulomatosis 443t
  embolic 437
  granulomatosis and 437
  infective 437
  systemic, Chapel Hill consensus classification 438b
Vasculogenesis 41
Vasidiobolus haptosporus 234
Vasoconstriction, pulmonary 22
Veins
  anatomy 2f
  bronchial 25–26
  see also Pulmonary veins
Veno-occlusive disease, pulmonary 427–429
  aetiology 428
  causes 428b
  pathology 428–429, 428f–429f
Ventilation, perfusion and 22, 26
Viral haemorrhagic agents 156
Viral infections 155–170, 156b, 156f
Viral pneumonia 157f

Viruses
  carcinogenesis and 535
  lung transplantation and 520–521, 520f–521f
Visceral giant cell angiitis, disseminated 444–446, 447t
Visceral larva migrans (ascariasis/toxocariasis) 257
Volcanic ash 372
Von Willebrand protein 24

W

Waldenstrom's macroglobulinaemia 668
Waterpipe tobacco smoking 373
Wegener's granulomatosis 438–442
  aetiology 438–442
  antineutrophil cytoplasmic antibodies (ANCA) 438–442, 439f, 439t
  clinical features 438–439
  differential diagnosis 441–442, 443t
  extrapulmonary lesions 441, 442f
  limited forms 442
  necrotising sarcoid angiitis and 443–444
  pathological features 439–441, 439f–442f
  sarcoidosis links 443–444
Weibel model of bronchial tree 3t
Weibel–Palade bodies 24, 171
Welder's lung 355
Welding 355, 355t
'Wheezy' bronchitis 100, 101t, 113
Whipple's disease 487
Whooping cough (pertussis) 96–97, 97f
Williams–Campbell syndrome 62
Woolsorter's disease (anthrax pneumonia) 187–188
World Health Organisation (WHO) 344–345
  classification
    adenocarcinoma 553–554
    adenosquamous carcinoma 564–566
    epithelial tumours 548t
    extranodal lymphomas 653
    histological typing 547–549
    lesions 522
    pulmonary adenocarcinoma 556b
    sarcomatoid carcinomas 566
    sclerosing haemangioma and 610
    squamous cell carcinomas 551
World Trade Center 372
'Worm cysts' (abscess cavities) 255, 255f
Wuchereria bancrofti 258, 460b

X

Xanthogranulomatosis 491–492

Y

Yeasts 223
Yellow-nail syndrome 77, 482, 709, 710f
Yersinia pestis (plague) 156, 187
Young's syndrome 69

Z

Zenker's pneumonokoniosis 327–328
Zeolite 337